Medicinal Chemistry and Drug Development

Medicinal Chemistry and Drug Development

Edited by

Gang Liu
School of Pharmaceutical Sciences, Tsinghua University, Beijing, P.R. China

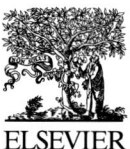

ELSEVIER

Elsevier
Radarweg 29, PO Box 211, 1000 AE Amsterdam, Netherlands
125 London Wall, London EC2Y 5AS, United Kingdom
50 Hampshire Street, 5th Floor, Cambridge, MA 02139, United States

Copyright © 2025 Tsinghua University Press Limited. Published by Elsevier Inc. All rights are reserved, including those for text and data mining, AI training, and similar technologies.

Publisher's note: Elsevier takes a neutral position with respect to territorial disputes or jurisdictional claims in its published content, including in maps and institutional affiliations.

No part of this publication may be reproduced or transmitted in any form or by any means, electronic or mechanical, including photocopying, recording, or any information storage and retrieval system, without permission in writing from the publisher. Details on how to seek permission, further information about the Publisher's permissions policies and our arrangements with organizations such as the Copyright Clearance Center and the Copyright Licensing Agency, can be found at our website: www.elsevier.com/permissions.

This book and the individual contributions contained in it are protected under copyright by the Publisher (other than as may be noted herein).

Notices

Knowledge and best practice in this field are constantly changing. As new research and experience broaden our understanding, changes in research methods, professional practices, or medical treatment may become necessary.

Practitioners and researchers must always rely on their own experience and knowledge in evaluating and using any information, methods, compounds, or experiments described herein. In using such information or methods they should be mindful of their own safety and the safety of others, including parties for whom they have a professional responsibility.

To the fullest extent of the law, neither the Publisher nor the authors, contributors, or editors, assume any liability for any injury and/or damage to persons or property as a matter of products liability, negligence or otherwise, or from any use or operation of any methods, products, instructions, or ideas contained in the material herein.

ISBN: 978-0-443-27402-2

For Information on all Elsevier publications
visit our website at https://www.elsevier.com/books-and-journals

Publisher: Stacy Masucci
Acquisitions Editor: Glyn Jones
Editorial Project Manager: Naomi Robertson
Production Project Manager: Fahmida Sultana
Cover Designer: Mark Rogers

Typeset by MPS Limited, Chennai, India

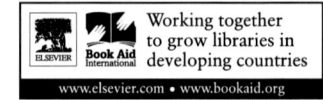

Contents

List of contributors	xv		1.9.4 Process chemistry of sitagliptin: application of asymmetric catalytic hydrogenation	14
About the editor	xvii			
Preface	xix			
Introduction	xxi		References	18
			Further reading	20

1. Medicinal chemistry and process development of the type 2 diabetes drug sitagliptin

Jinyou Xu and Guibai Liang

1.1 Introduction to the type 2 diabetes drug sitagliptin	1
1.2 Incretin and its degrading enzyme dipeptidyl peptidase-4	2
1.3 Property-based drug design	3
1.4 Common factors influencing the ADME/T properties of drugs	4
1.5 Early pharmacological and toxicological studies of dipeptidyl peptidase IV inhibitors	6
1.5.1 Early pharmacological effects of dipeptidyl peptidase IV inhibitors	6
1.5.2 Early toxicity studies of dipeptidyl peptidase IV inhibitors	7
1.5.3 Optimization strategies for DPP-4 inhibitors	8
1.6 Confirmation of lead compounds	8
1.6.1 What constitutes an ideal lead compound?	8
1.6.2 α-Amino acid-derived dipeptidyl peptidase-4 inhibitors	8
1.6.3 Identification of β-amino acid series of lead compounds	9
1.7 Optimization of the β-amino acid series lead compounds	10
1.8 Clinical studies of the new drug sitagliptin	11
1.9 Process chemistry of sitagliptin	12
1.9.1 What is process chemistry?	12
1.9.2 Efficiency of chemical reactions	13
1.9.3 Medicinal chemistry synthesis of sitagliptin: application of chiral auxiliaries	14

2. The developmental history of insulin pharmaceuticals

Hai Qian and Binbin Kou

2.1 Introduction to diabetes and insulin	21
2.1.1 Diabetes mellitus	21
2.1.2 Discovery history of insulin [1–3]	21
2.1.3 The structure of insulin	22
2.1.4 The mechanism of action of insulin	25
2.1.5 Insulin clearance mechanism	26
2.2 Development of insulin pharmaceuticals	26
2.2.1 The development process of insulin medications	27
2.2.2 Structural modification strategies for insulin analogs	28
2.3 Summary and outlook	37
References	38

3. The developmental trajectory of GLP-1 receptor agonists

Binbin Kou and Hai Qian

3.1 Glucagon-like peptide-1 (GLP-1)	41
3.1.1 Brief introduction to glucagon-like peptide-1 (GLP-1)	41
3.1.2 The development of GLP-1 medications	41
3.1.3 GLP-1 structure and physiology	42
3.2 The development of GLP-1 therapeutics	43
3.2.1 The limitations of native GLP-1 as a therapeutic agent	43
3.2.2 The strategies for extending GLP-1 analogs time action	44
3.3 The unsuccessful case in GLP-1 drug R&D and the implications and lessons	49
3.4 Summary and outlook	50
References	51

4. Antidiabetic drugs based on sodium-glucose cotransporter 2 inhibitors
Youhong Niu and Xinshan Ye

4.1 Overview of diabetes mellitus and antidiabetic drugs — 55
    4.1.1 Definition, classification, and current status of diabetes mellitus — 55
    4.1.2 Factors related to the onset of diabetes — 55
    4.1.3 Clinical anti-diabetic medications, and their targets and mechanisms — 56

4.2 Sodium-glucose cotransporter 2 (SGLT2) inhibitors as anti-diabetic drugs — 59
    4.2.1 Biological basis of SGLT2 as a therapeutic target for diabetes — 59
    4.2.2 SGLT2 inhibitors and successful development of dapagliflozin — 60
    4.2.3 Synthetic process of dapagliflozin — 65
    4.2.4 Efficacy and action of dapagliflozin — 67
    4.2.5 Other drugs based on SGLT2 inhibitors — 67

4.3 Successful experience in the development of dapagliflozin — 67
References — 69

5. Cholesterol-lowering drug atorvastatin
Zhi-Shu Huang, Jia-Heng Tan and Shuo-Bin Chen

5.1 Hypercholesterolemia and cardiovascular diseases — 71
    5.1.1 Lipid metabolism — 71
    5.1.2 Cholesterol metabolic regulation and hypercholesterolemia — 72

5.2 Atorvastatin, the cholesterol-lowering drug — 76
    5.2.1 Discovery of atorvastatin — 76
    5.2.2 Mechanism of action, clinical indications, and safety of atorvastatin — 80

5.3 Medicinal chemistry of atorvastatin — 81
    5.3.1 Target of statin drugs—HMG-CoA reductase — 81
    5.3.2 Structure-activity relationship of statin drugs inhibiting HMG-CoA reductase — 82
    5.3.3 Interaction of statins with HMG-CoA reductase — 89
    5.3.4 In vivo structure-activity, structure-metabolism, and structure-toxicity relationships of statin drugs — 92
    5.3.5 The total synthesis of atorvastatin — 95

5.4 Summary and outlook — 103
    5.4.1 Chapter summary — 103
    5.4.2 Knowledge expansion: novel molecules targeting HMG-CoA reductase — 103
    5.4.3 Knowledge expansion: additional effects of statins — 105
    5.4.4 Knowledge expansion: other cholesterol-lowering drugs and their targets — 106
References — 107

6. Angiotensin II receptor antagonists for treatment of hypertension: the discovery of losartan and its analogs
Jianmin Fu

6.1 Brief introduction of hypertension and commonly used medications for the treatment of hypertension — 109
6.2 The renin-angiotensin system — 110
6.3 Angiotensin II receptor antagonists — 113
6.4 Discovery of losartan — 114
    6.4.1 Evolution of lead compounds in the early stage — 114
    6.4.2 Lead optimization — 116
    6.4.3 Discovery of losartan — 117
    6.4.4 Metabolites of losartan and its corresponding pro-drugs — 123
    6.4.5 The safety profile of losartan — 125
    6.4.6 The properties and actions of losartan — 127
    6.4.7 The synthesis of losartan — 128
    6.4.8 Brief summary of the discovery of losartan — 130

6.5 Discovery of losartan analogs — 131
References — 136

7. Antithrombotic drug—apixaban
Yafei Liu, Yao Wu and Hong Shen

7.1 What is thrombosis? — 141
    7.1.1 The dangers of thrombosis — 141
    7.1.2 The pathogenesis of thrombosis — 141

7.2 Treatment of thrombosis — 143
    7.2.1 Commonly used antithrombotic drugs and their mechanisms of action — 143
    7.2.2 The specificity and advantages of selective FXa inhibitor — 144

7.3 The medicinal chemistry of apixaban — 146
    7.3.1 Discovery of hit compound — 146
    7.3.2 Optimization of lead compound — 147

	7.3.3 The binding model of apixaban and FXa	153
	7.3.4 The synthetic routes of apixaban	154
7.4	Clinical indications of apixaban	**158**
7.5	Postclass requirements and references	**158**
References		**159**

8. Development of the anticoagulant drug fondaparinux sodium

Zhongtang Li and Zhongjun Li

8.1	Thrombotic disorders	**161**
	8.1.1 Thrombotic disorders and their hazards	161
	8.1.2 Factors and mechanisms of thrombosis formation	162
	8.1.3 Functions of factor Xa	163
8.2	Treatment of thrombotic disorders	**163**
	8.2.1 Antiplatelet agents, anticoagulants, and thrombolytics	163
	8.2.2 Anticoagulants: the past and present of heparin	164
	8.2.3 Unfractionated heparin	165
	8.2.4 Low-molecular-weight heparin	166
	8.2.5 Ultra-low-molecular-weight heparins	168
8.3	Discovery and history of anticoagulant drug: fondaparinux sodium	**168**
	8.3.1 Lead compound: discovery of the heparin pentasaccharide sequence	168
	8.3.2 The genesis of fondaparinux sodium: structure-activity relationship studies based on the heparin pentasaccharide sequence	170
	8.3.3 Mechanism of action of fondaparinux sodium	176
	8.3.4 Pharmacokinetics and safety of fondaparinux sodium	176
8.4	Chemical process of fondaparinux sodium	**178**
	8.4.1 Synthesis challenges of fondaparinux sodium	178
	8.4.2 Chemical synthesis of fondaparinux sodium	179
	8.4.3 Chemo-enzymatic synthesis of fondaparinux sodium	179
8.5	Summary	**182**
	8.5.1 Development strategy for fondaparinux sodium	182
	8.5.2 Development trends in heparin-like anticoagulants	183
	8.5.3 Development of small-molecule carbohydrate drugs	183
References		**183**

9. Development of the nucleotide antiviral drug sofosbuvir for the hepatitis C virus

Jiamin Zheng, Dong Ding and Hong Shen

9.1	Hepatitis C and hepatitis C virus	**185**
	9.1.1 Hepatitis C: symptoms, causes, and transmission	185
	9.1.2 An overview of the epidemiology and genotyping of hepatitis C	186
	9.1.3 The discovery of hepatitis C and the development of its therapeutic drugs	186
9.2	Hepatitis C virus biology	**187**
	9.2.1 The structure of the hepatitis C virus	187
	9.2.2 The structure of the hepatitis C virus NS5B protein	187
9.3	Discovery of sofosbuvir	**189**
	9.3.1 Mechanism of nucleoside antiviral drugs	189
	9.3.2 Structure-activity relationship of the nucleoside scaffold: the birth of PSI-6130	190
	9.3.3 Pharmacokinetic study of PSI-6130: design and application of prodrugs	194
	9.3.4 The synthesis of sofosbuvir	201
9.4	Clinical studies of sofosbuvir	**203**
	9.4.1 Preclinical studies of sofosbuvir	203
	9.4.2 Clinical trial results of sofosbuvir	203
	9.4.3 Treatment regimens with sofosbuvir	204
9.5	Summary and outlook	**205**
	9.5.1 Summary	205
	9.5.2 Further reading: ProTide technology	206
References		**208**

10. The first HIV-1 integrase inhibitor, raltegravir

Xiaoqing Wang, Xiaowen Wei and Hong Shen

10.1	AIDS and HIV	**211**
	10.1.1 Discovery, transmission, and current status of AIDS	211
	10.1.2 Structure and replication of HIV	212
10.2	Anti-HIV drugs	**213**
	10.2.1 Classification of anti-HIV drugs	213
	10.2.2 Drug resistance to HIV	214
10.3	The discovery journey of raltegravir	**215**
	10.3.1 Structure and mechanism of action of HIV-1 integrase	215
	10.3.2 Discovery and optimization of hit compounds	216

10.3.3　Optimization of 1,6-naphthyridine
　　　　　　 lead compound　221
　　　10.3.4　Optimization of dihydroxy
　　　　　　 pyrimidine lead compound　226
　　　10.3.5　Clinical investigation of
　　　　　　 raltegravir　232
10.4　Research on the synthetic process of
　　　raltegravir　234
　　　10.4.1　Synthetic route in medicinal
　　　　　　 chemistry　234
　　　10.4.2　Optimization of the
　　　　　　 first-generation synthetic process　234
　　　10.4.3　Optimization of the second-
　　　　　　 generation synthetic process　236
10.5　Summary and knowledge expansion　239
　　　10.5.1　Summary of the discovery
　　　　　　 journey of raltegravir　239
　　　10.5.2　Knowledge expansion　241
References　242

11. Discovery and development of the human immunodeficiency virus protease inhibitor Saquinavir

Daoyuan Chen and Xianzhang Bu

11.1　Overview of virus　245
　　　11.1.1　Virus structure and its
　　　　　　 biological functions　245
　　　11.1.2　Classification and nomenclature
　　　　　　 of viruses　246
　　　11.1.3　Viral infection and pathogenic
　　　　　　 properties　246
　　　11.1.4　The human antiviral warfare　247
11.2　Human immunodeficiency virus and
　　　acquired immunodeficiency
　　　syndrome　247
　　　11.2.1　HIV and AIDS　247
　　　11.2.2　Structure of HIV　248
　　　11.2.3　Mechanisms of HIV infection
　　　　　　 and HIV life cycle　248
11.3　HIV protease and inhibitor saquinavir　249
　　　11.3.1　Structural characteristics of
　　　　　　 HIV proteases　249
　　　11.3.2　The design of HIV protease
　　　　　　 inhibitors　250
　　　11.3.3　Design and discovery of
　　　　　　 saquinavir　251
　　　11.3.4　Pharmacokinetic properties and
　　　　　　 deficiencies of saquinavir　253
11.4　Further development of Saquinavir　254
　　　11.4.1　Enhancement of pharmacokinetic
　　　　　　 properties　254
　　　11.4.2　The discovery of the Darunavir　256

11.5　Anti-HIV/AIDS drugs and novel
　　　treatment strategies　260
　　　11.5.1　Classification of anti-HIV/AIDS
　　　　　　 drugs　260
　　　11.5.2　New strategies for HIV/AIDS
　　　　　　 prevention and treatment　261
References　263

12. Baloxavir: an antiinfluenza drug with a novel mechanism of action

Peng Zhan, Kai Tang and Xinyong Liu

12.1　Influenza virus　265
　　　12.1.1　Transmission and status quo of
　　　　　　 influenza virus　265
　　　12.1.2　Structure, function, and
　　　　　　 classification of influenza viruses　265
　　　12.1.3　Life cycle of influenza virus　266
12.2　Antiinfluenza drugs　268
　　　12.2.1　M2 ion channel blockers　268
　　　12.2.2　Neuraminidase inhibitors　268
　　　12.2.3　Broad-spectrum antiviral drugs　268
　　　12.2.4　Influenza virus inhibitors
　　　　　　 targeting the polymerase complex　269
12.3　Development of baloxavir　270
　　　12.3.1　The structure and function of
　　　　　　 endonuclease　270
　　　12.3.2　Discovery of baloxavir　271
　　　12.3.3　Synthesis of baloxavir　279
　　　12.3.4　Clinical study of baloxavir　283
　　　12.3.5　Inspiration from the study of
　　　　　　 baloxavir　284
References　285

13. Paclitaxel: a natural antitumor agent

Yi Dong, Yao Ma and Gang Liu

13.1　Discovery and development of taxol　287
　　　13.1.1　Discovery of paclitaxel　287
　　　13.1.2　The antitumor action of
　　　　　　 mechanism　288
　　　13.1.3　The clinical research on
　　　　　　 paclitaxel　288
　　　13.1.4　The application limitations of
　　　　　　 injectable paclitaxel　289
　　　13.1.5　Other commercially available
　　　　　　 taxanes for anticancer therapy　292
　　　13.1.6　Other taxane-based drug
　　　　　　 candidates that have been
　　　　　　 studied in clinical trials　293
　　　13.1.7　The method of obtaining
　　　　　　 natural paclitaxel　296
13.2　The pharmaceutical chemistry of
　　　paclitaxel　297

- 13.2.1 The total synthesis of paclitaxel — 297
- 13.2.2 The semisynthesis of paclitaxel — 300
- 13.2.3 Study on the structure-activity relationship of paclitaxel — 302
- 13.3 Design strategy for paclitaxel prodrugs — 310
  - 13.3.1 A prodrug utilizing hydrophilic small molecule moieties as carriers — 310
- 13.4 Summary and outlook — 320
- References — 321

14. Antitumor drug eribulin
Yefeng Tang, Tianwen Sun and Hai Shang

- 14.1 Introduction — 327
- 14.2 Antitumor mechanism of eribulin — 328
  - 14.2.1 Structure and function of microtubules — 328
  - 14.2.2 Tubulin inhibitors — 329
  - 14.2.3 The mechanism of action of eribulin — 329
- 14.3 The development process of eribulin — 330
  - 14.3.1 Discovery and chemical synthesis of antitumor natural product halichondrin B — 330
  - 14.3.2 Study on the structure-activity relationship of halichondrin B - discovery process of eribulin — 333
  - 14.3.3 Study on the process chemistry of eribulin — 336
- 14.4 Pharmacological characteristics of eribulin — 342
  - 14.4.1 Pharmacodynamics of eribulin — 342
  - 14.4.2 Pharmacokinetics and toxicology of eribulin — 343
- 14.5 Clinical research and safety evaluation of eribulin — 343
  - 14.5.1 Clinical research of eribulin — 343
  - 14.5.2 Adverse effects of eribulin — 344
- 14.6 Conclusion — 345
- References — 346

15. Targeted protein kinase inhibitor imatinib
Lijie Peng and Ke Ding

- 15.1 Protein kinases (PKs) and protein kinase inhibitors (PKIs) as antineoplastic agents — 349
  - 15.1.1 Introduction — 349
  - 15.1.2 Protein kinases — 350
  - 15.1.3 Composition and catalytic mechanism of protein kinase — 350
  - 15.1.4 Classifications and design of PKIs — 354
- 15.2 Medicinal chemistry of imatinib — 362
  - 15.2.1 Bcr-Abl and CML — 362
  - 15.2.2 Molecular design and structure optimization — 363
  - 15.2.3 Structure-activity relationship — 366
  - 15.2.4 Synthesis of imatinib — 367
  - 15.2.5 Pharmacokinetics and pharmacodynamics of imatinib — 369
  - 15.2.6 Drug safety and drug-drug interaction — 370
  - 15.2.7 Clinical efficacy and expansion of indications — 371
- 15.3 Imatinib resistance and solutions — 373
  - 15.3.1 Clinical mechanisms of imatinib resistance — 373
  - 15.3.2 Next-generation drugs to overcome imatinib resistance — 374
- 15.4 Summary — 382
- References — 382

16. A case study of the irreversible covalent epidermal growth factor receptor (EGFR) inhibitor—afatinib
Yongping Yu and Wenteng Chen

- 16.1 Preface — 387
- 16.2 Epidermal growth factor receptor and quinazoline-based small molecule inhibitors — 388
  - 16.2.1 Epidermal growth factor receptor — 388
  - 16.2.2 Quinazoline-based small molecule epidermal growth factor receptor inhibitors — 388
  - 16.2.3 Resistance mutations for epidermal growth factor receptor — 390
- 16.3 Drug design based on covalent inhibition strategies — 390
  - 16.3.1 Introduction to covalent inhibition strategies — 390
  - 16.3.2 Covalent strategies based on the mechanism of Michael reaction [16] — 392
  - 16.3.3 Covalent strategies based on addition-elimination or oxidation mechanisms — 392
  - 16.3.4 Covalent strategies based on reversible covalent mechanisms — 392
- 16.4 Development of covalent irreversible EGFR inhibitor – afatinib — 393
  - 16.4.1 The application of covalent strategy in the development of small molecule EGFR inhibitors [26−28] — 393

16.4.2 The discovery of the covalent irreversible EGFR inhibitor — afatinib ... 402
16.4.3 The pharmacokinetics, pharmacodynamics, and adverse reactions of afatinib [49,50] ... 406
16.4.4 Summary of structure-activity relationship of covalent EGFR inhibitor ... 407
16.5 Synthesis of afatinib ... 408
16.5.1 Mitsunobu reaction ... 408
16.5.2 Dimroth rearrangement ... 409
16.5.3 The Horner-Wadsworth-Emmons reaction ... 409
16.5.4 Laboratory medicinal chemical synthetic route-modular synthesis approach ... 409
16.5.5 Commercial synthetic route-sequential synthesis approach ... 411
16.6 Summary and knowledge expansion ... 411
16.6.1 Summary of this chapter ... 411
16.6.2 Knowledge expansion ... 411
References ... 415

17. Medicinal chemistry and process development of the antibreast cancer drug tamoxifen

Hai-Bing Zhou and Xiaoyu Ma

17.1 Estrogen receptors and breast cancers ... 419
17.1.1 Breast cancer ... 419
17.1.2 Estrogens and estrogen receptors ... 420
17.1.3 Estrogen receptor-positive breast cancer and drug targets ... 422
17.1.4 Selective estrogen receptor modulators ... 422
17.2 The medicinal chemistry of the selective estrogen receptor modulator tamoxifen ... 423
17.2.1 Discovery of tamoxifen — serendipity and opportunity ... 423
17.2.2 The mechanism of action and structure-activity relationship of tamoxifen ... 425
17.2.3 Structure-activity relationship of tamoxifen ... 427
17.2.4 In vivo metabolic characteristics of tamoxifen ... 432
17.2.5 Tamoxifen drug interactions ... 435
17.2.6 Synthesis and process of tamoxifen ... 435
17.3 Clinical investigations of tamoxifen ... 438
17.3.1 Clinical indications of tamoxifen ... 438
17.3.2 Studies on tamoxifen resistance ... 439
17.3.3 Adverse reactions of tamoxifen ... 442
17.4 Summary, knowledge expansion, and references ... 442
17.4.1 Historical significance of tamoxifen ... 442
17.4.2 Other drugs targeting estrogen receptor pathway for breast cancer treatment ... 443
References ... 445

18. Triazole antifungal drug—fluconazole

Jie Tu and Chunquan Sheng

18.1 Overview of fungal infections ... 449
18.1.1 Human pathogenic fungi ... 449
18.1.2 Fungal cell structure and pathogenic mechanisms ... 450
18.1.3 Current status and challenges of fungal infections ... 451
18.2 Overview of antifungal drugs ... 452
18.2.1 Antifungal antibiotics ... 452
18.2.2 Azole antifungal drugs ... 453
18.2.3 Allylamine antifungal drug ... 454
18.2.4 Echinocandin antifungal drugs ... 454
18.3 The developmental history of fluconazole ... 455
18.3.1 The discovery of lead compounds: from imidazoles to triazoles ... 455
18.3.2 Optimizing lead compounds: elucidating the pharmacophore of "triazole-difluorophenyl-tertiary alcohol" ... 457
18.3.3 Mechanism of action of azole antifungal agents ... 457
18.3.4 Protein binding mode and structure-activity relationships of fluconazole ... 458
18.3.5 Research on the synthesis process of fluconazole ... 459
18.3.6 Clinical application of fluconazole ... 460
18.3.7 Drug resistance of fluconazole ... 460
18.4 Structure optimization of fluconazole: development of new generation triazole antifungal drugs ... 461
18.4.1 Development of voriconazole ... 461
18.4.2 Development of isavuconazole ... 462
18.4.3 The future development of triazole drugs: from triazoles to tetrazoles? ... 463
References ... 463

19. Discovery of the antibacterial drug Linezolid and its synthetic technology research

Hong Liu and Xuewu Liang

19.1	Development of antibacterial agents	465
19.2	Discovery of the antibacterial drug Linezolid	467
19.3	Bioactivity and pharmacokinetics of antibacterial drug Linezolid	472
	19.3.1 Antibacterial activity of Linezolid in vitro	472
	19.3.2 Antibacterial activity of Linezolid in vivo	474
	19.3.3 Pharmacokinetic properties of Linezolid	475
	19.3.4 The clinical efficacy of Linezolid	476
19.4	The antibacterial mechanisms of Linezolid	477
19.5	Study on structure-activity relationship of oxazolidinone antibiotics	479
19.6	Research on the synthesis process of Linezolid	484
19.7	Conclusion	486
References		486
Further reading		487

20. Carbapenem antibiotic meropenem

Li Zhuorong and Cui Along

20.1	Introduction	489
	20.1.1 Overview of bacterial infections	489
	20.1.2 Commonly used antibacterial medications	491
20.2	Bacterial resistance and special use level antibacterial drugs	493
	20.2.1 Bacterial resistance	493
	20.2.2 Special use level antibacterial drugs	495
20.3	Case of meropenem	495
	20.3.1 Discovery of carbapenem antibiotics	497
	20.3.2 Structural optimization of carbapenem antibiotics	497
	20.3.3 Discovery and structural features of meropenem	499
	20.3.4 Mechanism of action of meropenem	500
	20.3.5 Pharmacodynamics and pharmacokinetics of meropenem	500
	20.3.6 Process synthesis of meropenem	500
20.4	The progress on other carbapenem antibiotics	502
	20.4.1 Recently marketed carbapenem antibiotics	502
	20.4.2 Chemical structure features and structure-activity relationship of carbapenem antibiotics	505
	20.4.3 Mechanisms of carbapenem antibiotic resistance	506
	20.4.4 Research features of carbapenem antibiotics	506
References		507

21. Antiparasitic drug praziquantel

Fuli Zhang and Zhezhou Yang

21.1	Parasitic diseases	509
	21.1.1 Parasitic diseases	509
	21.1.2 Antiparasitic drugs	510
21.2	Antiparasitic drug praziquantel	510
	21.2.1 A brief history of antischistosomal drugs	510
	21.2.2 The insecticidal mechanism of action of praziquantel	513
	21.2.3 Dosage and treatment duration of praziquantel	513
	21.2.4 Resistance to praziquantel	514
21.3	Medicinal chemistry of praziquantel	514
	21.3.1 Structure-activity relationship of praziquantel	514
	21.3.2 Levopraziquantel	515
	21.3.3 Pharmacokinetics of praziquantel and deuterated praziquantel	517
21.4	Green process for praziquantel and its levoisomer	518
	21.4.1 Green chemistry	518
	21.4.2 Synthesis of praziquantel	519
	21.4.3 Synthesis of levorotatory praziquantel	522
21.5	Green chemistry future	526
References		527

22. A case study on the proton pump inhibitor omeprazole

Maosheng Cheng, Jian Wang and Rui Wen

22.1	Peptic ulcer	531
	22.1.1 Pathogenesis of peptic ulcer	531
	22.1.2 Classification and clinical applications of antiulcer medications	535
22.2	Why is omeprazole	538
	22.2.1 Physiological functions and structural characteristics of proton pumps	538

22.2.2 The development process of omeprazole ... 539
22.2.3 The mechanism of action of omeprazole ... 545
22.3 Medicinal chemistry of omeprazole ... 546
  22.3.1 The structural characteristics of omeprazole ... 546
  22.3.2 The synthesis process of omeprazole ... 546
  22.3.3 Structure-activity relationship of proton pump inhibitors ... 549
22.4 Clinical applications of omeprazole ... 550
  22.4.1 The clinical indications and safety of omeprazole ... 550
  22.4.2 Omeprazole and esomeprazole ... 551
22.5 Summary and knowledge expansion ... 553
  22.5.1 Chapter summary ... 553
  22.5.2 Expansion of knowledge: the patent portfolio of omeprazole ... 553
References ... 554

23. The inhibitors of phosphodiesterase type 5A effectively treat erectile dysfunction

Lei Guo and Hai-Bin Luo

23.1 The nitric oxide-cyclic guanosine monophosphate signaling pathway associated with penile erectile function ... 557
  23.1.1 Physiological mechanisms of penile erection ... 557
  23.1.2 Molecular biological mechanisms of priapism ... 558
  23.1.3 Phosphodiesterase protein structure and mechanism of action ... 558
23.2 Sildenafil for the management of male erectile dysfunction ... 559
  23.2.1 The discovery of sildenafil (UK-92480) and its structure-activity relationship study ... 562
  23.2.2 Unexpected findings of sildenafil in clinical trials: improvement in erectile dysfunction ... 565
23.3 The approval of second and third-generation highly selective phosphodiesterase type 5A inhibitors ... 565
  23.3.1 Second-generation selective phosphodiesterase type 5A inhibitor: vardenafil ... 565
  23.3.2 Tadalafil, a third-generation selective phosphodiesterase type 5A inhibitor ... 568
  23.3.3 Phosphodiesterase type 5A inhibitor activity, PK properties, and efficacy ... 572
23.4 Synthesis of selective phosphodiesterase type 5A inhibitors ... 576
  23.4.1 Synthesis of sildenafil citrate ... 576
  23.4.2 Synthesis of vardenafil hydrochloride ... 576
  23.4.3 Synthesis of tadalafil ... 577
23.5 Molecular mechanisms of phosphodiesterase type 5A inhibitors ... 578
  23.5.1 Protein structure of phosphodiesterase type 5A ... 578
  23.5.2 Molecular mechanisms of interaction between sildenafil or vardenafil and phosphodiesterase type 5A proteins ... 579
23.6 Summary and prospect ... 581
References ... 582

24. GABA$_A$ receptor agonists: discovery of the general anesthetic propofol and its analogs

Bowen Ke and Wei Zheng

24.1 Introduction to anesthesia ... 585
24.2 Common drugs in clinical anesthesia ... 586
  24.2.1 Inhalation anesthetics ... 586
  24.2.2 Intravenous anesthetics ... 587
  24.2.3 Local anesthetics ... 587
24.3 Medicinal chemistry of the general intravenous anesthetic propofol and its analogs ... 588
  24.3.1 The GABA$_A$ receptor and the GABAergic system: the first step to decipher the general anesthesia ... 589
  24.3.2 GABA$_A$ receptor agonists: finding a way to general anesthesia ... 593
  24.3.3 The story of propofol: the unexpected birth of the king ... 595
  24.3.4 Phenolic compounds: a new starting point ... 596
  24.3.5 Optimization of the candidate: a process of constant tradeoffs ... 600
  24.3.6 Propofol analogs: the emergence of ciprofol and fospropofol disodium ... 603
  24.3.7 Pharmaceutical manufacturing technology: the key link to realize industrial production ... 611
  24.3.8 Clinical application and metabolism of propofol in vivo ... 615
References ... 616

25. The discovery of risperidone: a case of multiple target antipsychotic drug

Zhiyu Li and Xiaoke Guo

25.1	Antipsychotic drugs	619
	25.1.1 Classical antipsychotic drugs	619
	25.1.2 Atypical antipsychotic drugs	620
	25.1.3 Multiple target drug design	621
25.2	Medicinal chemistry of risperidone	623
	25.2.1 The pharmacological basis of risperidone	623
	25.2.2 Discovery of risperidone	624
	25.2.3 The synthesis of risperidone	626
25.3	Characteristics of risperidone's effects	627
	25.3.1 Pharmacological characteristics of risperidone	627
	25.3.2 Pharmacokinetics of risperidone [13,17]	629
	25.3.3 Drug-drug Interaction of risperidone and others	629
	25.3.4 Progress of risperidone	630
	25.3.5 Conclusion and perspective	631
References		631

26. A case study on the first-in-class antirenal anemia drug roxadustat

Xiaojin Zhang and Qidong You

26.1	Renal anemia and its pathogenesis	633
	26.1.1 Introduction to renal anemia	633
	26.1.2 Proteolytic degradation and degron	633
	26.1.3 Hypoxia-inducible factor and prolyl hydroxylase	634
26.2	Medications for the treatment of renal anemia	636
	26.2.1 Commonly used drugs for renal anemia treatment	636
	26.2.2 Prolyl hydroxylase inhibitors	638
26.3	Development process of roxadustat	639
	26.3.1 Structure and mechanism of prolyl hydroxylase	639
	26.3.2 Identification and optimization of hit compounds	643
	26.3.3 Lead discovery and optimization of prolyl hydroxylase domain inhibitors	643
	26.3.4 Clinical research on roxadustat	645
	26.3.5 Synthetic process of roxadustat	647
26.4	Conclusion	648
References		648

27. Function, pharmaceutical, and pharmacological research and development of natural tetracyclic dipyranocoumarin (+)-calanolide A and its analogs

Tao Ma, Purong Zheng, Xueyuan Li, Xiaoqiao Hong and Gang Liu

27.1	Discovery and structural diversity of natural tetracyclic dipyranocoumarins	651
27.2	Natural nonnucleoside reverse transcriptase inhibitors	654
	27.2.1 Anti-HIV-1 activity of calanolides	654
	27.2.2 Anti-HIV-1 activity of inophyllums	656
	27.2.3 Anti-HIV-1 activity of cordatolides	657
	27.2.4 Investigation of 1 in clinical trial	657
27.3	Anti-HIV-1 activity of improved calanolides	658
	27.3.1 Total synthesis of ($\pm$)-1	658
	27.3.2 Enantioselective total synthesis of optical 1	659
	27.3.3 Other representative calanolide analogs	659
27.4	(+)-Calanolide A and its derivatives inhibit replicating and non-replicating *Mycobacterium tuberculosis*	666
	27.4.1 Natural product 1 as an anti-*Mycobacterium tuberculosis* compound	666
	27.4.2 Preliminary structural modifications [53]	667
	27.4.3 The discovered and optimized tetrahydropyranocoumarins derived from the nitrofuran moiety exhibit potent activity against both R-*Mycobacterium tuberculosis* and NR-*Mycobacterium tuberculosis* [54]	668
	27.4.4 Mechanism of antibacterial activity of tetrahydrobenzopyran nitrofuran derivatives	670
27.5	Fluorescent activity of nitrofuran derivatives: a revelatory outcome	672
	27.5.1 Relationship between structure and molecular fluorescence activity	672
	27.5.2 How do nitrofuran compounds interact with Rv2466c and mycothiol (160)	674
	27.5.3 The action of mycothiol (MSH, 160)	675
	27.5.4 Utilization of compound 125 as an innovative fluorescent diagnostic reagent for drug sensitivity	

	testing in tuberculosis diagnosis [59]	677
	27.5.5 Implementing single-cell diagnostic technology for nitrofuran compounds	678
27.6	Summary and outlook	683
References		685
Further reading		687

28. Bisphosphonates: a targeted therapeutic medication for skeletal system

Shuai Han and Yonghui Zhang

28.1	Unveiling the saga of bisphosphonates	689
	28.1.1 Pyrophosphate and hypophosphatasia	689
	28.1.2 Discovery of bisphosphonate compounds and their biological functions	691
	28.1.3 Historical progression of bisphosphonate drug development	691
28.2	Elucidating the mechanisms of action of bisphosphonate drugs	692
	28.2.1 Osteoporosis and bisphosphonates	692
	28.2.2 Isoprenoid biosynthesis pathway and farnesyl pyrophosphate synthase	693
	28.2.3 Molecular mechanisms of action of bisphosphonates on osteoclasts	694
28.3	Medicinal chemistry of nitrogen-containing bisphosphonates	696
	28.3.1 Farnesyl pyrophosphate synthase as the molecular target of nitrogen-containing bisphosphonates	696
	28.3.2 Structure-activity relationships of nitrogen-containing bisphosphonates	698
	28.3.3 Design and development of next-generation lipophilic bisphosphonate inhibitors	703
	28.3.4 In vivo distribution and metabolism of bisphosphonates	705
28.4	Novel applications of bisphosphonate inhibitors	706
	28.4.1 Bisphosphonate drugs and inhibitors in anticancer therapy	706
	28.4.2 Development of lipophilic bisphosphonate inhibitors as vaccine adjuvants	707
References		707

29. Celecoxib targets cyclooxygenase in nonsteroidal antiinflammatory drugs

Yong Wang and Ya-qiu Long

29.1	Nonsteroidal antiinflammatory drugs and cyclooxygenase	711
	29.1.1 Introduction to nonsteroidal antiinflammatory drugs	711
	29.1.2 Mechanism of action of nonsteroidal antiinflammatory drugs	712
29.2	Selective cyclooxygenase-2 inhibitor celecoxib	715
	29.2.1 Cyclooxygenase inhibitors	715
	29.2.2 Cyclooxygenase-2 selective inhibitor celecoxib	716
29.3	Other representative coxib drugs	731
29.4	Summary and perspective	732
References		732

30. Case study of antisense oligonucleotides for duchenne muscular dystrophy

Xinyang Zhou, Yufei Pan and Zhenjun Yang

30.1	Introduction	735
30.2	Duchenne muscular dystrophy	737
	30.2.1 Introduction to duchenne muscular dystrophy	737
	30.2.2 Treatment and exon skipping in duchenne muscular dystrophy	737
30.3	Mechanism of action of antisense oligonucleotide drugs	739
	30.3.1 RNase H	739
	30.3.2 Alternative mechanisms	740
	30.3.3 Exon skipping	740
30.4	The developmental trajectory of antisense oligonucleotide therapeutics targeting the DMD gene	741
	30.4.1 Chemical modifications of antisense oligonucleotides	742
	30.4.2 Oligonucleotide delivery techniques	745
	30.4.3 Exon skipping therapy for DMD by ASO	749
30.5	Summary and outlook	752
References		752

Index 755

List of contributors

Cui Along Institute of Medicinal Biotechnology, Peking Union Medical College, Beijing, P.R. China

Xianzhang Bu School of Pharmaceutical Sciences, Sun Yat-Sen University, Guangzhou, P.R. China

Daoyuan Chen School of Bioengineering, Zhuhai Campus of Zunyi University, Zhuhai, Guangdong, P.R. China; School of Pharmaceutical Sciences, Sun Yat-Sen University, Guangzhou, P.R. China

Shuo-Bin Chen School of Pharmaceutical Sciences, Sun Yat-Sen University, Guangzhou, P.R. China

Wenteng Chen College of Pharmaceutical Sciences, Zhejiang University, Hangzhou, Zhejiang Province, P.R. China

Maosheng Cheng School of Pharmaceutical Engineering, Shenyang Pharmaceutical University, Shenyang, P.R. China

Dong Ding Department of Medicinal Chemistry, China Innovation Center of Roche (CICoR), Shanghai, P.R. China

Ke Ding College of Pharmacy, Jinan University, Guangzhou, P.R. China; Shanghai Institute of Organic Chemistry, Chinese Academy of Sciences, Shanghai, P.R. China

Yi Dong Institute of Materia Medica, Chinese Academy of Medical Science, Beijing, P.R. China

Jianmin Fu Pharmaron Beijing Co., Ltd., BDA, Beijing, P.R. China

Lei Guo School of Pharmaceutical Sciences, Sun Yat-Sen University, Guangzhou, P.R. China

Xiaoke Guo China Pharmaceutical University, Nanjing, Jiangsu Province, P.R. China

Shuai Han WuXi AppTec Co., Ltd., Pudong New Area, Shanghai, P.R. China

Xiaoqiao Hong School of Pharmaceutical Sciences, Tsinghua University, Beijing, P.R. China

Zhi-Shu Huang School of Pharmaceutical Sciences, Sun Yat-Sen University, Guangzhou, P.R. China

Bowen Ke Department of Anesthesiology, Laboratory of Anesthesia and Critical Care Medicine, National-Local Joint Engineering Research Centre of Translational Medicine of Anesthesiology, West China Hospital, Sichuan University, Chengdu, P.R. China

Binbin Kou Eccogene, Inc., Cambridge, MA, United States

Xueyuan Li Institute of Basic Medical Sciences, Chinese Academy of Medical Sciences, Beijing, P.R. China

Zhiyu Li China Pharmaceutical University, Nanjing, Jiangsu Province, P.R. China

Zhongjun Li State Key Laboratory of Natural and Biomimetic Drugs, School of Pharmaceutical Sciences, Peking University, Beijing, P.R. China

Zhongtang Li State Key Laboratory of Natural and Biomimetic Drugs, School of Pharmaceutical Sciences, Peking University, Beijing, P.R. China

Guibai Liang SHEO Pharmaceutical, Shanghai, P.R. China

Xuewu Liang State Key Laboratory of Drug Research, Shanghai Institute of Materia Medica, Chinese Academy of Sciences, Shanghai, P.R. China

Gang Liu School of Pharmaceutical Sciences, Tsinghua University, Beijing, P.R. China

Hong Liu State Key Laboratory of Drug Research, Shanghai Institute of Materia Medica, Chinese Academy of Sciences, Shanghai, P.R. China

Xinyong Liu Department of Medicinal Chemistry, School of Pharmaceutical Sciences, Shandong University, Jinan, Shandong, P.R. China

Yafei Liu Department of Medicinal Chemistry, China Innovation Center of Roche (CICoR), Shanghai, P.R. China

Ya-qiu Long College of Pharmaceutical Sciences, Soochow University, Suzhou, P.R. China

Hai-Bin Luo School of Pharmaceutical Sciences, Hainan University, Haikou, P.R. China

Tao Ma School of Chinese Materia Medica, Beijing University of Chinese Medicine, Beijing, P.R. China

Xiaoyu Ma Department of Hematology, Zhongnan Hospital of Wuhan University, Wuhan, P.R. China;

School of Pharmaceutical Sciences, Wuhan University, Wuhan, P.R. China

Yao Ma Institute of Materia Medica, Chinese Academy of Medical Science, Beijing, P.R. China

Youhong Niu School of Pharmaceutical Sciences, Peking University, Beijing, P.R. China

Yufei Pan School of Pharmaceutical Sciences, Peking University, Beijing, P.R. China

Lijie Peng College of Pharmacy, Jinan University, Guangzhou, P.R. China

Hai Qian Center of Drug Discovery, China Pharmaceutical University, Nanjing, Jiangsu, P.R. China

Hai Shang Institute of Medicinal Plant Development, Chinese Academy of Medical Sciences and Peking Union Medical College, Beijing, P.R. China

Hong Shen China Innovation Center of Roche (CICoR), Shanghai, P.R. China

Chunquan Sheng Naval Medical University, Shanghai, P.R. China

Tianwen Sun Jiangsu Simcere Pharmaceutical Co., Ltd., Nanjing, Jiangsu, P.R. China

Jia-Heng Tan School of Pharmaceutical Sciences, Sun Yat-Sen University, Guangzhou, P.R. China

Kai Tang Department of Medicinal Chemistry, School of Pharmaceutical Sciences, Shandong University, Jinan, Shandong, P.R. China

Yefeng Tang School of Pharmaceutical Sciences, Tsinghua University, Beijing, P.R. China

Jie Tu Naval Medical University, Shanghai, P.R. China

Jian Wang School of Pharmaceutical Engineering, Shenyang Pharmaceutical University, Shenyang, P.R. China

Xiaoqing Wang Roche Innovation Center Shanghai, Shanghai, P.R. China

Yong Wang School of Medicine and Pharmacy, Key Laboratory of Marine Drugs, Chinese Ministry of Education, Ocean University of China, Shandong, P.R. China; Laboratory for Marine Drugs and Bioproducts, Pilot National Laboratory for Marine Science and Technology, Qingdao, P.R. China

Xiaowen Wei WuXi AppTec, Shanghai, P.R. China

Rui Wen School of Pharmaceutical Engineering, Shenyang Pharmaceutical University, Shenyang, P.R. China

Yao Wu Department of Medicinal Chemistry, China Innovation Center of Roche (CICoR), Shanghai, P.R. China

Jinyou Xu SHEO Pharmaceutical, Shanghai, P.R. China

Zhenjun Yang School of Pharmaceutical Sciences, Peking University, Beijing, P.R. China

Zhezhou Yang Shanghai Institute of Pharmaceutical Industry Co., Ltd., Shanghai, P.R. China

Xinshan Ye School of Pharmaceutical Sciences, Peking University, Beijing, P.R. China

Qidong You China Pharmaceutical University, Nanjing, P.R China

Yongping Yu College of Pharmaceutical Sciences, Zhejiang University, Hangzhou, Zhejiang Province, P.R. China

Peng Zhan Department of Medicinal Chemistry, School of Pharmaceutical Sciences, Shandong University, Jinan, Shandong, P.R. China

Fuli Zhang Shanghai Institute of Pharmaceutical Industry Co., Ltd., Shanghai, P.R. China

Xiaojin Zhang China Pharmaceutical University, Nanjing, P.R China

Yonghui Zhang School of Pharmaceutical Sciences, Tsinghua University, Haidian District, Beijing, P.R. China

Jiamin Zheng Department of Medicinal Chemistry, China Innovation Center of Roche (CICoR), Shanghai, P.R. China

Purong Zheng Ningbo Combireg Pharmaceutical Technology Co. Ltd., Ningbo, Zhejiang, P.R. China

Wei Zheng Haisco Pharmaceutical Group Co. Ltd., Chengdu, P.R. China

Hai-Bing Zhou Department of Hematology, Zhongnan Hospital of Wuhan University, Wuhan, P.R. China; School of Pharmaceutical Sciences, Wuhan University, Wuhan, P.R. China

Xinyang Zhou School of Pharmaceutical Sciences, Peking University, Beijing, P.R. China

Li Zhuorong Institute of Medicinal Biotechnology, Peking Union Medical College, Beijing, P.R. China

About the editor

Gang Liu, born in August 1963, has been engaged in research in the fields of medicinal chemistry and chemical biology for over 30 years. He studied abroad at The Scripps Research Institute and the University of California, Davis. In October 2000, he returned to China as a "Changjiang Scholar" Distinguished Professor and established an independent research group at the Institute of Materia Medica, Chinese Academy of Medical Sciences, serving as the director of the Department of Synthetic Medicinal Chemistry. Since 2011, he has been appointed as a "Hundred Talents Program" Professor at Tsinghua University, serving as the Vice Dean of the School of Medicine and responsible for the establishment of the Department of Pharmaceutical Sciences (now the School of Pharmaceutical Sciences). He was appointed as the first Director of the Department of Pharmaceutical Sciences at Tsinghua University. Professor Liu is currently a Tenured Professor and Doctoral Supervisor at the School of Pharmaceutical Sciences, Tsinghua University.

Professor Gang Liu received the first prize of the 14th China Pharmaceutical Association Science and Technology Award. He currently serves as a member of the 25th Council of the China Pharmaceutical Association and a member of the Organizing Committee. He is also a member of the Teaching Steering Committee for Pharmaceutical Majors in Higher Education Institutions under the Ministry of Education, a member of the Pharmaceutical Education Professional Committee of the China Pharmaceutical Association, a member of the Chemical Biology Professional Committee of the Chinese Chemical Society, a member of the Medicinal Chemistry Professional Committee of the China Pharmaceutical Association, and a people's juror of the Beijing Intellectual Property Court.

Preface

Medicinal chemistry is a specialized branch within the field of chemistry. Researchers and educators in this field not only require a strong research background in organic chemistry and practical skills but also the ability to design and synthesize chemical (organic) molecules with specific biological activities or drug-like properties. Competent medicinal chemists must have a deep understanding of and proficiency in biology, pharmacology, molecular pharmacokinetics, and the pharmacodynamics of specific drug targets, as well as relevant medical knowledge. Additionally, they need to study and master knowledge related to drug formulation (or delivery), drug analysis, quality control, and other relevant areas. Of course, individuals in this field also need to have a thorough understanding of safety assessment as related to drugs.

To date, medicinal chemistry, and even pharmaceutical sciences, remain a partly empirical discipline. Medicinal chemists must have a keen sense of the drug-likeness of molecules, a high level of resilience in the face of setbacks and failures in drug development, and be prepared to make long-term efforts to achieve their goals, so as not to miss out when that low chance of luck comes their way! Therefore successful medicinal chemists are used to continually learn and accumulate relevant knowledge throughout their careers, and they considered the drug-likeness of molecules from an experimental, practical perspective in the long term. The drug development process is a continual process of summarizing three relationships, including the structure–activity relationship, the structure–metabolism relationship, and the structure–safety relationship, to ultimately meet the three essential elements necessary for drugs used in clinical diagnosis, treatment, and prevention: safety, efficacy, and controllability.

After more than 20 years of collaboration involving scientists worldwide, the Human Genome Project was completed. For the first time, humanity was able to read the entire human genome and predict the amino acid sequences of all proteins. This led to the discovery of a growing number of life substances related to diseases, such as proteins, nucleic acids, and glycosylated compounds, as well as genes, receptors, enzymes, ion channels, signaling pathways, and metabolic pathways. Unfortunately, only a small fraction of these have been successfully developed as drug targets so far. However, in today's rapidly advancing state of the art biotechnology, more and more biological molecules that were previously considered unlikely to become drug targets are being developed as effective drug targets. Clearly, with the development of biology, medicinal chemistry has also been developing and progressing in practice, and its role in new drug development has become increasingly important!

Since the early 1990s, when I began studying medicinal chemistry, I have been involved in related research for over 30 years. Like all researchers in the field of medicinal chemistry (such as all the authors of this book), I have always maintained a strong interest in medicinal chemistry throughout the "dream-chasing" process. I have had the privilege of experiencing the entire process of national major research project solicitation, planning, and the complete implementation of three 5-year plans for the creation of new drugs in China. I have witnessed the process of drug research and development in China from initial generic imitation to following and now thriving independent innovation. On the journey of pursuing my dreams, I enthusiastically participated in various research and development projects related to innovative drugs. During this period, I increasingly felt the inadequacy of knowledge and the dullness of teaching methods in the teaching process. As a result, I conceived the idea of using drug development cases to assist in teaching the course "Medicinal Chemistry." In the subsequent practical process, I organically integrated the ideological and political education of medicinal chemistry with specific drug development cases, experiencing the interest and significance of teaching and research growing together.

In 2005 I was deeply moved when I read a brief introduction to 46 drugs that impact human health in *Chemical and Engineering News*. Since then, I have been inspired to write a textbook using key events that have influenced drug development to reflect the wisdom and perseverance shown by humanity in the process of drug development. It was not until August 2019, during the Chengdu China Pharmaceutical Chemistry Academic Conference and Sino-European Pharmaceutical Chemistry Seminar, that I discussed this idea with several friends and received their enthusiastic support and encouragement. Dr. Jian Li, Dr. Hong Shen, Dr. Hua Yang, and Dr. Jianmin Fu, in particular, provided timely and constructive suggestions and practical support, enabling the writing plan for this book to be smoothly launched!

Subsequently, we invited more than 70 experts, professors, and researchers with experience in drug development and teaching courses from domestic and foreign countries to participate in writing. They are all outstanding workers and educators who have long been engaged in medicinal chemistry research and drug development, providing excellent support for this book. The main difficulty we faced at the beginning of writing this book was the lack of a suitable template for reference. However, our idea was quite clear: each chapter had to tell a story about medicinal chemistry and focus on describing and introducing key events and roles of medicinal chemistry in the discovery of lead compounds, optimization of drug candidates, and the process of drug development, even including the target confirmation by proof of concept in clinic. Fortunately, Dr. Jinyou Xu and Dr. Guibai Liang, who were involved in the research and development of the "Medicinal chemistry and process development of the anti-type 2 diabetes drug sitagliptin" (Chapter 1), and Professor Zhi-Shu Huang, who has rich teaching experience, provided the drafts for "Cholesterol-lowering drug atorvastatin" (Chapter 5) quickly. The former, from the perspective of a drug development witness, tells the story of developing a best-in-class drug and addresses various issues related to drug-likeness and late-stage chemical process of production. The latter provides a detailed and comprehensive summary and introduction to the discovery, medicinal chemistry, and drug–drug interactions of a small-molecule drug (Lipitor, with annual sales of $12–15 billion at the moment), which was once the world's best-selling drug. These two chapters have clear and reasonable content, making them easy to learn and remember, and were therefore used as templates for writing the chapters of this book.

This book has been written over a span of more than 4 years, with the hope of playing a positive role in the cultivation of medicinal chemistry talent!

This marks the end of the preface.

Gang Liu

Introduction

What are pharmaceutical sciences? To address this question, we must first grasp the rationale behind the necessity of drug therapy for humans. What defines the essence of drug therapy? From my personal perspective, the fundamental life processes in the human body, such as mental activity, respiratory function, and metabolism, etc are achieved through the harmonious operation of normal signaling pathways (receptors), biochemical reactions (enzymes), metabolic processes, and immune regulation, and so on. Any disruption in these processes can lead to clinical symptoms or an increased risk of clinical events, resulting in the onset of diseases. Consequently, medications are required to readjust these fundamental regulatory pathways to a state of acceptable equilibrium, thereby maintaining the capacity and standard of normal human health. The latest definition by the China National Medical Products Administration stipulates that drugs are substances utilized for the prevention, treatment, and diagnosis of human diseases. They are designed to deliberately regulate human physiological functions and are prescribed based on specific indications or main therapeutic effects, usage guidelines, and dosages. This includes a variety of substances such as Chinese herbal medicine, chemical compounds, and biological products. Hence, drugs should only be administered when specific indications are present.

Medicinal chemistry is integral to all stages of drug development, including the discovery of active compounds, research on the drug-likeness of molecules, target validation, and drug synthesis processes. Drug development is an extremely arduous and risky process, encompassing the synthesis and practical application of knowledge from multiple interdisciplinary fields. At each stage of development before a candidate drug reaches the market, there is a risk of failure due to various factors, including but not limited to insufficient foundational research in medical biology, safety window issues caused by multiple factors, inadequate patient benefit (unmet medical needs), ethical issues in medicine, and market-driven research and development processes. Because drug development involves the comprehensive influence of multiple disciplines, including biology, chemistry, pharmacology, toxicology, formulation science, pharmacokinetics/pharmacodynamics, drug analysis and control, pharmaceutical technology, bioinformatics, drug management (regulations and laws), clinical and basic medicine, statistics, and market considerations, some have likened the development of an innovative drug to be even more challenging than launching a satellite!

From a chemical perspective, medicinal chemists must have a deep and detailed understanding of the spatial structure of organic molecules with carbon-carbon bonds as the main structural framework. They need to be aware of the low-energy orientations of rigid compound structures and their surface-polar groups and must accurately predict the conformational changes of flexible molecules in different environments. Medicinal chemists also need to have a sufficient understanding of the noncovalent interactions between small molecular compounds and their target molecules, such as proteins and nucleic acids, including the driving force mainly based on nondirectional hydrophobic effects and specific binding composed of directional forces such as salt bridges, hydrogen bonds, and dipole−dipole interactions. Additionally, medicinal chemists must have a deep understanding of the reactivity and specificity of modern binding and/or covalent drug molecules. Chemical drugs, due to their advantages of high stability, convenience of use, good availability, low production cost, and affordability, remain the mainstay of global innovative drug research and development. Since the invention of sulfonamides and penicillin antibiotics, looking back at the experiences and lessons behind various successful cases, chemical drugs have made an indelible contribution to human medicine history in all areas. Of note, the most important contribution is establishing the general methods and requirements for drug development, making "safety, efficacy, and controllability" the basic conditions for the development of drugs.

The original intention behind starting the writing of this book was to highlight the narrative of medicinal chemistry, focusing on describing and introducing key events and roles of medicinal chemistry in the discovery of lead compounds, optimization of drug candidates, and the process of drug development in late stage. The goal was to ensure that the users and readers of the textbook would not find the learning process dull and repetitive. It is hoped that students and other readers would develop an interest in medicinal chemistry and engage in the field of medicinal chemistry research. Additionally, the aim was to see more innovative drugs developed, providing effective treatments for patients.

This book ultimately collected 30 cases, which can be roughly categorized into anticancer drugs, antibiotics and antiparasitic drugs, antimetabolic disorder drugs, psychotropic drugs, antiviral drugs, drugs for cardiovascular and cerebrovascular diseases, drugs for osteoporosis, and orphan drugs, among others. If categorized by the characteristics of chemical structures, they can be further divided into small-molecule heterocyclic drugs, natural product drugs, peptide drugs, sugar drugs, nucleic acid drugs, etc. The prominent feature of this book is to introduce the drug-likeness of molecules as the focus of each chapter, emphasizing the narrative and practicality. It includes basic knowledge related to pharmaceutical sciences, especially medicinal chemistry, as well as extended knowledge. However, due to space limitations, it is not possible to cover everything. When necessary, readers can conduct literature research through some keywords to gain a deeper understanding of the role of medicinal chemistry in the drug development process.

In the process of writing this book, with the idea of learning for practical use, we invited experts from Pharmaron Beijing Co., Ltd., BDA, Beijing, China, Ningbo Combireg Pharmaceutical Technology Co., Ltd., and Roche R&D (China) Co., Ltd. to participate in the writing of this book. We introduced cases of representative Chinese enterprises in drug research and innovation. At the same time, they also provided some financial support, making this book a model of school-enterprise cooperation. We sincerely thank them for their support!

This book covers a wide range of content, so mistakes or inaccuracies are inevitable. These may be due to differences in individual understanding, misunderstandings, the editor's limited knowledge, or oversight during the organization process. Readers are encouraged to point out and correct any errors promptly!

This book is suitable for senior students and graduate students majoring in pharmaceutical sciences.

Finally, sincere thanks to all colleagues and friends who participated in the writing and provided suggestions!

Gang Liu
Tsinghua University
December 2024

Chapter 1

Medicinal chemistry and process development of the type 2 diabetes drug sitagliptin

Jinyou Xu and Guibai Liang
SHEO Pharmaceutical, Shanghai, P.R. China

Chapter outline

1.1 Introduction to the type 2 diabetes drug sitagliptin	1
1.2 Incretin and its degrading enzyme dipeptidyl peptidase-4	2
1.3 Property-based drug design	3
1.4 Common factors influencing the ADME/T properties of drugs	4
1.5 Early pharmacological and toxicological studies of dipeptidyl peptidase IV inhibitors	6
1.5.1 Early pharmacological effects of dipeptidyl peptidase IV inhibitors	6
1.5.2 Early toxicity studies of dipeptidyl peptidase IV inhibitors	7
1.5.3 Optimization strategies for DPP-4 inhibitors	8
1.6 Confirmation of lead compounds	8
1.6.1 What constitutes an ideal lead compound?	8
1.6.2 α-Amino acid-derived dipeptidyl peptidase-4 inhibitors	8
1.6.3 Identification of β-amino acid series of lead compounds	9
1.7 Optimization of the β-amino acid series lead compounds	10
1.8 Clinical studies of the new drug sitagliptin	11
1.9 Process chemistry of sitagliptin	12
1.9.1 What is process chemistry?	12
1.9.2 Efficiency of chemical reactions	13
1.9.3 Medicinal chemistry synthesis of sitagliptin: application of chiral auxiliaries	14
1.9.4 Process chemistry of sitagliptin: application of asymmetric catalytic hydrogenation	14
References	18
Further reading	20

1.1 Introduction to the type 2 diabetes drug sitagliptin

Glucose-dependent insulin secretion, also known as glucose-stimulated insulin secretion, is a new strategy for controlling blood sugar levels. It has received high attention from the academic and pharmaceutical communities in recent years and has made breakthrough progress in the research and development of new drugs for the treatment of type 2 diabetes. For instance, drugs such as gliptins (-gliptin) belong to dipeptidyl peptidase-4 (DPP-4) inhibitors. They mainly slow down the degradation of incretin, an important member of which is glucagon-like peptide-1 (GLP-1), to promote the synthesis and secretion of insulin after meals, achieving the purpose of regulating blood sugar levels. Compared with existing antidiabetic drugs such as sulfonylureas, this class of drugs can significantly reduce the risk of inducing hypoglycemia.

In October 2006, the US Food and Drug Administration (FDA) officially approved the first efficient and highly selective gliptin drug developed by Merck & Co., Inc., sitagliptin, as a new drug for the treatment of type 2 diabetes (Fig. 1.1). This opened up a new path for effective control, slowing down, and treatment of type 2 diabetes, bringing new hope to approximately 240 million diabetes patients worldwide. Sitagliptin peaked at annual sales of over 7 billion USD after its launch, making it a truly "blockbuster" drug.

This chapter is set against the backdrop of important milestones in the development of sitagliptin. It introduces the role of incretins in regulating blood sugar levels, as well as the pharmaceutical chemistry research of DPP-4 inhibitors,

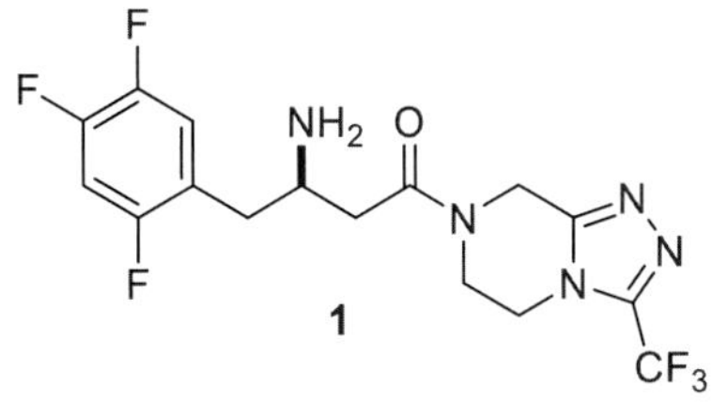

FIGURE 1.1 Sitagliptin (compound 1).

including the incretin effect, lead compound discovery and optimization, pharmacokinetics (PK) and pharmacodynamics (PD) evaluation, and novel inhibitor design. Finally, this chapter briefly discusses the chemical process of synthesis research and development of sitagliptin.

1.2 Incretin and its degrading enzyme dipeptidyl peptidase-4

Incretins are a group of hormones extracted from the mucosa of the intestine that regulate blood glucose levels. The two primary members of this group are GLP-1 and glucose-dependent insulinotropic polypeptide (GIP), and their secretion, function, and degradation mechanisms are shown in Fig. 1.2.

When secreted, incretins activate their respective receptors, such as the GIP and GLP-1 receptors on pancreatic β-cells. Activation of these receptors leads to a rapid increase in the concentration of intracellular cyclic adenosine monophosphate, resulting in insulin secretion [1]. Simultaneously, biosynthesis of insulin and proliferation of β-cells also occur and increase [2]. Additionally, activation of GLP-1 receptors helps to suppress the secretion of glucagon, reducing food intake and slowing gastric emptying [3]. Synthesis, secretion, and activation of the receptors for GIP and GLP-1 only occur when blood glucose levels are high after a meal, hence their classification as "glucose-dependent insulin biosynthesis and secretion." When GIP and GLP-1 levels are normal, they do not affect glucagon secretion. Furthermore, inhibition of glucagon secretion only occurs during the high blood glucose phase after a meal. Therefore, these drugs almost never cause hypoglycemia [4].

In healthy individuals, fasting GLP-1 level typically ranges between 5 and 10 pmol/L, but after a meal, it quickly rises to 15–50 pmol/L, which promotes insulin synthesis and secretion and accelerates glucose absorption in the blood. However, circulating levels of GIP and GLP-1 do not remain elevated after a meal and are quickly degraded by peptidases, becoming inactive GLP-1 and inactive GIP (Fig. 1.2). DPP-4 is the primary enzyme responsible for this degradation.

DPP-4 was first discovered in the liver of rats in the 1960s [5]. Subsequent research has shown that DPP-4 is widely expressed in various organs of the human body, such as the liver, pancreas, placenta, thymus, and lymphatic tissues, but its concentration is higher in the kidneys, intestines, and bone marrow. Since the 1990s, the role of DPP-4 in energy homeostasis has gained significant attention from the scientific and pharmaceutical industries. DPP-4 with enzymatic activity exists in the blood plasma in a soluble form, suggesting to scientists that it could be targeted to develop antidiabetic drugs. Inhibiting DPP-4 activity can prolong the half-life of GLP-1 and GIP in human plasma, thereby promoting insulin synthesis and secretion.

DPP-4 is a cell surface serine protease, also known as serine protease, which belongs to the prolyl oligopeptidase family and is sensitive to proline and alanine. In other words, DPP-4 can catalyze the hydrolysis of X-proline or X-alanine dipeptide residues from the *N*-terminus of peptides. Here, X represents any natural amino acid residue in proteins or peptides. Therefore, DPP-4 can degrade a variety of important protein and peptide substrates, including growth factors, chemokines, neuropeptides, and vasoactive peptides.

The protein crystal structure of DPP-4 was published in 2003 and is a membrane-bound homodimer, with each monomer having a molecular weight of 110–150 kDa. GIP and GLP-1 are natural substrates of DPP-4 in humans, which can be rapidly degraded into inactive GIP and GLP-1 by DPP-4 (essentially enzyme-catalyzed hydrolysis products).

Due to the rapid degradation of DPP-4, the half-life of incretin hormones in the biological system (including humans) is usually short. For instance, the half-life of GIP is about 10 minutes, while the half-life of GLP-1 is even shorter, only about 1 minute. This limits the direct application of incretin hormones in the clinical treatment of type 2 diabetes. Experimental results have shown that only about 10%–20% of the active substance remains after GLP-1 is injected intravenously or subcutaneously and is degraded by DPP-4. This cannot achieve the goal of reducing the high concentration of blood glucose (mainly glucose) in diabetic patients by promoting insulin synthesis and secretion.

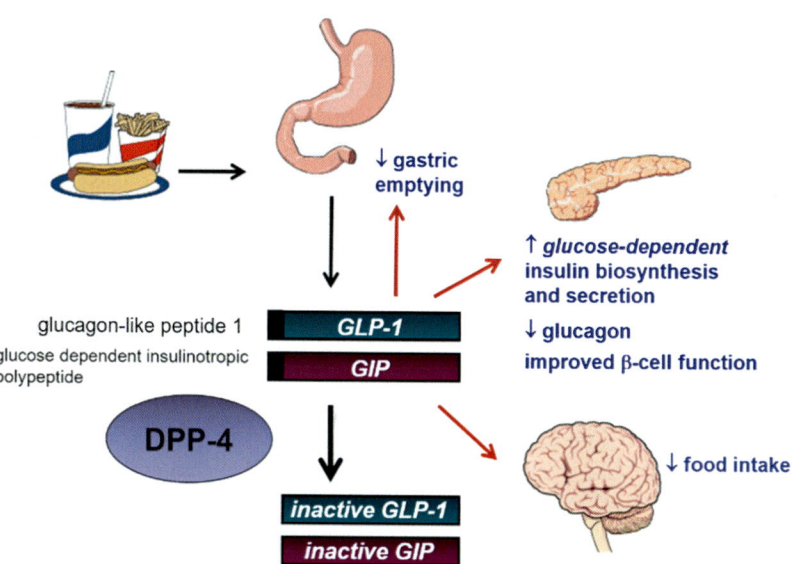

FIGURE 1.2 Secretion, function, and degradation of intestinal proinsulin.

Therefore, scientists proposed a concept and strategy for developing new antidiabetic drugs: by inhibiting the activity of DPP-4, the circulation time and concentration of GLP-1 in the human body can be extended and increased, thus restoring the incretin effect in type 2 diabetic patients, increasing insulin synthesis and secretion, and enhancing β-cell function, thereby achieving the goal of controlling postprandial blood sugar. After continuous exploration and efforts, scientists first confirmed this concept in animals in 1996 and identified DPP-4 as a potential drug target for antidiabetic drug development. Since then, major pharmaceutical companies have begun to develop DPP-4 inhibitors, opening a new era in the treatment of type 2 diabetes.

1.3 Property-based drug design

Designing a small molecule compound into a safe and effective drug is a lengthy and challenging process of multiparameter optimization. Common drug properties that require optimization include biological activity, target selectivity or specificity, compound solubility, cellular permeability, metabolic stability, oral bioavailability, plasma protein binding capacity, cytochrome P450 (CYP) enzyme inhibition or induction ability, human Ether-à-go-go-Related Gene (hERG) channel inhibition, and toxicity caused by compound promiscuity.

Medicinal chemistry is a semiempirical discipline, and every exceptional medicinal chemist must undergo long-term practice to become a true medicinal chemist. In optimizing lead compounds for their biological activity, selectivity, PK, and PD, medicinal chemists must also focus on avoiding potential toxicity and clinical adverse reactions related to both on-target and off-target effects. Therefore, optimizing lead compounds into a drug candidate is a continuous process of achieving the optimal balance between activity, oral bioavailability, and various adverse drug reactions, because, when optimizing a specific property of a compound, minor structural changes cannot be ignored, as even subtle modifications can affect other properties of the molecule and then introduce new issues for optimization after solving one problem.

Each optimization cycle of chemical drug development involves hypothesis, synthesis and/or preparation, in vitro and in vivo biological testing, and data analysis, therefore, it is lengthy and capital-intensive. Experienced drug designers begin the molecular design with careful consideration, taking into account various potential issues and alternative approaches, and clearly defining the purpose of synthesizing each compound. Typically, during the lead identification stage, a diverse set of compounds with varying structures needs to be synthesized for investigation and confirmation of structure-activity relationships. However, during the lead optimization, which involves fine-tuning the properties of the molecule, it is crucial to consider the impact of subtle structural changes on the overall drug properties and avoid introducing new problems. For example, to address the off-target activity of a drug candidate, medicinal chemists often introduce polar groups into the molecule to reduce its promiscuity that may affect its permeability to the target, while this can also make the molecule a substrate for efflux transporters such as P-glycoprotein (P-gp), leading to its extracellular transport and affecting drug absorption capability [6].

In the early 1970s, with the rapid development of protein crystallography and nuclear magnetic resonance spectroscopy, testing the three-dimensional structure of protein-ligand complexes became a routine technique. As a result, structure-based drug design and computer-aided drug design techniques experienced significant advancements, opening a new chapter in drug design. However, due to the lack of high-quality experimental data and limited understanding of factors influencing compound absorption, distribution, metabolism, excretion, and toxicity (ADME/T), early computer-aided drug design was primarily used to assist medicinal chemists in discovering active compounds and partially optimizing lead compounds.

It was not until the 1990s, with the development of related disciplines, particularly computer chemistry, physiology, biochemistry, drug metabolism, pharmacokinetics, drug transportation, and the study of drug behaviors in different organisms, that drug design entered a new era. Scientists developed various rational drug design models and technologies and actively participated in the process of drug discovery and development.

The development process of sitagliptin serves as a successful case study in understanding how drug molecule properties impact druggability. The project team members, including the authors of this chapter, employed a property-based drug design approach. They focused on the structure of lead compounds or candidate drugs and designed and optimized molecular pharmacokinetic properties to achieve desirable characteristics such as good oral absorption, targeted tissue distribution, controllable metabolism, reduced elimination rate, and decreased side effects. Currently, an increasing number of pharmaceutical companies require medicinal chemists to assess the ADME/T properties of compounds before synthesis, aiming to control failure factors during the lead discovery and optimization stages and minimize issues that may arise in later stages of drug development, such as clinical trials.

1.4 Common factors influencing the ADME/T properties of drugs

Several factors influence the drug-like properties of molecules, including molecular weight, solubility, lipophilicity, number of hydrogen bond donors, number of hydrogen bond acceptors, number of rotatable bonds, polar surface area (PSA), and number of aromatic rings (Table 1.1). These factors directly impact the ADME/T properties of drugs [7]. Consequently, drug designers face high demands, requiring them to possess a profound understanding and knowledge of various factors influencing the drug-like properties of candidate drug molecules, the physiological processes of candidate drug molecules in the body, and the biological activity characteristics of target biomolecules such as proteins.

Molecular weight is one of the key factors to consider in designing drug molecules as it can influence drug solubility, permeability, metabolic pathways, and toxicity. In 1997, Dr. Christopher Lipinski, a medicinal chemist at Pfizer, conducted a study comparing the characteristics of marketed oral drugs and those that failed in phase II/III clinical trials. He published the renowned "Lipinski's rule of five" for oral small-molecule drugs [8,9]. According to this rule, a compound is considered favorable for oral absorption if it satisfies the following criteria: molecular weight less than

TABLE 1.1 Common physicochemical properties of molecules that impact drug absorption, distribution, metabolism, excretion, and toxicity (ADME/T).

Physicochemical properties of molecules	Ideal values for oral drug
Molecular weight (Da)	<500
Lipophilicity	A clogP value between 2.0 and 3.0
Polar Surface Area (PSA) is the total surface area of a molecule that is occupied by polar atoms such as oxygen and nitrogen, including the hydrogen atoms bonded to them.	For nonCNS drugs, a PSA value of less than 120 is generally desirable. For CNS drugs, an optimal range for PSA is around 60–70. (When the PSA of a molecule exceeds 120, its cellular permeability tends to decrease. In the case of drugs that need to cross the blood-brain barrier, a PSA value in the range of 60–70 is considered favorable.)
Hydrogen bond acceptor	<10
Hydrogen bond donor	<2
Number of intramolecular rotatable bonds	<10
Number of the aromatic ring	<2

500, no more than five hydrogen bond donors, no more than ten hydrogen bond acceptors, and a calculated octanol-water partition coefficient (clogP) below 5. It is also believed that if a compound fails to meet at least two of these criteria, it is less likely to be an orally active drug. However, with the continuous advancement of modern technology and scientists' deeper understanding of intestinal absorption mechanisms, there have been exceptions to this rule, and some orally administered drugs have surpassed these limitations.

Molecular lipophilicity significantly impacts various properties of drugs, including water solubility, intestinal absorption, cell permeability, plasma protein binding, metabolism in the liver and other organs, and toxicity. Generally, a compound with a logP value between 2 and 3 is considered ideal, as it achieves a balance between solubility, permeability, and toxicity. Compounds with low logP values exhibit poor permeability, while compounds with high logP values (logP > 5) tend to have poor water solubility and higher susceptibility to metabolism by cytochrome P450 enzymes, resulting in high hepatic clearance, which in turn affects drug absorption and oral bioavailability. Furthermore, high logP values can increase the binding of drugs to plasma proteins, reducing the concentration of free drugs in the bloodstream and leading to a disconnection between PK and PD in clinical settings. Excessive logP values may also lead to increased promiscuity, thereby increasing the risk of off-target activities and adverse reactions.

The oral bioavailability of a drug presents a significant challenge for drug designers, as it is primarily associated with drug absorption and metabolism. Common factors influencing drug absorption include solubility, permeability, intestinal first-pass metabolism, liver first-pass metabolism, and whether the drug is a substrate for efflux transporters such as P-gp. Drug permeability is influenced by factors such as molecular weight, lipophilicity, the number of rotatable bonds within the molecule, shape, and PSA (Table 1.1). As mentioned earlier, controlling the logP value (lipophilicity) of a drug within the range of 2−3 can provide optimal permeability and solubility. Recent research indicates that, compared to lipophilicity, the PSA of a molecule can more accurately reflect its permeability and has become a commonly used design parameter. Typically, drugs with fewer than 10 rotatable bonds and a PSA less than 120 Å^2 exhibit good permeability and oral bioavailability. For drugs targeting the brain, the PSA is generally recommended to be less than 90 Å^2, with values ranging from 60 to 70 Å^2 being ideal [10].

To maximize oral absorption of a drug, in addition to having good permeability, drug molecules should avoid efflux by transporters such as P-gp and also need to evade rapid oxidative metabolism by cytochrome P450 enzymes in the intestine or liver cells. Transporters located on the cell membrane are essential functional membrane proteins present in various biological membranes, including the intestine, liver, kidneys, and blood-brain barrier. They have a multifaceted impact on drug absorption, distribution, and excretion processes. Transporters involved in drug efflux include P-gp, multidrug resistance-associated proteins, and breast cancer resistance protein (BCRP), among others. The effective absorption surface area in the human small intestine is approximately 200 m^2. To prevent the entry of toxic substances into the body through the intestinal tract, numerous efflux transporters, including P-gp and BCRP, are distributed on the intestinal surface. Together with cytochrome P450 enzymes, they play a role in restricting the penetration of drugs into the bloodstream [11].

The plasma protein binding capacity of a drug molecule is also an important indicator for evaluating PK and toxicity. High plasma protein binding affinity was an important issue encountered during the development of Sitagliptin. Because only free drug molecules, unbound to plasma proteins, can directly interact with drug targets, high plasma protein binding ability not only affects drug distribution, metabolism, and excretion but also influences drug efficacy. The extent of drug binding to plasma proteins can be influenced by factors such as patient age, disease status, and concurrent use of other medications. The FDA now requires additional safety studies for compounds with high plasma protein binding affinity [12].

Severe adverse reactions in clinical settings are often the key factors leading to the failure of drug development. During the development of sitagliptin, off-target activities and toxicity of the compounds led the project team to abandon many candidates with good biological activity and pharmacokinetic properties. Common drug toxicities include cytotoxicity, hepatotoxicity, genotoxicity, carcinogenicity, and cardiac toxicity, among others. Drug designers must strive to avoid factors in the molecular structure that can lead to these toxicities during the design phase [13]. However, the causes of these adverse effects or clinical adverse reactions are not solely attributed to the properties of the candidate drug molecules themselves. Sometimes, they can also result from the toxic effects of their metabolites or adverse reactions caused by drug-drug interactions (DDIs).

The CYP superfamily enzymes in the human body are the major enzymes responsible for drug metabolism. They are primarily monooxygenases (oxidases) predominantly present in the liver and intestines, located on the endoplasmic reticulum, and catalyze the oxidative metabolism of various endogenous and exogenous substances, including most clinical drugs. Inhibiting or inducing cytochrome P450 enzymes can affect the levels of metabolized drugs, endogenous hormones, and toxins in patients, thereby impacting the oxidative metabolism of all substances that may enter the body, including various toxic substances. Therefore, maintaining normal levels and functionality of cytochrome P450 enzymes is crucial for overall health. In particular, many patients with chronic or multiple diseases require the administration of multiple drugs or long-term combination therapy. Drugs that inhibit or induce cytochrome P450 enzymes can affect the PK of other drugs, alter drug concentrations in the plasma, result in DDIs, and cause adverse reactions, sometimes leading to severe adverse effects. Preventing drug-induced DDIs is, therefore, an important aspect that drug designers must consider [14].

The greatest challenge encountered in the development of DPP-4 inhibitors is addressing the issue of the compound's hERG activity. The hERG gene is expressed in various tissues of the human body, including the heart, brain, liver, and spleen, with the highest expression observed in cardiac tissue. Inhibition of the hERG potassium ion channel-mediated current across the cell membrane can lead to prolonged QT interval (a measurement made on an electrocardiogram used to assess some of the electrical properties of the heart) syndrome, causing severe cardiac arrhythmias and potentially life-threatening conditions. Currently, the assessment of a compound's interaction with the hERG potassium ion channel is a requirement by the FDA for new drug approval, aiming to mitigate the risk of cardiac toxicity associated with medications [15].

If a compound exhibits good activity, selectivity, PK, and PD properties, extensive off-target activity and toxicity studies should be conducted before it is selected as a preclinical candidate. This is done to avoid wasting substantial human, material, and financial resources. Molecular promiscuity has emerged as an important concept in recent years, used by many pharmaceutical companies to assess the selectivity and safety of drugs. Promiscuity refers to a compound's ability to interact with multiple targets, including various unknown targets, which may result in therapeutic effects but also potential toxic side effects. Through the analysis of the relationship between known compounds and off-target activities and toxicities, researchers have found that compounds with higher $clogP$ values tend to exhibit higher promiscuity, indicating that highly lipophilic molecules are more prone to binding with multiple targets [6].

1.5 Early pharmacological and toxicological studies of dipeptidyl peptidase IV inhibitors

Early clinical trial results have demonstrated that the use of DPP-4 inhibitors can indeed reduce the postprandial blood glucose elevation in patients with diabetes, providing proof-of-concept (POC) evidence of their efficacy. However, concurrently, early DPP-4 inhibitors have also exhibited certain toxic side effects or clinical adverse reactions.

1.5.1 Early pharmacological effects of dipeptidyl peptidase IV inhibitors

Merck & Co. initiated the development of DPP-4 inhibitors in 1999, preceded by two pharmaceutical companies that had already entered the clinical trial phase with their DPP-4 inhibitor candidates. For instance, the Phase I clinical trial results of DPP728 (Compound 2, Fig. 1.3) by Novartis Pharmaceuticals and P32/98 (Compound 3, Fig. 1.3) by the former East German Probiodrug company showed no significant adverse reactions in healthy volunteers. The plasma levels of active GLP-1 were also increased, and there was a noticeable reduction in the postprandial blood glucose elevation following a meal or direct glucose intake, similar to the results observed in animal experiments.

In 2002, Novartis Pharmaceuticals reported preliminary results from Phase II clinical trials of DPP-4 inhibitors. In a four-week trial involving 93 patients with type 2 diabetes, compared to the control group receiving a placebo, patients treated with the DPP-4 inhibitor showed a significant decrease in postprandial blood glucose elevation, fasting blood glucose levels, and 24-hour blood glucose levels following meals or direct glucose intake. This provided direct evidence that small-molecule DPP-4 inhibitors could be used as antidiabetic agents [16]. This milestone event is referred to as "clinical proof of concept" (cPOC). However, due to the compound's short half-life of 15 minutes in rats and less than 1 hour in humans, Novartis Pharmaceuticals ultimately decided to discontinue further clinical trials of this compound.

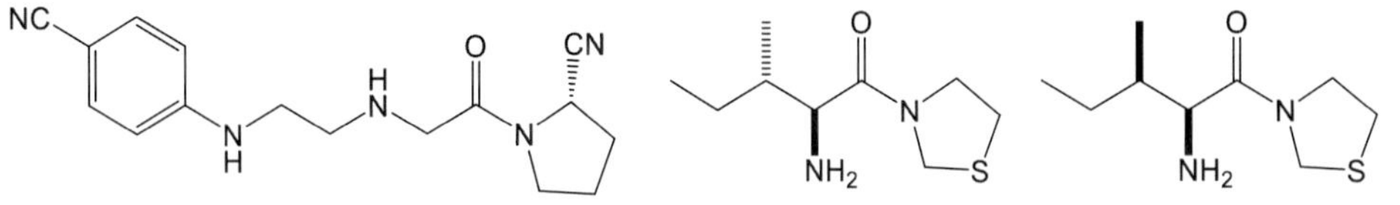

FIGURE 1.3 Early dipeptidyl peptidase-4 inhibitors.

1.5.2 Early toxicity studies of dipeptidyl peptidase IV inhibitors

In 2000, Merck & Co. acquired the rights to develop DPP-4 inhibitor compounds 3 and 4 from Probiodrug company. During the preclinical safety evaluation of compounds 3 and 4, the project team observed adverse symptoms in experimental rats, including anemia and decreased platelet counts, which ultimately led to the death of the rats. Additionally, significant side effects of acute gastrointestinal bleeding were observed in dog experiments [17]. The project team promptly conducted a thorough analysis of these adverse effects, which became one of the key factors in successfully developing DPP-4 inhibitors as drugs. It is crucial to analyze and determine whether the observed animal toxicities are related to DPP-4 inhibition itself, known as mechanism-based toxicity. If the toxicity is DPP-4-related, then DPP-4 cannot be a druggable target, and further development of DPP-4 inhibitors as new drugs would not be possible.

To identify the source of the animal toxicities caused by compounds 3 and 4, the project team conducted in-depth studies on their off-target activities. Off-target activities are typically assessed through counter screening, which can be categorized as specific counter screening or global counter screening. Specific counter screening is usually focused on evaluating protein family members closely related to the target or subtypes within the same family. On the other hand, global counter screening assesses the compound's effects on various known protein family members. Because the latter involves a large number of proteins and requires substantial resources, it is generally performed on a limited number of structurally representative compounds, such as the preferred candidates for clinical trials. In a comprehensive counter screening experiment conducted by MDS Pharma Services (a CRO company providing global counter screening for pharmaceutical companies), compounds 3 and 4 showed low promiscuity, as no off-target activities with IC_{50} values below 40 μM were found. However, during specific counter screening, compounds 3 and 4 exhibited relatively strong inhibitory activities against DPP-8 and DPP-9 (Fig. 1.4).

Analysis of the animal toxicity experiments on compound 3 (threo isomer) and its isomer, compound 4 (allo isomer) led researchers to hypothesize that the toxic side effects of these compounds are unrelated to DPP-4 inhibition. Despite exhibiting almost identical DPP-4 inhibitory activity in both in vitro and in vivo experiments, compounds 3 and 4 displayed significant differences in toxicity during animal studies. By calculating the administered dosage and measured blood drug concentrations in animals, it was observed that the toxicity of allo-isomer compound 4 was approximately 10 times stronger than that of compound 3, indicating that the toxicity is not directly related to their respective DPP-4 inhibitory activity. Thus, the possibility of mechanism-related toxicity was largely eliminated [17]. It is highly likely that the molecular-based toxicity arises from the early DPP-4 inhibitors' interaction with off-target enzymes within the acyl-peptidase family, such as nonspecific inhibition of DPP-8/9.

To further validate this hypothesis, the research team conducted comparative toxicology studies in rats using compound 5 and compound 6, which had similar PK parameters in rats but differed in their activity selectivity [compound 5 (Fig. 1.4) selectively inhibited DPP-8/9, while compound 6 (Fig. 1.4) selectively inhibited dipeptidyl peptidase-7 (DPP-7) or quiescent cell proline peptidase (QPP)]. The two-week toxicology experiment revealed that compound 5, which specifically inhibited DPP-8/9, exhibited toxicity similar to allo-isomer compound 4 in rats. However, compound 6, which

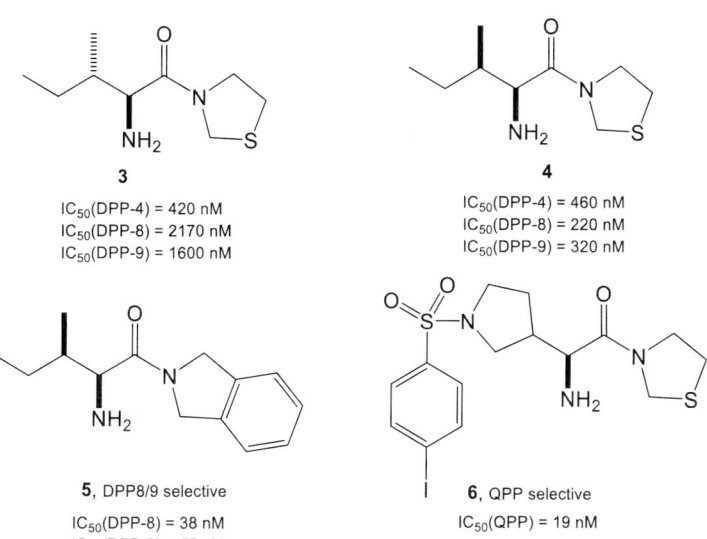

FIGURE 1.4 Selectivity of early dipeptidyl peptidase-4 inhibitors.

specifically inhibited QPP, showed no significant toxicity except at very high doses. Additionally, no apparent lesions were observed with the DPP-4-specific inhibitor [17]. These findings strongly support the research team's hypothesis and emphasize the importance of compound selectivity in the development of dipeptidyl peptidase IV inhibitors.

1.5.3 Optimization strategies for DPP-4 inhibitors

The project team at Merck Pharmaceuticals initially aimed to discover a best-in-class (BIC) drug for DPP-4 inhibition. To be considered a BIC drug, the drug candidate not only needs to exhibit excellent activity, PK, and PD properties but also requires exceptional selectivity and safety. In reality, only a few compounds with optimal biological activity can qualify as BIC drugs. Therefore, the project team believes that a safe and effective DPP-4 inhibitor must possess not only high DPP-4 inhibitory activity but also more than 1000-fold selectivity over other members of the acyl-peptidase family, with particular emphasis on selectivity toward DPP-8 and DPP-9.

Furthermore, because diabetes is a chronic disease requiring long-term medication, drugs should not interfere with other biologically significant protein families. For example, various ion channels play a crucial role in the normal functioning of the heart and should not be disrupted by the drug. Additionally, cytochrome P450 enzymes are vital metabolic enzyme families, and compounds that inhibit or induce cytochrome P450 enzymes can disrupt normal drug metabolism, leading to DDIs and potentially severe consequences. Therefore, molecules that interact with ion channels and cytochrome P450 enzymes must be screened out.

1.6 Confirmation of lead compounds

1.6.1 What constitutes an ideal lead compound?

In medicinal chemistry research, the correct selection and design of lead compounds is a crucial first step toward successful drug development. During the process of optimizing lead compounds into drugs, it is often necessary to simultaneously optimize 7–9 different parameters. Therefore, the synthetic route of the compounds should be as simple as possible. As the molecular weight and lipophilicity of compounds increase during the optimization of activity and permeability, it is preferable for lead compounds to have a smaller molecular weight and lipophilicity (*clogP* value).

1.6.2 α-Amino acid-derived dipeptidyl peptidase-4 inhibitors

Before the discovery of animal multiorgan toxicity associated with DPP-8/9 inhibition, early lead compounds for DPP-4 inhibitors (Fig. 1.5) were derived from α-amino acids. For example, compound 8 was an ideal lead compound with simple synthesis, rigid structure, excellent pharmacological and PK properties, and favorable safety data. However, further testing revealed that compound 8 lacked sufficient selectivity for DPP-8 and DPP-9. To address the selectivity issue, the project team performed significant scaffold modifications to compound 8 and discovered several compounds (such as 9 and 10) with excellent activity. However, these compounds still lacked sufficient selectivity for DPP-8 and DPP-9. At this stage, employing high-throughput screening technology, the project team identified a completely new series of compounds derived from β-amino acids that exhibited some selectivity for DPP-8 and DPP-9. Consequently, the decision was made to suspend research on α-amino acid derivatives and shift focus toward optimizing the β-amino acid derivative series (as described below).

Drug development is a complex process where issues can arise at any stage before the final drug approval. Pharmaceutical companies typically select a high-quality and structurally diverse backup compound as a contingency plan. After the discovery of sitagliptin (a β-amino acid derivative), the project team conducted further research on α-amino acid-derived DPP-4 inhibitors before initiating clinical studies. They observed that the only difference between compounds 3 and 4 was the stereochemical isomerism at the β-position, resulting in a 10-fold difference in inhibitory activity against DPP-8. Building upon compound 3, the project team optimized its selectivity toward DPP-8/9 and synthesized compound 11 (Fig. 1.6). Biological activity testing revealed excellent selectivity of compound 11 for DPP-8 and DPP-9, but its activity was not ideal.

Analyzing the data of previous α-amino acid-derived DPP-4 inhibitors, the project team hypothesized that the introduction of different substituents on the phenyl ring could enhance the biological activity of this compound series. For example, by introducing a 4-fluorophenyl group at the 4-position of the phenyl ring in compound 11 (IC_{50} = 1400 nM), they obtained compound 12 (IC_{50} = 64 nM), which showed a 20-fold increase in activity while maintaining high selectivity for DPP-8 and DPP-9. Compound 12 also exhibited favorable drug metabolism and pharmacokinetics properties. However, further research revealed that compound 12 had high plasma protein binding capability and poor selectivity

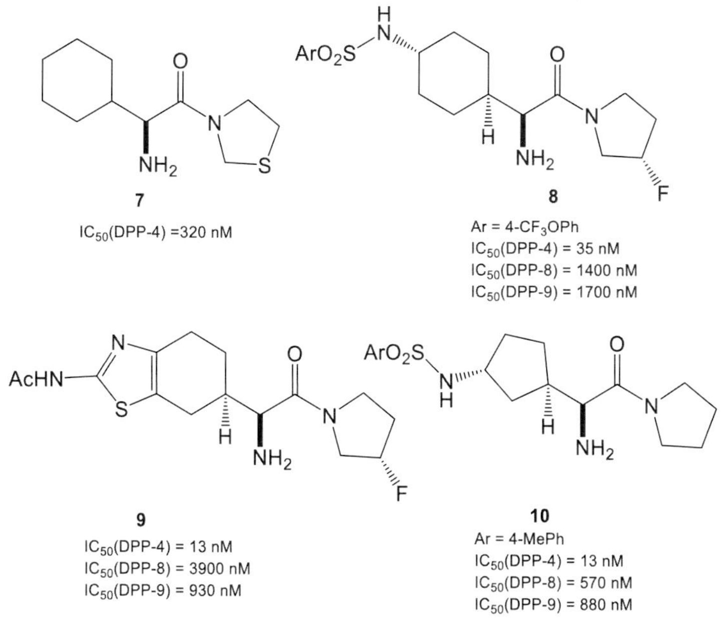

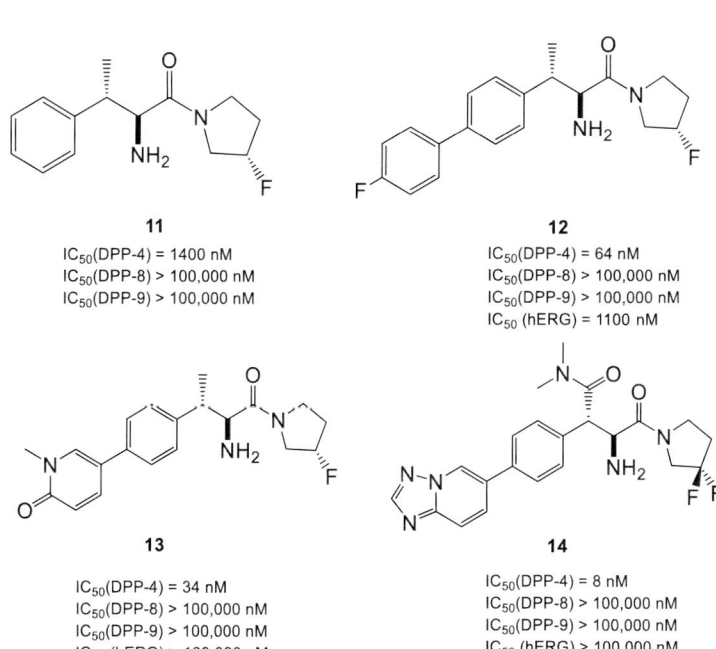

FIGURE 1.5 Early α-amino acid-derived dipeptidyl peptidase-4 inhibitors.

FIGURE 1.6 Optimization of α-amino acid-derived dipeptidyl peptidase-4 inhibitors.

for hERG. To fine-tune the properties of compound 12, the project team reduced its lipophilicity and introduced polar functional groups, resulting in the pyridone compound 13 (Fig. 1.6) [18,19]. Subsequent optimization led to the triazole compound 14, which exhibited excellent activity, selectivity, and ADME/T properties. Ultimately, compound 14 was chosen as the backup compound for Sitagliptin [20]. From the discovery of compound 11 to the identification of compound 14, the project team synthesized just over 300 compounds, demonstrating the highly efficient strategy of property-based drug design.

1.6.3 Identification of β-amino acid series of lead compounds

With the advancement of high-throughput screening technology, the project team identified novel β-amino acid-derived compounds, 15 and 16 (Fig. 1.7), which exhibited certain selectivity toward DPP-8 and DPP-9. However, upon

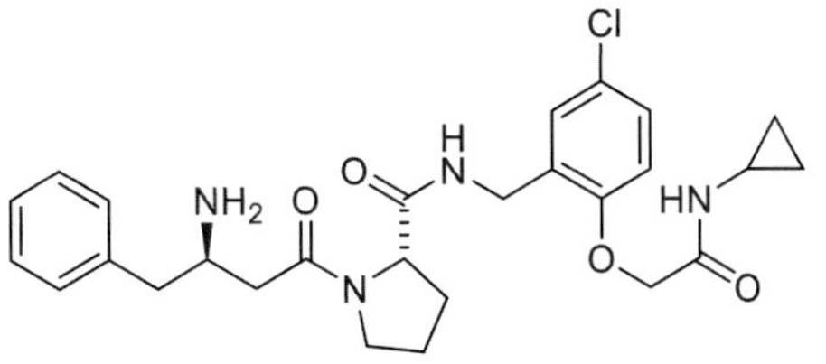

15
IC$_{50}$ DPP-4 = 1900 nM

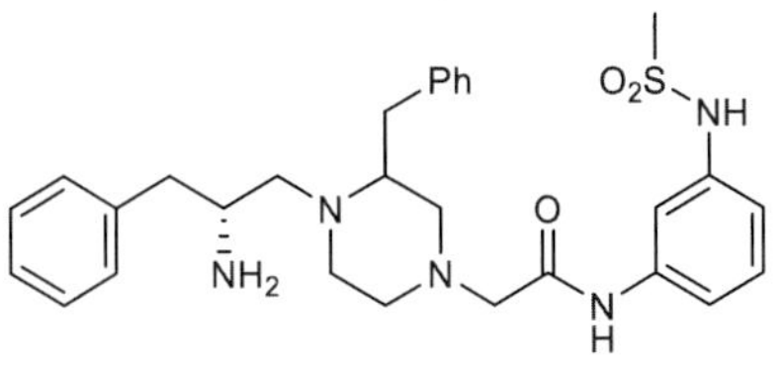

16
IC$_{50}$ DPP-4 = 11,000 nM

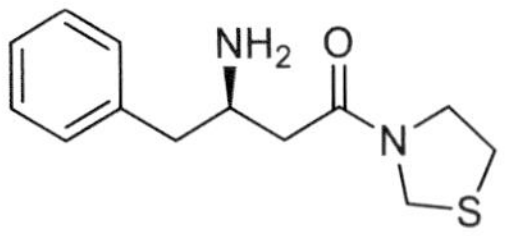

17
IC$_{50}$ DPP-4 = 3000 nM
IC$_{50}$ DPP-8 = 2000 nM
IC$_{50}$ DPP-9 = 23,200 nM

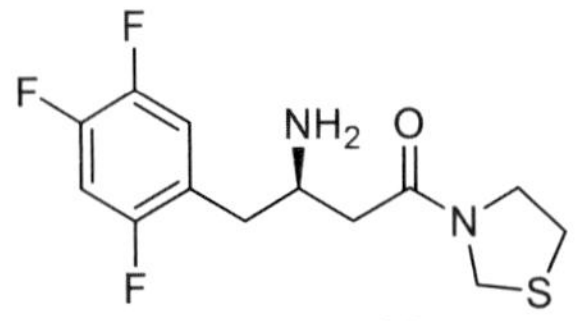

18
IC$_{50}$ DPP-4 = 119 nM
IC$_{50}$ DPP-8 = 2700 nM
IC$_{50}$ DPP-9 = 19,400 nM

FIGURE 1.7 Discovery and optimization of hit compounds in high-throughput screening.

analyzing the molecular properties of these lead compounds, it was determined that compounds 15 and 16 were highly unfavorable. Additionally, the oral bioavailability of this compound series was found to be very poor. To address these challenges, the team undertook simplification of compound 15, leading to the discovery of compound 17, which demonstrated comparable activity to compound 15 while exhibiting a substantially reduced molecular weight (MW = 250). This provided a solid foundation for further optimization of β-amino acid derivatives. Through an extensive investigation of substituents on the phenyl moiety, the project team identified a 2,4,5-trifluoro derivative, compound 18 (IC$_{50}$ = 119 nM) [21].

Although compound 18 exhibited promising activity, its selectivity toward DPP-8 and DPP-9 remained suboptimal. Further structure-activity relationship studies led to the discovery of a novel lead compound, 19 (Fig. 1.8) [22]. Compound 19 possessed desirable characteristics such as low molecular weight (MW = 355), high activity (IC$_{50}$ = 140 nM), good selectivity, and ease of modification, thereby providing essential prerequisites for further optimization efforts.

1.7 Optimization of the β-amino acid series lead compounds

Lead compounds often undergo significant transformations before becoming clinical candidates. Taking lead compound 19 as an example, researchers discovered that in animal models, the 2-fluorophenyl ring formed adducts with glutathione. Additionally, the presence of a piperazine ring exhibited poor metabolic stability due to oxidation, leading to undesirable PK properties such as low oral bioavailability.

To address the issue of piperazine oxidation and enhance the metabolic stability of DPP-4 inhibitors while maintaining selectivity toward DPP-8/9 and hERG, the research and development team conducted a series of chemical design studies. Among these, the most successful approach was the bicyclic strategy (Fig. 1.9) [23,24].

In the subsequent synthesis of bicyclic piperazine derivatives, the project team discovered several highly potent and selective DPP-4 inhibitors, such as the bicyclic triazole-piperazine compounds 21–23. Compound 21 (IC$_{50}$ = 460 nM) exhibited significantly improved activity compared to the nonbicyclic piperazine analog 20 (IC$_{50}$ = 3100 nM). In terms of drug metabolism studies, the ethyl-substituted derivative 22 (IC$_{50}$ = 230 nM) confirmed that the bicyclic triazole-piperazine moiety enhanced in vivo stability against oxidative metabolism. However, its oral bioavailability remained suboptimal [24]. Compound 22 demonstrated poor permeability, and it was observed that increasing the compound's lipophilicity could improve its permeability. The trifluoromethyl-substituted derivative 23 (IC$_{50}$ = 130 nM) not only improved DPP-4 inhibitory activity but also exhibited favorable metabolic stability and oral bioavailability (rat F = 44%). Further structure-activity relationship studies revealed that fluorine substitution on the "left-hand side" phenyl ring further enhanced compound activity. By combining these findings, a series of compounds, as shown in Fig. 1.10, was obtained. Among them, the 2,5-difluorinated derivative 24 (IC$_{50}$ = 27 nM) achieved 50% oral bioavailability in rats, while the 2,4,5-trifluorinated derivative 1 (IC$_{50}$ = 18 nM) demonstrated an even higher oral bioavailability of 76%. Compound 1 (sitagliptin) was ultimately developed as a novel BIC drug.

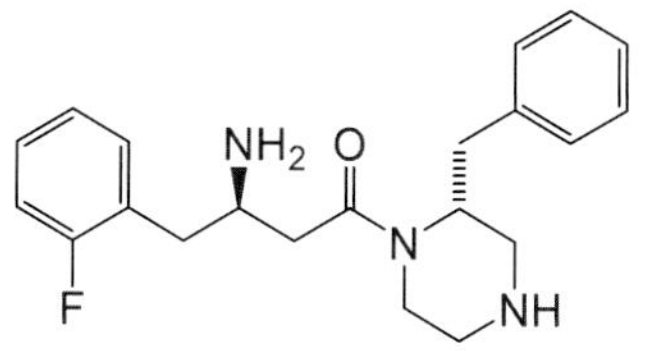

FIGURE 1.8 Lead compounds.

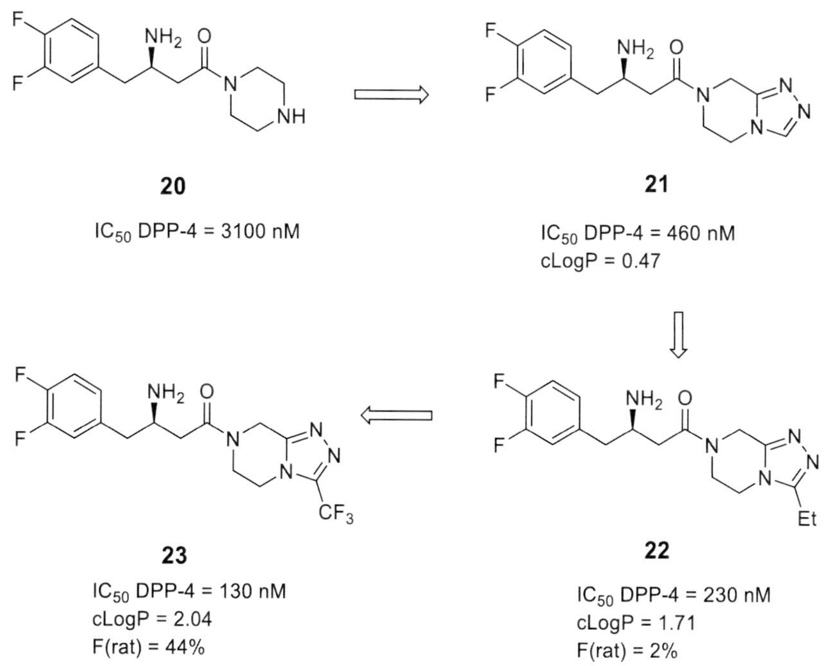

19
IC$_{50}$ DPP-4 = 139 nM
IC$_{50}$ DPP-8 > 100,000 nM
IC$_{50}$ DPP-9 = 41,700 nM

FIGURE 1.9 Strategies for optimizing compound metabolism, permeability, and bioavailability.

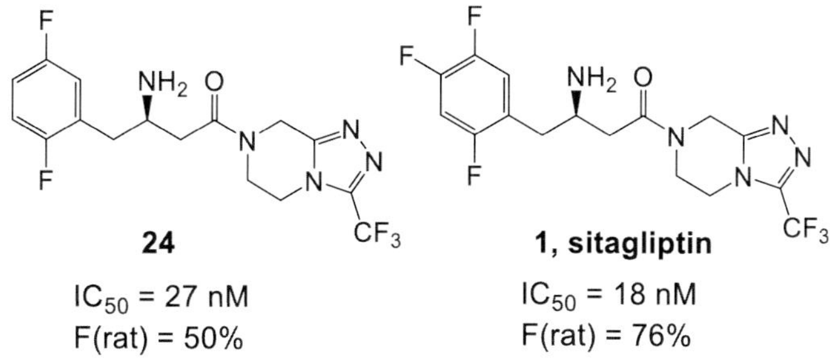

20
IC$_{50}$ DPP-4 = 3100 nM

21
IC$_{50}$ DPP-4 = 460 nM
cLogP = 0.47

23
IC$_{50}$ DPP-4 = 130 nM
cLogP = 2.04
F(rat) = 44%

22
IC$_{50}$ DPP-4 = 230 nM
cLogP = 1.71
F(rat) = 2%

FIGURE 1.10 Preclinical candidate compounds 24 and JANUVIA™ (sitagliptin).

24
IC$_{50}$ = 27 nM
F(rat) = 50%

1, sitagliptin
IC$_{50}$ = 18 nM
F(rat) = 76%

1.8 Clinical studies of the new drug sitagliptin

In the clinical studies of the new drug sitagliptin, which is derived from the lead compound 19, a series of β-amino acid-based DPP-4 inhibitors demonstrated good selectivity, with weak inhibition activity against DPP-8 and DPP-9 (IC$_{50}$ > 45 μM). Compounds 24 and 1, for example, exhibited over 1000-fold selectivity against DPP-8 and DPP-9, meeting the desired criteria.

In terms of off-target screening, compounds 24 and 1 also exhibited excellent selectivity. They showed no significant inhibition or induction effects on cytochrome P450 enzymes and did not display notable blockade of various ion channels. No significant off-target activities of concern or requiring further investigation were observed in vitro.

In efficacy experiments conducted in mice, compound 24 demonstrated slightly reduced inhibitory activity against mouse DPP-4 (IC_{50} = 100 nM). However, a significant reduction in blood glucose levels was achieved at an oral dose of 3 mg/kg with a corresponding blood drug concentration of 700 nM. In diabetic mice induced by a high-fat diet and streptozotocin, long-term administration of compound 24 resulted in a dose-dependent reduction in blood glucose levels, as confirmed by the levels of glycosylated hemoglobin (HbA1c) [25]. Histopathological examination revealed an increase in β-cells within the islets of these diabetic mice that received long-term treatment, providing evidence that DPP-4 inhibition contributes to the restoration of pancreatic and β-cell function and the normalization of islet morphology.

The two-week safety evaluation of compounds 1 and 24 showed no observable toxicity in rats and experimental dogs under the experimental conditions. However, in a canine cardiovascular model test, compound 24 caused adverse reactions such as decreased blood pressure, reduced heart rate, and increased intervals of P and R waves in the electrocardiogram at a dose of 10 mg/kg (plasma concentration of 46 μM). These phenomena were not observed at a dose of 1.0 mg/kg (plasma concentration of 6.5 μM), which is considered the "no effect level" (NOEL) in safety evaluation experiments. Compound 1, on the other hand, did not exhibit adverse reactions in the same cardiovascular model test, and its NOEL for safety was determined to be 10 mg/kg (plasma concentration of 59 μM), indicating a higher safety margin. Further safety evaluations confirmed that compound 1 was more suitable as a clinical candidate for further studies.

Subsequent clinical trial results have confirmed that Compound 1 (clinical code MK-0431, later named sitagliptin) exhibits dose-dependent inhibition of DPP-4. When administered orally at a single dose of 100 mg or higher, MK-0431 maintains over 80% inhibition of DPP-4 activity within 24 hours [26]. This level of inhibition is consistent with the maximum efficacy observed in preclinical animal experiments. The half-life of MK-0431 in the human body ranges from 8 to 14 hours, making it suitable for once-daily dosing (QD dosing), with a high oral bioavailability of 87% [27]. After administration to diabetic patients, the increase in blood glucose levels upon glucose intake is reduced, accompanied by elevated levels of the following biomarkers: active GLP-1, GIP, insulin, and C-peptide, while the biomarker glucagon is decreased [28].

In a 24-week Phase III clinical trial of monotherapy, compared to placebo, sitagliptin resulted in a reduction of 0.6%–0.8% in glycated hemoglobin (HbA1c) levels from a baseline of 8.0% in diabetic patients [29]. In patients with higher baseline HbA1c (>9%) in the diabetic population, sitagliptin led to a more significant decrease in HbA1c, reaching 1.52%. Both fasting and postprandial blood glucose levels of patients showed a decrease after treatment, and there were indications of β-cell function recovery. No side effects, such as hypoglycemia or weight gain, were observed during the clinical trials.

In addition to monotherapy, clinical trial results have also demonstrated the effective combination of MK-0431 with other antidiabetic drugs such as pioglitazone [30] or metformin [31]. In a 52-week comparative trial, diabetic patients receiving ≥1500 mg of metformin were treated with sitagliptin (100 mg) or the sulfonylurea drug glipizide (5–20 mg) in combination [32]. The entire diabetic patient group showed a reduction of 0.67% in HbA1c. Among diabetic patients with a total reduction in HbA1c below 7%, 63% were in the sitagliptin group and 59% were in the glipizide group, which was essentially equivalent. However, 32% of patients in the glipizide group experienced hypoglycemia, compared to only 4.9% in the sitagliptin group. Additionally, patients in the glipizide group had an average weight gain of 1.5 kg, while patients in the sitagliptin group had an average weight loss of 1.1 kg.

In October 2006, the U.S. FDA officially approved sitagliptin, developed by Merck & Co., Inc., as the first gliptin-class drug, a DPP-4 inhibitor, providing a new, safe, and effective treatment option for type 2 diabetes. In China, sitagliptin is approved for monotherapy to improve blood glucose control in patients with type 2 diabetes, in conjunction with diet control and exercise. Furthermore, a fixed-dose combination formulation of sitagliptin and metformin has also received approval and has been launched in the United States and European Union.

1.9 Process chemistry of sitagliptin

1.9.1 What is process chemistry?

In particular, process chemistry in the synthesis of small-molecule drugs refers to practical organic synthesis chemistry, encompassing three stages: laboratory-scale synthesis, pilot-scale up synthesis, and commercial-scale production.

The tasks and responsibilities of the process research department primarily include two aspects: (1) designing and developing scalable chemical processes that meet important criteria such as short synthetic routes, high atom economy, cost-effectiveness, technical reliability, and low environmental impacts; (2) preparing active pharmaceutical ingredients (also known as drug substances or APIs) that comply with standards, supporting the smooth progress of drug development throughout the entire clinical development stage of candidate drugs, and providing technical support for drug production after market approval [33].

In addition, the process development department needs to provide comprehensive documentation detailing reproducible production methods. In many pharmaceutical companies, the process department is also responsible for managing the entire lifecycle of the drug's commercial processes (life cycle management).

The synthesis of new compounds is initially carried out by the medicinal chemistry department. To improve efficiency and meet the needs of early screening, the first synthesis of new compounds is typically performed at the milligram scale, intended for in vitro biochemical experiments, preliminary screening, specificity counter-screening, and PK evaluations. As screening and optimization progress, the medicinal chemistry department usually needs to provide high-purity compounds at the scale of 1–100 grams for various animal model experiments and early toxicological evaluations.

Following these screening and evaluation steps, selected compounds enter the preclinical phase and undergo investigational new drug (IND)-enabling studies, requiring compound quantities in the kilogram range. In the majority of cases, the synthetic methods established by the medicinal chemistry department for early screening are no longer sufficient to meet the production needs at the kilogram scale. Therefore, the process chemistry department formally initiates process research for the project before entering IND, ensuring a seamless transition from medicinal chemistry to process chemistry and guaranteeing the smooth progress of the project.

Over the past few decades, the design and development of large-scale production processes for small-molecule drug synthesis have received significant attention. It has become fully integrated into the value chain of pharmaceutical research and development departments, being regarded as one of the core competencies of the pharmaceutical industry, requiring a high level of scientific literacy and expertise in chemical process experimentation.

The synthesis of sitagliptin, based on the initial synthesis conducted by the medicinal chemistry department, underwent iterative upgrades by the process department, ultimately achieving large-scale and sustainable production. It has received the prestigious Presidential Green Chemistry Challenge Award in the United States twice, making it a classic example in the field of pharmaceutical process chemistry.

1.9.2 Efficiency of chemical reactions

When discussing the efficiency of chemical reactions, the first thing that comes to mind is often the yield, which represents the conversion rate from reactants to products. It is an important parameter for measuring the efficiency of a chemical reaction and can be optimized by adjusting various conditions such as temperature, pressure, solvent, and reactants to achieve the desired yield. Apart from the actual yield obtained, there is another fundamental indicator for measuring the efficiency of a chemical reaction, known as atom economy. This concept was proposed by renowned American organic synthetic chemist Barry Trost in 1991 [34]. Trost suggested that the proportion of reactants that can ultimately be included in the desired products could be referred to as the atom economy. The highest level of atom economy is achieved when "two or more reactants combine solely to form the desired product using only a catalytic amount of any other reagent." He thus proposed the following formula for calculating the atom economy:

Atom economy (%) = (Molecular weight of the desired product)/(Sum of the molecular weights of all reactants and reagents required) × 100%

This parameter not only considers the conversion from reactants to products but also considers the generation of reaction waste. According to this calculation formula, some well-known chemical reactions, such as the Wittig reaction, have low atom economies because the stoichiometric equivalent of triphenylphosphine, a common reagent, cannot be included in the product molecule. Therefore, it is not suitable for large-scale chemical process workflows. In contrast, the Diels–Alder reaction, which only requires a catalyst to combine two reactants to form the product without generating any byproducts, exhibits a high atom economy. Students interested in this topic can use this formula to calculate the atom economy of chemical reactions they have studied and contemplate how to optimize the reaction conditions to achieve the best results while minimizing byproducts and waste.

Through simple calculations, it is evident that catalytic reactions have a significant advantage over stoichiometric reactions in terms of atom economy. The process research on sitagliptin started with the application of chiral auxiliaries in reactions and eventually evolved into an efficient catalytic reaction process, aligning with the principles of green and sustainable modern process chemistry.

From the perspective of organic synthesis, the molecular structure of sitagliptin is not overly complex, with only one chiral carbon atom. Establishing this chiral center naturally became the focus of process research. Due to space limitations, this section will focus on the synthesis process of chiral β-amino acids, excluding the synthesis process of the heterocyclic part. Students interested in the latter can refer to relevant literature for further study [35].

1.9.3 Medicinal chemistry synthesis of sitagliptin: application of chiral auxiliaries

The initial medicinal chemistry synthesis of sitagliptin employed the use of chiral auxiliaries, a mature asymmetric synthesis technique that is widely applicable for introducing various chemical functionalities [36]. During the early stages of medicinal chemistry development, time constraints and the relatively small quantities of compounds required make chiral auxiliaries an attractive and expedient choice due to their predictable induction effects.

There are many options available for chiral auxiliaries, with the most common ones including 8-phenylmenthol, oxazolidinone, pseudoephedrine sulfate, and tert-butylsulfinamide. These auxiliaries can be employed in a variety of chemical reactions, such as aldol condensation, alkylation, Diels–Alder cycloaddition, commonly used carbon-carbon bond-forming reactions, and the introduction of various heteroatoms.

Several methods have been extensively studied for the chiral synthesis of α-amino acids. Additionally, there are multiple well-established methods for the conversion of α-amino acids to β-amino acids. Therefore, Merck's medicinal chemistry team initially explored the diazotization reaction and alkylation reaction using chiral auxiliaries, both of which were successful (Fig. 1.11) [24]. In small-scale syntheses, the experimental results of these two routes were roughly comparable.

The conversion from α-amino acids to β-amino acids can be achieved through the Wolff rearrangement reaction (Fig. 1.12). This reaction offers mild conditions and high yields. However, it involves the use of highly toxic and explosive diazomethane, making it unsuitable for large-scale production processes.

The successful application of chiral auxiliaries provided an ample supply of sitagliptin for pharmaceutical chemistry research and early animal experiments, ensuring rapid progress in the project. However, in addition to the highly toxic and explosive diazo reagents mentioned earlier, the use of chiral auxiliaries introduces two additional linear synthesis steps for attachment and removal of the auxiliary group. This not only reduces efficiency but also significantly increases the consumption of chemical solvents and reagents, as well as energy consumption. The handling and disposal of liquid and solid waste are also affected. From the perspective of atom economy, one equivalent chiral auxiliary that cannot be incorporated into the product structure becomes waste; even if it can be recovered, it adds extra processing steps and costs.

1.9.4 Process chemistry of sitagliptin: application of asymmetric catalytic hydrogenation

Upon transfer to the Process Chemistry department, a thorough evaluation of the previous synthetic route for sitagliptin was conducted. It was determined that the use of this route for large-scale production in kilograms was not only time-consuming and inefficient but also had significant environmental impacts and safety concerns. Therefore, the Process Chemistry department decided to abandon the chiral auxiliary route and instead employ asymmetric catalytic hydrogenation to introduce the chiral center in β-amino acids.

Asymmetric catalytic hydrogenation is widely applied in organic synthesis and has been extensively studied [37]. The pioneers in the field of asymmetric catalytic hydrogenation are Japanese chemist Ryoji Noyori and American chemist William Knowles, who were jointly awarded the Nobel Prize in Chemistry in 2001.

Currently, a variety of chiral hydrogenation catalysts are available, typically composed of transition metals from the platinum group and chiral ligands. Common transition metals used include ruthenium (Ru), rhodium (Rh), palladium (Pd), and iridium (Ir), among others. The most commonly used chiral ligands are alkyl phosphine ligands, which can be employed in various hydrogenation reactions, including the reduction of carbon-carbon double and triple bonds, carbonyl compounds, and the hydrogenation of olefins and amines, among other commonly encountered reduction reactions.

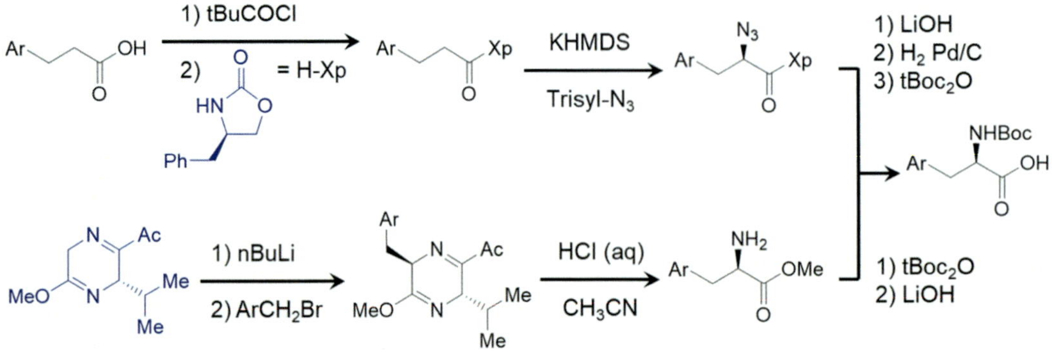

FIGURE 1.11 Application of chiral auxiliary in the drug synthesis pathway of sitagliptin.

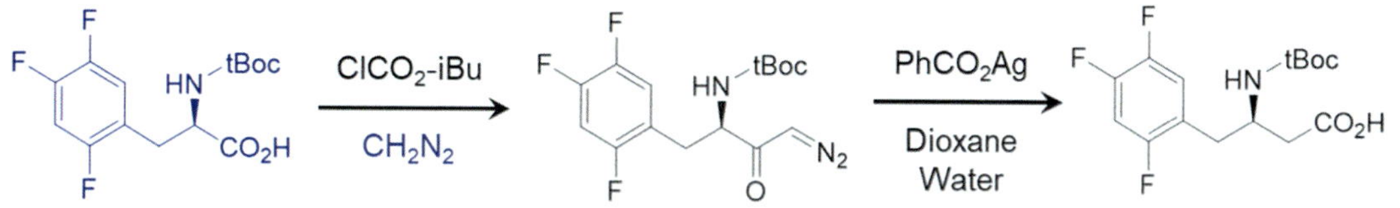

FIGURE 1.12 Conversion from α-amino acid to β-amino acid in the drug synthesis pathway of sitagliptin.

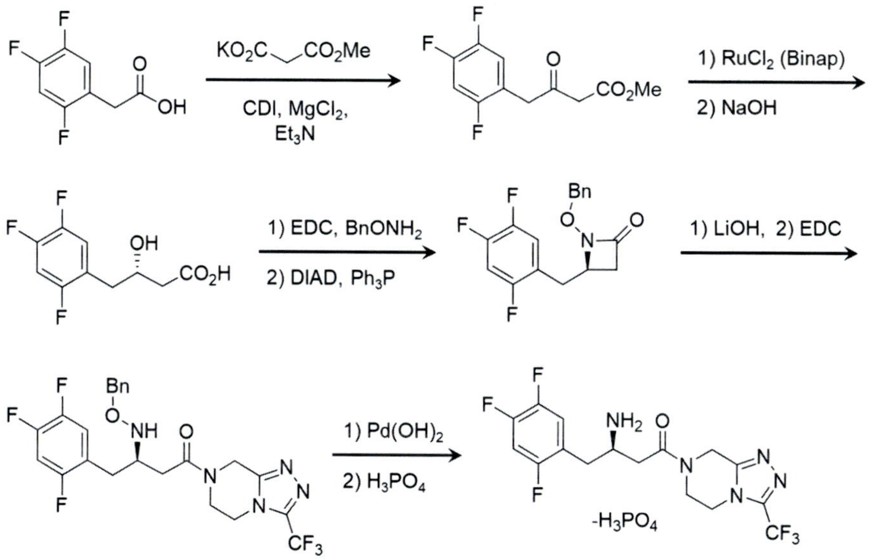

FIGURE 1.13 First-generation synthesis pathway of sitagliptin.

1.9.4.1 First generation process chemistry of sitagliptin: chiral hydrogenation process synthesis

The first-generation process chemistry focused on the asymmetric reduction of carbonyl compounds as the key reaction (Fig. 1.13). Starting from inexpensive carboxylic acids, the carbon chain was extended through esterification reactions to form chiral substrates, β-ketoesters, suitable for asymmetric hydrogenation. Subsequently, researchers systematically screened, selected, and optimized the catalysts (metal and ligand) and reaction conditions for the asymmetric hydrogenation. Eventually, a ruthenium complex with a chiral binaphthyl ligand was identified as the catalyst, with a catalyst loading below 0.1 mol.%. Upon hydrolysis, the carboxylic acid was obtained with a yield of 83% and a 94% enantiomeric excess (ee value) [35].

After the standard 1-Ethyl-3-(3-dimethylaminopropyl)carbodiimide (EDC) amide coupling reaction, a four-membered cyclic lactam was formed through the Mitsunobu reaction, accompanied by a configuration inversion at the chiral center. This step completed the asymmetric synthesis of chiral β-amino acids. The entire synthetic route involved nine linear steps and achieved a final yield of 52%, with an average yield of 93% per step. It was successfully applied to the synthesis of sitagliptin at a scale of 100 kg.

From the perspective of atom economy in organic synthesis, the reactions employed in this process, such as the Mitsunobu reaction and the EDC amide coupling reaction, require the addition of stoichiometric amounts of triphenylphosphine and Diisopropyl azodicarboxylate (DIAD), (in the Mitsunobu reaction) or EDC (in the amide coupling reaction) as reaction reagents. These reagents cannot be included in the structure of the final product, resulting in relatively low efficiency and generating a significant amount of waste. This has a considerable impact on the environment and is not favorable for large-scale production.

1.9.4.2 Second-generation sitagliptin process chemistry: chiral hydrogenation synthesis

To further improve synthesis efficiency and reduce environmental impact, Merck's Process Chemistry department continued to optimize the green process for precursor synthesis and successfully explored the first example of asymmetric catalytic hydrogenation of nonnitrogen-substituted enamines. This led to the development of the second-generation sitagliptin production process, with enantioselective hydrogenation of enamines as the core reaction.

16 Medicinal Chemistry and Drug Development

In the new precursor synthesis process, the application of malonic acid enabled a streamlined approach from carboxylic acid extension to preformed heterocyclic amine coupling, followed by enamine transformation, all in a one-pot synthesis. This significantly simplified the process flow. The main byproducts of the reaction were small, water-soluble molecules such as carbon dioxide, acetone, and tert-butanol, eliminating the need for a large amount of environmentally harmful chemical reagents (Fig. 1.14) [38].

After a systematic screening process, the Merck process team made a significant discovery of a highly efficient asymmetric enamine hydrogenation system based on rhodium metal as the catalyst core. This breakthrough was subsequently optimized and successfully implemented in industrial-scale production for the first time (Fig. 1.15) [37].

From the perspective of production costs and profits, this new process allows for the recovery of over 95% of the precious metal catalyst rhodium, significantly reducing catalyst costs. Moreover, the new process involves only three operational steps, resulting in a 70% cost reduction and a nearly 50% overall increase in profits. Additionally, the production process centered around asymmetric enamine hydrogenation has reduced industrial waste related to the production of sitagliptin's active pharmaceutical ingredient by 80%. As a result, this method was honored with the U.S. Presidential Green Chemistry Challenge Award in 2006. It is estimated that throughout the entire product life cycle of sitagliptin, this improvement has enabled Merck's production division to reduce chemical waste by approximately 150,000 tons, which is an astounding figure.

1.9.4.3 Third-generation sitagliptin process: enzyme catalysis application

In the aforementioned process, the asymmetric selectivity of the enamine hydrogenation reaction was only 95%, requiring an additional step of recrystallization with a free base to meet the required standard of 99.7% for the drug substance. Additionally, the hydrogenation reaction had to be conducted under high pressures of 15–20 atmospheres, necessitating special high-pressure reaction equipment. Furthermore, the recovery of the precious metal rhodium catalyst and the removal of residual traces of rhodium from the product also required additional process steps and production costs.

To further enhance asymmetric selectivity and simplify the process, the process department successfully developed a transaminase-catalyzed process. This new process replaces the precious metal-catalyzed hydrogenation reaction, eliminating the need for any metal (rhodium and iron) reagents and high-pressure reaction vessels, further significantly reducing resource consumption (Fig. 1.16).

Enzyme catalysis is a novel biotechnological process that has experienced rapid development in recent years, with the breakthrough technique of "directed evolution of enzymes" being the key [39]. In 2018, Frances Arnold, who made significant contributions to this research, was awarded the Nobel Prize in Chemistry.

The key to developing enzyme catalysis is the discovery or invention of suitable enzymes. The synthesis process of sitagliptin involved finding or developing a transaminase that exhibits high conversion rates and high selectivity and is applicable to large-scale industrial production.

Sitagliptin is a compound that is completely synthesized through artificial design. Initially, through screening, the collected transaminases did not exhibit any activity toward the conversion of enamines. Using the technique of "directed evolution of enzymes," and employing an "induced" approach, researchers started from the chemically similar

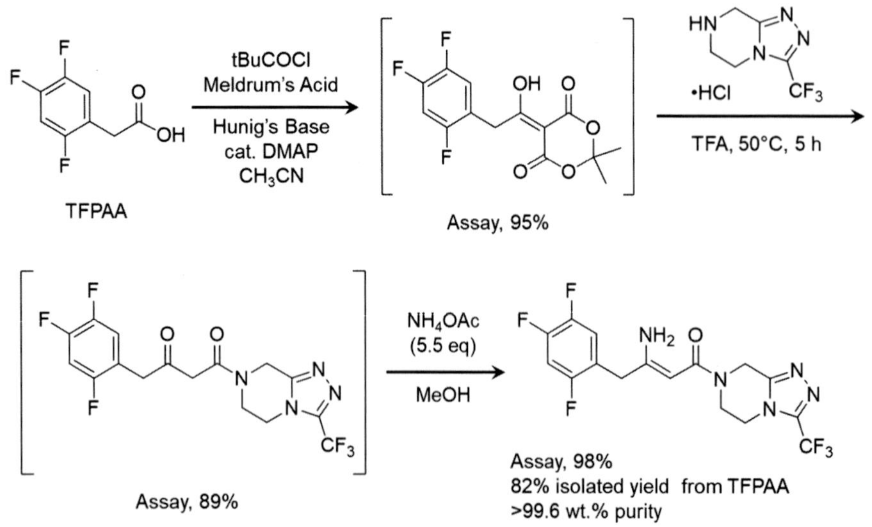

FIGURE 1.14 Second-generation sitagliptin process synthesis route: "one-pot" synthesis of hydrogenation precursor.

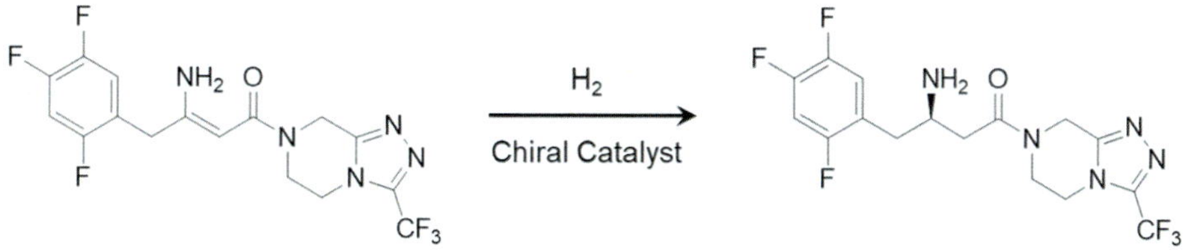

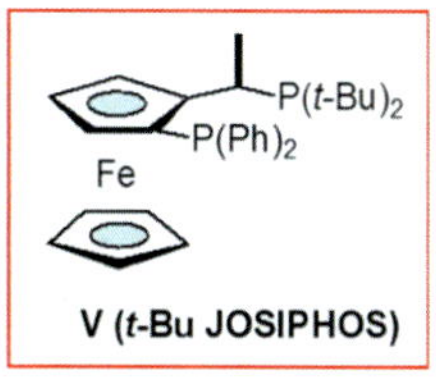

FIGURE 1.15 Key steps in the second-generation sitagliptin process synthesis route: screening of chiral hydrogenation catalysts.

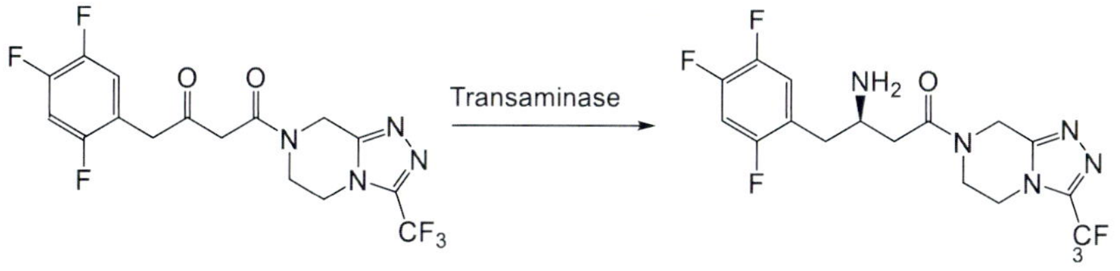

Metal	Ligand	% Conversion	% e.e.
Ir COD Cl	(R)-BINAP	65	4
	(S,S)-ChiraPhos	28	4
	(R,S)-JosiPhos	35	8
	(R,R)-Et BPE	33	4
Ru COD Cl	(R)-BINAP	18	-
	(R,S)-JosiPhos	16	-
Rh(COD)CF$_3$SO$_3$	(R)-BINAP	0	-
	(R,R)-Et BPE	40	38
	I	90	6
	II	>99	72
	III	99	86
	IV	>99	89
	V	99	95

V (t-Bu JOSIPHOS)

FIGURE 1.16 Third-generation synthesis route of sitagliptin: transaminase-mediated reductive amination.

aspects and synthesized several reaction transition state intermediates. Through a step-by-step "learning" process, the original transaminase gradually evolved into an enzyme with detectable conversion rates. However, at that time, the conversion rate of this enzyme was only 0.5% (Fig. 1.17).

The researchers persisted and used site-directed mutagenesis techniques to introduce random artificial mutations into the original transaminase. Through this process, they screened and selected for improved conversion rates, resulting in the discovery of "mutant enzymes." This marked the completion of one cycle of evolution for the transaminase. Using the newly evolved transaminase as a starting point, the second cycle began with additional rounds of random site-directed mutagenesis and screening, continuing until satisfactory results were achieved. In the screening and optimization process of the enamine-converting enzyme for sitagliptin synthesis, only 11 rounds of "mutation-selection" were performed. These cycles led to a remarkable improvement in the transaminase's conversion rate, increasing it from 0.5% to over 95%. The catalytic efficiency of the optimized transaminase after evolution was an astonishing 25,000 times higher than that of the original transaminase. Furthermore, throughout the entire evolution process of the transaminase, the asymmetric selectivity ratio remained consistently above 99.9% (Fig. 1.18) [40].

The transaminase-catalyzed new process significantly increased the productivity of existing equipment by 56% and improved the overall yield by 10%−13%. Furthermore, the process led to a reduction in overall waste generation by 19%. These impressive achievements were recognized when the new process received the U.S. Presidential Green Chemistry Challenge Award in 2010, highlighting its contributions to sustainable and environmentally friendly chemistry practices.

1.9.4.4 Green chemistry—a promising pathway toward sustainability

Green chemistry, also known as sustainable chemistry, is defined as the development of chemical processes that minimize or eliminate the use of hazardous substances. With the accelerated pace of global industrialization and the

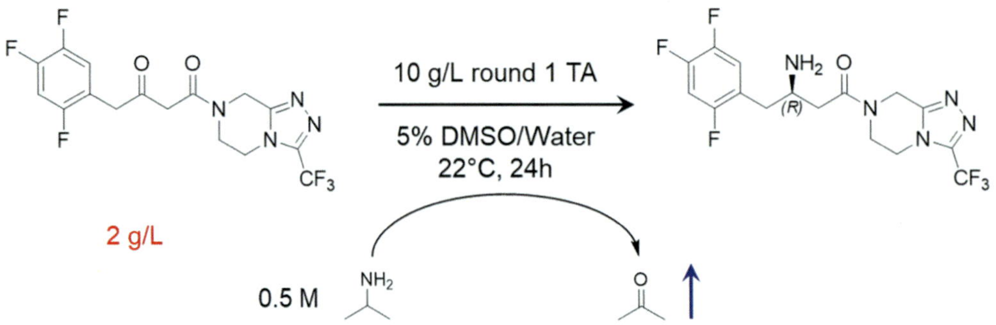

FIGURE 1.17 Third-generation synthesis route of sitagliptin: primary transaminase with a conversion rate of 0.5%.

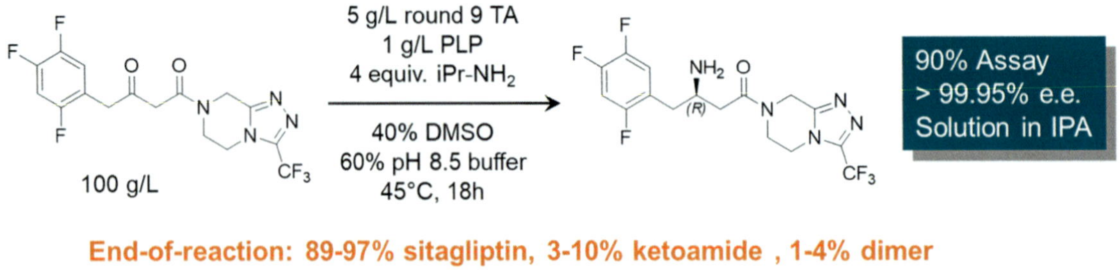

End-of-reaction: 89-97% sitagliptin, 3-10% ketoamide , 1-4% dimer

FIGURE 1.18 Third-generation synthesis route of sitagliptin: highly efficient transaminase after evolution.

increasing severity of climate change and resource depletion, there is a growing demand for green chemical processes and the elimination of harmful chemical products. The importance of green chemistry in process development is gaining increasing attention [41], as it plays a crucial role in shaping the future of our living environment.

In this chapter, we conclude by highlighting the application of green chemistry in the industrial synthesis of the antidiabetic drug sitagliptin. We aim to emphasize the significance of sustainable chemistry in pharmaceutical research and employ the perspective of atom economy to analyze the impact of chemical reactions on the human living environment. Moreover, we hope that the historical journey of Sitagliptin's process development will inspire more students and readers to contribute their knowledge, passion, and experiences toward the pursuit of more sustainable chemical processes. In closing, let us be reminded of the words of Nobel laureate Professor Ryōji Noyori, who encourages aspiring students, "Green chemistry is not merely a popular catchphrase; it is the key to human survival."

References

[1] Drucher DJ, Philippe J, Mosjsov S, et al. Glucagonlike peptide-I stimulates insulin gene-expression and increases cyclic-AMP levels in a rat islet cell-line. Proc Natl Acad Sci U S A 1987;84:3434–8.
[2] Drucker DJ. The biology of incretin hormones. Cell Metab 2006;3:153–65.
[3] Burcelin R, Da Costa A, Drucker D, et al. Glucose competence of the hepatoportal vein sensor requires the presence of an activated glucagon-like peptide-1 receptor. Diabetes 2001;50:1720–8.
[4] Nauck MA, Heimesaat MM, Behle K, et al. Effects of glucagon-like peptide 1 on counterregulatory hormone responses, cognitive functions, and insulin secretion during hyperinsulinemic, stepped hypoglycemic clamp experiments in healthy volunteers. J Clin Endocrinol Metab 2002;87:1239–46.
[5] Deacon CF, Nauck MA, Toftnielsen M, et al. Both subcutaneously and intravenously administered glucagon-like peptide-I are rapidly degraded from the Nh2-terminus in type-Ii diabetic-patients and in healthy-subjects. Diabetes 1995;44:1126–31.
[6] Young RJ, Leeson PD. Mapping the efficiency and physicochemical trajectories of successful optimizations. J Med Chem 2018;61:6421–67.
[7] Gleeson MP. Generation of a set of simple interpretable ADMET rules of thumb. J Med Chem 2008;51:817–34.
[8] Lipinski CA, Lombardo F, et al. Experimental and computational approaches to estimate solubility and permeability in drug discovery and development settings. Adv Drug Deliv Rev 2001;46:3–26.
[9] Degoey DA, Chen HJ, et al. Beyond the rule of 5: lessons learned from Abbvie's drugs and compound collection. J Med Chem 2018;61:2636–51.
[10] Veber DF, Johnson SR, Cheng H. Molecular properties that influence the oral bioavailability of drug candiates. J Med Chem 2002;45:2615–23.

[11] Raub TJ. P-Glycoprotein recognition of substrates and circumvention through rational drug design. and compound collection. Mol Pharm 2006;3:3−25.
[12] Bohnert T, Gan L. Plasma protein binding: from discovery to development. J Pharm Sci 2013;102:2953−4.
[13] Price DA, Blagg J, Jones L, et al. Physicochemical drug properties associated with in vivo toxicological outcomes: a review. Expert Opin Drug Metab Toxicol 2009;5:921−31.
[14] Malki MA, Pearson ER. Drug-drug-gene interactions and adverse drug reactions. Pharmacogen J 2020;20:355−66.
[15] Munawar S, Windley MJ, et al. Experimentally validated pharmacoinformatics approach to predict hERG inhibition potential of new chemical entities. Front Pharmacol 2018;9:1−20.
[16] Ahren B, Simonsson E, Larsson H, et al. Inhibition of dipeptidyl peptidase IV improves metabolic control over a 4-week study period in type 2 diabetes. Diabetes Care 2002;25:869−75.
[17] Lankas GR, Leiting B, Roy RS, et al. Dipeptidyl peptidase IV inhibition for the treatment of type 2 diabetes—potential importance of selectivity over dipeptidyl peptidases 8 and 9. Diabetes 2005;54:2988−94.
[18] Xu J, Wei L, Mathvink R, et al. Discovery of potent and selective phenylalanine based dipeptidyl peptidase IV inhibitors. Bioorg Med Chem Lett 2005;15:2533−6.
[19] Xu J, Wei L, Mathvink R, et al. Discovery of potent, selective and orally bioavailable pyridone based dipeptidyl peptidase IV inhibitors. Bioorg Med Chem Lett 2006;16:1346−9.
[20] Edmondson SD, Mastracchio A, Mathvink RJ, et al. (2S,3S)-3-Amino-4-(3,3-difluoropyrrolidin-1-yl)-N,N-dimethyl-4-oxo-2-(4-[1,2,4]triazole [1,5-a]pyridin-6-ylphenyl)butanamide: a selective α − amino amide dipeptidyl peptidase IV inhibitor for the treatment of type 2 diabetes. J Med Chem 2006;49:3614−27.
[21] Xu J, Ok HO, Gonzalez EJ, et al. Discovery of potent and selective β-homophenylalanine based dipeptidyl peptidase IV inhibitors. Bioorg Med Chem Lett 2004;14:4759−62.
[22] Brockunier LL, He JF, Colwell LF, et al. Substituted piperazines as novel dipeptidyl peptidase IV inhibitors. Bioorg Med Chem Lett 2004;14:4763−6.
[23] Ashton WT, Sisco RM, Hong D, et al. Dipeptidyl peptidase IV inhibitors derived from beta-aminoacylpiperidines bearing a fused thiazole, oxazole, isoxazole, or pyrazole. Bioorg Med Chem Lett 2005;15:2253−8.
[24] Kim D, Wang LP, Beconi M, et al. (2R)-4-Oxo-4-[3-(trifluoromethyl)-5,6-dihydro[1,2,4]triazolo[4,3-alpha]pyrazin-7(8H)-yl]-1-(2,4,5-trifluorophenyl)butan-2-amine: a potent, orally active dipeptidyl peptidase IV inhibitor for the treatment of type 2 diabetes. J Med Chem 2005;48:141−51.
[25] Mu J, Woods J, Zhou YP, et al. Chronic inhibition of dipeptidyl peptidase-4 with a Sitagliptin analog preserves pancreatic beta-cell mass and function in a rodent model of type 2 diabetes. Diabetes 2006;55:1695−704.
[26] Herman GA, Stevens C, Van Dyck K, et al. Pharmacokinetics and pharmacodynamics of Sitagliptin, an inhibitor of dipeptidyl peptidase IV, in healthy subjects: results from two randomized, double-blind, placebo-controlled studies with single oral doses. Clin Pharmacol Ther 2005;78:675−88.
[27] Vincent SH, Reed JR, Bergman AJ, et al. Metabolism and excretion of the dipeptidyl peptidase 4 inhibitor [C-14]Sitagliptin in humans. Drug Metab Dispos 2007;35:533−8.
[28] Herman GA, Bergman A, Stevens C, et al. Effect of single oral doses of Sitagliptin, a dipeptidyl peptidase-4 inhibitor, on incretin and plasma glucose levels after an oral glucose tolerance test in patients with type 2 diabetes. J Clin Endocrinol Metab 2006;91:4612−19.
[29] Aschner P, Kipnes MS, Lunceford JK, et al. Effect of the dipeptidyl peptidase 4 inhibitor Sitagliptin as monotherapy on glycemic control in patients with type 2 diabetes. Diabetes Care 2006;29:2632−7.
[30] Rossenstock J, Brazg R, Andryuk PJ, et al. Efficacy and safety of the dipeptidyl peptidase-4 inhibitor Sitagliptin added to ongoing pioglitazone therapy in patients with type 2 diabetes: a 24-week, multicenter, randomized, double-blind, placebo-controlled, parallel-group study. Clin Ther 2006;28:1556−68.
[31] Charbonnel B, Karasik A, Liu J, et al. Efficacy and safety of the dipeptidyl peptidase-4 inhibitor Sitagliptin added to ongoing metformin therapy in patients with type 2 diabetes inadequately controlled with metformin alone. Diabetes Care 2006;29:2638−43.
[32] Nauck MA, Meininger G, Sheng D, et al. Efficacy and safety of the dipeptidyl peptidase-4 inhibitor, Sitagliptin, compared with the sulfonylurea, glipizide, in patients with type 2 diabetes inadequately controlled on metformin alone: a randomized, double-blind, non-inferiority trial. Diabetes Obes Metab 2007;9:194−205.
[33] Federsel H-J. Chemical process research and development in the 21st century: challenges, strategies, and solutions from a pharmaceutical industry perspective. Acc Chem Res 2009;42:671−80.
[34] Trost BM. The atom economy—a search for synthetic efficiency. Science 1991;254:1471−7.
[35] Hansen KB, Balsells J, Dreher S, et al. First generation process for the preparation of the DPP-IV inhibitor sitagliptin. Org Proc Res Dev 2005;9:634−9.
[36] Munoz-Diaz G, Mirnda IL, Sartori SK, et al. Use of chiral auxiliaries in the asymmetric synthesis of biologically active compounds: a review. Chirality 2019;31:776−812.
[37] Ojima I, editor. Catalytic asymmetric synthesis. New York: Wiley-VCH; 2004.
[38] Hansen KB, Hsiao Y, Xu F, et al. Highly efficient asymmetric synthesis of Sitagliptin. J Am Chem Soc 2009;131:8798−804.
[39] Porter JL, Rusli RA, Ollis DL. Directed evolution of enzymes for industrial biocatalysis. ChemBioChem 2015;17:197−203.
[40] Savile CK, Janey JM, Mundorff EC, et al. Biocatalytic asymmetric synthesis of chiral amines from ketones applied to Sitagliptin manufacture. Science 2010;329:305−9.
[41] Cue BW, Zhang J. Green process chemistry in the pharmaceutical industry. Green Chem Lett Rev 2009;2:193−211.

Further reading

Murcko, 2018 Murcko MA. What makes a great medicinal chemist? A personal perspective. J MED Chem 2018;61:7419–24.

Parmee ER, He J, Mastracchio A, et al. 4-Amino cyclohexylglycine analogs as potent dipeptidyl peptidase IV inhibitors. Bioorg Med Chem Lett 2004;14:43–6.

Pauly RP, Demuth HU, Rosche F, et al. Improved glucose tolerance in rats treated with the dipeptidyl peptidase IV (CD26) inhibitor ile-thiazolidide. Metabolism 1999;48:385–9.

Rasmusseen HB, Branner S, Wiberg FC, et al. Crystal structure of human dipeptidyl peptidase IV/CD26 in complex with a substrate analog. Nat Struct Biol 2003;10:19–25.

Van De Waterbeemd H, Smith DA, et al. Property-based design: optimization of drug absorption and pharmacokinetics. J Med Chem 2001;44:1313–33.

Vilsboll and Holst, 2004 Vilsboll T, Holst JJ. Incretins, insulin secretion and Type 2 diabetes mellitus. Diabetologia 2004;47:357–66.

Chapter 2

The developmental history of insulin pharmaceuticals

Hai Qian[1] and Binbin Kou[2]

[1]Center of Drug Discovery, China Pharmaceutical University, Nanjing, Jiangsu, P.R. China, [2]Eccogene, Inc., Cambridge, MA, United States

Chapter outline

2.1 Introduction to diabetes and insulin	21
2.1.1 Diabetes mellitus	21
2.1.2 Discovery history of insulin [1–3]	21
2.1.3 The structure of insulin	22
2.1.4 The mechanism of action of insulin	25
2.1.5 Insulin clearance mechanism	26
2.2 Development of insulin pharmaceuticals	26
2.2.1 The development process of insulin medications	27
2.2.2 Structural modification strategies for insulin analogs	28
2.3 Summary and outlook	37
References	38

2.1 Introduction to diabetes and insulin

2.1.1 Diabetes mellitus

Diabetes mellitus is a heterogeneous metabolic disorder primarily characterized by chronic hyperglycemia. Common symptoms include increased thirst, polydipsia, polyuria, polyphagia, blurred vision, and weight loss. In severe cases, it can lead to ketoacidosis or a nonketotic hyperosmolar state. As diabetes progresses, patients are at a higher risk of developing chronic, progressive complications affecting the heart, brain, kidneys, retina, and nervous system, significantly impacting their overall health and quality of life.

The etiology and pathogenesis of diabetes are complex, but insufficient insulin secretion, increased hepatic glucose output, and decreased peripheral glucose utilization are considered core factors contributing to type 2 diabetes. As research on diabetes continues to advance, factors such as neural dysregulation in the brain, increased glucagon secretion, reduced gastric hormone secretion, enhanced renal reabsorption, and increased fat breakdown are also recognized as related to high blood sugar levels.

2.1.2 Discovery history of insulin [1–3]

The utilization of insulin as a therapeutic agent boasts a century-long history and has forged several pioneering chapters in the annals of pharmaceutical research. These include the distinction of being the inaugural biopharmaceutical product discovered and applied to the human body, the first semisynthetic biopharmaceutical, the trailblazing product crafted through genetic recombination, the premiere nonnatural sequence biopharmaceutical, and the preeminent biopharmaceutical in terms of annual consumption. Additionally, insulin analogs have secured numerous accolades in the realms of market dominance and sales, giving rise to several blockbuster medications. As of the present day, insulin-based pharmaceuticals maintain an unassailable lead in both consumption and sales on the global stage.

In 1890, scientists first discerned that dogs could develop diabetes following a complete pancreatectomy, thus irrefutably affirming the pancreas's pivotal role in regulating glucose metabolism. In 1894, the hypothesis that pancreatic islet tissue might exert an influence on blood glucose control was first articulated. In 1909, the secretions of pancreatic islet tissue were first named "insuline."

In 1920, Dr. Banting conceived a visionary notion: ligating the pancreatic duct in dogs, allowing the acinar tissue to atrophy, leaving only the islets of Langerhans, and then isolating the endocrine substance within to observe its therapeutic impact on diabetes. In May 1921, Dr. Banting and Dr. Best conducted experiments in the laboratory of Professor Macleod, conclusively demonstrating that crude pancreatic extracts could lower blood glucose levels in pancreatectomized dogs. Subsequently, Dr. Collip refined the purification process of insulin, and on January 23, 1922, he administered the first clinical trial on a young boy named Leonard Thompson, achieving resounding success. In 1923, Dr. Banting and Dr. Macleod were awarded the Nobel Prize in Physiology or Medicine, which they shared with Dr. Best and Dr. Collip.

Between 1923 and 1924, pharmaceutical companies such as Eli Lilly, Novo Nordisk, and Hoechst endeavored to convert extracts from bovine and porcine pancreases into medications for the treatment of human diabetes. However, the relative impurity of these pancreatic extracts was an enduring challenge. Subsequent research predominantly concentrated on the purification and crystallization of the active constituents in a quest to unravel the intricate chemical structure of insulin. These endeavors directly led to the emergence of crystalline insulin [4,5], ultimately confirming insulin's composition as a protein. In 1954, Sanger et al. reported the primary protein structure of insulin [6,7], an achievement that earned them the Nobel Prize in Chemistry in 1958.

Chinese scientists also made significant strides in the realm of synthetic bovine insulin. Beginning in 1958, a collaborative effort among three institutions—the Shanghai Institute of Biochemistry of the Chinese Academy of Sciences, the Shanghai Institute of Organic Chemistry of the Chinese Academy of Sciences, and the Department of Chemistry at Peking University—spearheaded by Wang Yinglai and featuring researchers such as Gong Yueting, Zou Chenglu, Du Yucang, Ji Aixue, Xing Qiyi, Wang You, and Xu Jiecheng—entered on a mission to synthetically produce insulin through chemical means. This groundbreaking endeavor culminated in the first total synthesis of crystalline bovine insulin on September 17, 1965. The synthetic process unfolded in three steps: first, natural insulin was disassembled into separate A and B chains, each synthesized individually. Subsequently, the artificial B chain was joined with the natural A chain. Lastly, the rigorously verified semisynthetic A and B chains were connected to form the complete insulin molecule. This achievement mirrored natural bovine insulin in terms of structure, biological activity, physical-chemical properties, and crystalline morphology. It represented the world's first artificial synthesis of a protein, a pivotal milestone in humanity's quest to fathom the mysteries of life. For this remarkable feat, Wang Yinglai was acclaimed by the distinguished British scholar Joseph Needham (1900–1995) as one of the founding figures of Chinese biochemistry.

In 1974, mankind accomplished the first complete chemical synthesis of human insulin, an intricate method comprising hundreds of reactions [6,8]. Subsequently, scientists delved into alternative pathways for insulin synthesis, including the conversion of porcine insulin into human insulin [8]. In 1976, Obermeier and Geiger undertook the pioneering effort of semisynthesis, albeit with a total yield of less than 10% [9]. In 1978, a groundbreaking revelation by Homandberg et al. showcased the potential for enzymatic catalysis in a mixture of water and organic solvents to facilitate large-scale production of human insulin [10]. This breakthrough ushered in several enzyme-mediated conversion methods, such as Markussen and colleagues' discovery that porcine insulin could be directly transformed into human insulin esters [11], achieving an impressive yield of 97%.

In the late 1980s, Eli Lilly and Genentech embarked on a transformative journey, employing recombinant deoxyribo nucleic acid (DNA) technology with Escherichia coli or yeast to biosynthesize human insulin [6]. The inaugural production of recombinant human insulin involved the separate production of A and B chains, followed by their chemical concatenation to yield the complete insulin molecule [8].

2.1.3 The structure of insulin

The medicinal chemistry of insulin must be grounded in a precise comprehension of its three-dimensional spatial structure. The primary structure of natural insulin (Fig. 2.1) consists of two chains, A and B, with the A chain comprising 21 amino acid residues and the B chain containing 30 amino acid residues. These two chains are linked by two pairs of disulfide bonds (A7–B7 and A20–B19), and the A chain itself possesses an additional intramolecular disulfide bond (A6–A11) [6]. Insulin monomers can be associated with divalent metal ions, with zinc ions (Zn^{2+}) being the most common ligands. Under the influence of Zn^{2+}, they can aggregate to form hexamers [12], and this polymerization process is pH-dependent.

The lengths of the A and B chains remain essentially constant across different species of animals, and the number and positions of cysteine residues are also conserved. Sequence comparisons reveal that among the 51 amino acids in vertebrate insulin, 10 amino acids (GlyA1, IleA2, ValA3, TyrA19, LeuB6, GlyB8, LeuB11, ValB12, GlyB23, and PheB24) are fully conserved,

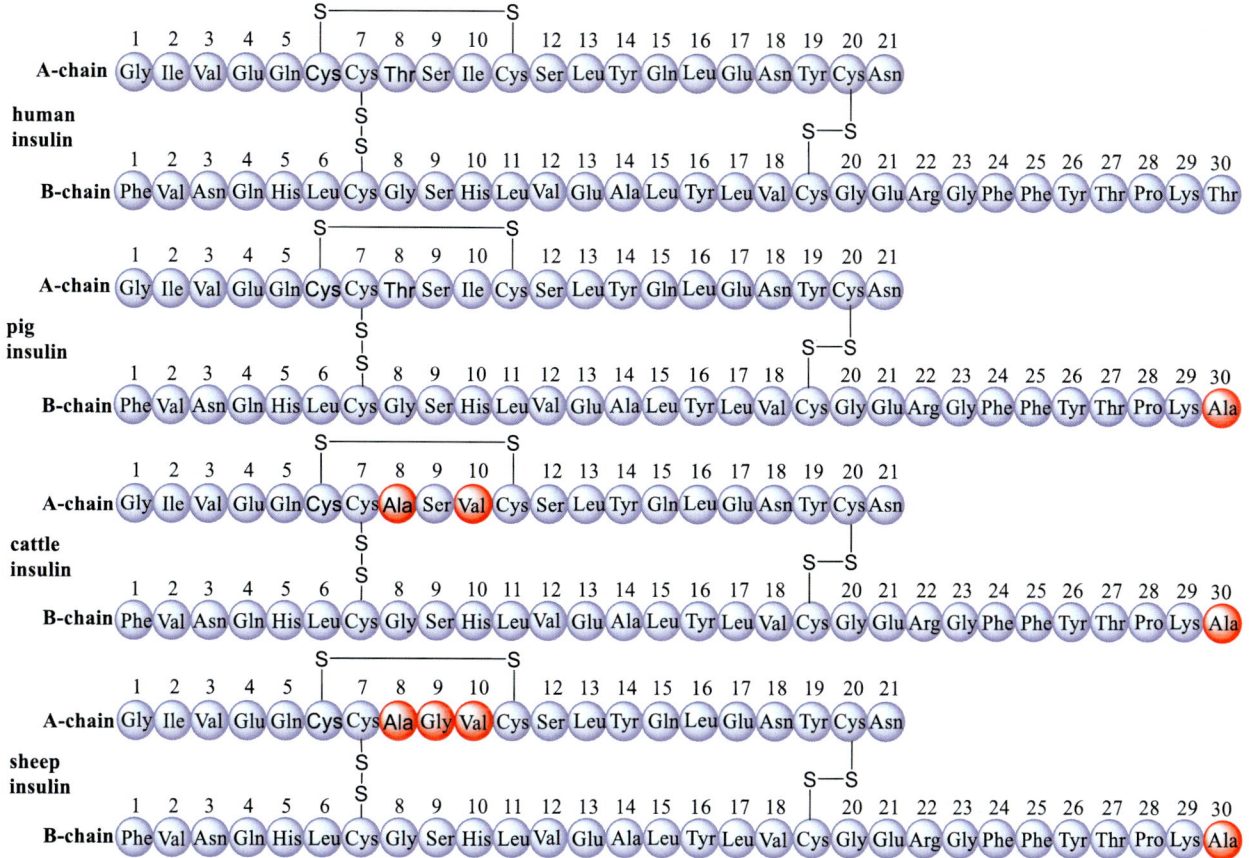

FIGURE 2.1 Displays the primary sequences of insulin from humans, pigs, cattle, and sheep.

with 5 of them (IleA2, ValA3, TyrA19, GlyB23, and Phe24) participating in interactions with the receptor, while the other 5 (LeuB6, GlyB8, LeuB11, GluB13, and PheB25) are involved in maintaining the conformation necessary for receptor binding [13]. In summary, three regions in the A chain are crucial for the structure and activity of insulin: A1–A3, A12–A17, and A19, while in the B chain, B8–B25 is of the utmost importance.

Insulin possesses a secondary structure that is relatively more intricate compared to a polypeptide but comparatively simpler than a protein (Fig. 2.2). The A chain comprises two shorter, antiparallel α-helical structures, A1–A8 and A12–A19. A9–A12 forms an atypical turn structure connecting the two α-helices and bringing the amino and carboxyl termini of the A chain in proximity. The B chain includes a relatively longer α-helical structure, B9–B19, two β-turn structures (B7–B10) and (B20–B23), and a β-strand structure (β-strand) B24–B28, relative to the α-helix B9–B19. B1–B5 constitutes relatively flexible regions. The β-turn of B7–B10 facilitates interactions with the imidazole ring of the histidine side chain in B5, forming disulfide bonds with A7 and B7, thereby stabilizing the conformation. The β-turn of B20–B23 guides the carboxyl terminus B23–B30 in a direction that is antiparallel and in close proximity to the α-helix of the B chain. These two structural segments (B9–B19 and B23–B30) and the side chains (B11 leucine, B15 isoleucine, B12 valine, B24 phenylalanine, and B26 tyrosine) stabilize the molecular conformation through hydrophobic interactions [14].

Insulin exists as a monomer under physiological conditions, and it can self-associate into dimers at elevated concentrations ($> 10^{-6}$ M). This process is primarily driven by hydrophobic interactions among the side-chain amino acids of the carboxyl terminus (B23–B28) of the B-chain. Altering the side-chain structure can disrupt these hydrophobic interactions, ultimately affecting dimer formation. Under the chelation of two divalent Zn^{2+} ions, three insulin dimers can form a stable insulin hexamer. The hexamer can be further divided into three distinct states (Fig. 2.3A and B), known as T_6, $T_3R_3^f$, and R_6, with the ability to interconvert. Fig. 2.4 illustrates the subtle differences in the conformations of the T and R states, primarily in two regions. The T state is closer to the conformation of insulin monomers. First, in the B1–B8 region, indicated by red dots representing the glycine at B8, B1–B5 adopts a more flexible and extended conformation. In contrast, the R state forms an α-helical structure from B1–B9, connecting to B9–B19 as a continuous α-helix. Second, in the case of

24 Medicinal Chemistry and Drug Development

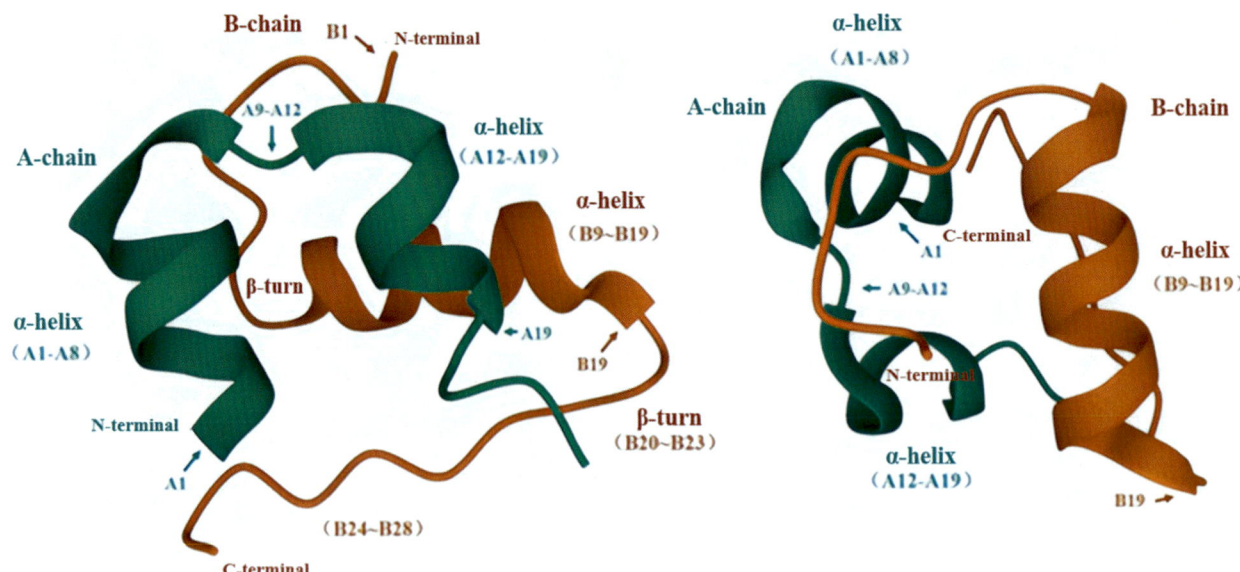

FIGURE 2.2 The three-dimensional structure of the insulin molecule shown in the left panel from the A-chain perspective and the right panel from the A-chain to the B-chain side. In this representation, the A-chain is in green, and the B-chain is in orange [6].

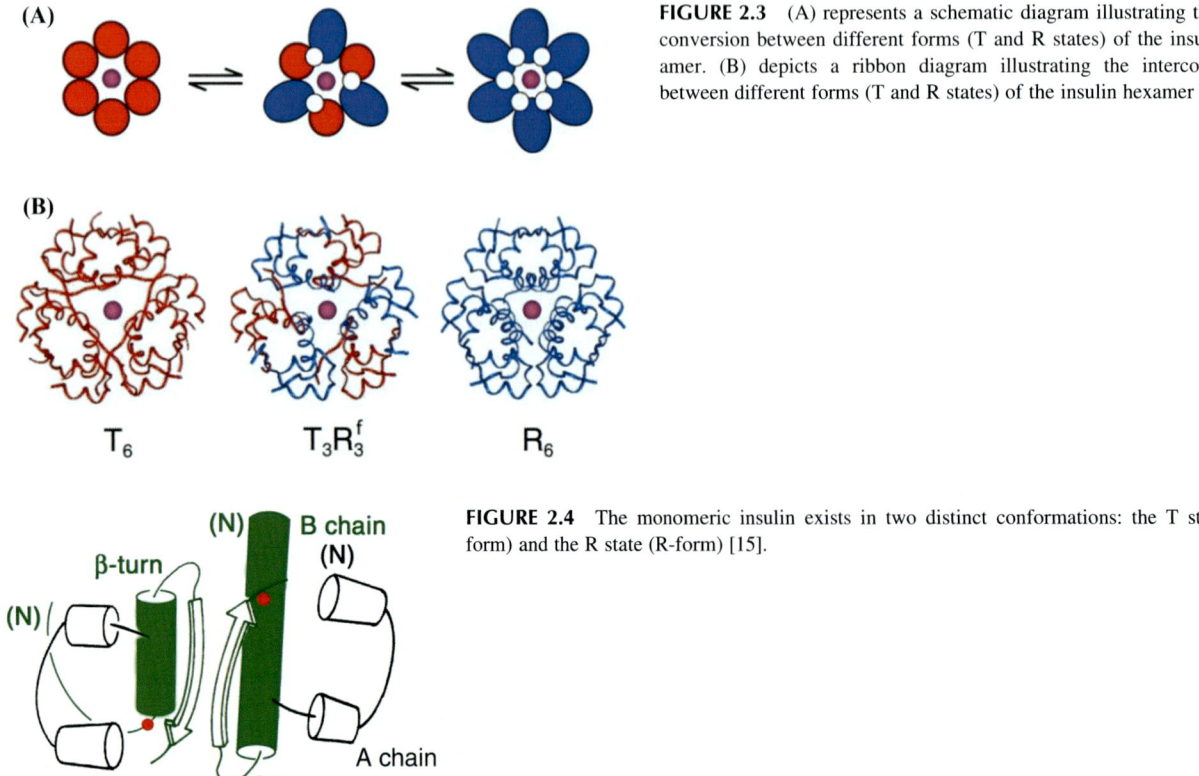

FIGURE 2.3 (A) represents a schematic diagram illustrating the interconversion between different forms (T and R states) of the insulin hexamer. (B) depicts a ribbon diagram illustrating the interconversion between different forms (T and R states) of the insulin hexamer [15].

FIGURE 2.4 The monomeric insulin exists in two distinct conformations: the T state (T-form) and the R state (R-form) [15].

B25 phenylalanine, the phenyl ring side chain in the T state is exposed on the protein surface and is considered an important binding site for the insulin receptor. Conversely, in the R state, the phenyl ring side chain of B25 folds inward, significantly reducing its binding affinity to the receptor. Therefore, the T state is generally regarded as more hydrophobic and more receptor-affine [15]. The chelation effect of divalent Zn^{2+} primarily occurs through a coordination bond between one Zn^{2+}

ion and the three histidine imidazole side chains at B10. If B10 histidine is mutated to other residues, this chelation effect is disrupted, preventing the formation of a stable hexamer [16]. Interfering with the formation of insulin dimers and hexamers has played a crucial role in the field of insulin drug chemistry, which will be elaborated upon in the subsequent chapters on insulin therapeutics.

The structure-activity relationship (SAR) studies were conducted through alanine scanning [17], as shown in Fig. 2.5, along with X-ray diffraction and nuclear magnetic resonance (NMR) research findings, which have revealed critical residues for insulin's binding to its receptor surface. These key residues include A1 glycine, A5 glutamine, A19 tyrosine, A21 asparagine, B12 valine, B16 tyrosine, B23 glycine, and B24 and B25 phenylalanine. Mutations in these residues lead to a significant reduction in the activity of insulin and its analogs [18]. It is evident that disulfide bonds are essential structural elements for maintaining the conformation of insulin. Any replacement of a disulfide bond results in a complete loss of insulin activity [19,20].

2.1.4 The mechanism of action of insulin

Insulin primarily activates two signaling pathways within cells: the phosphatidylinositide-3-kinase (PI3K) pathway and the mitogen-activated protein kinases (MAPKs) pathway, which subsequently regulate cellular metabolism. The initial step in the activation of these signaling pathways is the binding of insulin to the insulin receptor on the cell membrane of target tissues. The insulin receptor exhibits high specificity and widespread distribution, and it can only bind to insulin or proinsulin molecules containing insulin. It is a glycoprotein composed of two α-subunits and two β-subunits connected by disulfide bonds to form a tetramer. The two α-subunits are located on the extracellular side of the cell membrane, have a molecular weight of 130 kD, consist of 723 amino acid residues, and contain binding sites for insulin, insulin-like growth factor-I (IGF-I), and IGF-II. The two β-subunits are transmembrane proteins with a molecular weight of 95 kD, consisting of 620 amino acid residues and forming α-helices during transmembrane passage due to 23 hydrophobic amino acids. Each α-subunit has two insulin binding sites but can only bind to one insulin molecule. Insulin molecules have two binding sites located on the A and B chains, and they bind to different sites on the two α-subunits. The β-subunits possess tyrosine kinase activity, while the α-subunits can inhibit the tyrosine kinase activity of the β-subunits.

Upon binding insulin to the α-subunit, it rapidly induces a conformational change in the insulin receptor, leading to the activation of the tyrosine kinase domain of the β-subunits. This results in the phosphorylation of tyrosine residues on substrate proteins, such as insulin receptor substrates, initiating both the PI3K and MAPK pathways. Activation of PI3K generates phosphatidylinositol-3,4,5-triphosphate, which serves as a second messenger and activates phosphoinositide-dependent protein kinase-1 (PDK-1) and PDK-2. These kinases recruit protein kinase B (PKB) to the cell membrane, where PKB is phosphorylated and its kinase activity is activated. PKB subsequently phosphorylates numerous downstream signaling molecules, including phosphorylating glycogen synthase kinase-3. This leads to the translocation of glucose transporter-2 and glucose transporter-4 from the cytoplasm to the cell membrane, facilitating glucose uptake by the cell and inhibiting glycogen synthesis, ultimately achieving glucose-lowering effects.

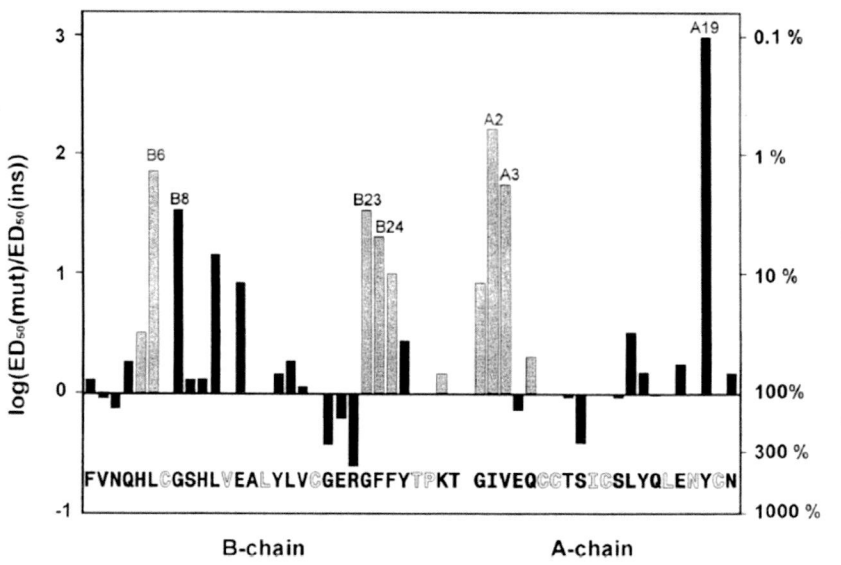

FIGURE 2.5 The structure-activity relationship (SAR) of insulin obtained through alanine scanning. All analogs involve a single alanine substitution, and the activity data are derived from binding experiments between insulin and its receptor. Blank spaces indicate the absence of experimental data [17].

2.1.5 Insulin clearance mechanism

Currently, the clearance mechanism of insulin in the internal environment has been elucidated quite comprehensively. Similar to other chemical substances, insulin clearance is primarily achieved through metabolic processes in the liver and filtration mechanisms in the kidneys, each contributing to approximately 50% of the clearance [21].

The metabolic processes in the liver are closely associated with the binding of insulin to its receptor and the subsequent exertion of its biological activity. Insulin receptors are predominantly distributed in the liver, with some presence in skeletal muscles. These receptors belong to the tyrosine kinase receptor family. When insulin binds to its receptor, it activates the tyrosine kinase domain, catalyzing the phosphorylation of tyrosine residues on substrate proteins. This activation initiates the PI3K and MAPK pathways. Simultaneously, the insulin-receptor complex undergoes endocytosis, entering the cells and forming endosomes during the process [21]. These endosomes contain a substantial amount of insulin-degrading enzymes (IDE), which constitute a family of enzymes, including disulfide bond isomerases and various peptidases responsible for insulin degradation. Insulin that remains undegraded is further transported to lysosomes, which are rich in acidic proteases, for additional degradation. A certain amount of insulin may also avoid degradation and be transferred back into the extracellular space, reentering the internal environment. Studies suggest that not more than 50% of intact insulin reenters the internal environment, meaning that over half of the insulin is cleared through its receptor-binding mechanism. Consequently, insulin analogs with high binding affinity and strong biological activity exhibit faster clearance rates, resulting in shorter plasma half-lives.

As our understanding of this receptor-mediated clearance mechanism becomes increasingly clear, the perspectives of medicinal chemists have evolved. After the 1970s, with the maturation of solid-phase peptide synthesis techniques, chemists could easily perform site-specific mutagenesis on the insulin sequence in a short period of time. They could even introduce D-amino acids and unnatural amino acids with diverse side chains, aiming to discover superinsulins through SAR studies. However, as biological science continues to elucidate how insulin interacts with its receptor and its clearance mechanism, along with deepening insights among clinical physicians regarding clinical insulin therapy, medicinal chemists have begun to explore other avenues to optimize insulin's drug properties in the last 20 years. This involves regulating the molecular aggregation and in vivo distribution of insulin, among other approaches, to address the therapeutic challenges encountered in clinical diabetes treatment.

Small-molecule drugs that enter the bloodstream initially bind to serum albumin. This binding is reversible and represents one of the primary mechanisms determining the half-life of small-molecule drugs. However, highly hydrophilic macromolecules like peptide hormones cannot bind to serum albumin. This makes them prone to renal filtration or uptake into cells through proximal tubular reabsorption, leading to subsequent degradation within lysosomes. Consequently, the plasma half-lives of the majority of peptide hormones are only a few minutes to a dozen minutes, or even shorter. Insulin is no exception to this phenomenon. It can also be subjected to glomerular filtration in the renal glomerulus as well as proximal tubular reabsorption, which involves endocytosis, transferring insulin into lysosomes where IDE facilitates degradation. The subtle distinction between renal and hepatic metabolism lies in the fact that insulin is primarily degraded *via* lysosomal pathways within the kidneys, whereas in the liver, it primarily undergoes intracellular degradation. The remaining fraction of insulin after hepatic metabolism proceeds for further degradation through renal processes. Both of these organs' metabolic activities constitute the overwhelming majority of insulin clearance, accounting for almost 100%. In conclusion, the purpose of this extensive discussion on insulin clearance is to introduce the concepts and directions of insulin's medicinal chemistry research.

2.2 Development of insulin pharmaceuticals

As mentioned earlier, insulin is a century-old medication used to control blood sugar and treat diabetes. Its progress and development, like other drugs, have been driven by in-depth clinical research, the continuous identification of various treatment needs, and their practical solutions, leading to the further optimization of insulin medications.

Clearly, the ultimate goal in blood sugar control is to achieve insulin therapy that can mimic the physiological secretion pattern of insulin, thereby restoring blood sugar levels to a normal physiological state [22]. Fig. 2.6 illustrates the physiological changes in human blood sugar throughout the day and the corresponding physiological insulin secretion patterns. Under physiological conditions, the dynamic range of blood sugar concentration in the human body remains within a very narrow and highly stable range, between 70–140 mg/dL or 3.8–7.8 mmol/L. This range can be further divided into the basal blood sugar range (70–100 mg/dL or 3.8–5.6 mmol/L) and the postmeal blood sugar range (100–140 mg/dL or 5.6–7.8 mmol). Correspondingly, there are basal insulin levels and postprandial bolus insulin levels. From this, it can be inferred and clinically confirmed that insulin has a relatively narrow therapeutic window.

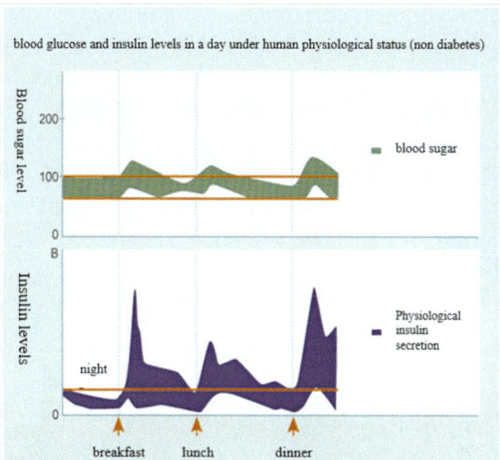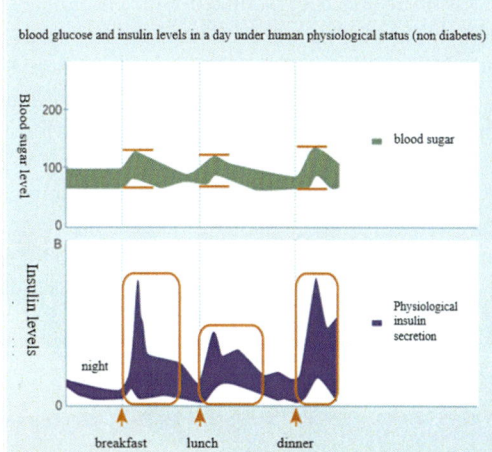

FIGURE 2.6 The left panel illustrates the physiological range of blood glucose concentration in the human body, with two orange lines denoting the basal blood glucose range of 70–100 mg/dL. In the lower section of the left panel, we observe basal insulin secretion levels in the physiological state. A single orange line signifies the basal insulin level. Moving to the right panel, it portrays the postprandial blood glucose concentration range within the human body, with two orange lines representing the postprandial blood glucose range of 70–140 mg/dL. In the lower-right graph, we can observe the pulsatile secretion of insulin in response to postprandial conditions. The orange region illustrates the rapid increase in insulin secretion followed by a subsequent decline to the basal level as part of the physiological process [23].

Although exogenous insulin can mimic the glucose-lowering effect of endogenous insulin in the human body and to some extent compensate for the inadequate insulin secretion in diabetic patients, it has a relatively short half-life, and its onset and peak effects are slow [22]. Moreover, exogenous insulin itself has two apparent defects, preventing it from completely mimicking the physiological secretion pattern of insulin. First, endogenous insulin exerts its glucose-lowering effect through the endocrine pathway in response to elevated blood sugar levels in the body, while exogenous insulin is delivered through external injection. Second, when a patient's blood sugar levels drop, exogenous insulin cannot regulate and inhibit its own levels through negative feedback, leading to hypoglycemia. For type 1 diabetes patients, the incidence rate of hypoglycemia can be as high as 36%. Even for type 2 diabetes patients with relatively good blood sugar control, the rate of hypoglycemia is close to 10% [24]. Hypoglycemic adverse reactions can cause patients to faint, experience decreased cognitive abilities, or even lose cognitive function, leading to a significantly reduced attention span, thereby increasing the likelihood of accidents and, in some cases, direct fatalities [25]. The development of insulin analogs aims to better mimic the secretion of endogenous insulin to achieve improved pharmacokinetic properties within the body, thereby maintaining blood sugar levels within the ideal range for diabetes patients.

2.2.1 The development process of insulin medications

Since its discovery and clinical application by Canadian scholars Banting and Best in 1921, insulin drugs have undergone several significant phases of development.

2.2.1.1 Phase one: 1921 to the late 1970s

As pioneers in the field of insulin, Eli Lilly Pharmaceuticals in the United States and Novo Nordisk Pharmaceuticals in Denmark jointly pioneered the method of extracting insulin from animal pancreas and applying it clinically. This innovation transformed diabetes from an incurable condition into one that could be effectively managed, saving millions of diabetic patients. As previously mentioned, insulin from different mammalian species bears strong sequence similarity to human insulin, with only a single residue differing in pig insulin (B30) [26]. Initially, insulin drugs were extracted and recrystallized from pig, cow, and sheep pancreas. During this phase, the main focus was on overcoming the short plasma half-life of insulin. Various approaches were employed to optimize insulin formulations, such as incorporating components like Zn^{2+}, phenol, and m-cresol into insulin preparations, promoting the formation of more R_6 hexamers [27]. When injected into the body, insulin underwent a reversible conversion to form T_6 hexamers, which were then dissociated into dimers or monomers, exerting its pharmacological effects. This physical dissociation process delayed insulin release and degradation, thereby extending the drug's duration of action. These formulation advancements continue to be utilized in long-acting basal insulin drugs. In 1950, Novo Nordisk introduced neutral protamine Hagedorn (NPH) insulin, which consisted of insulin cocrystallized with protamine, a positively charged protein rich in arginine. This interaction, under neutral conditions, delayed the dissociation of insulin into the bloodstream, prolonging its action. According to literature reports [28], NPH insulin had an onset time of 1–2 hours, a peak time of 4–8 hours, a duration of action of 8–14 hours, and a plasma half-life of approximately 4 hours—significant improvements compared to the 6-minute half-life of insulin monomers. NPH insulin allowed for twice-daily dosing and became the preferred insulin drug during this phase. However, it had notable drawbacks, including the risk of hypoglycemia due to individual variability and the inconvenience of precise individualized dose and timing adjustments, both for physicians and patients. Additionally, insulin during this period was primarily sourced from extracts of pig or cow pancreas. Even with purity levels exceeding 97% after crystallization, impurities and cross-immunogenic reactions between insulin from different species and the human body led to the production of insulin antibodies in over 90% of drug users [29], rendering the treatment less effective and safe.

2.2.1.2 Phase two: early 1980s to pre-approval of insulin lispro in 1996

During this phase, as gene recombinant technology rapidly advanced, human insulin produced through recombinant DNA technology gained Food and Drug Administration (FDA) approval in 1982, thanks to the efforts of Eli Lilly Pharmaceuticals and Genentech Pharmaceuticals. Human-sequence insulin drugs gradually replaced those produced through animal extraction and semisynthesis methods. This transition had two major advantages: First, human insulin significantly reduced cross-immunogenicity, substantially decreasing the production of antiinsulin antibodies. Second, it reduced the production cost of insulin (approximately 40% of the cost of animal extraction). While each insulin dose was only 3–10 mg (100–300 U), the global demand for insulin exceeded thousands of tons per year. At this point, production costs remained a crucial factor limiting insulin drug prices.

2.2.1.3 Phase three: since the FDA approval of insulin lispro in 1996

This phase, symbolized by the FDA approval of insulin lispro in 1996, marked a new era in insulin drug research. Insulin lispro, a rapid-acting insulin developed by Eli Lilly Pharmaceuticals, was the first nonnaturally occurring sequence protein biologic product to be introduced for clinical use. During its development and registration, insulin lispro sparked widespread controversy, centered around its nonnatural amino acid sequence. In the case of insulin lispro, the drug developers swapped the positions of B28 proline and B29 lysine, resulting in a peptide sequence never before detected in any animal species. Some researchers, particularly those in the industry, believed that hormones, bioactive peptides, and proteins had undergone millions of years of natural selection to reach optimal states. They argued that these sequences should remain unaltered, especially considering the immunogenicity issue. Consequently, they held a negative view of this development. We now know that this perspective was not entirely justified. Immunogenicity can be overcome, and even natural sequences can exhibit substantial differences between pharmacological and physiological states. Occasionally, resistance antibodies can arise under pharmacological conditions. In the author's view, this represented a clash of scientific concepts at the time, with the belief that science should always start with objective data and that practice is the only true standard for testing the truth. Fortunately, the project leader at Eli Lilly Pharmaceuticals persevered against objections, driving the project forward to its successful market introduction. This achievement marked the advent of the first insulin analog and ushered in a new era in insulin drug research.

2.2.2 Structural modification strategies for insulin analogs

As mentioned earlier, at high concentrations, exogenous insulin tends to self-associate into hexamers. Consequently, conventional human insulin injections into the body require a process of hexamer dissociation into monomers before they can take effect, which limits their onset time. Therefore, one of the key aspects of structural modification is the development of insulin analogs with release and onset durations closer to endogenous insulin.

Currently marketed therapeutic insulins (Table 2.1) are categorized based on their duration of action in the human body and include rapid-acting insulin, short-acting insulin, intermediate-acting insulin, long-acting insulin, and ultralong-acting insulin. Among these, only short-acting insulin is recombinant human insulin, while the others are insulin analogs.

The corresponding strategies for modifying insulin analogs are introduced one by one, as follows:

TABLE 2.1 Pharmacokinetic and pharmacodynamic characteristics of insulin and its analogs.

Insulin classification	Insulin name	Onset	T_{max}	Action time
Rapid-acting insulin	lispro insulin	~15 min	30–70 min	2–5 h
	insulin aspart	10–20 min	1–3 h	3–5 h
	insulin glulisine	10–20 min	55 min	~6 h
Short-acting insulin	human insulin	~30 min	1.5–3.5 h	7–8 h
NPH	NPH	1.5–4 h	2.8–13 h	~24 h
Long-acting insulin	insulin glargine	1–3 h	—	~24 h
	insulin detemir	1–2 h	6–8 h	~24 h
Ultra-long acting insulin	insulin degludec	0.5–1.5 h	—	~48 h

2.2.2.1 Amino acid substitution

The absorption and onset duration of insulin formulations hinge on the rate of their disintegration into monomers following subcutaneous injection. Consequently, it is conceivable to formulate insulin analogs with a more expeditious onset by reinforcing the charge-repulsion effect, thus mitigating the formation of dimers. The research elucidates that the B26–B30 region of the insulin molecule represents a nonessential portion for insulin receptor recognition but exerts influence over the self-aggregation process of insulin molecules [30]. The substitution of amino acids within this domain affords the attainment of rapid-acting insulin analogs.

Substantive findings disclose that the individual elimination of either ProB28 or LysB29 does not perturb the self-aggregation process of insulin monomers. Nevertheless, the concurrent removal of all amino acid residues within the B28-B30 domain results in a conspicuous reduction in the self-aggregation capacity of insulin monomers while preserving their biological activity. Substituting Pro28 with Asp28, Ala28, or Lys28 similarly engenders the inhibition of self-aggregation, with the lowest degree of self-aggregation observed when Pro28 is substituted with Asp28. Furthermore, it is noteworthy that supplementary substitution of Lys29 with Pro29 further attenuates its self-aggregation capacity, albeit without validation of its hypoglycemic activity through animal experimentation.

Lispro insulin diverges in molecular structure from conventional human insulin due to the reciprocal exchange of Pro28 and Lys29 positions within the B chain, as delineated in Fig. 2.7 [31,32]. This alteration leaves the entire insulin molecule's isoelectric point unaffected but does impart a change to the molecule's conformation. This shift results in the displacement of the typical binding of the C-terminus of the B chain, consequently inducing hexamer instability [32,33], facilitating the swift dissociation of hexamers into dimers and monomers. In comparison to human insulin, lispro insulin manifests an 84% affinity for the insulin receptor while concurrently sharing an identical dissociation rate [34]. Nonetheless, its dimerization capacity experiences a marked attenuation, amounting to merely 1/300th of that of human insulin [30]. Interestingly, it is worth noting that even in the presence of Zn^{2+} and phenol within the drug formulation, lispro insulin can persist in the formation of stable hexamers. Furthermore, lispro insulin is amenable to binding with protamine to yield intermediate-acting formulations, known as neutral protamine lispro. Protamine's predisposition to aggregate in solution results in the formation of an uneven suspension upon insulin binding, thereby extending subcutaneous absorption duration.

The molecular structure of insulin aspart (also known as NovoLog or NovoRapid) differs from regular human insulin by the substitution of Pro28 on the B chain with negatively charged Asp28 [31,35], as illustrated in Fig. 2.8. The principle behind its rapid-acting action involves disrupting the interactions between monomers, thereby inhibiting the formation of dimers and hexamers [30], allowing it to rapidly take effect upon entering the bloodstream. Compared to human insulin, its dimerization constant is reduced by 200- to 300-fold. Insulin aspart formulations include the addition of arginine and niacinamide, which accelerate the rate of monomer formation, thereby expediting absorption. Pharmacokinetic research data reveals that insulin aspart has a twice-faster absorption rate and peak concentration compared to human insulin but a shorter duration of action.

The molecular structure of insulin glulisine (also known as Apidra), in contrast to regular human insulin, exhibits differences in two key locations on the B chain. Specifically, Asn3 and Lys29 are replaced by Lys3 and Glu29 [31,36], as depicted

30 Medicinal Chemistry and Drug Development

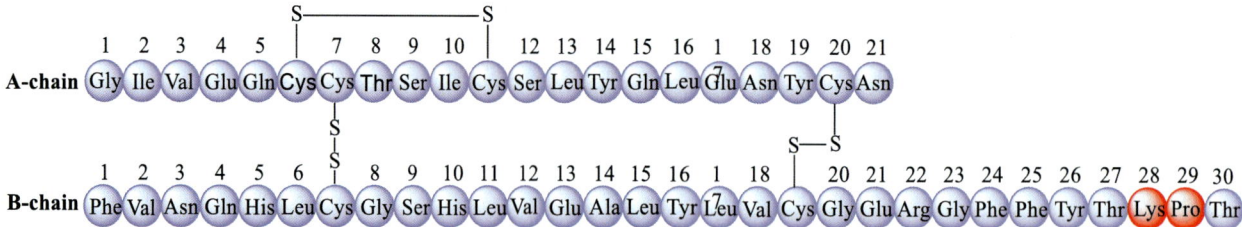

FIGURE 2.7 The molecular structure of lispro insulin.

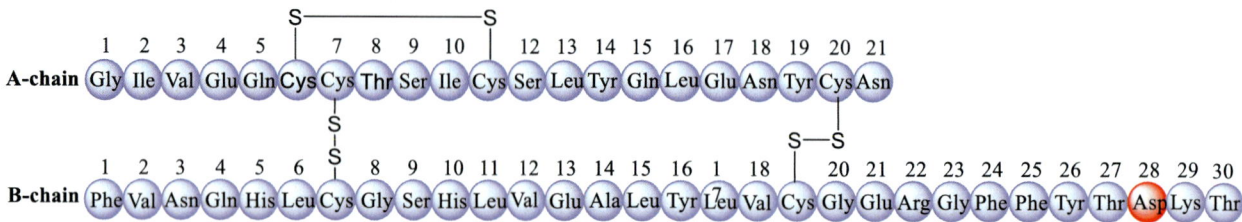

FIGURE 2.8 The molecular structure of insulin aspart.

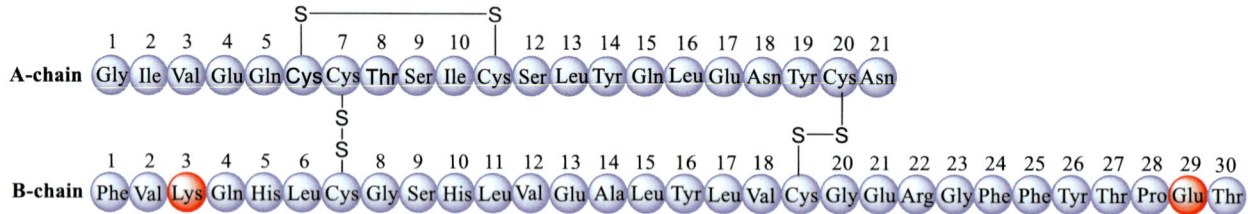

FIGURE 2.9 The molecular structure of insulin glulisine.

in Fig. 2.9. These amino acid substitutions lower the molecule's isoelectric point from 5.4 to 5.1, thereby enhancing its solubility under physiological pH conditions and accelerating its disintegration into monomers. Furthermore, replacing Lys29 with Glu29 not only reduces insulin dimerization but also enhances its physical stability [36].

Insulin glulisine's buffering system does not include the addition of Zn^{2+}. Instead, it incorporates polylysine20 as a stabilizer, preventing the formation of hexamers and further expediting its absorption rate.

Rapid-acting insulin analogs can mimic the physiological secretion of insulin during meals and act more quickly. They excel at controlling postmeal blood glucose levels and reducing the incidence of premeal hypoglycemia compared to regular human insulin. Insulin lispro, insulin aspart, and insulin glulisine achieve rapid action by replacing specific amino acid residues at the C-terminus of the insulin B chain to increase charge repulsion, thereby inhibiting self-association in solution. This is a common strategy for developing rapid-acting insulin analogs. The same approach can also be applied to the development of long-acting insulin analogs.

Incorporating positively charged amino acids into the insulin peptide chain raises its isoelectric point from 5.4 to a more neutral value, extending its duration of action [37]. Novosol Basal is the first long-acting insulin analog designed based on this principle (Fig. 2.10). It involves the substitution of AsnA21 with GlyA21, ThrB27 with ArgB27, and the conversion of the carboxyl group of ThrB30 to an amide group. While Novosol Basal prolongs the duration of action, it has not entered clinical studies due to significant individual variability and low in vivo bioavailability [38].

The molecular structure of insulin glargine (Lantus, depicted in Fig. 2.11) differs from regular human insulin in two key ways. First, it features the addition of two positively charged arginine (Arg) residues at the C-terminus of the B chain. Second, it replaces asparagine (Asn) at position 21 on the A chain with glycine (Gly) [31,39]. The addition of

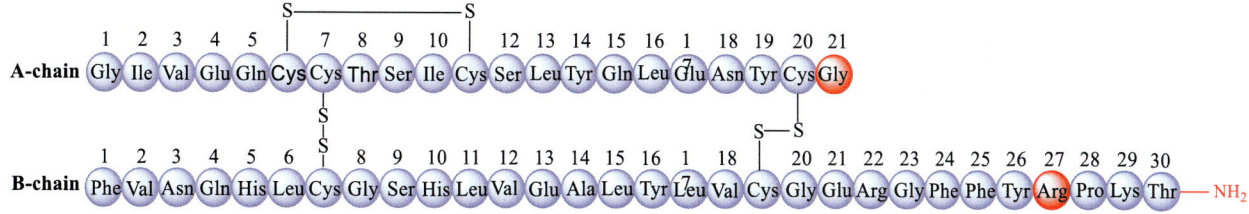

FIGURE 2.10 The molecular structure of Novosol Basal.

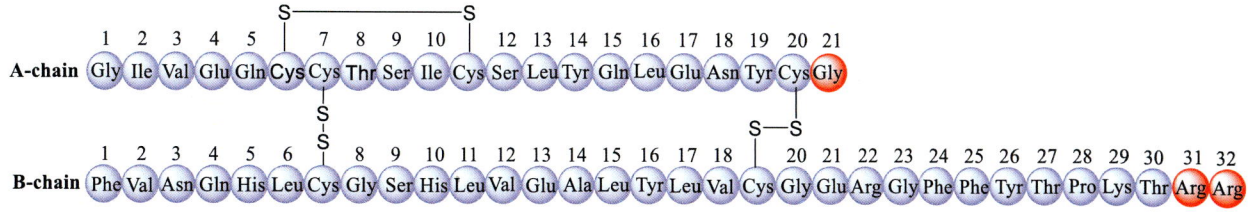

FIGURE 2.11 The molecular structure of insulin glargine.

two basic arginine residues on the B chain raises the molecule's isoelectric point from 5.4 to 6.7, reducing its solubility at physiological pH and slowing down its disintegration into monomers. However, since the formulation must be prepared under acidic conditions and asparagine at position 21 on the A chain is acid-sensitive and prone to deamidation and dimerization, replacing it with the neutral glycine can neutralize the molecule's charge and stabilize it under weakly acidic conditions [39].

Insulin glargine forms an amorphous precipitate upon subcutaneous injection, tightly aggregating in the subcutaneous tissue to create a reservoir, which leads to the slow release of the molecule. This characteristic delays the time-to-peak effect and significantly reduces the incidence of nocturnal hypoglycemia. Insulin glargine U300 is an improved version of insulin glargine U100, with the main difference being the concentration. The former precipitates at physiological pH and forms dense aggregates at the injection site, reducing the absorption surface area and extending absorption and duration of action. It also exhibits a 21% lower incidence of nocturnal hypoglycemia compared to the latter, which also precipitates at physiological pH but forms less dense aggregates, resulting in a relatively shorter duration of action.

Indeed, insulin glargine, as a long-acting insulin analog, is designed differently from rapid-acting insulin analogs. The former achieves its prolonged action by adding basic amino acids to raise its isoelectric point, and the role of amino acid substitution, in this case, is primarily to neutralize the molecule's charge rather than affecting its interaction with receptors. In contrast, rapid-acting insulin analogs achieve their quick action by replacing amino acids to increase charge repulsion inhibiting self-association in solution to attain rapid onset.

2.2.2.2 Conjugated long-chain fatty acids

The strategy of appending long-chain fatty acids represents an alternative approach to extending the duration of insulin action. The underlying principle hinges on the propensity of long-chain fatty acids to bind with human serum albumin (HSA). HSA, a multifunctional transport protein, exhibits the capacity to engage in reversible interactions with various endogenous substances and pharmaceutical agents. Consequently, the formation of albumin-drug complexes facilitates transmembrane transport. This modality offers an avenue for enhancing the pharmacokinetic properties of drugs by manipulating their affinity for albumin.

Insulin detemir (depicted as insulin detemir in Fig. 2.12) constitutes a derivational variant of human insulin. Its molecular distinctiveness from regular human insulin resides in the removal of Thr30 from the B chain, concomitant with the attachment of a 14-carbon myristic acid fatty chain to Lys29 [31]. The inclusion of this fatty acid moiety facilitates the self-association of insulin molecules at the injection site [40], resulting in the formation of strong hexamers despite the formation of weak dihexamers in the solution. Intriguingly, both at the injection site and within the bloodstream, insulin detemir demonstrates a propensity for reversible binding with albumin. This phenomenon has led to a substantial augmentation and prolongation of its absorption and duration of action. The binding between fatty acid-acylated insulin

32 Medicinal Chemistry and Drug Development

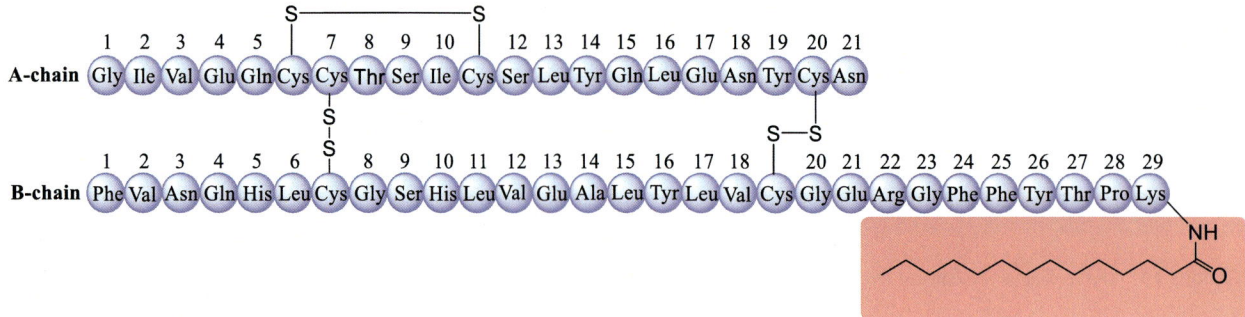

FIGURE 2.12 The molecular structure of insulin detemir.

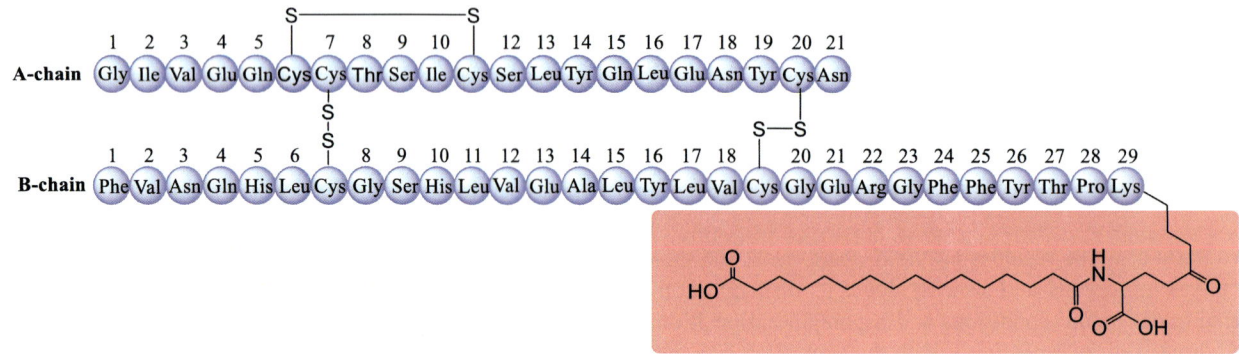

FIGURE 2.13 The molecular structure of insulin degludec.

and albumin arises as a consequence of both hydrophobic interactions and ionic bonding. To a certain degree, the strength of this interaction with albumin is contingent upon the number of carbon atoms present in the acyl chain. The increase from 10 to 14 carbon atoms in the acyl moiety results in an eightfold escalation in the association constant [41]. Furthermore, the removal of the B30 residue positions the negatively charged carboxyl group of the C-terminal amino acid (Lys) in closer proximity to the fatty acid chain linked to Lys29 on the B chain. This spatial orientation of charges, coupled with the association of nonpolar fatty acid chains, simulates the high affinity exhibited by albumin toward free fatty acids themselves [42].

Insulin degludec (also known as insulin degludec, as depicted in Fig. 2.13) is an ultra-long-acting insulin analog. Its molecular structure differs from regular human insulin by the removal of Thr30 from the B chain and the addition of a 16-carbon fatty acid chain, separated by an additional glutamic acid residue at Lys29 [31]. The design objective of insulin degludec is to maintain its solubility while enhancing its self-association ability after injection to achieve prolonged absorption. Insulin degludec operates through a unique mechanism of action: in the presence of phenol and Zn^{2+}, insulin degludec molecules can form stable and soluble dihexamers. However, after subcutaneous injection and the diffusion of phenol, it reverts to multihexamers, thus slowing its absorption [43]. Furthermore, within the bloodstream, insulin degludec can undergo reversible binding with albumin, further delaying its release. These characteristics contribute to a significantly extended duration of absorption and action for insulin degludec.

Conjugation with long-chain fatty acids is a commonly employed strategy to extend the duration of drug action, as discussed in Chapter Three of this book, particularly in the design of long-acting analogs of glucagon-like peptide-1. When compared to insulin glargine, the advantages of insulin detemir and insulin degludec extend beyond their longer duration of action. They can be formulated as neutral solutions, mitigating the skin irritability associated with injectable formulations.

In summary, existing long-acting insulin formulations primarily employ four mechanisms to slow down absorption and extend their duration of action (Table 2.2). These mechanisms include: (1) incorporating protamine to form NPH insulin, which interacts with insulin through charge interactions, resulting in coprecipitation under neutral conditions, leading to delayed release. (2) Adding high concentrations of zinc to limit or slow down hexamer disassociation, thus reducing the rate of insulin monomer absorption, as seen in zinc insulin suspensions. (3) Forming aggregates that

TABLE 2.2 Variations in absorption and onset rates exist among different insulin formulations [31].

	Insulin degludec	Insulin glargine U300	Insulin glargine U100	Insulin detemir	Human NPH insulin	Human routine insulin	Insulin lispr/aspart insulin/insulin glulisine	Quick-acting aspart insulin
In solution	Dihexamer	Hexamer	Hexamer	Dihexamer	Hexamer protamine	Hexamer	Hexamers and polymers	Hexamer
subcutaneous injection site	polyhexamer (<5000 KDa)	dense hexamer collective	Loose hexamer collective	hexamer albumin	hexamer protamine	hexamers and monomers	hexamers and monomers	Hexamers, dimers, and monomers
Absorption rate				Slow fast				
action time				Long short				

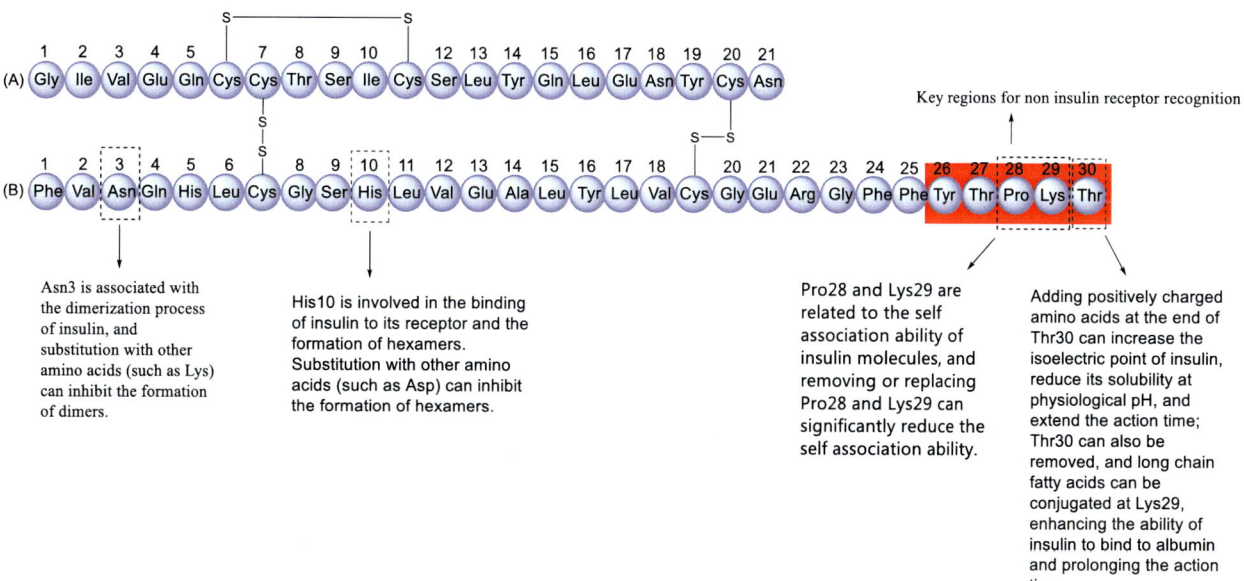

FIGURE 2.14 Structural modification strategies for insulin analogs.

precipitate at specific pH levels but release insulin at physiological pH, exemplified by insulin glargine. (4) Increasing the opportunities and capabilities for insulin to bind with HSA, achieving controlled release, as demonstrated by insulin detemir and others [40].

From a structural perspective, the design of insulin analogs primarily focuses on the B-chain. Whether it involves amino acid substitutions or the attachment of long-chain fatty acids, the aim is to modulate intermolecular forces to achieve the desired effect (Fig. 2.14).

2.2.2.3 Boronic glucose sensor

For the concept of glucose-sensitive insulin, envisioning insulin activity that can automatically adjust based on blood glucose concentration to prevent hypoglycemic side effects, while promising, presents formidable challenges [44]. As previously discussed, the physiological range of blood glucose in the human body is exceedingly narrow, ranging from 3.8 to 7.8 mmol. Even in pathological conditions, the range is only about threefold. Generally, levels below 3.5 mmol lead to hypoglycemic reactions, while values below 3.0 mmol pose life-threatening risks. To achieve the aforementioned objective, glucose-sensitive insulin must exhibit both sensitivity and reversible responsiveness to dynamic changes in blood glucose levels. However, based on the accumulated understanding of chemistry, typical chemical reactions cannot attain such precise dynamic ranges. The following section provides an example of the development of glucose-sensitive insulin.

Currently, one primary strategy to achieve glucose-sensitive insulin is the construction of boronic acid molecular glucose sensors. Boronic acid molecules can covalently bind to the multiple hydroxyl groups on sugar molecules, rapidly and reversibly forming boronates, akin to the formation of hemiacetal structures in organic chemistry. In general, the preparation of alkylboronic acid derivatives necessitates high-pH conditions. Nevertheless, the synthesis of aromatic boronic acid derivatives can be accomplished under physiological pH conditions. This strategy faces several key challenges: (1) the ability to control the dynamic range of blood glucose remains significantly broader than the physiological range, posing a substantial gap between practical glycemic control; (2) distinguishing between glucose and lactate molecules in the bloodstream, as they exhibit similar concentrations, may give rise to adverse reactions if not effectively differentiated; and (3) potential toxicity issues associated with boron compounds, especially concerning long-term medication for diabetes treatment, may present chronic accumulative toxicity concerns.

Novo Nordisk, a pharmaceutical company, has attempted various approaches using boronic acid derivatives, including (1) a strategy based on the hexamer formation of degludec insulin (Fig. 2.15). By utilizing insulin-derived polyol hydroxyl groups competing reversibly for binding with glucose's multiple hydroxyl groups, they aimed to achieve the transition between monomers and hexamers to regulate efficacy and loss of efficacy. Nevertheless, the primary challenge remains in controlling the dynamic range and kinetics of glucose responsiveness, which are still far from ideal [42]. (2) A strategy based on conformational switching: The N-terminus of the A chain and the C-terminus of the B chain of insulin precursor proinsulin are connected through the C-peptide segment; when structurally intact, there is no insulin activity. It is necessary to undergo enzymatic cleavage to remove the C-peptide segment, enabling the formation of fully active insulin. Scientists discovered that covalently linking the N-terminus of the A chain and the C-terminus of the B chain leads to the complete loss of insulin activity. Based on this feature, by linking the multihydroxyl structure to the B29 lysine side chain and the boronic acid glucose sensor to the N-terminus of the A chain, at low glucose concentrations, B29 covalently binds to A1, rendering the molecule inactive. At high glucose concentrations, high levels of glucose bind with B29 boronic acid, displacing the A chain, forming an open-chain active insulin, and achieving glucose-sensitive regulation. However, this method also failed to achieve the desired results and was ultimately halted at the research stage [42]. (3) A strategy based on the combination of fatty acids' high affinity with albumin and the reversible reaction of boronic acid with glucose (Fig. 2.16). The aforementioned fatty acids and connecting molecules can bind to plasma albumin with high affinity. The boronic acid reacts reversibly with glucose. Combining these two mechanisms, at low glucose concentrations, insulin exists as a fatty acid-modified molecule, serving as the active basal insulin. At high glucose concentrations, boronic acid binds with glucose, inhibiting the binding of fatty acids to albumin and leading to the rapid renal filtration and clearance of the drug molecule. Unfortunately, this strategy also did not achieve the envisioned objectives.

2.2.2.4 Competitive interference with the mannose receptor and lectin degradation strategy

Another strategy for achieving blood glucose-sensitive insulin is through competition with the mannose receptor and lectin degradation. In 2010, Merck Pharmaceuticals invested a substantial $500 million to acquire Smart Cells Inc., a preclinical drug company, for their Smart Insulin candidate, which is a blood glucose-sensitive insulin analog. It was later renamed MK-2640 (Fig. 2.17). This molecule is designed with four mannose molecules attached at insulin positions A1 and B29.

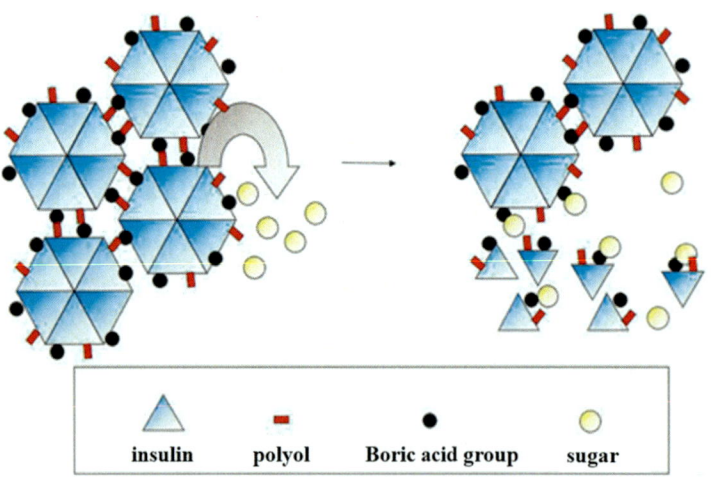

FIGURE 2.15 Glucose-sensitive deglutinin hexamer [45].

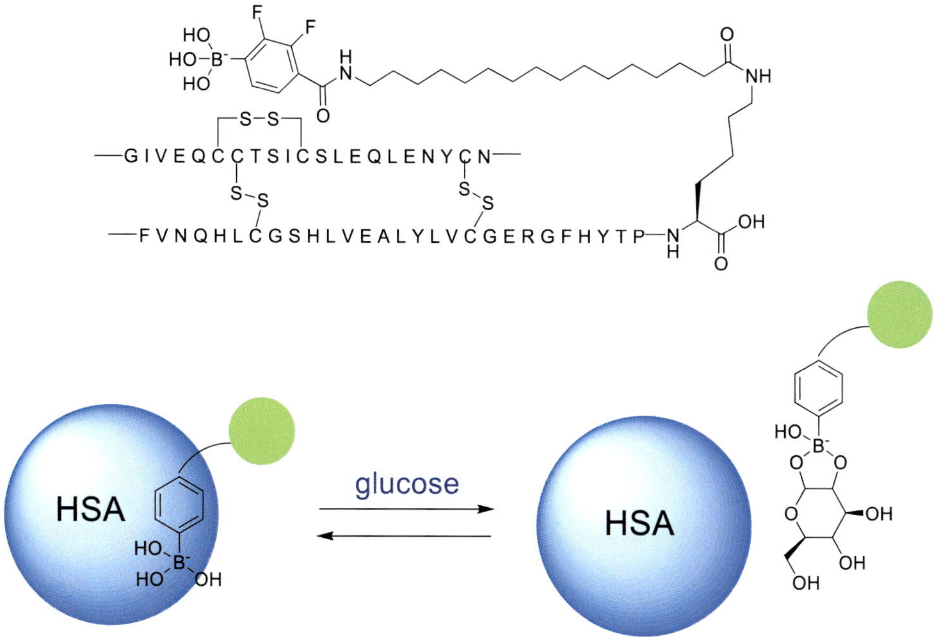

FIGURE 2.16 Glucose-sensitive insulin is based on the dual mechanisms of fatty acids and albumin, as well as boric acid and glucose [44].

Mannose receptors are widely present on lectin surfaces, which are part of the body's immune system defense. Soluble lectin molecules in the circulatory system identify foreign pathogens and transport them to lysosomes for degradation. When blood glucose is low, insulin modified with four mannose molecules binds to the mannose receptors on lectins, leading to its degradation. In contrast, when blood glucose is high, glucose competitively binds to the mannose receptors, preventing insulin from binding and allowing it to take effect. This strategy is more sensitive compared to boronic acid-based approaches. Following Merck's acquisition, a Phase 1 clinical trial was conducted, and the data analysis showed that the insulin candidate did increase the therapeutic window of natural insulin from 2.19 times to 2.9 times. However, it did not significantly improve blood glucose control, and the goal of true blood glucose-sensitive regulation was not achieved. Due to the candidate's low receptor affinity and inability to extend the duration of action, coupled with high production costs, Merck ultimately discontinued the project. It seems that the path to developing blood glucose-sensitive insulin remains challenging.

One of the current hot topics in insulin drug research is oral insulin. Due to the physical and chemical properties inherent in biological macromolecules, their oral bioavailability is extremely low. As a result, these molecules must currently be administered through injections. To ensure quality control, insulin and its derivatives must be formulated as liquid preparations and stored at temperatures between 2°C and 8°C, which presents significant inconveniences for patients and contributes to the high cost of these drugs.

The low oral bioavailability of peptides and protein-based molecules stems from their susceptibility to degradation by gastrointestinal proteases. This prevents their delivery to the small intestine, as their strong hydrophilic nature makes it difficult for them to traverse the mucosal epithelial cells of the digestive tract. Research has indicated several barriers that must be overcome for the absorption of peptide and protein drugs into the bloodstream [45]: (1) Chemical degradation in the highly acidic environment of the stomach, along with the action of gastric proteases like pepsin and pancreatic proteases like trypsin; (2) Protection by the mucin layer in the gastrointestinal mucosa. Mucins, consisting of over 20 different glycoproteins, provide lubrication and resistance to external pathogens. They also impede the passage of hydrophilic macromolecules.

In recent years, advancements in formulation technology have led to the development of a class of compounds known as transient permeation enhancers (TPEs; Fig. 2.18). TPEs are small molecules with amphiphilic properties, serving two key functions: (1) Their amphiphilic nature facilitates the temporary passage of large molecules across epithelial cell membranes, allowing them to enter the bloodstream *via* the transcellular pathway; (2) TPEs exert temporary effects on mucins, causing structural loosening between mucosal epithelial cells and creating relatively large channels. This temporary alteration allows large molecules to pass through into the bloodstream *via* the paracellular pathway [47].

Combining certain protease inhibitors to inhibit degradation during transport can significantly enhance the oral bioavailability of biologics, especially peptide drugs. Currently, there are FDA-approved oral medications like semaglutide

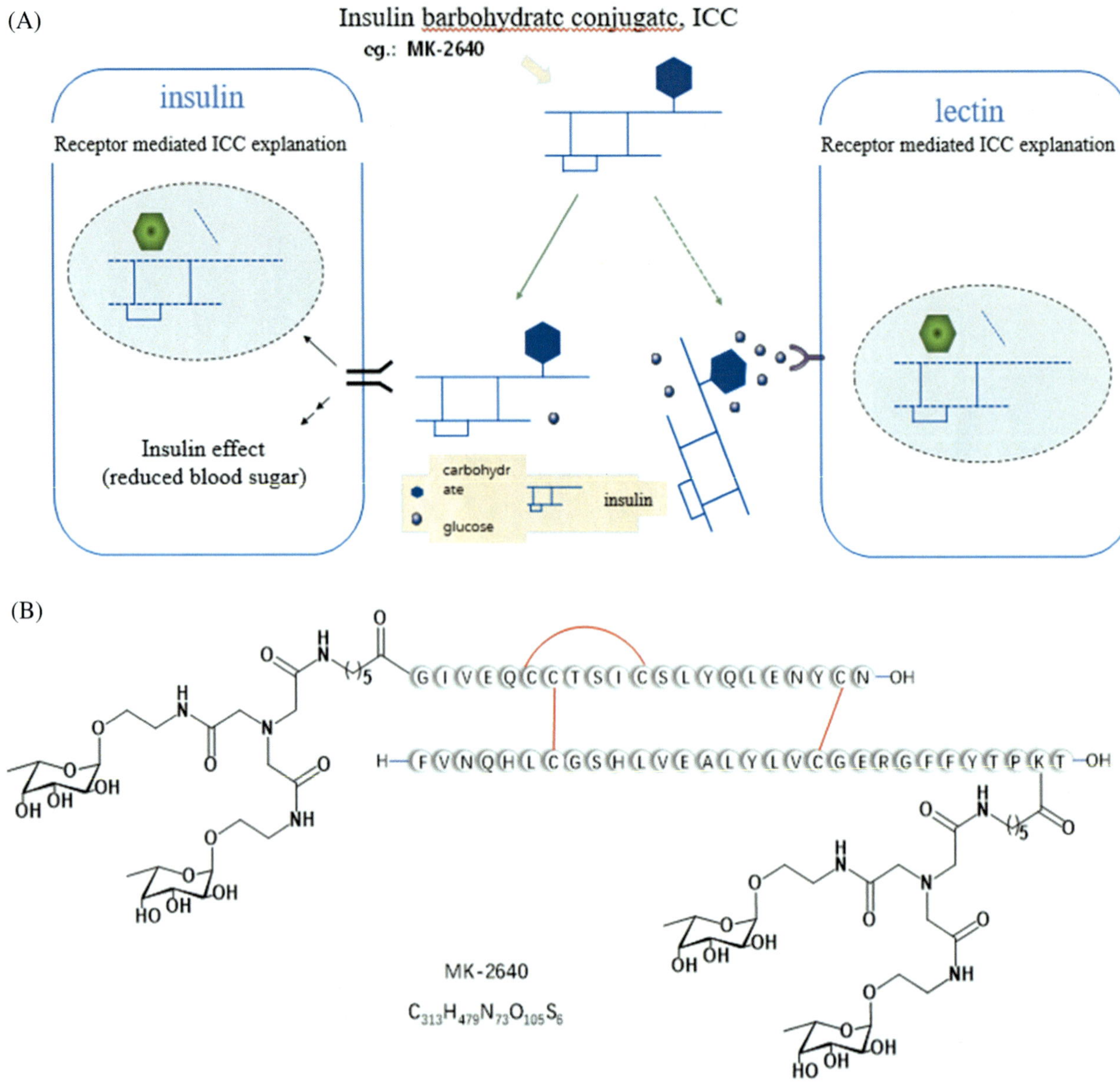

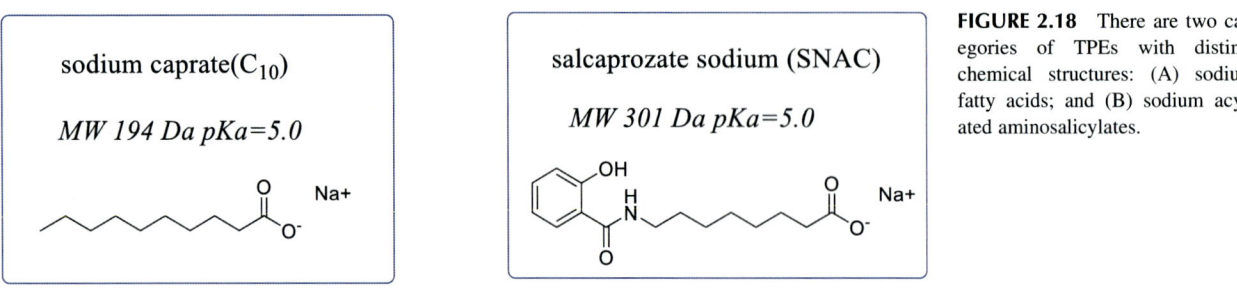

FIGURE 2.17 (A) The mechanism of action of blood glucose-sensitive insulin developed by Smart Cells Inc. (B) The molecular structure of MK-2640 [46].

FIGURE 2.18 There are two categories of TPEs with distinct chemical structures: (A) sodium fatty acids; and (B) sodium acylated aminosalicylates.

sodium caprate(C_{10})

MW 194 Da pKa=5.0

salcaprozate sodium (SNAC)

MW 301 Da pKa=5.0

(RYBELSUS) and octreotide (MYCAPSSA). Many more oral peptide and protein drugs are in various stages of clinical trials. Insulin, as the most widely used peptide protein drug globally, has naturally garnered more attention in terms of oral delivery research.

Novo Nordisk, for instance, has been conducting clinical research on a candidate molecule known as OI-338. It boasts a 70-hour half-life in the human body, more than tenfold resistance to degradation by gastrointestinal proteases, and an extremely low receptor clearance rate. When formulated together with TPE, its bioavailability reached 3.9% in canine experiments, a sixfold improvement compared to natural insulin. As a once-daily oral formulation, OI-338 completed phase 2a clinical trials. The results indicated that its pharmacokinetic profile was similar to that of short-acting insulins, with a peak during the absorption phase. However, it differed from subcutaneous basal insulin in having a flatter curve (see Fig. 2.19). It had a lower probability of causing hypoglycemia and, overall, could meet the clinical requirements for basal insulin. Nevertheless, Novo Nordisk decided to suspend the project after completing phase 2a trials for several reasons: (1) The drug's efficacy and pharmacokinetic results did not achieve the expected optimization. (2) Due to issues related to enzyme degradation and receptor clearance rates, chemists still considered that the oral bioavailability was relatively low. This necessitated the use of higher doses of insulin, significantly increasing production costs.

Other companies are also in the clinical trial phase for oral insulin molecules. For instance, Insulin Tregopil (IN-105) is currently undergoing Phase II clinical trials. It achieves oral bioavailability of approximately 1% through B29 glycerol derivatization along with TPE. Notably, Oramed Pharmaceuticals has developed ORM-D0801, which combines natural insulin with an undisclosed TPE and protease inhibitor. This formulation attains oral bioavailability ranging from 5% to 8%. When administered orally three times a day, it effectively maintains daily blood glucose control without significant hypoglycemic side effects [49]. This molecule is presently undergoing Phase IIa clinical trials in both the United States and China.

2.3 Summary and outlook

The forefront of insulin drug research has remained consistent in its primary objective: to serve diabetes patients by addressing evolving clinical needs and alleviating the suffering caused by the disease. Since the inception of insulin, scientists initially tackled the challenge of making diabetes manageable and proved that controlling the condition with insulin was possible—a groundbreaking achievement in the treatment of a major human ailment.

The development of animal insulin, semisynthetic insulin, and recombinant insulin substantially lowered production costs, making long-term treatment affordable for a broader range of patients. Basal insulins like NPH insulin and insulin glargine, which simulate the physiological secretion of insulin, have allowed for more precise diabetes management. They mitigate the inherent risk of hypoglycemia and weight gain associated with insulin therapy, providing patients with improved blood glucose control and significantly delaying the progression of diabetes complications. Additionally, these innovations have shown promise in assisting the treatment of other chronic conditions [50].

At present, all Phase III clinical trials for antidiabetic drugs must provide evidence to the FDA regarding their efficacy in treating cardiovascular diseases, nonalcoholic fatty liver disease, and chronic kidney disease. This evidence is used to assess the relative merits of these drugs when compared to others, ultimately influencing the approval process.

Rapid-acting insulins, which mimic the effects of physiological insulin, represent another pivotal aspect of diabetes treatment. The maturation and application of platforms such as fatty acylation and antibody Fc fusion technology in insulin drug development have extended drug half-lives, reduced concentration fluctuations, enhanced the efficacy of basal insulin, and improved patient convenience and compliance. This has become a prominent trend and necessity in

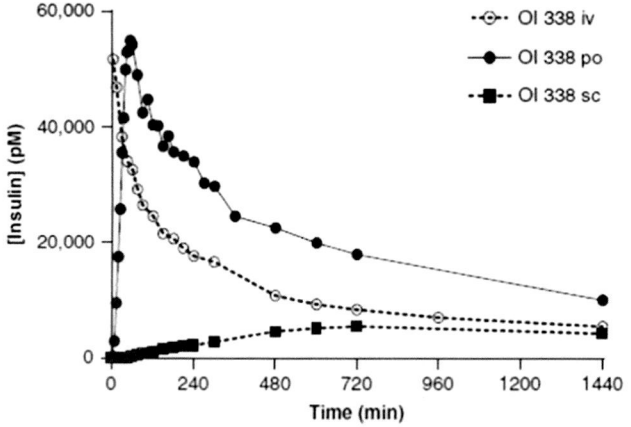

FIGURE 2.19 The pharmacokinetic profiles across different administration routes [48].

insulin drug development. Nevertheless, current insulin therapies continue to face challenges, including the risk of hypoglycemia and the discomfort and inconvenience associated with daily injections.

Future research directions will strive to address clinical demands for faster onset of action, longer duration of effect, flatter blood glucose control curves, and heightened safety and convenience. Successful development of more challenging glucose-responsive drugs may serve as a milestone in the advancement of next-generation insulin therapies. Furthermore, exploring alternative delivery methods for injection, such as inhalation, transdermal, and oral administration, holds significant promise.

In conclusion, the quest to improve insulin therapies remains an enduring commitment to alleviating the burden of diabetes on patients and providing them with enhanced treatment options.

References

[1] Rosenfeld L. Insulin: discovery and controversy. Clin Chem 2002;48(12):2270–88.
[2] Heller S, Kozlovski P, Kurtzhals P. Insulin's 85th anniversary-an enduring medical miracle. Diabetes Res Clin Pract 2007;78(2):149–58.
[3] Moroder L, Musiol HJ. Insulin-from its discovery to the industrial synthesis of modern insulin analogues. Angew Chem Int Ed Engl 2017;56(36):10656–69.
[4] Tom B, Guy D, Dorothy H, et al. Insulin: the structure in the crystal and its reflection in chemistry and biology. Adv Prote Chem 1972;26:279–402.
[5] Abel JJ. Crystalline insulin. Proc Natl Acad Sci USA 1926;12(2):132–6.
[6] Mayer JP, Zhang F, Dimarchi RD. Insulin structure and function. Biopolymers 2007;88(5):687–713.
[7] Brown H, Sanger F, Kitai R. The structure of pig and sheep insulins. Biochem J 1955;60(4):556–65.
[8] Rolf H, Gerhard S, Harald B, et al. The evolution of insulin glargine and its continuing contribution to diabetes care. Drugs 2014;74(8):911–27.
[9] Obermeier R, Geiger R. A new semisynthesis of human insulin. Hoppe-Seyler's Z Physiol Chem 1976;357(1):759–68.
[10] Homandberg GA, Mattis JA, Laskowski M, et al. Synthesis of peptide bonds by proteinases. Addition of organic cosolvents shifts peptide bond equilibria toward synthesis. Biochemistry 1978;17(24):5220–7.
[11] Markussen J, Damgaard U, Jrgensen KH, et al. Human monocomponent insulin. Chem Charact 1983;671:99–105.
[12] Meyts PD. Insulin and its receptor: structure, function and evolution. Bioessays 2004;26(12):1351–62.
[13] Conlon JM. Evolution of the insulin molecule: insights into structure-activity and phylogenetic relationships. Peptides 2001;22(7):1183–93.
[14] Derewenda U, Derewenda Z, Dodson GG, et al. Molecular structure of insulin: the insulin monomer and its assembly. Br Med Bull 1989;45(1):4–18.
[15] Weiss M, Steiner DF, Philipson LH. Insulin biosynthesis, secretion, structure, and structure-activity relationships. South Dartmouth, MA; 2000.
[16] Schwartz GP, Burke GT, Katsoyannis PG. A superactive insulin: [B10-aspartic acid]insulin(human). Proc Natl Acad Sci USA 1987;84(18):6408–11.
[17] Kristensen C, Kjeldsen T, Wiberg FC, et al. Alanine scanning mutagenesis of insulin. J Biol Chem 1997;272(20):12978–83.
[18] Pullen RA, Lindsay DG, Wood SP, et al. Receptor-binding region of insulin. Nature 1976;259(5542):369–73.
[19] Hua QX, Nakagawa SH, Jia W, et al. Hierarchical protein folding: asymmetric unfolding of an insulin analogue lacking the A7-B7 interchain disulfide bridge. Biochemistry 2001;40(41):12299–311.
[20] Hua QX, HU SQ, Frank BH, et al. Mapping the functional surface of insulin by design: structure and function of a novel A-chain analogue. J Mol Biol 1996;264(2):390–403.
[21] Duckworth WC, Bennett RG, Hamel FG. Insulin degradation: progress and potential. Endocr Rev 1998;19(5):608–24.
[22] Monnier L, Colette C. Target for glycemic control: concentrating on glucose. Diabetes Care 2009;32(Suppl 2):S199–204.
[23] Jacobs MA, Keulen ET, Kanc K, et al. Metabolic efficacy of preprandial administration of Lys(B28), Pro(B29) human insulin analog in IDDM patients. A comparison with human regular insulin during a three-meal test period. Diabetes Care 1997;20(8):1279–86.
[24] Frier BM. Hypoglycaemia in diabetes mellitus: epidemiology and clinical implications. Nat Rev Endocrinol 2014;10(12):711–22.
[25] Mccall AL. Insulin therapy and hypoglycemia. Endocrinol Metab Clin North Am 2012;41(1):57–87.
[26] Mann NP, Johnston DI, Reeves WG, et al. Human insulin and porcine insulin in the treatment of diabetic children: comparison of metabolic control and insulin antibody production. Br Med J (Clin Res Ed) 1983;287(6405):1580–2.
[27] Gualandi-Signorini AM, Giorgi G. Insulin formulations-a review. Eur Rev Med Pharmacol Sci 2001;5(3):73–83.
[28] Deckert T. Intermediate-acting insulin preparations: NPH and lente. Diabetes Care 1980;3(5):623–6.
[29] Heding LG, Marshall MO, Persson B, et al. Immunogenicity of monocomponent human and porcine insulin in newly diagnosed type 1 (insulin-dependent) diabetic children. Diabetologia 1984;27(Suppl):96–8.
[30] Brems DN, Alter LA, Beckage MJ, et al. Altering the association properties of insulin by amino acid replacement. Protein Eng 1992;5(6):527–33.
[31] Mathieu C, Gillard P, Benhalima K. Insulin analogues in type 1 diabetes mellitus: getting better all the time. Nat Rev Endocrinol 2017;13(7):385–99.

[32] Wilde I, Mctavish D. Insulin lispro: a review of its pharmacological properties and therapeutic use in the management of diabetes mellitus. Drugs 1997;54(4):597–614.
[33] IRL B, Hirsch MD. Insulin analogues. N Engl J Med 2005;174–83.
[34] Heller S. Insulin lispro: a useful advance in insulin therapy. Exp Opin Pharmacother 2003;4(8):1407–16.
[35] Gammeltoft S, Hansen BF, Dideriksen L, et al. Insulin aspart: a novel rapid-acting human insulin analogue. Expert Opin Investigat Drugs 1999;8(9):1431–42.
[36] Becker RH. Insulin glulisine complementing basal insulins: a review of structure and activity. Diabetes Technol Ther 2007;9(1):109–21.
[37] Rosskamp RH, Park G. Long-acting insulin analogs. Diabetes Care 1999;22(Suppl 2) B109-113.
[38] Vajo Z, Duckworth WC. Genetically engineered insulin analogs: diabetes in the new millenium. Pharmacol Rev 2000;52(1):1–9.
[39] Bolli GB, Di Marchi RD, Park GD, et al. Insulin analogues and their potential in the management of diabetes mellitus. Diabetologia 1999;42(10):1151–67.
[40] Svend H, Anne P, Ulla R, et al. The mechanism of protraction of insulin detemir, a long-acting, acylated analog of human insulin. Pharm Res 2004;21(8):1498–504.
[41] Kurtzhals P, Havelund S, Jonassen IB, et al. Albumin binding of insulins acylated with fatty acids: characterization of the ligand-protein interaction and correlation between binding affinity and timing of the insulin effect in vivo. Biochem J 1995;312(pt 3):725–31.
[42] Kurtzhals P. Pharmacology of insulin detemir. Endocrinol Metab Clin North Am 2007;36(Suppl 1):14–20.
[43] Jonassen I, Havelund S, Hoeg-Jensen T, et al. Design of the novel protraction mechanism of insulin degludec, an ultra-long-acting basal insulin. Pharm Res 2012;29(8):2104–14.
[44] Hoeg-Jensen T. Review: glucose-sensitive insulin. Mol Metab 2021;46:101107.
[45] Drucker DJ. Advances in oral peptide therapeutics. Nat Rev Drug Discov 2020;19(4):277–89.
[46] Kaarsholm NC, Lin S, Yan L, et al. Engineering glucose responsiveness into insulin. Diabetes 2018;67(2):299–308.
[47] Lemmer HJ, Hamman JH. Paracellular drug absorption enhancement through tight junction modulation. Expert Opin Drug Deliv 2013;10(1):103–14.
[48] Hubalek F, Refsgaard HHF, Gram-Nielsen S, et al. Molecular engineering of safe and efficacious oral basal insulin. Nat Commun 2020;11(1):3746.
[49] Eldor R, Neutel J, Homer KE, et al. Multiple oral insulin (ORMD-0801) doses elicit a cumulative effect on glucose control in T2DM patients. Diabetes 2018;67(Suppl 1) 982-P.
[50] Chaudhury A, Duvoor C, Reddy Dendi VS, et al. Clinical review of antidiabetic drugs: implications for type 2 diabetes mellitus management. Front Endocrinol (Lausanne) 2017;8:6.

Chapter 3

The developmental trajectory of GLP-1 receptor agonists

Binbin Kou[1] and Hai Qian[2]
[1]Eccogene, Inc., Cambridge, MA, United States, [2]Center of Drug Discovery, China Pharmaceutical University, Nanjing, Jiangsu, P.R. China

Chapter outline

3.1 Glucagon-like peptide-1 (GLP-1) 41
   3.1.1 Brief introduction to glucagon-like peptide-1 (GLP-1) 41
   3.1.2 The development of GLP-1 medications 41
   3.1.3 GLP-1 structure and physiology 42
3.2 The development of GLP-1 therapeutics 43
   3.2.1 The limitations of native GLP-1 as a therapeutic agent 43
   3.2.2 The strategies for extending GLP-1 analogs time action 44
3.3 The unsuccessful case in GLP-1 drug R&D and the implications and lessons 49
3.4 Summary and outlook 50
References 51

3.1 Glucagon-like peptide-1 (GLP-1)

3.1.1 Brief introduction to glucagon-like peptide-1 (GLP-1)

Glucagon-like peptide-1 (GLP-1), secreted from enteroendocrine L cells within the gastrointestinal tract, constitutes a polypeptide hormone to promote insulin secretion. In conjunction with another peptide hormone that shares a comparable functionality, namely glucose-dependent insulinotropic polypeptide (GIP), these hormones are collectively referred to as incretins. Both hormones stimulate or regulate postprandial insulin secretion, promote growth and differentiation of pancreatic β cells, reduce β cell apoptosis, inhibit glucagon secretion, slow gastric emptying, and suppress appetite [1,2]. Notably, although the discovery of GIP predates GLP-1 [3], there is still significant controversy pertaining to its physiological functions and mechanisms in blood glucose regulation.

3.1.2 The development of GLP-1 medications

The development of GLP-1 therapeutics has spanned over four decades. During this extensive period, it encompassed the discovery of its genetic and amino acid sequences, the confirmation of receptors and physiological functions, attempts at creating antidiabetic medications, the discovery of exenatide [4], the achievement of once-weekly injectable formulations [5], the successful development of orally administered treatments for type 2 diabetes, the recognition of its weight-reduction effects [6], the establishment of cardiovascular benefits associated with its therapy, the amelioration of nonalcoholic steatohepatitis, and the promotion of its utilization in the treatment of various chronic diseases (Fig. 3.1).

   1981−82: cloning of pufferfish glucagon complementary DNA (cDNA);
   1987: the discovery of GLP-1 stimulation of insulin secretion;
   2014: the GLP-1R agonist antiobesity medication, administered once daily.

Initially, scientists observed that oral glucose ingestion had a more potent effect in stimulating insulin secretion compared to glucose injection, suggesting the existence of a gastrointestinal hormone capable of regulating insulin secretion [8]. In the early

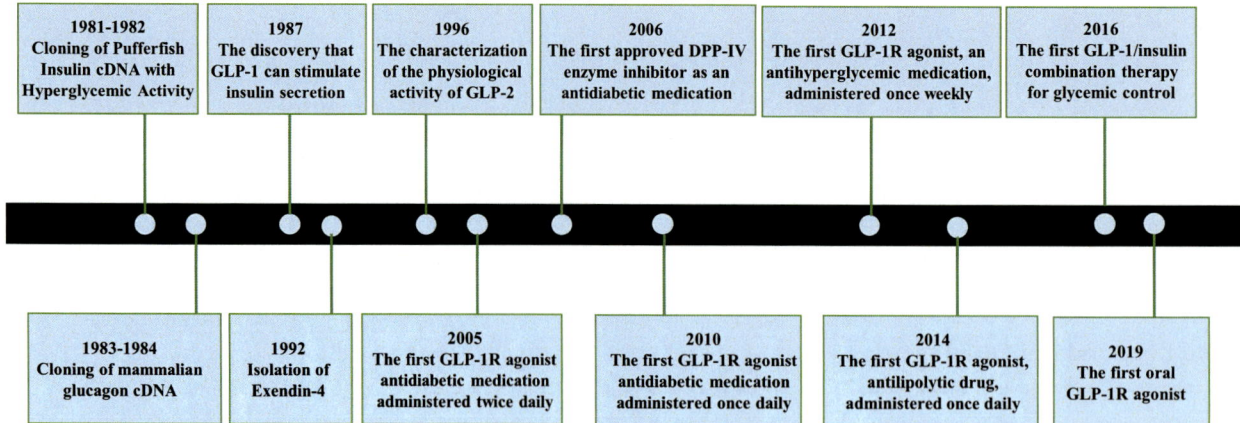

FIGURE 3.1 The key milestones in the historical progression of GLP-1 drug therapy [7].

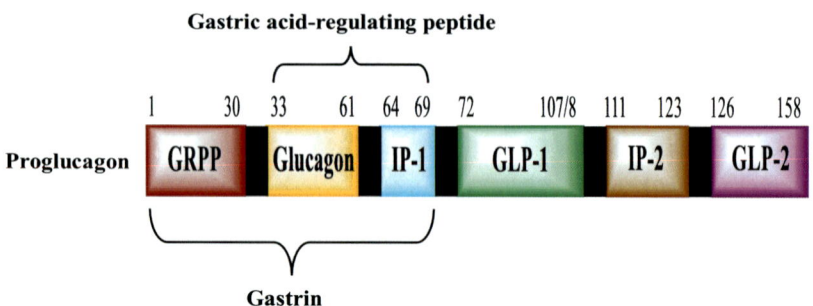

GRPP: Gastrin-Releasing Peptide; IP-1: Insertion Peptide-1

FIGURE 3.2 The proglucagon protein enzymatic cleavage mediated by converting enzymes, resulting in the generation of various biologically active peptide hormones.

1980s, scientists made a pivotal discovery of an intestinal hormone, subsequently named GLP-1. The discovery of GLP-1 was intimately linked to the development of DNA recombinant technology. Researchers, through decoding of cDNA library of messenger RNA, identified the amino acid sequence of proglucagon from various animal species. Proglucagon is a prohormone protein, following posttranslational selective enzymatic cleavage, which generates a repertoire of biologically active peptide hormones (Fig. 3.2), including GLP-1 and GLP-2, among others.

3.1.3 GLP-1 structure and physiology

When analyzing the enzymatic cleavage sites, GLP-1 was initially believed to be a peptide with either 37 amino acids of the carboxylic acid terminal (1–37 COOH) or a 36 amino acid amide terminal (1–36 NH_2) [9]. However, subsequent research revealed that the biologically active hormone sequences are indeed GLP-1 (7–37 COOH) and GLP-1 (7–36 NH_2) [10,11] (Fig. 3.3). The determination of these active structures was ultimately accomplished through solid-phase peptide chemical synthesis. It is worth noting that solid-phase peptide synthesis (SPPS) refers to the elongation of a peptide chain on a resin support, followed by cleavage and purification. American scientist Dr. Bruce Merrifield was awarded the Nobel Prize in Chemistry in 1984 for his contributions to SPPS. Further investigations by scientists demonstrated that enzymatic cleavage of proglucagon primarily occurs in the intestine rather than the pancreas, confirming the production of GLP-1 in the intestines and rightfully establishing it as an incretin hormone.

GLP-1 receptors belong to the G protein-coupled receptor family, widely distributed not only in the primary pancreatic islets and the central nervous system but also in organs such as the heart, kidneys, and gastrointestinal tract [12–14] (Table 3.1). When GLP-1 receptors located in pancreatic β-cells are activated, they stimulate the production of cyclic adenosine monophosphate (cAMP), which serves as a second messenger to initiate a cascade of biological responses. Elevated blood glucose levels, together with the second messenger, promote intracellular ATP synthesis. Consequently, ATP-dependent K^+ ion channels close, leading to membrane depolarization and an influx of Ca^{2+}. The increased intracellular Ca^{2+} concentration triggers the transcriptional regulation of insulin genes, thereby stimulating insulin secretion.

```
HDEFERHAEGTFTSDVSSYLEGQAAKEFIAWLVKGRG-OH     GLP-1(1-37 COOH)
      HAEGTFTSDVSSYLEGQAAKEFIAWLVKGRG-OH     GLP-1(7-37 COOH)
      HAEGTFTSDVSSYLEGQAAKEFIAWLVKGR-NH₂     GLP-1(7-36 Amide)
```

FIGURE 3.3 GLP-1 related peptide amino acid sequence.

TABLE 3.1 The physiological and pharmacological effects of GLP-1 in various organs [15].

	Physiological actions of GLP-1	Pharmacological actions of GLP-1Ras
Brain	Appetite reduction and increased satiety	Partially preventing neurodegeneration
Heart	Improving endothelial function	Decreased blood pressure; increased heart rate; increased myocardial contractility; elevated diastolic pressure; and enhanced cardiac protection
Gastrointestinal tract	Delayed gastric emptying and reduced gastric acid secretion	N/A
Pancreas	Increased insulin secretion and decreased glucagon secretion	Stimulates β-cell proliferation
Adipose tissue	N/A	Promotes fat breakdown and increases glucose uptake
Renal	Promotes sodium excretion	N/A
Muscle	Promotes glycogen synthesis and glucose oxidation	N/A

Because the GLP-1-induced enhancement of insulin secretion is glucose-dependent, its action diminishes in hypoglycemic conditions [16]. Due to this distinctive effect, GLP-1 rarely causes adverse reactions related to hypoglycemia [13].

Notably, neurons in the human brain also produce proglucagon, and therefore, GLP-1 receptors are widely distributed in the brain, primarily concentrated in the hypothalamus. When centrally produced GLP-1 acts on these receptors, it elicits appetite suppression and reduces food intake [17,18]. Peripherally, GLP-1 can slow down gastrointestinal motility and emptying. Furthermore, GLP-1 is a hydrophilic peptide that can hardly penetrate the blood-brain barrier and has an exceedingly short half-life in circulation, lasting only 1–2 minutes. Therefore, theoretically, peripheral administration of GLP-1 cannot attain effective drug concentrations in the central nervous system. However, both animal experiments and clinical trials have consistently demonstrated the appetite-suppressing and weight-reducing effects of peripheral GLP-1 administration [19,20], serving as another notable characteristic of GLP-1 therapeutics [21].

3.2 The development of GLP-1 therapeutics

3.2.1 The limitations of native GLP-1 as a therapeutic agent

With the discovery of GLP-1 and extensive research into its physiological and pharmacological activities, scientists have recognized its immense potential in the field of type 2 diabetes treatment. However, the results of GLP-1 in animal studies and human clinical trials were unsatisfactory at the beginning. There are two major reasons: firstly, GLP-1 is rapidly cleared by renal filtration, and secondly, it is highly susceptible to degradation and inactivation by dipeptidyl peptidase-4 (DPP-4), resulting in the production of inactive metabolites such as GLP-1 9–37 COOH or 9–36 NH₂. Moreover, these inactive metabolites themselves act as antagonists of GLP-1 receptors [22]. Under physiological conditions, the metabolic degradation of GLP-1 is essential for regulating hormone levels [23]. However, under pharmacological conditions, injected GLP-1 rapidly degrades into inactive products, significantly diminishing its therapeutic efficacy [24]. At that point, a GLP-1 analog molecule called exenatide (exenatide-4) emerged in scientists' vision [25].

3.2.2 The strategies for extending GLP-1 analogs time action

As previously mentioned, the primary challenges in the clinical application of GLP-1 are rapid renal clearance and enzymatic degradation in the circulation. Therefore, medicinal chemists have focused on extending the duration of action of GLP-1 analogs. The main strategies employed include (1) site-specific modifications on the peptide backbone to reduce the enzymatic cleavage at specific sites by peptidase and (2) conjugation of the peptide with long chain fatty acids, human serum albumin, antibody Fc fragments, or polyethylene glycol segments to increase the relative molecular mass of the peptide and reduce renal filtration clearance of the peptide.

3.2.2.1 Amino acid mutation of peptide backbone

Exendin-4 was initially extracted and isolated from the saliva of the Gila monster, a venomous lizard native to the Americas. In 1992, Dr. John Eng, a renowned endocrinologist, and his research team first purified exendin-4 using a reversed-phase C18 high-performance liquid chromatography. They employed mass spectrometry and enzymatic cleavage of peptide fragments to further determine its natural peptide sequence, naming it exexdin-4 [26]. Subsequent research revealed that exendin-4 shares a 53% sequence similarity with GLP-1 (Fig. 3.4). Furthermore, both molecules exhibit similar physiological activities, as exendin-4, upon activating its receptors, also triggers the generation of the cAMP second messenger [27].

Indeed, scientists ultimately confirmed that the receptor of exendin-4 is the GLP-1 receptor. While exendin-4 biological activity is similar to that of GLP-1, its structure and mechanism of action on the GLP-1 receptor differ. Exendin-4 consists of 39 amino acids and adopts a secondary structure characterized by an α-helical region from the 11th amino acid (Ser11) from the N-terminus to the 27th amino acid (Lys27), which is the binding site for the GLP-1 receptor (Fig. 3.5, left). The first 10 amino acids at the N-terminus form an irregularly coiled structure and do not interact with the receptor. A turn structure is formed at positions 28−30, and the 30−39 region constitutes a polyproline structure, interacting with the 25th amino acid, tryptophan, forming a miniature three-dimensional structure known as the "Trp cage." This structure plays a stabilizing role in maintaining the α-helical structure from residues 11−27 [28, 29]. The primary amino acid residues involved in the interaction between exendin-4 and the GLP-1 receptor are in positions 19−27; however, any deletion or substitution of amino acids within the 1−10 region results in a molecule that only retains the ability to bind to the GLP-1 receptor, losing its receptor activation and becoming a receptor antagonist [30] (Fig. 3.5, right). The carboxylic terminal structure from 30 to 39 helps stabilize the α-helical structure, enhancing its binding affinity with the receptor. Compared to GLP-1, exendin-4 exhibits a much stronger binding affinity to the GLP-1 receptor, approximately 400 times stronger (K_d value of 6 vs. >500 nmol/L) [31]. This is one of the reasons why the exenatide clinical dose is significantly lower than GLP-1 analogs.

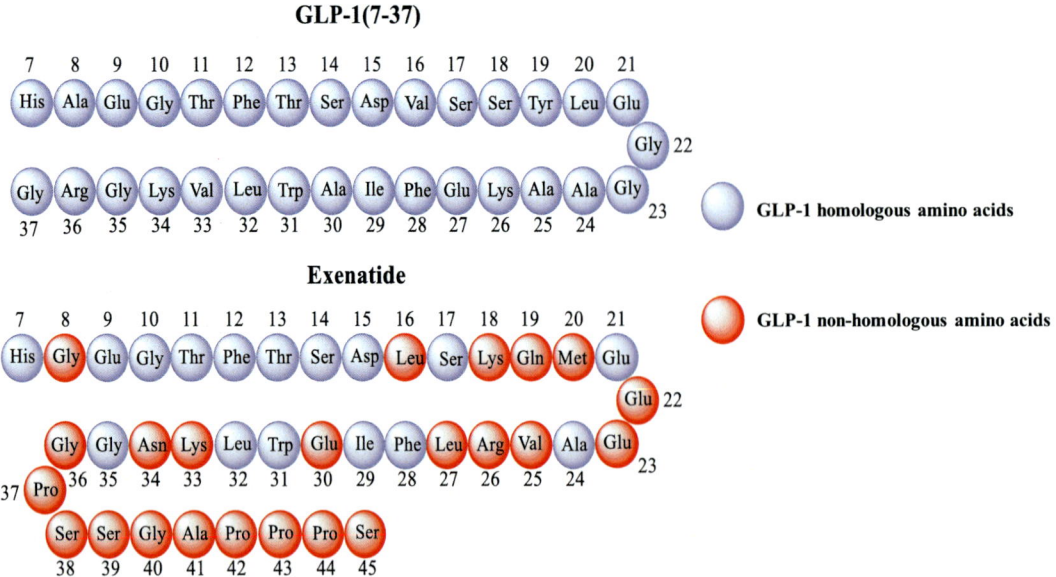

FIGURE 3.4 Comparison of sequence similarity between exendin-4 and GLP-1.

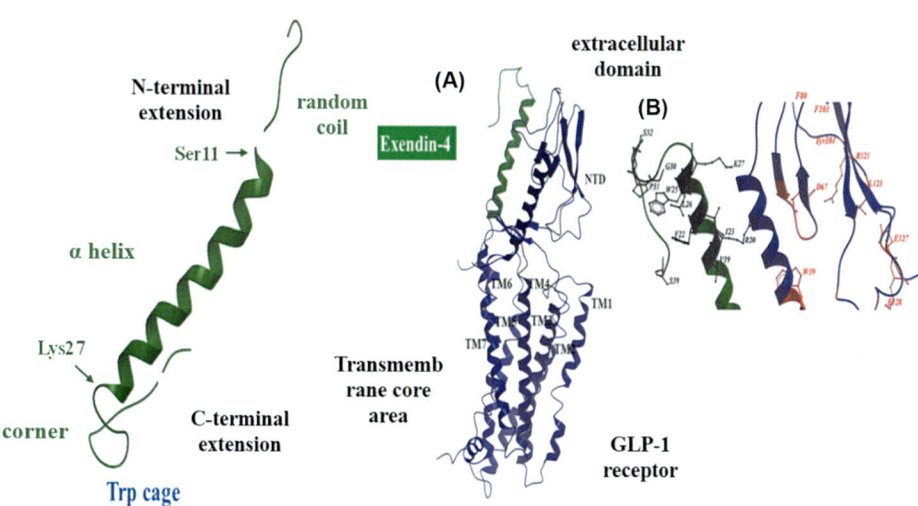

FIGURE 3.5 (A) The secondary structure of exendin-4 (represented by a green-ribbon diagram). (B) The interaction between the extracellular domain (ECD) (represented by a blue-ribbon diagram) of the GLP-1 receptor and exendin-4 (green ribbon).

Exendin-4 is also subject to degradation and inactivation by DPP-4, but it differs from GLP-1 in that the second amino acid from the N-terminus is glycine (Gly) rather than alanine (Ala). Studies on DPP-4 have revealed significant differences in its catalytic capacity toward different amino acid substrates [32]. DPP-4 exhibits the strongest catalytic hydrolysis activity on sequences with proline and Ala as the second amino acid [33]. Exendin-4 DPP-4 cleavage site is Gly, leading to significantly lower hydrolysis activity than GLP-1 Ala. Its plasma half-life can reach 2.4 hours, much longer than GLP-1's 1—2 minutes [34,35]. Initially, this unique feature of exendin-4 did not attract enough researchers' interest because it is not a naturally human sequence but rather originates from reptiles, posing potential immunogenicity risks. However, preclinical and clinical trials later discovered that exendin-4 exhibited the same expected pharmacological effects as GLP-1, along with superior pharmacokinetic properties. It demonstrated confirmed efficacy in treating type 2 diabetes, as well as weight control effects, with low titers of antidrug antibody. Therefore, in 2005, the FDA approved exenatide for the treatment of type 2 diabetes. As the first GLP-1 receptor agonist (GLP-1RA) drug to be marketed, exenatide offers the dual benefit of controlling both blood glucose level and body weight, overcoming the issue encountered with most previous antidiabetic drugs, weight gain and consequently worsening of the disease condition [36]. Subsequently, it was also proven that exenatide had beneficial effects on cardiovascular, chronic liver, and kidney diseases. GLP-1-based drugs have gradually become the first line of type 2 diabetes treatment, with exenatide being a pioneer among them. Unfortunately, despite the tremendous success of various GLP-1RA drugs that followed, exenatide did not achieve sales exceeding one billion dollars at its peak year and did not become a "blockbuster drug." The main reasons include its relatively short plasma half-life, which, although significantly improved compared to native GLP-1, still cannot achieve once-daily dosing administration, necessitating twice-daily administration. Moreover, due to its characteristics as a large biomolecule, it must be administered by injection, which leads to poor patient compliance due to this twice-daily dosing. Although formulation improvements resulted in the introduction of Bydureon, a once-weekly dosage form, in 2012, by that time it had already been eclipsed by liraglutide, which was approved by the FDA in 2010 [37].

3.2.2.2 Fatty acid conjugation (lipidation)

3.2.2.2.1 liraglutide

As mentioned earlier, due to the extremely short plasma half-life of GLP-1, it has not become a prominent antidiabetic drug for a long time. GLP-1's mechanism of action on its receptor is similar to that of exendin-4, but there are also some differences. Conventionally, GLP-1 is referred to as 7—37 (or 7—36 NH_2), with histidine at the N-terminus being designated as position 7. Therefore, the following GLP-1 sequence is based on this convention, with threonine (Thr) at so-called position 13 being the 7th residue. The secondary structure of GLP-1 primarily consists of a continuous α-helix structure from Thr at position 13 to valine (Val) at position 33. The region from Ala at position 24 to Val at position 33 interacts with the extracellular domain of the receptor through the inherent hydrophobic and hydrophilic surfaces of the α-helix structure [38] (Fig. 3.6). Similar to exendin-4, its N-terminus does not participate in receptor binding; however, mutations in the first six amino acids or removal of the dipeptide by DPP-4 almost completely abolish its agonistic activity, transforming GLP-1 (9—39) into a receptor antagonist [30].

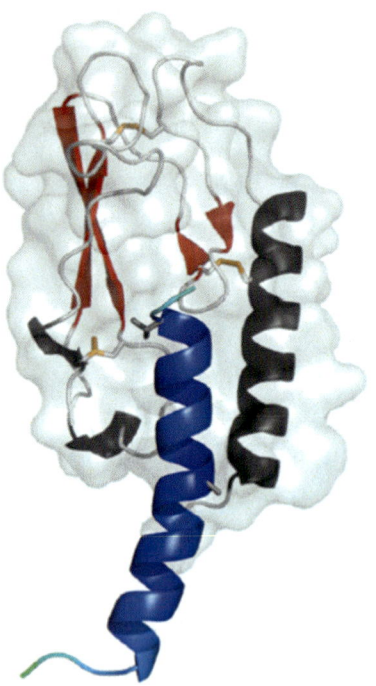

FIGURE 3.6 Schematic representation of the interaction between the secondary structure of GLP-1 (blue ribbon) and the extracellular domain (ECD) of the GLP-1 receptor, with the black and blue ribbon representing the α-helix region of the receptor's ECD involved in the interaction with GLP-1 [38].

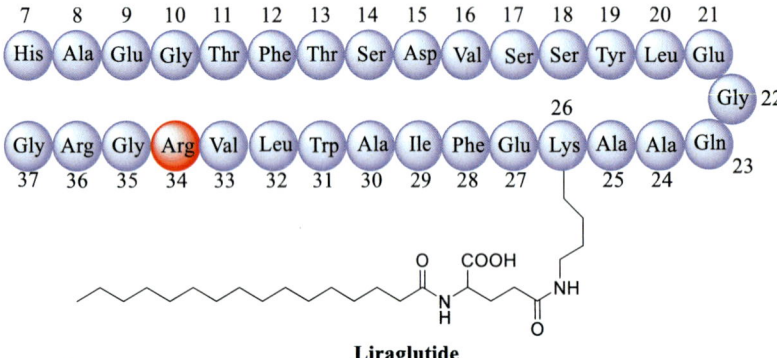

FIGURE 3.7 The structure of liraglutide.

In the insulin pharmaceuticals cases outlined in Chapter 2, it is noteworthy that as we entered the 21st century, there has been substantial progress in long-acting peptide and protein technologies. Platforms such as pegylation, fatty acid acylation, antibody-Fc conjugation, and albumin fusion have sequentially emerged and matured [39]. Fatty acid acylation, in particular, has exhibited multifaceted attributes in enhancing the pharmacokinetic properties of macromolecular therapeutics. This encompasses the extension of drug half-life, modulation of drug hydrophilicity and lipophilicity to augment drug-receptor binding affinity and cellular membrane permeability, as well as reduction in immunogenicity [39].

Fatty acylation has significantly ameliorated the physicochemical characteristics of GLP-1-based pharmaceuticals, gradually proved clinical significance, and heralded the advent of two pivotal medications for type 2 diabetes. The first one is liraglutide, which obtained FDA approval for market entry in 2010 [40]. Novo Nordisk played a pioneering role in the design of fatty-acylated pharmaceuticals, with the inaugural member of this category being insulin detemir, bearing a 14-carbon monocarboxylic acid as a fatty acid moiety on its side chain. Through noncovalent reversible binding interactions with albumin, this modification prolonged the half-life of insulin from a mere 6 minutes to approximately 6 hours. In contrast, liraglutide bears a 16-carbon monocarboxylic acid side chain appended with a γ-glutamic acid linker molecule (see Fig. 3.7), boasting binding affinity to albumin several-fold greater than that of the 14-carbon monocarboxylic acid. Liraglutide exhibits 97% sequence homology with GLP-1 [41], diverging only at position 34, where a lysine (Lys) in GLP-1 is replaced with arginine (Arg). This substitution, motivated by selective modification considerations, retains a hydrophilic positively charged moiety at position 34 while ensuring selectivity for side chain modification reactions [41].

The term "peptide" generally pertains to molecules comprised of fewer than 50 amino acids, sharing similar properties to proteins yet distinct in significant aspects. Research indicates that peptides trigger considerably weaker immunogenic responses than protein therapeutics, thereby tolerating greater mutations of natural sequence, consequently diminishing the likelihood of developing high-titer antidrug antibodies [42]. However, there are exceptions within the realm of GLP-1-based pharmaceutical research, which will be expounded upon subsequently. Presently, the utilization of in silico software in the prediction of immunogenicity augments the capacity of medicinal chemists to engage in targeted mutagenesis for drug design, thereby reducing the probability of clinical trial failures [43].

Following subcutaneous administration, liraglutide enters the bloodstream in a complex form with albumin, accounting for more than 98% of its presence [41]. This association serves to mitigate renal filtration, while the drug-albumin complexes also resist enzymatic degradation by DPP-IV [44]. Furthermore, the fatty acid side chain imparts the ability for liraglutide to form heptameric structures in the drug formulation [45,46]. Post-administration, these heptameric structures gradually dissociate into monomers, thus facilitating a sustained-release effect. The cumulative impact of these factors extends the plasma half-life of liraglutide to approximately 13 hours [41,47], with a subcutaneous bioavailability of 55% [48], thereby realizing the goal of once-daily dosing. Liraglutide exerts a pronounced reduction in the average glycated hemoglobin (HbA1c) levels in diabetic patients, effectively controlling blood glucose levels. It also demonstrates a noteworthy effect on weight reduction and an exceedingly low incidence of hypoglycemic adverse events [49,50].

3.2.2.2.2 Semaglutide

Novo Nordisk Inc. introduced the next-generation acylated GLP-1 medication known as semaglutide, receiving FDA approval in 2017. Structurally similar to liraglutide, semaglutide features a Lys at position 26, which is attached to two polyethylene glycol molecules and γ-glutamic acid (2OEG-γGlu), linking with an 18-carbon dicarboxylic acid fatty acid moiety (see Fig. 3.8). The connection molecule and its associated negative charges on the fatty acid side chain enhance its binding affinity to albumin by nearly 20-fold compared to liraglutide. Semaglutide retains the Arg at position 34 while substituting the naturally occurring Ala at position 8 of the GLP-1 sequence with α-aminoisobutyric acid (Aib). This substitution further reduces susceptibility to degradation by DPP-IV enzymes [51]. Sequence homology with native GLP-1 remains high at 94% [52], and its half-life in the human body reaches an astonishing 165 hours [41,52], with a 2−3 times higher in vitro activity on the GLP-1 receptor than the natural sequence [49]. Currently, semaglutide demonstrates outstanding glycemic control and notably promotes weight loss [53], as well as reduces the risks of cardiovascular diseases [54]. Due to its exceptionally extended half-life, it allows for once-weekly dosing [54].

From the above introduction, it becomes evident that fatty acylation exerts a profoundly impactful role in extending the plasma half-life of GLP-1-based pharmaceuticals. For biologic therapeutic agents similar to GLP-1 that require injectable administration, it greatly reduces the frequency of injections, significantly reduces patient discomfort, and greatly improves the convenience and compliance of medication.

An oral formulation of semaglutide known as RYBELSUS was successfully introduced to the market toward the end of 2018. This achievement was made possible through the application of the transient permeation enhancer oral

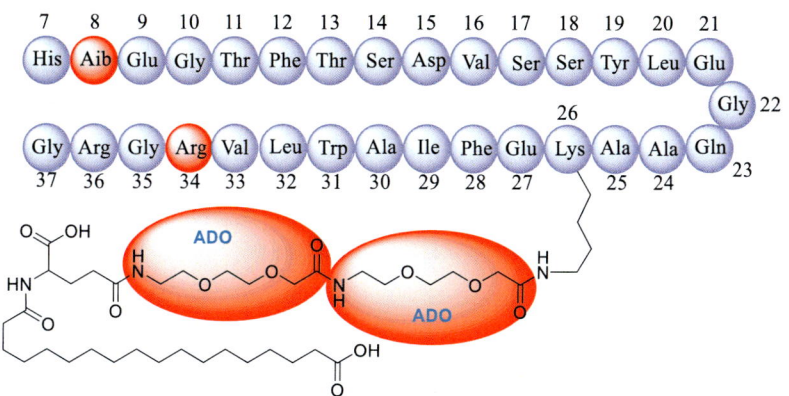

FIGURE 3.8 The structure of semaglutide.

formulation technology mentioned in Chapter 2. In the case of RYBELSUS, semaglutide is coformulated with an eight-carbon amino salicylate sodium compound known as SNAC (sodium N-[8-(2-hydroxybenzoyl)amino]caprylate). Upon oral administration, this formulation disintegrates in the stomach, allowing semaglutide to exist in its monomeric form, which is then absorbed through the gastric wall [55]. This innovative approach has led to a substantial increase in the oral bioavailability of semaglutide ($F = 1.5\%$). Furthermore, by optimizing the oral dosage, satisfactory therapeutic outcomes have been achieved [56].

3.2.2.3 Antibody Fc segments fusion

As mentioned earlier, over the past two decades, there has been a notable emergence of the Fc-fusion technology, which utilizes the fragment crystallizable (Fc) region of human immunoglobulin G (IgG) to achieve covalent linkage with GLP-1. This modification alters the molecular diameter and weight of the drug, consequently reducing renal filtration clearance and enzymatic degradation. This, in turn, prolongs the drug's half-life, ultimately achieving the goal of extended duration of action.

The Fc segment of IgG constitutes part of human IgG (Fig. 3.9, left). IgG (broadly referred to as antibodies) serves as a critical molecule in immune defense against exogenous pathogens and is primarily composed of variable regions (Fab) and constant regions (Fc). Fab is responsible for binding pathogens, while Fc can bind to the neonatal Fc receptor (FcRn) on immune effector cells, leading to the internalization and processing of the IgG-pathogen complex inside the immune cells [58]. Under weakly acidic conditions inside the cells (pH = 6.5), the pathogen and antibody complex dissociates. FcRn and IgG are then recycled to the cell surface for reuse. This entire process is known as FcRn-mediated IgG recycling [59] (Fig. 3.9, right). This process extends the plasma half-life of IgG to approximately 22–23 days and can be leveraged to enhance the drug's circulating half-life.

Eli Lilly and Company utilized the Fc segment, employing protein recombinant technology to covalently link GLP-1 with Fc (Fig. 3.10). Due to Fc being a dimer connected by a pair of disulfide bonds, each Fc molecule can link two GLP-1 analogs. The GLP-1 portion of this construct features three amino acid mutations: first, Ala at position 8 is mutated to Gly to reduce susceptibility to degradation by DPP-IV; second, Gly at position 22 is changed to glutamic acid (Glu) to enhance receptor binding affinity; and third, Arg at position 36 is substituted with Gly to mitigate potential immunogenicity [60].

Through covalent binding with Fc and the amino acid mutations in GLP-1, the molecular weight of dulaglutide reaches approximately 60 kDa. This modification reduces renal clearance and enhances resistance to DPP-IV degradation, ultimately extending its half-life to approximately 120 hours, enabling once-weekly dosing [60]. Furthermore, due to FcRn-mediated recycling, lower drug dosages are achieved. Compared to semaglutide, the molar dosage of

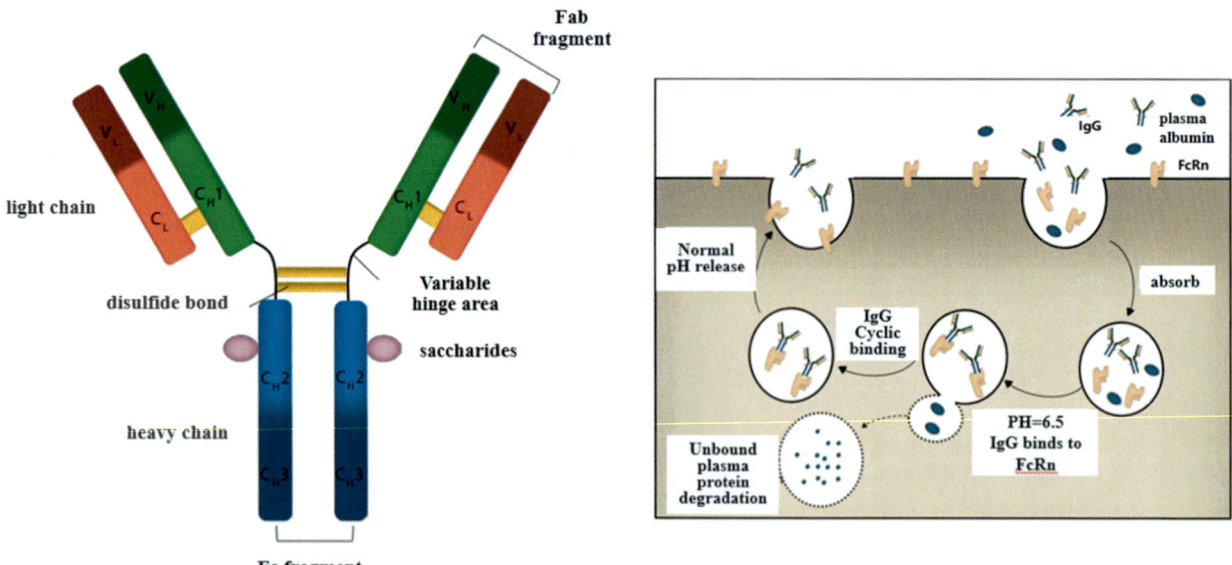

FIGURE 3.9 On the left is the structure of the IgG antibody, where the red and green regions represent the variable regions (Fab), and the blue region represents the constant region (Fc). On the right is an illustrative diagram of FcRn-mediated IgG recycling [57].

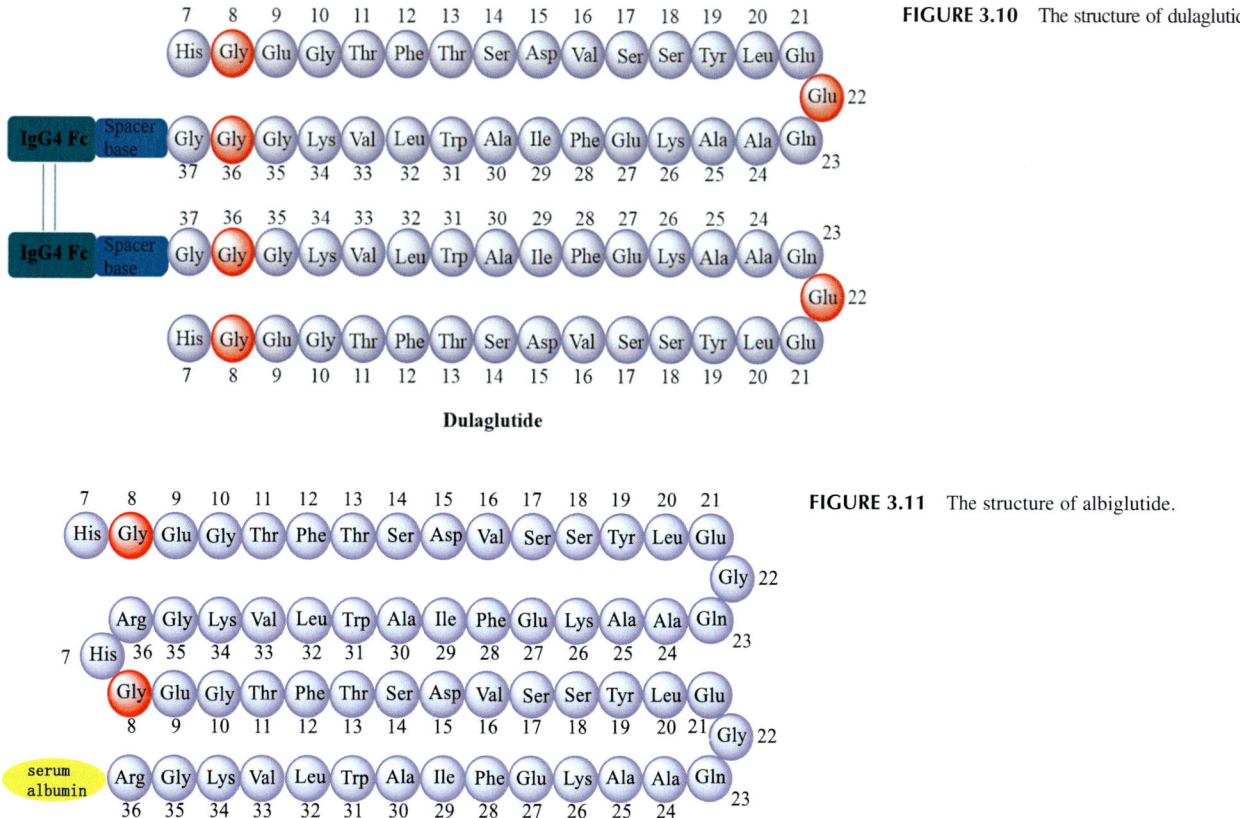

FIGURE 3.10 The structure of dulaglutide.

FIGURE 3.11 The structure of albiglutide.

dulaglutide is approximately one-tenth, reducing the occurrence of adverse effects for patients on chronic medication and improving the safety profile for long-term use.

3.2.2.4 Human serum albumin fusion

Albumin is one of the major proteins that constitute the human body, accounting for approximately 60% of total plasma proteins. It has a half-life of 2–3 weeks and is nearly nonimmunogenic, making it an excellent candidate for drug carriers to achieve extended drug action. The core design principle and key factor in using human serum albumin fusion to achieve drug longevity is the selection of fusion sites. These sites can include amino or carboxyl termini of albumin, or any region within the protein sequence (achieved through chemical modification rather than recombinant expression). The primary consideration is to minimize the reduction of drug activity [61].

Albiglutide is an example of the fusion with human serum albumin achieved through protein recombinant technology. In albiglutide, two GLP-1 (7–36) molecules are connected at the C-terminus of GLP-1 to the N-terminus of human serum albumin (see Fig. 3.11). This fusion results in a conjugated molecule with a molecular weight of 73 kDa. It significantly reduces renal filtration clearance [41], decreases DPP-IV degradation of GLP-1 [62,63], and extends its half-life to approximately 120 hours [64]. Albiglutide received FDA approval in 2014; however, its efficacy in blood glucose control is moderate compared to other similar drugs. It is less effective than dulaglutide and semaglutide in terms of HbA1c lowering, weight reduction, and cardiovascular risk management. As a result, it was recommended as an adjunctive treatment for type 2 diabetes. In 2018, its development company, GlaxoSmithKline, withdrew it from the global market [64].

3.3 The unsuccessful case in GLP-1 drug R&D and the implications and lessons

Now, let's discuss one of the most regrettable failures in GLP-1 drug development, which highlights the issues encountered in the development of GLP-1 drugs. Taspoglutide, developed by Roche Pharmaceuticals, was a GLP-1 analog.

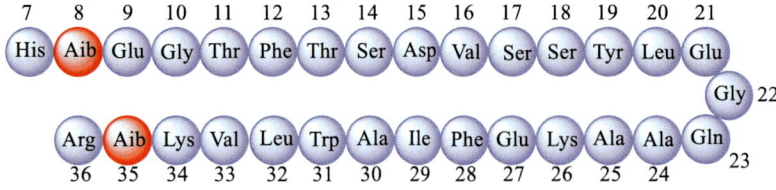

FIGURE 3.12 The structure of taspoglutide.

The molecule was a GLP-1 (7−36 NH_2), with two critical mutations at positions 8 and 35, where Ala were mutated to Aib (see Fig. 3.12). These mutations were primarily designed to enhance resistance to DPP-IV (mutation at position 8) and plasmin and kallikrein enzymes, thereby extending its half-life. Combining with formulation technology, it achieved once-weekly dosing, pioneering long-acting administration in GLP-1 applications. This drug showed good efficacy in blood glucose control for type 2 diabetes, along with significant weight reduction effects. However, it was ultimately terminated in 2010 after phase III clinical trials. This decision also partially led to the closure of Roche's research center in the United States.

Several factors contributed to its failure: (1) Significant gastrointestinal adverse effects, including nausea, vomiting, and gastrointestinal flatulence, were more observed compared to other GLP-1 control drugs. (2) Injection site discomfort reactions were significantly higher compared to other GLP-1 control drugs. (3) There was a notable increase in hypersensitivity reactions, leading to the development of antidrug antibodies in some patients, which even caused allergic reactions. Consequently, some patients had to prematurely withdraw from clinical trials [65]. These clinical adverse reactions highlight general safety concerns in GLP-1 drug development. While GLP-1 analogs are highly effective in blood glucose control, weight reduction, and improvement in cardiovascular disease, their inherent adverse effects or side effects must be identified and resolved in early-stage research to increase the success rate of drug development.

The adverse reactions associated with GLP-1 analogs include [66]: (1) Gastrointestinal side effects, such as nausea, vomiting, and slowed gastrointestinal motility, which often occur along with their blood glucose and weight control functions. (2) Pancreatic hyperplasia and pancreatitis, as the activation of GLP-1 receptors promotes pancreatic beta cell differentiation and proliferation, stimulating insulin secretion. GLP-1 analogs tend to keep beta cells in an active state for extended periods, potentially leading to pancreatic hyperplasia and even necrosis. This phenomenon has been observed in animal and clinical trials and must be addressed during drug development. (3) Allergic reactions caused by the development of antidrug antibodies. Although GLP-1 is an endogenous substance, its analogs possess amino acid mutations and covalent conjugation with long-acting carriers. Under high-concentration pharmacological conditions, all currently clinically used GLP-1 drugs produce antidrug antibodies. Exenatide analogs, in particular, have a significantly higher ability to induce antidrug antibodies than other GLP-1 analogs. The generation of antidrug antibodies not only reduces drug efficacy (as they can bind to the drug) but also raises concerns about allergic reactions, significantly increasing the safety risks. (4) Injection site reactions. Although all large molecule drugs administered by injection carry this risk, the types of reactions and their severity can vary widely among drugs. In the drug development process, meticulous attention must be paid to these potential adverse reactions, taking them into account early to ensure patient compliance and develop safer and more effective drugs.

In addition to the GLP-1 analog drugs mentioned earlier, there are other notable drugs in this category. Sanofi Pharmaceuticals introduced lixisenatide in 2016 (see Fig. 3.13A) and polyethylene glycol-loxenatide (PEG-loxenatide), among others (see Fig. 3.13B) [67]. Lixisenatide is a GLP-1 analog that originated from the exenatide sequence and is used as a second-line treatment for type 2 diabetes [68]. Polyethylene glycol (PEG) is a polymer composed of repeating ethylene oxide units. It is chemically inert and of low toxicity. It has been approved by the U.S. FDA for the development of oral, intravenous administration, and dermatological drug formulations [69]. As an effective long-acting carrier, PEG has been extensively researched and utilized. However, it has some safety concerns related to immunogenicity and potential brain accumulation [70]. In the past decade, it has lost its strong attraction for chronic disease treatment, but it can still be utilized in long-acting antiinfective drugs or immunotherapy medications.

3.4 Summary and outlook

From Dr. John Eng's discovery and research on exendin-4 in 1992 to the present day, spanning three decades, GLP-1 class drugs have evolved from their early stages to matured and highly effective frontline treatments for type 2 diabetes. It began with twice-daily injections of exenatide, progressing to once-daily liraglutide, and further to long-acting once-

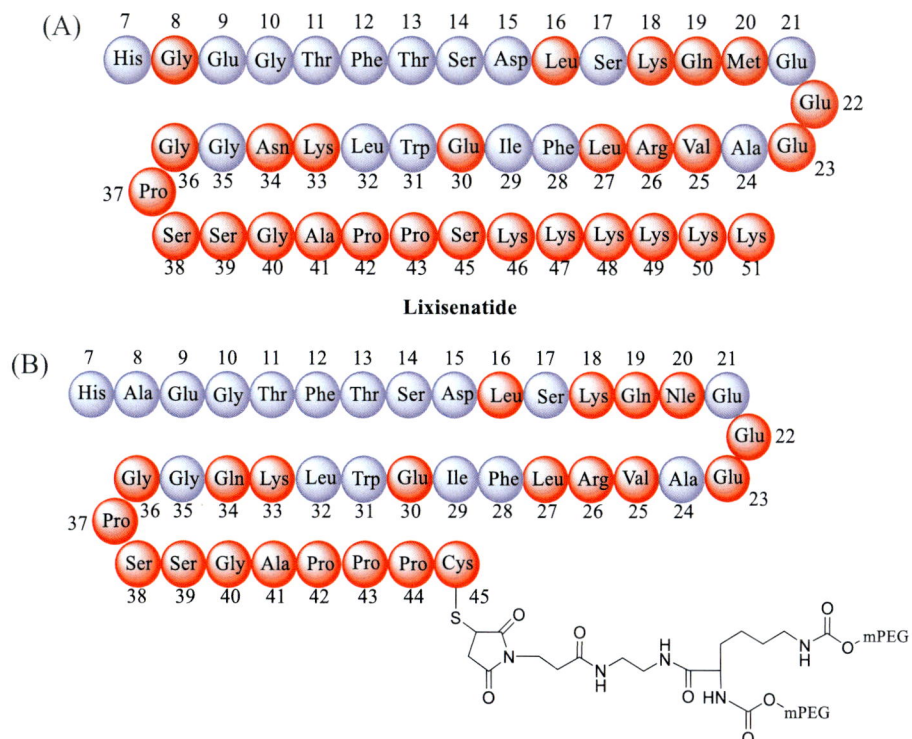

FIGURE 3.13 (A) Structure of lixisenatide. (B) Structure of PEG-loxenatide.

weekly formulations, dulaglutide and semaglutide, and the latest development of oral semaglutide. In 2020, the annual sales of dulaglutide injections exceeded $5 billion, while semaglutide injections and oral tablets reached approximately $3.7 billion, with a rapidly growing rate [71].

Compared to other antidiabetic medications, GLP-1 class drugs offer advantages such as a lower risk of hypoglycemia, weight reduction, and improvements in cardiovascular, chronic liver, and kidney diseases [72]. Currently, the research focus for developing newer GLP-1 class drugs is centered on targeting some specific areas. One key area is the development of combination formulations with insulin. As discussed in Chapter 2 regarding insulin medications, one of the side effects of long-term insulin use is the total weight and fat mass gain, which is particularly disadvantageous for chronic disease patients. Even though the latest basal insulin has better weight control compared to traditional insulin, it remains an important issue in insulin therapy. GLP-1 class drugs are known for their ability to reduce weight and complement insulin therapy effectively, enhancing the overall treatment outcome of diabetes [73,74]. Lixisenatide, mentioned earlier, is an example developed by Sanofi specifically for use in combination with prandial insulin. Another prominent research area is centered on the use of agonists targeting multiple brain-gut hormone receptors. It includes, but is not limited to, dual agonists targeting both GLP-1 and GIP receptors, such as tirzepatide, which is currently in phase III clinical trial by Eli Lilly. Phase III clinical data show an even more excellent effect in reducing HbA1c and body weight [75]. There are also triple agonists targeting the GLP-1, GIP, and glucagon receptors, which are currently in the clinical trial research stage. GLP-1 and GIP have blood glucose-lowering and appetite-suppressing effects, while glucagon can slightly increase blood glucose while accelerating energy expenditure and promoting glycogen and fat consumption, thus enhancing the weight loss effect and improving metabolic comorbidities risk factors [76,77]. Research is also being conducted on other agonists targeting other brain-gut peptide receptors as well.

References

[1] Holst JJ. Extrapancreatic glucagons. Digestion 1978;17(2):168—90.
[2] Donnelly D. The structure and function of the glucagon-like peptide-1 receptor and its ligands. Br J Pharmacol 2012;166(1):27—41.
[3] Brown JC, Dryburgh JR. A gastric inhibitory polypeptide. II. The complete amino acid sequence. Can J Biochem 1971;49(8):867—72.
[4] Shah M, Vella A. Effects of GLP-1 on appetite and weight. Rev Endocr Metab Disord 2014;15(3):181—7.

[5] Sheahan KH, Wahlberg EA, Gilbert MP. An overview of GLP-1 agonists and recent cardiovascular outcomes trials. Postgrad Med J 2020;96 (1133):156−61.

[6] Seghieri M, Christensen AS, Andersen A, et al. Future perspectives on GLP-1 receptor agonists and GLP-1/glucagon receptor co-agonists in the treatment of NAFLD. Front Endocrinol (Lausanne) 2018;9:649.

[7] Drucker DJ, Habener JF, Holst JJ. Discovery, characterization, and clinical development of the glucagon-like peptides. J Clin Invest 2017;127 (12):4217−27.

[8] Mcintyre N, Holdsworth CD, Turner DS. new interpretation of oral glucose tolerance. Lancet 1964;2(7349):20−1.

[9] Holst JJ, Orskov C, Nielsen OV, et al. Truncated glucagon-like peptide I, an insulin-releasing hormone from the distal gut. FEBS Lett 1987;211 (2):169−74.

[10] Steiner DF. The proprotein convertases. Curr Opin Chem Biol 1998;2(1):31−9.

[11] Orskov C, Wettergren A, Holst JJ. Biological effects and metabolic rates of glucagonlike peptide-1 7-36 amide and glucagonlike peptide-1 7-37 in healthy subjects are indistinguishable. Diabetes 1993;42(5):658−61.

[12] Eldred WD, Ammermuller J, Schechner J, et al. Quantitative anatomy, synaptic connectivity and physiology of amacrine cells with glucagon-like immunoreactivity in the turtle retina. J Neurocytol 1996;25(5):347−64.

[13] Holst JJ. The physiology of glucagon-like peptide 1. Physiol Rev 2007;87(4):1409−39.

[14] Franek E, Gajos G, Gumprecht J, et al. The role of glucagon-like peptide 1 in glucose homeostasis and in other aspects of human physiology. Polskie Archiwum Medycyny Wewnetrznej 2009;119(11):743−51.

[15] Andersen A, Lund A, Knop FK, et al. Glucagon-like peptide 1 in health and disease. Nat Rev Endocrinol 2018;14(7):390−403.

[16] Meloni AR, De Young MB, Lowe C, et al. GLP-1 receptor activated insulin secretion from pancreatic β-cells: mechanism and glucose dependence. Diabetes Obes Metab 2013;15(1):15−27.

[17] Goke R, Larsen PJ, Mikkelsen JD, et al. Distribution of GLP-1 binding sites in the rat brain: evidence that exendin-4 is a ligand of brain GLP-1 binding sites. Eur J Neurosci 1995;7(11):2294−300.

[18] Turton MD, O'Shea D, Gunn I, et al. A role for glucagon-like peptide-1 in the central regulation of feeding. Nature 1996;379(6560):69−72.

[19] Gutzwiller JP, Goke B, Drewe J, et al. Glucagon-like peptide-1: a potent regulator of food intake in humans. Gut 1999;44(1):81−6.

[20] Larsen PJ, Holst JJ. Glucagon-related peptide 1 (GLP-1): hormone and neurotransmitter. Regul Pept 2005;128(2):97−107.

[21] Hira T, Pinyo J, Hara H. What is GLP-1 really doing in obesity? Trends Endocrinol Metab 2020;31(2):71−80.

[22] Knundsen LB, Pridal L. Glucagon-like peptide-1-(9-36) amide is a major metabolite of glucagon-like peptide-1-(7-36) amide after in vivo administration to dogs, and it acts as an antagonist on the pancreatic receptor. Eur J Pharmacol 1996;318(2-3):429−35.

[23] Drucker DJ, Philippe J, Mojsov S, et al. Glucagon-like peptide I stimulates insulin gene expression and increases cyclic AMP levels in a rat islet cell line. Proc Natl Acad Sci U S A 1987;84(10):3434−8.

[24] Deacon CF, Nauck MA, Toft-Nielsen M, et al. Both subcutaneously and intravenously administered glucagon-like peptide I are rapidly degraded from the NH2-terminus in type II diabetic patients and in healthy subjects. Diabetes 1995;44(9):1126−31.

[25] Yap MKK, Misuan N. Exendin-4 from Heloderma suspectum venom: from discovery to its latest application as type II diabetes combatant. Basic Clin Pharmacol Toxicol 2019;124(5):513−27.

[26] Eng J, Kleinman WA, Singh L, et al. Isolation and characterization of exendin-4, an exendin-3 analogue, from Heloderma suspectum venom. Further evidence for an exendin receptor on dispersed acini from guinea pig pancreas. J Biol Chem 1992;267(11):7402−5.

[27] Raufman JP, Singh L, Singh G, et al. Truncated glucagon-like peptide-1 interacts with exendin receptors on dispersed acini from guinea pig pancreas. Identification of a mammalian analogue of the reptilian peptide exendin-4. J Biol Chem 1992;267(30):21432−7.

[28] Neidigh JW, Fesinmeyer RM, Prickett KS, et al. Exendin-4 and glucagon-like-peptide-1: NMR structural comparisons in the solution and micelle-associated states. Biochemistry 2001;40(44):13188−200.

[29] Jensen L, Helleberg H, Roffel A, et al. Absorption, metabolism and excretion of the GLP-1 analogue semaglutide in humans and nonclinical species. Eur J Pharm Sci 2017;104:31−41.

[30] Montrose-Rafizadeh C, Yang H, Rodgers BD, et al. High potency antagonists of the pancreatic glucagon-like peptide-1 receptor. J Biol Chem 1997;272(34):21201−6.

[31] Lopez de Maturana R, Willshaw A, Kuntzsch A, et al. The isolated N-terminal domain of the glucagon-like peptide-1 (GLP-1) receptor binds exendin peptides with much higher affinity than GLP-1. J Biol Chem 2003;278(12):10195−200.

[32] Liao S, Liang Y, Zhang Z, et al. In vitro metabolic stability of exendin-4: pharmacokinetics and identification of cleavage products. PLoS One 2015;10(2):e0116805.

[33] Mulvihill EE, Drucker DJ. Pharmacology, physiology, and mechanisms of action of dipeptidyl peptidase-4 inhibitors. Endocr Rev 2014;35 (6):992−1019.

[34] Bhavsar S, Mudaliar S, Cherrington A. Evolution of exenatide as a diabetes therapeutic. Curr Diabetes Rev 2013;9(2):161−93.

[35] Kolterman OG, Kim DD, Larry S, et al. Pharmacokinetics, pharmacodynamics, and safety of exenatide in patients with type 2 diabetes mellitus. Am J Health-System Pharm 2005;62(2):173−81.

[36] Heine RJ, Van Gaal LF, Johns D, et al. Exenatide versus insulin glargine in patients with suboptimally controlled type 2 diabetes: a randomized trial. Ann Intern Med 2005;143(8):559−69.

[37] Aroda VR, De Young MB. Clinical implications of exenatide as a twice-daily or once-weekly therapy for type 2 diabetes. Postgrad Med 2011;123(5):228−38.

[38] Underwood CR, Garibay P, Knudsen LB, et al. Crystal structure of glucagon-like peptide-1 in complex with the extracellular domain of the glucagon-like peptide-1 receptor. J Biol Chem 2010;285(1):723–30.

[39] Menacho-Melgar R, Decker JS, Hennigan JN, et al. A review of lipidation in the development of advanced protein and peptide therapeutics. J Control Rel 2019;295:1–12.

[40] Garber A, Henry R, Ratner R, et al. Liraglutide versus glimepiride monotherapy for type 2 diabetes (LEAD-3 Mono): a randomised, 52-week, phase III, double-blind, parallel-treatment trial. Lancet 2009;373(9662):473–81.

[41] Lund A, Knop FK, Vilsboll T. Glucagon-like peptide-1 receptor agonists for the treatment of type 2 diabetes: differences and similarities. Eur J Intern Med 2014;25(5):407–14.

[42] Yin L, Chen X, Vicini P, et al. Therapeutic outcomes, assessments, risk factors and mitigation efforts of immunogenicity of therapeutic protein products. Cell Immunol 2015;295(2):118–26.

[43] Grime KH, Barton P, Mcginnity DF. Application of in silico, in vitro and preclinical pharmacokinetic data for the effective and efficient prediction of human pharmacokinetics. Mol Pharm 2013;10(4):1191–206.

[44] Jacobsen LV, Flint A, Olsen AK, et al. Liraglutide in type 2 diabetes mellitus: clinical pharmacokinetics and pharmacodynamics. Clin Pharmacokinet 2016;55(6):657–72.

[45] Frederiksen TM, Sonderby P, Ryberg LA, et al. Oligomerization of a glucagon-like peptide 1 analog: bridging experiment and simulations. Biophys J 2015;109(6):1202–13.

[46] Wang Y, Lomakin A, Kanai S, et al. Transformation of oligomers of lipidated peptide induced by change in pH. Mol Pharm 2015;12(2):411–19.

[47] Russell-Jones D. Molecular, pharmacological and clinical aspects of liraglutide, a once-daily human GLP-1 analogue. Mol Cell Endocrinol 2009;297(1-2):137–40.

[48] Elbrond B, Jakobsen G, Larsen S, et al. Pharmacokinetics, pharmacodynamics, safety, and tolerability of a single-dose of NN2211, a long-acting glucagon-like peptide 1 derivative, in healthy male subjects. Diabetes Care 2002;25(8):1398–404.

[49] Pi-Sunyer X, Astrup A, Fujioka K, et al. A randomized, controlled trial of 3.0 mg of liraglutide in weight management. N Engl J Med 2015;373(1):11–22.

[50] Blonde L, Russell-Jones D. The safety and efficacy of liraglutide with or without oral antidiabetic drug therapy in type 2 diabetes: an overview of the LEAD 1-5 studies. Diabetes Obes Metab 2009;11(Suppl 3):26–34.

[51] Lau J, Bloch P, Schaffer L, et al. Discovery of the once-weekly glucagon-like peptide-1 (GLP-1) analogue semaglutide. J Med Chem 2015;58(18):7370–80.

[52] Gotfredsen CF, Molck AM, Thorup I, et al. The human GLP-1 analogs liraglutide and semaglutide: absence of histopathological effects on the pancreas in nonhuman primates. Diabetes 2014;63(7):2486–97.

[53] Pratley RE, Aroda VR, Lingvay I, et al. Semaglutide versus dulaglutide once weekly in patients with type 2 diabetes (SUSTAIN 7): a randomised, open-label, phase 3b trial. Lancet Diabetes Endocrinol 2018;6(4):275–86.

[54] Marso SP, Holst AG, Vilsboll T. Semaglutide and cardiovascular outcomes in patients with type 2 diabetes. N Engl J Med 2017;376(9):891–2.

[55] Buckley ST, Baekdal TA, Vegge A, et al. Transcellular stomach absorption of a derivatized glucagon-like peptide-1 receptor agonist. Sci Transl Med 2018;10(467) eaar7047.

[56] Bucheit JD, Pamulapati LG, Carter N, et al. Oral semaglutide: a review of the first oral glucagon-like peptide 1 receptor agonist. Diabetes Technol Ther 2020;22(1):10–18.

[57] V P, Ca K, Perez Le G, et al. A new approach to drug therapy: fc-fusion technology. Prim Health Care Open Access 2017;07(01):1–5.

[58] Hogarth PM, Pietersz GA. Fc receptor-targeted therapies for the treatment of inflammation, cancer and beyond. Nat Rev Drug Discov 2012;11(4):311–31.

[59] Ober RJ, Martinez C, Vaccaro C, et al. Visualizing the site and dynamics of IgG salvage by the MHC class I-related receptor, FcRn. J Immunol 2004;172(4):2021–9.

[60] Glaesner W, Vick AM, Millican R, et al. Engineering and characterization of the long-acting glucagon-like peptide-1 analogue LY2189265, an Fc fusion protein. Diabetes Metab Res Rev 2010;26(4):287–96.

[61] Rogers B, Dong D, Li Z, et al. Recombinant human serum albumin fusion proteins and novel applications in drug delivery and therapy. Curr Pharm Des 2015;21(14):1899–907.

[62] Matthews JE, Stewart MW, De Boever EH, et al. Pharmacodynamics, pharmacokinetics, safety, and tolerability of albiglutide, a long-acting glucagon-like peptide-1 mimetic, in patients with type 2 diabetes. J Clin Endocrinol Metab 2008;93(12):4810–17.

[63] Muller TD, Finan B, Bloom SR, et al. Glucagon-like peptide 1 (GLP-1). Mol Metab 2019;30:72–130.

[64] Bush MA, Matthews JE, De Boever EH, et al. Safety, tolerability, pharmacodynamics and pharmacokinetics of albiglutide, a long-acting glucagon-like peptide-1 mimetic, in healthy subjects. Diabetes Obes Metab 2009;11(5):498–505.

[65] Rosenstock J, Balas B, Charbonnel B, et al. The fate of taspoglutide, a weekly GLP-1 receptor agonist, versus twice-daily exenatide for type 2 diabetes: the T-emerge 2 trial. Diabetes Care 2013;36(3):498–504.

[66] Filippatos TD, Panagiotopoulou TV, Elisaf MS. Adverse effects of GLP-1 receptor agonists. Rev Diabet Stud 2014;11(3-4):202–30.

[67] Yang GR, Zhao XL, Jin F, et al. Pharmacokinetics and pharmacodynamics of a polyethylene glycol (PEG)-conjugated GLP-receptor agonist once weekly in Chinese patients with type 2 diabetes. J Clin Pharmacol 2015;55(2):152–8.

[68] Bain SC. The clinical development program of lixisenatide: a once-daily glucagon-like Peptide-1 receptor agonist. Diabetes Ther 2014;5(2):367–83.

[69] Park EJ, Choi J, Lee KC, et al. Emerging PEGylated non-biologic drugs. Expert Opin Emerg Drugs 2019;24(2):107−19.
[70] Shiraishi K, Yokoyama M. Toxicity and immunogenicity concerns related to PEGylated-micelle carrier systems: a review. Sci Technol Adv Mater 2019;20(1):324−36.
[71] Romera I, Cebrian-Cuenca A, Alvarez-Guisasola F, et al. A review of practical issues on the use of glucagon-like peptide-1 receptor agonists for the management of type 2 diabetes. Diabetes Ther 2019;10(1):5−19.
[72] Hollander PA, Krasner A, Klioze S, et al. Body weight changes associated with insulin therapy: a retrospective pooled analysis of inhaled human insulin (Exubera) versus subcutaneous insulin in five controlled Phase III trials. Diabetes Care 2007;30(10):2508−10.
[73] Nuffer W, Guesnier A, Trujillo JM. A review of the new GLP-1 receptor agonist/basal insulin fixed-ratio combination products. Ther Adv Endocrinol Metab 2018;9(3):69−79.
[74] Vora J. Combining incretin-based therapies with insulin: realizing the potential in type 2 diabetes. Diabetes Care 2013;36(Suppl 2):S226−32.
[75] Frias JP, Davies MJ, Rosenstock J, et al. Tirzepatide versus semaglutide once weekly in patients with type 2 diabetes. N Engl J Med 2021;385(6):503−15.
[76] Finan B, Ma T, Ottaway N, et al. Unimolecular dual incretins maximize metabolic benefits in rodents, monkeys, and humans. Sci Transl Med 2013;5(209) 209ra151.
[77] Finan B, Yang B, Ottaway N, et al. A rationally designed monomeric peptide triagonist corrects obesity and diabetes in rodents. Nat Med 2015;21(1):27−36.

Chapter 4

Antidiabetic drugs based on sodium-glucose cotransporter 2 inhibitors

Youhong Niu and Xinshan Ye
School of Pharmaceutical Sciences, Peking University, Beijing, P.R. China

Chapter outline

4.1 Overview of diabetes mellitus and antidiabetic drugs 55
    4.1.1 Definition, classification, and current status of diabetes mellitus 55
    4.1.2 Factors related to the onset of diabetes 55
    4.1.3 Clinical anti-diabetic medications, and their targets and mechanisms 56
4.2 Sodium-glucose cotransporter 2 (SGLT2) inhibitors as anti-diabetic drugs 59
    4.2.1 Biological basis of SGLT2 as a therapeutic target for diabetes 59
    4.2.2 SGLT2 inhibitors and successful development of dapagliflozin 60
    4.2.3 Synthetic process of dapagliflozin 65
    4.2.4 Efficacy and action of dapagliflozin 67
    4.2.5 Other drugs based on SGLT2 inhibitors 67
4.3 Successful experience in the development of dapagliflozin 67
References 69

4.1 Overview of diabetes mellitus and antidiabetic drugs

4.1.1 Definition, classification, and current status of diabetes mellitus

Diabetes mellitus is an endocrine metabolic disorder characterized by chronic hyperglycemia caused by abnormalities in insulin secretion, insulin action, or both, affecting the metabolism of glucose, lipids, and proteins [1,2]. The international diabetes federation classifies diabetes into three main categories: (1) Type 1 diabetes. This type of diabetes accounts for approximately 10% of all diabetes cases, is primarily caused by an autoimmune attack on insulin-producing cells, leading to reduced or even no insulin secretion, thereby developing glycosuria symptoms. Type 1 diabetes is commonly observed in children and adolescents. (2) Type 2 diabetes. The most prevalent form, accounting for approximately 90% of diabetes cases, is characterized by insulin resistance. These patients are generally older and have a familial inheritance. (3) Gestational diabetes. Gestational diabetes, often overlooked, refers to elevated blood glucose levels during pregnancy, which return to normal after childbirth. Gestational diabetes can also give rise to various complications, posing risks to both the mother and the child. Furthermore, it increases the risk of developing Type 2 diabetes in affected individuals [3,4].

Prolonged hyperglycemia can lead to vascular and microvascular damage, posing risks to organs such as the heart, brain, kidneys, peripheral nerves, eyes, and feet, resulting in a multitude of complications. Diabetes complications encompass over 100 different conditions [5–7], making it the chronic disease with the highest number of known complications. These include cardiovascular diseases, peripheral neuropathy, diabetic nephropathy, retinopathy, diabetic eye disease, neuropathic damage, diabetic foot disorders, and an increased susceptibility to infections.

4.1.2 Factors related to the onset of diabetes

The occurrence and progression of diabetes involve a multifactorial and polygenic process with a complex pathogenesis that is not yet fully elucidated [8]. However, it is widely believed to be associated with the following factors: (1) Hereditary factors. Genetic studies have shown a significant difference in the incidence of diabetes between blood relatives and non-blood relatives, with approximately a fivefold higher rate among the former. The importance of genetic factors varies noticeably between Type 1 and Type 2 diabetes, constituting approximately 50% in Type 1 diabetes and exceeding 90% in Type 2 diabetes. Here, "genetic" refers to susceptibility rather than inherited diabetes. (2) Psychosocial factors. Since the beginning of the new century, researchers, domestic and abroad, have confirmed the role of psychosocial factors in the occurrence and development of diabetes. Psychological stress, emotional excitement, and various stressful conditions are believed to induce the excessive secretion of hormones such as growth hormone, epinephrine, glucagon, and adrenal cortex hormones, leading to elevated blood glucose levels. (3) Obesity factors. Currently, obesity is considered an important factor in triggering diabetes. The research has shown that 60%−80% of adult diabetes patients are obese before the onset of the disease, and the incidence of diabetes is directly proportional to the degree of obesity. (4) Prolonged overeating factor. Excessive and uncontrolled dietary intake, resulting in nutritional excess, imposes an excessive burden on the already compromised pancreatic β-cells responsible for insulin secretion, thereby triggering diabetes. (5) Viral infection. There is a significant relationship between early-onset diabetes and viral infections. Infection itself will not induce diabetes, but it can make asymptomatic diabetes explicit. (6) Pregnancy. Studies have discovered an association between the number of pregnancies and the onset of diabetes, with multiple pregnancies being more likely to induce diabetes. (7) Genetic factors. Current research suggests that diabetes is caused by several genetic impairments. Type 1 diabetes is attributed to damage to the HLA-D gene on the short arm of the sixth pair of human chromosomes. Type 2 diabetes is caused by impairments in insulin genes, insulin receptor genes, glucose lyase genes, and mitochondrial genes. It has been confirmed that maturity-onset diabetes of the young (MODY), which manifests during adolescence and resembles adult-onset diabetes, results from a single-gene genetic mutation [9,10].

4.1.3 Clinical anti-diabetic medications, and their targets and mechanisms

Currently, the treatment of diabetes mainly involves the administration of insulin injections and oral anti-diabetic medications. According to their action mechanisms [11−13], these medications can be broadly classified into the following categories:

4.1.3.1 Insulin and insulin analogs
See below.

4.1.3.2 Insulin secretagogues
Type 2 diabetes patients are often accompanied by secondary β-cell dysfunction, leading to insufficient insulin secretion. Insulin secretagogues can stimulate pancreatic β-cells to secrete more insulin to lower blood glucose levels. The reason that these drugs induce insulin secretion is by inhibiting ATP-dependent potassium channels, leading to the efflux of K^+ ions, β-cell depolarization, influx of Ca^{2+} ions, and subsequent insulin secretion. In addition, this type of drug can augment the effect of insulin by enhancing the binding ability of insulin to its receptors.

According to their chemical structures, insulin secretagogues can be divided into two types, including sulfonylureas and non-sulfonylureas. The representative structures of sulfonylurea secretagogues are shown in Table 4.1, wherein the substituents R and R_1 are different, leading to different hypoglycemic action times and intensities.

Despite the fact that the chemical structures of non-sulfonylurea drugs being different from those of sulfonylurea drugs, these type of secretagogues shares a similar action mechanism [14] a sulfonylurea drugs. Non-sulfonylurea secretagogues can directly improve the deficiency in early insulin secretion and have unique advantages in lowering postprandial blood glucose levels. The currently approved drugs of non-sulfonylurea type for clinical use are listed in Fig. 4.1, including repaglinide, nateglinide, and mitiglinide, which is used as a mixture of enantiomers.

4.1.3.3 Biguanides
This class of medications reduces blood glucose mainly through mechanisms such as promoting glucose uptake by peripheral tissues, inhibiting gluconeogenesis, decreasing hepatic glycogen output, and delaying glucose absorption in the intestine. Representative drugs include metformin and phenformin (Fig. 4.2). Metformin is currently the first-line medication used in clinical practice, characterized by low toxicity, no hypoglycemic effect in normal individuals, and minimal risk of inducing hypoglycemia. In addition, metformin has the effect of increasing insulin receptor sensitivity, reducing insulin resistance, improving lipid metabolism and fibrinolysis, and alleviating platelet aggregation. Therefore, metformin is beneficial in mitigating the occurrence and progression of cardiovascular complications.

TABLE 4.1 Sulfonylurea secretagogues.

Drug	R	R₁	In vivo half-life (h)	In vivo action time (h)
First generation				
Tolbutamide	CH₃–	–nC₄H₉	4.5~6.5	6~12
Chlorpropamide	–Cl	–nC₄H₉	36	>60
Tolazamide	CH₃–	(azepane)	7	12~14
Acetohexamide	CH₃CO–	(cyclohexyl)	6~8	12~18
Second generation				
Glyburide	5-Cl, 2-OCH₃-C₆H₃-C(O)NHCH₂CH₂–	(cyclohexyl)	1.5~3.0	>24
Glipizide	5-methylpyrazine-2-C(O)NHCH₂CH₂–	(cyclohexyl)	4	>24
Gliclazide	CH₃–	(octahydrocyclopenta[c]pyrrolyl)	10~12	>24
Glimepiride	3-ethyl-4-methyl-2-oxo-3-pyrrolin-1-yl-C(O)NHCH₂CH₂–	4-methylcyclohexyl	2~3	>24
Gliquidone	7-methoxy-4,4-dimethyl-1,3-dioxo-isoquinolin-2-yl-CH₂CH₂–	(cyclohexyl)	1.5	16~24
Glisoxepide	5-methylisoxazol-3-yl-C(O)NHCH₂CH₂–	(azepane)		

4.1.3.4 α-Glucosidase inhibitors

α-Glucosidase inhibitors are the current first-line anti-diabetic medication used in clinical practice. These drugs can lower or alleviate postprandial blood glucose levels by competitively inhibiting the activity of α-glucosidase, thus decreasing the rate of polysaccharide breakdown and subsequent glucose production and delaying glucose absorption. Studies demonstrated that the glycated hemoglobin concentration of most patients drops after long-term use of α-glucosidase inhibitors. α-Glucosidase inhibitors currently used in clinical practice are the mimics of monosaccharide or oligosaccharide, and representative drugs include acarbose, voglibose [15], and miglitol [16] as shown in Fig. 4.3.

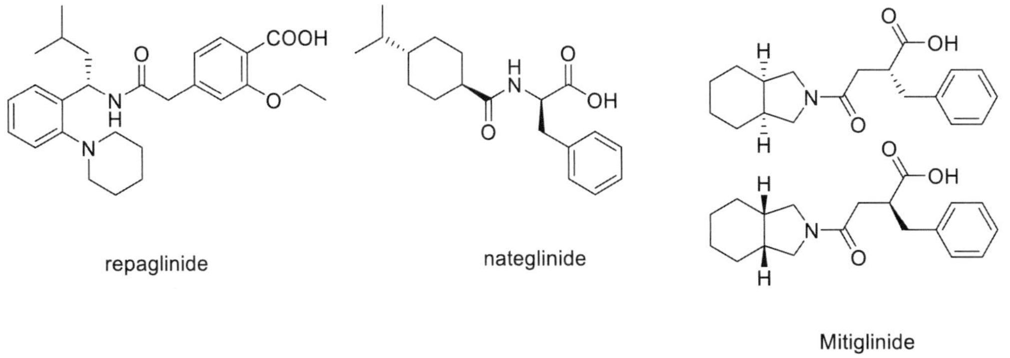

FIGURE 4.1 Nonsulfonylurea secretagogues.

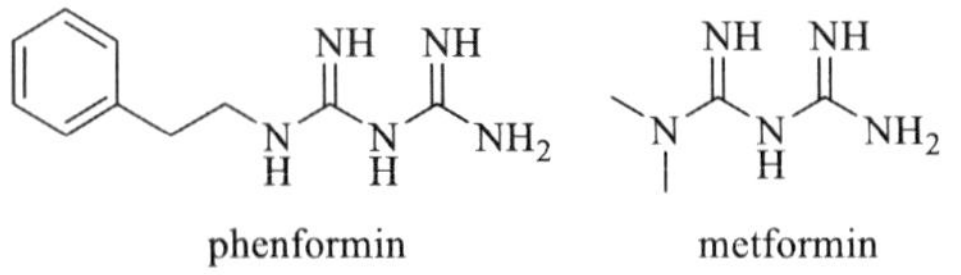

FIGURE 4.2 The structures of phenformin and metformin.

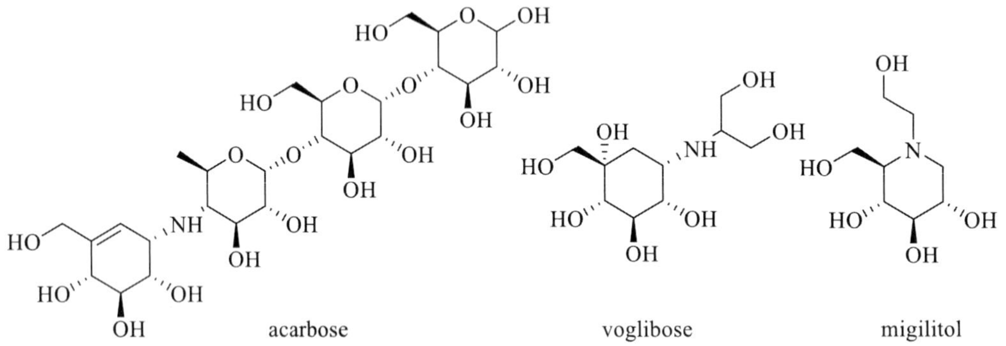

FIGURE 4.3 The structures of representative drugs of α-glucosidase inhibitors.

4.1.3.5 Insulin sensitizers

The glucose-lowering effects of insulin sensitizer medications are mediated by increasing the sensitivity of target tissues to insulin and the utilization of insulin, facilitating glucose metabolism, thus resulting in effectively reducing fasting and postprandial blood glucose levels. Insulin sensitizers are mainly thiazolidinediones, including rosiglitazone, pioglitazone, troglitazone, and ciglitazone (Fig. 4.4). These drugs, when used alone, do not cause hypoglycemia and are often combined with other types of oral antidiabetic drugs, resulting in a significant synergistic effect. Rosiglitazone and pioglitazone exhibit more pronounced glucose-lowering effects and higher safety profiles.

4.1.3.6 GLP-1 receptor agonists
See below.

4.1.3.7 Dipeptidyl peptidase-4 (DPP-4) inhibitors

Incretin is a type of peptide hormone produced by intestinal L cells, mainly including two peptides such as GLP-1 and GIP, in the human body (see Chapter 1 of this book where the partial contents were discussed). After binding to GLP-1 receptors, GLP-1 can stimulate insulin secretion from pancreatic beta cells in a glucose-dependent manner, exerting its effect on lowering blood glucose. It also regulates pancreatic beta cell regeneration, proliferation, and survival. However, GLP-1 is easily hydrolyzed by dipeptidyl peptidase-4 (DPP-4) present on the cell surface, leading to its

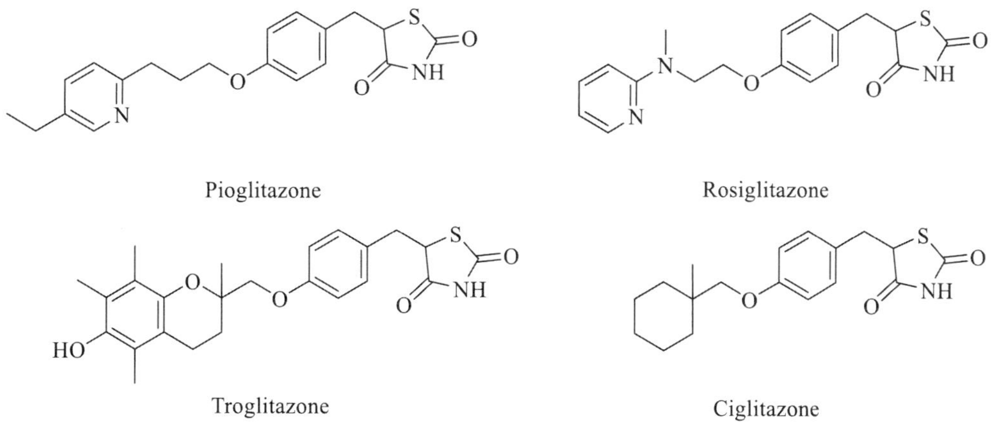

FIGURE 4.4 The representative structures of thiazolidinedione medications.

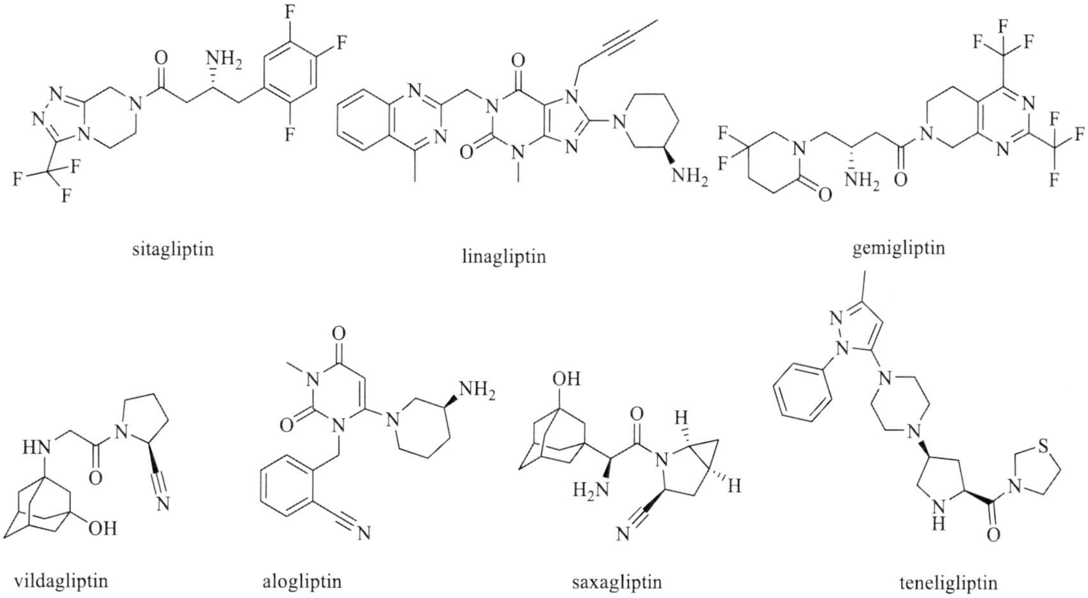

FIGURE 4.5 The chemical structures of DPP-4 inhibitors.

inactivation. Therefore, inhibition of DPP-4 enzyme activity leads to reduced degradation of GLP-1 and elevated GLP-1 concentration in the blood, which exerts its role in glycemic control.

Since 2006, seven DPP-4 inhibitors have been developed for the treatment of type 2 diabetes, including sitagliptin, linagliptin, saxagliptin, vildagliptin, alogliptin, gemigliptin, and trelagliptin (Fig. 4.5) [17–20].

4.2 Sodium-glucose cotransporter 2 (SGLT2) inhibitors as anti-diabetic drugs

4.2.1 Biological basis of SGLT2 as a therapeutic target for diabetes

The maintenance of glucose homeostasis is the collective outcome of the involvement of various organs and tissues, including the gastrointestinal tract, liver, pancreas, kidneys, adipose tissue, and muscle tissue. Different types of antidiabetic medications exert their control over blood glucose levels by targeting the respective regulatory tissues and organs involved in glucose metabolism, as illustrated in Fig. 4.6 [21]. The kidneys are one of the most important organs in maintaining blood glucose balance, achieving their roles in controlling blood glucose balance through glomerular filtration and tubular reabsorption of blood glucose within the renal glomeruli and tubules. Approximately 162 g (900 mmol) of glucose is filtered by the kidneys daily, and when blood glucose levels fall below 10 mmol/L, the filtered glucose is entirely reabsorbed by the renal tubules, helping to maintain normal fasting blood glucose levels

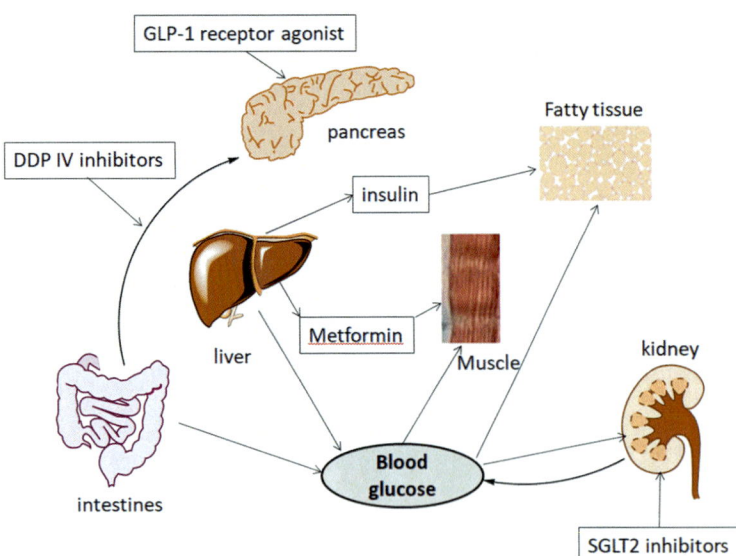

FIGURE 4.6 Vital organs and tissues of regulating blood glucose balance, drugs and corresponding targets for treatment of diabetes.

(3.9−6.0 mmol/L). However, if blood glucose is more than 10 mmol/L (renal glucose threshold), exceeding the maximum reabsorption capacity of the kidney, the part of glucose that has not been reabsorbed will be excreted in the urine to form glucose in the urine, preventing excessive elevation of blood glucose levels.

Glucose, a polar molecule, cannot freely traverse cell membranes, and its transport into cells relies on two types of carrier proteins: SGLTs and glucose transporters (GLUTs) [22−24]. SGLTs can facilitate the transport of glucose against its concentration gradient into the cell and are encoded by genes belonging to the SLC5A family, mainly including SGLT1, SGLT2, SGLT3, SGLT4, and SGLT5. On the other hand, GLUTs are passive carrier proteins that transport glucose along its concentration gradient, and they are encoded by genes of the SLC2A family, which mainly include GLUT1, GLUT2, GLUT3, GLUT4, etc., and are primarily distributed in various tissues and organs such as red blood cells, liver, brain, kidneys, pancreas, and muscle. GLUTs serve as vital energy supply channels for cellular metabolism [25].

SGLT1 is a high-affinity, low-capacity transport protein predominantly expressed in the S3 segment of renal tubules. It is responsible for the reabsorption of approximately 10% of glucose filtered by the renal glomeruli. SGLT2, on the other hand, is a low-affinity, high-capacity transport protein mainly expressed in the S1 segment of renal tubules. It is responsible for the reabsorption of approximately 90% of the filtered glucose in the renal glomeruli [26]. At the molecular level (Fig. 4.7) [27], the transport of one glucose molecule by SGLT1 requires the coordinated transport of two sodium ions to provide energy. In contrast, the transport of one glucose molecule by SGLT2 only requires the coordinated transport of one sodium ion to provide energy. However, both processes rely on the maintenance of sodium-potassium ion concentration gradients across the cell basolateral membrane by the sodium-potassium ATPase pump. The renal reabsorption of filtered glucose is primarily accomplished by the SGLT2 carrier protein [28].

The mechanism of renal-controlling blood glucose levels is abnormal in individuals with diabetes. Studies have demonstrated an elevation in the expression and activity of SGLT-2 in individuals with familial diabetes. Under persistent chronic hyperglycemic conditions, the kidneys exhibit an increased maximum capacity for glucose reabsorption, known as renal glucose threshold elevation. This allows for the continued reabsorption of higher levels of glucose, leading to sustained elevation of blood glucose levels. Sustained hyperglycemia, in turn, exacerbates glucose reabsorption, leading to a vicious cycle of high glucose toxicity. In a chronic hyperglycemic state, SGLT-2 can mediate increased glucose transport, resulting in a greater extent of reabsorption and ultimately contributing to persistent hyperglycemia in patients. Therefore, the development of SGLT2 inhibitors as novel therapeutic agents for diabetes has garnered significant attention [29].

4.2.2 SGLT2 inhibitors and successful development of dapagliflozin

At first, the studies on SGLT2 inhibitors primarily focused on structural modifications of phlorizin (**1**, Fig. 4.8) [30,31], aiming to enhance the selective inhibition of SGLT2 over SGLT1 and improve its metabolic stability in vivo. Phlorizin is a glucoside of dihydrochalcone and is found in various fruits. As early as 1835, French scientists isolated phlorizin from apple bark and discovered its antipyretic effect, leading to its use in the treatment of malaria. In 1886, von Mering

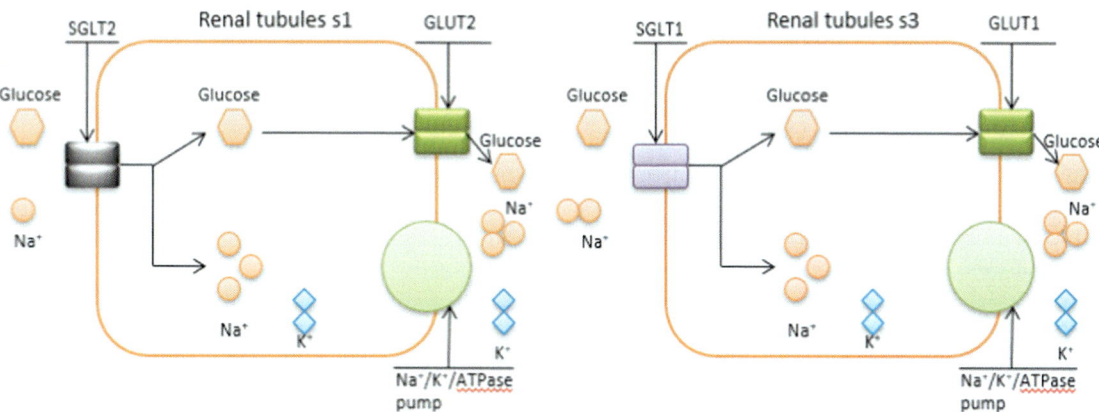

FIGURE 4.7 The molecular mechanisms underlying the glucose absorption by sodium-glucose co-transporter 1 (SGLT1) and sodium-glucose co-transporter 2 (SGLT2).

1

2 : T-1095A (R = H)
3 : T-1095 (R = COOMe)

4 : Sergliflozin (R = H)
5 :Sergliflozin-A (R = COOEt)

Sergliflozin

Pseudo-serglifozin **6**

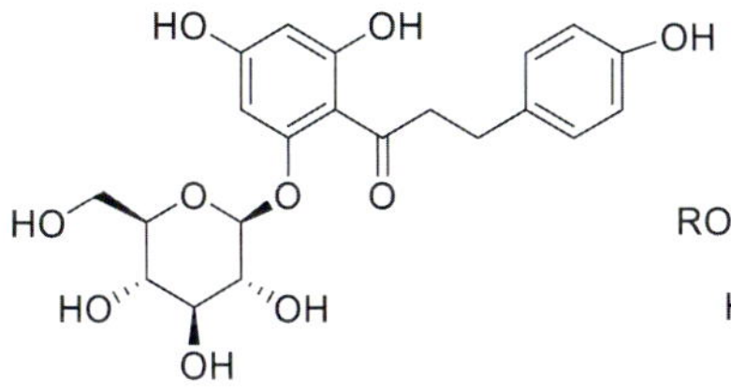

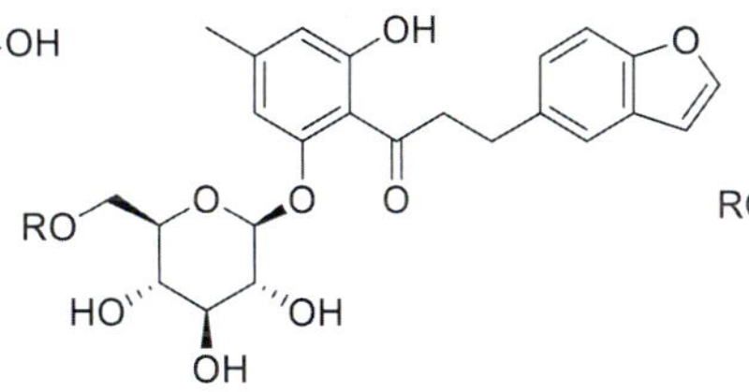

FIGURE 4.8 Phlorizin and its structural modifications.

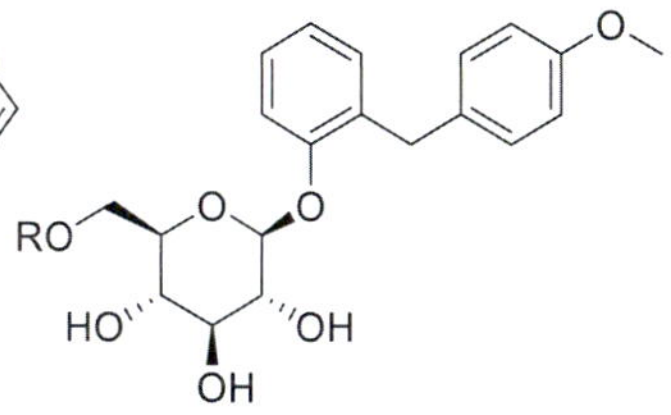

observed in animal experiments that doses greater than 1 g of phlorizin could induce glucose in urine, making it a valuable tool for creating diabetes models and studying renal function. Furthermore, it was found that long-term administration of phlorizin to dogs not only caused glucose in urine but also induced polyuria and weight loss. Since 1950, researchers began to investigate the mechanism underlying phlorizin-induced glucose in urine at the cellular and molecular levels and eventually revealed that phlorizin is able to inhibit sodium-dependent glucose transporter proteins (sodium-dependent glucose transporters, SGLTs) on the cell surface, including inhibition of SGLT2 and SGLT1, but without selectivity. The subsequent animal experiments demonstrated that administration of phlorizin can lead to severe adverse reactions and the even death of experimental animals. Further investigations revealed that the cause of these adverse reactions is the non-selective inhibition of SGLT1 by phlorizin. In 1987, for the first time, Rossetti et al. confirmed that phlorizin could alleviate glucose toxicity and aid in the restoration of insulin sensitivity by reducing blood glucose levels. However, the non-selective inhibitory effects of phlorizin on both SGLT2 and SGLT1, as well as its susceptibility to degradation by ß-glucosidase in the intestine, resulting in reduced bioavailability, make it a failure to be applied in clinical practice. As a result, chemists from major pharmaceutical companies and drug research institutions initiated the structural modifications of phlorizin to accomplish the following objectives: (1) enhancing the compound specificity for SGLT2 inhibition; (2) improving compound stability resistant to degradation by glucosidase to ensure their in vivo activity; (3) meeting the requirements for oral administration.

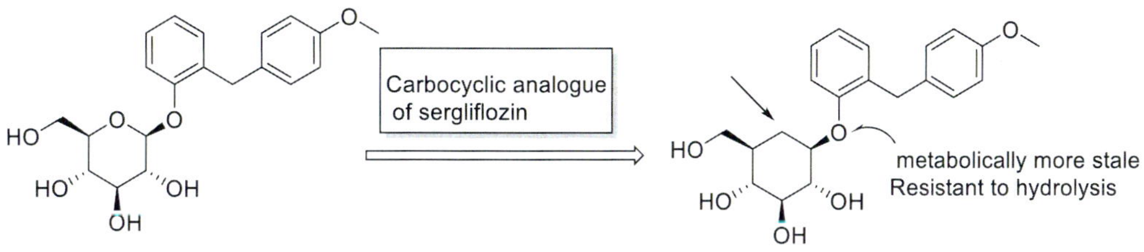

Between 1997 and 2004, researchers at Johnson Pharmaceuticals made structural modifications to phlorizin, specifically focusing on the aromatic ring portion farthest from the sugar moiety and the linker between the two aromatic rings. This led to the discovery of a phlorizin analog **2** (T-1095A, Fig. 4.8). In T-1095A, the *para*-hydroxyphenyl group of phlorizin was replaced by a benzofuran moiety, and one hydroxyl group on the benzene ring linking to the sugar moiety was substituted with a methyl group. Further introduction of an ester group at the 6-position of the sugar moiety in T-1095A yielded the prodrug **T-1095** (Compound **3**). Studies using various models, such as n-STZ rats, Goto-Kakizaki rats, ZDF rats, KKAy mice, and db/db mice, demonstrated that T-1095 effectively lowered blood glucose levels without causing hypoglycemic side effects. It reduced insulin resistance in peripheral tissues, including the liver and skeletal muscles, thereby preventing the decline of pancreatic β-cells. Additionally, its improved insulin secretion and sensitivity by alleviating glucotoxicity, showing potential for alleviating diabetic complications. T-1095 advanced to phase II clinical trials and became one of the most promising molecules among *O*-glycoside SGLT2 inhibitors, in addition to phlorizin [32–39]. Unfortunately, the *O*-glycosidic bond in T-1095 remained intolerant to β-glucosidase, preventing its development into a drug. However, these research findings laid a solid foundation for the subsequent development of novel, metabolically more stable drugs.

During the same period, Kissei Pharmaceutical Co. Ltd. in Japan discovered a selective SGLT2 inhibitor called sergliflozin (**4**) and converted it to a prodrug, sergliflozin-A, in the form of ethyl carbonate (**5**) for in vivo activity studies [40,41]. Additionally, Shing et al. synthesized a sergliflozin analog (**6**), but the specific activity results have not been disclosed or published [42].

Medicinal chemists from Bristol-Myers Squibb Pharmaceuticals have also conducted extensive and in-depth research on SGLT2 inhibitors. Initially, they focused on synthesizing SGLT2 inhibitors based on *O*-glucoside derivatives of glucose (depicted in Fig. 4.9), including *O*-arylglucosides (**7**) [43], *O*-benzamide glucosides (**8**) [44], and *O*-pyrazole glucosides (**9**) [45], etc., from which remogliflozin (compound **10**, Fig. 4.9) was discovered. Remogliflozin is a highly selective inhibitor of SGLT2 with a completely new structure (the benzene ring attached to the glucose in phlorizin is replaced by a pyrazole ring, and the benzene ring should be considered as the supporting structure of this type of inhibitor). In vitro studies demonstrated that remogliflozin exhibited inhibition of human SGLT2 and SGLT1 with EC_{50} values of 12.4 and 4520 nM, respectively. In 2013, its prodrug (remogliflozin etabonate, **11**) was approved for clinical trial [46]. Additionally, research indicated that WAY123783 (**12**) possessed activity in increasing glucosuria and

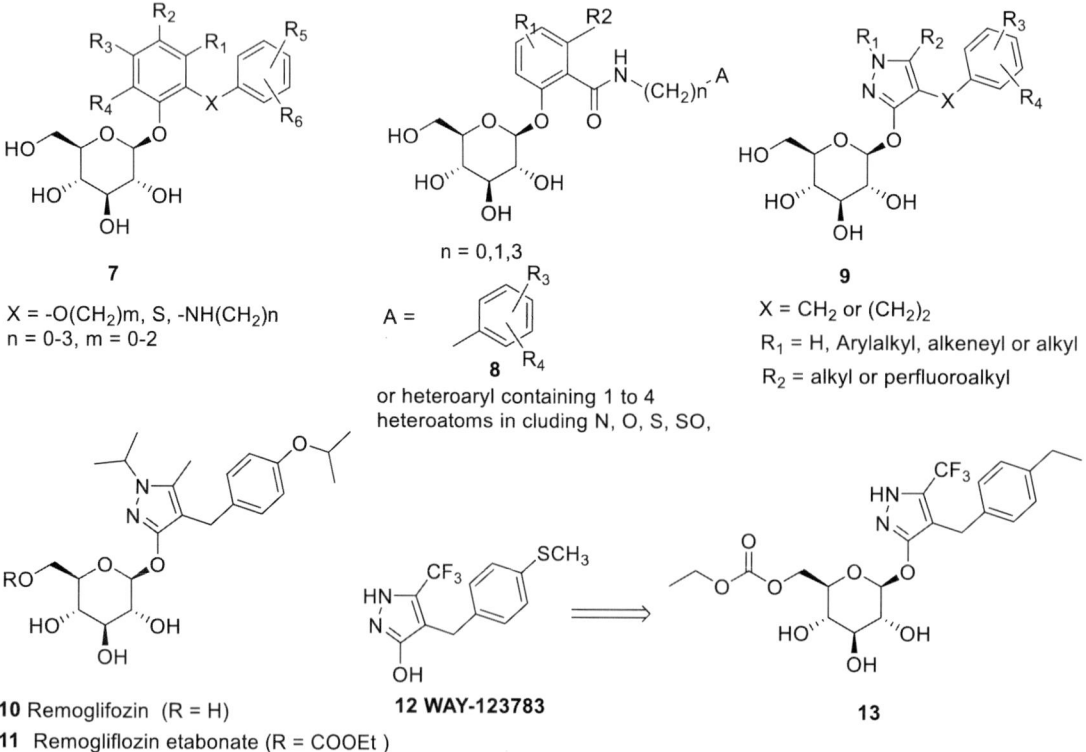

FIGURE 4.9 SGLT2 inhibitors of *O*-glucosides.

reducing blood glucose levels, suggesting its potential as an SGLT2 inhibitor. Based upon this finding, researchers, including Koji Ohsumi at Ajinomoto Co., Inc., synthesized pyrazole glucoside **13** (depicted in Fig. 4.9). This compound exhibited an 84% inhibition rate of rat renal SGLT2 at a concentration of 10 μM, whereas T-1095 demonstrated a 90% inhibition rate at the same concentration. Compound **13** also induced glucosuria, resulting in the excretion of 63 g of urinary glucose at a dosage of 3 mg/kg, whereas T-1095 produced 300 g of urinary glucose at the same dosage [47].

Although the previous efforts on modifications of phlorizin yielded some promising *O*-glucoside derivatives for glucose-lowering purposes, they all shared a common drawback. Namely, they were susceptible to degradation by glucosidases in vivo or hydrolysis under acidic conditions, leading to the loss of their glucose moiety and consequently losing their glucose-lowering activity. Nonetheless, these studies provided valuable insights into the structure-activity relationships; they have been summarized as follows: (1) The sugar moiety is essential for glucose-lowering activity, as compounds lacking the glycosyl portion exhibit significantly reduced or abolished SGLT2 inhibitory activity; (2) The aromatic group adjacent to the glycosyl moiety plays a crucial role in SGLT2 inhibition.

C-Glycosides are an important class of glycosides, characterized by the attachment of the sugar moiety to the aglycone portion through a carbon-carbon bond at the 1-position (anomeric site) (Fig. 4.10). These compounds also exist in the structures of many biologically active natural products, characterized by their resistance to glycosidases and their stability to be degraded by these enzymes. Moreover, from a medicinal chemistry perspective, the anomeric carbon serves as a bioisosterism of oxygen atoms, making *C*-glycosides potential analogs of *O*-glycosides and capable of exerting biological effects. Based on the aforementioned information and according to the principles of bioisosterism, researchers from Bristol-Myers Squibb Pharmaceuticals synthesized the aryl-*C*-glucoside **14** for the first time (Fig. 4.11), a derivative of phlorizin, with an EC_{50} value of 1.3 μM.

This *C*-glycoside compound exhibited very high stability against β-glucosidase. Choosing compound **14** as a template and based on the structure-activity relationships of the *O*-glucoside inhibitors mentioned above, the researchers performed systematic structural modifications and optimization of the aglycone while retaining the glucose moiety, resulting in a series of derivatives (**15**, Fig. 4.11). Continuing on further diversification and substitution at the 4-position and 4'-position of the two benzene rings, namely the R and X groups, researchers finally discovered that *C*-glucoside **16** (Fig. 4.12), bearing an *ortho*-substituted arylmethyl aglycone, is a superior skeletal structure for SGLT2 inhibition [48]. Further diversification and modification of the R and X groups led to the identification of the marketed drug compound **17** (dapagliflozin) [49].

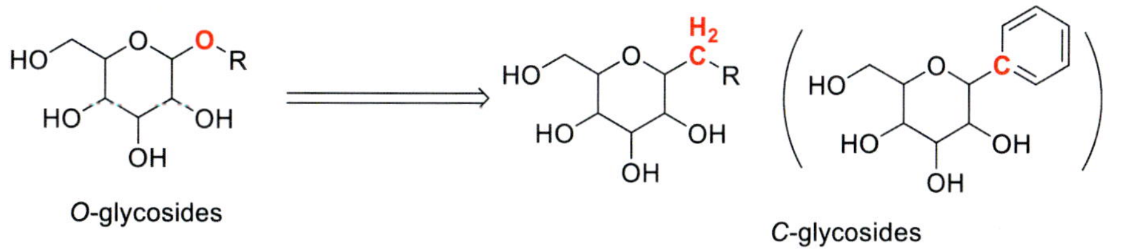

FIGURE 4.10 Structural features of *O*-glycosides and *C*-glycosides.

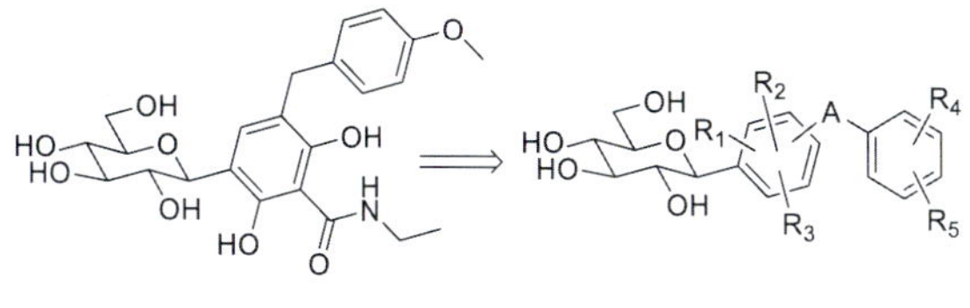

FIGURE 4.11 *C*-Glucosides exhibiting SGLT2 inhibitory activity.

R_1 and R_2, R_3 and R_2, R_4 and R_5 are connected to each other by a five-, six-, or seven-membered carbon ring or heterocycle.

R_4 and R_5 can be H, OH, OAryl, OCH_2Aryl, CF_3, $-OCHF_2$, $-OCF_3$, halogen, -CN, $-CO_2R$, -COR, CH(OH)R, -CH(OR)R, -CONRR, -NHCOR, $-NHSO_2R$, $-NHSO_2Aryl$, -SR, SOR, or SO_2R; or R_3 and R_4 can be connected to each other by a five-, six-, or seven-membered carbon ring or heterocycle.

A can be S, NH, O, CH_2, CH_2CH_2, or $CH_2CH_2CH_2$.

The aforementioned R groups represent short alkyl chains.

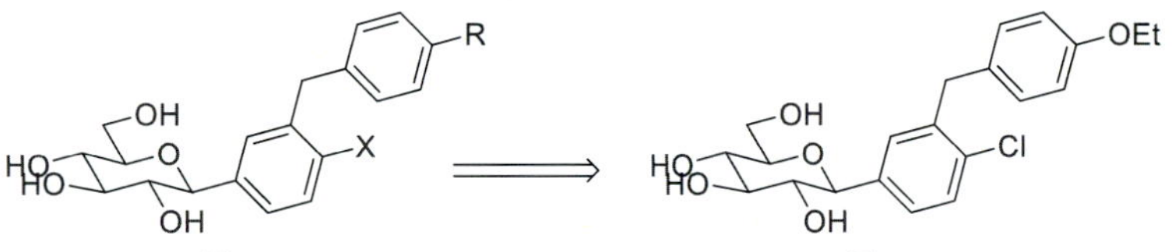

FIGURE 4.12 Discovery of compound 17 (dapagliflozin).

TABLE 4.2 The inhibitory activity of compounds 2, 4, 14, and 17 on hSGLT2 and hSGLT1.

No.	hSGLT2 EC$_{50}$ (nM)	hSGLT1 EC$_{50}$ (nM)	Selectivity vs hSGLT1 (fold)
2	6.6 ± 0.7 (n = 3)	211 ± 29 (n = 3)	30
4	9.2 ± 0.8 (n = 3)	>8000 (n = 2)	>90
14	1300 ± 600 (n = 3)	>8000 (n = 2)	>10
17	1.1 ± 0.06 (n = 18)	1390 (n = 16)	1200

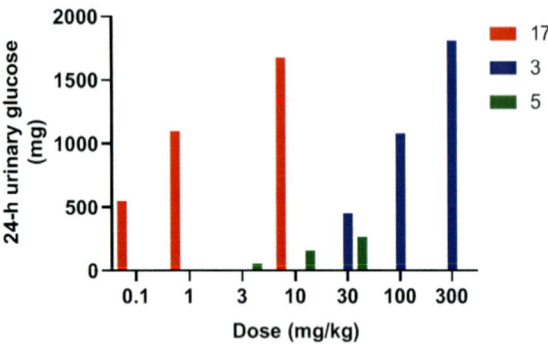

FIGURE 4.13 Dose-dependent glycosuria changes in normal mice after oral administration of compound 17 at 24 h.

Compound **17** exhibited remarkable potency and excellent selectivity as an SGLT2 inhibitor. Compared with compounds **2**, **4**, and **14**, it showed significant improvements in both SGLT2 inhibitory activity and selectivity (Table 4.2). In vitro, studies revealed that compound **17** displays EC$_{50}$ values of 3.0 nM and 1.1 nM for inhibiting rat-derived rSGLT2 and human-derived hSGLT2, respectively. Moreover, it exhibited EC$_{50}$ values of 1.4 and 1.39 μM for inhibiting rat-derived rSGLT1 and human-derived hSGLT1, respectively. Oral administration of compound **17** to normal Sprague-Dawley rats resulted in a statistically significant dose-dependent glucosuria within 24 hours. Compared to the solvent control group, mice treated with the compound **17** showed an increase in glucose excretion ranging from 1000 to 10000-fold (Fig. 4.13). In rats, a single oral dose of 0.1, 1.0, and 10 mg/kg leads to the excretion of 550, 1100, and 1900 mg of glucose within 24 hours. These findings collectively emphasize the crucial role of C-glucosidic stability in facilitating glucose excretion by compound **17**.

Compound **17**, also known as dapagliflozin, possesses a C-glucoside chemical structure that is resistant to hydrolysis by ß-glucosidases in the small intestine. This characteristic ensures its stability upon oral administration and contributes to favorable pharmacokinetic properties, including a relatively long half-life and duration of action. Peak plasma concentrations of compound **17** are reached approximately 2 hours after oral administration following fasting, with an average half-life ranging from 11.2 to 16.6 hours. In general, a once-daily dosage is sufficient. Within the therapeutic dose range, both the maximum plasma concentration (C_{max}) and the area under the concentration-time curve (AUC) increase proportionally with the dose. The oral administration of 10 mg of dapagliflozin results in a bioavailability of 78%. When compared to fasting conditions, a high-fat diet decreases C_{max} by 50% and prolongs T_{max} by approximately 1 hour, with no effect on AUC. The plasma protein binding rate of dapagliflozin is 91%, remaining unchanged in patients with liver or kidney impairment. The primary metabolic pathway for dapagliflozin involves UGT1AG, with minimal involvement of CYP-mediated metabolism in the human body. Metabolism studies using [^{14}C]-labeled dapagliflozin reveal that it is primarily metabolized into inactive 3-O-glucuronide metabolites. Both dapagliflozin and its metabolites are predominantly eliminated via renal excretion.

In vitro studies demonstrated that compound **17** does not inhibit CYP1A2, 2C9, 2C19, 2D6, or 3A4, and it has a weak interaction with P-glycoprotein (P-gp). However, its metabolite, 3-O-glucuronide, acts as a substrate for OAT3 (organic anion transporter 3). Neither compound **17** nor its 3-*O*-glucuronide metabolite affect the pharmacokinetic properties of P-gp, OCT2 (organic cation transporter 2), OAT1 (organic anion transporter 1), or OAT3 substrates. When co-administered with metformin, pioglitazone, sitagliptin, glimepiride, voglibose, hydrochlorothiazide, bumetanide, simvastatin, rifampicin, sodium phenylbutyrate, warfarin, and digoxin, dapagliflozin does not exhibit any significant changes in C_{max} or AUC. Therefore, no dose adjustment is required when dapagliflozin is co-administered with these drugs.

Clinical trials have demonstrated that dapagliflozin, when used alone or in combination with other drugs such as metformin and sulfonylureas, can significantly reduce blood glucose levels and HbA1c levels while also promoting weight loss. Furthermore, it does not display adverse effects such as hypoglycemia. Based on its favorable activity, selectivity, and pharmacokinetic data, compound **17** was named as dapagliflozin [50] and became the first SGLT2 inhibitor approved for the treatment of type 2 diabetes. It was approved for marketing in China in May 2017. The discovery of dapagliflozin laid the foundation for the development of other aryl-*C*-glucoside SGLT2 inhibitors and has become an important therapeutic option in the treatment of diabetes. Dapagliflozin exhibits efficacy similar to that of other novel anti-diabetic agents, such as dipeptidyl peptidase-4 inhibitors, and it also has a mild blood pressure-lowering and weight-reducing effect. Pharmacokinetic studies conducted in healthy subjects have shown the rapid absorption of dapagliflozin after oral administration, with a T_{max} of 1–2 hours. The plasma protein binding rate is 91%, and the oral bioavailability is approximately 78%. The terminal half-life in plasma is 12.9 hours. After oral administration, dapagliflozin is primarily metabolized in the liver through uridine diphosphate-glucuronosyltransferase 1A9 (UGT1A9) into inactive metabolites, with a minor fraction undergoing metabolism by P450 enzymes, which does not exhibit inhibitory or inducer effects on these enzymes.

4.2.3 Synthetic process of dapagliflozin

Dapagliflozin [51], developed by Bristol-Myers Squibb, received its first approval for market authorization from the European Commission on November 12, 2012, and was subsequently approved by the U.S. FDA in 2014 under the trade name Farxiga.

The chemical systematic name for dapagliflozin is (2*S*,3*R*,4*R*,5*S*,6*R*)-2-[4-chloro-3-(4-ethoxy-benzyl) phenyl]-6-hydroxymethyl-tetrahydron-2*H*-pyran-3,4,5-triol. Its molecular formula is $C_{21}H_{25}ClO_6$, molecular weight is 408.13, and CAS number is 461432-26-8.

Several patents and papers describe the synthesis of dapagliflozin, and its major synthetic routes can be summarized as follows: [52–54] The glycosyl moiety is derived from D-glucuronic acid-δ-lactone (**22**), which is protected by trimethylchlorosilane to furnish 2,3,4,6-tetra-*O*-trimethylsilyl-D-glucuronic acid-δ-lactone (**23**). The aglycone moiety is derived from 5-bromo-2-chlorobenzoic acid (**18**), which is first converted to the benzoyl chloride derivative **19** using oxalyl chloride, and then it is subjected to the Friedel-Crafts acylation reaction with ethoxybenzene in the presence of aluminum chloride. The *ortho* or *para* selectivity is 1:7, and the desired product, the *para*-substituted diphenyl ketone derivative **20**, is obtained in 65% yield through recrystallization with ethanol. The ethoxy diphenylmethane **21** is then obtained by reducing the ketone carbonyl group with boron trifluoride etherate and triethylsilane. Intermediate **21** is treated with *n*-butyllithium or *sec*-butyllithium as base at −78°C to prepare lithium reagent **A**, which undergoes addition with 2,3,4,6-tetra-*O*-trimethylsilyl-D-glucuronic lactone at −70°C to afford the intermediate, which is directly treated with methane sulfonic acid/methanol, providing the key intermediate **24**. Reduction of **24** with triethyl silane/boron trifluoride etherate yields a mixture of the desired product, furan ring isomers, and anomeric α-isomer. This mixture, after multiple co-crystallizations with various organic small molecules to remove impurities, yields the dapagliflozin co-crystal substance **17**. The commonly used co-crystalline small molecule compounds include proline and other organic small molecules such as 1,4-butyne diol [52] (Fig. 4.14).

The aforementioned drawbacks of the purification method for the target compound involve the necessity of multiple recrystallization steps, resulting in a significant loss of the desired product. To overcome this limitation, researchers from BMS and Princeton have made improvements to the synthetic process of dapagliflozin (Fig. 4.15). After demethoxylation of intermediate **24** using triethyl silane/boron trifluoride etherate, they directly conducted acetylation of hydroxyl groups in the obtained intermediate to afford the fully acetylated intermediate **25**, which is followed by recrystallization with ethanol, yielding product **26** with a high optical purity. Finally, complete deacetylation of compound **26** affords dapagliflozin **17** in a total yield of up to 40% [54].

Overall, the production route for dapagliflozin is commendable. However, certain steps still exhibit notable deficiencies. For instance, the intermediate 2,3,4,6-tetra-*O*-trimethylsilyl-D-glucopyranosiduronic lactone (**23**) assumes a syrupy consistency, which hampers its quality control and operational feasibility for industrial-scale production. Furthermore, the formation of furan rings and isomeric impurities during the anomeric etherification and removal

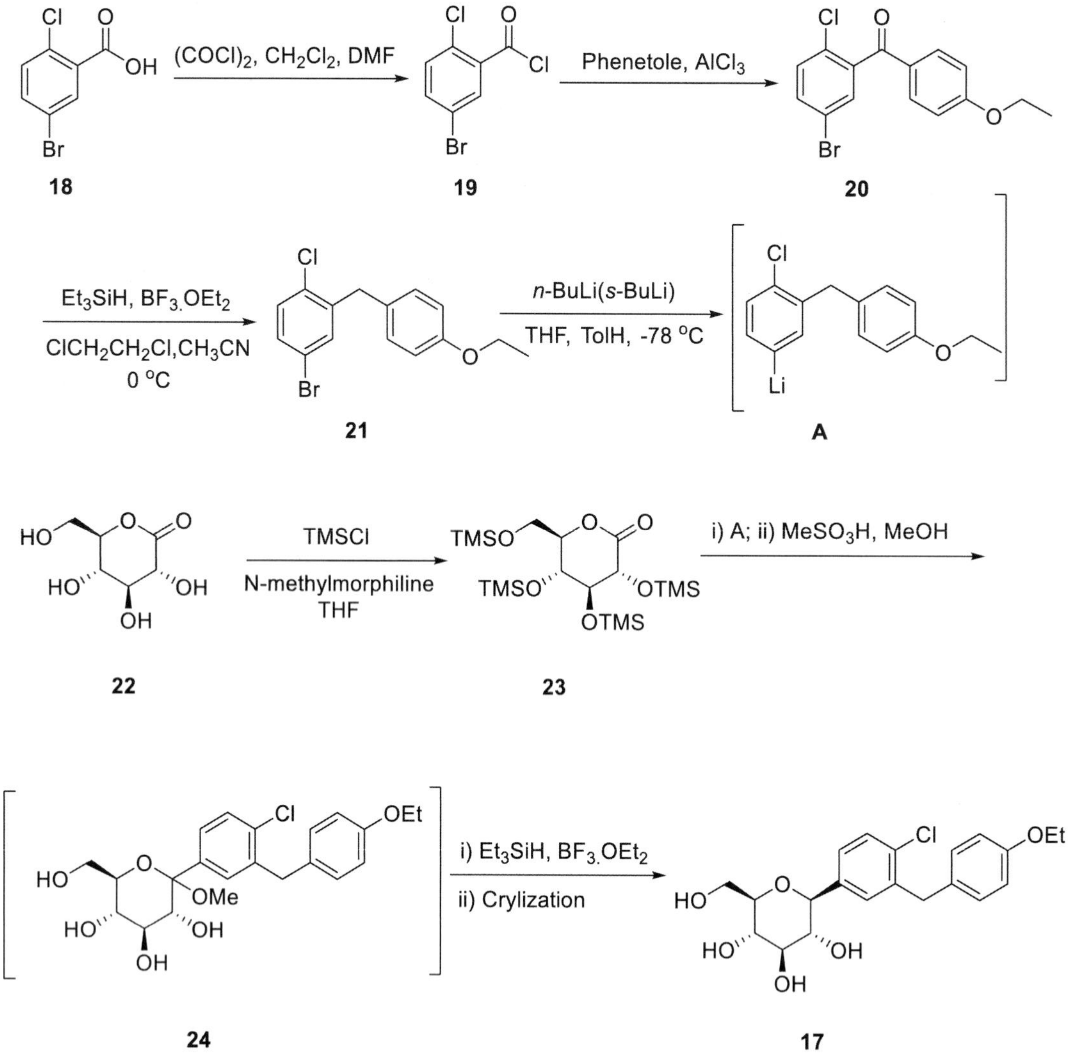

FIGURE 4.14 The initial synthetic route for dapagliflozin.

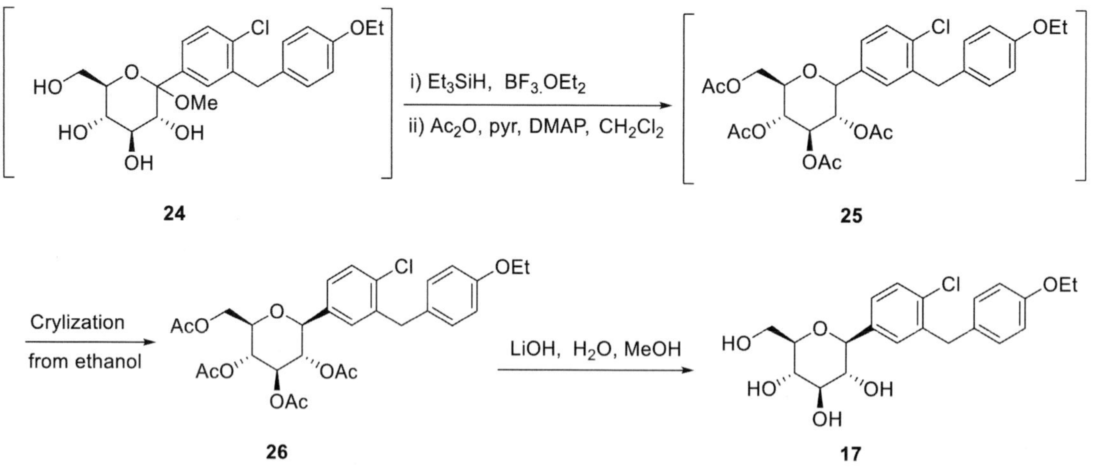

FIGURE 4.15 The optimized synthetic route for dapagliflozin.

of trimethylsilyl protecting groups need multiple recrystallizations in subsequent stages to effectively eliminate the impurities, thereby affecting the overall yield.

In addition to the aforementioned synthetic routes, several research institutions in our country have also explored the synthesis of dapagliflozin [55–61]. However, these improvements have not yet been applied to practical production. Upon reviewing multiple synthetic routes, it is apparent that the production process of dapagliflozin invariably involves the use of *n*-butyllithium, a hazardous and flammable chemical reagent. Furthermore, the synthetic conditions are stringent, making the operation cumbersome. To date, this issue has not been effectively resolved and requires further optimization.

4.2.4 Efficacy and action of dapagliflozin

Dapagliflozin exerts its hypoglycemic effects by inhibiting the renal reabsorption of glucose. Additionally, dapagliflozin has been found to have other effects: [62]

Weight reduction. Dapagliflozin increases urinary glucose excretion by 50–80 g/day, equivalent to an energy expenditure of 200–320 kcal/day. Continuous use for 3–6 months can lead to a weight reduction of approximately 1.5–3.5 kg.

Blood pressure reduction. Dapagliflozin decreases sodium absorption and promotes sodium ion excretion, resulting in a decrease in plasma volume. Data analysis has shown that SGLT inhibitors can lead to an average systolic blood pressure reduction of 3.77 mmHg.

Uric acid reduction. Research indicates that SGLT2 inhibitors can lower blood uric acid levels by accelerating its excretion in the urine. Whether used as monotherapy or in combination with other antidiabetic agents, dapagliflozin effectively reduces blood uric acid levels.

Renal protection. One of the mechanisms through which dapagliflozin protects the kidneys is by reducing intraglomerular pressure, resulting in a restoration of glomerular filtration rate (GFR) and a decrease in proteinuria. The increased levels of sodium ions and glucose in the tubular fluid, due to their passage through the juxtaglomerular apparatus (JGA), lead to tubuloglomerular feedback, causing afferent arteriolar vasoconstriction and a subsequent reduction in renal pressure.

Cardiovascular benefits. Dapagliflozin exhibits cardiovascular-protective effects. For patients with type 2 diabetes and concomitant cardiovascular disease, SGLT2 inhibitors, including dapagliflozin, can reduce the risks of cardiovascular and all-cause mortality (referring to the combined mortality from cardiovascular disease-related factors, such as stroke, coronary heart disease, or death resulting from other cardiovascular complications), as well as the risk of heart failure hospitalization. Therefore, SGLT2 inhibitors can be considered as a first-line treatment option for patients with cardiovascular comorbidities and type 2 diabetes.

Dapagliflozin is associated with adverse reactions, including diabetic ketoacidosis, acute kidney injury and renal impairment, urosepsis and pyelonephritis, hypoglycemia when used in combination with insulin or insulin secretagogues, genital fungal infections, and elevated low-density lipoprotein cholesterol (LDL-C) levels.

4.2.5 Other drugs based on SGLT2 inhibitors

In addition to dapagliflozin, seven antidiabetic drugs based on SGLT2 inhibitors have been approved globally (Table 4.3). These medications are all *C*-aryl-glycosides, characterized by the sugar moiety linked to the aryl group B, which is connected to the aryl ring C through a methylene bridge. The distinguishing feature among them lies in the variations of the substituents on the two aryl rings [63,64].

Therefore, there are currently a total of eight SGLT2 inhibitors approved worldwide. Among them, canagliflozin (Johnson & Johnson), dapagliflozin (AstraZeneca), empagliflozin (Boehringer Ingelheim/Eli Lilly), and ertugliflozin (Merck) have been approved and launched in China, with the first three also included in the 2019 National Medical Insurance Category B List through negotiations.

4.3 Successful experience in the development of dapagliflozin

As a novel therapeutic target for type 2 diabetes, SGLT2 inhibitors have gained increasing market share in oral antidiabetic medications due to their unique mechanism of action. These medications offer several advantages over other oral hypoglycemic agents, including a reduced risk of hypoglycemia, renal protection, moderate weight loss potential, and improved pancreatic β-cell function.

TABLE 4.3 Other drugs based on SGLT2 inhibitors.

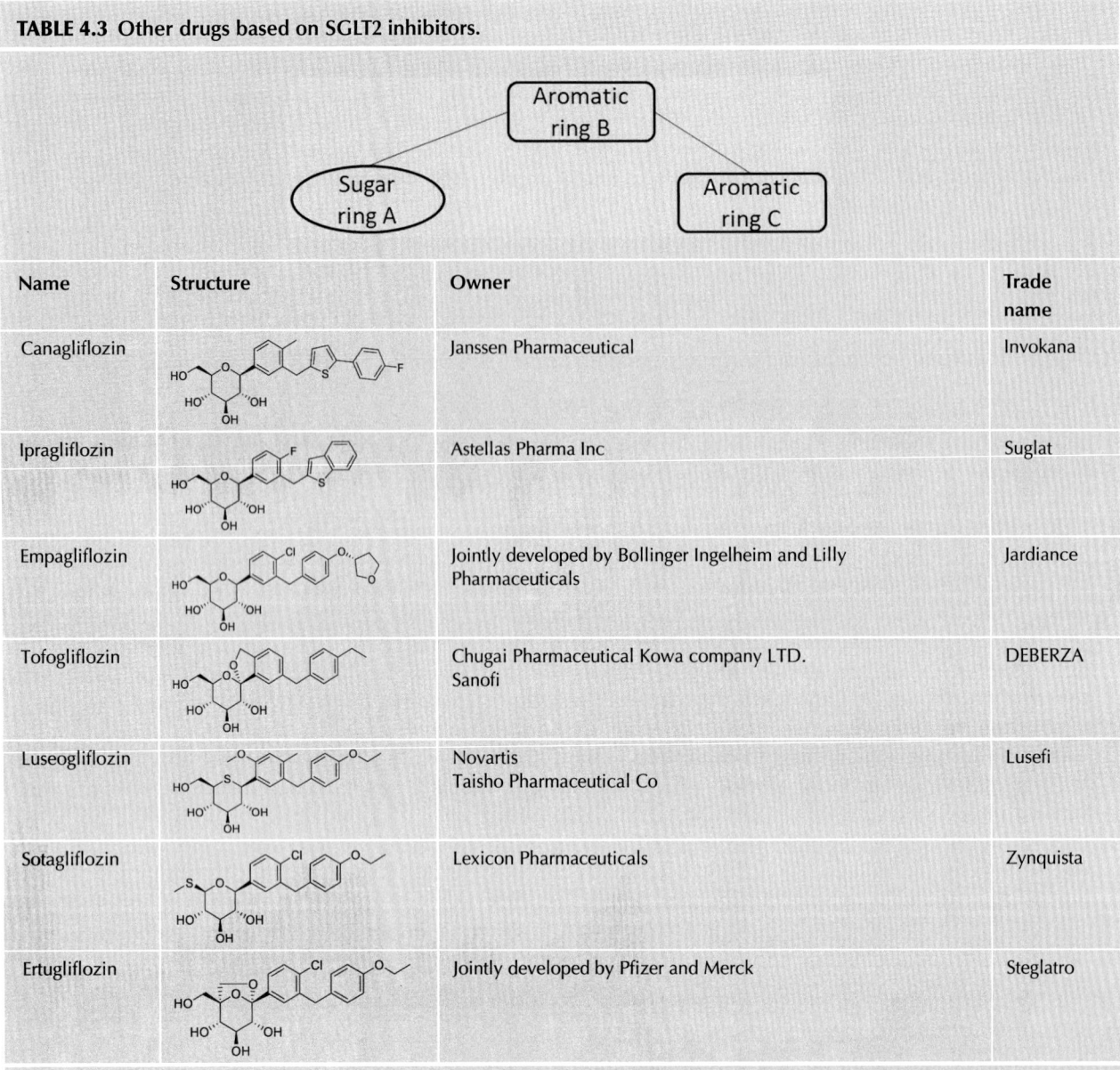

Name	Structure	Owner	Trade name
Canagliflozin		Janssen Pharmaceutical	Invokana
Ipragliflozin		Astellas Pharma Inc	Suglat
Empagliflozin		Jointly developed by Bollinger Ingelheim and Lilly Pharmaceuticals	Jardiance
Tofogliflozin		Chugai Pharmaceutical Kowa company LTD. Sanofi	DEBERZA
Luseogliflozin		Novartis Taisho Pharmaceutical Co	Lusefi
Sotagliflozin		Lexicon Pharmaceuticals	Zynquista
Ertugliflozin		Jointly developed by Pfizer and Merck	Steglatro

The development process of dapagliflozin (Fig. 4.16) serves as a typical case study that demonstrates the transition from chemical biology to medicinal chemistry, specifically the transformation from "a chemical small-molecule probe" to a drug entity. As early as the 19th century, the diuretic effect of phlorizin, a naturally occurring chemical compound, was discovered. Further research on the mechanisms underlying the diuretic effect of phlorizin revealed that its promotion of glucose excretion was attributed to the inhibition of the sodium-glucose co transporter (SGLT1/2) on the surface of the proximal tubule cells. This mechanism prevents the reabsorption of excess glucose into the bloodstream, leading to improved blood glucose levels without increasing insulin secretion. Consequently, SGLT2 was validated as a potential novel target for antidiabetic drug development.

Subsequent pivotal modifications and structural transformations of phlorizin, along with the accumulation of structure-activity relationship (SAR) information, enabled medicinal chemists to design and synthesize structurally diverse O-aryl-glycosides. These efforts resulted in the discovery of new, promising compounds. However, the selective inhibition of SGLT2 without affecting SGLT1 and the enzymatic instability of the O-glucosides posed significant challenges in developing an oral drug (considered the optimal route for chronic diseases). To overcome these obstacles, medicinal chemists adopted the C-aryl-glycoside derivation strategy and developed efficient synthetic chemistry for the

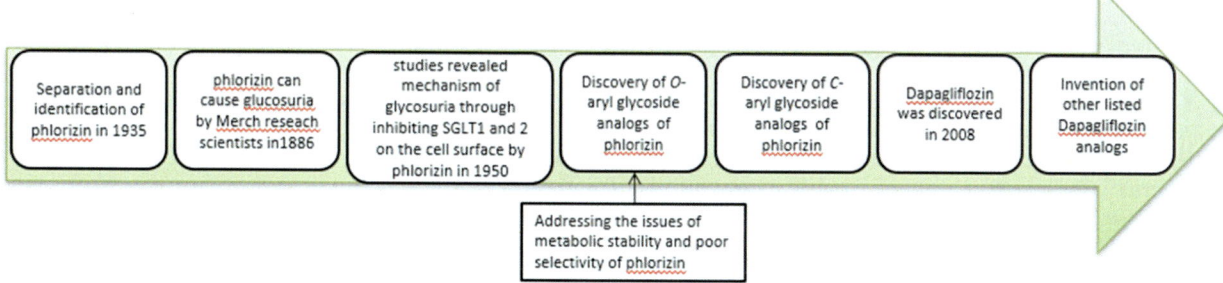

FIGURE 4.16 The development process of dapagliflozin.

construction of relevant *C*-aryl-glycosides. Eventually, dapagliflozin was successfully developed, exhibiting both high selectivity for SGLT2 and favorable stability against glucosidases. This achievement laid the foundation for the subsequent development of a new class of anti-diabetic drugs with similar mechanisms of action. The journey from isolating phlorizin from tree bark to the successful development of dapagliflozin is a lengthy process, representing a deepening understanding of the phenomenon from surface to core and serving as a classical case study in chemical biology and medicinal chemistry textbooks.

References

[1] Zimmet P, Alberti K, Shaw J. Global and societal implications of the diabetes epidemic. Nature 2001;414:782−7.
[2] Eckel RH, Grundy SM, Zimmet PZ. The metabolic syndrome. Lancet 2005;365:1415−28.
[3] https://www.idf.org/aboutdiabetes/what-is-diabetes.html.
[4] Zimmet PZ, Magliano DJ, Herman WH, et al. Diabetes: a 21st century challenge. Lancet Diabetes Endocrinol 2014;2(1):56−64.
[5] Moliinaro R, Dauscher C. Complications resulting from uncontrolled diabetes. MLO Med Lab Obs 2017;49(2):20−2.
[6] Gebel E. An overview of what diabetes can do to your body (and what you can do to prevent it). Diabetes Forecast 2008;61(12):45−6.
[7] Cole JB, Florez JC. Genetics of diabetes mellitus and diabetes complications. Nat Rev Nephrol 2020;16(7):377−90.
[8] Stumvoll M, Goldstein BJ, Van Haeften TW. Type 2 diabetes: principles of pathogenesis and therapy. Lancet 2005;365:1333−46.
[9] Lebovitz HE. Etiology and pathogenesis of diabetes mellitus. Pediatr Clin North Am 1984;31(3):521−30.
[10] Long R, Yang Y. Research progress on pathogenesis, prevention and treatment of adult onset diabetes in adolescents. Word Last Med Inf 2019;19(99):43−4.
[11] Krentz AJ, Bailey CJ. Oral antidiabetic agents: current role in type 2 diabetes mellitus. Drugs 2005;65:385−411.
[12] Moller DE. New drug targets for type 2 diabetes and the metabolic syndrome. Nature 2001;414:821−7.
[13] Nourparvar A, Bulotta A, Di Mario U, Perfetti R. Novel strategies for the pharmacological management of type 2 diabetes. Trends Pharmacol Sci 2004;25(2):86−91.
[14] Tian Q, Hong T-P. Role of non-sulfonylurea insulin secretagogues in blood glucose management in patients with type 2 diabetes. Chin J Diabet 2016;24(16):245−6.
[15] Kaku K. Efficacy of voglibose in type 2 diabetes. Expert Opin Pharmacother 2014;15(8):1181−90.
[16] Sugimoto S, Nakajima H, Kosaka K, Hosoi H. Review: miglitol has potential as a therapeutic drug against obesity. Nutr Metab (Lond) 2015;12:51−7.
[17] Deacon CF. Dipeptidyl peptidase-4 inhibitors in the treatment of type 2 diabetes: a comparative review. Diabetes ObesMetab 2011;13:7−18.
[18] Gallwitz B. Small molecule dipeptidylpeptidase IV inhibitors under investigation for diabetes mellitus therapy. Exp Opin Invest Drugs 2011;20:723−32.
[19] Weber AE. Dipeptidyl peptidase IV inhibitors for the treatment of diabetes. J Med Chem 2004;47:4135−41.
[20] Gai K-K, Duan R, Li Z-X. Clinical research progress of dipeptidyl peptidase-4 inhibitors. Chin Hos Pharm J 2016;36(17):1529−34.
[21] Bailey CJ. Renal glucose reabsorption inhibitors to treat diabetes. Trends Pharmacol Sci 2011;32(2):63−71.
[22] Abdul-Ghani MA, Norton L, Defronzo RA. Role of sodium-glucose cotransporter 2 (SGLT 2) inhibitors in the treatment of type 2 diabetes. Endocr Rev 2011;32(4):515−31.
[23] Wright EM, Loo DD, Hirayama BA. Biology of human sodium glucose transporters. Physiol Rev 2011;91(2):733−94.
[24] Hirayama BA, Loo DD, Diez-Sampedro A, et al. Sodium-dependent reorganization of the sugar-binding site of SGLT1. Biochemistry 2007;46(46):13391−406.
[25] Scheepers A, Joost HG, Schurmann A. The glucose transporter families SGLT and GLUT: molecular basis of normal and aberrant function. JPEN J Parenter Enter Nutr 2004;28(5):364−71.
[26] Chen LH, Leung PS. Inhibition of the sodium glucose co-transporter-2: its beneficial action and potential combination therapy for type 2 diabetes mellitus. Diabetes ObesMetab 2013;15(5):392−402.

[27] Loo DD, Jiang X, Gorraitz E, et al. Functional identification and characterization of sodium binding sites in Na symporters. Proc Natl Acad Sci USA 2013;110(47):E4557−66.
[28] Ferrannini E, Solini A. SGLT2 inhibition in diabetes mellitus: rationale and clinical prospects. Nat Rev Endocrinol 2012;8(8):495−502.
[29] Chao EC, Henry RR. SGLT2 inhibition−a novel strategy for diabetes treatment. Nat Rev Drug Discov 2010;9(7):551−9.
[30] Rossetti L, Smith D, Shulman GI, Papachristou D, Defronzo RA. Correction of hyperglycemia with phlorizin normalizes tissue sensitivity to insulin in diabetic rats. J Clin Invest 1987;79(5):1510−15.
[31] Ehrenkranz JR, Lewis NG, Kahn CR, Roth J. Phlorizin: a review. Diabetes Metab Res Rev 2005;21(1):31−8.
[32] Arakawa K, Ishihara T, Oku A, et al. Improved diabetic syndrome in C57BL/KsJ-db/db mice by oral administration of the Na(+)-glucose cotransporter inhibitor T-1095. Br J Pharmacol 2001;132(2):578−86.
[33] Oku A, Ueta K, Arakawa K, et al. Antihyperglycemic effect of T-1095 via inhibition of renal Na^+-glucose cotransporters in streptozotocin-induced diabetic rats. Biol Pharm Bull 2000;23:1434−7.
[34] Saito A, Seiyaku T, Tsujihara K. SGLT inhibitor (T-1095). Nihon Rinsho 2002;60(Suppl 9):588−93.
[35] Adachi T, Yasuda K, Okamoto Y, Shihara N, et al. T-1095, a renal Na^+-glucose transporter inhibitor, improves hyperglycemia in streptozotocin-induced diabetic rats. Metabolism 2000;49:990−5.
[36] Tsujihara K, Hongu M, Saito K, et al. Na(+)-glucose cotransporter(SGLT) inhibitors as antidiabetic agents. Synthesis and pharmacological properties of 4′-dehydroxyphlorizin derivatives substituted on the B ring. J Med Chem 1999;42:5311−24.
[37] Oku A, Ueta K, Nawano M, et al. Antidiabetic effect of T-1095, an inhibitor of Na(+)-glucose cotransporter, in neonatally streptozotocin-treated rats. Eur J Pharmacol 2000;391:183−92.
[38] Nawano M, Oku A, Ueta K, et al. Hyperglycemia contributes insulin resistance in hepatic and adipose tissue but not skeletal muscle of ZDF rats. Am J Physiol Endocrinol Metab 2000;278:535−43.
[39] Dudash Jr J, Zhang XY, Zeck RE, et al. Glycosylated dihydrochalcones as potent and selective sodium glucose co-transporter 2 (SGLT2) inhibitors. Bioorg Med Chem Lett 2004;14(20):5121−5.
[40] Katsuno K, Fujimori Y, Takemura Y, et al. Sergliflozin, a novel selective inhibitor of low-affinity sodium glucose cotransporter (SGLT2), validates the critical role of SGLT2 in renal glucose reabsorption and modulates plasma glucose level. J Pharmacol Exp Ther 2007;320(1):323−30.
[41] Fujimori Y, Katsuno K, Ojima K, et al. Sergliflozin etabonate, a selective SGLT2 inhibitor, improves glycemic control in streptozotocin-induced diabetic rats and Zucker fatty rats. Eur J Pharmacol 2009;609(1-3):148−54.
[42] Shing TKM, Ngw L, Chan JYW, et al. Design, syntheses, and SAR studies of carbocyclic analogues of sergliflozin as potent sodium-dependent glucose cotransporter 2 inhibitors. Angew Chem Int Ed 2013;52:8401−5.
[43] Washburn W.N., Sher P.M., Wu G. Preparation of O-aryl glucosides as antidiabetic agents and SGLT2 inhibitors. US Patent 6,683,056, 2004; Chem Abstr, 2001, 135, 273163.
[44] Washburn W.N. Preparation of *O*-glucoside benzamides as antidiabetic agents and SGLT2 inhibitors. US Patent 6,555,519, 2003; Chem Abstr 2001, 135, 273164.
[45] Washburn W.N., Preparation of O-pyrazole glucoside SGLT2 inhibitors as antidiabetic agents. PCT Int ApplWO2003020737, 2003; Chem Abstr 2003, 138, 221784.
[46] Mikail N. Remogliflozin etabonate: a novel SGLT2 inhibitor for treatment of diabetes mellitus. Expert Opin Investig Drugs 2015;24(10):1381−7.
[47] Ohsumi K, Matsueda H, Hatanaka T, et al. Pyrazole-*O*-glucosides as novel Na(+)-glucose cotransporter (SGLT) inhibitors. Bioorg Med Chem Lett 2003;13(14):2269−72.
[48] Meng W, Ellsworth BA, Nirschl AA, et al. Discovery of dapagliflozin: a potent, selective renal sodium-dependent glucose cotransporter 2 (SGLT2) inhibitor for the treatment of type 2 diabetes. J Med Chem 2008;51(5):1145−9.
[49] Ellsworth B., Washburn W.N., Sher P.M., et al. *C*-Aryl glycoside SGLT2 inhibitors and method, US 6515117 B2, 2003.
[50] Albarran OG, Ampudia-Blasco FJ. Dapagliflozina, el primer inhibidor SGLT2 eneltratamiento de la diabetes tipo 2(Dapagliflozin, the first SGLT-2 inhibitor in the treatment of type 2 diabetes). Med Clin (Barc) 2013;141(Suppl 2):36−43.
[51] Dhillon S. Dapagliflozin: a review in type 2 diabetes. Drugs 2019;79:1135−46.
[52] Gougoutas J.Z., Lobinger H., Ramakrishnan S., et al. Crystal structures of SGLT2 inhibitors and processes for preparing same. US 7919598 B2, 2011.
[53] Desgbde P.P., Ellsworth B.A., Singh J., et al. Methods of producing C-aryl glucoside SGLT2 inhibitors. US 7932379 B2, 2011.
[54] Mundla M.V., Malyala S., Narani C.P., et al. Processes for the preparation of SGLT-2 inhibitors, Intermeidates thereof. US 10703772 B2, 2020.
[55] Luo H-R, Gu R-L, Tan C-R, et al. Synthesis of dapagliflozin. Spec Petrochem 2019;36(4):53−7.
[56] Huang K, Jiang H-L, Wu Y-L, et al. Synthesis of dapagliflozin. Chin J Pharm 2015;46(7):680−2.
[57] Zhang S-Y, Xu B, Wang D-C. Graphical synthetic routes of dapagliflozin. Chin J Pharm 2014;45(12):1192−5.
[58] Yu Y-K, Ji Y-F. Synthesis of dapagliflozin. Chin J Pharm 2011;42(02):84−7.
[59] Shao H, Zhao G-L, Liu W, et al. Total synthesis of SGLT2 Inhibitor dapagliflozin. Chin J Synth Chem 2010;18(3):389−92.
[60] Liu W-J, Chen L, Shi K, et al. Synthesis of dapaliflozin. Chem Res App 2016;28(4):530−3.
[61] Chen Y., Lv H.-H., Wang Y.-J. Preparation method of dapagliflozin CN105294624A, 2016.
[62] Rosentstock J, Voco M, Li W, et al. Effects of dapagliflozin, an SGLT2 inhibitor, on HbA1c, body weight, and hypoglycemia risk in patients with type 2 diabetes inadequately controlled on pioglitazone monotherapy. Diabetes Care 2012;35:1473−8.
[63] Vivian EM. Sodium-glucose co-transporter 2 (SGLT2) inhibitors: a growing class of antidiabetic agents. Drugs Context 2014;3:212−64.
[64] Washburn WN. Sodium glucose co-transporter 2 (SGLT2) inhibitors: novel antidiabetic agents. Exp Opin Ther Pat 2012;22:483−94.

Chapter 5

Cholesterol-lowering drug atorvastatin

Zhi-Shu Huang, Jia-Heng Tan and Shuo-Bin Chen

School of Pharmaceutical Sciences, Sun Yat-Sen University, Guangzhou, P.R. China

Chapter outline

- 5.1 Hypercholesterolemia and cardiovascular diseases 71
  - 5.1.1 Lipid metabolism 71
  - 5.1.2 Cholesterol metabolic regulation and hypercholesterolemia 72
- 5.2 Atorvastatin, the cholesterol-lowering drug 76
  - 5.2.1 Discovery of atorvastatin 76
  - 5.2.2 Mechanism of action, clinical indications, and safety of atorvastatin 80
- 5.3 Medicinal chemistry of atorvastatin 81
  - 5.3.1 Target of statin drugs—HMG-CoA reductase 81
  - 5.3.2 Structure-activity relationship of statin drugs inhibiting HMG-CoA reductase 82
  - 5.3.3 Interaction of statins with HMG-CoA reductase 89
  - 5.3.4 In vivo structure-activity, structure-metabolism, and structure-toxicity relationships of statin drugs 92
  - 5.3.5 The total synthesis of atorvastatin 95
- 5.4 Summary and outlook 103
  - 5.4.1 Chapter summary 103
  - 5.4.2 Knowledge expansion: novel molecules targeting HMG-CoA reductase 103
  - 5.4.3 Knowledge expansion: additional effects of statins 105
  - 5.4.4 Knowledge expansion: other cholesterol-lowering drugs and their targets 106
- References 107

5.1 Hypercholesterolemia and cardiovascular diseases

5.1.1 Lipid metabolism

Lipids are a broad class of water-insoluble natural substances widely present in animals and plants. They mainly include triglycerides (TG), phospholipids, and cholesterol (CHL). Lipid metabolism plays a vital role in life processes, serving not only as an energy source but also, upon metabolism, producing various bioactive substances with critical physiological functions, such as vitamins and hormones. Dysregulation in lipid metabolism can lead to several severe metabolic diseases, including cardiovascular diseases.

In the human body, lipid metabolism primarily involves the metabolism of four types of lipids: TG, phospholipids, CHL, and plasma lipoproteins. This process is intricately regulated by numerous factors, including insulin, glucagon, dietary nutrition, and enzymatic activity. Fats ingested from food are digested and absorbed in the small intestine and enter the circulatory system, from where they are transported to various tissues and organs for catabolism and anabolism. The liver, adipose tissue, and small intestine are significant sites for fat synthesis, with the liver being the most potent synthesizer. In the liver, synthesized fats combine with apolipoproteins and CHL to form very-low-density lipoproteins (VLDLs). Once in the bloodstream, these are transported to extrahepatic tissues for storage or utilization. During this transport, they further transform into lipoproteins of varying densities, including intermediate-density lipoproteins (IDL), low-density lipoproteins (LDL), and high-density lipoproteins (HDL) (Table 5.1).

Apolipoproteins as proteins in lipoproteins play a vital role in determining the size and stability of the lipoprotein particle. They are also involved in lipid transport, receptor recognition, and activation of lipid metabolism enzymes. The most common apolipoproteins include apoA, apoB, apoC, and apoE. Although the structure of various lipoproteins is similar, their types of apolipoproteins and the relative proportion of lipids to apolipoproteins vary (Table 5.1).

The primary function of lipoproteins is to transport lipids and lipophilic substances throughout the body. LDL, for instance, primarily transports CHL to peripheral (nonhepatic) tissues (Fig. 5.1). The apolipoprotein apoB100 on the LDL surface can be recognized by the low-density lipoprotein receptor (LDLR) on the cell surface, facilitating the

TABLE 5.1 Physicochemical parameters of various plasma lipoproteins.

	Chylomicrons	Very-low-density lipoproteins	Intermediate-density lipoproteins	Low-density lipoproteins	High-density lipoproteins
Molecular weight ($\times 10^{-6}$)	> 400	10~80	5~10	2~3	0.18~0.36
Density (g/cm^3)	< 0.95	0.95~1.006	1.006~1.019	1.019~1.063	1.063~1.210
Type of apolipoprotein	apoA				apoA
	apoB48	apoB100	apoB100		apoC
	apoC	apoC	apoC	apoB100	apoD
	apoE	apoE	apoE		apoE
Chemical composition (%)					
Protein	2	10	18	25	33
Triglycerides	85	50	31	10	8
Cholesterol	4	22	29	45	30
Phospholipids	9	18	22	20	29

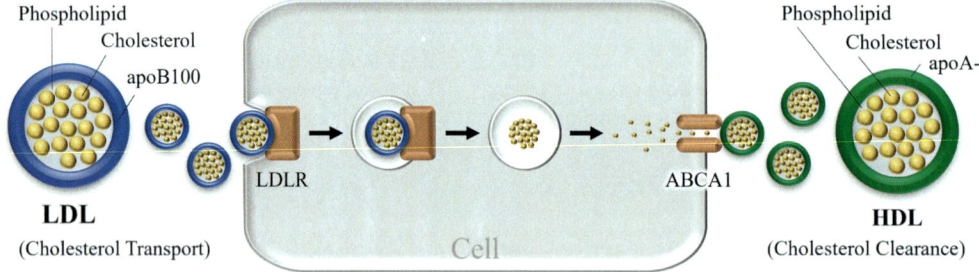

FIGURE 5.1 The role of LDL and HDL in cholesterol metabolism.

cellular uptake of LDL via receptor-mediated endocytosis. High plasma levels of LDL cholesterol (LDL-C, often termed "bad cholesterol") and apoB, along with defects in LDLR function, can lead to the accumulation of LDL in the arterial intima, contributing to atherosclerosis. Consequently, LDL is also referred to as an atherogenic factor. On the other hand, HDL is another CHL-rich lipoprotein. The interaction of apolipoprotein apoA-I on its surface with the transmembrane ABCA1 transporter (ATP-binding cassette A1 transporter) captures CHL, i.e., HDL cholesterol (HDL-C, often termed "good cholesterol"), producing nascent HDL particles (Fig. 5.1). This CHL clearance mediated by HDL is termed reverse CHL transport. Because HDL modulates the transfer of excess CHL from arterial macrophages and releases it into the liver for metabolism and excretion, its increased levels are inversely associated with atherosclerotic risk. Thus, HDL is also termed an antiatherogenic factor.

5.1.2 Cholesterol metabolic regulation and hypercholesterolemia

CHL is an essential biomolecule (Fig. 5.2). It not only constitutes a critical component of the cell membranes of eukaryotes but also serves as a precursor molecule for the synthesis of vitamin D, bile acids, and steroid hormones. For the human body, CHL plays a dual role. While it is indispensable for growth and development, it is also closely associated with numerous diseases. High concentrations of CHL can induce macrophage foam cell formation and apoptosis, leading to the establishment of atherosclerotic plaques and the formation of necrotic cores, making it a primary factor in atherosclerosis and cardiovascular diseases. Additionally, CHL is linked to conditions like fatty liver, gallstones, and diabetes.

The level of CHL in biological systems is regulated through a series of intricate and interlinked biochemical mechanisms. In a healthy organism, a delicate balance exists between CHL biosynthesis, utilization, and transport, minimizing its deleterious deposition.

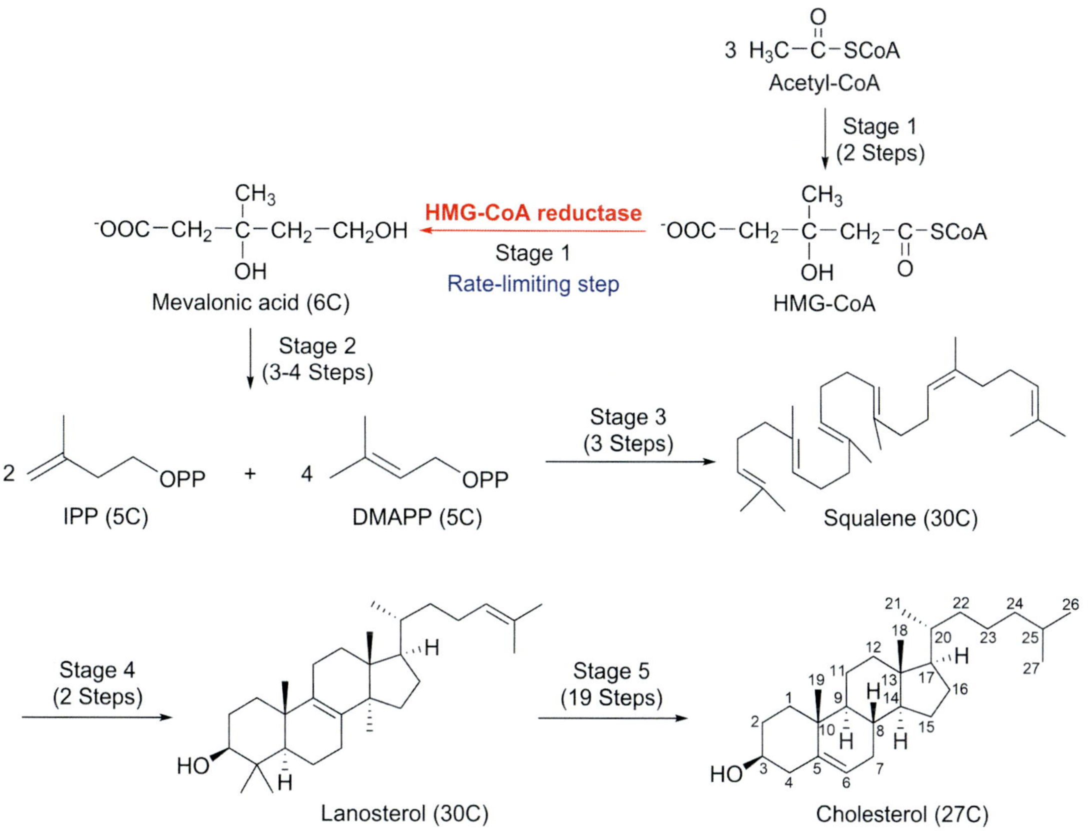

FIGURE 5.2 Biosynthesis of cholesterol.

5.1.2.1 Cholesterol biosynthesis and its regulation

Nearly every animal cell possesses the capability to synthesize CHL autonomously. In the human circulatory system, approximately one-fifth of CHL originates from dietary intake, while the remaining four-fifths is derived from endogenous synthesis, primarily in the liver. Isotopic tracing studies have demonstrated that all carbon atoms in CHL are derived from acetyl coenzyme A (acetyl-CoA). The entire biosynthetic pathway for CHL encompasses 31 steps of chemical reactions, categorized into five stages. As depicted in Fig. 5.2:

1. The initial stage involves the condensation of three molecules of acetyl-CoA in 2 steps to form 3-hydroxy-3-methylglutaryl coenzyme A (HMG-CoA). Subsequently, under the catalysis of HMG-CoA reductase, HMG-CoA is reduced to mevalonic acid (or mevalonate).
2. In the second stage, mevalonic acid undergoes 3 and 4 steps of reactions to respectively synthesize isopentenyl pyrophosphate (IPP) and dimethylallyl pyrophosphate (DMAPP). Both IPP and DMAPP are essential structural building blocks in the biosynthesis of terpenes.
3. In the third stage, two molecules of IPP and four molecules of DMAPP combine to produce the triterpene compound squalene through 3 steps of reactions.
4. In the fourth stage, squalene undergoes 2 steps of reactions to be transformed into the tetracyclic triterpene compound lanosterol.
5. Finally, in the fifth stage, lanosterol, through approximately 19 steps of reactions, undergo the removal of three methyl groups and the migration of a double bond to positions 5 and 6, yielding a CHL molecule comprising 27 carbon atoms.

Throughout the entire biosynthetic pathway of CHL, HMG-CoA reductase acts as the rate-limiting enzyme, regulating the synthesis rate of CHL. The activity of HMG-CoA reductase is susceptible to short-term modulation, such as competitive inhibition, allosteric effects, and reversible phosphorylation, making it a crucial target in drug research [1]. Additionally, HMG-CoA reductase is subject to long-term feedback regulation, primarily involving two CHL-negative feedback mechanisms: the sterol regulatory element binding protein (SREBP) pathway and the HMG-CoA reductase degradation pathway [2]. As depicted in Fig. 5.3, when CHL levels rise, on one hand, CHL can bind to the SREBP cleavage-activating protein (SCAP) and suppress the expression of CHL synthesis genes at the transcriptional level via the SCAP-SREBP pathway. On the other hand, lanosterol, an intermediate in CHL synthesis, can promote the degradation of HMG-CoA reductase, thereby reducing CHL synthesis. Moreover, CHL can also be converted into CHL esters by acyl CoA-CHL acyltransferase. Thus, the human body employs a multifaceted regulatory approach to maintain steady-state CHL levels, ensuring that tissues or organs are not damaged due to excessive CHL.

5.1.2.2 Cholesterol transport and its regulation

As shown in Fig. 5.4, CHL in human blood originates from both exogenous and endogenous sources. Exogenous CHL (from food) undergoes digestion and absorption in the small intestine and finally enters the blood circulation system in the form of chylomicrons via the lymphatic system. The endogenous CHL is synthesized by the liver, where CHL ester is produced. Under the action of the liver microsomal triglyceride transfer protein (MTTP), CHL is assembled with TG and apolipoproteins into newly formed VLDL particles. This is then converted into LDL. LDL is the main form that transports hepatically synthesized endogenous CHL into extrahepatic tissues. There are LDL receptors on the surface of the liver and other cell membranes. The ligand-binding region of LDL receptors binds to apoB100 on the LDL particles, forming an endocytosis complex with LDLR adaptor protein 1. This gets internalized into the cell and undergoes degradation in the lysosomes, releasing LDL CHL. Meanwhile, the LDL receptor recycles back to the cell surface to function anew. The LDL-derived free CHL can suppress the cell's further synthesis of CHL and reduce its further uptake of LDL, maintaining intracellular CHL levels. If LDL CHL levels in the blood rise, intracellular CHL levels will increase. This activates the expression of proprotein convertase subtilisin/kexin 9 (PCSK9). PCSK9 is synthesized in the endoplasmic reticulum and processed in the Golgi apparatus before being secreted into the plasma. Upon binding to the LDL endocytosis complex, PCSK9 leads to the degradation of all components, including the LDL receptor, affecting the normal circulation of the LDL receptor and thereby reducing the metabolic rate of LDL degradation [3]. This suggests that an increase in LDL CHL levels further intensifies the disruption in CHL transport mediated by the LDL receptor.

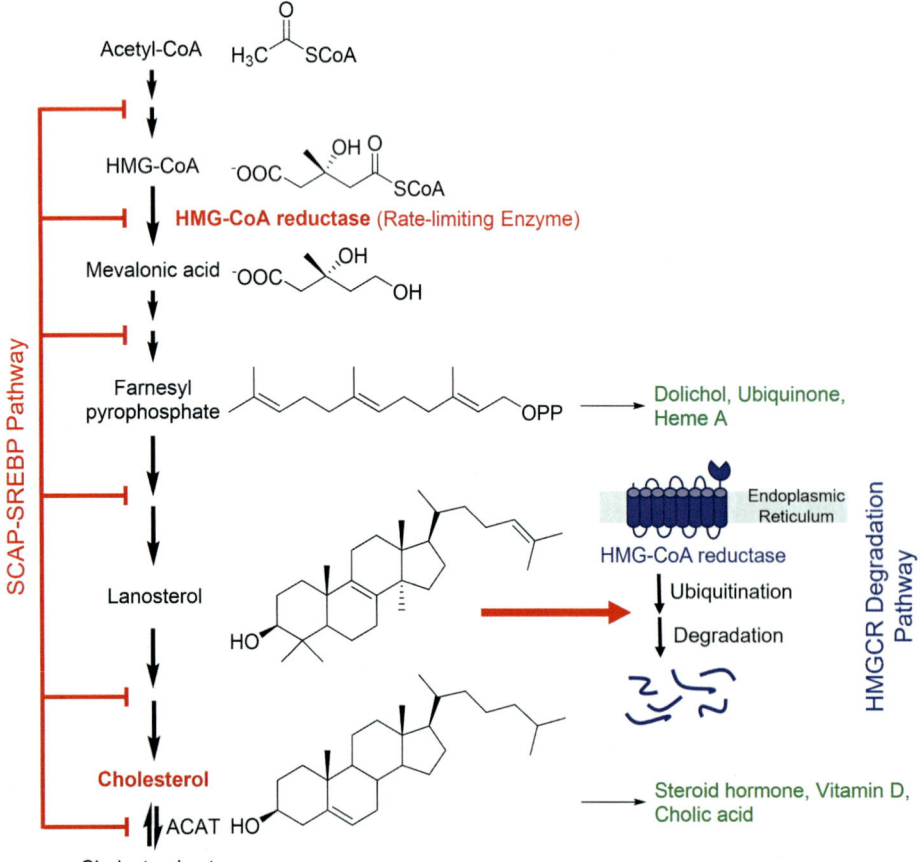

FIGURE 5.3 Regulation of cholesterol biosynthesis.

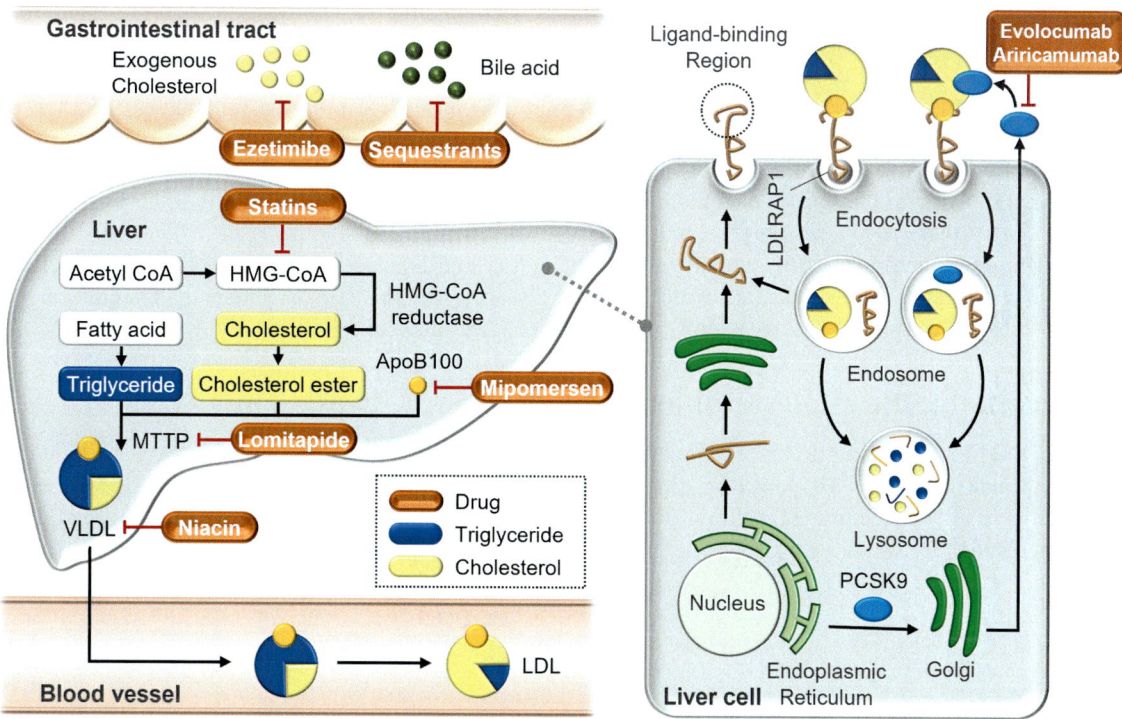

FIGURE 5.4 Cholesterol transport and its regulation [3].

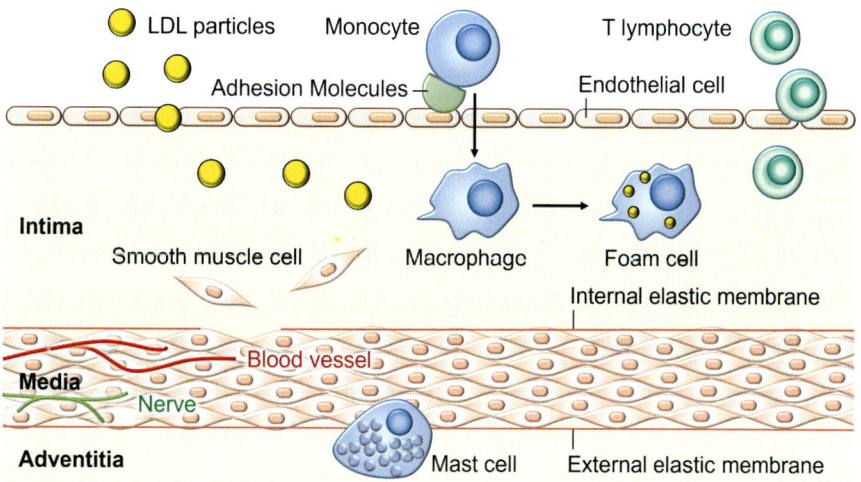

FIGURE 5.5 Formation and progression of atherosclerosis. In the early stages of the disease, low-density lipoprotein (LDL) particles accumulate in the arterial intima and undergo oxidative modification. Monocytes from the blood circulation enter the arterial intima by binding to adhesion molecules of activated endothelial cells. These monocytes then differentiate into macrophages, which uptake the oxidatively modified LDL particles, forming foam cells. This process contributes to the formation of atherosclerotic plaques. T lymphocytes can also infiltrate the intima, modulating the functions of endothelial cells, smooth muscle cells, and other cells in the vicinity.

5.1.2.3 Pathogenesis of hypercholesterolemia

Hypercholesterolemia refers to an excessively high CHL content in the blood. Excessive CHL gradually accumulates on the arterial walls forming plaques, known as "atherosclerotic plaques" (Fig. 5.5). The accumulation of CHL in the arterial walls leads to the narrowing of the arteries, causing obstruction in the flow of blood. This can result in symptoms like elevated blood pressure and ischemia in organs. Over time, it also leads to hardening of the arterial walls, decreasing their elasticity and making them prone to rupture. When these plaques rupture, it can trigger inflammation and the formation of blood clots, or thrombi. If these thrombi block the arteries supplying the heart or brain, it can lead to cardiac events or strokes, respectively.

Defects in the LDL receptor are a primary cause of hypercholesterolemia [4]. Individuals with familial hypercholesterolemia (FH, a genetic disorder) typically (in over 85% of cases) have defects in the function of the LDL receptor. The impaired function of the LDL receptor leads to a reduced clearance rate of LDL from the circulation, resulting in elevated plasma LDL CHL levels. Moreover, high intracellular CHL concentrations, in turn, suppress the synthesis of the LDL receptor, leading to the retention of more LDL particles in the plasma. Consequently, a long-term diet high in fats and CHL can also lead to hypercholesterolemia.

Understanding the mechanism of hypercholesterolemia and its consequences is essential in devising strategies for the prevention and treatment of associated cardiovascular diseases. Effective management and monitoring of CHL levels can significantly reduce the risk of atherosclerosis and its associated complications.

5.2 Atorvastatin, the cholesterol-lowering drug

Atorvastatin is the fifth statin drug to hit the market globally, developed by Pfizer and first approved by the US FDA in 1997. As a safe and effective CHL-lowering drug, it is used for cardiovascular protection and lipid-lowering. With annual sales consistently exceeding $12 billion for several years, it dominated as the world's top-selling drug, truly a blockbuster medication.

Chemical Name: (3R,5R)-7-(2-(4-fluorophenyl)-5-isopropyl-3-phenyl-4-(phenylcarbamoyl)-1H-pyrrol-1-yl)-3,5-dihydroxyheptanoic acid

Molecular Formula: $C_{33}H_{35}FN_2O_5$
Molecular Weight: 558.65
Melting Point: 176°C–178°C

Trade Name: Lipitor (generic name: atorvastatin calcium tablet. Every two atorvastatin molecules chelate with one Ca^{2+} and combine with three molecules of water, having a molecular weight of 1209.42).

5.2.1 Discovery of atorvastatin

During the 1950s and 60s, it was recognized that elevated plasma CHL was one of the major risk factors for coronary heart disease, prompting the search for drugs that could lower CHL. One approach was to inhibit the biosynthesis of CHL, and as HMG-CoA reductase was the rate-limiting enzyme in the CHL biosynthesis pathway, it became a potential target. Starting in the 1970s, the development of lipid-lowering drugs based on HMG-CoA reductase inhibitors became a major focus. Nine statin drugs or candidates were developed, with seven eventually being approved for marketing, and classified according to their origin: the naturally derived lovastatin, simvastatin, and pravastatin as first-generation (Type I) statins, and the fully synthetic drugs as second-generation (Type II) statins (Table 5.2) [5–7].

5.2.1.1 Mevastatin: the beginning of statins

Discovered in the 1970s by Japanese researchers from *Penicillium citrium* [8], it effectively reduced total CHL in experimental dogs and monkeys. However, during clinical phase I and II studies, long-term toxicity tests in dogs showed carcinogenic effects, halting clinical trials. However, it did introduce the statin suffix in pharmacology.

TABLE 5.2 Development overview of statin drugs.

	Pharmaceutical designation (trade name)	Chemical structure and identifier	Source serum	LDL-C reduction rate (at 40 mg oral dosage)	Market introduction date	Developing corporation
First generation	Mevastatin		Natural (*Penicillium citrium*)	—	Not Marketed	Sankyo
	Lovastatin (Mevacor, Altocor, and Altoprev)		Natural (*Penicillium terreus*)	34%	1987	Merck
	Simvastatin (Zocor and Lipex)		Natural chemical modification	41%	1988	Merck
	Pravastatin (Pravachol, Selektine, and Lipostat)		Natural bioconversion	34%	1989	Sankyo
Second generation	Fluvastatin (Lescol)		Total synthesis	24%	1994	Sandoz

(*Continued*)

TABLE 5.2 (Continued)

	Pharmaceutical designation (trade name)	Chemical structure and identifier	Source serum	LDL-C reduction rate (at 40 mg oral dosage)	Market introduction date	Developing corporation
	Atorvastatin (Lipitor and Torvast)		Total synthesis	50%	1997	Warner-Lambert; Pfizer
Second generation	Cerivastatin (Lipobay and Baycol)		Total synthesis	28%	1997 (Caused rhabdomyolysis and was withdrawn from the market in 2001)	Bayer
	Rosuvastatin (Crestor)		Total synthesis	63%	2003	Shionogi; AstraZeneca
	Pitavastatin (Livalo and Pitava)		Total synthesis	48%	2003	Kowa

5.2.1.2 Lovastatin: the first marketed drug

Discovered in 1978 by Merck researchers from *Penicillium terreus* [9]. It became the first successfully marketed statin drug, approved in 1987.

5.2.1.3 Simvastatin and pravastatin: simple modification of natural product

Simvastatin was developed by introducing a methyl group into the side chain of lovastatin. Pravastatin was developed by introducing a hydroxyl group into the hexahydronaphthalene ring and opening the lactone ring of mevastatin. They were approved in Sweden in 1988 and Japan in 1989, respectively.

5.2.1.4 Fluvastatin: replacement of the hexahydronaphthalene ring

Developed by Sandoz Pharmaceuticals, the first fully synthetic statin was created by replacing the hexahydronaphthalene ring with an indole ring, and the hydrophobic groups, such as methylbutanoate and methyl groups on the ring are also replaced by fluorophenyl and isopropyl groups. Fluvastatin was first approved in the UK in 1994.

5.2.1.5 Atorvastatin: the blockbuster drug

The Roth research group at the University of Rochester started synthesizing and investigating the structure-activity relationship (SAR) of statin compounds in 1981 [10–12]. They synthesized a series of derivatives starting from 1,2,5-trisubstituted pyrroles. The promising compounds they identified could not fit well into the enzyme's active pocket. They then designed a series of pentasubstituted derivatives, identifying a highly active atorvastatin prodrug. Eventually, the Warner-Lambert company selected the (+)-3R,5R isomer, successfully bringing it to market in 1997 (Fig. 5.6, Table 5.3).

5.2.1.6 Cerivastatin, rosuvastatin, and pitavastatin

Cerivastatin: Developed and launched by Bayer in 1997. However, its use was associated with a significant risk of rhabdomyolysis, a condition where skeletal muscle deteriorates, leading to potential kidney failure. Due to this adverse effect, Bayer voluntarily withdrew cerivastatin from the market in 2001. *Rosuvastatin:* Developed jointly by Yamanouchi and AstraZeneca and introduced to the market in 2003. This drug was developed as a more potent alternative to other statins and has since proven to be a highly effective treatment for hypercholesterolemia. *Pitavastatin:* Developed by Japanese company Kowa and introduced to the market in 2003.

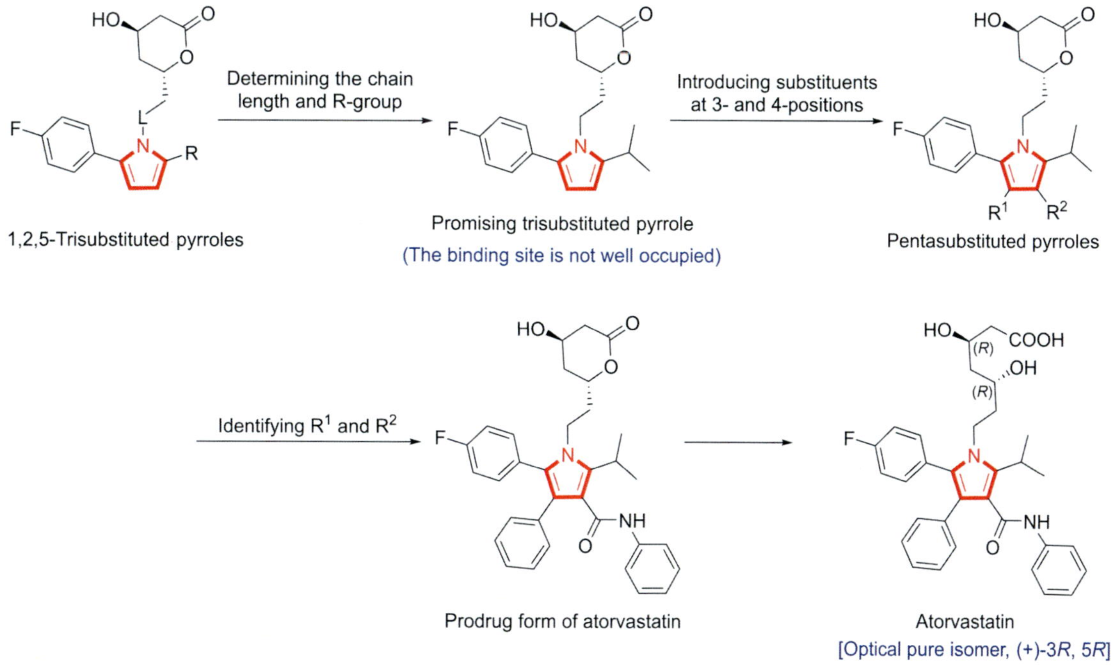

FIGURE 5.6 The discovery journey of atorvastatin.

TABLE 5.3 Major milestones in the development of atorvastatin.

Time	Events
1959	Discovery of the rate-limiting enzyme in cholesterol biosynthesis.
1973	Sankyo discovers the first HMG-CoA reductase inhibitor—mevastatin.
1978	Merck identifies Lovastatin.
1980	Due to suspected carcinogenic outcomes associated with mevastatin, clinical trials for both mevastatin and lovastatin are halted.
1982	Merck restarts lLovastatin clinical trials.
1985	Bruce Roth first synthesizes atorvastatin calcium.
1986	Warner–Lambert files patent to protect racemic Atorvastatin.
1987	The first statin drug, lovastatin, is launched.
1989	Atorvastatin enters Phase I clinical trials.
1991	Warner–Lambert files a patent to protect the (+)-3R,5R optically pure atorvastatin
1996	Warner–Lambert and Pfizer jointly conduct Phase III clinical studies; efficacy significantly surpasses other products in the same category.
1996	In July, Warner–Lambert files a patent for the Atorvastatin crystal form.
1996	In December, the FDA approves atorvastatin for market launch, with Pfizer overseeing market development under the trade name "Lipitor."
1999	Pfizer acquires Warner–Lambert for 90 billion USD.
2003	ASCOT[a] confirms Lipitor significantly reduces the risk of fatal and nonfatal cardiac events and stroke.
2004	The FDA approves new indications for Lipitor to reduce the risk of cardiac events, revascularization, and angina.
2004	Lipitor becomes the first drug in history to achieve annual sales exceeding 10 billion USD, maintaining this level for seven consecutive years.
2005	The FDA approves Lipitor for reducing the risk of stroke and cardiac events in type 2 diabetes patients without heart disease.
2006	The Heart Association releases new guidelines recommending Lipitor as a secondary prevention treatment to reduce LDL cholesterol.
2007	The FDA approves new indications for Lipitor to reduce the risk of nonfatal myocardial infarction, fatal and nonfatal stroke, revascularization, hospitalization due to congestive heart failure, and angina in heart disease patients.
2014	*The New England Journal of Medicine* reflects on 200 years of modern medicine, highlighting the significance of Lipitor.

[a]ASCOT, Anglo-Scandinavian cardiac outcome trial.

5.2.2 Mechanism of action, clinical indications, and safety of atorvastatin

5.2.2.1 Mechanism of action

Atorvastatin acts as a selective and competitive inhibitor of the rate-limiting enzyme HMG-CoA reductase in CHL biosynthesis, thereby suppressing hepatic CHL synthesis [13]. In animal models, atorvastatin not only inhibits hepatic HMG-CoA reductase, reducing CHL biosynthesis, but also increases the number of LDLRs on the liver cell surface. This augments the hepatic uptake and catabolism of LDL, leading to decreased plasma CHL and lipoprotein levels.

5.2.2.2 Clinical indications

1. Cardiovascular Disease Prevention

    In adult patients with multiple coronary heart disease risk factors (e.g., age, smoking, hypertension, elevated LDL CHL, or a family history of early-onset coronary disease) but without overt clinical symptoms, atorvastatin can reduce the risk of myocardial infarction, stroke, revascularization procedures, and angina. In patients with type 2 diabetes or those with multiple coronary heart disease risk factors (e.g., retinopathy, proteinuria, smoking, or hypertension) but no overt clinical symptoms, this medication can decrease the risk of myocardial infarction and stroke. In patients exhibiting overt clinical symptoms of coronary heart disease, atorvastatin can mitigate the risk of nonfatal myocardial infarction, fatal and nonfatal stroke, revascularization procedures, hospitalization due to congestive heart failure, and angina.

2. Hyperlipidemia Treatment

As a dietary adjunct, atorvastatin can lower elevated levels of total CHL, LDL CHL, apoB, and TG, while also elevating HDL CHL levels in patients with primary hypercholesterolemia and mixed dyslipidemia. It can treat patients with elevated serum triglyceride levels and is effective for primary β-lipoproteinemia patients unresponsive to dietary management. Additionally, it can lower total and LDL CHL in homozygous FH patients unresponsive to other lipid-lowering treatments. Furthermore, in cases where, despite appropriate dietary management, LDL cholesterol remains ≥ 190 mg/dL or LDL CHL is ≥ 160 mg/dL combined with a positive family history of premature cardiovascular disease or the presence of two or more cardiovascular risk factors in pediatric patients, atorvastatin can lower total CHL, LDL CHL, and apoB levels in heterozygous familial males aged 10−17 and postpartum females.

5.2.2.3 Safety

Adverse effects of atorvastatin include myopathy/rhabdomyolysis, hepatic insufficiency, endocrine disturbances, central nervous system toxicity, and worsening conditions in patients with recent strokes or transient ischemic attacks. Common side effects comprise hemorrhagic stroke, joint pain, diarrhea, and nasopharyngitis. Other side effects encompass urinary tract infections, insomnia, limb pain, muscle spasms, musculoskeletal pain, myalgia, and nausea.

5.3 Medicinal chemistry of atorvastatin

5.3.1 Target of statin drugs—HMG-CoA reductase

The gene encoding HMG-CoA reductase (EC1.1.1.34) is located on q13.3-q14 of human chromosome 5. Its promoter region contains sterol-responsive elements, estrogen response elements, and cAMP response elements (CRE).

Phylogenetic analysis suggests there are two classes of HMG-CoA reductases. Eukaryotes and some archaea possess Class I enzymes, while prokaryotes and certain archaea have Class II enzymes. In eukaryotes, the HMG-CoA reductase is anchored to the endoplasmic reticulum, whereas in prokaryotes, it is soluble. Although both classes exhibit similar maximum reaction rates and Michaelis constants, statin drugs display vastly differing inhibitory capabilities, often showing 3−5 orders of magnitude greater inhibition toward Class I enzymes. In mammals, the HMG-CoA reductase plays a pivotal role in maintaining cellular CHL homeostasis, it has multiple regulatory mechanisms at the transcriptional, translational, and posttranslational levels.

Human HMG-CoA reductase is a tetramer consisting of four identical subunits. Each subunit contains 888 amino acid residues with an approximate molecular weight of 97 kD. The enzyme is divided into an N-terminal nonconservative transmembrane domain, a highly conserved C-terminal catalytic domain, and an intermediary connecting arm. The catalytic domain encompasses three subdomains: N domain, L domain, and S domain. The N domain resides between the L domain and the connecting arm. The L domain, consisting of two peptide segments, binds the substrate HMG-CoA, while the S domain binds the coenzyme NADP(H). The serine residue at position 872 is a phosphorylation site that can modulate enzyme activity through reversible phosphorylation (phosphorylation leads to decreased enzyme activity). Glu559, Lys691, Asp767, and His866 are four crucial amino acid residues involved in catalysis. Additionally, a cis-loop formed by peptide segments 683−693 is a unique structural feature of human HMG-CoA reductase (Fig. 5.7).

HMG-CoA reductase is among the few enzymes to undergo a 4-electron oxidation-reduction reaction, catalyzing the reductive deacylation of substrate (S)-HMG-CoA to product (R)-mevalonic acid (Fig. 5.8). This involves three stages: Stages 1 and 3 are reduction reactions facilitated by the reduced coenzyme NADPH, while stage 2 is the hydrolysis of an aldehyde from a hemiacetal. Mevaldehyde formed during the process is not released by the enzyme but proceeds through either the forward reaction of stage 3 or the reverse reaction back to (S)-HMG-CoA. Mevalonic acid can also be oxidized back to (S)-HMG-CoA catalyzed by the HMG-CoA reductase [14].

Enzyme kinetics studies with mutant proteins and crystal structure analysis confirm that the four amino acid residues (histidine, lysine, aspartate, and glutamate) in the active site play pivotal roles in catalysis. The function of histidine is to promptly provide a proton for the departing CoA sulfhydryl anion, preventing it from attacking the generated mevaldehyde and ensuring the forward progression of the reaction. Lysine, aspartate, and glutamate interact with the HMG moiety of HMG-CoA, establishing a hydrogen bond network. Mutational studies indicate that aspartate plays a crucial role in every reaction stage, serving as the core of the hydrogen bond network and possibly participating in proton shuttling. Although glutamate influences every reaction stage, it predominantly functions as a general base in stage 3 (making proton removal

82 Medicinal Chemistry and Drug Development

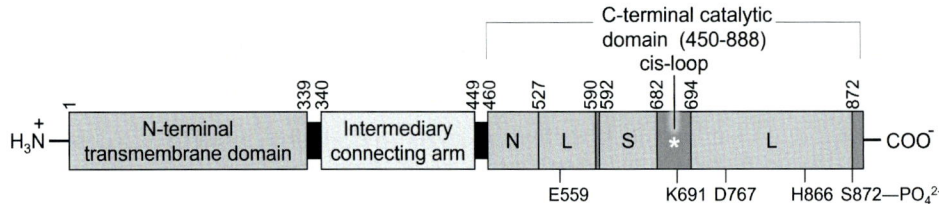

FIGURE 5.7 Structural representation of human HMG-CoA reductase.

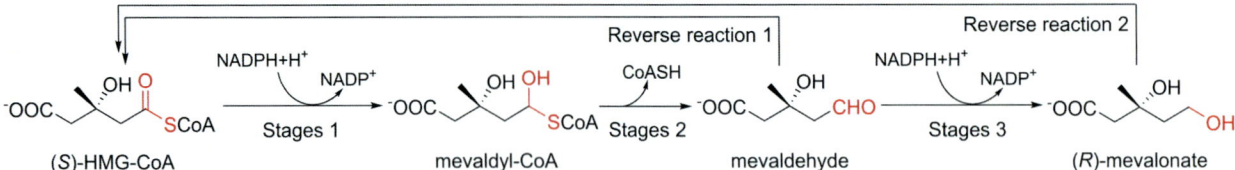

FIGURE 5.8 Catalytic steps of HMG-CoA reductase.

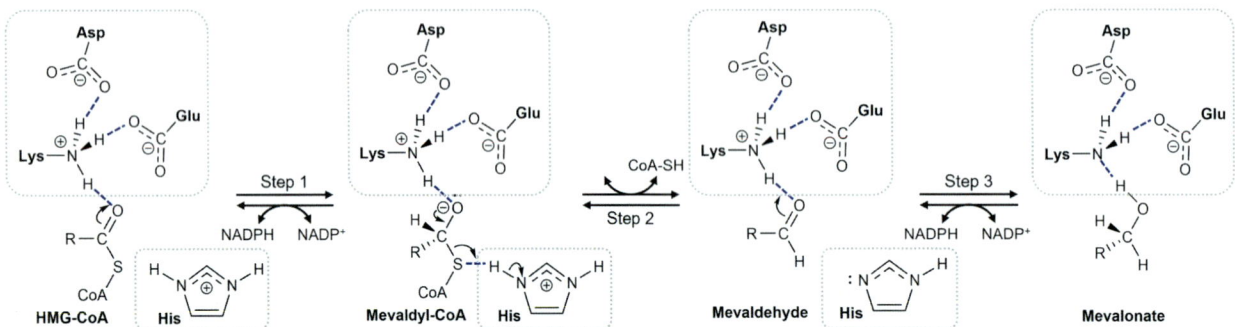

FIGURE 5.9 Catalytic mechanism of HMG-CoA reductase [14].

from lysine's N more facile). Protonated lysine (positively charged) stabilizes the product mevaldehyde-CoA anion and provides a proton in the 3rd step. Ultimately, all protons originate from the reduced coenzyme NADHP (Fig. 5.9).

5.3.2 Structure-activity relationship of statin drugs inhibiting HMG-CoA reductase

The overarching strategy in developing statin drugs was target-based drug design, initiating from the function of the target, progressing through screening, molecular interaction studies, SAR analysis, structural optimization, in vivo evaluations, and finally determining drug candidates.

The activity evaluation of statin compounds often employs two in vitro evaluation models:

Cholesterol synthesis inhibition (CSI) screening: Evaluates compound's inhibition of cholesterol synthesis.

$$[^{14}C]\text{-Acetc acid} \xrightarrow{\text{Rat liver homogenate}} [^{14}C]\text{-Cholesterol}$$

CoA reductase (COR) inhibition screening: Assesses the compound's inhibition of HMG-CoA reductase.

$$\text{D,L-}[^{14}C]\text{HMG-CoA} \xrightarrow{\text{Purified rat liver microsomal enzymes}} [^{14}C]\text{-Mevalonic acid}$$

Both evaluation models use IC_{50}-CSI and IC_{50}-COR (the concentration at which the compound inhibits 50% of the theoretical product generation) as activity indices. Analyses reveal a moderate correlation between the IC_{50} values of the two models.

Fig. 5.10 displays the chemical structures and enzyme inhibitory activity data for nine representative statin drug molecules. It is discernible that the molecular structure of statin drugs can broadly be divided into three parts: (1) Dihydroxypentanoic acid side chain, an indispensable pharmacophore mimicking the HMG part of the enzyme's substrate HMG-CoA, is vital for competitive inhibition and is irreplaceable. It exists in the form of lactone in molecules **1~3** and is hydrolyzed in vivo by esterase to generate the open-chain carboxylic acid, so it can be regarded as the prodrug form. (2) A hydrophobic structural segment, which binds to the hydrophobic pocket produced after enzyme allostery, is imperative for strong binding affinity of inhibitors. Because the hydrophobic pocket structure has strong flexibility and plasticity, it can accommodate a variety of structures with different sizes and shapes, so it can be modified and optimized on this part of the structure of inhibitors. It can be found that the hydrophobic fragments contain a central ring and two substituents (R^1 and R^2) adjacent to the side chain of dihydroxypentanoic acid. (3) A connecting chain links the above segments, with its length strictly limited, with two-carbon ethylidene ($-CH_2CH_2-$) or trans vinylidene ($-CH=CH-$) being the best.

The first-generation statins (1~4) have a hexahydronaphthalene central ring, with 1−2 methyl substituents and a methylbutanoate substituent. Notably, from the activity of lovastatin (2) and pravastatin (4), it is evident that a methyl substituent at the 6-position of the hexahydronaphthalene ring offers higher activity than a hydroxyl substituent, underlining the significance of hydrophobic structures.

The second-generation statins (5~9) are characterized by a nonchiral hydrophobic aromatic core. This core has at least two lipophilic substituents, one being a *para*-fluorophenyl group and the other being an isopropyl group (or cyclopropyl in the case of compound 9).

In summary, a straightforward SAR can be deduced: Statin drugs consist of a fundamental pharmacophore (dihydroxypentanoic acid) connected to a basic scaffold (central ring) via a two-carbon linkage, and other substituents interact with the enzyme through induced-fit mechanisms.

5.3.2.1 Substitutions of the central ring—eliminating unnecessary chiral centers

The hexahydronaphthalene central ring of the first-generation statins introduced 5 chiral centers, which is unfavorable for chemical synthesis and industrial production. Scientists aimed to eradicate these unnecessary chiral centers. Fortuitously, replacing the hexahydronaphthalene with nonchiral aromatic rings yielded numerous potent inhibitors, including four approved drugs (fluvastatin, atorvastatin, rosuvastatin, and pitavastatin). Fig. 5.10 clearly indicates that the central ring tolerates diverse structures, from monocyclic rings such as benzene, pyridine, pyrazine, and pyrrole to fused rings such as indole and quinoline. This shows that the hydrophobic segment binding the enzyme does not require chiral control.

5.3.2.2 Optimization of structures with pyrrole as central ring—the emergence of atorvastatin

The medicinal chemistry of atorvastatin is exemplary and can be referred to in references 10, 15, and 16 [10,15,16]. Here, we will focus on the development process of atorvastatin through the optimization of structures with a pyrrole central ring.

1. SAR of the 2-Position Substituent

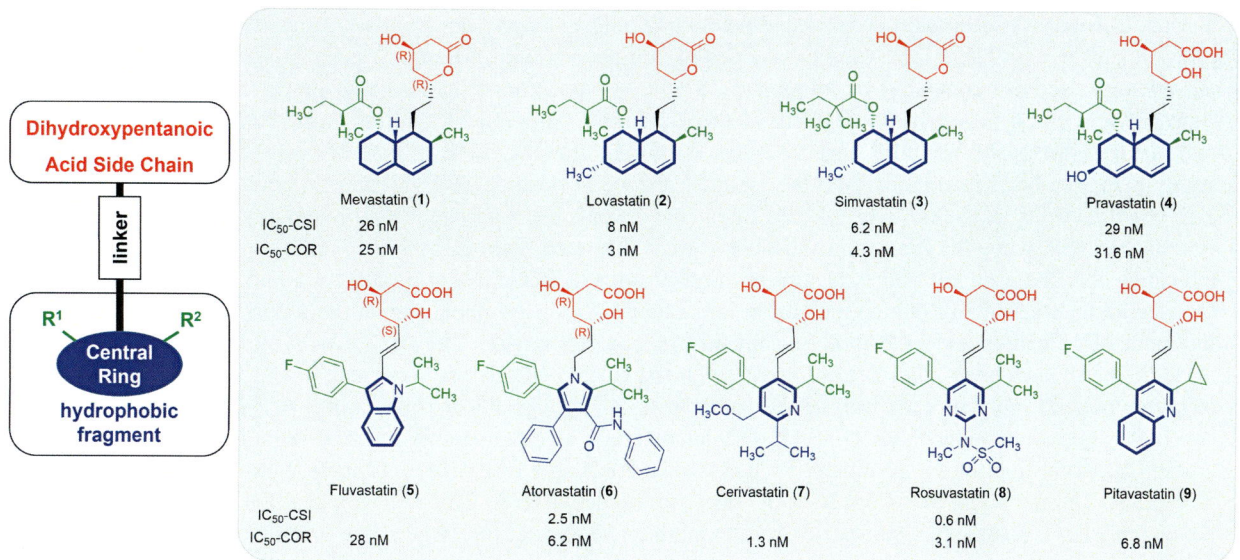

FIGURE 5.10 Structure and activity data of representative statin drugs.

From the basic molecular skeleton, the pyrrole ring serves a supporting role for the pharmacophore. Its 2-position substituent is analogous to the methylbutanoate part in natural statin molecules (Fig. 5.10). Molecular simulations suggest that this segment binds to the enzyme's hydrophobic cavity, crucial for enhancing inhibitor-enzyme interaction. With the connecting chain fixed as ethenyl and methyl at the 5-position, changing the 2-position substituent yielded various inhibitors (**10**~**27**). The activity data in Table 5.4 indicates that all compounds have markedly lower activity than mevastatin (**1**). The most active compound, compound **16**, only has about 1/20 of mevastatin's activity. Different aromatic substituents have certain effects on activity. The position and electron-donating/electron-withdrawing properties on the phenyl group do not significantly impact activity. Compounds with a 4-substituted phenyl group (**16**~**20**) show varied activities. 4-fluoro substitution (**16**) exhibits the highest activity, while 4-methoxy (**18**), 4-chloro (**19**), and 4-phenyl (**20**) substitutions reduce activity, suggesting that the 4-position fluorine atom on the phenyl group enhances activity. Compounds with a benzyl (**21**) and naphthyl (**22, 23**) group also significantly reduce activity. Compounds with a cycloaliphatic (**24**) or bridged ring (**25**~**27**) retain some activity. Evidently, the preliminary SAR suggests that the 4-position fluorine atom of 2-substituted phenyl is involved in the interaction with the target.

2. Structure-Activity Relationship of the 5-Position Substituents

   With the preferred 4-fluorophenyl group fixed at the 2-position and varying the 5-position substituents to different saturated hydrocarbon groups, the following observations were made (Table 5.5):
   1. Compounds with substituents being isopropyl (**28**) and trifluoromethyl (**34**) showed slightly stronger activity than the compound **16** with a methyl substituent. The enhanced activity observed for the trifluoromethyl substitution over the methyl substitution may be attributed to the electron-withdrawing effect of the trifluoromethyl group, which reduces the electron cloud density of the pyrrole ring, favoring binding to the enzyme. Analogous to the frequent substitution of hydrogen atoms with fluorine, trifluoromethyl groups often replace methyl groups in medicinal chemistry studies, exploring the impact of strong electron-withdrawing groups on activity.
   2. With larger substituents at the 5-position, such as *tert*-butyl (**29**) and 2-ethylpropyl (**30**), there is a notable decrease in activity, indicating that the enzyme's binding pocket imposes stringent constraints on the size of the 5-position substituent.
   3. Substitution with cycloalkanes of different ring sizes distinctly impacts activity. From cyclopropyl (**31**) to cyclobutyl (**32**) and then to cyclohexyl (**33**) substitutions, as the substituent ring size increases sequentially, there is a marked decrease in activity, even to the point of eradication, further emphasizing the enzyme binding pocket's specific limitations concerning the 5-position substituent's volume.

   After optimization, the 5-position was chosen to have an isopropyl substitution.

3. Further Exploration of the Structure-Activity Relationship of the 2-Position Substituent

   Small molecule compounds and large biomolecular targets bind through mutually induced fitting conformations, which is often the result of a combination of multiple factors. As previously discussed, preliminary findings suggest that the 5-isopropyl substituent is favorable for maintaining relatively good activity. Scientists then revisited the 2-position substituent (Table 5.6). Clearly, a series of compounds with different 2-position substituents (**35**~**44**) displayed lower activity compared to compound **28** with a 2-position 4-fluorophenyl group, further highlighting the superiority of the 4-fluorophenyl segment at the 2-position. Subsequent studies on the interaction of atorvastatin with the enzyme crystal structure (Fig. 5.12) also confirmed that the fluorine atom of the 4-fluorophenyl group has a strong hydrogen bond interaction with the arginine residue at position 590. In contrast, compounds substituted with 2-fluorophenyl (**35**) or 3-fluorophenyl (**36**) might have weakened hydrogen bond interactions due to distance constraints. Notably, when the 2-position substituent was a saturated hydrocarbon (**44**), the activity was completely lost, indicating that the aromatic ring structure at the 2-position is beneficial for activity. Some literature suggests that the guanidine group of Arg590 has a cation-π interaction with the aromatic ring at the 2-position.

4. Influence of 2-Position and 5-Position Substituent Sizes on Activity

   Utilizing molecular simulation techniques, scientists calculated the lengths of the R^1 and R^2 substituents in some of the compound molecules, as well as the width from R^1 through the pyrrole ring to R^2 (Table 5.7). It is evident that highly active compounds ($IC_{50} < 1.6\ \mu M$) have certain size constraints for their substituents. Specifically, the length (d_1) of the 2-position substituent R^1 is less than 5.8 Å, the length (d_2) of the 5-position substituent R^2 is less than 3.3 Å, and the width (d_3) from R^1 to R^2 does not exceed 10.6 Å. This indicates that the hydrophobic pocket of the enzyme has certain size requirements for the inhibitor molecule; too large a size is unfavorable for their binding.

TABLE 5.4 Activity of compounds with a fixed 5-methyl group and varied 2-position substituents.[a]

Compounds	R	IC$_{50}$-CSI (μM)	Relative activity (%)[b]	IC$_{50}$-COR (μM)
Lovastatin		0.026	100	0.025
10	C$_6$H$_5$	1.4	0.4	13
11	2-HO-C$_6$H$_4$	2.5	1.1	30
12	2-CH$_3$O-C$_6$H$_4$	2.1	0.9	25
13	3-HO-C$_6$H$_4$	1.9	1.4	12
14	3-CH$_3$O-C$_6$H$_4$	2.5	0.8	11
15	3-F$_3$C-C$_6$H$_4$	1.5	0.3	5.4
16	4-F-C$_6$H$_4$	0.51	0.9	2.8
17	4-HO-C$_6$H$_4$	2.6	1.0	6.3
18	4-CH$_3$O-C$_6$H$_4$	12	0.1	28
19	4-Cl-C$_6$H$_4$	10	0.2	3.2
20	4-Ph-C$_6$H$_4$	23	0.1	23
21	Ph$_2$CH	13	0.1	8.9
22	1-naphthyl	1.8	0.7	4.0
23	2-naphthyl	16	0.1	3.6
24	cyclohexyl	0.69	0.5	2.2
25	norbornyl	1.4	1.1	5.8
26	norbornyl	1.3	1.6	3.2
27	norbornyl	2.3	1.1	2.3

[a] The test compound samples must undergo hydrolysis with alkali (0.1N NaOH) to form an open-ring structure; the same applies below.
[b] Relative activity (%) = (lovastatin IC$_{50}$ - CSI / Test compound IC$_{50}$ - CSI) × 100. The activity of lovastatin is measured simultaneously each time a compound is evaluated; the same applies below. Due to systematic errors in activity measurement, the IC$_{50}$ and relative activity of compounds are not proportional, but the ratios between them are comparable in the context of medicinal chemistry.

TABLE 5.5 Activity of compounds with a fixed 2-(4-fluorophenyl) and varied 5-position substituents.

Compounds	R	IC$_{50}$-CSI (μM)	Relative activity (%)[a]	IC$_{50}$-COR (μM)
16	CH$_3$	0.51	0.9	2.8
28	(CH$_3$)$_2$CH	0.40	30.3	0.23
29	(CH$_3$)$_3$C	1.6	1.7	1.8
30	(C$_2$H$_5$)$_2$CH	20	0.1	32
31	cyclopropyl	2.2	1.3	2.6
32	cyclobutyl	17	0.2	—
33	cyclohexyl	>100	<0.01	>100
34	CF$_3$	0.25	8.0	0.63

[a]Relative activity = (Lovastatin IC$_{50}$-COR / Test compound IC$_{50}$-COR) × 100, to be measured concurrently.

TABLE 5.6 Activity of compounds with a fixed 5-isopropyl and varied 2-position substituents.

Compounds	R	IC$_{50}$-CSI (μM)	Relative activity (%)[a]	IC$_{50}$-COR (μM)
28	4-F-C$_6$H$_4$	0.40	30.3	0.23
35	2-F-C$_6$H$_4$	3.2	0.9	1.8
36	3-F-C$_6$H$_4$	1.3	1.8	2.6
37	2,4-F$_2$-C$_6$H$_3$	1.6	1.5	2.6
38	2-CH$_3$O-C$_6$H$_4$	2.2	1.0	5.6
39	2,6-(CH$_3$O)$_2$-C$_6$H$_3$	19	0.2	87
40	2,5-(CH$_3$)$_2$-C$_6$H$_3$	12	0.2	16
41	2-(CH$_3$)$_2$CH-C$_6$H$_4$	3.2	0.9	—
42	2-Cl-C$_6$H$_4$	3.2	0.5	9.1
43	2-methoxynaphthyl	9.6	0.2	25
44	(CH$_3$CH$_2$)$_2$CH	>100	<0.01	—

[a]Relative activity = (Lovastatin IC$_{50}$-COR / Test compound IC$_{50}$-COR) × 100, to be measured concurrently.

5. Structure-Activity Relationship of 3-Position and 4-Position Substituents

From the results presented above, it is clear that compound **28**, with a 1-position linker of ethyl or ethenyl, a 2-position 4-fluorophenyl, and a 5-position isopropyl, exhibited relatively high activity, with an IC_{50}-COR of 230 nM. However, its activity, when compared to lovastatin, still differs by an order of magnitude. Scientists, therefore, initiated optimization studies on the 3-position and 4-position of the pyrrole ring (Table 5.8).

The initial work introduced a single substituent at the 3-position or 4-position (compounds **45~49**), adopting aromatic (**45, 46**) and heteroaromatic (**47~49**) substitution strategies. Encouragingly, the heteroaromatic compounds at the 3-position (**47, 48**) displayed activity comparable to lovastatin, operating at the same order of magnitude in activity. When halogen atoms were introduced at both the 3-position and 4-position (**52, 53**), their activity slightly surpassed that of lovastatin, suggesting that dual substitution at both the 3-position and 4-position enhances molecular activity. The specific SAR is summarized as:

1. A decrease in the electron cloud density of the pyrrole ring (introduction of electron-withdrawing groups) augments activity. For instance, the activity of 3-position 2-pyridyl substituted **47** and 3-pyridyl substituted **48** was notably superior to the unsubstituted **28** and phenyl substituted **46**. However, the 4-pyridyl substituted **49** did not exhibit improved activity, possibly due to the hydrophilic nature of the 4-pyridyl group.
2. Reduced hydrophobicity (introduction of hydrophilic groups) is unfavorable for enhanced activity. For example, the activity of the trifluoroacetyl substituted **50** diminished, perhaps owing to its pronounced polarity (reduced

TABLE 5.7 Size of 2-position and 5-position substituents and compound activity.

Compounds	R^1	R^2	IC$_{50}$-CSI (μM)	d$_1$ (Å)	d$_2$ (Å)	d$_3$ (Å)
1			0.026	5.66	1.50	8.81
16	4-F-C$_6$H$_4$	CH$_3$	0.51	5.58	1.50	7.66
19	4-Cl-C$_6$H$_4$	CH$_3$	10	5.89	1.50	9.33
25a	(norbornyl)	CH$_3$	1.4	3.64	1.50	7.22
25b	(norbornyl)	CH$_3$	1.4	4.27	1.50	7.87
28	4-F-C$_6$H$_4$	(CH$_3$)$_2$CH	0.40	5.58	2.48	10.12
29	4-F-C$_6$H$_4$	(CH$_3$)$_3$C	1.6	5.58	2.48	10.20
30	4-F-C$_6$H$_4$	(C$_2$H$_5$)$_2$CH	20	5.58	3.47	10.99
32	4-F-C$_6$H$_4$	cyclobutyl	17	5.58	3.35	10.62
33	4-F-C$_6$H$_4$	cyclohexyl	>100	5.58	4.33	11.92

TABLE 5.8 Activity of compounds with varied 3-position and 4-position substituents.

Compounds	R^1	R^2	IC$_{50}$-COR (μM)	Relative activity (%)^a
1 (Lovastatin)			0.030	100
28	H	H	0.23	10.9
45	H	C$_6$H$_5$	0.12	36.3
46	C$_6$H$_5$	H	0.35	12.5
47	2-pyridyl	H	0.046	76
48	3-pyridyl	H	0.071	9.4
49	4-pyridyl	H	0.31	2.1
50	CF$_3$CO	H	0.80	8.8
51	CH$_3$	CH$_3$	0.14	16
52	Cl	Cl	0.028	78.6
53	Br	Br	0.028	78.6
54	CH$_3$OCO	CH$_3$OCO	0.18	14.3
55	C$_2$H$_5$OCO	C$_2$H$_5$OCO	0.35	2.8
56	C$_2$H$_5$OCO	C$_6$H$_5$	0.050	100
57	C$_6$H$_5$	C$_2$H$_5$OCO	0.20	35.5
58	4-CN-C$_6$H$_4$	C$_2$H$_5$OCO	0.28	16.2
59	C$_6$H$_5$	C$_6$H$_5$CH$_2$OCO	0.040	24.0
60 (±)	C$_6$H$_5$	C$_6$H$_5$NHCO	0.025	81.4
60 (+)	C$_6$H$_5$	C$_6$H$_5$NHCO	0.007	500
60 (−)	C$_6$H$_5$	C$_6$H$_5$NHCO	0.44	13.9

^{a}Relative activity = (Lovastatin IC$_{50}$-COR / Test compound IC$_{50}$-COR) × 100, to be measured concurrently.

lipophilicity). As methyl is a weak electron-donating group (hyperconjugation effect) with lipophilicity, the 3,4-dimethyl substituted **51** displayed slightly better activity than **28**.
3. Reducing the electron cloud density of the pyrrole ring while enhancing hydrophobicity significantly bolsters activity. For instance, the 3,4-dichloro or dibromo substituted compounds **52** and **53** achieved 79% of the activity of lovastatin. However, compound **53**, which underwent further clinical trials, was terminated due to toxicity concerns.
4. The introduction of a phenyl ring augments activity. In the 3,4-dual substituted series, the inclusion of one or two phenyl rings (compounds **56~60**) generally heightened activity.
5. Introducing an electron-withdrawing cyano group at the para-position of the 3-position phenyl (**58**) marginally reduced activity.

In summary, compounds **59** and **60**, with a 3-position phenyl and 4-position benzyloxycarbonyl or phenylcarbamoyl, respectively, exhibited heightened activity. The racemic compound **60** reached 81% of lovastatin's activity, while its dextrorotatory form (+)-**60** (3′R, 5′R) showcased activity five times that of lovastatin. The activity of levorotatory form (−)-**60** (3′R, 5′S) is significantly weaker, suggesting that the binding between molecules has the requirement of spatial orientation.

1. Overall Structure-Activity Relationship (Fig. 5.11)
2. Approval of Atorvastatin for Market Release

Through the detailed SAR studies, it was eventually discovered that (+)-**60** is a potent inhibitor of HMG-CoA reductase, with an IC_{50} value of 0.6 nM for rat liver cell HMG-CoA reductase. This is stronger than previously marketed lovastatin (IC_{50} = 2.7 nM) and pravastatin (IC_{50} = 5.5 nM). Radiolabeled isotope studies indicated that 2 hours after administration, atorvastatin distribution in the rat liver was 28–254 times higher than in other tissues [19], demonstrating good liver tissue selectivity. Preclinical pharmacological studies further confirmed: (1) In a hypercholesterolemia rabbit model fed with casein-based feed, this compound at low (1 mg/kg), medium (3 mg/kg), and high (10 mg/kg) doses all showed significant CHL-lowering activity, markedly superior to lovastatin [20]; (2) In a hypertriglyceridemia rat model, this compound at a dose of 1 mg/kg significantly reduced plasma TG, while the same dose of lovastatin had a less pronounced effect [21]. Ultimately, scientists identified (+)-**60** as a drug candidate and named it atorvastatin. Its calcium salt form is used as the drug, with the brand name "Liptor."

Clinical research results indicated that atorvastatin's efficacy in lowering CHL and TG was significantly better than the first four statins that had been approved for the market (lovastatin, pravastatin, simvastatin, and fluvastatin). Starting from the project initiation in 1982 to the completion of preclinical studies in 1989, and then to the completion of Phase III clinical trials in 1996, it took 14 years for atorvastatin to gain market approval. Phase IV clinical trials further confirmed the remarkable efficacy of atorvastatin, making it the best-in-class CHL-lowering drug. Coupled with Pfizer's successful commercial operations, it became a blockbuster drug with annual sales exceeding ten billion for seven consecutive years.

5.3.3 Interaction of statins with HMG-CoA reductase

5.3.3.1 Interaction modes

Fig. 5.12A displays a tetrameric structure of the catalytic domain of human HMG-CoA reductase (PDB ID: 1DQA). Crystal structure studies of the statins complexed with HMG-CoA reductase revealed [18,22]: (1) The structurally similar portion of the inhibitor molecule to HMG (dihydroxypentanoic acid side chain moiety) occupies the enzyme's substrate-binding pocket (Fig. 5.12B), competing with the HMG part of substrate molecule; (2) There is a noticeable change in the pocket where the enzyme binds with the CoA part of the substrate, exposing a relatively shallow hydrophobic pocket, facilitating strong hydrophobic interactions with the bulky hydrophobic structures in the inhibitor molecules. In fact, not

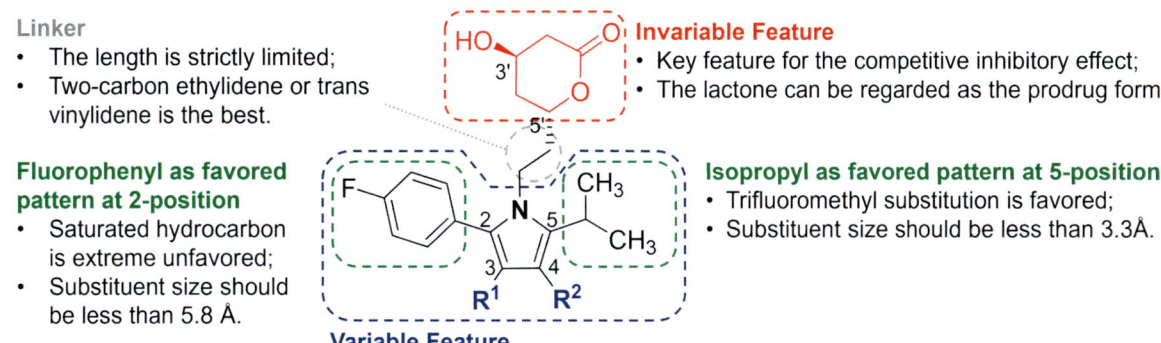

FIGURE 5.11 Structure-activity relationship of statins centered around the pyrrole ring.

only can the C-terminal portion of the enzyme's active pocket adjust its conformation to accommodate the large hydrophobic groups in the statin ligand molecules, but the statin molecules themselves can also adjust their conformations to achieve optimal binding with the enzyme's hydrophobic cavity, effectively blocking the interaction between the substrate and the enzyme. This excellent induced fit between the enzyme and the inhibitor results in a highly complementary interaction, achieving extremely low (nanomolar level) inhibition constants (Table 5.9).

Specifically, from Fig. 5.12C and D, it is evident that the 3′,5′-dihydroxypentanoic acid segment of atorvastatin binds to the position in the enzyme where the substrate HMG resides. The amino acid residues interacting with them are essentially the same. For instance, the terminal carboxyl group similarly interacts with Lys^{735} and Ser^{684} of the enzyme and also interacts with Lys^{692}; the 3′-hydroxyl group forms hydrogen bonds with Arg^{590} and Asp^{690}; and the 5′-hydroxyl group forms a hydrogen bond network with Lys^{691}, Glu^{559}, and Asn^{755}. Additionally, the hydrophobic segment in the atorvastatin molecule significantly contributes to its strong binding with the enzyme. Notably, the fluorine atom on the fluorophenyl group forms a clear hydrogen bond with the ε-NH of the Arg^{590} residue's side chain guanidine group, effectively increasing the drug's affinity for the enzyme. Compared to other statin molecules, the most distinct feature of atorvastatin's binding to the enzyme lies in its 4-position amide segment. The carbonyl oxygen in its amide forms a hydrogen bond with the hydroxyl group of Ser^{565}, further enhancing affinity and significantly boosting atorvastatin's inhibitory potency against the enzyme.

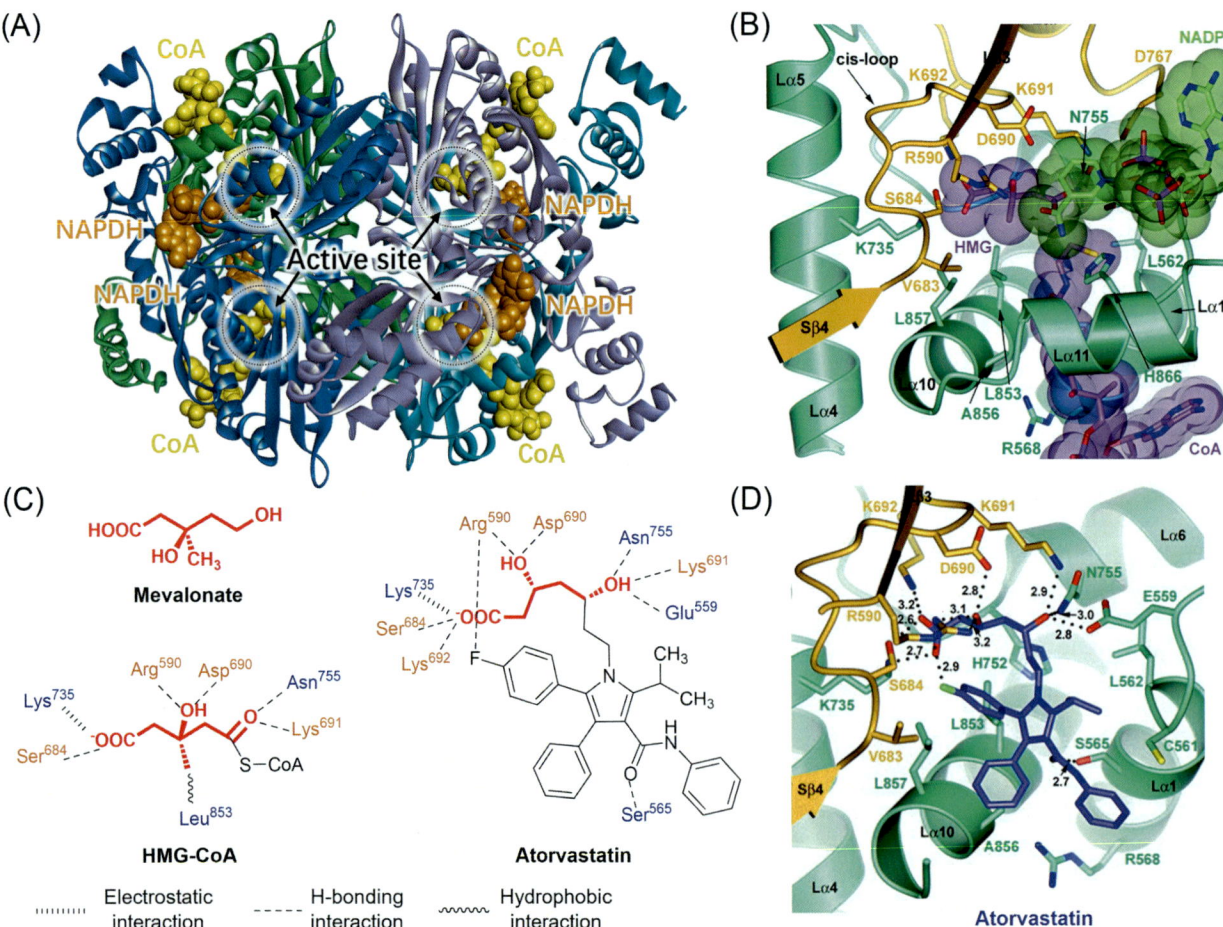

FIGURE 5.12 (A) A tetrameric structure of the catalytic domain of human HMG-CoA reductase (PDB ID: 1DQA). The four identical subunits are marked in different colors. (B) The active site of human HMG-CoA reductase in complex with its natural substrate HMG-CoA and NADP is located at the interface between two monomers. (C) Parts of the atorvastatin structure that are similar to the substrate HMG-CoA and the product mevalonic acid (in red) and their binding mode with the enzyme's active pocket. (D) Binding of atorvastatin (in blue) to the active site of HMG-CoA reductase [17,18].

TABLE 5.9 Parameters related to the interaction of four statin drugs with HMG-CoA reductase [23].

	Fluvastatin	Pravastatin	Atorvastatin	Rosuvastatin
K_i (nM)[a]	256	103	5.7	3.1
ΔG (kcal/mol)[b]	-9.0 ± 0.4	-9.7 ± 0.4	-10.9 ± 0.8	-12.3 ± 0.7
ΔH (kcal/mol)[b]	~ 0	-2.5 ± 0.1, 25.8%[c] (42%)[d]	-4.3 ± 0.1, 39.5%[c] (57%)[d]	-9.3 ± 0.1, 75.6%[c] (100%)[d]
$-T\Delta S$ (kcal/mol)[b]	~ -9.0	-7.2 ± 0.4	-6.6 ± 0.6	-3.0 ± 0.7
$DSASA_{polar}$ (Å^2)	291	–	323	341
$DSASA_{nonpolar}$ (Å^2)	593	–	692	512
Number of hydrogen bonds in the hydrophobic region	0	–	1	1
Number of rotatable bonds in hydrophobic regions	4	–	9	6

[a]Enzyme inhibition constant measured at 37°C.
[b]Thermodynamic parameters measured at 25°C using ITC.
[c]Percentage of enthalpy change in binding free energy at 25°C.
[d]Percentage of enthalpy change in binding free energy at 37°C.

5.3.3.2 Affinity and thermodynamic characteristics

Most drugs interact with their targets through noncovalent binding, forming a dynamic equilibrium between the complex, free drug, and target. The strength of this noncovalent interaction (affinity, such as dissociation constant K_d or enzyme inhibition constant K_i) is closely related to the in vitro activity demonstrated by the drug molecule (e.g., EC_{50} or IC_{50}) and is a primary metric to evaluate compound quality in early phases. The affinity between a ligand and its target can be translated into binding free energy (ΔG), and thermodynamic methods can further decompose this energy into contributions from enthalpy and entropy. During structural optimization, by measuring a compound's free energy, change in enthalpy (ΔH), and change in entropy ($-T\Delta S$), one can understand the effects on activity and the trends in these changes at a more microscopic level—based on atom and group properties, orientations, positions, and distances. Combined with the structural biology features of the ligand-target complex, it is possible to delve deeper into the essence of ligand-target binding and the inherent nature of the exhibited activity, thus discerning the influence of structural changes on activity from the variations in enthalpy and entropy. Therefore, studies on affinity and thermodynamic behavior are effective means to elucidate the mechanism of drug action and guide molecular design [17]. Table 5.9 lists the affinity and thermodynamic parameters associated with the interaction of four statin molecules—fluvastatin, pravastatin, atorvastatin, and rosuvastatin—with HMG-CoA reductase.

From Table 5.9, it is evident that the affinity of statin drugs binding to the enzyme falls within the nanomolar range, significantly higher than the natural substrate ($K_m = 4$ μM). This suggests that not all groups in the natural substrate molecule interact effectively with the enzyme, which might be beneficial for the smooth release of the reduction product mevalonic acid. Among them, rosuvastatin has the strongest affinity for HMG-CoA reductase, and its binding free energy is the lowest, followed by atorvastatin.

Typically, due to differences in chemical structures, the contributions of enthalpy and entropy to the binding energy of analogs to the same target vary. It is generally believed that binding mainly driven by enthalpy is characterized by specific interactions, such as hydrogen bonds, electrostatic interactions, and van der Waals forces (shape complementarity). In contrast, binding primarily driven by entropy is often due to hydrophobic interactions and is relatively less specific [24].

Interestingly, when statin drugs are arranged in order of their market release, a trend emerges: newer statin compounds not only show enhanced inhibition of HMG-CoA reductase but also display increasing contributions from enthalpy, suggesting increased specificity in their enzyme binding. For instance, the four representative statins—fluvastatin, pravastatin, atorvastatin, and rosuvastatin—show increasing potencies. Thermodynamic values obtained through isothermal titration calorimetry indicate that fluvastatin's binding is purely entropy-driven, with $\Delta H \approx 0$. Although pravastatin has some enthalpic contribution, it is still entropy-favored. The enthalpic contribution for atorvastatin increases further, while for rosuvastatin, the enthalpic contribution reaches 75.6%. At physiological temperature (37°C), the enthalpy changes for all statin molecules increase, especially for rosuvastatin, where binding is entirely determined by enthalpy.

In fact, the variability in the hydrophobic segments of statin molecules largely determines their different thermodynamic behaviors. The variation in solvent contact surfaces before and after the interaction, represented by the change in solvent-accessible surface area, includes both polar and nonpolar surfaces and reflects the desolvation effect post-interaction. As listed in Table 5.9, different statins have varying polar and nonpolar surfaces when binding to HMG-CoA reductase. On the one hand, atorvastatin and rosuvastatin, when binding to the enzyme, result in a greater burial of solvent-accessible polar surface area (respectively 323 and 341 $Å^2$) than fluvastatin (291 $Å^2$). This increase in polar region burial relates to the ability of statin molecules to form hydrogen bonds in the hydrophobic region, and the number of these bonds thus primarily reflecting the contribution of enthalpy. The stronger and more numerous the hydrogen bonds, the greater the burial of the polar region, and the more significant the contribution of enthalpy during binding.

On the other hand, during binding, the exclusion of solvent (manifested as an increase in solvent entropy) and the reduction in conformational freedom (manifested as a decrease in conformational entropy) are the primary factors causing entropy differences in statin drug binding. For instance, atorvastatin, having the largest hydrophobic region, shows the greatest nonpolar surface area burial (692 $Å^2$). This results in the maximum solvent entropy contribution to atorvastatin's binding. However, the hydrophobic region of atorvastatin also has as many as nine rotatable bonds, leading to a relatively significant loss in conformational entropy. The two effects counteract each other, making the entropy change for atorvastatin not particularly prominent. In contrast, for fluvastatin, which has the fewest rotatable bonds, the increase in solvent entropy clearly outweighs the loss in conformational entropy, making its binding almost entirely entropy-driven.

In summary, a relatively larger hydrophobic region (expanded ring structure) results in more nonpolar interactions, reflecting an increase in the entropy contribution. At the same time, the presence of oxygen (or nitrogen) groups in the hydrophobic region will increase the number of hydrogen bond interactions, reflecting an increase in the enthalpy contribution. This ultimately manifests as an increase in binding free energy, thus enhancing the in vitro activity of the inhibitor.

5.3.4 In vivo structure-activity, structure-metabolism, and structure-toxicity relationships of statin drugs

The chemical structure of drug molecules determines not only their pharmacological activity but also their druglikeness. On the one hand, because drug molecules often bind to targets through multipoint interactions, this means that multidimensional matching between the drug molecule and the target is key to achieving high activity and selectivity. Therefore, the activity of a drug molecule is determined by its detailed structure. On the other hand, the physicochemical properties of a drug molecule, such as its lipophilicity/hydrophilicity, significantly impact in vivo efficacy as well as absorption, distribution, metabolism, excretion, and even safety. The lipophilic/hydrophilic nature of a molecule is determined by its chemical structure. Here, fluvastatin, pravastatin, atorvastatin, and rosuvastatin are used as representative drugs for summarization (Table 5.10) [25–27].

5.3.4.1 Hydrophilicity/lipophilicity and in vivo efficacy, pharmacokinetics, and adverse effects
1. Hydrophilicity/Lipophilicity

   From log$D$ values in Table 5.10, the order of lipophilicity among the four representative compounds is atorvastatin > fluvastatin > rosuvastatin > pravastatin. The presence of a fluorophenyl group in both fluvastatin and atorvastatin gives them decent lipophilicity while also exhibiting varying degrees of hydrophilicity. Due to atorvastatin's larger hydrophobic ring system, its lipophilicity stands out. The presence of a hydroxyl group on pravastatin and a sulfonyl amide group on rosuvastatin makes these two drug molecules exhibit stronger hydrophilicity (with negative log$D$ values).
2. Pharmacological effects

   Because the liver is the main organ for CHL synthesis, the body also needs nonhepatic tissue cells to produce CHL to maintain normal physiological activities. Therefore, the selectivity of HMG-CoA reductase inhibitors for liver tissue is undoubtedly a key factor in achieving their in vivo pharmacological effects and reducing adverse effects. It is also an important indicator for evaluating whether such inhibitors can become effective drugs.

   The liver extraction rates of the four drugs in Table 5.10 are all above 50%, indicating that they have high content in liver tissue, ensuring the exertion of their in vivo pharmacological effects. Consistent with the in vitro enzyme inhibition activity of the drugs, among the four statins, rosuvastatin has the strongest pharmacological effect, with a 63% decrease in low-density lipoprotein CHL (LDL-C) levels at a dose of 40 mg. This is followed by atorvastatin, which can achieve a reduction of 50%.

TABLE 5.10 Hydrophilicity/lipophilicity and human pharmacokinetic characteristics of four representative statin drugs [25,26].

Properties		Fluvastatin	Pravastatin	Atorvastatin	Rosuvastatin
Lipophilicity/ Hydrophilicity	Lipophilic/hydrophilic	Amphiphilic	Hydrophilic	Lipophilic	Hydrophilic
	Solubility in water	2 mg/mL (sodium salt)	19 mg/mL (sodium salt)	0.6 mg/mL (sodium salt)	
	pK_a	4.72	4.31	4.39	4.25
	$logP^a$	3.62	1.44	4.13	0.42
	$logD$ (pH 7.4)^a	1.0 ~ 1.25	−0.84	1.5 ~ 1.75	−0.33
Pharmaceutical effect	Serum LDL-C decreasing (%)*	24	34	50	63
	Serum HDL-C increasing (%)*	8	12	6	10
	Serum TG decreasing (%)*	10	24	29	28
Absorption	Absorptivity (%)	98	34	30	50
	T_{max} (h)*	<1	1 ~ 1.5	1 ~ 2	3 ~ 5
	C_{max} (ng/mL)*	200 ~ 400	45 ~ 66	13 ~ 67	19
	AUC (ng·h/mL)*	320 ~ 570	110 ~ 140	58 ~ 620	176
	Oral bioavailability (%)*	24	17	14	20
Distribution	Protein binding rate (%)*	98	50	98	88
	Hepatic extraction rate (% of absorbed dose)	>70	46 ~ 66	>70	55 ~ 71
Metabolism	CYP_{450} metabolism and isoenzyme	2C9	no	3A4	limited, 2C9
	Active metabolites	no	no	yes	yes(minor)
Excretion	$t_{1/2}$ (h)*	0.5 ~ 2.3	1.3 ~ 2.8	14	19
	Fecal excretion rate (%)*	90	71	70	90
	Renal excretion rate (%)*	6	20	2	10

pK_a is the dissociation constant; $logP$ is the logarithmic value of the oil-water partition coefficient of the octanol-water system, which refers to the distribution equilibrium of the undissociated molecule between the oil phase and the aqueous phase; $logD$ refers to the distribution equilibrium of all forms (ions and molecules) of the compound between the oil phase and the aqueous phase, which is pH-dependent. $LogD$ (pH 7.4) is usually used to express the apparent distribution coefficient of the drug in the intestinal environment; T_{max} is the time to reach the peak concentration; C_{max} is the maximum concentration; *40 mg oral dose.

3. Pharmacokinetics
   a. Absorption: From the pharmacokinetic data in Table 5.10, it can be seen that the four statins are rapidly absorbed after administration, reaching their peak within 4 hours, with absorption rates ranging from 30% to 98%. Pravastatin and rosuvastatin have good water solubility and can quickly dissolve in the gastrointestinal tract, but are not easily transported through passive diffusion across membranes. Therefore, they are mainly actively transported into cells through transporter-mediated pathways. The amphiphilic property of fluvastatin (both lipophilic and hydrophilic) gives it a certain solubility and allows it to pass through membranes by passive diffusion, showing a high absorption rate (98%) in the jejunum. Because the jejunum does not have corresponding transporters, fluvastatin is mainly absorbed into cells through passive transport. Atorvastatin has poor solubility and is mainly absorbed into cells through passive diffusion across membranes. Its permeability in the jejunum is low, resulting in a lower absorption rate. In addition, although the liver extraction rates of all four drugs are high (>46%), their cytochrome P450 (CYP_{450}) metabolic pathways are weak. They are mainly excreted through the bile pathway and feces, and their oral bioavailability is not high (14%−24%).
   b. Distribution: The hydrophilic/lipophilic nature of statins determines the degree of plasma protein binding. Compounds with strong lipophilicity (such as atorvastatin and fluvastatin) are easy to bind to plasma proteins, showing a higher plasma protein binding rate (Table 5.10). If a large amount of drug binds to plasma proteins in the body,

the amount of free drug in the plasma will inevitably decrease, limiting the distribution and accumulation of the drug in peripheral tissues and organs and causing the drug to selectively distribute in the liver tissue. Pravastatin, which has the strongest hydrophilicity, has the lowest plasma protein binding rate (50%); however, due to the lack of effective transporters in peripheral tissues, it cannot enter peripheral tissues and selectively enters liver tissue.

On the other hand, the liver extraction rate of statins also reflects the selective distribution of drugs in the liver to a certain extent. After oral administration, the drug first enters the liver through the portal vein. Whether the drug is extracted by the liver and concentrated in the liver depends on the lipophilicity of the drug. Relatively speaking, the uptake rate of hydrophilic statins by liver cells is lower than that of lipophilic drugs, so their systemic exposure is greater than that of lipophilic drugs.

In summary, regardless of whether statins are hydrophilic or lipophilic, although their ways of entering cells are different, they all have good liver tissue selectivity.

c. Metabolism: Generally, lipophilic statins are more easily metabolized by the CYP_{450} system. Pravastatin and rosuvastatin are relatively hydrophilic drugs, and their metabolism by CYP_{450} enzymes is relatively insignificant. Therefore, they may be safer statins, and because they cannot or only partially be metabolized by the CYP_{450} system, they are mainly excreted in the form of essentially unmodified parent drugs through the renal system.

Atorvastatin is metabolized by CYP_{450}-3A4 and other metabolic enzymes to form hydroxyl and beta-oxidation derivatives, among which the two major primary metabolites—ortho-hydroxy atorvastatin PD152873 and para-hydroxy atorvastatin PD142542—have been identified and exhibit HMG-CoA reductase inhibition activity that is comparable to that of the parent drug. It is precisely because of the persistent presence of these active metabolites that the half-life of atorvastatin in plasma is 14 hours, and the half-life of its inhibition of HMG-CoA reductase in the human body can reach 20–30 hours.

PD152873   **PD142542**

d. Excretion: The plasma half-life of pravastatin, which is derived from fungal metabolites, is relatively short at 1.8 hours. In contrast, the plasma half-lives of fluvastatin, atorvastatin, and rosuvastatin, which are fully synthetic, vary widely from 1.2 to 19 hours, with atorvastatin (14 hours) and rosuvastatin (19 hours) being cleared more slowly from the plasma compared to other statins.

As shown in Table 5.10, the metabolic products of statins are mainly excreted through the bile pathway in the feces, with low renal excretion. Generally, highly lipophilic drugs are reabsorbed by the kidney, and only metabolites that become hydrophilic can be excreted through the renal system.

4. Adverse Effects

Because mevalonic acid and its products, including CHL, play important roles in the formation and maintenance of cellular homeostasis, drugs that inhibit the generation of mevalonic acid and its products at high doses may produce various adverse effects in many different tissues.

Most statins demonstrate good tolerance and safety. However, a small number of patients may experience myalgia due to the effect of statins on muscle tissue. In clinical trials, myalgia occurred in 2%–7% of patients, and this proportion increased with increasing drug dosage, leading to poor adherence to treatment in some patients. The most serious consequence of this side effect is rhabdomyolysis, which can be fatal. The mechanism of statin-induced myalgia is complex, and part of the reason involves statins' ability to inhibit HMG-CoA reductase in extrahepatic tissue (especially in muscle), thereby interfering with the posttranslational modification of proteins (such as isoprenylation) and the biosynthesis of important isoprenoid biomolecules (such as ubiquinone) involved in electron transfer. Evidence suggests that by increasing the liver-targeting specificity of HMG-CoA reductase inhibitors and limiting their exposure to extrahepatic tissues, it may be possible to reduce the likelihood of statin-induced myalgia.

Therefore, achieving selective inhibition of HMG-CoA reductase in the liver is an important direction for the development of HMG-CoA reductase inhibitors [28,29].

Generally, lipophilic statins have greater exposure in extrahepatic tissues, whereas statins with stronger hydrophilicity exhibit greater selectivity for liver tissue. Therefore, from a medicinal chemistry perspective, it is possible to regulate the selectivity of inhibitors for liver tissue by controlling their lipophilicity [30]. This involves introducing enthalpy-driven structural fragments (hydrophilic fragments) into the molecule to reduce its lipid solubility, thereby increasing its liver-targeting selectivity. For example, rosuvastatin (Fig. 5.10), which was marketed after atorvastatin, has a sulfonic acid group in its molecule that interacts electrostatically with arginine at position 568 of the enzyme, significantly increasing the contribution of enthalpy change to free energy change [24]. The presence of a polar methylsulfonyl amino group makes the drug less lipophilic, reducing its passive diffusion ability and making it difficult to enter extrahepatic tissues, thereby demonstrating selective distribution and acting on HMG-CoA reductase in liver tissue cells. Moreover, its relative water solubility also enables it to avoid CYP_{450} metabolism before elimination, greatly reducing the probability of interaction with other drugs.

5.3.4.2 Drug–drug interactions of atorvastatin

Atorvastatin is metabolized by CYP_{450}-3A4 [13,26]. Therefore, when used with other drugs, the possibility of drug–drug interactions should be considered first. When statins must be used in combination with CYP_{450}-3A4 inhibitors, inducers, or substrates, it is recommended to prioritize the use of fluvastatin, pravastatin, rosuvastatin, and pitavastatin to reduce the occurrence of drug-drug interactions.

Specific drug–drug interactions of atorvastatin are as follows:

1. Strong inhibitors of CYP_{450}-3A4: When atorvastatin is used in combination with strong CYP_{450}-3A4 inhibitors, it can lead to an increase in plasma atorvastatin concentration. The degree of interaction depends on the different effects on CYP_{450}-3A4, including the combined use of clarithromycin, protease inhibitors (such as ritonavir and saquinavir), and itraconazole.
2. Grapefruit juice: It contains one or more components that inhibit CYP_{450}-3A4, especially when consumed in excess (more than 1.2 L per day), which can increase the plasma concentration of atorvastatin.
3. Cyclosporine: Atorvastatin and its metabolites are substrates of OATP1B1 transporter. OATP1B1 inhibitors (such as cyclosporine) can increase the bioavailability of atorvastatin.
4. Rifampin or other CYP_{450}-3A4 inducers: Atorvastatin used in combination with CYP_{450}-3A4 inducers (such as efavirenz and rifampin) can lead to a decrease in plasma atorvastatin concentration. Given the interaction mechanism of rifampin, it is generally recommended to administer atorvastatin and rifampin simultaneously. If atorvastatin is given after rifampin, its plasma concentration will be significantly reduced.
5. Digoxin: When multiple doses of atorvastatin and digoxin are used in combination, the steady-state plasma digoxin concentration increases by approximately 20%.
6. Oral contraceptives: When atorvastatin is used in combination with oral contraceptives, it increases the area under the blood concentration-time curve (AUC) of norethindrone and ethinyl estradiol, thereby increasing the exposure of the drugs in the body.

Clinical studies have shown that rosuvastatin is the most effective drug for lowering LDL CHL, followed by atorvastatin. In general, statins are well tolerated, and the incidence of serious adverse events (such as rhabdomyolysis) is low. Understanding the differences between statins can help with clinical rational drug use.

5.3.5 The total synthesis of atorvastatin

The structure of atorvastatin can be divided into two parts: one is a five-substituted pyrrole ring and the other is a 3,5-dihydroxyheptanoic acid side chain with two chiral centers. Therefore, the key to synthesizing this molecule is how to construct the multisubstituted pyrrole ring and introduce two chiral centers on the side chain. Currently, the main methods for synthesizing atorvastatin include the Paal–Knorr synthesis, [3 + 2] cycloaddition, and asymmetric synthesis. These methods involve important organic chemical reactions such as follows:

1. Paal–Knorr pyrrole synthesis reaction

It is a classic pyrrole synthesis reaction that synthesizes pyrrole derivatives from 1,4-dicarbonyl compounds and amine compounds under acidic catalysis. The reaction conditions are mild.

2. Condensation reactions
   a. Aldol condensation reaction: Aldehydes or ketones with α-hydrogen atoms form enolate anions under certain conditions, which then undergo additional reactions with another molecule of carbonyl compound to form β-hydroxy carbonyl compounds. The reaction equation for two aldehyde molecules undergoing this type of reaction is as follows:

   b. Claisen condensation reaction: Esters with α-active hydrogen atoms undergo condensation under strongly basic conditions such as sodium alcohol to lose one molecule of alcohol and form β-keto esters.

   c. Knoevenagel condensation reaction: Compounds with active methylene groups (such as malonate, β-keto esters, cyanoacetate, and nitroacetate) undergo hydroxyl aldehyde condensation and dehydration with aldehydes or ketones in the presence of ammonia, amines, or their carboxylate salts to form α,β-unsaturated compounds.

3. [3 + 2] Cycloaddition reaction (1,3-dipolar cycloaddition reaction)
   It is a type of cycloaddition reaction that occurs between 1,3-dipoles and alkenes, alkynes, or their corresponding derivatives, resulting in a five-membered heterocyclic compound. German chemist Rolf Huisgen first extensively used this type of reaction to prepare five-membered heterocyclic compounds, hence it is also called the Huisgen reaction.

4. Stetter reaction
   Under the catalysis of cyanide or thiazolium salts, aldehyde carbonyl carbons undergo 1,4-addition with α,β-unsaturated compounds, generating 1,4-dicarbonyl compounds and their analogs. This reaction is also known as the Michael–Stetter reaction.

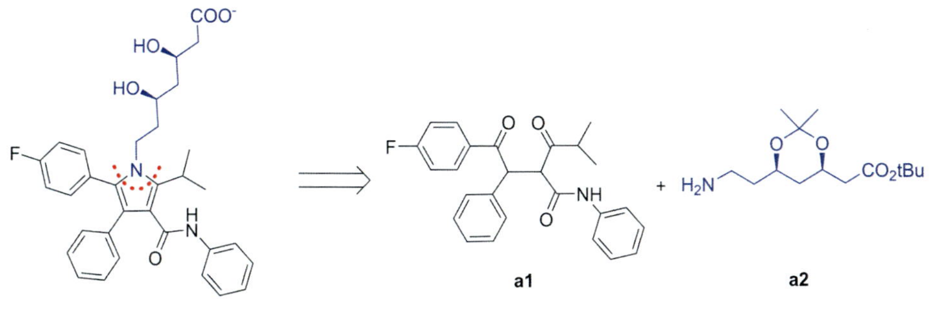

FIGURE 5.13 Retro-synthesis analysis of Paal–Knorr pyrrole synthesis.

5.3.5.1 Paal–Knorr pyrrole synthesis

According to the retro-synthesis analysis shown in Fig. 5.13, atorvastatin can be obtained from intermediates **a1** and **a2** through the Paal–Knorr pyrrole synthesis reaction [31,32].

1. Synthesis of intermediate **a1**

    Starting from isobutyrylacetic acid methyl ester **a1−1** and aniline, isobutyrylacetanilide **a1−2** is obtained via an amine-ester exchange reaction. **a1−2** is then condensed with benzaldehyde through the Knoevenagel reaction to obtain intermediate **a1−3**, which is then subjected to a Stetter reaction to produce the key intermediate **a1** (as shown in the figure below). This route has relatively mild reaction conditions, simple operation, no involvement of hazardous metal reagents, and readily available raw materials. The yield is high, making it a commonly used method for **a1** synthesis.

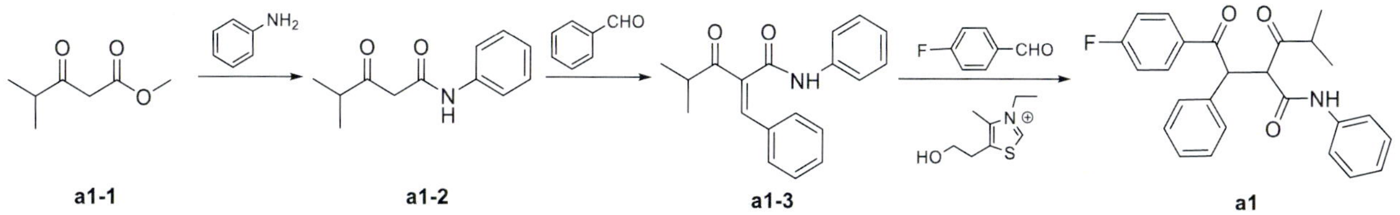

2. Synthesis of intermediate **a2**

    Using chiral reagent **a2−1** and *tert*-butyl acetate as starting materials, intermediate **a2−2** with two additional carbons in the carbon chain is obtained through Claisen ester condensation, and then stereoselectively reduced with NaBH4 to obtain the *erythro*-1,3-diol intermediate **a2−3**. The diol groups of **a2−3** are protected to form **a2−4**, which is then reduced to a primary amine by Raney nickel-catalyzed hydrogenation of the cyano group to obtain intermediate **a2** (as shown in the figure below).

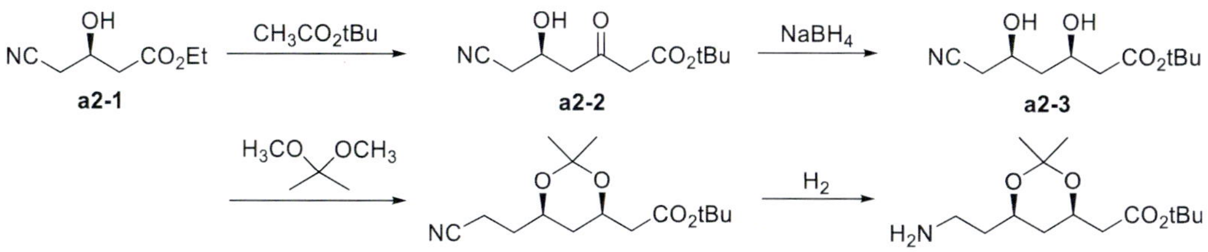

3. Synthesis of the target compound

    Intermediates **a1** and **a2** are refluxed with trimethyl acetic acid as catalyst in a mixed solvent of toluene-*n*-hexane-tetrahydrofuran (1:4:1, volume ratio) to undergo the Paal–Knorr pyrrole synthesis reaction, resulting in the important ring-closure intermediate **a1a2**. After deprotection, atorvastatin can be obtained, which can then be prepared into dosage forms such as calcium salt (as shown in the figure below). This synthetic method has simple operation and high yield and is the most commonly used method in industry. A highly efficient method for converting **a1a2** into high-purity atorvastatin calcium has also been developed, in which ethyl acetate is used for extraction in the preparation of the calcium salt, and after evaporation, a product with a purity exceeding 95% can be obtained [33].

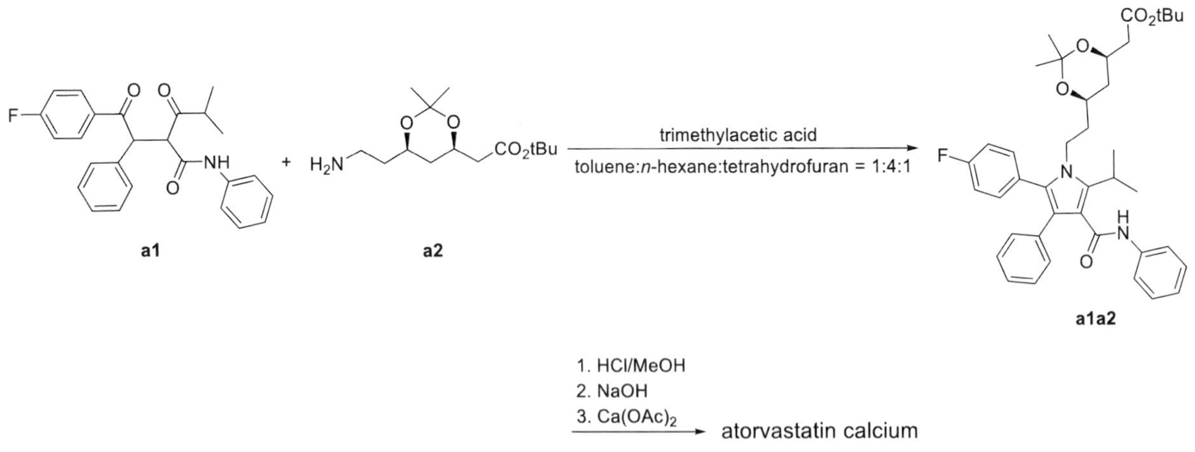

5.3.5.2 [3 + 2] Cycloaddition pyrrole synthesis

The construction of pyrrole rings can also be achieved through [3 + 2] cycloaddition reactions using $-\overset{|}{\underset{|}{C}}=\overset{\oplus}{N}-\overset{\ominus}{\underset{|}{C}}-$ dipoles and alkynes [15], which is shown in Fig. 5.14. Two routes can be taken: one is to construct the target molecule structure through intermediates **b1**, **b2**, and **b3**, and then obtain optically pure target products through chiral separation in the later stage; the other is to first construct chiral intermediate **b4** through chiral introduction, and then obtain the target product through [3 + 2] cycloaddition reaction with alkyne intermediate **b1**.

1. Chiral separation method

    The synthesis of key intermediate **b2** starts with **b2−1**, which reacts with 2-(2-aminoethyl)-1,3-dioxolane to form intermediate **b2−2** through nucleophilic substitution, followed by reaction with isobutyryl chloride to obtain intermediate **b2−3**. Finally, **b2** is obtained through ester hydrolysis.

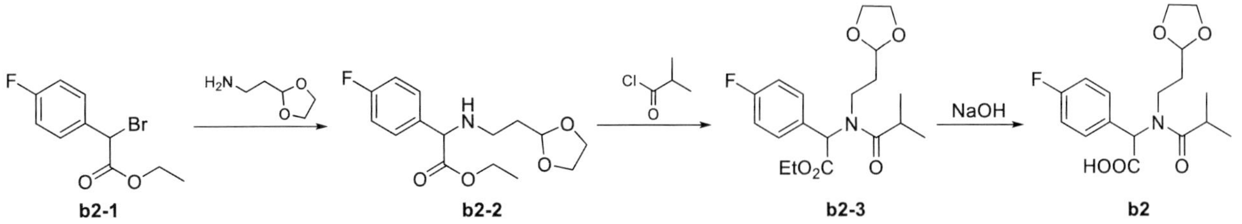

    Alkyne intermediate **b1** undergoes [3 + 2] cycloaddition reaction with **b2** to produce the pentasubstituted pyrrole compound **b1b2−1**, which is then condensed with aldehyde and deprotected to obtain the key intermediate **b1b2−2**. **b1b2−2** undergoes aldol condensation with methyl acetoacetate (**b3**) to produce compound **b1b2b3−1**, which is then reduced with NaBH4 to produce diol compound **b1b2b3−2**. The atorvastatin lactone **b1b2b3−3** with a trans-configuration as the main product (trans: cis = 9:1) is obtained by refluxing with xylene as a solvent, and the almost single trans-configuration product can be obtained after recrystallization with toluene-ethyl acetate. As the trans-configuration product still consists of enantiomers, chiral separation is necessary. (R)-2-methylbenzylamine can be used as a separation agent to obtain a single chiral product **b1b2b3−4**, which can be converted to atorvastatin calcium through the subsequent action of NaOH and CaCl$_2$, as shown in Fig. 5.15. Since this synthetic route is relatively cumbersome and a part of the product will inevitably be lost through chiral separation, the yield is low, and the cost is high.

2. Chiral introduction method

    The chiral introduction method involves placing the [3 + 2] cycloaddition reaction step after the construction of a chiral side chain. This route first involves synthesizing an intermediate **b4** with a chiral side chain. Using 4-fluorophenylacetic acid (**b4−1**) as a starting material, **b4−2** is synthesized via esterification and bromination, which is then substituted with chiral amine **a2** (synthesis route described earlier) to generate **b4−3**. The intermediate

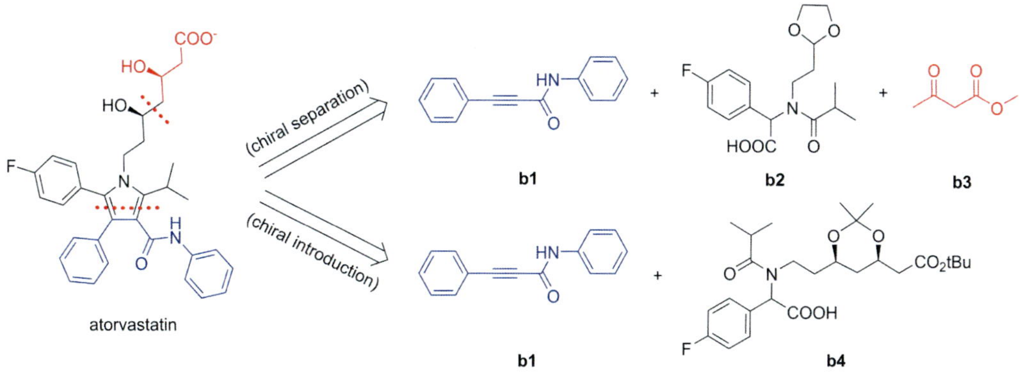

FIGURE 5.14 Retro-synthesis analysis of [3 + 2] cycloaddition pyrrole synthesis.

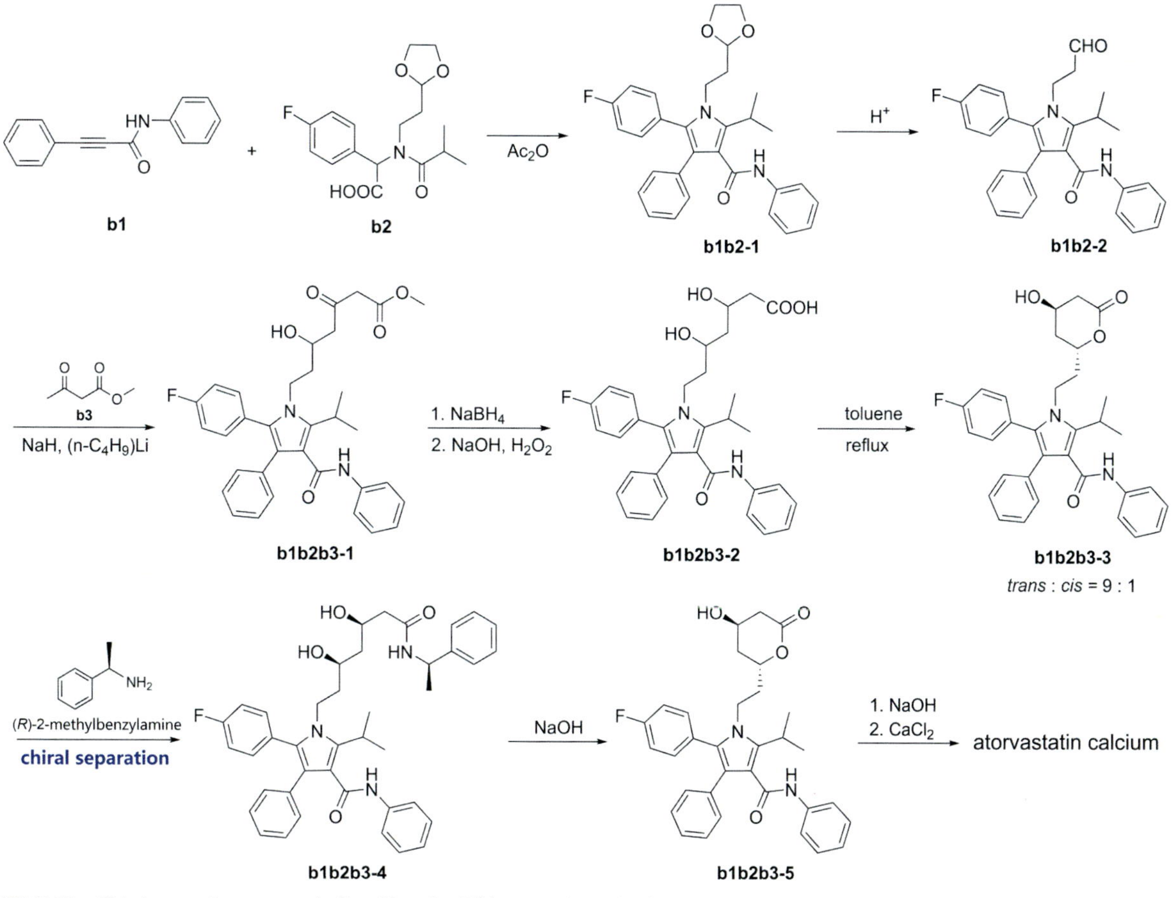

FIGURE 5.15 Chiral separation strategy in [3 + 2] cycloaddition pyrrole synthesis.

is then acylated with isobutyryl chloride to produce amide intermediate **b4−4**, which is further alkaline hydrolyzed to obtain **b4**. The reaction of **b4** with alkyne intermediate **b1** via [3 + 2] cycloaddition produces intermediate **b1b4** (same as **a1a2**). Finally, the deprotection of HCl and NaOH, followed by the reaction with Ca(OAc)$_2$, yields atorvastatin calcium (Fig. 5.16). The disadvantage of this route is that column chromatography purification is required for the preparation of critical intermediate **b4**, which is not conducive to industrial production.

5.3.5.3 Asymmetric side chain synthesis methods

In addition to the two methods mentioned above that focus on the construction of the five-substituted pyrrole ring [34−36], some asymmetric synthesis methods have been developed to address the construction of chiral side chains. Here, we introduce two representative synthetic routes based on the number of carbon units introduced to the chiral

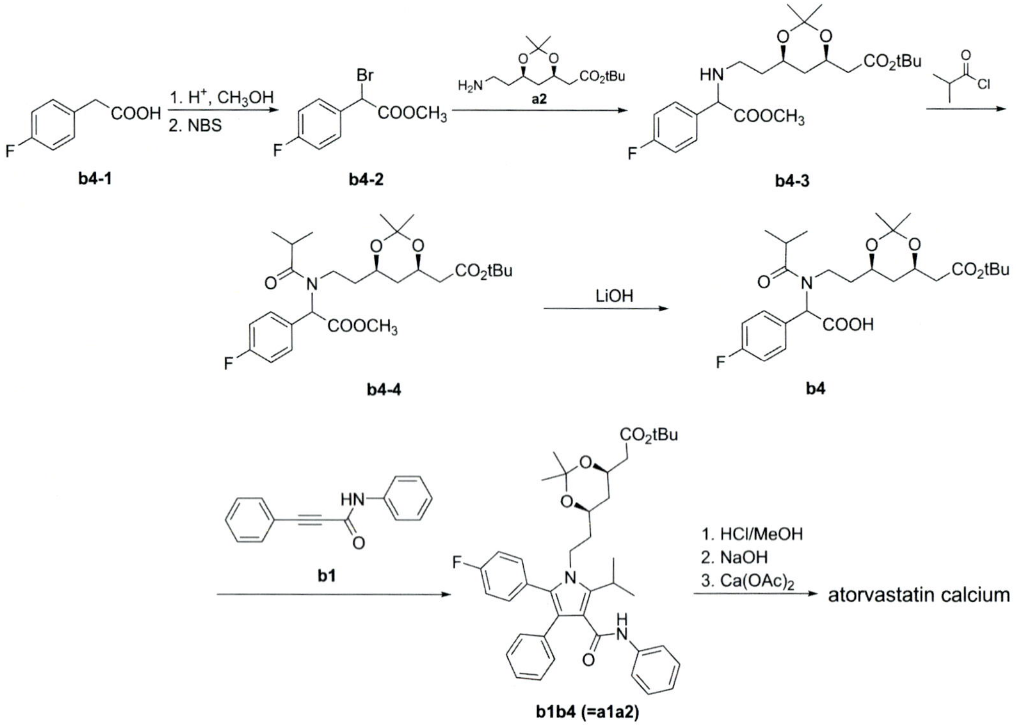

FIGURE 5.16 Chiral introduction strategy in [3 + 2] cycloaddition pyrrole synthesis.

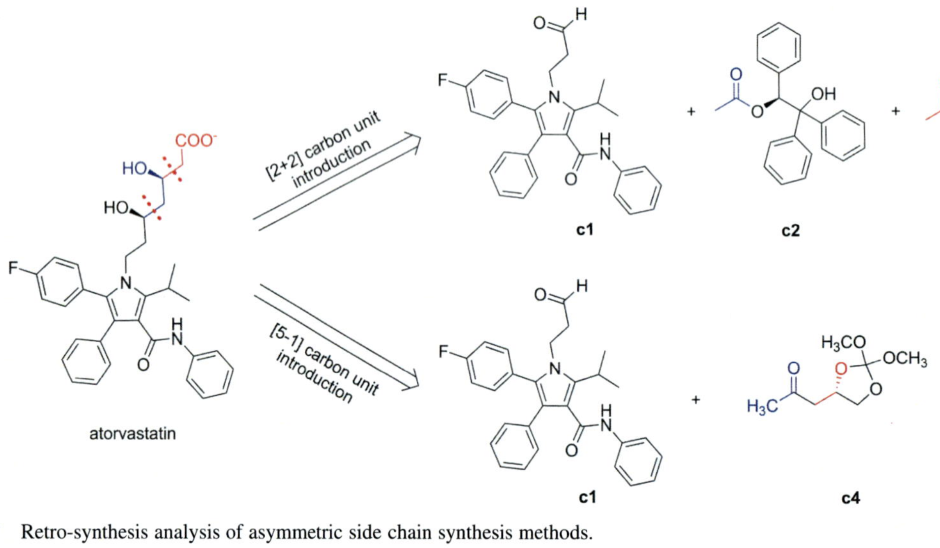

FIGURE 5.17 Retro-synthesis analysis of asymmetric side chain synthesis methods.

center. The retro-synthesis analysis in Fig. 5.17 shows that after obtaining the intermediate **c1** with a five-substituted pyrrole ring, the side chain can be extended and four carbons can be added through asymmetric synthetic means. One route involves introducing two carbons twice separately through intermediates **c2** and **c3**, respectively, while the other involves introducing five carbon atoms at once through intermediate **c4**, followed by removing one carbon atom.

1. [2 + 2] carbon unit introduction method

In this synthesis method, the first step is to synthesize chiral ester **c2**. **c2** can be obtained using an asymmetric synthesis method by reacting acetyl chloride (**c2−1**) with (S)-(+)-1,1,2-triphenyl-1,2-ethanediol (**c2−2**). The chiral intermediate **c1c2−1** with a side chain lengthened by two carbon atoms can be obtained by nonenantioselective aldol condensation of the chiral **c2** with intermediate **c1**, followed by the generation of methyl ester intermediate **c1c2−2** under the action of methanol sodium. Subsequently, Claisen ester condensation reaction with ester **c3** under the action of LDA is performed to obtain intermediate **c1c2c3−1** with a further lengthened side chain by two carbon atoms. The intermediates are then stereoselectively reduced with NaBH4 to generate **c1c2c3−2** with two chiral centers. After ester hydrolysis and $CaCl_2$ treatment, atorvastatin calcium can be obtained (Fig. 5.18). However, this route has poor regioselectivity in the aldol condensation reaction and uses organic lithium reagents, which have harsh conditions and low yields.

2. [5−1] carbon unit introduction method

The key to this method is synthesis of intermediate **c1c4−1**, which has a side chain lengthened by five carbon atoms, through an aldol condensation reaction of pyrrole aldehyde intermediate **c1** with chiral ketone reagent **c4** in the presence of an organoboron reagent to achieve remote 1,5-trans asymmetric induction synthesis. Intermediate **c1c4−2** is obtained by stereoselectively reducing **c1c4−1** with NaBH4, followed by acid hydrolysis and recrystallization to obtain highly optically pure critical intermediate **c1c4−3**. After oxidation and cleavage by sodium periodate, one carbon atom is removed to generate intermediate **c1c4−4**, which is then oxidized by manganese dioxide to obtain atorvastatin lactone. Finally, atorvastatin calcium is obtained (Fig. 5.19). This method has a relatively short synthesis process and a high overall yield.

Of the three representative synthesis methods, the Paal−Knorr pyrrole synthesis method first separately prepares critical intermediates **a1** and **a2** and then obtains optically active atorvastatin calcium through cyclization and deprotection steps. This method has the advantage of being convergent, with independent synthesis steps for **a1** and **a2**, fewer

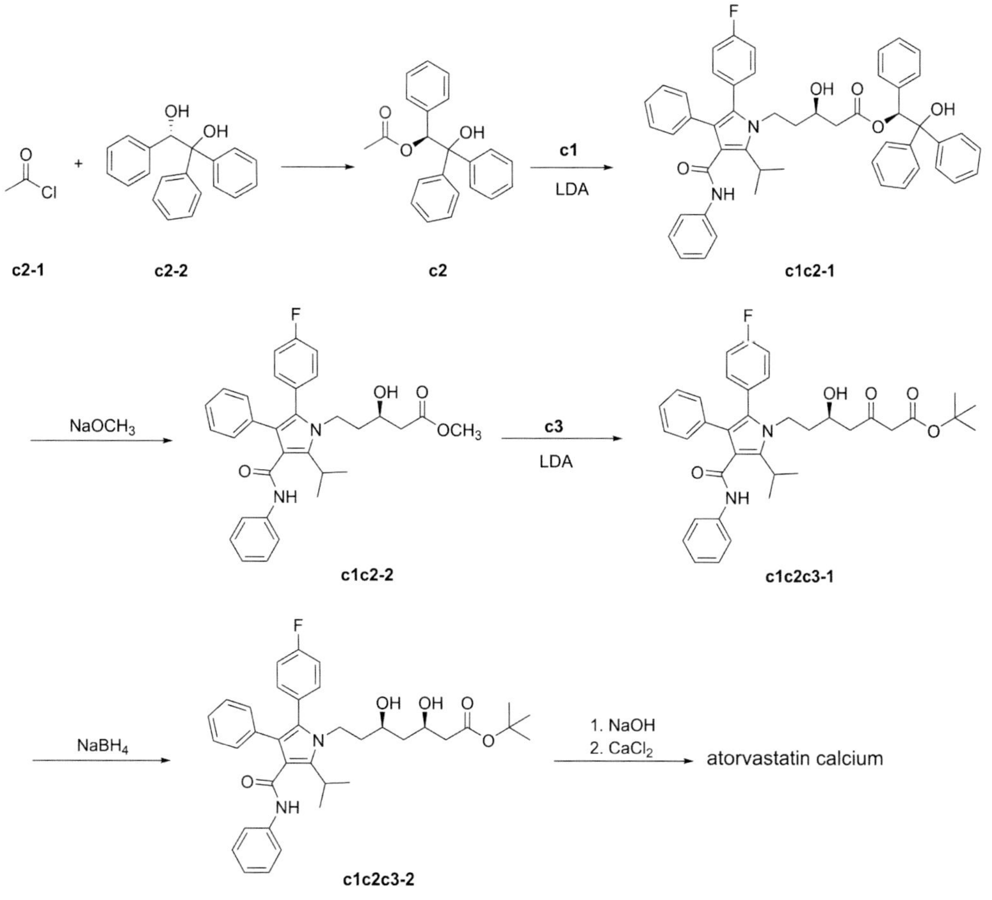

FIGURE 5.18 [2 + 2] carbon unit introduction strategy in asymmetric side chain synthesis methods.

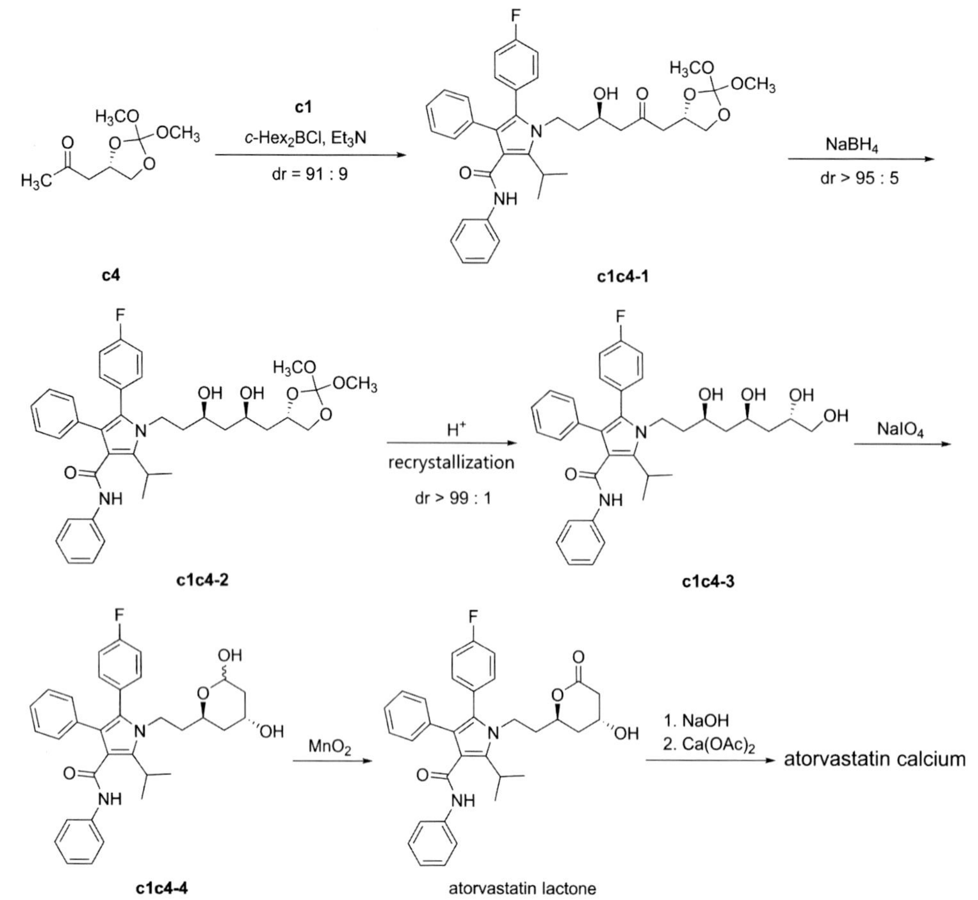

FIGURE 5.19 [5−1] carbon unit introduction strategy in asymmetric side chain synthesis methods.

intermediate steps, and a high overall yield. In the [3 + 2] cycloaddition pyrrole synthesis method, the chiral separation strategy involves a linear synthesis with multiple steps and low yield. Moreover, chiral separation means that some products are wasted, making them unsuitable for industrial production. Although the chiral introduction strategy does not belong to a completely linear synthesis, the synthesis of chiral intermediate **b4** requires more steps and column chromatography separation, which is not conducive to industrial production. The asymmetric side chain synthesis method requires the construction of intermediate **c1** with a five-substituted pyrrole ring first and involves multiple low-temperature reactions, resulting in low conversion yield and making industrialization difficult.

In addition, it is worth mentioning biocatalytic methods. Research has shown that chiral pure critical intermediate (R)-4-cyano-3-hydroxybutyrate can be efficiently synthesized from 4-chloroacetoacetic acid ethyl ester through ketone reductase and halohydrin dehalogenase catalysis, thereby constructing chiral side chain fragments efficiently [37].

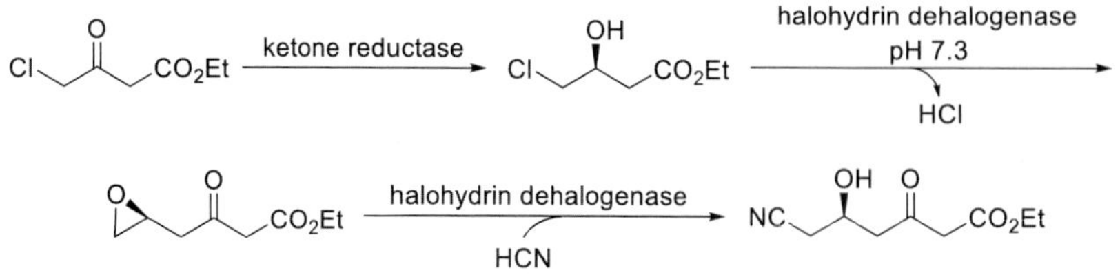

5.4 Summary and outlook
5.4.1 Chapter summary

As lifestyles evolve, there is an ascending trend in the number of patients suffering from hypercholesterolemia. Heart diseases such as atherosclerosis and coronary, emanating from hypercholesterolemia, gravely imperil human health and safety. Statin drugs, by inhibiting the rate-limiting enzyme HMG-CoA reductase in the CHL biosynthesis pathway, reduce CHL synthesis in the liver and consequently lower the levels of LDL-C (bad cholesterol), exerting a lipid-lowering effect. Indeed, the mechanism by which statins reduce LDL-C is much more intricate than merely inhibiting the HMG-CoA reductase enzyme. A salient feature is that these drugs upregulate liver LDL receptors, thus augmenting the clearance of LDL from the plasma.

Atorvastatin, the fifth commercially available statin, is developed under the "fast-follow" or "me-too" paradigm for known targets. Through the relentless endeavors and judicious decisions of pharmaceutical companies, it was unequivocally demonstrated in clinical trials, bolstered by comprehensive data, that Atorvastatin is the paragon within its class.

Atorvastatin was identified during SAR studies of polysubstituted pyrrole derivatives. Early investigations of activity-based small molecule inhibitors elucidated the fundamental principles of enzyme-inhibitor interactions, laying the groundwork for the design of novel inhibitors. The discovery journey of atorvastatin underscores the quintessence of in-depth SAR studies. Concurrently, the elucidation of the structure of inhibitor-enzyme complexes furnishes insights into their interaction modalities, offering theoretical guidance for designing superior inhibitors.

Various methodologies have been developed for the synthesis of atorvastatin. From an industrial manufacturing perspective, considerations include the length of the synthetic route, reaction conditions, yields, and the simplicity or complexity of the preparation processes.

Despite atorvastatin's commendable hepatic selectivity and good tolerability and safety profiles, adverse reactions, such as myalgia, persist. Moreover, given its metabolism via CYP_{450}-3A4, caution is warranted regarding adverse reactions stemming from drug−drug interactions.

5.4.2 Knowledge expansion: novel molecules targeting HMG-CoA reductase

Given the nonnegligible side effects associated with inhibiting other enzymes, HMG-CoA reductase remains a compelling pharmaceutical target in CHL biosynthesis. The pursuit of developing novel inhibitors for this enzyme has not stopped, resulting in emergent molecules with potential therapeutic promise. These entities comprise structurally modified statins and a few novel scaffolds, including terpenoids, sterols, and peptide molecules, but unfortunately, none of these new skeleton molecules can achieve nanomolar levels of inhibitory activity.

5.4.2.1 Novel HMG-CoA reductase inhibitors

1. Statin-based

    The recent discovery of HMG-CoA reductase inhibitors predominantly features statin derivatives [38]. Building upon existing statin structures and modifying specific moieties aims to yield superior compounds. Notably, several literature sources contend that the cyclic form of the statin side chain (lactone prodrug form) is the less active form, while the open-chain (dihydroxypentanoic acid form) possesses higher activity. However, recent in vitro inhibitory studies reveal that the cyclic form of atorvastatin slightly outperforms its open-chain counterpart. Fig. 5.20 delineates two enzyme inhibitors exhibiting greater activity than current drugs, highlighting the introduction of bulky substituents on the existing drug's side chain semialdehyde ring.

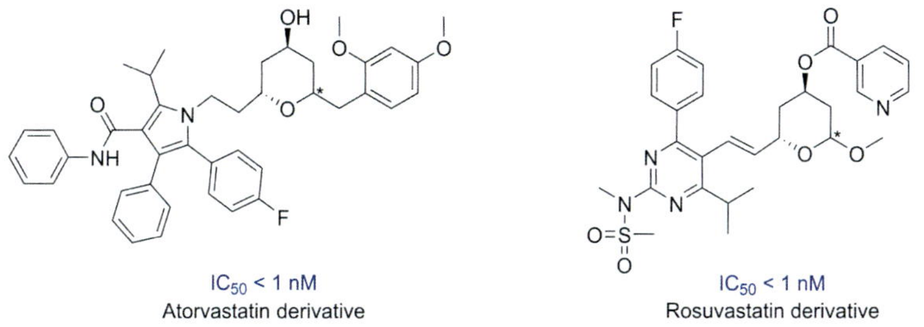

FIGURE 5.20 Chemical structures of potent novel statin molecules.

2. Others

Research corroborates certain natural sterols and pentacyclic triterpenes from plants as moderate inhibitors of HMG-CoA reductase. Fig. 5.21 illustrates the chemical structures of two sterol compounds isolated from rice by Monascus fermentation and the primary component, euscaphic acid, from *Amelanchier alnifolia* berries. Both demonstrate some inhibitory activity against HMG-CoA reductase.

Considering the reduced cardiovascular disease incidence in Asians consuming soy products compared to Western diets, certain enterprises are investigating peptides extracted from plant proteins, which show potential for CHL reduction. Both animal and human clinical studies suggest that soy proteins can lower LDL CHL without affecting high-density lipoprotein CHL (good cholesterol). Some studies posit that the CHL-lowering effects of soy are chiefly attributed to glycinin and β-conglycinin, and the peptides resulting from their proteolytic degradation exhibit CHL-lowering activity. For instance, the 24-peptide LRVPAGTTFYVVNPDNDENLRMIA, derived from glycinin digestion, has been shown to increase LDL uptake in human HepG2 cells by 41%.

5.4.2.2 Combination therapy of statins with other agents

While statins are highly efficacious in CHL reduction, cardiovascular diseases often entail a plethora of complex risk factors. Multifaceted therapeutic interventions are pivotal for effective disease management. For instance, alongside CHL reduction, it is crucial to decrease triglyceride levels, inhibit intestinal CHL absorption, and reduce blood pressure. Studies have demonstrated the benefits of multitarget therapeutic strategies for cardiovascular diseases and other chronic conditions such as type 2 diabetes, viral infections, and cancers. Combining atorvastatin with calcium channel blockers like amlodipine has shown positive outcomes in treating cardiovascular diseases. Drugs paired with statins mainly include omega-3 fatty acids (long-chain polyunsaturated fatty acids) and niacin that reduce blood triglyceride levels by inhibiting diacylglycerol acyltransferase-2, renin-angiotensin system antihypertensive drugs, bile acid sequestrants, CHL absorption inhibitors, PCSK9 inhibitors, platelet aggregation inhibitors, calcium channel blockers, fibrates, panthenols, atherosclerotic plaque emulsifiers, CHL ester transfer protein inhibitors, MTP inhibitors, and more.

5.4.2.3 HMG-CoA reductase degradants

It is observed that statin use leads to a compensatory increase in HMG-CoA reductase due to negative feedback mechanisms [39], which might attenuate the lipid-lowering effects and elevate the risk of adverse reactions. Inspired by CHL intermediates triggering reductase degradation, an alternative strategy targets HMG-CoA reductase inhibition by identifying its degradants, thus reducing its accumulation in vivo, leading to diminished CHL biosynthesis (Fig. 5.22). SAR analysis of sterol analogs unveiled the small molecule HMG449 as a potential effective degradant (its structure is illustrated in Fig. 5.22). This degradant stimulates ubiquitination and degradation of the enzyme, significantly reducing protein accumulation induced by various statins. In mice, HMG449 can act alone or synergize with statins to lower CHL and mitigate atherosclerotic plaque formation. These findings suggest that inducing HMG-CoA reductase degradation through its degradants, either alone or in combination with statins, might be a novel strategy for treating cardiovascular diseases.

The inhibition rate was 29.4% at 80 μg/mL
(The inhibition rate of lovastatin at 80 μg/mL was 54.4%)

The inhibition rate was 31.4% at 100 μg/mL
(The inhibition rate of lovastatin at 40 μg/mL was 42.3%)

The inhibition rate was 91% at 3 μM
(The inhibition rate of 3 μM lovastatin was 100%)

Sterols isolated from rice by monascus fermentation

Euscaphic acid

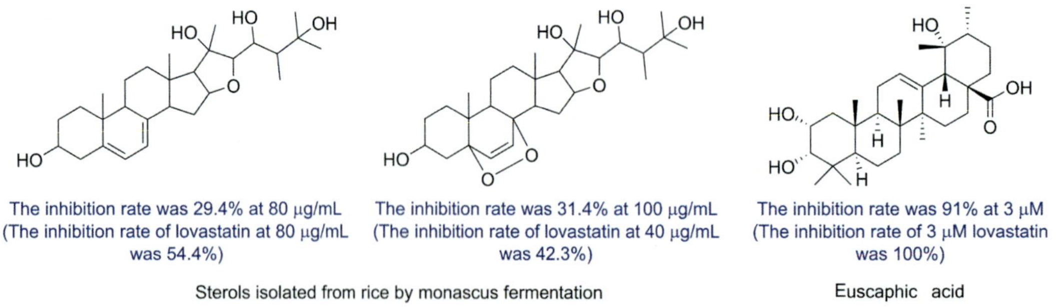

FIGURE 5.21 Chemical structures of natural sterol and triterpene molecules with HMG-CoA reductase inhibitory activity.

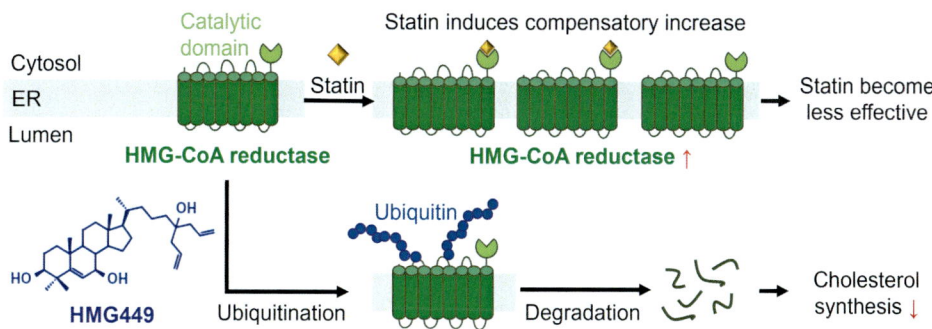

FIGURE 5.22 Mechanism of action of the HMG-CoA reductase degradant HMG449.

5.4.3 Knowledge expansion: additional effects of statins

The inhibition of HMG-CoA reductase not only curtails CHL synthesis in the liver but also disrupts the production of several nonsterol isoprenoid compounds [38,40], which are derived from mevalonate. These include ubiquinones essential in the mitochondrial respiratory chain and isoprenyl groups crucial for protein posttranslational modifications. As these compounds play a pivotal role in the functioning of numerous cell signaling proteins such as Ras, Rac, and Rho, they serve as molecular switches governing a myriad of signaling pathways and cellular functions such as maintenance of cell shape, motility, factor secretion, differentiation, and proliferation. Recent studies have unearthed potential applications of statins in treating an array of disorders, including inflammation, autoimmune diseases, various cancers, diabetes, asthma, bone regeneration, neurodegenerative diseases, and neurodevelopmental disorders.

5.4.3.1 Inflammation and autoimmune diseases

Statins possess extensive antiinflammatory properties across various tissues, inhibiting vascular and myocardial inflammation, effectively controlling vascular and myocardial redox states, and augmenting nitric oxide bioavailability. Some propositions suggest that statins can ameliorate endothelial cell apoptosis, leading to vascular functional alterations and potentially reducing the risk of posttransplant strokes and vascular lesions. Research indicates that combined therapy of statins with antidiabetic agents such as metformin could significantly enhance the treatment outcomes for vascular, autoimmune (such as multiple sclerosis), and inflammatory conditions.

5.4.3.2 Cancer

Recently, statins have been spotlighted as potential prophylactic agents against cancer development. They exhibit prospective therapeutic activity against various cancers, including breast, stomach, pancreas, lung, colorectal, ovarian, prostate, neuroblastoma, melanoma, mesothelioma, and acute myeloid leukemia cells. Their modus operandi encompasses (1) Proapoptotic actions: Inducing cell death across various sensitivity thresholds. (2) Antiangiogenic actions: Downregulating angiogenic factors, inhibiting angiogenesis, and diminishing endothelial cell proliferation; further hindering cellular adhesion by disrupting cell adhesion molecules. (3) Immune modulation: Regulating genes encoding pivotal molecules involved in antigen presentation or downregulating transcription factors closely related to immune modulation, such as NF-κB.

5.4.3.3 Diabetes and metabolic disorders

Type 2 diabetes is characterized by hyperglycemia, insulin resistance (leading to lipid abnormalities), or insulin deficiency. This metabolic disorder, accompanied by hyperlipidemia, culminates in elevated cardiovascular incidents. Since statins primarily act by reducing LDL CHL levels, with minimal effects on other lipoproteins, they are recommended only for diabetic patients with regular LDL CHL levels. Nevertheless, recent studies suggest that statins might harbor risks of inducing diabetes in patients at cardiovascular risk. In 2012, the US FDA revised the safety labels for statins, indicating potential elevations in glycated hemoglobin and fasting blood glucose levels. The adverse effects of statins in diabetes may transpire through various mechanisms, such as downregulating GLUT4 expression on adipocytes, resulting in decreased insulin-mediated cellular glucose uptake.

5.4.3.4 Respiratory disorders such as asthma

Statins exhibit pleiotropic effects in alleviating oxidative stress and inflammation. Research indicates that statins may mitigate airway inflammation in asthmatic patients, especially smokers and obese individuals with a suboptimal response to primary antiinflammatory medications. However, they do not significantly enhance lung function. Recent studies posit that certain combinatorial formulations containing statins might treat respiratory disorders, such as asthma, with rosuvastatin being the preferred drug.

5.4.3.5 Bone regeneration

Another remarkable pleiotropy of statins is their therapeutic potential in bone regeneration, periodontal disease, and bone tissue engineering. During the osteoarthritis progression, statins may act as protective agents against chondrocyte aging and articular cartilage degradation, possibly inhibiting inflammatory arthritis. Some scholars believe statins can inhibit IL-1β induced cartilage matrix degradation by metalloproteinases-1 and -13 and suppress chondrocyte aging. In fact, statins can significantly improve bone turnover and regeneration processes, making them a potential therapeutic strategy for inflammatory-induced cartilage damage in orthopedics, such as osteoarthritis.

5.4.3.6 Neurodegenerative diseases

Statins might exhibit therapeutic effects against neurodegenerative diseases (although epidemiological studies do not support this notion), such as dementia (including Alzheimer's and Parkinson's) as well as neurodevelopmental disorders/autism spectrum disorders (like Rett syndrome, Fragile X syndrome, neurofibromatosis, and tuberous sclerosis). Moreover, statins might possess antidepressant properties. Interestingly, based on the minimal impact of statins on brain CHL levels, this treatment does not compromise other CHL functions.

5.4.4 Knowledge expansion: other cholesterol-lowering drugs and their targets

While statins have made significant strides in managing CHL, they have certain limitations [41]. On one hand, at conventional starting doses (rosuvastatin 5 mg; pravastatin, simvastatin, and atorvastatin 10 mg; and fluvastatin and lovastatin 20 mg), statins can reduce LDL-CHL by 20%~39%. Doubling the dose thereafter only yields an approximate additional 6% reduction, known as the "statin 6 rule." On the other hand, increasing the dosage of statins (excluding rosuvastatin) also heightens the risk of muscle pain and potential liver complications. Therefore, in scenarios where raising the statin dose alone does not achieve therapeutic targets, combination therapy is often necessary to enhance CHL-lowering effects.

Beyond statins, there has been a surge in the development of CHL-lowering drugs targeting other pathways. Based on their mechanism of action, CHL-lowering drugs can be categorized into seven types as follows:

5.4.4.1 HMG-CoA reductase inhibitors

Represented by statins, they can lower LDL-CHL by up to 60%.

5.4.4.2 Intestinal cholesterol absorption inhibitors

Ezetimibe is a prime example (Fig. 5.23), reducing LDL-CHL by approximately 20%. By inhibiting CHL absorption in the intestines, it reduces CHL delivery to the liver, decreases liver CHL content, and upregulates liver LDL receptors. Ezetimibe serves as an effective adjunctive treatment for patients with insufficient statin therapy or those intolerant to statins, with minimal side effects.

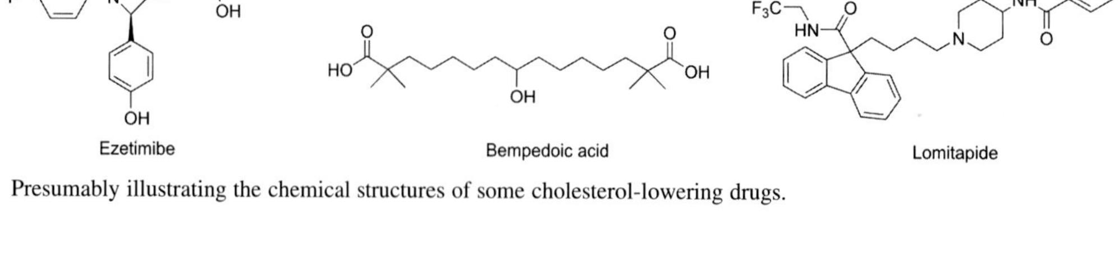

FIGURE 5.23 Presumably illustrating the chemical structures of some cholesterol-lowering drugs.

5.4.4.3 Bile acid sequestrants

These agents can reduce LDL-CHL by 10%~30%. Notable drugs include cholestyramine and colestipol. They primarily work by reducing intestinal bile acid absorption, stimulating CHL to be converted into bile acids, ultimately decreasing liver CHL, and upregulating liver LDL receptors. However, due to decreased absorption of multiple drugs, increased TG, constipation, and other gastrointestinal side effects, their use is limited.

5.4.4.4 PCSK9 monoclonal antibodies

By binding to PCSK9, they can lower LDL-CHL by 50%−60%. PCSK9 is a liver-derived secreted serine protease that lowers LDL receptors on the surface of liver cells by binding to and degrading them, which in turn reduces the ability of liver cells to clear LDL-CHL particles, resulting in CHL being elevated. PCSK9 inhibitors are especially suitable for statin-intolerant, resistant, and FH patients with minimal side effects. Notable drugs are alirocumab and evolocumab.

5.4.4.5 ATP-citrate lyase inhibitors

Bempedoic acid (Fig. 5.23) is a representative drug, capable of reducing LDL-CHL by 15%~25%. In the presence of ATP and HSCoA, ATP citrate lyase catalyzes the cleavage of citric acid into acetyl CoA and oxaloacetic acid, and acetyl CoA is the raw material for the synthesis of fatty acids and sterols. Therefore, during lipid formation, the inhibition of this enzyme actually blocks the upstream of the HMG-CoA reductase. It has demonstrated safety and efficacy, suitable for patients who do not achieve LDL-CHL goals with max-tolerated statin therapy or those intolerant to statins.

5.4.4.6 Apolipoprotein antisense oligonucleotides

Mipomersen is an example. It is an antisense oligonucleotide approved by the FDA for homozygous FH. By targeting the mRNA coding region of apoB-100 protein, mipomersen hinders the translation of apoB-100, which leads to decreased LDL-CHL and total CHL levels while increasing HDL-CHL levels. However, its hepatotoxicity should be noted.

5.4.4.7 Microsomal triglyceride transfer protein inhibitors

Lomitapide is a representative drug (Fig. 5.23). MTTP is a crucial lipid transfer protein in hepatocytes and intestinal cells. Lomitapide directly binds and inhibits MTTP, thereby preventing the assembly of apoB-containing lipoproteins in enterocytes and hepatocytes, inhibiting chylomicron and VLDL synthesis. Lomitapide also carries a risk of hepatotoxicity.

References

[1] Tavormina PA, Gibbs MH, Huff JW. The utilization of β-hydroxy-β-methyl-δ-valerolactone in cholesterol biosynthesis. J Am Chem Soc 1956;78:4498−9.
[2] Liu T-F, Song B-L. Mechanisms of negative feedback regulation of cholesterol biosynthesis. Chin J Cell Biol 2013;35:11−19.
[3] Defesche JC, Gidding SS, Harada-Shiba M, Hegele RA, Santos RD, Wierzbicki AS. Familial hypercholesterolaemia. Nat Rev Dis Prim 2017;3:17093.
[4] Goldstein JL, Brown MS. The LDL receptor. Arterioscl Throm Vasc Biol 2009;29:431−8.
[5] Endo A. A historical perspective on the discovery of statins. Proc Jpn Acad Ser B 2010;86:484−93.
[6] Stossel TP. The discovery of statins. Cell 2008;134:903−5.
[7] Tobert JA. Lovastatin and beyond: the history of the HMG-CoA reductase inhibitors. Nat Rev Drug Discov 2003;2:517−26.
[8] Endo A, Kuroda M, Tanzawa K. Competitive inhibition of 3-hydroxy-3-methylglutaryl coenzyme A reductase by ML-236A and ML-236B fungal metabolites, having hypocholesterolemic activity. FEBS Lett 1976;72:323−6.
[9] Alberts A, Chen J, Kuron G, Hunt V, Huff J, Hoffman C, et al. Mevinolin: a highly potent competitive inhibitor of hydroxymethylglutaryl-coenzyme A reductase and a cholesterol-lowering agent. Proc Natl Acad Sci 1980;77:3957−61.
[10] Guo Z-R. The lipid-lowering drug atorvastatin come from behind and win. Acta Pharmaceut Sin 2017;52:1970−4.
[11] Bai D-L, Shen J-K. Case studies on drug discovery and development − the way from bench to market of star drugs. Chemical Industry Press; 2014. Chapter 4.
[12] Roth BD. The discovery and development of atorvastatin, a potent novel hypolipidemic agent. Prog Med Chem 2002;40:1−22.
[13] Pfizer. Lipitor (atorvastatin calcium) tablets, 2019. accessdata.fda.gov.
[14] Friesen JA, Rodwell VW. The 3-hydroxy-3-methylglutaryl coenzyme-A (HMG-CoA) reductases. Genome Biol 2004;5:1−7.

[15] Roth BD, Blankley C, Chucholowski A, Ferguson E, Hoefle M, Ortwine D, et al. Inhibitors of cholesterol biosynthesis. 3. Tetrahydro-4-hydroxy-6-[2-(1H-pyrrol-1-yl) ethyl]-2H-pyran 2-one inhibitors of HMG-CoA reductase. 2. Effects of introducing substituents at positions three and four of the pyrrole nucleus. J Med Chem 1991;34:357−66.
[16] Roth BD, Ortwine D, Hoefle M, Stratton C, Sliskovic D, Wilson M, et al. Inhibitors of cholesterol biosynthesis. 1. trans-6-(2-pyrrol-1-ylethyl)-4-hydroxypyran-2-ones, a novel series of HMG-CoA reductase inhibitors. 1. Effects of structural modifications at the 2-and 5-positions of the pyrrole nucleus. J Med Chem 1990;33:21−31.
[17] Guo Z-R. Enthalpy and entropy in drug optimization. Chin J Med Chem 2012;22:310−22.
[18] Istvan ES, Deisenhofer J. Structural mechanism for statin inhibition of HMG-CoA reductase. Science 2001;292:1160−4.
[19] Bocan TM, Ferguson E, Mcnally W, Uhlendorf PD, Mueller SB, Dehart P, et al. Hepatic and nonhepatic sterol synthesis and tissue distribution following administration of a liver selective HMG-CoA reductase inhibitor, CI-981: comparison with selected HMG-CoA reductase inhibitors. Biochim Biophys Acta (BBA)-Lipids Lipid Metab 1992;1123:133−44.
[20] Auerbach BJ, Krause BR, Bisgaier CL, Newton RS. Comparative effects of HMG-CoA reductase inhibitors on apo B production in the casein-fed rabbit: atorvastatin versus lovastatin. Atherosclerosis 1995;115:173−80.
[21] Krause BR, Newton RS. Lipid-lowering activity of atorvastatin and lovastatin in rodent species: triglyceride-lowering in rats correlates with efficacy in LDL animal models. Atherosclerosis 1995;117:237−44.
[22] Istvan ES, Palnitkar M, Buchanan SK, Deisenhofer J. Crystal structure of the catalytic portion of human HMG-CoA reductase: insights into regulation of activity and catalysis. EMBO J 2000;19:819−30.
[23] Carbonell T, Freire E. Binding thermodynamics of statins to HMG-CoA reductase. Biochemistry 2005;44:11741−8.
[24] Guo Z-R. The first in class drug lovastatin and its successors. Acta pharmaceutica Sin 2015;50:123−6.
[25] Li D-D, Tao T. Influence of chemical structures and physicochemical properties of statins on their pharmacodynamics and pharmacokinetics. Chin J Pharm 2012;43:497−502.
[26] Schachter M. Chemical, pharmacokinetic and pharmacodynamic properties of statins: an update. Fundament Clin Pharmacol 2005;19:117−25.
[27] Murphy C, Deplazes E, Cranfield CG, Garcia A. The role of structure and biophysical properties in the pleiotropic effects of statins. Int J Mol Sci 2020;21:8745.
[28] Sarver RW, Bills E, Bolton G, Bratton LD, Caspers NL, Dunbar JB, et al. Thermodynamic and structure guided design of statin based inhibitors of 3-hydroxy-3-methylglutaryl coenzyme A reductase. J Med Chem 2008;51:3804−13.
[29] Singh N, Tamariz J, Chamorro G, Medina-Franco JL. Inhibitors of HMG-CoA reductase: current and future prospects. Mini Rev Med Chem 2009;9:1272−83.
[30] Hamelin BA, Turgeon J. Hydrophilicity/lipophilicity: relevance for the pharmacology and clinical effects of HMG-CoA reductase inhibitors. Trends Pharmacol Sci 1998;19:26−37.
[31] Baumann KL, Butler DE, Deering CF, Mennen KE, Millar A, Nanninga TN, et al. The convergent synthesis of CI-981, an optically active, highly potent, tissue selective inhibitor of HMG-CoA reductase. Tetrahedron Lett 1992;33:2283−4.
[32] Brower PL, Butler DE, Deering CF, Le TV, Millar A, Nanninga TN, et al. The synthesis of (4R-cis)-1, 1-dimethylethyl 6-cyanomethyl-2, 2-dimethyl-1, 3-dioxane-4-acetate, a key intermediate for the preparation of CI-981, a highly potent, tissue selective inhibitor of HMG-CoA reductase. Tetrahedron Lett 1992;33:2279−82.
[33] Novozhilov YV, Dorogov MV, Blumina MV, Smirnov AV, Krasavin M. An improved kilogram-scale preparation of atorvastatin calcium. Chem Cent J 2015;9:1−4.
[34] Dias LC, Vieira AS, Barreiro EJ. The total synthesis of calcium atorvastatin. Org Biomol Chem 2016;14:2291−6.
[35] Lee HT, Woo PW. Atorvastatin, an HMG-COA reductase inhibitor and effective lipid-regulating agent. Part II. Synthesis of side-chain-labeled [14C] atorvastatin. J Label Compd Radiopharm Off J Int Isotope Soc 1999;42:129−33.
[36] Braun M, Devant R. (R)-and (S)-2-acetoxy-1, 1, 2-triphenylethanol-effective synthetic equivalents of a chiral acetate enolate. Tetrahedron Lett 1984;25:5031−4.
[37] Fox RJ, Davis SC, Mundorff EC, Newman LM, Gavrilovic V, Ma SK, et al. Improving catalytic function by ProSAR-driven enzyme evolution. Nat Biotechnol 2007;25:338−44.
[38] Oliveira EF, Santos-Martins D, Ribeiro AM, Brás NF, Cerqueira NS, Sousa SF, et al. HMG-CoA Reductase inhibitors: an updated review of patents of novel compounds and formulations (2011-2015). Expert Opin Ther Pat 2016;26:1257−72.
[39] Jiang S-Y, Li H, Tang J-J, Wang J, Luo J, Liu B, et al. Discovery of a potent HMG-CoA reductase degrader that eliminates statin-induced reductase accumulation and lowers cholesterol. Nat Commun 2018;9:5138.
[40] Bifulco M, Endo A. Statin: new life for an old drug. Pharmacol Res 2014;88:1−2.
[41] Kenneth R, Feingold M. Cholesterol lowering drugs, 2024. https://www.ncbi.nlm.nih.gov/books/NBK395573/.

Chapter 6

Angiotensin II receptor antagonists for treatment of hypertension: the discovery of losartan and its analogs

Jianmin Fu
Pharmaron Beijing Co., Ltd., BDA, Beijing, P.R. China

Chapter outline

6.1 Brief introduction of hypertension and commonly used medications for the treatment of hypertension	109
6.2 The renin-angiotensin system	110
6.3 Angiotensin II receptor antagonists	113
6.4 Discovery of losartan	114
6.4.1 Evolution of lead compounds in the early stage	114
6.4.2 Lead optimization	116
6.4.3 Discovery of losartan	117
6.4.4 Metabolites of losartan and its corresponding pro-drugs	123
6.4.5 The safety profile of losartan	125
6.4.6 The properties and actions of losartan	127
6.4.7 The synthesis of losartan	128
6.4.8 Brief summary of the discovery of losartan	130
6.5 Discovery of losartan analogs	131
References	136

6.1 Brief introduction of hypertension and commonly used medications for the treatment of hypertension

Hypertension is a common chronic disease characterized by persistently high arterial blood pressure above normal levels. The situation in China is similar to the global scenario, with approximately one out of three adults being affected by hypertension. Additionally, one out of four deaths is attributed to high blood pressure. Hypertension can also lead to complications such as cerebrovascular diseases, ischemic heart disease, and heart and kidney failures. It is evident that hypertension is a major disease directly impacting human health and quality of life. Therefore, finding new drugs for the treatment and control of hypertension remains a driving force for the global community.

Blood pressure measurement is important in diagnosing and monitoring hypertension. By measuring blood pressure, we can determine whether a person's blood pressure is normal. Using a blood pressure monitor is a standard method for measurement. Through the measurement, a physician will provide us with the maximum and minimum values of the blood pressure. The maximum value represents the systolic pressure (high pressure), while the minimum value represents the diastolic pressure (low pressure). More than two thousand years ago, our wise ancestors described the phenomenon of elevated arterial pressure in the "Huangdi Neijing". It stated, "By measuring the size, observing the floating and sinking, and assessing the smoothness and frequency, one can understand the origin of the disease. Treatment should not go beyond what is necessary, while diagnosis should be accurate. By examining the balance of yin and yang and distinguishing between softness and hardness, one can understand the heart, which is the source of life, and the transformation of spirit. Its radiance is reflected on the face, and its abundance is manifested in the blood vessels. Therefore, excessive consumption of salty food leads to a thickened and discolored pulse." This historical perspective highlights the long-standing interest in understanding and managing health conditions such as hypertension. The modern history of hypertension research began with the understanding of the cardiovascular system, based on the description of the circulatory system in William Harvey's book "De Motu Cordis" (On the Motion of the Heart and Blood). In 1733, the British clergyman Stephen Hales

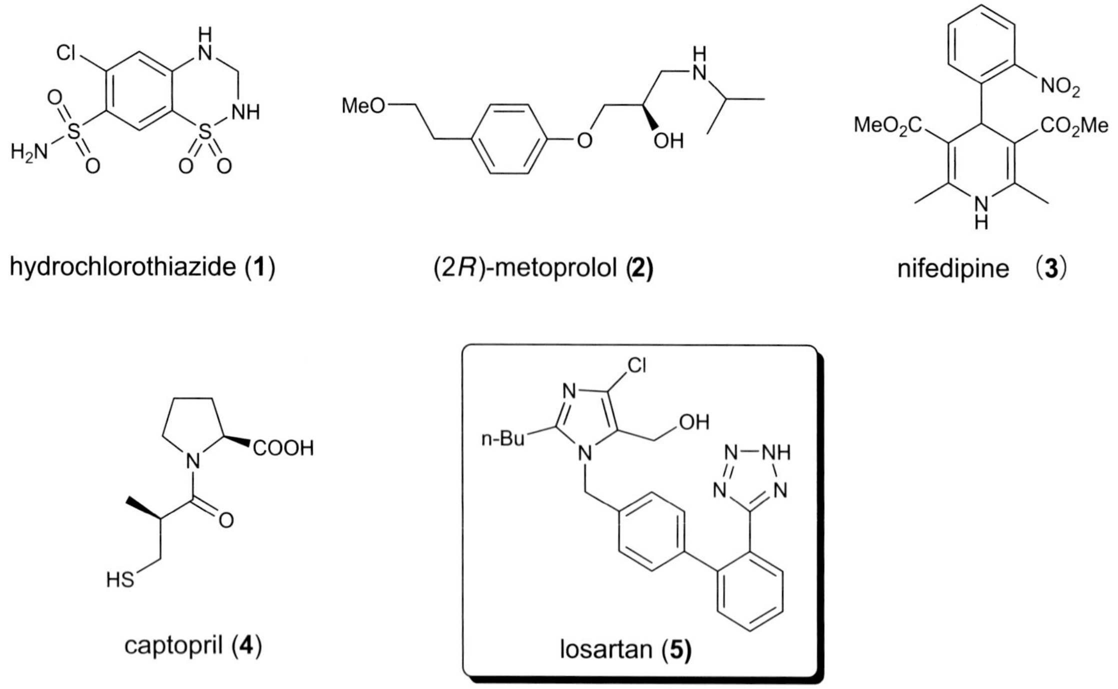

FIGURE 6.1 Structures of commonly used medications for the treatment of hypertension.

published the first blood pressure measurements. Later, the French physician Jean Louis Marie Poiseuille constructed a glass tube filled with mercury to measure blood pressure, which was modified into the armband sphygmomanometer by Italian doctor Scipione Riva-Rocci. Finally, the Russian physician Nikolai Korotkoff was the first to use a stethoscope as an aid in measuring blood pressure, allowing for the measurement of systolic and diastolic pressures. This method of blood pressure measurement, known as the Korotkoff sounds, has been used ever since. These advancements in understanding and measuring blood pressure have played a crucial role in diagnosing and managing hypertension and monitoring the effectiveness of treatment interventions.

For most adults, normal blood pressure falls between 100–130 mmHg systolic and 60–80 mmHg diastolic. Without the use of any antihypertensive medications, a diagnosis of hypertension is made if blood pressure measurements on three separate occasions (not on the same day) are consistently higher than the normal range, specifically systolic blood pressure ≥ 140 mmHg and/or diastolic blood pressure ≥ 90 mmHg. Based on the magnitude of blood pressure elevation, hypertension can be categorized into three risk levels: Level 1 hypertension: blood pressure ranging from 140–159 mmHg systolic and/or 90–99 mmHg diastolic. This is considered low-risk. Level 2 hypertension: blood pressure ranging from 160–179 mmHg systolic and/or 100–109 mmHg diastolic. This is categorized as moderate risk (or Level 1 hypertension with the presence of 1–2 other risk factors). Level 3 hypertension: blood pressure ≥ 180 mmHg systolic and/or ≥ 110 mmHg diastolic. This is considered-high risk (or Level 1 or 2 hypertension with the presence of ≥ 3 other risk factors). These classifications effectively help healthcare professionals assess the severity of hypertension and guide treatment decisions to manage and reduce the associated risks.

The first-line medications for treating hypertension can be classified into five categories (Fig. 6.1): (1) thiazide diuretics (e.g., hydrochlorothiazide (**1**)); (2) β-blockers (e.g., metoprolol (**2**)); (3) calcium channel blockers (e.g., nifedipine (**3**)); (4) angiotensin-converting enzyme (ACE) inhibitors (e.g., captopril (**4**)); and (5) angiotensin II receptor blockers (ARBs) (e.g., losartan (**5**)). This chapter will focus on the discovery and development of the fifth category, ARBs, which includes the first Ang II receptor blocker introduced to the market, losartan, as well as other similar drugs within the sartan class.

6.2 The renin-angiotensin system

In 1897, Professor Robert Tigerstedt, a physiologist at the Karolinska Institute in Sweden, along with his student Per Bergman, found that injecting extracts from the kidneys into rabbits caused a significant increase in blood pressure. Based on this observation, they hypothesized that the kidneys produce a protein named "renin" that raises blood pressure, thereby initiating research into the relationship between renin and hypertension. Later experiments confirmed that renin is an aspartic protease; it plays a pivotal role as the initiating enzyme in the renin-angiotensin system (RAS), which affects the elevation of blood pressure. In humans, renin cleaves a series of cascading peptide bonds, ultimately regulating the frequency of extracellular fluid (plasma, lymph, and interstitial fluid) and arterial vasoconstriction. The resulting effects help regulate the average arterial blood pressure [1].

As shown in Fig. 6.2, (1) when blood pressure decreases, the kidneys start secreting renin. Its function is to cleave its currently known substrate, angiotensinogen, which is produced in the liver, leading to the formation of a decapeptide called angiotensin I (Ang-I). This step is considered rate-limiting in the process. (2) The biologically inactive Ang-I is further cleaved by an enzyme called ACE, which is produced in the lungs, into the endogenous octapeptide angiotensin II (Ang-II) [2].

In humans, four subtypes of angiotensin receptors have been discovered, including angiotensin type 1 receptor (AT1), angiotensin type 2 receptor (AT2), angiotensin type 3 receptor (AT3), and angiotensin type 4 receptor (AT4). AT1 receptors have the highest expression in humans, while AT2 receptors have lower levels. Currently, there is limited understanding of AT3 and AT4 receptors. When Ang-II binds to AT1 receptors, it initiates a series of physiological effects, such as vasoconstriction and the reabsorption of sodium and water by the kidneys. These actions increase fluid volume and ultimately lead to a net increase in blood pressure. Ang-II can also bind to AT2 receptors, leading to cell

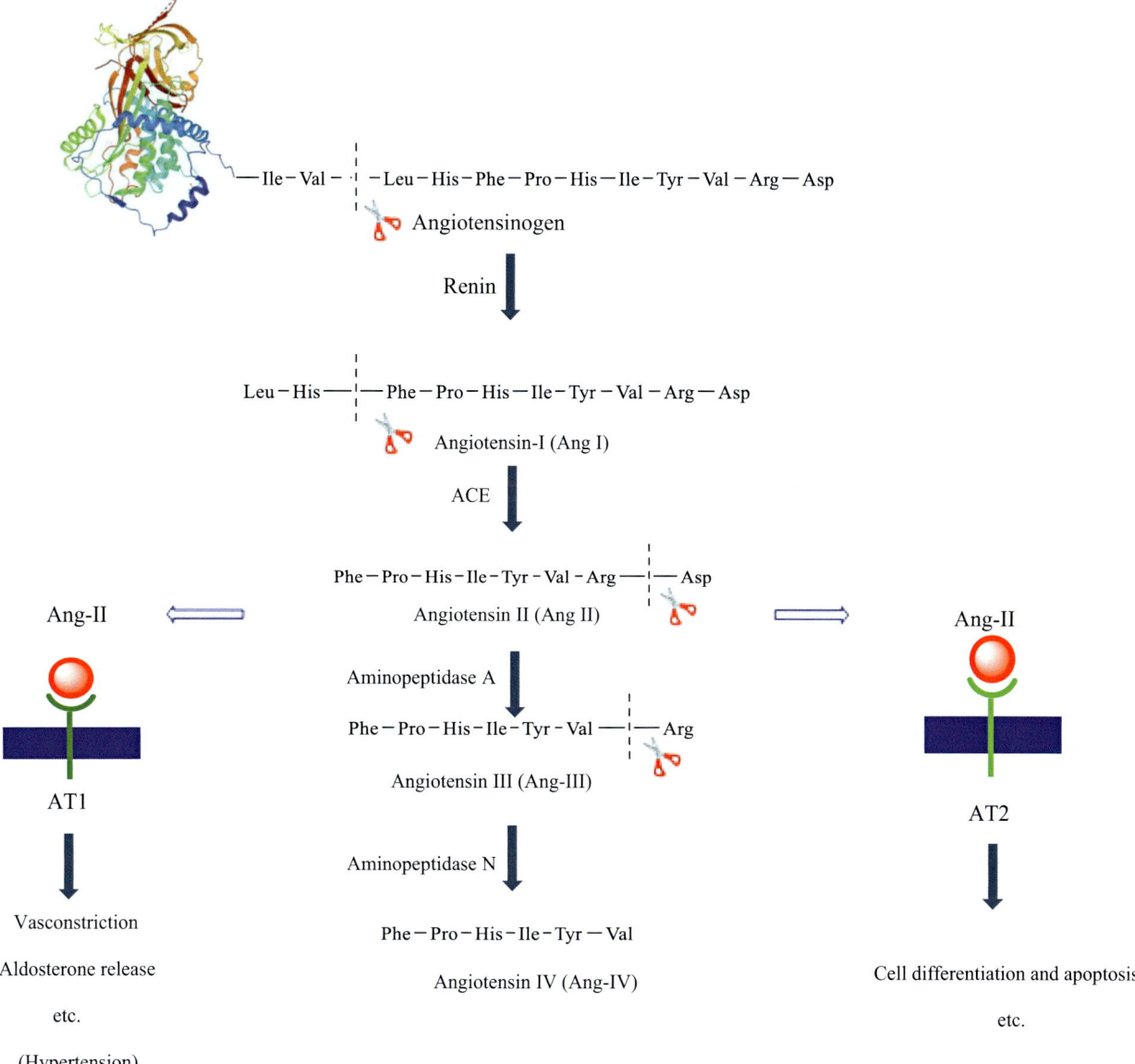

FIGURE 6.2 The relationship between the renin-angiotensin system (RAS) and the elevation of blood pressure.

differentiation and apoptosis. It may also have vasodilatory effects. In addition, AT2 receptors have been studied as a therapeutic target for the treatment of idiopathic pulmonary fibrosis [3]; this topic is out of the scope of the current discussion. Recent studies have found that Ang-II can be further cleaved by aminopeptidase A into angiotensin III (Ang-III) and then by aminopeptidase N into angiotensin IV (Ang-IV). Ang-III and Ang-IV are associated with central nervous system diseases. Currently, research on Ang-III and Ang-IV is still in the early stages.

In the 1970s, researchers began studies using small-molecule inhibitors of the RAS to reduce blood pressure. After 30 years of relentless efforts, they finally discovered a peptide-like drug called aliskiren (Fig. 6.3, **6**), with a certain degree of oral bioavailability [4]. This drug was discovered by Novartis and was approved in 2007. It is currently the only renin inhibitor used for treating hypertension. However, its adverse effects on the kidneys have limited its use, especially for patients with type 2 diabetes.

Along with the research on renin inhibitors, scientists also began to develop ACE inhibitors [5]. Initially, it was found that components isolated from the venom of the South American lancehead snake could lower blood pressure by inhibiting ACE. Inspired by this discovery, scientists developed a series of ACE inhibitors [6]. The first drug, captopril (Fig. 6.1, **4**), was approved for the treatment of hypertension in 1980 [7]. This was followed by the introduction of enalapril in 1984 [8]. Subsequently, thirteen other similar drugs were developed. Table 6.1 lists the name and launch time of a series of ACE inhibitors. These drugs have achieved tremendous success in treating hypertension and congestive heart failure.

Although ACE inhibitors can be used to treat or control hypertension, they still cannot achieve satisfactory treatment results. Scientists have also noted that ACE is a nonspecific protease that can also degrade bradykinin and other peptides, such as substance P and enkephalin (Fig. 6.4).

When ACE is inhibited, the degradation of these related peptides is reduced, leading to their accumulation in the body. Therefore, the use of ACE inhibitors can cause some adverse effects [9]. For example, in the hypertensive population being treated with ACE inhibitors, approximately 5% to 10% of patients experience dry cough and rare angioedema, both of which are caused by the increased accumulation of bradykinin in the body [10]. A recent study has revealed that the use of ACE inhibitors may also increase the incidence of lung cancer [11]. Data shows that the risk of developing cancer increases by 22% in patients taking ACE inhibitors for 5 years and by 31% in hypertensive patients taking them for 10 years. Although there is currently no definitive scientific evidence directly linking the use of ACE inhibitors to the incidence of lung cancer, the results of this investigation are enough to sound the alarm for patients

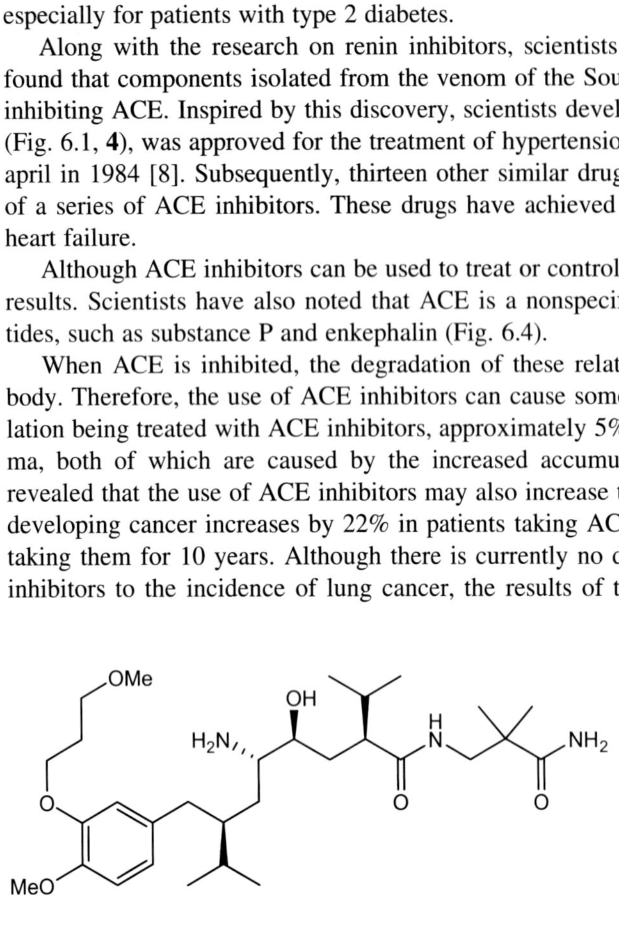

FIGURE 6.3 Structure of aliskiren (**6**).

aliskiren (**6**)

TABLE 6.1 Name and launched time of a list of ACE inhibitors.

Name	Launched time	Name	Launched time	Name	Launched time
Captopril	1980	Ramipril	1989	Trandolapril	1993
Enalapril	1984	Benazepril	1990	Temocapril	1994
Lisinopril	1987	Cilazapril	1990	Spirapril	1995
Perindopril	1988	Fosinopril	1991	Moexipril	1995
Quinapril	1989	Imidapril	1993	Zofenopril	2000

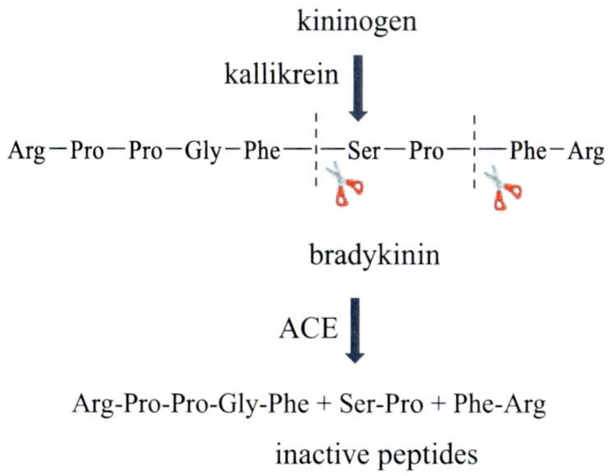

kininogen

kallikrein ↓

Arg—Pro—Pro—Gly—Phe—┆—Ser—Pro—┆—Phe—Arg

bradykinin

ACE ↓

Arg-Pro-Pro-Gly-Phe + Ser-Pro + Phe-Arg

inactive peptides

FIGURE 6.4 The conversion of bradykinin by ACE.

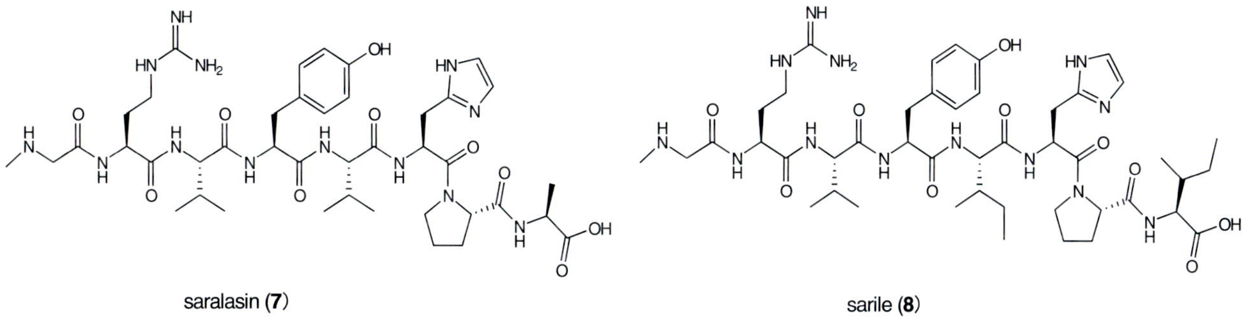

saralasin (**7**)

sarile (**8**)

FIGURE 6.5 Structures of saralasin (**7**) and sarile (**8**).

who continue to take ACE inhibitors to lower their blood pressure. It is worth mentioning that in the RAS, ACE converts Ang I into Ang II. However, research has also found that chymase CAGE (chymostatin-sensitive angiotensin II-generating enzyme), cathepsin G, and elastase can also generate angiotensin II, apart from ACE.

6.3 Angiotensin II receptor antagonists

The above issue prompted researchers to think about whether it is possible to achieve selective inhibition of downstream processes in the RAS, such as blocking the activation of Ang II receptors, without affecting ACE. This could potentially help avoid adverse effects caused by increased levels of bradykinin, such as dry cough or angioedema, during the use of Ang II receptor antagonists [12]. In fact, research on Ang II receptor antagonists began even before the emergence of ACE inhibitors. In 1971, through modifications to the peptide structure of Ang II, researchers discovered saralasin (**7**) and sarile (**8**) (Fig. 6.5). These two peptides were compounds obtained by chemically modifying the terminals of Ang II and exhibited antagonistic effects on Ang II receptors. As the first specific peptide antagonists of Ang II [13], although both saralasin and sarile reduced arterial pressure in hypertensive patients in clinical trials, their therapeutic potential was greatly limited due to poor oral bioavailability, short duration of action, and significant Ang II-like stimulatory properties [14].

In the 1960s and 1970s, significant efforts had been devoted to discovering nonpeptide Ang II receptor antagonists, but the results were minimal. It was not until 1982 that Takeda Chemical Industries, Ltd. disclosed a series of imidazole-5-acetic acid derivatives (Fig. 6.6, **9**, and **10**) with Ang II antagonistic activity in two patents [15]. These imidazole-5-acetic acids were initially used for studying their antiinflammatory effects but were unexpectedly found to possess antagonistic activity against Ang II receptors. Although there was no information about the selectivity of these compounds at that time, it marked the beginning of a new era in the research of nonpeptide Ang II receptor antagonists. Since then, a series of nonpeptide small molecule Ang II receptor antagonists have been developed for the treatment of hypertension, and through these drug molecules, researchers have gained a thorough understanding of the mechanisms by which the RAS affects blood pressure at various stages.

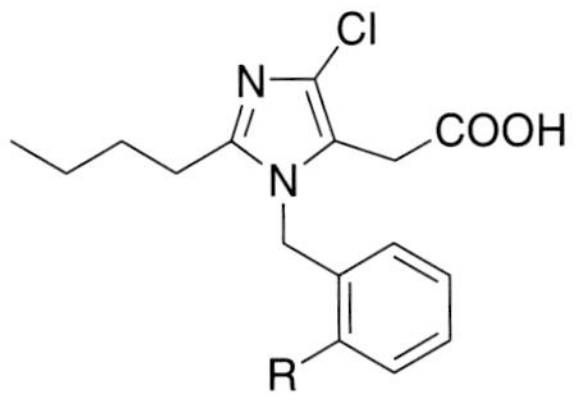

R = H (**9**) , R = Cl (**10**)

FIGURE 6.6 Structures of hit compounds discovered at Takeda.

6.4 Discovery of losartan

6.4.1 Evolution of lead compounds in the early stage

The former DuPont Pharmaceuticals (now part of Bristol Myers Squibb) was a pioneer in the discovery of nonpeptide small-molecule Ang II receptor antagonists. Losartan (Fig. 6.1, **5**) was the first nonpeptide small-molecule Ang II receptor antagonist to be successfully marketed for the treatment of hypertension.

In the early 1980s, when DuPont Pharmaceuticals began to search for Ang II receptor antagonists, the ACE inhibitor captopril had just been introduced to the market. Captopril was designed based on the peptide structure of ACE. Naturally, inspired by this, the initial strategy for designing Ang II receptor antagonists also started with the modification of the peptide structure of Ang II, attempting to find small peptide molecules with fewer than four amino acid residues (which are not easily degraded by gastric proteases). However, over the course of about a year, the synthesized short peptides did not exhibit significant biological activity. It was later proven that maintaining peptide molecules with activity equivalent to Ang II requires at least six to eight amino acid residues, making it difficult to meet the requirements for developing orally bioavailable nonpeptide drugs. Meanwhile, scientists at DuPont Pharmaceuticals also screened approximately 10,000 compounds in their chemical library, but unfortunately, no promising hit compound was identified.

Good drug targets always attract different laboratories simultaneously conducting similar research. Therefore, during the process of drug discovery, researchers usually keep track of the progress and directions of other laboratories' studies. While advancing their own project, the researchers at DuPont noticed, through routine patent searches, two patents disclosed by Takeda regarding Ang II receptor antagonists, which were nonpeptide small molecules [15]. They immediately synthesized these compounds and tested their antagonistic activity against the Ang II receptor. Clearly, another important aspect of the drug development process is establishing reliable biological screening and evaluation methods to help medicinal chemists assess the reliability of reported compounds in the literature. The researchers at DuPont first synthesized the promising imidazole analog (Fig. 6.6, **10**) from Takeda's patent. Although they found that this compound was a weak antagonist in vitro (IC_{50} = 40 μM) [16], they decided to evaluate its in vivo efficacy tests in rats. The researcher conducting this study lacked experience, as he had just graduated from university and entered the industry. The compound was administered at a relatively high dose (100 mg/kg), and the desired antihypertensive effect was observed, confirming that compound **10** was a selective antagonist of the Ang II receptor without excitatory effects [16]. This result encouraged the researchers at DuPont to continue the optimization of this series of compounds, eventually leading to the discovery of losartan.

The subsequent work was to improve the activity of compound **10** toward the Ang II receptor. This is where computer-aided drug design (CADD) comes into play. Since the 1980s, CADD has been widely used in the design of new drugs, particularly for enhancing activity and selectivity in the early stages. For information on the conformation of compound **9** established using computer modeling and the docking results of compound **9** with Ang II in the model, please refer to the literature cited in reference [17].

Fig. 6.7 shows the overlapping image of compound **9** with Ang II. Experience gained from peptide compound studies suggests that the carboxyl-terminal fragment of Ang II is a critical site for binding to the receptor's positively charged region. When the carboxylic acid group at the C-terminus was transformed into an ester or amide, the molecular binding affinity significantly decreased. Therefore, scientists initially manually docked the carboxylic acid group of Takeda compound **9** with the carboxylic acid group at the C-terminus of Ang II in the model, allowing the imidazole ring of compound **9** to overlap with the histidine imidazole ring in Ang II. The hydrophobic n-butyl group at the 2-position of the imidazole was directed toward the isoleucine side chain of Ang II. Meanwhile, the benzyl group of compound **9** extended toward the N-terminus of Ang II. In comparison, the structure of compound **9** is much smaller than that of the endogenous peptide, providing possibilities for enlarging the size of small molecules. The most promising site for extension in

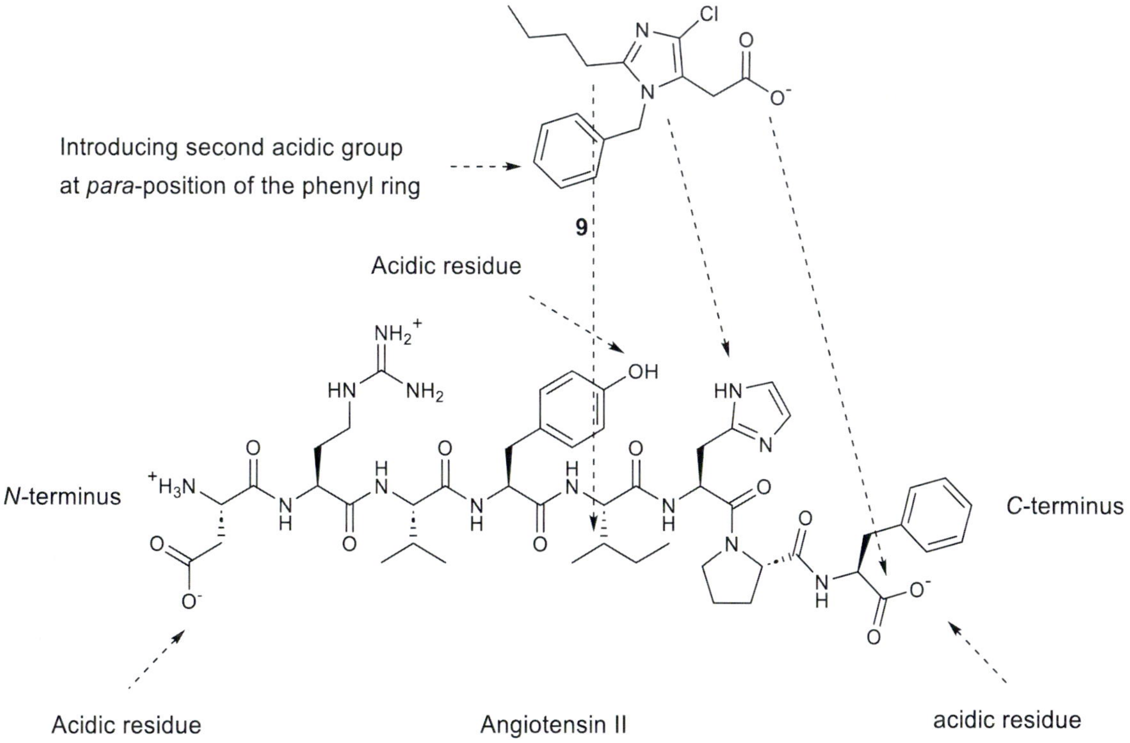

FIGURE 6.7 Overlapping hypothesis of compound **9** with Ang II.

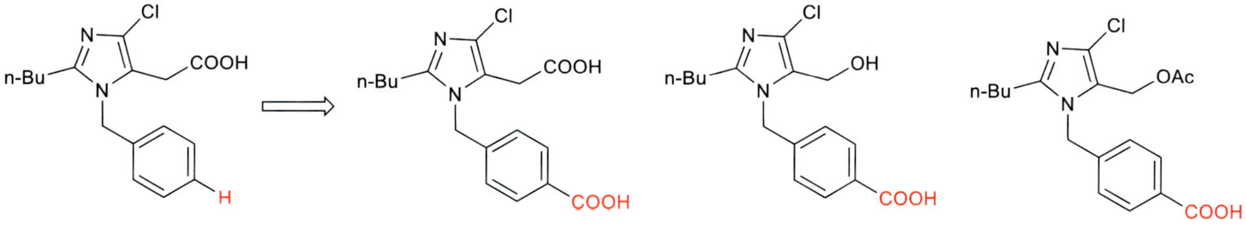

9 IC_{50}: 150 μM **11** IC_{50}: 1.2 μM **12** IC_{50}: 1.7 μM **13** IC_{50}: 5.3 μM

FIGURE 6.8 Evolution of *para*-carboxylated *N*-benzyl derivatives.

compound **9** was the *para*-position of the phenyl ring. Therefore, scientists started to consider what functional group to introduce at the *para*-position of the phenyl ring. Considering that the *N*-terminus of Ang II has two acidic groups in the amino acid residues, one being the phenolic hydroxyl group of tyrosine and the other being the carboxyl group of aspartic acid, the researchers at DuPont speculated that introducing a second acidic group at the *para*-position of the phenyl ring would help improve the activity. As expected, the antagonistic activity of a simple 4-carboxylic acid derivative **11** (Fig. 6.8) was 125-fold higher than that of the lead compound **9** [17]. This promising start provided strong momentum for the progress of this project.

Due to the need to synthesize compounds with as many different substituents as possible for structure-activity relationship (SAR) studies, medicinal chemists often synthesize all the compounds they can think of, which are not too complex to synthesize and test, to fully understand the detailed SAR. Therefore, researchers at DuPont quickly found that the 5-acetic acid group on the imidazole ring could be replaced. When it was replaced with CH_2OH (**12**), the IC_{50} value was 1.7 μM, a slight decrease in activity. When CH_2OH was further converted to the corresponding acetic ester group CH_2OAc (**13**), removing the hydrogen bond donor effect, the activity did not significantly decrease (IC_{50} = 5.3 μM). This SAR suggested that the carboxylic acid group in the *para*-position of the benzyl phenyl ring contributed the most to the activity. Subsequent efforts focused on the modification of the carboxylic acid group on

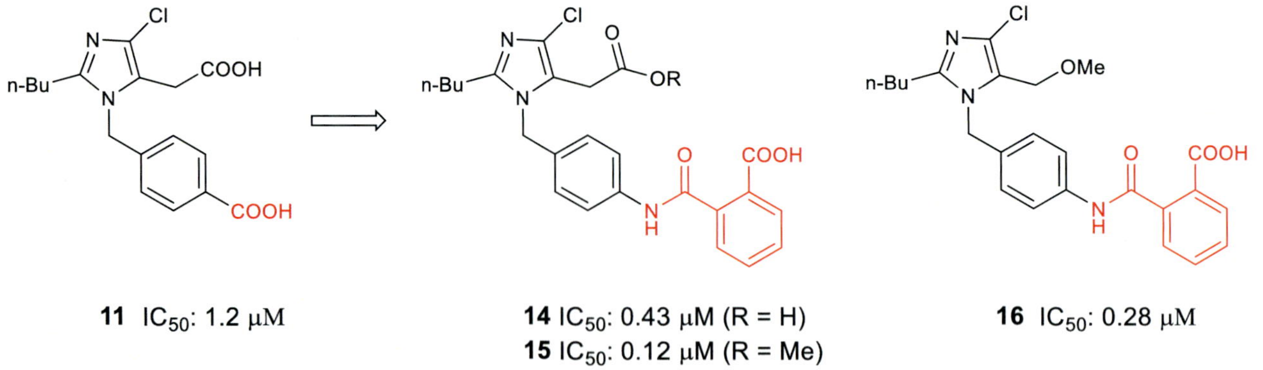

116 Medicinal Chemistry and Drug Development

FIGURE 6.9 Evolution of *N*-benzyl *para*-amide analogs.

the *para*-position of the phenyl ring. It was thought that extending the molecule further may better simulate the biological function of Ang II. Therefore, the key structural modification was to address how to maintain a carboxylic acid group while extending the molecular length. Due to the amino group being in the *para*-position of the phenyl ring, after generating the benzamide, the carboxylic acid on the second phenyl ring at the far end remains in the *para*-position of the benzyl group, but at a further distance. As expected, compounds **14** and **15** obtained from this modification exhibited 2.8-fold and 10-fold increases in antagonistic activity against the Ang II receptors compared to compound **11**. On the other hand, when the carboxylic acid group at the 5-position of compound **14** was replaced with an ester group to obtain compound **15**, its activity was not reduced but instead enhanced, with the IC_{50} value decreasing from 0.43 μM to 0.12 μM. To further demonstrate the nonessential nature of the carboxylic acid group at the 5-position of the imidazole, the chemists synthesized methoxy compound **16**, which also cannot provide a hydrogen bond donor, and it also showed slightly improved activity (IC_{50} = 0.28 μM). This SAR suggested that the carboxylic acid group at the 5-position of the imidazole was not crucial for in vitro activity (Fig. 6.9).

The results of the in vivo pharmacological evaluation of compound **15** showed that its oral bioavailability was poor; therefore, its antihypertensive effect (ED_{30} = 11 mg/kg) could only be observed when administered intravenously in renal hypertensive rats (RHR) [17]. However, since the in vitro activities of compounds **14** and **15** as well as **16** had already met the desired level, it could be claimed as a milestone achievement that the first class of nonpeptide lead compounds had successfully been discovered. The next goal was to optimize the lead compounds, aiming to improve their oral bioavailability to obtain orally active nonpeptide antihypertensive drug candidates.

6.4.2 Lead optimization

Further analysis of compound **15** suggested that the carboxylic acid group (highlighted in red) on the distal phenyl ring might be responsible for its poor oral bioavailability. The carboxylic acid group is a hydrophilic polar pharmacophore, and in general, reducing their polarity is necessary to improve the oral bioavailability of carboxylic acid-containing compounds. However, the carboxylic acid group is an essential group for activity on Ang II receptors. Therefore, medicinal chemists decided to investigate the bioisosteres of the carboxylic acid group. The concept of bioisosterism involves replacing a functional group with another one that has similar physicochemical properties but different structural features. In this case, the carboxylic acid group in compound **15** was first replaced with sulfonamide bioisosteres to investigate their impact on compounds' activities and oral bioavailabilities since the acidity of the N-H in some sulfonamides is comparable to that of carboxylic acid. Unfortunately, as shown in Fig. 6.10, replacing the carboxylic acid in compound **15** with more lipophilic sulfonamide bioisosteres such as CH_3SO_2NH- (**17**) and CF_3SO_2NH- (**18**) was unsuccessful. Both compounds **17** (IC_{50} = 2.3 μM) and **18** (IC_{50} = 0.5 μM) showed lower antagonistic activity compared to their precursor **15** (IC_{50} = 0.12 μM). Compound **18**, in particular, did not show any improvement in oral efficacy [17].

The unsuccessful attempts to improve oral bioavailability by replacing the carboxylic acid group with sulfonamide bioisosteres at the distal phenyl ring highlighted the complexity of optimizing the benzyl *para*-amide compounds and the challenges in balancing activity and oral bioavailability. Further explorations shifted toward replacing the amide linker between the two phenyl rings with less polar connecting groups. To systematically investigate the impact of the linker between the two phenyl rings on the activity, compounds were designed with a varying number of atoms in the linker, ranging from 2 to 1, and ultimately to 0. These compounds included connecting units different from the amide,

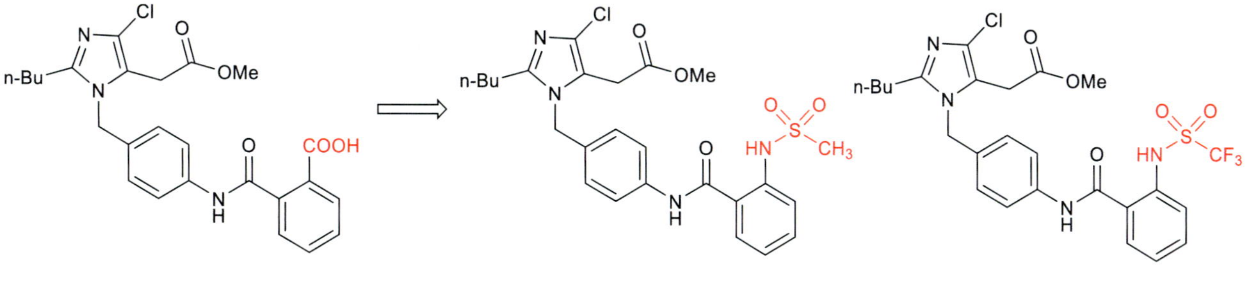

15 IC$_{50}$: 0.12 μM   **17** IC$_{50}$: 2.3 μM   **18** IC$_{50}$: 0.5 μM

FIGURE 6.10 Representative sulfonamides as carboxylic acid bioisosteres.

such as -OCH$_2$- and *trans*-CH=CH-, as well as compounds with one connecting atom, such as -CO-, -O-, and -S-, and compounds with zero connecting atoms, known as biphenyl compounds (Fig. 6.11). Results revealed that the activity significantly decreased when the amide was replaced with other connecting units containing two atoms, such as -OCH$_2$- (compounds **19** and **20**) and *trans*-CH=CH- (compound **21**). It was speculated that the more flexible -OCH$_2$- unit compared to the amide conformation might be the reason for the decreased activity in compounds **19** and **20**. Assuming that the methoxymethyl and hydroxymethyl groups at the 5-position of the imidazole ring contributed equally to the activity, researchers further speculated that the amide group in compound **16** could induce a *trans* conformation of the two phenyl rings, leading to the synthesis of a similar *trans*-stilbene derivative **21**. However, unexpectedly, compound **21** exhibited a 19-fold reduced activity (IC$_{50}$ = 5.4 μM) compared to compound **16**. These results were frustrating.

Compounds having a single connecting atom, such as compound **22**, a dibenzyl ketone derivative, compound **23**, a diaryl ether derivative, and compound **24**, a diaryl sulfide derivative, exhibited activities like those of compound **16** [18]. This suggested that the choice of a connecting group could have an impact on the compound's activity. This finding led DuPont's medicinal chemists to synthesize biphenyl compounds without connecting atoms, aiming to further explore the SAR and potentially discover compounds with enhanced activity.

Here, it is important to emphasize that during the optimization of lead compounds, more focus is placed on the drug-like nature of the molecules, especially when there is a strong need to selectively synthesize certain compounds with specific structures. This approach is significantly different from the random synthetic strategy employed in the earlier stage of discovering lead compounds, as well as from the traditional methods of organic synthesis used in studying synthetic routes for organic molecules. In the initial stages of lead compound discovery, diverse molecules can be designed freely to establish SAR, often resulting in the synthesis of as many compounds as possible. Therefore, the parallel synthesis approach used in combinatorial chemistry is well-utilized at this stage. However, during the lead optimization phase, specific structures of new molecules need to be designed and synthesized based on the specific requirements. This involves addressing targeted issues, and as a result, the molecules that need to be synthesized are often highly challenging. Sometimes, it may even require the development of new synthetic methods to meet these requirements, leading to the discovery of exciting novel molecular structures.

6.4.3 Discovery of losartan

The key breakthrough in the discovery of losartan occurred after the synthesis of biphenyl compounds. By completely removing the amide bond that connects the two phenyl rings and reducing the number of atoms connecting the rings to zero, compound **25** (Fig. 6.12) showed slightly lower in vitro activity (IC$_{50}$ = 0.23 μM) compared to compound **15** (IC$_{50}$ = 0.12 μM). However, it exhibited good oral efficacy, with an ED$_{30}$ value of 11 mg/kg in RHR [19]. This discovery gave scientists a glimpse of the potential for oral antihypertensive drugs. Subsequent research focused on further exploring the SAR based on the imidazole-biphenyl core structure to enhance the in vivo activity and drug-like properties of the compounds.

The optimization of the more advanced lead compound **25** began with the variation of the carboxylic acid group on the terminal phenyl ring (Fig. 6.12). When the carboxylic acid group (R^1) of compound **25** was moved to different positions along the terminal phenyl ring, including the *meta*- and *para*-positions, compounds **26** and **27** were obtained. Compound **26**, with the carboxylic acid group at the *meta*-position, showed an IC$_{50}$ of 0.49 μM, slightly lower than compound **25**, but it completely lost its *in vivo* activity in animals. It was believed that compound **25** had greater steric hindrance compared to **26**, resulting in a different conformation. The neighboring carboxylic acid group of **25** could be

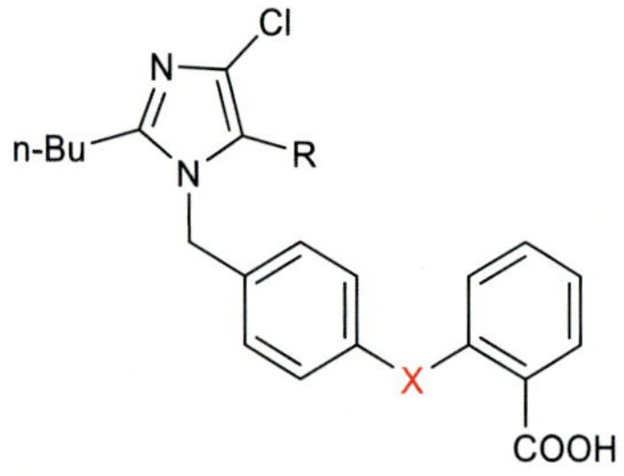

FIGURE 6.11 SAR of different connecting groups between two phenyl rings.

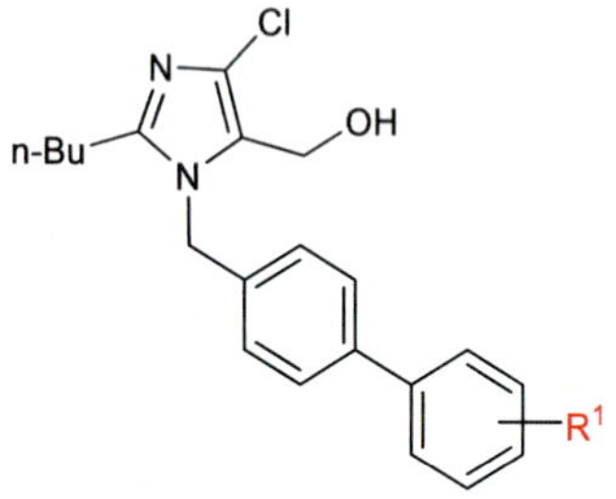

Compound	R	X	IC$_{50}$ (µM)
15	CH$_2$COOMe	-NHC(O)-	0.12
16	CH$_2$OMe	-NHC(O)-	0.28
19	CH$_2$OMe	-OCH$_2$-	1.2
20	CH$_2$OH	-OCH$_2$-	0.92
21	CH$_2$OH	trans-CH=CH-	5.4
22	CH$_2$OH	-C(O)-	0.16
23	CH$_2$OH	-O-	0.4
24	CH$_2$OH	-S-	0.4

Compound	R^1	In vitro IC$_{50}$ (µM)	In vivo iv/po ED$_{30}$ (mg/kg)
25	2-COOH	0.23	3.0/11
26	3-COOH	0.49	No activity
27	4-COOH	11.0	No activity

FIGURE 6.12 Impact of different positions of the carboxylic acid group on the terminal phenyl ring on activity.

more deeply buried in the lipophilic biphenyl system, leading to higher metabolic stability. However, the physicochemical properties of the two compounds, such as similar logP values (clogP = 1.17 for **25** and clogP = 1.38 for **26**), could not fully explain the significant difference in oral efficacy. This discrepancy highlighted the challenges and excitement in the field of medicinal chemistry, which is a semiempirical discipline. Unexpected situations and problems arise during the discovery and optimization process of each drug molecule, and they cannot be solved solely based on ideal human thinking, imagination, or experience. It is worth noting that the biological system of the human body is a complex system that surpasses human control. In this example, when the carboxylic acid group was placed at the *para*-position, the regioisomer **27** exhibited very low activity with an IC_{50} of 11.0 μM. This was likely because the *para*-carboxylic acid group was not in the correct orientation to interact effectively with the positive charges in the Ang II receptor. Thus, the carboxylic acid group on the terminal phenyl ring was locked in the optimal *ortho*-position.

Following the strategy for optimizing the amide compound **15** (Fig. 6.10), researchers at DuPont performed a systematic and in-depth investigation of bioisosteres with an acidity similar to carboxylic acids but with slightly higher lipophilicity. Fig. 6.13 shows the SAR of representative bioisosteric analogs of the carboxylic acid **25**. Through persistent efforts, they eventually discovered that the tetrazole analog **5** met all the desired criteria. The following is a brief overview of the discovery process for compound **5**.

Because they all have an acidic proton, amides, sulfonamides, triazoles, and tetrazoles have been used as bioisosteres of carboxylic acid. However, it is necessary to determine the acidity of each bioisostere's acidic proton, i.e., whether the pKa value is related to its activity. As shown in Fig. 6.13, the in vitro antagonistic activity of analogs with these acidic functional groups was indeed closely related to their pKa values. The stronger the acidity, the higher the activity. Amide compound **28**, which lacks acidity, exhibited very weak activity (IC_{50} = 35 μM). When electron-withdrawing groups

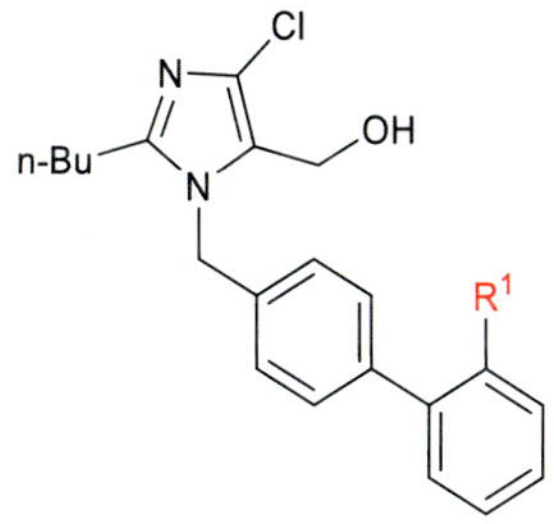

Compound	R¹	pKa	*In vitro* IC_{50} (μM)	*In vivo* iv/po ED_{30} (mg/kg)
28	-CONH₂	23	35.0	nd/nd
29	-CONHOMe	10.9	2.9	10/inactive
30	-CONHSO₂Ph	8.44	0.14	>3/nd
31	-NHCOCF₃	9.5	6.3	10/inactive
32	-NHSO₂CF₃	4.5	0.083	10/100
33	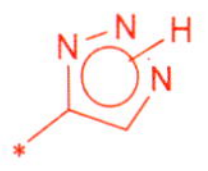 triazole	9	9.6	nd/nd
34	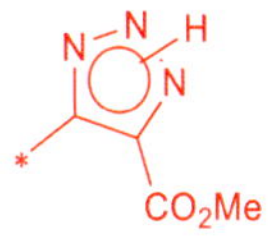 triazole-CO₂Me	7	0.26	>1/>10
5	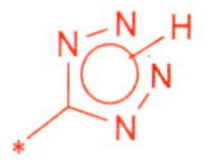 tetrazole	5-6	0.019	0.8/0.59

FIGURE 6.13 SAR of representative bioisosteric analogs of carboxylic acid.

were introduced to the amide moiety to enhance the acidity of the N-H bond, the activity increased. Comparing amides **29** and **30**, the pKa value decreased from 10.9 to 8.44, and the IC_{50} values decreased from 2.9 μM to 0.14 μM, indicating an improvement in Ang II receptor antagonistic activity. The same trend was observed in *trans*-amide compounds, where the IC_{50} value of analog **32** was 0.083 μM (pKa = 4.5), while the IC_{50} value of analog **31** was 6.3 μM (pKa = 9.5). Unfortunately, compounds **30** and **32**, although showing better in vitro activity than **25**, did not exhibit improved oral efficacy. The simple 1,2,3-triazole analog **33** is undoubtedly not acidic enough (pKa = 9). To enhance acidity, an electron-withdrawing group such as CO_2Me (**34**) was introduced, and its pKa value was reduced to 7. As a result, compound **34** exhibited antagonistic activity (IC_{50} = 0.26 μM) similar to the parent carboxylic acid **25**. However, its oral activity had still not been improved. The tetrazole analog **5** seemed to fall within the ideal range. Its in vitro IC_{50} value was 0.019 μM, indicating that tetrazole **5** was 12-fold more potent than carboxylic acid **25**, and its oral efficacy (ED_{30} = 0.59 mg/kg) in RHR was 19-fold higher than that of carboxylic acid **25** [19]. Pharmacokinetic studies in animals had shown that compound **5** had good oral bioavailability and a longer elimination half-life, with an oral bioavailability (F) of 33% and a half-life ($t_{1/2}$) of 2 hours in rats [20]. In addition to the similarity in acidity between the tetrazole group and the typical carboxylic acid group, the tetrazole group might allocate for better interaction with the positive charges on the Ang II receptor by distributing the negative charge over the four nitrogen atoms. Another possibility was that the tetrazole group could induce a conformation of the linked aryl ring to be more favorable for binding to the Ang II receptor.

After the discovery of the tetrazole bioisostere, researchers at DuPont continued extensive SAR studies. Despite significant efforts and the synthesis of numerous different compounds, the data from various aspects was ultimately considered, leading to the selection of compound **5** as the drug candidate for clinical development. This decision paved the way for the first Ang II receptor antagonist, losartan, to be brought to the market. Subsequently, successful clinical trial results further validated the rightness of this selection.

Based on compound **5** as an example of medicinal chemistry research, we will provide a detailed overview of the systematic SAR studies conducted around the biphenyl imidazole scaffold. We hope that readers will find inspiration from this and benefit from further studying medicinal chemistry.

While fixing the tetrazole moiety at the *ortho*-position of the terminal phenyl ring and introducing substituents on the terminal phenyl ring of compound **5**, including a methoxy group at the 4-position and 5-position and introducing a cyano group at the 6-position, this resulted in analogs **35**, **36**, and **37**, respectively (Fig. 6.14). Comparing the biological activities of these compounds with compound **5**, which lacks any substituent, it was found that the introduction of substituents led to a decrease in activity [20]. This suggested that the terminal phenyl ring, once occupied by the tetrazole moiety, already exhibited effective binding to the hydrophobic pocket of the receptor. Therefore, there was limited or no additional room available on the terminal phenyl ring to accommodate other groups without a negative impact on the compound's activity. This finding highlighted the importance of the structural features and the impact of the substituent on the terminal phenyl ring in the biphenyl imidazole scaffold.

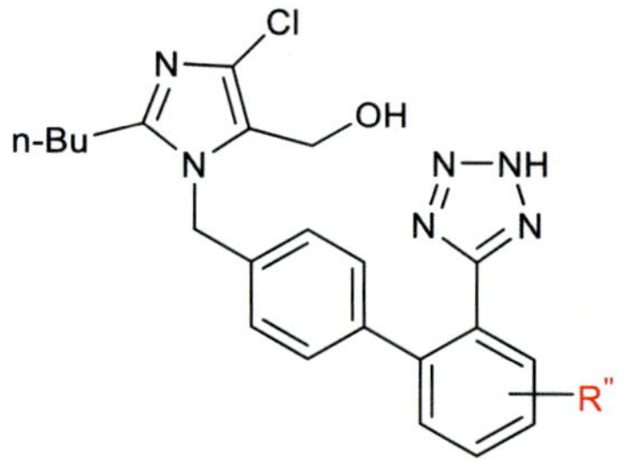

Compound	R″	In vitro IC_{50} (μM)	In vivo iv/po ED_{30} (mg/kg)
35	4-OMe	0.58	1.75/>10
36	5-OMe	0.12	6.03/>10
37	6-CN	0.51	3/>10

FIGURE 6.14 Impact of different substituents on the terminal phenyl ring on activity.

In parallel to the search for carboxylic acid-based bioisosteres on the terminal phenyl ring, medicinal chemists synthesized compounds **38–42** (Fig. 6.15) with different substituents, replacing the *n*-butyl in compound **25** at the 2-position of the imidazole ring while keeping the carboxylic acid functional group at the *ortho*-position of the terminal phenyl ring. Compared to compound **25**, compounds (**38–42**) containing liner alkyl groups displayed favorable in vitro antagonistic activity, with 3–4 carbon atoms being optimal (**25, 39**). This suggested that alkyl chains of appropriate length could better fit into a hydrophobic pocket of the Ang II receptor. However, if an aromatic group, such as in compound **42** (R^2 = Ph), was introduced, the activity was essentially lost (IC_{50} = 24 μM). Although compound **39** with an *n*-propyl group had a slightly lower IC_{50} value (IC_{50} = 0.16 μM) compared to compound **25** with an *n*-butyl group (IC_{50} = 0.23 μM), compound **25** exhibited better in vivo efficacy [19], indicating that compound **25** had superior properties. Medicinal chemists further transferred these findings obtained from carboxylic acid compounds to tetrazole compounds, with the substituent at the 2-position of the imidazole ring being locked as *n*-butyl.

When the substituent at the 4-position of the imidazole ring was changed to H, Br, I, and CF_3 (Fig. 6.16, **43-46**), there was no significant change in the in vitro activity. This suggested that the precise spatial or electronic properties at the 4-position of the imidazole ring did not have a significant impact on the activity. However, these compounds were found to have high melting points (>200°C) and significantly reduce oral bioactivity [19]. Additionally, compounds containing Br and I often have poor stability. Taking these factors into consideration, the best substituent at the 4-position of the imidazole ring was selected as Cl.

As shown in Fig. 6.17, analogs **47–52** provided further insight into the impact of the substituent at the 5-position of the imidazole ring on activity. It was found that in addition to the hydroxymethyl group, as long as there is a hydrogen bond acceptor substituent at the 5-position of the imidazole ring, compounds such as methoxymethyl (**47**), methyl amino formate ester (**48**), oxime (**49**), sulfonyl oxime (**50**), and secondary alcohol (**51**) all exhibited good in vitro antagonistic activity [20]. However, it can still be noted that the size of the substituent at this position has a certain sensitivity to the activity. As the size of the substituent increased, the antagonistic activity decreased. This SAR suggested that a large group in this position might have some influence on achieving the optimal conformation of the biphenyl. When the substituent at the 5-position of the imidazole ring was a carboxyl group, compound **52** showed a significant improvement in antagonistic activity (IC_{50} = 0.0013 μM) [21]. This unexpected result suggested the presence of an additional positive charge on the Ang II receptor, and the carboxylate negative charge at the 5-position of the imidazole ring could form a strong interaction with it, leading to a significant increase in the binding affinity with the Ang II receptor.

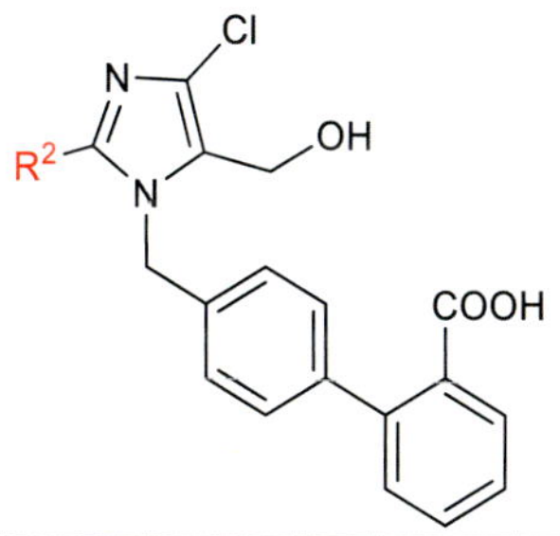

Compound	R^2	In vitro IC_{50} (μM)	In vivo iv/po ED_{30} (mg/kg)
38	Et	1.70	10/100
39	*n*-Pr	0.16	3/30
25	*n*-Bu	0.23	3/11
40	*n*-Pentyl	0.98	3/>10
41	*n*-Hexyl	1.30	10/inactive
42	Ph	24	10/100

FIGURE 6.15 Impact of different substituents at the 2-position of the imidazole ring on activity.

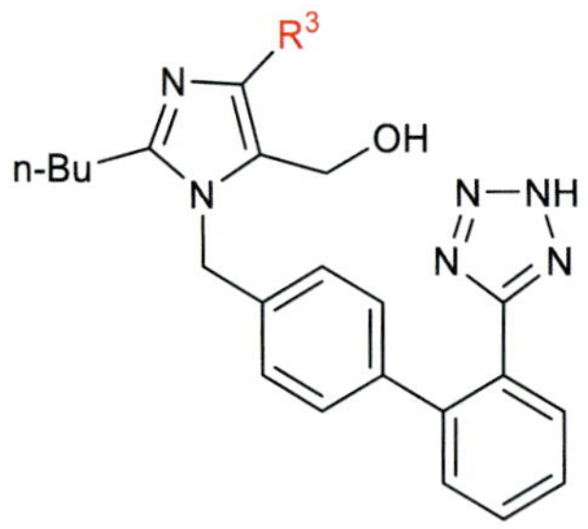

Compound	R³	In vitro IC₅₀ (µM)	In vivo iv/po ED₃₀ (mg/kg)
43	H	0.029	nd/nd
5	Cl	0.019	0.80/0.59
44	Br	0.019	0.3/3
45	I	0.020	1/10
46	CF₃	0.012	0.53/>3

FIGURE 6.16 Impact of different substituents at the 4-position of the imidazole ring on activity.

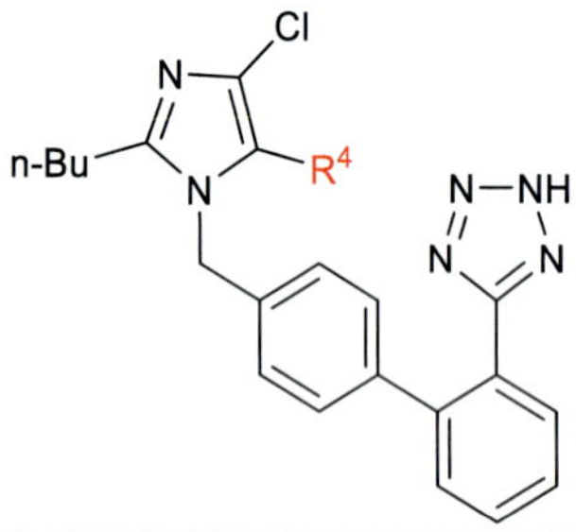

Compound	R⁴	In vitro IC₅₀ (µM)	In vivo iv/po ED₃₀ (mg/kg)
5	-CH₂OH	0.019	0.80/0.59
47	-CH₂OMe	0.032	1/3
48	-CH₂NHCO₂Me	0.06	1/>10
49	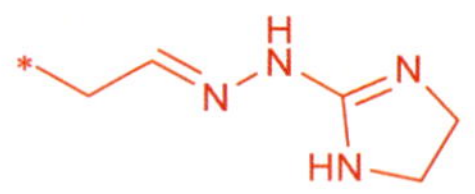 (imidazoline hydrazone structure)	0.29	3/30
50	-CH=N-NHSO₂Ph	0.66	3/30
51	-CH(OH)Ph	0.41	3/>30
52	-COOH	0.0013	0.038/0.66

FIGURE 6.17 Impact of different substituents at the 5-position of the imidazole ring on activity.

6.4.4 Metabolites of losartan and its corresponding pro-drugs

Compound **52** showed excellent in vitro antagonistic activity, nearly 15-fold higher compared to losartan (**5**). Following intravenous administration in RHR, it effectively decreased arterial pressure with an ED_{30} value of 0.038 mg/kg [21]. However, its oral efficacy did not improve (ED_{30} = 0.66 mg/kg for **52** compared to ED_{30} = 0.59 mg/kg for **5**). As mentioned earlier, the oral bioavailability (F) of losartan was 33%, which was also not optimal. Therefore, researchers at DuPont analyzed the efficacy results of the intravenous dosing studies for losartan and found that it exhibited a biphasic pharmacological effect. This meant that with the prolongation of the drug's duration in the body, there were two peaks of pharmacological effect. They speculated that the initial pharmacological effect was caused by the prototype drug losartan, and the secondary pharmacological effect was caused by its metabolites. It was inferred that compound **52** might be a metabolite of losartan in the body and be responsible for the secondary pharmacological effect. Subsequently, this hypothesis was confirmed when analyzing the metabolites of losartan in rat plasma [21]. Furthermore, researchers also observed that the in vivo efficacy of losartan varied among different animal species, indicating that the pharmacological differences in animal species are caused by the varying extent (speed) of losartan metabolism in the body, leading to different levels of metabolites. At this point, researchers had unanimously believed that a portion of losartan's efficacy came from its metabolite, compound **52**. Clearly, this result was an unexpected discovery that researchers had made through rigorous study, careful observation, thoughtful analysis, and strict adherence to the laws of scientific research. From the perspective of a medicinal chemist, it can be said that they often face tremendous pressure throughout the entire drug research and development process, but these pressures are often released through such unexpected findings. Without exaggeration, medicinal chemists are a group of great, humble, and selfless scientists who make significant contributions to the field of life science industry.

Due to the superior efficacy of compound **52** when dosed intravenously compared to losartan (**5**) (ED_{30} = 0.038 mg/kg for **52**, ED_{30} = 0.8 mg/kg for **5**), the researchers at DuPont decided to perform structural modification of compound **52**. Eventually, the substitute at the 5-position on the imidazole ring was changed to a carboxylic acid group, hoping to improve the oral bioavailability by changing the functional groups in other regions. Their goal was to develop an antihypertensive drug that was superior to losartan, which is often referred to as the second generation of losartan.

As a part of systematic lead optimization, researchers at DuPont Pharmaceuticals explored the effects of various substituents at the 4-position of the imidazole ring, primarily focusing on the investigation of straight-chain and branched alkyl substitutions ranging from one carbon to four carbons (Fig. 6.18, compounds **53–62**). To ensure an optimal balance between activity and lipophilicity, *n*-propyl was chosen as the substituent at the 2-position of the imidazole ring instead of *n*-butyl. SAR revealed that compound **54** with an ethyl substitution at the 4-position of the imidazole ring exhibited the best oral activity (ED_{30} = 0.03 mg/kg). When the chain length was kept the same and fluorine atoms were introduced (fluorine atoms are common electron-withdrawing groups that often enhance the metabolic stability of drugs), the electronic properties of the compound changed from electron-donating to electron-withdrawing. Comparing compounds **53** and **61**, as well as compounds **54** and **62**, compounds with electron-donating groups showed better in vitro activity than compounds with electron-withdrawing groups when the chain length was the same. In fact, compound **54** was the most effective oral antihypertensive compound identified in DuPont Pharmaceuticals' Ang II receptor antagonist project. Despite its low bioavailability (F = 8%), its oral potency was 20 times higher than that of losartan (**5**), which was another surprising finding [22].

To improve the oral bioavailability of compound **54**, medicinal chemists naturally considered the possibility of converting it into a pro-drug. For example, compound **54** could be transformed into ester pro-drugs **63** and **64** (Fig. 6.19). Although the oral bioavailability of compound **63** increased from 8% to 47% compared to the parent compound **54**, its oral potency did not surpass that of compound **54**. On the other hand, compound **64** exhibited weaker efficacy than the parent compound **54** [22d]. Therefore, this strategy was not pursued further at DuPont. However, this approach provided significant opportunities for other companies and led to many drugs in this class being successfully marketed as pro-drugs, particularly allisartan isoproxil (the pro-drug of compound **52**), which has been launched in China.

Metabolism studies of losartan in animals and humans indicated that losartan was primarily metabolized in the liver through the oxidation of two cytochrome P450 enzyme subtypes, CYP2C9 and CYP3A4, which is referred to as phase I metabolism. This was followed by a glucuronidation reaction to complete phase II metabolism [23]. Compound **52** was the major metabolite resulting from the oxidation of the 5-hydroxymethyl group of losartan's imidazole moiety, accounting for 10% of the total metabolites in humans. Due to the cumulative pharmacological effects and extended half-life of metabolite **52**, losartan appeared to act as a pro-drug. However, its pharmacological effects in humans were the combined result of the activities of both compounds [21,23]. Numerous studies have demonstrated that grapefruit juice is an inhibitor of cytochrome P450 3A4, so it is possible that grapefruit juice may affect the metabolism of losartan, leading to delayed or reduced formation of metabolite **52**, which could potentially impact the efficacy of losartan [24].

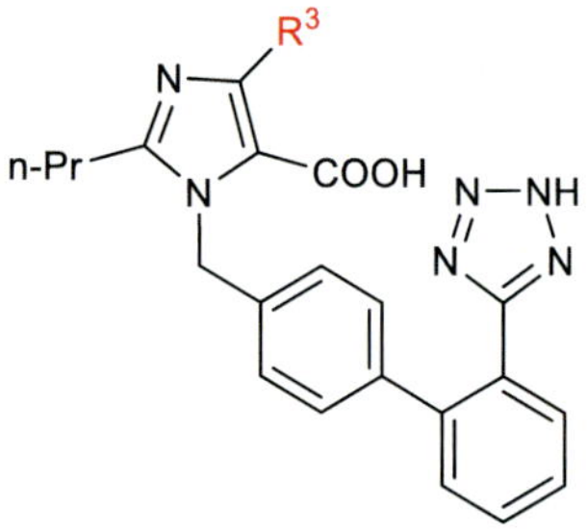

Compound	R³	*In vitro* IC₅₀ (µM)	*In vivo* iv/po ED₃₀ (mg/kg)
53	Me	nd	nd/0.19
54	Et	0.006	0.005/0.03
55	n-Pr	nd	nd/0.63
56	i-Pr	nd	nd/0.01
57	n-Bu	nd	nd/1.3
58	i-Bu	nd	nd/0.87
59	s-Bu	nd	nd/0.46
60	t-Bu	nd	nd/0.35
61	CF₃	nd	0.01/0.79
62	CF₂CF₃	0.0031	0.042/0.21

FIGURE 6.18 The impact of substituent at the 4-position of the imidazole ring on activity.

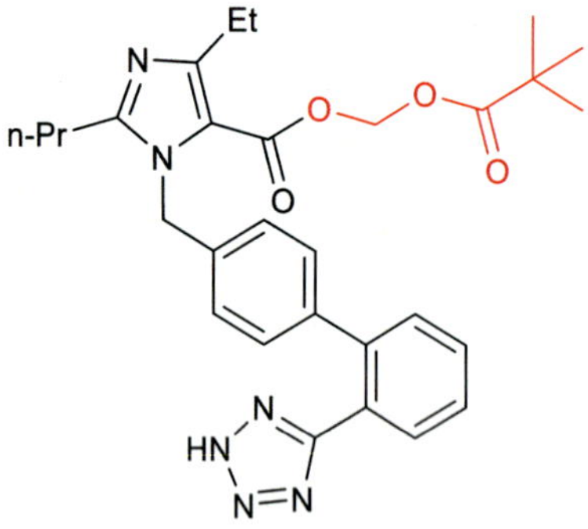

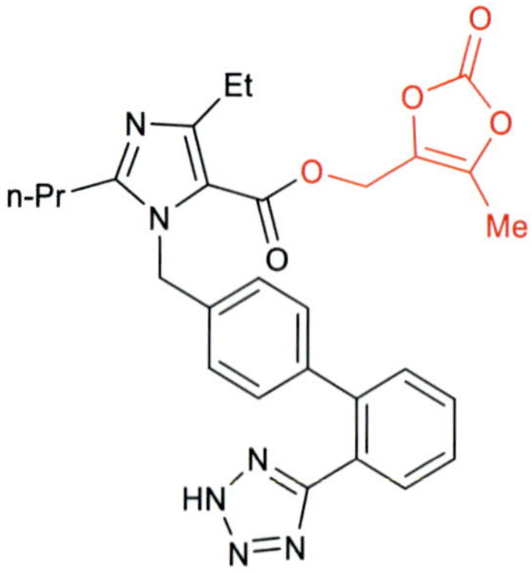

FIGURE 6.19 Structures of compounds **63** and **64**.

TABLE 6.2 Properties of losartan (5) and compound 52.

Compound	Caco-2 ($\times 10^{-6}$ cm/s) B-A, A-B (B-A/A-B)	PPB	CLr (mL/min)	$t_{½}$(h)	Vss(L/kg)	Tmax(h)
5	5.17, 0.63 (8.2)	98.7%	56	2	34	0.9
52	1.12, 0.19 (5.9)	99.8%	20	6~9	12	3.5

Compound **52** is a selective, long-acting, and noncompetitive Ang II receptor antagonist. Its antihypertensive effects have been confirmed to be associated with the inhibition of the RAS. It can be eliminated through both renal and nonrenal pathways, but compared to the parent compound, losartan (**5**), compound **52** is cleared from the body at a much slower rate. In cytotoxicity experiments, compound **52** showed no observed lactate dehydrogenase release in human mesangial cells within the range of 1 to 100 μM, and its inhibition of neutral red uptake was also normal, indicating that compound **52** has a good safety profile [25].

After confirming that compound **52** was the major metabolite of losartan, clinical trials were also conducted on its antihypertension effects. In patients with primary hypertension, continuous intravenous infusion of compound **52** for four hours resulted in a decrease in both systolic and diastolic blood pressures, with no abnormal changes in heart rate. The peak concentration of compound **52** was reached between 3.5 and 4 hours after the infusion, but the antihypertensive effect appeared 6–8 hours after the injection [23c]. However, as oral losartan became the main formulation marketed, DuPont did not further conduct in-depth clinical trials on compound **52**.

Table 6.2 lists various properties of losartan and compound **52**. The cellular permeability of losartan from the apical (A) to basolateral (B) direction (0.63×10^{-6} cm/s) was lower than the permeability from B to A (5.17×10^{-6} cm/s), which seemed contrary to our usual expectations for a new drug. In general, researchers hope that the permeability of Caco-2 cells (the Caco-2 cell model is a human cloned colon adenocarcinoma cell line that has a similar structure and function to differentiated small intestinal epithelial cells, including microvilli and enzymes associated with the brush border epithelium of the small intestine; it is commonly used to simulate the ability of drugs to be transported in the intestines) is greater than 2×10^{-6} cm/s in the A to B direction, with an efflux ratio less than 2. Additionally, losartan was a substrate of P-glycoprotein (P-gp) and possibly other transport proteins, while compound **52** was not [26]. This may be one of the reasons for the lower oral bioavailability of losartan. However, this case also provided scientists with a hint from another perspective. Although in vitro data can provide guidance for compound design and the priority order of studies, it is sometimes unnecessary to overly rely on in vitro data. Ultimately, in vivo efficacy results are the most important, and the discovery of losartan is a good example of this.

6.4.5 The safety profile of losartan

In general, during the preclinical stage of drug development, the primary focus is on the efficacy and safety of the compounds. The previous discussion provided a detailed introduction to the SAR of imidazole biphenyl compounds as Ang-II receptor antagonists, as well as an overview of the discovery process of losartan. Now, let us briefly discuss the safety profile of losartan (**5**).

Drug-drug interactions are important safety factors to consider for oral medications. Therefore, it is necessary to test the inhibitory activity of drug candidates on cytochrome P450 (CYP450) enzymes and identify which specific CYP450 enzyme subtype is responsible for oxidative metabolism. CYP450 enzymes are primarily distributed in the liver and intestines, which are the main metabolic organs for drugs. As monooxygenases, CYP450 enzymes primarily oxidize drug molecules to increase the water solubility of the resulting oxidized metabolites (phase I metabolism), making them easier to eliminate through urine. If a drug candidate inhibits these CYP450 enzymes, they would not be able to carry out the metabolism of other drugs simultaneously, leading to an increase in the concentration of another drug in the body, potentially exceeding its safety threshold and causing adverse reactions. Nowadays, the inhibition of drug molecule on CYP450 enzymes is generally controlled to be $IC_{50} > 10$ μM. Table 6.3 lists the inhibitory activity of losartan on some CYP450 enzyme subtypes, with IC_{50} values greater than 81 μM. Therefore, losartan is unlikely to cause significant drug-drug interactions [27].

TABLE 6.3 Inhibitory activity of losartan on certain CYP450 enzymes.

	CYP1A2	CYP2A6	CYP2C9	CYP2C19	CYP2D6	CYP2E1	CYP3A4
$IC_{50}(\mu M)$	524	>1000	81	138	>1000	>1000	210

Cardiovascular safety is another important concern in drug development. With the development of drug research techniques, it has been recognized that cardiovascular safety is mainly associated with a potassium ion (K^+) channel known as hERG (the human Ether-a-go-go-Related Gene) or the KCNH2 gene. The protein encoded by this gene is a potassium ion channel, Kv11.1. Research has shown that when the ability of Kv11.1 to mediate current across the cell membrane is inhibited by a drug, it can affect the cardiac repolarization process, leading to a potentially life-threatening condition called QT interval (the electrical activity that occurs between the Q and T waves in the heart's ventricles) prolongation syndrome, which can cause arrhythmias. Around 2002, regulatory agencies such as the U.S. Food and Drug Administration and the European Medicines Agency began to require preclinical evaluation of hERG safety for new drugs. Since the development of losartan was completed before this requirement was implemented, it did not undergo hERG safety evaluation during the development phase. However, later research yielded interesting results. Losartan had a certain inhibitory effect on the hERG channel, but its major metabolite, **52**, increased the current through the hERG channel. Therefore, taking losartan does not impact the hERG channel or cause cardiovascular safety issues. On the contrary, losartan has potential benefits for treating ventricular arrhythmias and heart failure caused by arrhythmias. This may be related to the phosphorylation of the Ang II receptor and its downstream protein kinase C (PKC), which acts as a G-protein-coupled receptor. Studies have shown that PKC can inhibit the hERG channel through self-phosphorylation, meaning that Ang II can inhibit the hERG channel by stimulating its receptor. As an Ang II receptor antagonist, losartan can regulate the repolarizing K^+ current produced by hERG through this pathway, leading to therapeutic effects in heart failure [28,29].

Finally, a comprehensive preclinical safety evaluation is necessary for drug candidates to fully understand the potential adverse reactions that researchers predict may occur after entering clinical trials and to have certain treatment measures in case of serious adverse events. Preclinical safety evaluation is generally conducted in rodent species (mice or rats) and nonrodent species (dogs or monkeys). It mainly includes clinical observations, biochemical data analysis, and anatomical experiments to observe pathological changes. Based on the results of acute toxicity experiments, the injection LD_{50} (lethal dose for 50% of the population) of losartan potassium salt in mice was 2248 mg/kg, and the oral median lethal dose was 2000 mg/kg. The dose at which the drug was tolerated was close to 1000 mg/kg. In dogs, the oral tolerance dose range of losartan potassium salt was 160–320 mg/kg, indicating higher sensitivity compared to mice. When administered intraperitoneally, the metabolite **52** of losartan had an LD_{50} value of 441 mg/kg in mice. The long-term toxicological studies of losartan potassium salt were conducted in rats, dogs, and monkeys. In rats, toxicity experiments were carried out for 5, 14, and 53 weeks, with doses of 0, 15, 45, and 135 mg/kg/day. During the studies, slight increases in body weight and decreased food intake were observed. There were also minor reductions in red blood cells and triglycerides, slight increases in serum chloride, glucose, sodium, and potassium levels, as well as elevated cholesterol levels, urine alkalization, decreased urinary protein, increased blood urea nitrogen, and parathyroid cell hyperplasia. Additionally, a slight decrease in heart weight and focal erosion of the gastric gland mucosa were observed. In dogs, toxicity experiments were conducted for 5, 14, and 53 weeks with doses of 0, 15, 45, and 135 mg/kg/day. Adverse reactions in the gastrointestinal system, such as vomiting, abnormal feces, and positive fecal occult blood, were observed. No drug-related deaths, changes in body weight, food intake, or eye-related changes were observed. Only slight changes in red blood cell parameters were noted. Urine analysis, serum biochemical or hematological parameters, and electrocardiograms showed no significant changes, although a slight decrease in heart weight was observed. A 14-week safety evaluation study was conducted in monkeys with daily doses of 0, 20, 100, and 300 mg/kg. No drug-related deaths, changes in body weight, food intake, or eye-related changes were observed. Decreased red blood cell parameters and reduced blood urea nitrogen were noted, but urine analysis showed no changes. The stomach and small intestine exhibited red spots, and organ weights remained unchanged. In addition, in male and female rats, losartan potassium salt did not affect fertility or reproductive capacity (genetic toxicity) when administered at daily doses of 150 and 300 mg/kg. However, in teratogenicity studies conducted on rats, losartan potassium salt was found to have adverse effects on fetuses and newborns, including decreased body weight, renal toxicity, and death. Analysis of rat milk revealed significant levels of losartan and its metabolite compound **52**, indicating a certain degree of exposure to these substances during pregnancy and lactation. Therefore, it is contraindicated for pregnant women to take losartan. In carcinogenicity studies conducted on rodents, it was found that administration of losartan potassium salt at a daily dose of 200 mg/kg for a duration of 92 weeks in mice and 270 mg/kg for a duration of 105 weeks in rats did not show any carcinogenic effects. Moreover, the results of microbial mutagenicity and V-79 mammalian cell mutation tests for losartan potassium salt were negative. There were no observed chromosomal abnormalities in bone marrow cells at tolerated doses of up to 1500 mg/kg per day. Its metabolite compound **52** also did not exhibit genotoxicity or the ability to induce microbial mutagenicity and chromosomal abnormalities. In conclusion, losartan potassium salt was considered generally safe and had been approved for marketing.

6.4.6 The properties and actions of losartan

After completing the safety assessment and obtaining clear and necessary data, the registration application for clinical trial research of new drugs, known as investigational new drug, can be submitted to the regulatory authorities of various countries. Once permission is granted, the drug can proceed to the clinical trial phase. The clinical trial phase is generally divided into four stages. Phase I trials are primarily conducted to determine the drug's tolerability and study its pharmacokinetic properties in the human body. For nononcology drugs, healthy male volunteers are usually recruited. Phase II trials aim to preliminarily evaluate the drug's efficacy and safety in patients with the intended indications, building upon the results obtained from Phase I trials. These trials can provide initial evidence of effectiveness and safety within a shorter timeframe. Phase III trials further validate the drug's efficacy and safety in larger populations with statistical significance. This stage involves longer-term trials conducted in a larger number of clinical patients with the expectation of obtaining significant differences in efficacy (or noninferiority). Phase IV trials are postmarketing studies conducted to further monitor the drug's efficacy and safety after it has been approved and launched. The entire process of developing a new drug, from preclinical research to market entry, generally takes around ten years. Based on current estimates, the average cost of developing a new drug is approximately 2 billion US dollars.

Based on the comprehensive analysis of losartan's characteristics, during its initial development stage, it showed a high probability of becoming a viable drug. However, according to the estimates at that time, its clinical research would require several years and hundreds of millions of dollars in funding, which posed a significant burden for DuPont Pharmaceuticals. At the same time, DuPont's management also considered that ACE inhibitors had already successfully captured the market for antihypertensive drugs, and losartan had a similar mechanism of action. Taking into account the economic and market factors, as well as the rich experience accumulated by Merck and Co. in the development and marketing of the ACE inhibitor enalapril, DuPont ultimately decided to form a partnership with Merck and Co. in 1991 to jointly develop and market losartan. Losartan was eventually developed as its potassium salt and received approval for marketing in the United States in 1995 and in China in 1998.

Losartan potassium is a white, crystalline substance. It is soluble in water and alcohols and slightly soluble in acetonitrile and methyl ethyl ketone.

Losartan is a selective antagonist of the Ang II receptor subtype 1 (AT1) with an IC_{50} of 0.019 μM, and it has virtually no antagonistic activity against the AT2 receptor subtype (IC_{50} = 100 μM) [30]. Clearly, losartan is a competitive antagonist of Ang II at the AT1 receptor, without the partial agonist properties of peptide antagonists such as saralasin [31]. It has no inhibitory effect on ACE and no binding or blocking activity with known hormone receptors involved in cardiovascular regulation. In RHR, losartan showed antihypertensive activity with an ED_{30} of 0.80 mg/kg when dosed intravenously and an ED_{30} of 0.59 mg/kg when dosed orally. The antihypertensive effect can last for more than 24 hours without affecting heart rate [32].

The trade name of losartan potassium is Cozaar. It is primarily used for the treatment of hypertension. It is also used for patients with type 2 diabetes accompanied by left ventricular hypertrophy (enlarged heart muscle), heart failure, and renal impairment. It has been found to have a beneficial effect on slowing the progression of kidney disease in patients with type 2 diabetes. Additionally, research has shown that losartan, as a specific inhibitor of the urate transporter 1, can prevent uric acid from entering cells, allowing more uric acid to be filtered and excreted through the kidneys, making losartan potassium also useful in the treatment of uremia [33].

The initial dose of losartan potassium for the treatment of hypertension is usually 50 mg per day, and the typical maintenance dose ranges from 25 to 100 mg per day. The maximum impact on blood pressure usually occurs within 3−6 weeks after administration. Losartan potassium can be used as a monotherapy or in combination with hydrochlorothiazide. One-third of patients with severe hypertension may have a better response to combination therapy. Food does not affect the efficacy of losartan potassium.

Common adverse reactions to losartan potassium include dizziness, muscle cramps, back pain, nasal congestion, cough, hyperkalemia (high potassium levels), and anemia. Severe adverse reactions may include vascular edema, hypotension (low blood pressure), and kidney problems.

6.4.7 The synthesis of losartan

The development of a new drug typically involves research on the drug's chemical synthesis route and the final production synthesis route. Although both routes aim to synthesize the same compound, their starting points and requirements can be significantly different, leading to different strategies. In the early stages of chemical drug discovery, the goal is to synthesize as many compounds as possible for biological testing and to identify active compounds as quickly as possible. At this stage, the focus is often on synthesizing common intermediates and using them to derive numerous analogs to establish valuable SAR. The yield of the products is not the primary concern at this phase, as long as purified compounds (typically with a purity >95%) can be obtained. Therefore, the early-stage synthesis usually yields milligram quantities of the compounds, and column chromatography is commonly used for compound purification. However, during the later stages of scale-up production, kilogram quantities of the active pharmaceutical ingredient are required for various studies in the development phase, and all synthetic activities at this stage must be conducted under Good Manufacturing Practice conditions. Since the focus is now on synthesizing a single pure compound, similar to the total synthesis of natural products, the main concerns are how to improve yield and efficiency to reduce costs. Additionally, there is a need to avoid the use of highly hazardous reagents and reactions and to address environmental pollution issues. Importantly, column chromatography is generally not suitable for purifying kilogram quantities of compounds due to the high cost of the stationary phase, such as silica gel, and the generation of a large amount of waste. Therefore, recrystallization of intermediates and final products often becomes a necessary method.

Here is a comparison of two synthetic routes for losartan. Scheme 6.1 shows the medicinal chemistry synthesis route [19]. Disconnection of the structure of losartan revealed that the key step in its synthesis lies in the construction of the biphenyl portion. Since the discovery of the losartan project began in the early 1980s, the Suzuki reaction for constructing biphenyls had not been broadly exploited at that time. Chemists at DuPont used Meyers' method to construct the biphenyl moiety. Grignard reagent **65** underwent aromatic nucleophilic substitution with oxazolinone compound **66**, resulting in the

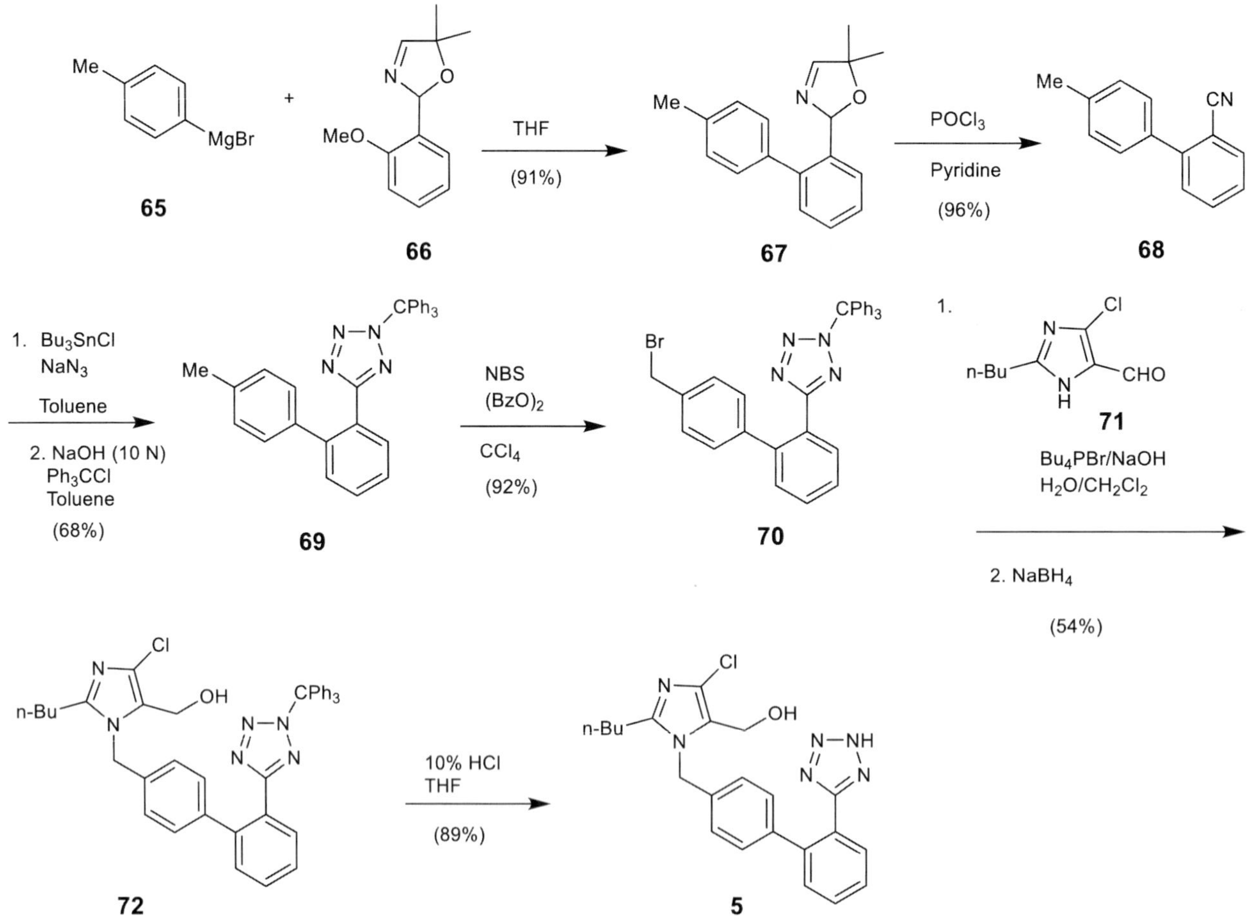

SCHEME 6.1 Medicinal chemistry synthesis route of losartan.

formation of biphenyl compound **67**. After treatment with phosphorus oxychloride, the oxazolinone group in **67** was converted into a CN group. The formation of tetrazole in compound **69** was achieved under standard conditions employing sodium azide. Subsequently, bromination of **69** with *N*-bromosuccinimide (NBS) provided compound **70**. Alkylation of the imidazole ring and reduction of the aldehyde provided compound **72**. The removal of the triphenylmethyl protection group from the tetrazole resulted in losartan (**5**) with an overall yield of 26%, which was considered very reasonable.

The process route for the production of losartan by DuPont/Merck is shown in Scheme 6.2 [34]. This route benefits from the widely used Suzuki coupling reaction. This sequence started with the protection of phenyltetrazole **73** to form triphenylmethyl phenyltetrazole **74**. Lithiation of **74** was followed first by treatment with triisopropyl borate, then with ammonium chloride solution to generate boronic acid **75** for the Suzuki coupling reaction.

Another coupling partner (**79**) for the Suzuki coupling reaction was prepared in 3 steps, starting with the construction of the imidazole ring. Treatment of methyl pentanimidate **76** with glycine in a methanol/water mixture afforded

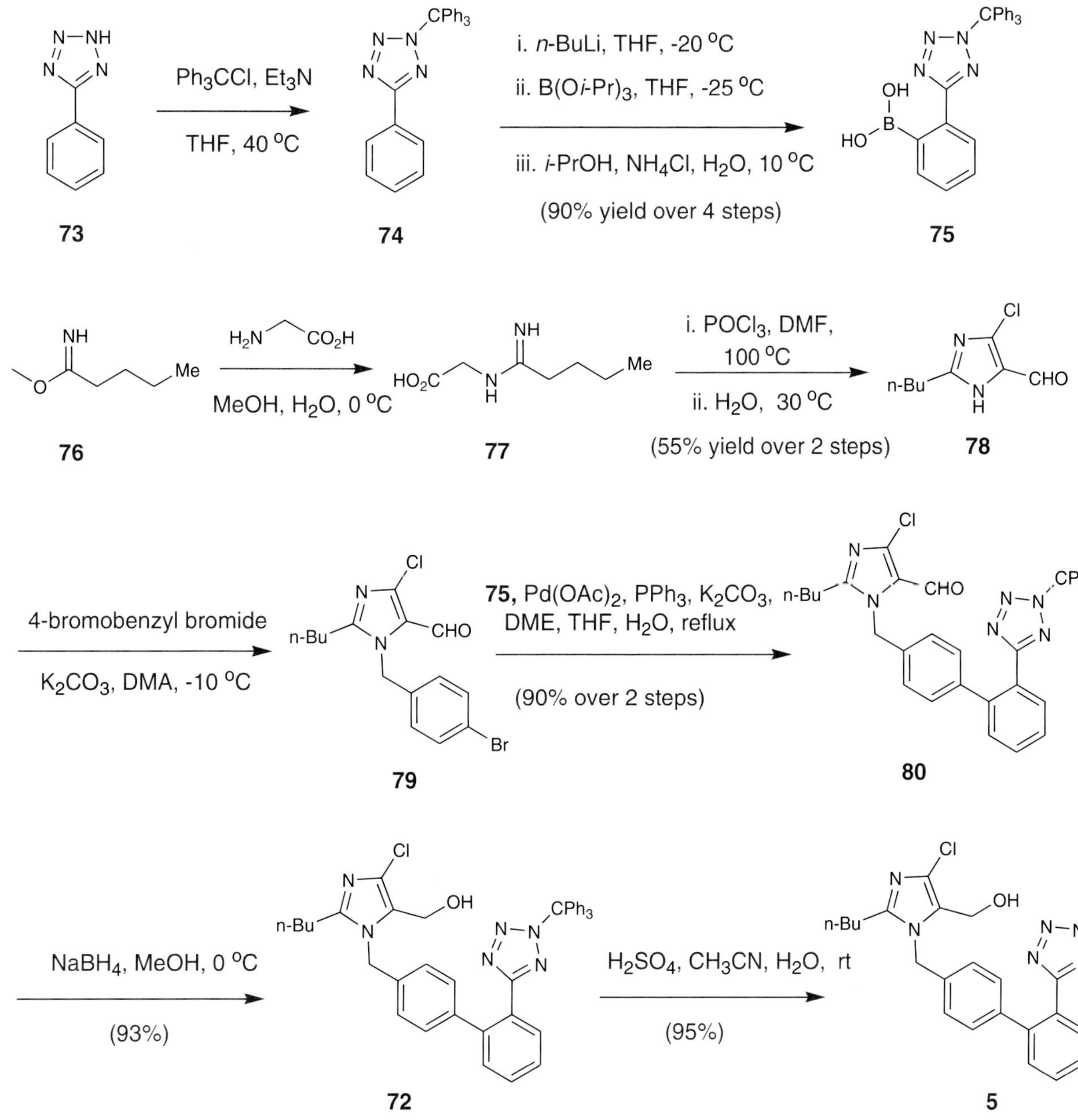

SCHEME 6.2 Process route for production of losartan.

130 Medicinal Chemistry and Drug Development

(pentanamido)acetic acid **77**. Compound **77** then underwent the Vilsmeier reaction, followed by hydrolysis to afford imidazole-5-aldehyde **78**, with a yield of 55% for two steps. Alkylation of **78** with 4-bromobenzyl bromide in the presence of potassium carbonate provided compound **79**. Subsequently, the bromophenyl compound **79** was subjected to a Suzuki coupling reaction with boronic acid **75** to yield biphenyl compound **80**, and the aldehyde group was reduced with sodium borohydride to form alcohol **72**. The triphenylmethyl protection group was removed using dilute sulfuric acid, resulting in the formation of losartan (**5**). Compared to the medicinal chemistry synthesis route, this production process route utilized a more efficient Suzuki coupling reaction to construct the biphenyl portion, achieving an overall yield of 72%, thereby significantly improving the production efficiency.

6.4.8 Brief summary of the discovery of losartan

To summarize, the successful discovery of losartan involved several key breakthroughs (Fig. 6.20). (1) Prompt literature alert, synthesis, and evaluation: scientists at DuPont Pharmaceuticals promptly found in the patent literature the nonpeptide small molecule Ang II receptor antagonists disclosed by Takeda Pharmaceuticals and immediately synthesized and evaluated the activity and selectivity of compound **10**. (2) Lead compound discovery: through CADD and medicinal chemistry experience, lead compound **11** was discovered by adding a carboxylic acid group at the *para*-position of the phenyl ring as the second functionality, resulting in improved in vitro activity but not sufficient. Therefore, compound **11** was optimized, and a 10-fold more potent compound **15** was quickly discovered by extending the spatial orientation of the benzyl group. Although compound **15** exhibited significantly improved in vitro activity, it was not orally active. (3) Improved oral activity: to improve oral bioavailability, the main strategy adopted by the medicinal chemists at DuPont was to reduce the polarity of the compound. By removing the polar amide bond that connects the two phenyl rings, they discovered the biphenyl compound **25**, which marked a key breakthrough. Although compound **25** exhibited slightly lower in vitro activity than compound **15**, it demonstrated good oral activity in animal studies. (4) Enhancement of oral efficacy: the

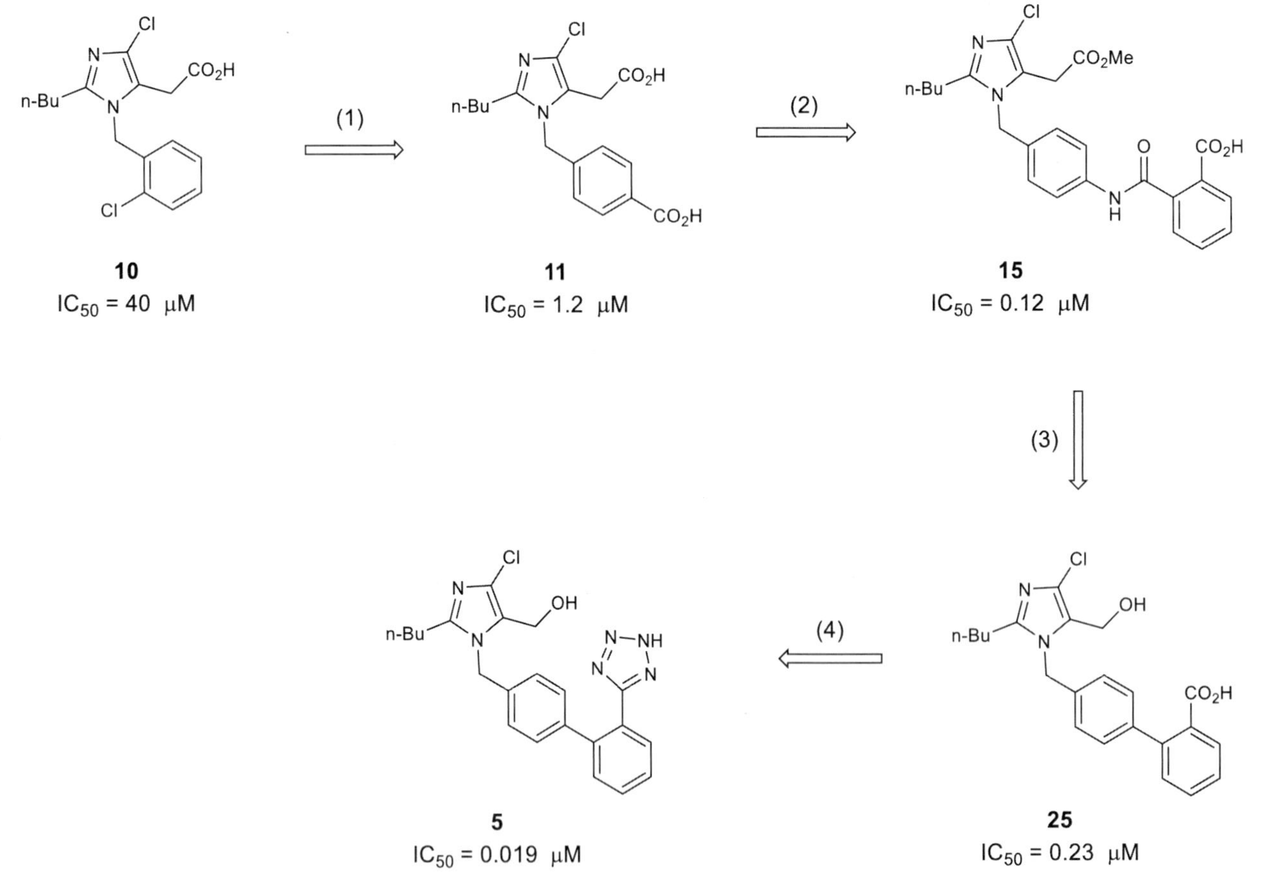

FIGURE 6.20 Key breakthroughs in the discovery of losartan.

polar carboxylic acid group was replaced with a lipophilic bioisostere tetrazole, leading to a significant improvement in oral efficacy. This modification resulted in the successful discovery of losartan (**5**).

The preclinical research on losartan took nearly four years [35]. Several years later, Dr. Duncia, the inventor of losartan, and his colleagues provided a detailed account of the discovery process in their review article [20], which interested readers can refer to for further information.

6.5 Discovery of losartan analogs

The successful development of losartan made it the world's first selective Ang II receptor antagonist for the treatment of hypertension. After the disclosure of the early encouraging results of losartan from DuPont, a number of other pharmaceutical companies, including some small biopharmaceutical companies, began their fast follow-up research to pursue novel nonpeptide Ang II receptor antagonists. The renowned journal "Bioorganic and Medicinal Chemistry Letters" dedicated its first issue in 1994 to the research achievements of nonpeptide Ang II receptor antagonists. Among numerous "me-too" projects, nine new nonpeptide Ang II receptor antagonists were successfully brought to the market, collectively known as "Ang II receptor blockers" (ARBs), a class of antihypertensive drugs. The discovery of these drugs allows for further exploration of their potential in treating various medical conditions related to the RAS and provides physicians with additional options for treating hypertension. Most of the drugs that were subsequently launched on the market, apart from eprosartan, resulted from the modification of losartan (**5**) or its active metabolite **52**. Based on the properties of this class of compounds, some molecules were successfully developed as ester pro-drugs to improve oral bioavailability. The following is a brief introduction to the sequence of these ARBs that were marketed, with a focus on the key structural modifications of each compound. The purpose is to provide readers with examples of "me-too" as a strategy in drug discovery.

Among numerous competitors, the most agile company was Ciba-Geigy (now part of Novartis). Just one year after the launch of losartan in 1996, they introduced the first analog, valsartan (Fig. 6.21, **81**), to the market, with an astonishingly fast response. Valsartan is the only compound among the losartan analogs that retains the biphenyl backbone while replacing the imidazole ring with a nonheterocyclic moiety, where the imidazole ring is substituted with an acylated amino acid. The design of valsartan was credited to the use of a three-dimensional model. Scientists at Ciba-Geigy superimposed the key C-terminal pentapeptide (Tyr-Ile-His-Pro-Ile) part of sarile (Fig. 6.5, **8**) with losartan (**5**) and found that the imidazole ring could potentially serve as a linker for an amide bond in the peptide (Fig. 6.22A). Based on this observation, they designed a series of acylated amino acid derivatives and screened their activity on Ang II receptors, which led to the most potent compound, valsartan (**81**). They hypothesized two completely opposite overlap orientations of the pentapeptide: losartan (Fig. 6.22A) and valsartan (Fig. 6.22B). As shown in Fig. 6.22A, the acidic tetrazole moiety was hypothesized to mimic the carboxylic acid group of isoleucine (Ile) of the pentapeptide, while in Fig. 6.22B, the tetrazole moiety was hypothesized to mimic the less acidic phenolic hydroxyl group of tyrosine (Tyr), and the valine fragment was assumed to mimic the Ile in the pentapeptide [36*a*]. If readers are interested in specific or more in-depth information about the overlap patterns between those molecules, it is recommended that they refer to reference [36*a*]. Recently, Novartis combined valsartan with the neprilysin inhibitor sacubitril as a combination drug called Entresto (sacubitril/valsartan) to use for the treatment of heart failure [36*b*].

Eprosartan (Fig. 6.23, **82**) is the only nonbiphenyl Ang II receptor antagonist and was introduced by SmithKline Beecham (now part of GlaxoSmithKline, GSK) in 1997. Its design was guided by conformational analysis of Takeda's compound **10** and the Ang II pentapeptide. The starting point for the design was to orientate the acetic acid moiety toward the C-terminus of Ang II and introduce a *trans*-acrylic acid to mimic the carboxylic acid moiety at that position. A benzyl group was introduced at the 2-position of the acrylic acid to ensure overlap with the side chain of

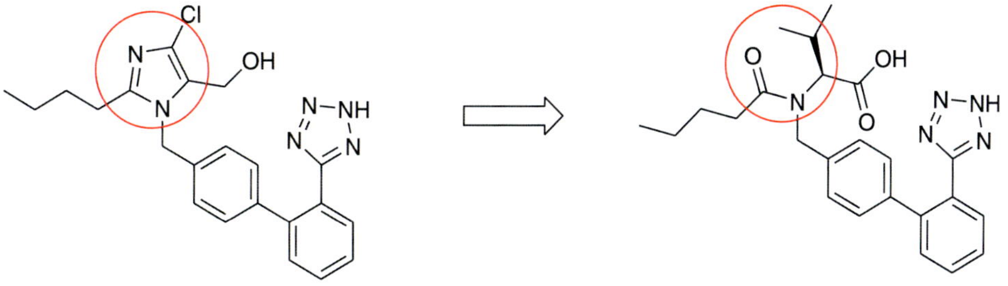

FIGURE 6.21 Structures of losartan (**5**) and valsartan (**81**).

losartan (**5**)   valsartan (**81**)

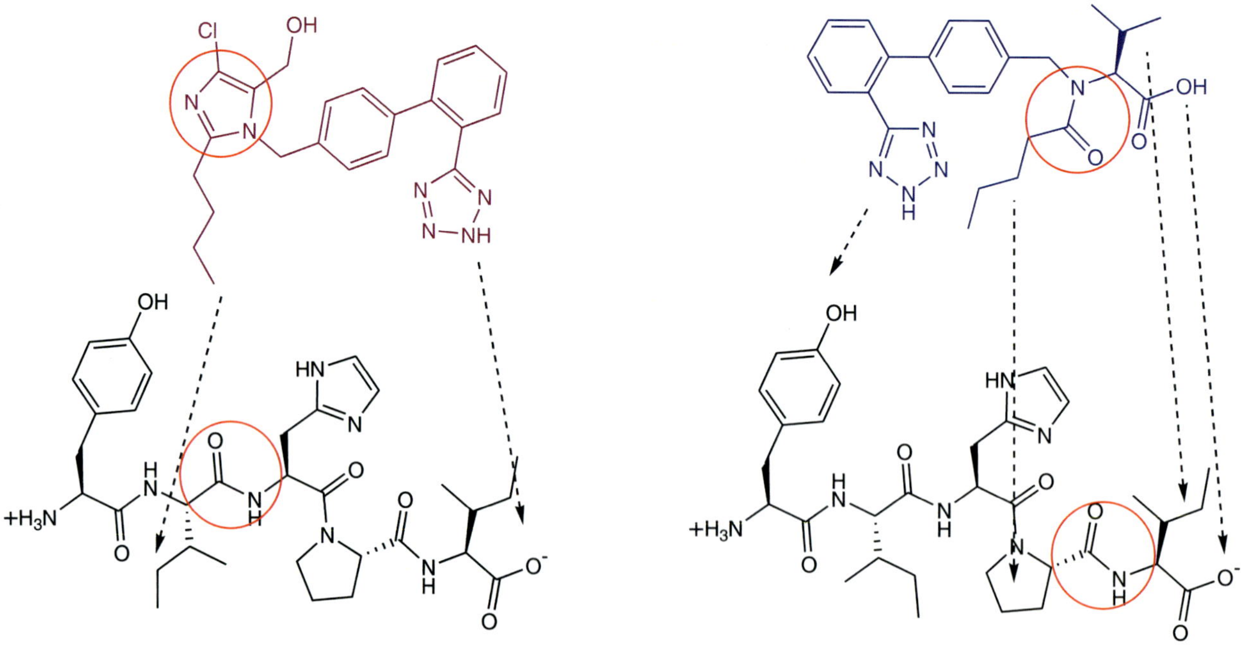

132 Medicinal Chemistry and Drug Development

FIGURE 6.22 Overlap hypotheses of the C-terminal pentapeptide (Tyr-Ile-His-Pro-Ile) part of sarile (Fig. 6.5, **8**) with losartan (**5**) and valsartan (**81**).

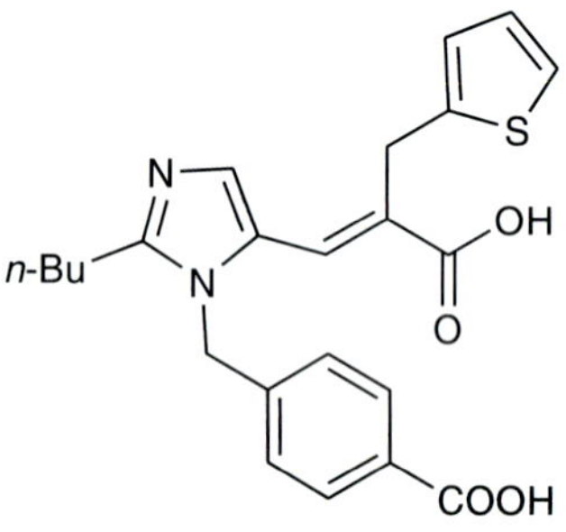

FIGURE 6.23 Structure of eprosartan (**82**).

eprosartan (**82**)

phenylalanine 8 (Phe8) in the Ang II pentapeptide. It was found that replacing the phenyl ring in the benzyl group with a benzene bioisostere thiophene ring improved the activity. The *n*-butyl group aligned with the side chain of isoleucine 5 (Ile5) in the angiotensin II pentapeptide. The carboxylic acid group at the 4-position of the imidazole benzyl moiety mimicked the phenolic hydroxyl group of tyrosine 4 (Tyr4) in the angiotensin II pentapeptide. The double bond between the imidazole ring and the acrylic acid moiety corresponded to the amide bond in the angiotensin II pentapeptide. Guided by this model, eprosartan (**82**) was designed, and it eventually exhibited excellent in vitro activity (IC_{50} = 1 nM), 40,000-fold more potent than compound **10** [37].

Irbesartan (Fig. 6.24, **83**) was introduced to the market in 1997 by Sanofi. The discovery of irbesartan was based on the modification of the imidazole ring of losartan (**5**). The SAR of the imidazole ring in losartan indicated the need for a hydrogen bond acceptor at the 5-position of the imidazole ring. The design rationale was shown in Fig. 6.24; researchers at Sanofi first reduced the hydroxymethyl group of losartan by one carbon atom, allowing the hydroxyl group to directly attach to the imidazole ring. This arrangement also allowed the hydroxyl group to exist in its keto-tautomeric form. However, when the 5-position of the imidazole ring exists in keto form, the carbon atom at the 4-position of the imidazole ring becomes unstable. The SAR of losartan also revealed that the chlorine atom at the 4-position of the imidazole ring interacted with a hydrophobic pocket of the receptor. By replacing the chlorine atom with two alkyl groups, the imidazoline ring becomes more stable while retaining the lipophilic interaction at the 4-position of the imidazole

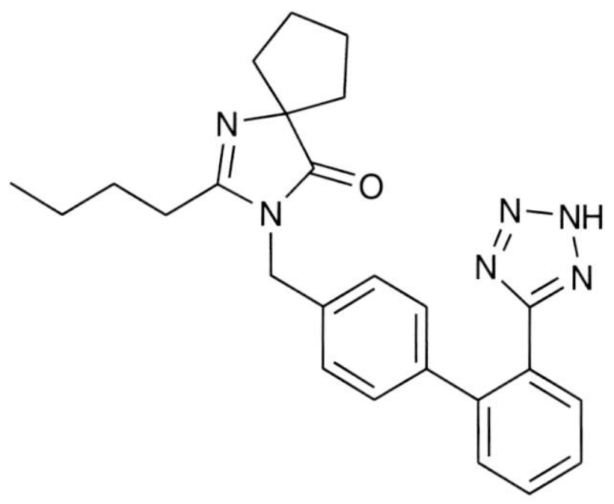

irbesartan (**83**)

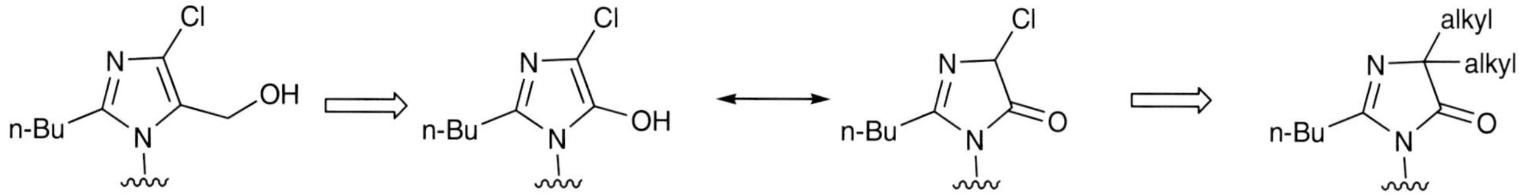

FIGURE 6.24 Structure of irbesartan (**83**) and design rationale.

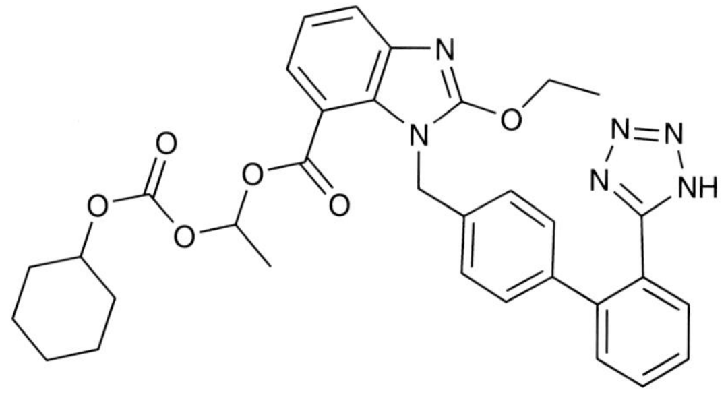

candesartan cilexetil (**84**)

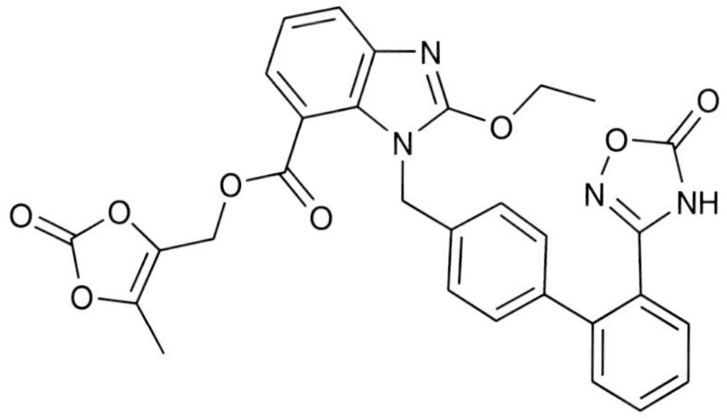

azilsartan medoxomil (**85**)

FIGURE 6.25 Structures of candesartan cilexetil (**84**) and azilsartan medoxomil (**85**).

ring. Subsequently, Sanofi's medicinal chemists synthesized a series of bis-alkylated compounds at the 4-position of the imidazole ring and discovered a series of spiro-ring compounds formed by combining two alkyl groups, leading to the discovery of a series of losartan analogs containing a spiro-ring imidazolinone moiety, including irbesartan (**83**) [38].

In the losartan series, the introduction of various functional groups at the 4- and 5-positions of the imidazole ring showed that these substituents could form a fused ring on the imidazole. 1-(Biphenylmethyl)benzimidazole was studied comprehensively and successfully utilized by several research groups, including candesartan, azilsartan, and telmisartan, which will be mentioned below.

As it has been shown, the entire class of sartan drugs was discovered based on the imidazole carboxylic acid compounds disclosed by Takeda in 1982. After the discovery of these compounds, Takeda made significant efforts to modify their structures but failed to improve their activity [39], so they had to temporarily abandon the project. Takeda must have felt regretful when DuPont Pharmaceuticals seized the opportunity and successfully discovered losartan. After the disclosure of losartan, Takeda scientists also adopted a "me-too" strategy by incorporating the biphenyl structure in losartan into their design and eventually discovered two new drugs in their own field: candesartan cilexetil (**84**) and azilsartan medoxomil (**85**) (Fig. 6.25). Both compounds are pro-drugs, with the carboxylic acid at the 7-position of the benzimidazole ring converted into an ester to enhance oral efficacy.

Takeda's focus was on the modification of the imidazole ring. Since the chlorine atom at the 4-position of the imidazole ring interacts with the receptor's lipophilic pocket, it was expected that the lipophilic benzene ring would also have a similar effect. Considering the importance of the carboxylic acid group for activity, compounds needed to retain this group, and thus the pro-drug of candesartan was designed [40]. In candesartan's benzimidazole ring, the original butyl group on the imidazole ring was replaced with an ethoxy group, and the carboxylic acid group was positioned at the 7-position of the benzimidazole [41], based on quantitative structure-activity relationship calculations. Although the parent compound of candesartan exhibited excellent in vitro activity, its in vivo efficacy did not correspondingly manifest. After exploration to introduce pro-drug groups on the tetrazole and carboxylic acid groups, Takeda found that esters introduced at the 7-position of the benzimidazole showed better in vivo activity. Among them, candesartan cilexetil, with a cyclohexylcarbonyloxy group, exhibited the best in vivo activity, characterized by its fast onset of action. The oral bioavailability of candesartan cilexetil in rats increased from 5% to 33.4% [42]. In 1998, candesartan cilexetil was successfully approved for marketing.

The design of azilsartan was primarily focused on the replacement of the tetrazole portion of candesartan, as the tetrazole exhibited certain deficiencies in synthesis, metabolism, and properties. For example, the synthesis of tetrazole unavoidably involved the use of relatively hazardous azide reagents. The nitrogen at the 2-position of the tetrazole could undergo glucuronidation, which accelerated its metabolism. Additionally, the presence of two polar and acidic groups on both the imidazole and biphenyl rings in these sartans also affected their oral bioavailability. Therefore, Takeda scientists decided to replace the tetrazole moiety with biphenyl to improve bioavailability. Through the evaluation of a series of five-membered heterocyclic compounds, a less acidic oxadiazole ring was found to effectively replace the tetrazole ring in candesartan, resulting in azilsartan. Although azilsartan was approximately fourfold less potent than candesartan, its better oral bioavailability (fourfold higher than candesartan) led to comparable in vivo efficacy [43]. Azilsartan medoxomil was also approved as a pro-drug in 2011. Both candesartan cilexetil and azilsartan medoxomil have stronger antihypertensive effects compared to losartan [44].

Another benzimidazole antihypertensive drug is telmisartan (Fig. 6.26, **86**), which was introduced by Boehringer Ingelheim in 1999. The design of telmisartan was also based on the modification of the imidazole ring in losartan. Similar to candesartan, scientists at Boehringer Ingelheim used a benzimidazole to replace the imidazole. Through systematic studies on the benzimidazole ring, they found that the C6-position was optimal when introducing the same substituent, such as amino, amide, and urea groups, at different positions of the benzimidazole ring. Subsequent SAR on the C6-position revealed that compounds containing amide and sulfonamide groups exhibited excellent in vitro activity with IC_{50} values in the low nanomolar range. However, their poor water solubility resulted in inferior oral activity. Furthermore, results from this study also confirmed an observation made during the research on losartan, which was that only one hydrogen bond acceptor was needed at the hydroxymethyl position of losartan. In search of compounds with improved oral activity, researchers at Boehringer Ingelheim introduced nitrogen-containing heterocycles as hydrogen bond acceptors at the C6-position of the benzimidazole. The results showed that a compound with an additional benzimidazole ring at the C6 position exhibited the best activity. A more significant finding was that a compound with two benzimidazole rings only required a carboxylic acid group on the biphenyl portion without the need to convert it to a tetrazole moiety (**87**), as the carboxylic acid **86** (IC_{50} = 3 nM) demonstrated better activity than the corresponding tetrazole analog **87** (IC_{50} = 13 nM) [45]. It is also worth noting that the substitute at the C2-position of the central benzimidazole could be *n*-propyl rather than *n*-butyl. In addition, introducing a methyl group at the C4-position had little impact on the activity, but this modification could avoid the regioselectivity issue in preparation when introducing the biphenyl group. Telmisartan is approximately 100-fold more potent than losartan in terms of blood pressure reduction, with a long half-life of approximately 24 hours [46].

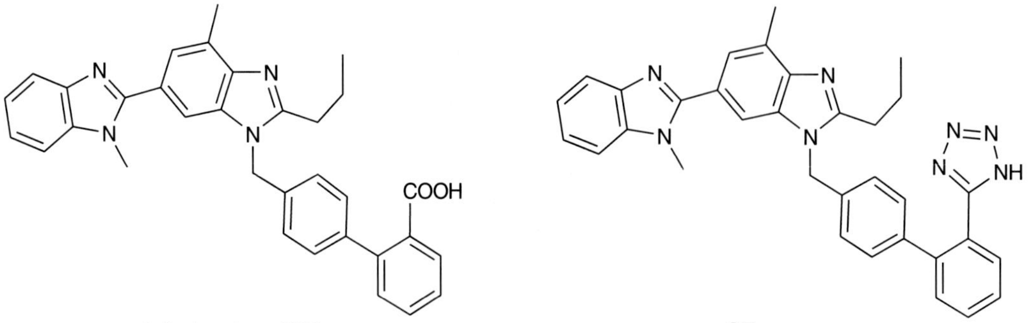

FIGURE 6.26 Structures of telmisartan (**86**) and compound **87**.

Olmesartan (Fig. 6.27, **88**) is the structurally closest analog of the metabolite **52** of losartan. It was discovered by Sankyo Pharmaceutical Co., Ltd. (now a subsidiary of Daiichi Sankyo Co., Ltd.). Olmesartan was obtained through exploration of the 4-substituent of the imidazole ring in compound **52**. SAR showed that a simple alkyl group could be used to replace the chlorine atom while retaining its in vitro activity, and introducing a hydrophilic hydroxyl group could compensate for the high lipophilicity of a pure alkyl group. As a result, the hydroxyisopropyl group emerged as a replacement for the chlorine atom. Furthermore, it was found that the *n*-butyl group at the 2-position of the imidazole ring could be replaced with a less lipophilic *n*-propyl group without affecting the activity. To improve oral bioavailability, olmesartan was ultimately formulated as the ester pro-drug olmesartan medoxomil [47]. As a result, olmesartan medoxomil was approved for the treatment of hypertension in 2002.

In fact, analogs with an alkyl substituent instead of a chlorine atom at the 4-position of the imidazole ring (Fig. 6.18, **53–62**) had been investigated by researchers at DuPont. Olmesartan and compound **56** from DuPont differ only by a hydroxyisopropyl group at the 4-position of the imidazole ring in olmesartan and an isopropyl group in compound **56**. It is remarkable how such a subtle change could lead to improved efficacy; most possibly, the hydroxyl of the hydroxyisopropyl group could form intramolecular hydrogen bonds with the carboxylic acid group at the 5-position of the imidazole ring, resulting in reduced polarity, thereby leading to improved oral activity. It is worth noting that compounds of this nature are beyond the scope of DuPont Pharmaceuticals' patent protection, another surprise of medicinal chemistry.

Fimasartan (Fig. 6.28, **90**) is a novel Ang II receptor antagonist discovered and marketed by Boryung Pharmaceuticals Co., Ltd. of South Korea in 2010. Fimasartan is a losartan derivative with a pyrimidine-4(3*H*)-one core replacing the imidazole ring of losartan. The lipophilic thioamide group on the pyrimidine-4(3*H*)-one ring plays a role similar to the chlorine atom on the imidazole ring of losartan [48]. Fimasartan has higher potency, a longer half-life, and faster and more effective antihypertensive effects compared to losartan. Fimasartan is rapidly absorbed; a daily dose range of 60–120 mg demonstrates antihypertensive effects within 24 hours after oral administration; and no drug accumulation has been observed after continuous administration for 7 days [49].

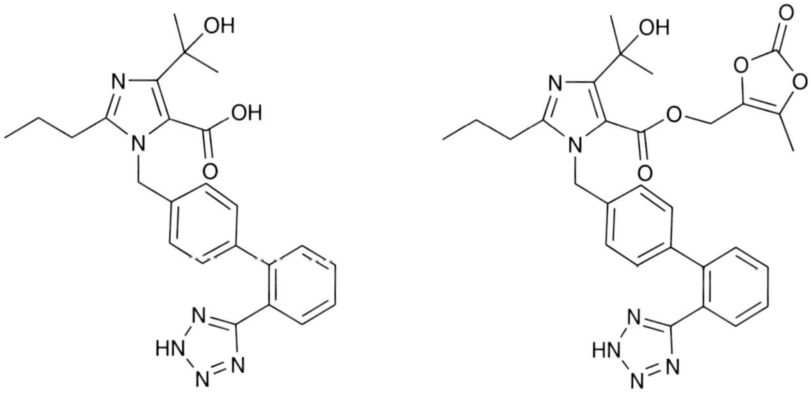

FIGURE 6.27 Structures of olmesartan (**88**) and olmesartan medoxomil (**89**).

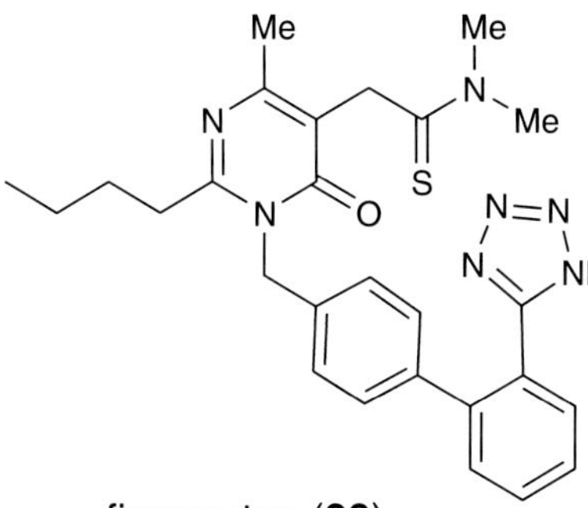

FIGURE 6.28 Structure of fimasartan (**90**).

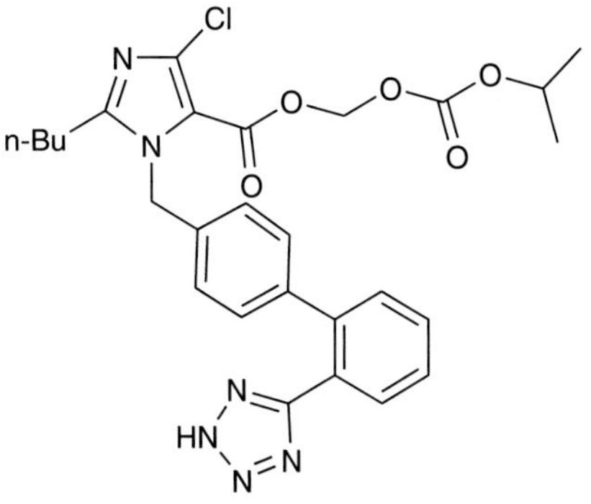

FIGURE 6.29 allisartan isoproxil (**91**).

allisartan isoproxil (**91**)

In the research on ARBs for hypertension, Chinese scientists have also made significant contributions. Allisartan isoproxil (Fig. 6.29, **91**), a first-class 1.1 innovative drug for hypertension developed independently in China, was discovered by Shanghai Allist Pharmaceuticals, which was approved in China in 2013. Allisartan isoproxil was a pro-drug of compound **52**, a metabolite of losartan with improved in vivo activity. This pro-drug exhibited enhanced oral bioavailability compared to the parent molecule **52**; it could be rapidly hydrolyzed to generate the active compound **52**, which reached peak concentration in the blood within 1.5−2.5 hours, and the exposure increased when the dosage increased [50].

The success of allisartan isoproxil embodies the wisdom and hard work of a group of elites in the field of new drug research and development in China; it also reflects the tremendous potential of China in this field. Dr. Jianhui Guo, the inventor and developer of allisartan isoproxil, passed away at an early age due to illness, just over a month after approval of allisartan isoproxil by the Chinese Food and Drug Administration. Dr. Guo's dedication to the development of new drugs in China deserves our admiration as a role model.

In summary, these case stories indicate that once a good drug target emerges, it will attract the interest of many pharmaceutical companies. It also reflects the current situation in new drug development, where many companies often target the same drug target, leading to unnecessary resource waste. At the same time, the development of numerous "sartan"-class drugs serves as a warning to drug developers. When applying for a patent, it is advisable to broaden the scope of coverage to prevent competitors from taking advantage of the me-too approach. However, no matter how thorough your protection might have been at the time, others could still find loopholes in the patent. This is because the field of pharmaceutical science is constantly advancing, and new research findings continually open new perspectives that could be applied in the process of drug development.

References

[1] (a) MacGregor GA, Markandu ND, Roulston JE, Jones JC, Morton JJ. Maintenance of blood pressure by the renin-angiotensin system in normal man. Nature 1981;291:329−31.
(b) Aurell M. The renin-angiotensin system: the centenary jubilee. Blood Pressure 1998;7(2):71−5.

[2] (a) Wolny A, Clozel JP, Rein J, Mory P, Vogt P, Turino M, et al. Functional and biochemical analysis of angiotensin II-forming pathways in the human heart. Circ Res 1997;80(2):219−27.
(b) Fukami H, Okunishi H, Miyazaki M. Chymase: its pathophysiological roles and inhibitors. Curr Pharm Des 1998;4(6):439−53.

[3] Larhed M, Hallberg M, Hallberg A. Nonpeptide AT2 receptor agonists. Med Chem Rev 2016;51:69−82.

[4] Maibaum J, Stutz S, Göschke R, Rigollier P, Yamaguchi Y, Cumin F, et al. Structural modification of the P2' position of 2,7-dialkyl-substituted 5(S)-amino-4(S)-hydroxy-8-phenyl-octanecarboxamides: The discovery of Aliskiren, a potent nonpeptide human renin inhibitor active after once daily dosing in marmosets. J Med Chem 2007;50:4832−44.

[5] Ondetti MA, Cushman DW. Inhibition of the renin angiotensin system: a new approach to the therapy of hypertension. J Med Chem 1981;24:355−61.

[6] McAreavey D, Robertson JIS. Angiotensin converting enzyme inhibitors and moderate hypertension. Drugs 1990;40(3):326−45.

[7] (a) Ondetti MA, Rubin A, Cushman DW. Design of specific inhibitors of angiotensin-converting enzyme: new class of orally active antihypertensive agents. Science 1977;196(4288):441−4.
(b) Cushman DW, Ondetti MA. Hypertension 1991;17(4):589−92.

[8] Patchett AA, Harris E, Tristram EW, Wyvratt MJ, Wu MT, Taub D, et al. A new class of angiotensin-converting enzyme inhibitors. Nature 1980;288:280−3.

[9] Skidgel RA, Erdoes EG. The broad substrate specificity of human angiotensin I converting enzyme. Clin Exp Hypertens A 1987;9(2−3):243−59.

[10] (a) Lindgren BR, Andersson RGG. Angiotensin-converting enzyme inhibitors and their influence on inflammation, bronchial reactivity and cough. Med Toxicol Adverse Drug Exp 1989;4(5):369−80.

(b) Chin HL, Buchan DA. Severe angioedema after long-term use of an angiotensin-converting enzyme inhibitor. Ann Intern Med 1990;112(4):312−13.

(c) Levens NR, de Gasparo M, Wood JM, Bottari SP. Could the pharmacological differences observed between angiotensin II antagonists and inhibitors of angiotensin converting enzyme be clinically beneficial? Pharmacol Toxicol 1992;71(4):241−9.

[11] Hicks BM, Filion KB, Yin H, Sakr L, Udell JA, Azoulay L. Angiotensin converting enzyme inhibitors and risk of lung cancer: population-based cohort study. Br Med J 2018;363:k4209.

[12] (a) Johnson AL, Carini DJ, Chiu AT, Duncia JV, Price WA, Wells Jr GJ, et al. Nonpeptide angiotensin II receptor antagonist. Drug News Perspect 1990;3:337−51.

(b) Timmermans PBMWM, Wong PC, Chiu A, Herblin WF. Nonpeptide angiotensin II receptor antagonists. Trends Pharmacol Sci 1991;12(2):55−62.

(c) Wexler RR, Greenlee WJ, Irvin JD, Goldberg MR, Prendergast K, Smith RD, et al. Nonpeptide angiotensin II receptor antagonists: the next generation in antihypertensive therapy. J Med Chem 1996;39:625−56.

[13] (a) Pals DT, Masucci FD, Denning Jr. GS. A specific competitive antagonist of the vascular action of angiotensin II. Circ Res 1971;29:664−72.

(b) Pals DT, Masucci FD, Denning Jr GS, Sipos F, Fessler DC. Role of the pressor action of angiotensin II in experimental hypertension. Circ Res 1971;29:673−81.

[14] (a) Brunner HR, Gavras H, Laragh JH, Keenan R. Angiotensin II blockade in man by SAR^1-ALA^8-angiotensin II for understanding and treatment of high blood pressure. Lancet 1973;302(7837):1045−8.

(b) Pals DT, Denning Jr GS, Keenan RE. Historical development of Saralasin. Kidney Int Suppl 1979;9:S7−10.

(c) Moore AF, Fulton RW. Angiotensin II antagonists-saralasin. Drug Dev Res 1984;4:331−49.

(d) Hata T, Ogihara T, Mikami H, Nakamura M, Maruyama A, Mandai T, et al. Comparison of the biological effects of two angiotensin II analogues in hypertensive patients with sodium depletion. Life Sci 1978;22(21):1955−62.

[15] (a) Furukawa Y, Kishimoto S, Nishikawa K. Hypotensive imidazole derivatives. U.S. Patent No 1982; US 4,340,598, July 20.

(b) Furukawa Y, Kishimoto S, Nishikawa K. Hypotensive imidazole-5-acetice acid derivatives. U.S. Patent No 1982; US 4,355,040, October 19.

[16] Wong PC, Chiu AT, Price WA, Thoolen MJ, Carini DJ, Johnson AL, et al. Nonpeptide angiotensin II receptor antagonists. I. Pharmacological characterization of 2-n-butyl-4-chloro-1-(2-chlorobenzyl) imidazole-5-acetic acid, sodium salt (S-8307). J Pharmacol Exp Ther 1988;247:1−7.

[17] Duncia JV, Chiu AT, Carini DJ, Gregory GB, Johnson AL, Price WA, et al. The Discovery of potent nonpeptide angiotensin II receptor antagonists: a new class of potent antihypertensives. J Med Chem 1990;33:1312−29.

[18] Carini DJ, Duncia JV, Johnson AL, Chiu AT, Price WA, Wong PC, et al. Nonpeptide angiotensin II receptor antagonists: N-[(benzyloxy)benzyl]imidazoles and related compounds as potent antihypertensives. J Med Chem 1990;33:1330−6.

[19] Carini DJ, Duncia JV, Aldrich PE, Chiu AT, Johnson AL, Pierce ME, et al. Nonpeptide angiotensin II receptor antagonists: the discovery of a series of N-(biphenylylmethyl)imidazoles as potent, orally active antihypertensives. J Med Chem 1991;34:2525−47.

[20] Duncia JV, Carini DJ, Chiu AT, Johnson AL, Price WA, Wong PC, et al. The discovery of DuP 753, a potent, orally active nonpeptide angiotensin II antagonist. Med Res Rev 1992;12(2):149−91.

[21] (a) Wong PC, Price WA, Chiu AT, Duncia JV, Carini DJ, Wexler RR, et al. Nonpeptide angiotensin II receptor antagonists. XI. Pharmacology of EXP3174: an active metabolite of DuP 753, an orally active antihypertensive agent. J Pharmacol Exp Ther 1990;255(1):211−17.

(b) Tamaki T, Nishiyama A, Kimura S, Aki Y, Yoshizumi M, Houchi H, et al. EXP3174: the major active metabolite of losartan. Cardiov Drug Rev 1997;15(2):122−36.

[22] (a) Carini DJ, Chiu AT, Wong PC, Johnson AL, Wexler RR, Timmermans PBMWM. The preparation of (perfluoroalkyl)imidazoles as nonpeptide angiotensin II receptor antagonists. Bioorg Med Chem Lett 1993;3:895−8.

(b) Chiu AT, Carini DJ, Duncia JV, Leung KH, McCall DE, Price Jr WA, et al. DuP 532: a second generation of nonpeptide angiotensin II receptor antagonists. Biochem Biophys Res Commun 1991;177:209−17.

(c) Wong PC, Hart SD, Chiu AT, Herblin WF, Carini DJ, Smith RD, et al. Pharmacology of DuP 532, a selective and noncompetitive AT1receptor antagonist. J Pharmacol Exp Ther 1991;259:861−70.

(d) Carini DJ, Ardeckly RJ, Ensinger CL, Pruitt JR, Wexler RR, Wong PC, et al. Nonpeptide angiotensin II receptor antagonists: the discovery of DMP581 and DMP811. Bioorg Med Chem Lett 1994;4:63−8.

(e) Wong PC, Huang S-M, Ardeckly RJ, Carini DJ, Chiu AT, Price Jr WA, et al. Pharmacology and pharmacokinetics of a novel nonpeptide angiotensin II receptor antagonist - DMP 811. Clin Exp Hypertens 1995;17:1233−56.

[23] (a) Stearns RA, Miller RR, Doss GA, Chakravarty PK, Rosegay A, Gatto GJ, et al. The metabolism of DuP 753, a nonpeptide angiotensin II receptor antagonist, by rat, monkey, and human liver slices. Drug Metab Dispos 1992;20(2):281−7.

(b) Chiu SH. The use of in vitro metabolism studies in the understanding of new drugs. J Pharmacol Toxicol Methods 1993;29(2):77−83.

(c) Sweet CS, Bradstreet DC, Berman RS, Saenz NJA, Weidler DJ. Pharmacodynamic activity of intravenous E-3174, an angiotensin II antagonist, in patients with essential hypertension. Am J Hypertens 1994;7:1035−40.

(d) Sterns RA, Chakravarty PC, Chen R, Chiu SH. Biotransformation of losartan to its active carboxylic acid metabolite in human liver microsomes. Drug Metab Dispos 1995;23(2):207−15.

(e) Lo MW, Goldberg MR, McCrea JB, Lu H, Furtek CI, Bjornsson TD. Pharmacokinetics of losartan, an angiotensin ☒ receptor antagonist, and its active metabolite EXP 3174 in humans. Clin Pharmacol Ther 1995;58(6):641–9.

(f) Kazierad DJ, Martin DE, Blum RA, Tenero DM, Ilson B, Boike SC, et al. Clin Pharmacol Ther 1997;62(4):417–25.

(g) Schmidt B, Schieffer B. Angiotensin II AT1 receptor antagonists. Clinical implications of active metabolites. J Med Chem 2003;46:2261–70.

[24] Zaidenstein R, Soback S, Gips M, Avni B, Dishi V, Weissgarten Y, et al. Effect of grapefruit juice on the pharmacokinetics of losartan and its active metabolite E3174 in healthy volunteers. Ther Drug Monit 2001;23(4):369–73.

[25] Chansel D, Badre L, Czekalski S, Vandermeersch S, Cambar J, Ardaillou R. Intrinsic properties of the nonpeptide angiotensin ☒ antagonist losartan in glomeruli and mesangial cells at high concentrations. J Pharmacol Exp Ther 1993;265(3):1534–43.

[26] Soldner A, Benet LZ, Mutschler E, Christians U. Active transport of the angiotensin-☒antagonist losartan and its main metabolite EXP 3174 across MDCK-MDR1 and Caco-2 cellmonolayers. Br J Pharmacol 2000;129(6):1235–43.

[27] Taavitsainen P, Kiukaanniemi K, Pelkonen O. In vitro inhibition screening of human hepatic P450 enzymes by five angiotensin-☒receptor antagonists. Eur J Clin Pharmacol 2000;56(2):135–40.

[28] Caballero R, Delpón E, Valenzuela C, Longobardo M, Tamargo J. Losartan and its metabolite E3174 modify cardiac delayed rectifier K^+ currents. Circulation 2000;101(10):1199–205.

[29] Wang YH, Shi CX, Dong F, Sheng JW, Xu YF. *Inhibition of the rapid component of the delayed rectifier potassium current in ventricular myocytes by angiotensin☒ via the AT_1 receptor*. Br J Pharmacol 2008;154(2):429–39.

[30] Chiu AT, Herblin WF, McCall DE, Ardeckly RJ, Carini DJ, Duncia JV, et al. Identification of angiotensin II receptor subtypes. Biochem Biophys Res Commun 1989;165(1):196–203.

[31] (a) Chiu AT, McCall DE, Price WA, Wong PC, Carini DJ, Duncia JV, et al. Nonpeptide angiotensin II receptor antagonists. VII. Cellular and biochemical pharmacology of DuP 753, an orally active antihypertensive agent. J Pharmacol Exp Ther 1990;252(2):711–18.

(b) Wong PC, Price WA, Chiu AT, Duncia JV, Carini DJ, Wexler RR, et al. Nonpeptide angiotensin II receptor antagonists. VIII. Characterization of functional antagonism displayed by DuP 753, an orally active antihypertensive agent. J Pharmacol Exp Ther 1990;252(2):719–25.

[32] (a) Wong PC, Price WA, Chiu AT, Duncia JV, Carini DJ, Wexler RR, et al. Nonpeptide angiotensin II receptor antagonists. IX. Antihypertensive activity in rats of DuP 753, an orally active antihypertensive agent. J Pharmacol Exp Ther 1990;252(2):726–32.

(b) Wong PC, Price WA, Chiu AT, Duncia JV, Carini DJ, Wexler RR, et al. Hypotensive action of DuP 753, an angiotensin II antagonist, in spontaneously hypertensive rats. Nonpeptide angiotensin II receptor antagonists. X Hypertension 1990;15(5):459–68.

[33] Hamada T, Ichida K, Hosoyamada M, Mizuta E, Yanagihara K, Sonoyama K, et al. Uricosuric action of losartan via the inhibition of urate transporter 1 (URAT 1) in hypertensive patients. Am J Hypertens 2008;21(10):1157–62.

[34] (a) Larsen RD, King AO, Chen CY, Corley eg,, Foster BS, Roberts FE, et al. Efficient synthesis of Losartan, A nonpeptide angiotensin II receptor antagonist. J Org Chem 1994;59:6391–4.

(b) Griffiths GJ, Hauck MB, Imwinkelried R, Kohr J, Roten CA, Stucky GC, et al. Novel syntheses of 2-butyl-5-chloro-3*H*-imidazole-4-carbaldehyde: a key intermediate for the synthesis of the angiotensin II antagonist Losartan. J Org Chem 1999;64:8084–9.

[35] (a) Wexler RR, Carini DJ, Duncia JV, Johnson AL, Wells GJ, Chiu AT, et al. Rationale for the chemical development of angiotensin II receptor antagonists. Am J Hypertens 1992;5(12):209S–20S.

(b) Bhardwaj G. How the antihypertensive losartan was discovered. Expert Opin Drug Discov 2006;1(6):609–18.

[36] Bühlmayer P, Furet P, Criscione L, Gasparo M, Whitebread S, Schmidlin T, et al. Combined angiotensin receptor antagonism and neprilysin inhibition. Circulation 2016;133(11):1115–24.

[37] (a) Weinstock J, Keenan RM, Samanen JM, Hempel J, Finkelstein JA, Franz RG, et al. 1-(Carboxybenzyl)imidazole-5-acrylic acids: potent and selective angiotensin ☒ receptor antagonists. J Med Chem 1991;34:1514–17.

(b) Keenan RM, Weinstock J, Finkelstein JA, Franz RG, Gaitanopoulos DE, Girard GR, et al. Imidazole-5-acrylic acids: potent nonpeptide angiotensin ☒ receptor antagonists designed using a novel peptide pharmacophore model. J Med Chem 1992;35:3858–72.

(c) Keenan RM, Weinstock J, Finkelstein JA, Franz RG, Gaitanopoulos DE, Girard GR, et al. Potent nonpeptide angiotensin ☒ receptor antagonists. 2. 1-(Carboxybenzyl)imidazole-5-acrylic acids. J Med Chem 1993;36:1880–92.

[38] Bernhart CA, Perreaut PM, Ferrari BP, Muneaux YA, Assens JLA, Clement J, et al. A new series of imidazolones: highly specific and potent nonpeptide AT1 angiotensin II receptor antagonists. J Med Chem 1993;36:3371–80.

[39] (a) Nishikawa K, Shibouta Y, Inada Y, Terashita Z-I, Kawazoe K. Nonpeptide angiotensin II receptor Antagonists: pharmacological studies on imidazoleacetic acid derivatives. J Takeda Res Labs 1991;50:56–74.

(b) Nishikawa K, Shibouta Y, Inada Y, Terashita Z-I, Kawazoe K. Nonpeptide angiotensin II receptor antagonists: pharmacological studies on imidazoleacetic acid derivatives. J Takeda Res Labs 1991;50:75–98.

[40] Kubo K, Inada Y, Kohara Y, Sugiura Y, Ojima M, Itoh K, et al. Nonpeptide angiotensin II receptor antagonists. Synthesis and biological activity of benzimidazoles. J Med Chem 1993;36:1772–84.

[41] Kubo K, Kohara Y, Imamiya E, Sugiura Y, Inada Y, Furukawa Y, et al. Nonpeptide angiotensin II receptor antagonists. Synthesis and biological activity of benzimidazolecarboxylic acids. J Med Chem 1993;36:2182–95.

[42] Kubo K, Kohara Y, Yoshimura YE, Inada Y, Shibouta Y, Furukawa Y, et al. Nonpeptide angiotensin II receptor antagonists. Synthesis and biological activity of potential prodrugs of benzimidazole-7-carboxylic acids. J Med Chem 1993;36:2343–9.

[43] (a) Kohara Y, Imamiya E, Kubo K, Wada T, Inada Y, Naka T. A new class of angiotensin II receptor antagonists with a novel acidic bioisostere. Bioorg Med Chem Lett 1995;5:1903—8.
(b) Kohara Y, Kubo K, Imamiya E, Wada T, Inada Y, Naka T. Synthesis and angiotensin II receptor antagonistic activities of benzimidazole derivatives bearing acidic heterocycles as novel tetrazole bioisosteres. J Med Chem 1996;39:5228—35.

[44] (a) McClellan KJ, Goa KL. Candesartan cilexetil. A review of its use in essential hypertension. Drugs 1998;56(5):847—69.
(b) Perry CM. Azilsartanmedoxomil: a review of its use in hypertension. Clin Drug Investig 2012;32(9):621—39.

[45] Ries UJ, Mihm G, Narr B, Hasselbach KM, Wittneben H, Entzeroth M, et al. 6-Substituted benzimidazoles as new nonpeptide angiotensin II receptor antagonists: synthesis, biological activity, and structure activity relationships. J Med Chem 1993;36:4040—51.

[46] Wienen W, Entzeroth M, van Meel JCA, Stangier J, Busch U, Ebner T, et al. A review on Telmisartan: a novel, long-acting angiotensin II-receptor antagonist. Cardiov Drug Rev 2000;18(2):127—54.

[47] (a) Yanagisawa H, Amemiya Y, Kanazaki T, Fujimoto K, Shimoji Y, Fujimoto Y, et al. Angiotensin II receptor antagonists: imidazole and pyrroles bearing hydroxymethyl and carboxy substituents. Bioorg Med Chem Lett 1994;4:177—82.
(b) Yanagisawa H, Amemiya Y, Kanazaki T, Shimoji Y, Fujimoto K, Kitahara Y, et al. Nonpeptide angiotensin II receptor antagonists: synthesis, biological activities, and structure-activity relationships of imidazole-5-carboxylic acids bearing alkyl, alkenyl, and hydroxyalkyl substituents at the 4-position and their related compounds. J Med Chem 1996;39:323—8.

[48] Kim TW, Yoo BW, Lee JW, Kim JH, Lee K-T, Chi YH, et al. Synthesis and antihypertensive activity of pyrimidin-4(3*H*)-one derivatives as losartan analogue for new angiotensin II receptor type 1 (AT1) antagonists. Bioorg Med Chem Lett 2012;22:1649—54.

[49] Lee H-Y, Oh B-H. Fimasartan: a new angiotensin receptor blocker. Drugs 2016;76(10):1015—22.

[50] (a) Guo J, An D. The salts of imidazole-5-carboxylic acid derivatives, preparation methods and use thereof. International patent No 2008; WO 2008/067687 A1, June 12.
(b) Wu M-Y, Ma X-J, Yang C, Tao X, Liu A-J, Su D-F, et al. Effects of allisartan, a new AT1 receptor blocker, on blood pressure and end-organ damage in hypertensive animals. Acta Pharmacol Sin 2009;30(3):307—13.

Chapter 7

Antithrombotic drug—apixaban

Yafei Liu[1], Yao Wu[1] and Hong Shen[2]

[1]*Department of Medicinal Chemistry, China Innovation Center of Roche (CICoR), Shanghai, P.R. China,* [2]*China Innovation Center of Roche (CICoR), Shanghai, P.R. China*

Chapter outline

7.1 What is thrombosis?	141
7.1.1 The dangers of thrombosis	141
7.1.2 The pathogenesis of thrombosis	141
7.2 Treatment of thrombosis	143
7.2.1 Commonly used antithrombotic drugs and their mechanisms of action	143
7.2.2 The specificity and advantages of selective FXa inhibitor	144
7.3 The medicinal chemistry of apixaban	146
7.3.1 Discovery of hit compound	146
7.3.2 Optimization of lead compound	147
7.3.3 The binding model of apixaban and FXa	153
7.3.4 The synthetic routes of apixaban	154
7.3.4.1 Route 1	155
7.3.4.2 Route 2	157
7.3.4.3 Route 3	157
7.3.4.4 Route 4	158
7.4 Clinical indications of apixaban	158
7.5 Postclass requirements and references	158
References	159

7.1 What is thrombosis?

Thrombosis[1] refers to the process that the components of normally circulating blood (such as fibrin, platelets, and red blood cells) aggregate within the blood vessels to form clots under certain conditions, causing partial or complete blockage of blood vessels, restricting blood flow, and thus causing obstacles of blood supply to the corresponding areas [1]. The clots formed during this process are known as thrombus.

According to the type of blood vessels where the thrombosis occurs, thrombosis can be classified into arterial thrombosis, venous thrombosis, and microvascular thrombosis.

7.1.1 The dangers of thrombosis

Thrombosis can occur in the blood vessels anywhere in the body, so it can cause serious damage to any part of the body. For example, when it occurs in the lungs, it may lead to pulmonary embolism (PE); when it occurs in the brain, it may cause stroke; and when it occurs in the myocardium, it may lead to infarction.

Thrombosis is not only a major factor in the onset and death of arterial diseases (such as stroke and infarction), but also the main culprit in venous thromboembolism (VTE), such as deep vein thrombosis and PE. VTE is the third leading cause of cardiovascular-associated death, after myocardial infarction and stroke [2]. Approximately 12 million people die from cardiovascular and cerebrovascular diseases such as cerebral thrombosis, cerebral infarction, myocardial infarction, coronary heart disease, and arteriosclerosis worldwide every year, accounting for nearly a quarter of the world's total deaths. Therefore, there is a huge market demand for drugs to prevent and treat thrombotic diseases both domestically and internationally.

7.1.2 The pathogenesis of thrombosis

There are two types of substances related to thrombosis in human body: one is **coagulant** substances [3,4], such as adenosine diphosphate, thromboxane A_2, fibrin, and calcium, which can cause the aggregation of platelets to form thrombus, thereby achieving the purpose of hemostasis; the other is **anticoagulant** substances, such as fibrinolytic enzymes and prostacyclin, which play a role in anticoagulation and prevent thrombus formation. Under normal conditions, the coagulant and anticoagulant substances are in dynamic equilibrium, ensuring that the body can maintain normal blood flow [5].

When the balance is disrupted by factors such as aging, surgery, limited movement, and trauma, the body is prone to thrombosis [5]. Especially, as age increases, the concentration of certain coagulation factors (such as FV, FVII, FVIII, and FIX) and platelets in the plasma will gradually increase; therefore, the elderly are susceptible or the main group to cardiovascular diseases. In addition, under normal circumstances, the endothelium of human blood vessels plays an important role in hemostasis. However, changes in the structure and function of the vascular wall during aging increase the risk of thrombotic diseases in the elderly, especially atherosclerotic thrombosis.

The introduction of coagulation factors is shown in Table 7.1, and the coagulation cascade involving coagulation factors is shown in Fig. 7.1 [6,7]. Activated coagulation factors are indicated by adding "a" after the Roman numerals of the corresponding coagulation factor. The coagulation pathways are divided into intrinsic and extrinsic pathways. The extrinsic pathway is as follows: under normal circumstances, there is no coagulation factor III (tissue factor) in the plasma of the human body. However, when tissue inflammation, infection, and other traumas occur, the synthesis and expression of coagulation factor III will be promoted and released into the plasma. Then, coagulation factor III will further activate coagulation factor VII, and the activated coagulation factor VIIa can further activate coagulation factor X, thereby obtaining activated coagulation factor Xa (FXa). In the intrinsic pathway, factor XII can be activated after

TABLE 7.1 Introduction of coagulation factors.

Code	English name
FI	Fibrinogen
FII	Prothrombin
FIII	Tissue thromboplastin
FIV	Ca^{2+}
FV	Proaccelerin
FVII	Proconvertin
FVIII	Antihemophilic factor
FIX	PTC
FX	Stuart-Prower factor
FXI	PTA
FXII	Contact factor
FXIII	Fibrin-stabilizing

Coagulation Cascade

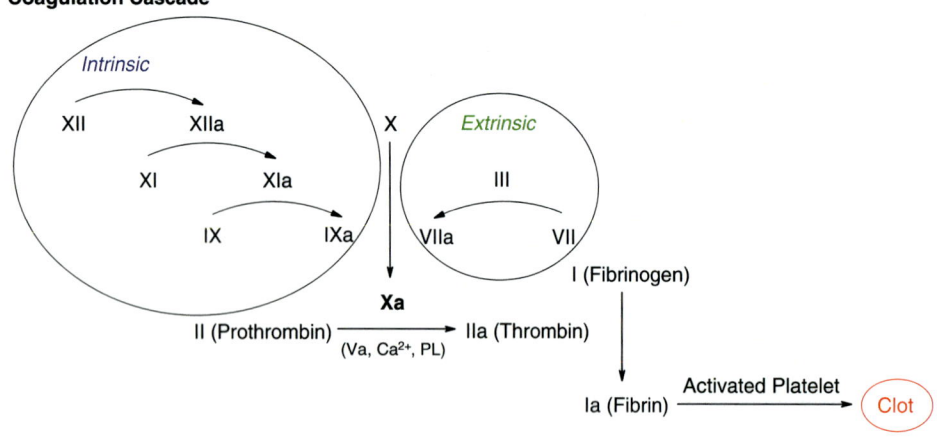

FIGURE 7.1 The coagulation cascade.

damage to the interior of the blood vessel. The activated coagulation factor XIIa can continue to activate the downstream coagulation factor XI. The resulting activated factor XIa can further activate coagulation factor IX, and the produced activated factor IXa can also activate coagulation factor X to obtain FXa. FXa produced by both the intrinsic and extrinsic pathways can go through the same process to produce a thrombus. That is, FXa activates prothrombin FII, which interacts with activated procoagulant globulin Va, calcium ions, and phospholipids to obtain activated thrombin FIIa. Thrombin FIIa can continue to activate fibrinogen FI to obtain fibrin FIa, and then fibrin FIa combines with activated platelets, leading to the formation of blood clots, that is, thrombus.

7.2 Treatment of thrombosis

Medications for treating thrombosis can be divided into three categories: anticoagulant drugs, antiplatelet drugs, and thrombolytic drugs [2].

7.2.1 Commonly used antithrombotic drugs and their mechanisms of action

Anticoagulant drugs (Fig. 7.2) inhibit specific coagulation factors and prolong the clotting time, making the blood less likely to coagulate, thereby reducing or preventing the formation of thrombus. Including (1) indirect thrombin inhibitors [8], such as unfractionated heparin and low molecular weight heparin; (2) vitamin K-dependent anticoagulants [9], such as warfarin; (3) direct thrombin inhibitors [10–12], such as Pradaxa, apixaban, and rivaroxaban. In comparison, direct thrombin inhibitors can reduce the risk of bleeding, decrease the frequency of monitoring coagulation function, increase the speed of onset of action, and weaken interactions with other foods or drugs.

Heparin is a glycosaminoglycan produced by the mast cells of mammals [8]. Heparin contains a unique pentasaccharide compound that can enhance the activity of the protease inhibitor antithrombin III in inactivating various key proteases (especially coagulation FXa and thrombin IIa) in the coagulation cascade. As an anticoagulant, heparin has been widely used in clinical, but it still has the following shortcomings: (1) heparin has low bioavailability, and it is difficult to monitor and control the quality of heparin produced in different batches; (2) heparin is a byproduct of animals, so there is a potential risk for patients to be infected by animal pathogens; (3) high molecular weight heparin (10–15 kDa) cannot be administered orally and must be injected intravenously; (4) the clinical dose-response curve for heparin is steep [13], with a narrow safety window, which requires continuous monitoring of the patient's plasma coagulation time to avoid drug overdosing and bleeding complications. In attempts to overcome the challenges related to heparin, low molecular weight (400–6500) heparin formulations have been developed, which maintained the original activity of heparin while reducing the probability of heparin-induced bleeding complications, and due to the reduced molecular size, the bioavailability is improved and they can be administered subcutaneously.

Because the synthesis of coagulation factors FII, FVII, FIX, and FX all require the participation of vitamin K [14], vitamin K antagonists can effectively inhibit the coagulation cascade. As a vitamin K antagonist, warfarin (Fig. 7.2A) is the first oral anticoagulant drug in the past 50 years and is widely used for the prevention of thromboembolic diseases. The antithrombotic effect of warfarin is clear and reliable; however, it also has some shortcomings [13], e.g., narrow therapeutic window, the need for frequent monitoring of the patient's coagulation function (initially measuring INR values weekly, then once a month after stabilization), greatly varied treatment effect among individuals, sensitivity to food and drugs, and slow onset and offset effect.

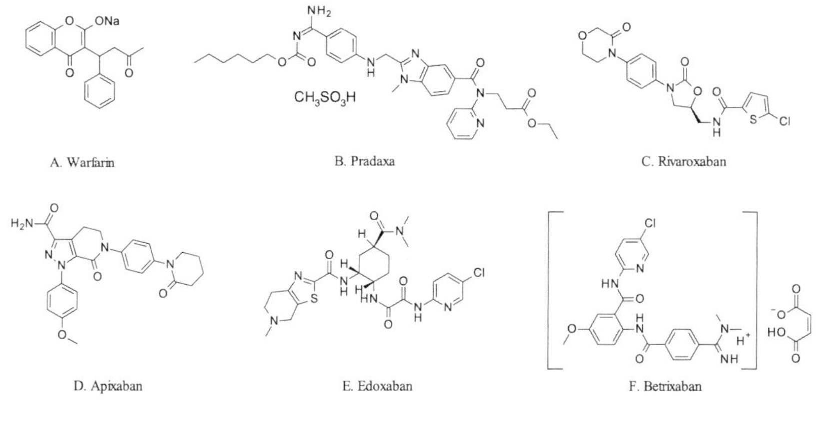

FIGURE 7.2 Commonly used anticoagulant drugs.

Pradaxa (Fig. 7.2B) belongs to the class of β-alanine coagulation enzyme inhibitors. As the prodrug of dabigatran, it is a new direct thrombin inhibitor [15,16]. The original research company is Boehringer Ingelheim from Germany. It is used to prevent stroke and thrombosis in patients with nonvalvular atrial fibrillation (NVAF). Pradaxa was first launched in Germany in 2008 and then approved by FDA in October 2010. The mechanism of action (MOA) is as follows: after oral administration, Pradaxa is absorbed by the gastrointestinal tract and converted to dabigatran, which could bind to the active site of thrombin FIIa, resulting in directly inhibiting the activity of thrombin, thus inhibiting the conversion of FI to FIa. In addition, Pradaxa can also inhibit FVa, FVIIIa, FIXa, FXIIIa, and platelet kinase-activated receptors, thereby blocking the final steps of the coagulation cascade and preventing thrombus formation. As for adverse effects (AEs), Pradaxa would inevitably cause bleeding during treatment, and high-dose medication will also increase the probability of bleeding.

Rivaroxaban (brand name Xarelto, Fig. 7.2C) is an oral highly selective direct FXa inhibitor [17]. It was jointly developed by Bayer Pharmaceuticals and Johnson & Johnson for the use of preventing the formation of venous thrombosis in adult patients undergoing elective hip [18] or knee [19] replacement surgery. Rivaroxaban was first launched in European Union and Canada in 2008 and then approved in China in June 2009. Rivaroxaban was also approved for the treatment of PE in April 2017 and has been marketed in more than 50 countries worldwide by now. The MOA is as follows: it could inhibit FXa to interrupt both intrinsic and extrinsic pathways of the coagulation cascade, resulting in inhibiting thrombin formation and thrombosis. In addition, rivaroxaban neither inhibit FIIa nor affect platelets. Rivaroxaban ranked tenth in global drug sales in 2020 with sales of $6.93 billion.

Apixaban (brand name Eliquis, Fig. 7.2D) is a direct, reversible, and highly selective FXa inhibitor [20]. It was jointly developed by Bristol-Myers Squibb and Pfizer. Apixaban binds to the active site of FXa in a highly complementary manner, thereby blocking the conversion of prothrombin to thrombin in the coagulation cascade. Apixaban does not affect thrombin activity, thus preserving the hemostatic function of thrombin. In addition, apixaban can also inhibit platelet aggregation indirectly by inducing thrombin. As the global small molecule sales champion in 2018, apixaban has the best-in-class clinical trial results, with better efficacy and safety effects. It could also significantly reduce the risk of bleeding and is currently the most widely used anticoagulant drug [21]. With sales of $9.17 billion, apixaban ranked fourth in global drug sales in 2020.

Edoxaban (Fig. 7.2E) is a selective inhibitor of FXa [22], developed by Daiichi Sankyo. It is used to reduce the potential risk of stroke and thrombosis in patients with NVAF, as well as for the treatment of deep vein thrombosis and PE. Edoxaban was approved for marketing in Japan in 2011 and then approved by the FDA and European Union in 2015.

Betrixaban (Fig. 7.2F) is an FXa inhibitor developed by Portola Pharmaceuticals [23]. It is used to prevent the formation of VTE. Betrixaban was approved by the FDA in June 2017. It is currently the first anticoagulant drug that can be administered long-term to adult patients who are acutely hospitalized, during both the inpatient stay and the subsequent treatment phase, to prevent VTE due to reduced mobility [24].

Antiplatelet aggregation drugs [25,26], as the name implies, prevent blood clot formation by reducing or inhibiting platelet aggregation. They are used in the prevention and treatment of arterial thrombotic diseases. These drugs cannot prevent the formation of deep vein thrombosis and pulmonary thrombosis. The first generation is COX enzyme inhibitors, such as aspirin; the second generation is platelet ADP receptor antagonists, such as ticlopidine, clopidogrel; and the third generation is platelet glycoprotein (GP) IIb/IIIa receptor antagonists, such as abciximab.

Thrombolytic drugs, administered through intravenous infusion or local delivery via catheter, can re-establish blood flow [27]. This class of drugs works by activating plasminogen to break the arginine-lysine bonds in fibrin, breaking down fibrin into soluble substances, thereby dissolving the thrombus. Widely used thrombolytics include streptokinase (SK), urokinase, alteplase, and reteplase.

7.2.2 The specificity and advantages of selective FXa inhibitor

FX is a vitamin K-dependent serine protease, synthesized by the liver with a half-life of 40−45 hours [7]. The activated FXa can hydrolyze the peptide bonds of prothrombin to active thrombin (Fig. 7.3).

As shown in Fig. 7.4, FXa has four active sites, S1, S2, S3, and S4 (the groups occupying the S1, S2, S3, and S4 pockets are marked as P1, P2, P3, and P4, respectively). S1 is a deep hydrophobic pocket, which contributes significantly to the binding activity and selectivity; the S2 pocket is smaller and shallower; the S3 pocket is located at the edge of the S1 pocket and is exposed to the solvent area; and the S4 pocket has three regions that provide ligand binding, including the hydrophobic area, the cationic cavity, and the water molecule. Among these, the S1 and S4 pockets are the main pockets for drug binding. The FXa inhibitors are typically "L"-shaped molecules, with P1 located in the

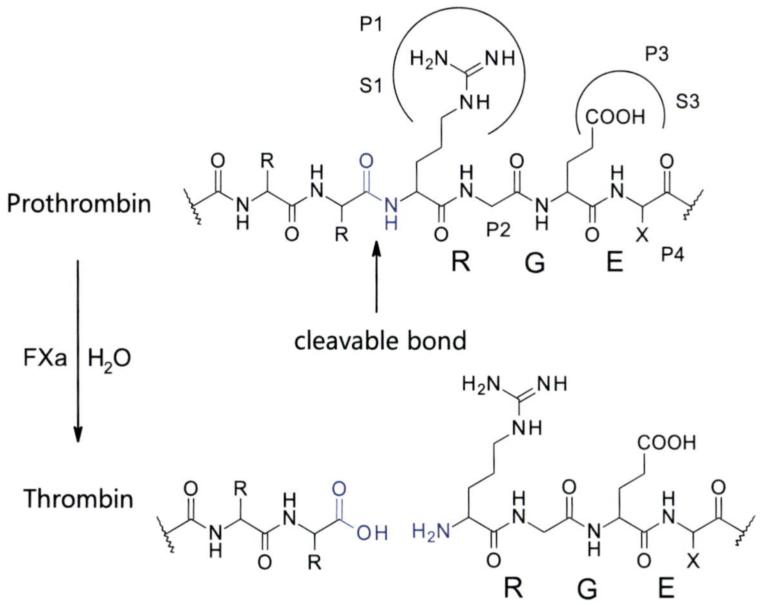

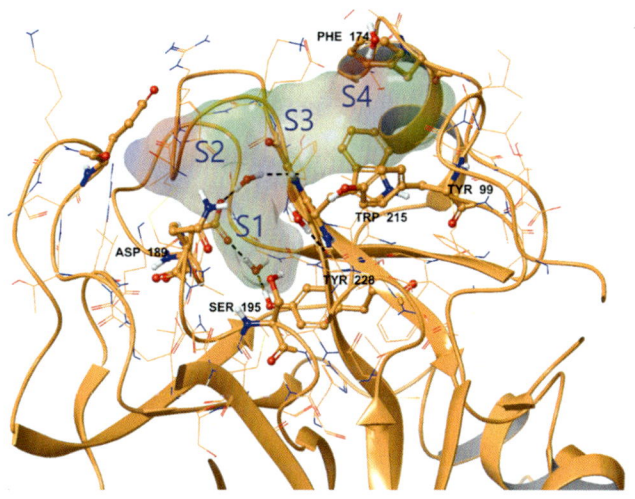

FIGURE 7.3 Activation of prothrombin by FXa. *R*, arginine; *G*, glycine; *E*, glutamate.

FIGURE 7.4 The structure of FXa protein. *PHE*, phenylalanine; *ASP*, aspartic acid; *SER*, serine; *TYR*, tyrosine, *TRP*, tryptophan.

S1 pocket formed by residues Asp189, Ser195, and Tyr228, and P4 located in the S4 pocket formed by residues Tyr99, Phe174, and Trp215. P1 and P4 are connected by a relatively rigid scaffold.

As shown in the coagulation cascade (Fig. 7.1), FXa is at the center of the coagulation cascade and can be activated by both intrinsic and extrinsic coagulation pathways. Therefore, effective inhibition of FXa activity can simultaneously suppress both intrinsic and extrinsic pathways of coagulation [28], and also prolong the clotting times of the intrinsic pathway (activated partial thromboplastin time, APTT) and the extrinsic pathway (prothrombin time, PT) [29]. In addition, the concentration of FXa in the body is lower than that of thrombin, and one molecule of FXa can catalyze the generation of nearly 1000 thrombin molecules. Therefore, compared with FIIa inhibitors, lower doses of FXa inhibitors can effectively prevent the formation of thrombin [30]. Preclinical research results have shown that the risk of bleeding of FXa inhibitors is significantly lower than that of FIIa inhibitors. Moreover, orally active FXa inhibitors have demonstrated more significant advantages in preventing the formation of thrombin [31,32].

To be effective antithrombotic drugs, selective FXa inhibitors must demonstrate both good potency and high selectivity. In the initial evaluation of selectivity, the activities of thrombin (selectivity within the coagulation cascade) and trypsin (selectivity against other serine proteases) were tested. This ensures that the inhibitor targets FXa without significantly affecting other serine proteases that are important for various physiological processes, thereby reducing potential side effects and increasing the therapeutic index.

7.3 The medicinal chemistry of apixaban

The research and development of apixaban mainly went through the following processes (Fig. 7.5): (1) screening of the GPIIb/IIIa compound library and rational drug design provided a dual-basic lead compound containing guanidine groups for the FXa inhibitor project; (2) optimization of the isoxazoline series and retaining one basic center led to the identification of less-basic compounds SF303 and SK509; (3) removal of the chiral center in isoxazoline ring resulted in planar isoxazole series, among which SA862 demonstrated subnanomolar binding affinity for FXa; (4) modification of the core isoxazole structure led to the discovery of a new type of five-membered heterocyclic series, which can act as effective FXa inhibitors with substitution of amidine; (5) further optimization of the pyrazole series resulted in SN429 with picomolar-level FXa binding affinity; (6) reducing basicity led to benzylamine-substituted DPC423 with improved oral bioavailability; (7) optimization of P1 substitutions resulted in razaxaban with improved selectivity for trypsin; (8) bicyclic series was developed to inhibit the formation of aromatic amine metabolites and solve related safety concerns, ultimately leading to apixaban.

7.3.1 Discovery of hit compound

Initially, by screening DuPont-Merck's compounds library [33], scientists discovered that a series of isoxazole derivatives such as compound **1** showed weak FXa binding affinity (Fig. 7.6). These compounds were previously designed as GPIIb/IIIa receptor antagonists by mimicking Arg-Gly-Asp (RGD) tripeptide sequence. The RGD sequence is quite

FIGURE 7.5 Key compounds during the development of apixaban.

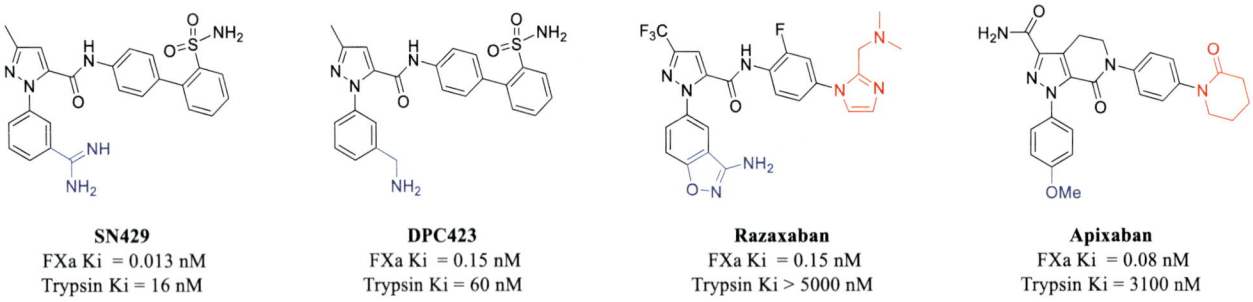

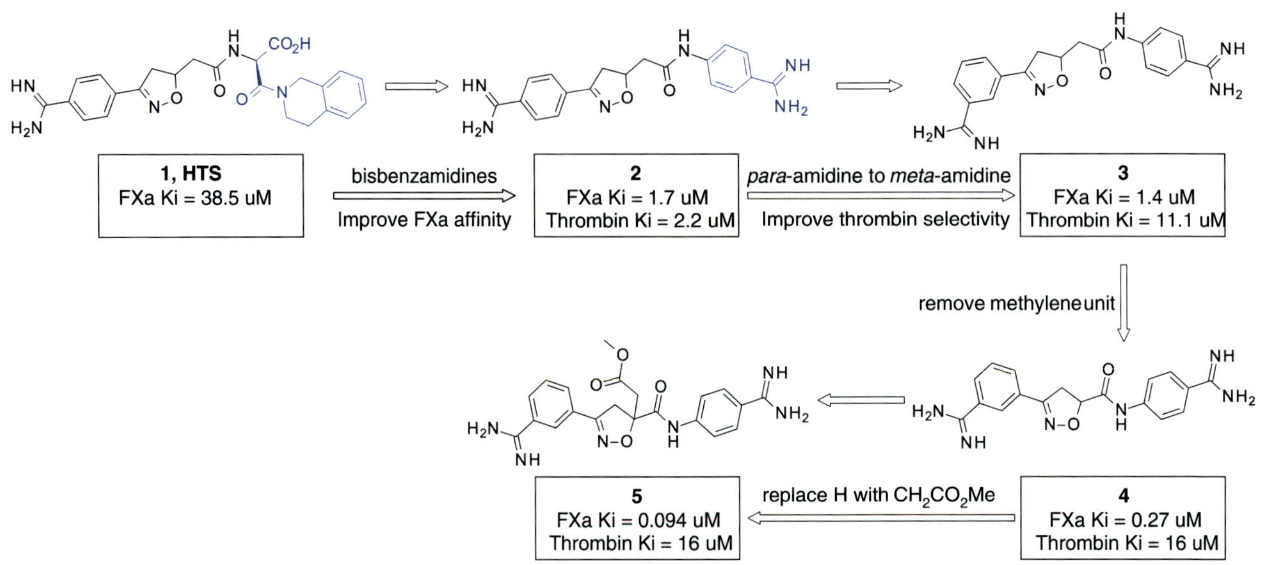

FIGURE 7.6 Optimization from HTS to diamidine compound.

similar to the Glu-Gly-Ar (EGR) of the active site of thrombin. Besides, there was some literature about diamidine compounds showing FXa binding affinity. Therefore, the project team decided to keep the amidinoisoxazole as the core structure. Diamidine compound **2** was obtained by replacing the right site of compound **1** with benzamidine, which showed 22-fold higher binding potency. Compound **3** demonstrated improved selectivity by shifting the *para*-amidine substitution on the left of compound **2** to the *meta* position. When the methylene unit between isoxazole and amide in compound **3** was removed, racemic compound **4** was obtained with a five folds better binding affinity. After replacing the hydrogen substituent on the isoxazole with methyl acetate substitution, the FXa binding affinity of compound **5** was further improved, and it had nearly 170-fold selectivity for thrombin. In addition, **5** showed in vivo efficacy with an ID_{50} value of 1.6 mg/kg/h in a rat vena cava thrombosis model (dosed via intravenous infusion).

7.3.2 Optimization of lead compound

As a dibasic compound, compound **5** did not exhibit sufficient oral bioavailability in pharmacokinetics [34]. To reduce its basicity, researchers replaced one of the amidine groups with a neutral substituent such as a biphenyl moiety, which may interact with the aromatic residues in the S4 pocket (Fig. 7.7). Compared to compound **5**, compound **6** showed two folds lower binding affinity, but it provided opportunities to introduce substituents on P4 (the biphenyl aromatic ring). It was found that substitutions at the 2'-position demonstrated better binding potency than the 3'-position by exploring substitutions on the terminal aromatic ring (**7** vs. **8**). The insertion of sulfonyl amide group (compound **8**) or methyl sulfone (compound **9**) at 2'-position improved potency by 35-fold (**8** and **9** vs. **6**).

The ester group in the side chain of compound **8** (**SF303**) could be hydrolyzed by esterases (widely present in the human body), resulting in poor in vivo metabolic stability. A large amount of esterase metabolite (compound **10**) was detected in rabbit plasma samples by mass spectrometry analysis, and the content of the carboxylic acid metabolite **10** continued to increase over time. To improve the in vivo antithrombotic efficacy, it is necessary to find alternative groups for the ester (Fig. 7.8) [35]. The most direct approach is to hydrolyze the ester group to obtain the carboxylic acid derivative **10**. The FXa binding affinity of compound **10** decreased by nearly three-fold, but its selectivity relative to thrombin was improved, which may be attributed to the electrostatic repulsion between the carboxylate group and thrombin's Glu192 residue. Surprisingly, compound **11** also showed similar FXa binding potency to **SF303** by directly removing the side chain ester group.

In order to further improve potency, scientists changed the connection site of the amide and aromatized the isoxazoline core, resulting in a more planar isoxazole ring, while also eliminating all chiral centers, yielding compound **12** with further increased potency (Fig. 7.9) [36]. Then the structure-activity relationship (SAR) of five-membered ring scaffolds directly connecting through a nitrogen atom to benzamidine was further explored [31]. When choosing a pyrazole

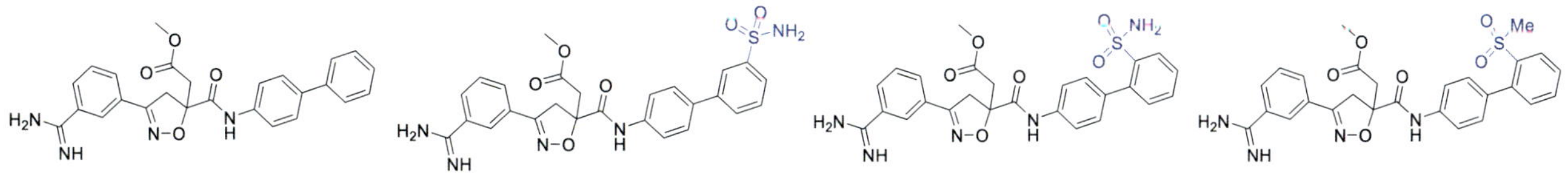

6
FXa Ki = 220 nM
Thrombin Ki = 3500 nM

7
FXa Ki = 68 nM
Thrombin Ki = 3100 nM

8 (SF303)
FXa Ki = 6.3 nM
Thrombin Ki = 3100 nM

9
FXa Ki = 4.2 nM
Thrombin Ki = 600 nM

FIGURE 7.7 Optimization of substitutions on the terminal aromatic ring of biphenyl group.

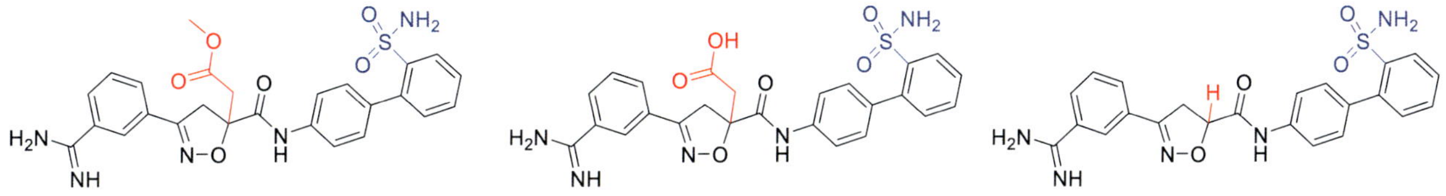

8 (SF303)
FXa Ki = 6.3 nM
Thrombin Ki = 3100 nM

10
FXa Ki = 20 nM
Thrombin Ki > 21000 nM

11
FXa Ki = 7.2 nM
Thrombin Ki = 3900 nM

FIGURE 7.8 Optimization of substitutions on isooxazoline.

12 (SA862)
FXa Ki = 0.15 nM
Thrombin Ki = 2000 nM

13
FXa Ki = 0.16 nM
Thrombin Ki = 900 nM

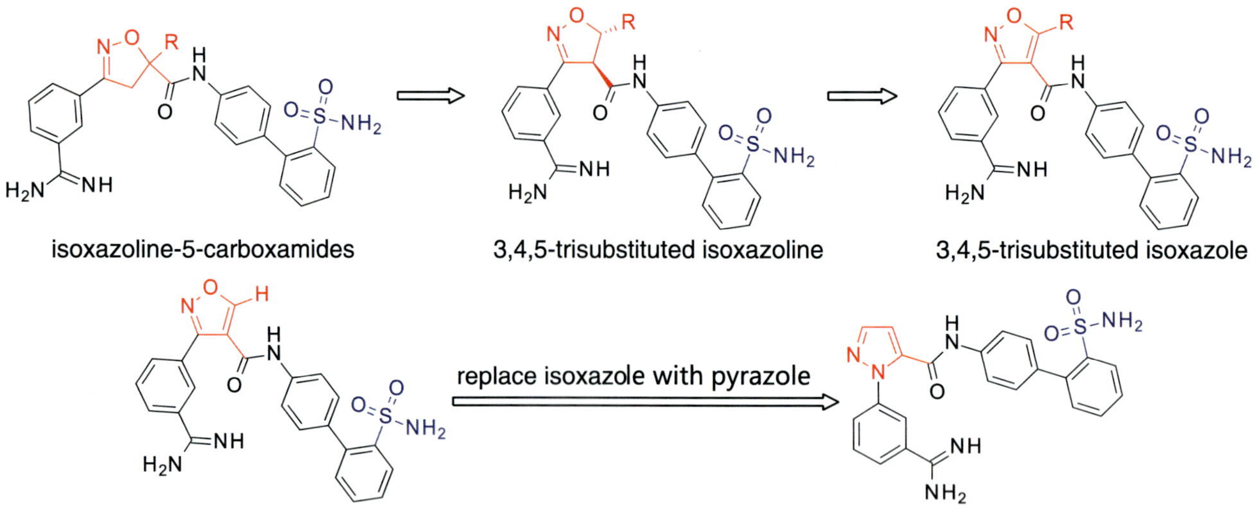

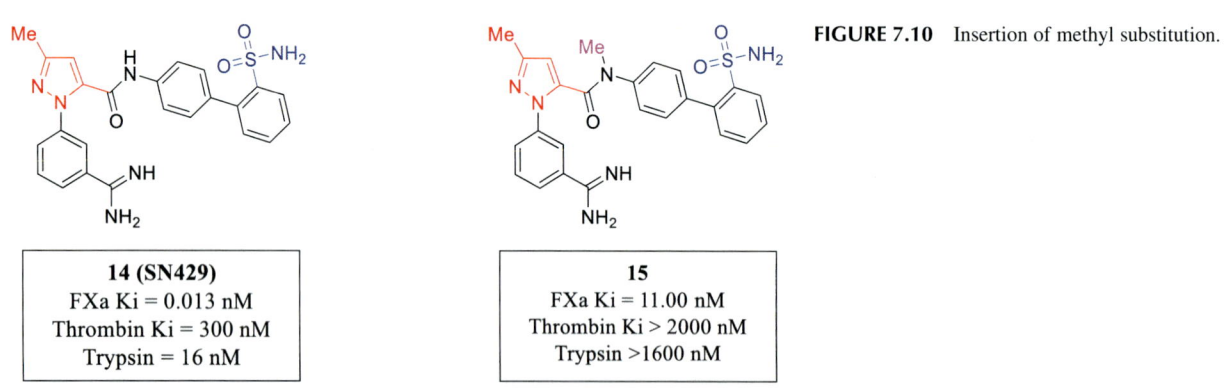

FIGURE 7.9 Scaffold hopping of core structure.

14 (SN429)
FXa Ki = 0.013 nM
Thrombin Ki = 300 nM
Trypsin = 16 nM

15
FXa Ki = 11.00 nM
Thrombin Ki > 2000 nM
Trypsin >1600 nM

FIGURE 7.10 Insertion of methyl substitution.

scaffold to mimic the isoxazole ring, compound **13** was obtained [37]. The introduction of pyrazole provided the possibility to introduce substituents at the 3-position to modulate the molecular potency, selectivity, and physicochemical properties. It was found that the pyrazole compound **13** gave comparable potency to the isoxazole compound **12**, but its selectivity for thrombin was reduced.

Compound **14** (**SN429**) was obtained by introducing a methyl group at the 3-position of the pyrazole ring of compound **13**, which demonstrated improved FXa binding potency by 10-fold than compound **13**, and it also showed more than 1000 times selectivity over thrombin and trypsin. However, after introducing a methyl group to the amide nitrogen of compound **14**, the FXa binding potency of compound **15** decreased by nearly 800 times (Fig. 7.10), which is likely due to the introduction of the *N*-methyl substitution altered the amide conformation.

The pharmacokinetic properties in dog of compound **14** are shown in Table 7.2 (IV, 1 mg/kg; PO, 4 mg/kg). As we can see, compound **14** exhibited a low in vivo clearance rate (clearance = 0.67 L/kg/h), moderate half-life ($t_{1/2}$ = 0.82 h), and low volume of distribution (V_{dss} = 0.29 L/kg). However, its oral bioavailability is quite poor ($F\%$ = 4), which may be due to the presence of an amidine group, resulting in a high basic p*K*a value of 10.7, which made the molecule to be more likely to exist in a positively charged form in plasma, which is unable to pass through cell membranes, leading to very poor permeability. This is also confirmed by the low apparent permeability rate in the in vitro Caco-2 permeability assay. In addition, compound **14** exhibited in vivo antithrombotic efficacy with an ID_{50} value of 0.02 μmol/kg/h in a rabbit arterio-venous shunt thrombosis model (rabbit A-V shunt model) [37].

TABLE 7.2 Pharmacokinetic properties of compound 14 in dogs.

Cl (L/kg/h)[a]	V_{dss} (L/kg)[a]	$t_{1/2}$ (h)[a]	F% (PO)[b]	Caco-2 Papp*10^{-6} cm/s	rabbit A-V shunt ID_{50} (μmol/kg/h)
0.67	0.29	0.82	4	0.30	0.02

[a]IV dose of 1 mg/kg.
[b]Oral dose of 4 mg/kg.

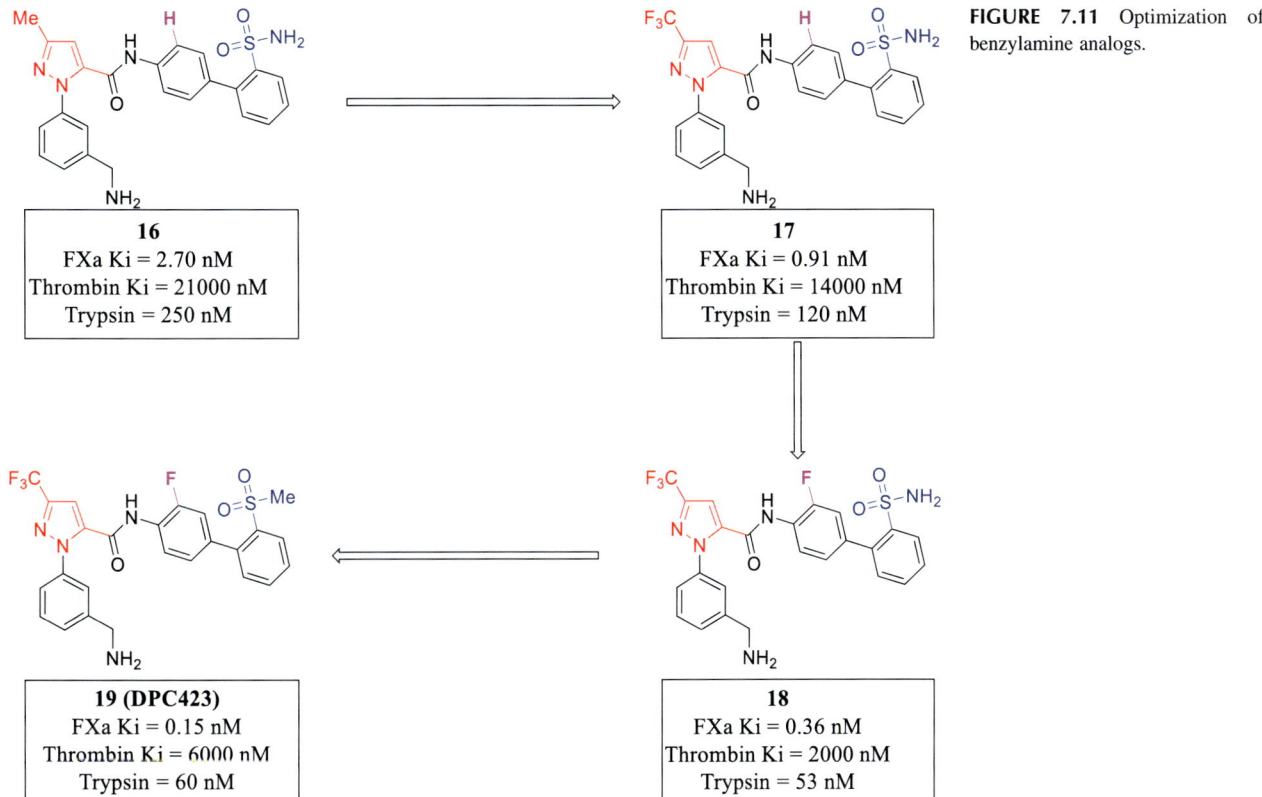

FIGURE 7.11 Optimization of benzylamine analogs.

In order to improve oral bioavailability, researchers attempted to replace the benzamidine substitution with a less basic moiety (Fig. 7.11). One of their first benzamidine replacements was benzylamine moiety (pKa ∼ 8.8). Compound **16** showed nearly 200 times lower binding potency than the corresponding benzamidine analog (compound **14**); however, after replacing the methyl substituent at the 3-position of the pyrazole with trifluoromethyl, they obtained compound **17** with improved binding potency. By introducing a fluorine atom at the proximal 2-position of the biaryl substituent, compound **18** was obtained with improved binding potency. By replacing the sulfonamide with methanesulfonyl group, the binding potency of compound **19** was further improved.

Besides, researchers investigated the pharmacokinetic properties of compound **19** in dogs (Table 7.3). Compared to the benzamidine analog **14**, the benzylamine-substituted **19** showed a lower in vivo clearance rate (Cl = 0.24 L/kg/h), longer half-life ($t_{1/2}$ = 7.50 h), appropriate volume of tissue distribution (V_{dss} = 0.90 L/kg), and moderate oral bioavailability (F% = 57%). In vitro, the Caco-2 assay also indicated that it has good membrane permeability. In addition, compound **19** effectively inhibited the formation of thrombosis (ID_{50} = 1.1 μmol/kg/h) in a dose-dependent manner in the rabbit A-V shunt model. Therefore, **DPC423** [38], the crystalline nonhygroscopic hydrochloride salt form of compound **19**, was selected for clinical development.

Although DPC423 demonstrated over 1000-fold selectivity for thrombin and other serine proteases, its selectivity for pancreatic protease is only 400-fold. Because the clinical use of such drugs is long-term oral administration, it is necessary to avoid long-term inhibition of pancreatic protease to avoid related AEs. Therefore, researchers carried out

TABLE 7.3 Pharmacokinetic properties of compound 19 in dog.

Cl (L/kg/h)[a]	V_{dss} (L/kg)[a]	$t_{1/2}$ (h)[a]	F% (PO)[b]	Caco-2 Papp*10^{-6} cm/s	HPB[c]	rabbit A-V shunt ID_{50} (µmol/kg/h)
0.24	0.90	7.50	57	4.86	89%	1.1

[a]IV dose of 0.5 mg/kg.
[b]Oral dose of 0.2 mg/kg.
[c]Human plasma protein binding.

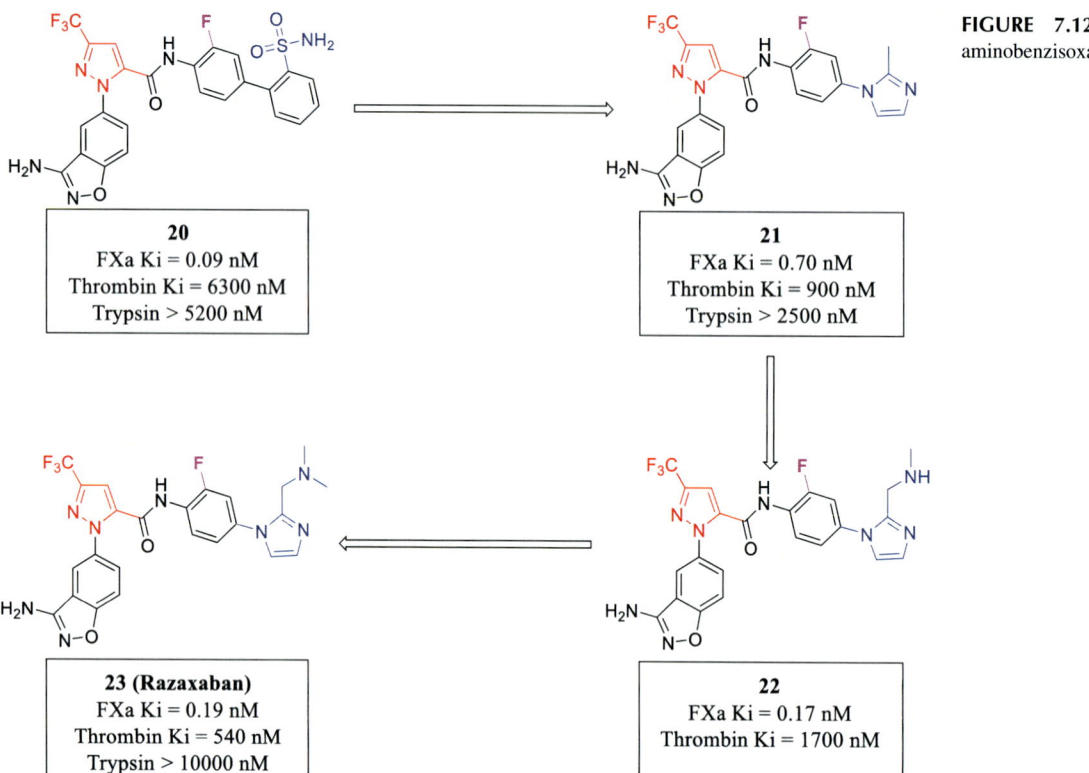

FIGURE 7.12 Optimization of aminobenzisoxazole series.

further optimization of DPC423 [32]. Because FXa has a larger S1 pocket than other pancreatic proteases, researchers systematically examined the benzylamine mimics at the P1 position through molecular recognition analysis and structure-based drug design (SBDD), and they found that compounds with aminobenzisoxazole, such as compound **20**, could maintain excellent binding potency and selectivity [39]. In particular, the selectivity for pancreatic protease was significantly improved. Unfortunately, compound **20** showed poor membrane permeability (the apparent permeability coefficient measured by Caco-2 assay was lower than 0.1×10^{-6} cm/s) and low solubility (<0.0001 mg/mL), resulting in low oral bioavailability (F% = 2%) in dogs with an oral dose of 0.2 mg/kg.

Keeping the aminobenzisoxazole substitution, researchers investigated the distal aromatic ring of the biaryl substituent (Fig. 7.12) [40]. By introducing soluble heterocycles, such as 2-methylimidazole-1-yl, the membrane permeability of compound **21** was greatly improved (7.41×10^{-6} cm/s), but the activity was reduced. When an alkylamine group was introduced into the newly added imidazole ring and a methyl or dimethyl group on the nitrogen atom could both enhance its binding potency (compounds **22** and **23**).

Pharmacokinetic properties of compounds **22** and **23** in dogs are shown in Table 7.4. As we can see they showed almost the same in vivo clearance rates; however, compound **23** had significantly better membrane permeability and oral bioavailability (F% = 84%) than **22** (F% = 27%). They also gave low plasma protein binding (PPB) rates. Compound **23** exhibited good dose-response [ID_{50} = 1.6 mg/(kg·h)] in the rabbit A-V shunt thrombosis model by

TABLE 7.4 Pharmacokinetic properties of compounds 22 and 23 in dogs.

Compound	PPB	Caco-2 Papp*10^{-6} cm/s	Cl (L/kg/h)[a]	$t_{1/2}$ (h)[a]	V_{dss} (L/kg)[a]	F% (PO)[b]
22	85.6%	0.2	1.1	3.7	4.6	27
23	90.5%	5.56	1.1	3.4	5.3	84

[a]IV dose of 0.4 mg/kg.
[b]Oral dose of 0.2 mg/kg.

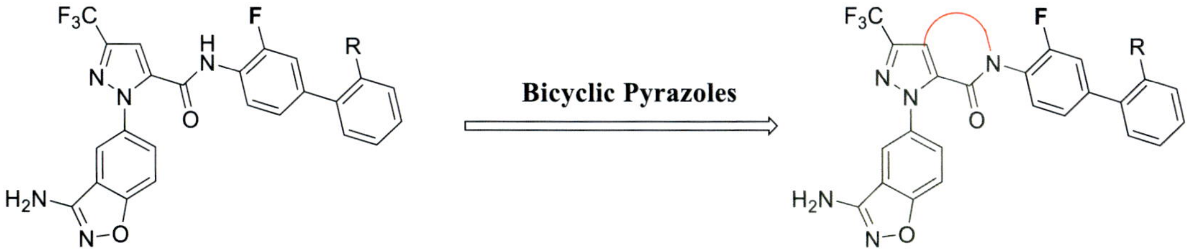

FIGURE 7.13 Bicyclic pyrazoles to reduce the probability of amide hydrolysis.

intravenous administration [41]. The hydrochloride salt form of compound 23 (razaxaban, DPC906, and BMS-562389) is the second compound to enter clinical trial studies.

In compounds of DPC423, DPC602, and razaxaban, there is a 5-pyrazole amide linker, which is susceptible to hydrolysis by numerous proteolytic enzymes in the body. During the long-term administration of the drug, there may be an accumulation of aromatic amine fragments that are potentially mutagenic (Ames positive). Medicinal chemists decided to optimize this fragment to de-risk the potential Ames positive issue, and they employed an amide bond cyclization strategy, resulting in bicyclic pyrazole series (Fig. 7.13) [42].

Compared with razaxaban, most compounds with a bicyclic scaffold retained nanomolar-level FXa binding potency (Fig. 7.14). However, the ring size of the bicyclic scaffold had a significant effect, and the six-membered ring lactam scaffold is superior to that of the seven-membered ring lactam scaffold (24 vs. 26, 25 vs. 27). Compound 24 showed better FXa binding potency than razaxaban by five folds. In the nonbicyclic compounds, the introduction of a fluorine atom ("F") at the proximal 2'-position of the biaryl group is helpful in improving binding potency. However, in the bicyclic series, a similar SAR effect was not observed; that is, the introduction of a fluorine atom did not effectively improve the binding potency (24 vs. 25, 26 vs. 27, 28 vs. 29). The introduction of double bond into the azepananone ring had no significant impact on potency (26 vs. 28, 27 vs. 29). Although these compounds all exhibited subnanomolar binding potency, it did not translate into good in vivo coagulation activity [42].

In order to further optimize compound 24, medicinal chemists investigated the biaryl substituents and their pharmacokinetic properties in dogs (Fig. 7.15) [37,42]. After removing one methyl substituent on the nitrogen atom, compound 30 showed decreased binding potency and in vivo metabolic stability (clearance rate increased). When the substituent on the terminal aromatic ring was replaced with pyrrolidine, compound 31 also showed reduced binding potency. However, after introducing an R-OH group at the 3-position of pyrrolidine, compound 32 showed comparable binding potency with compound 24, improved in vivo metabolic stability with a clearance rate value of 0.35 L/kg/h, and better oral bioavailability (F% = 82%), resulting in good pharmacokinetic profiles. While it is not the same with S-OH at the 3-position (compound 33 did not exhibit such good activity and properties as compound 32). After introducing a fluorine atom at the 2'-position of the proximal phenyl ring of P4 in compound 32, compound 34 demonstrated improved permeability, but its binding potency decreased. When replacing the methyl substituent at the 3-position of the pyrazole of compound 32 with methyl group, compound 35 exhibited decreased binding potency. Introducing a fluorine atom at the 2'-position of the biaryl group of compound 35 did not improve the binding potency. Due to good permeability and pharmacokinetic properties, this series of compounds generally have high oral bioavailability. Among them, compounds 32 and 34 had relatively lower in vivo clearance and distribution volumes, as well as moderate half-lives and high oral bioavailability. Compound 32 showed the strongest in vivo activity with an IC$_{50}$ value of 135 nmol/L in the rabbit A-V shunt thrombosis model. No metabolites resulting from amide bond cleavage were detected by stability analysis of compound 32. Therefore, BMS-740808, the crystalline hydrochloride salt form of compound 32, was selected for further preclinical studies and evaluation.

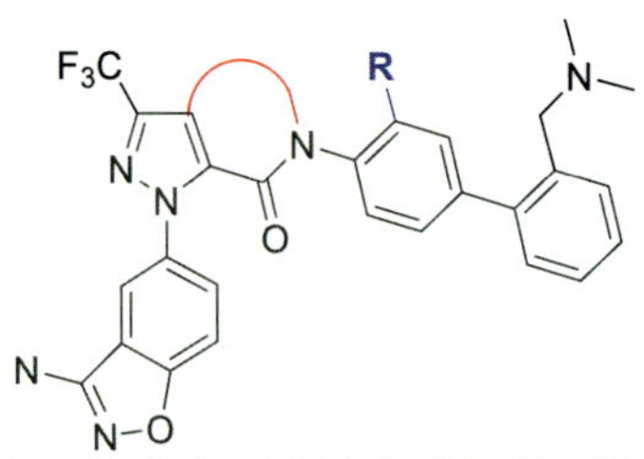

Compound	Scalffold	R	fXa Ki (nM)	PT EC$_2$x (uM)
24	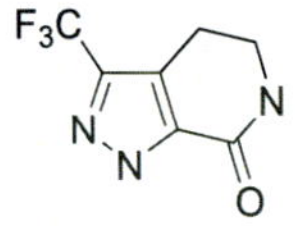 F$_3$C-pyrazole-piperidinone (6,6)	H	0.04	2.7
25	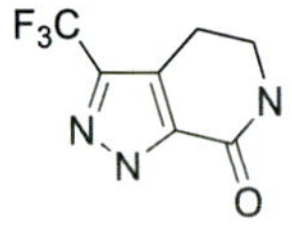 F$_3$C-pyrazole-piperidinone (6,6)	F	0.13	5.6
26	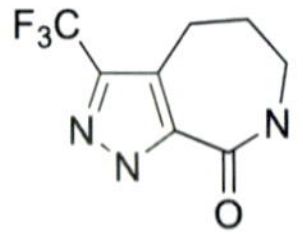 F$_3$C-pyrazole-azepanone (6,7)	H	0.81	4.0
27	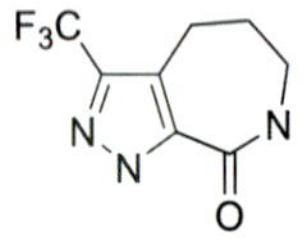 F$_3$C-pyrazole-azepanone (6,7)	F	0.85	8.5
28	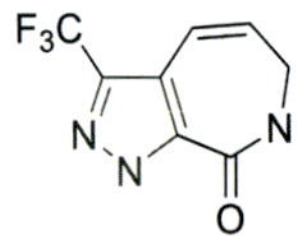 F$_3$C-pyrazole-dihydroazepinone	H	0.60	6.9
29	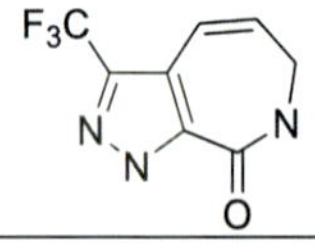 F$_3$C-pyrazole-dihydroazepinone	F	0.60	15

FIGURE 7.14 Exploration of the bicyclic scaffold.

The discovery of the bicyclic scaffold in BMS-740808 resulted in good pharmacokinetic properties in dogs, such as low in vivo clearance rates and distribution volumes, while maintaining good potency. However, the structure is not so significantly diversified from razaxaban (low structure diversity), which made it less attractive for further development.

In order to increase structure diversity, medicinal chemists further explored the 3-position substituent of pyrazole (Fig. 7.16) [20]. When the 3-position substituent is trifluoromethyl (**37**), methylsulfonyl (**38**), amide (**39**), cyano (**40**), or dimethylamino (**44**), all yielded subnanomolar binding potency. Compared with trifluoromethyl-substituted compound **37**, compound **39** showed significant improvement in both binding potency and coagulation efficacy. Ester-substituted compound **41** and carboxylic acid-substituted compound **42** gave reduced potency. When the C$_3$ position was substituted with an amino group, N,N-dimethylamino-substituted compound **44** showed better binding potency than amino-substituted compound **43**. In summary, when the 3-position substituent of pyrazole was amide, compound **39** showed the best binding potency and coagulation efficacy.

Compound **39** exhibited a low clearance rate, a moderate volume of distribution, and a half-life of 5.6 hours in the PK studies in dogs. The good membrane permeability resulted in excellent oral bioavailability ($F = 100\%$) (Table 7.5).

At the same time, while maintaining the trifluoromethyl substitution at the 3-position of the pyrazole and the bicyclic structure in BMS-740808, medicinal chemists also investigated the R substituent of P4 part connected to the benzene ring with a nitrogen atom (Fig. 7.17 [20]). The introduction of an amino substituent significantly reduced the FXa binding potency of compound **46**. Further introducing methyl substituent to the amino group improved the FXa binding potency of compounds **47** and **48**. Based on compound **49** with an N-acetyl substituent, further introduction of a methyl group led to the N-methylacetamide-substituted compound **50**, which exhibited good FXa binding potency and

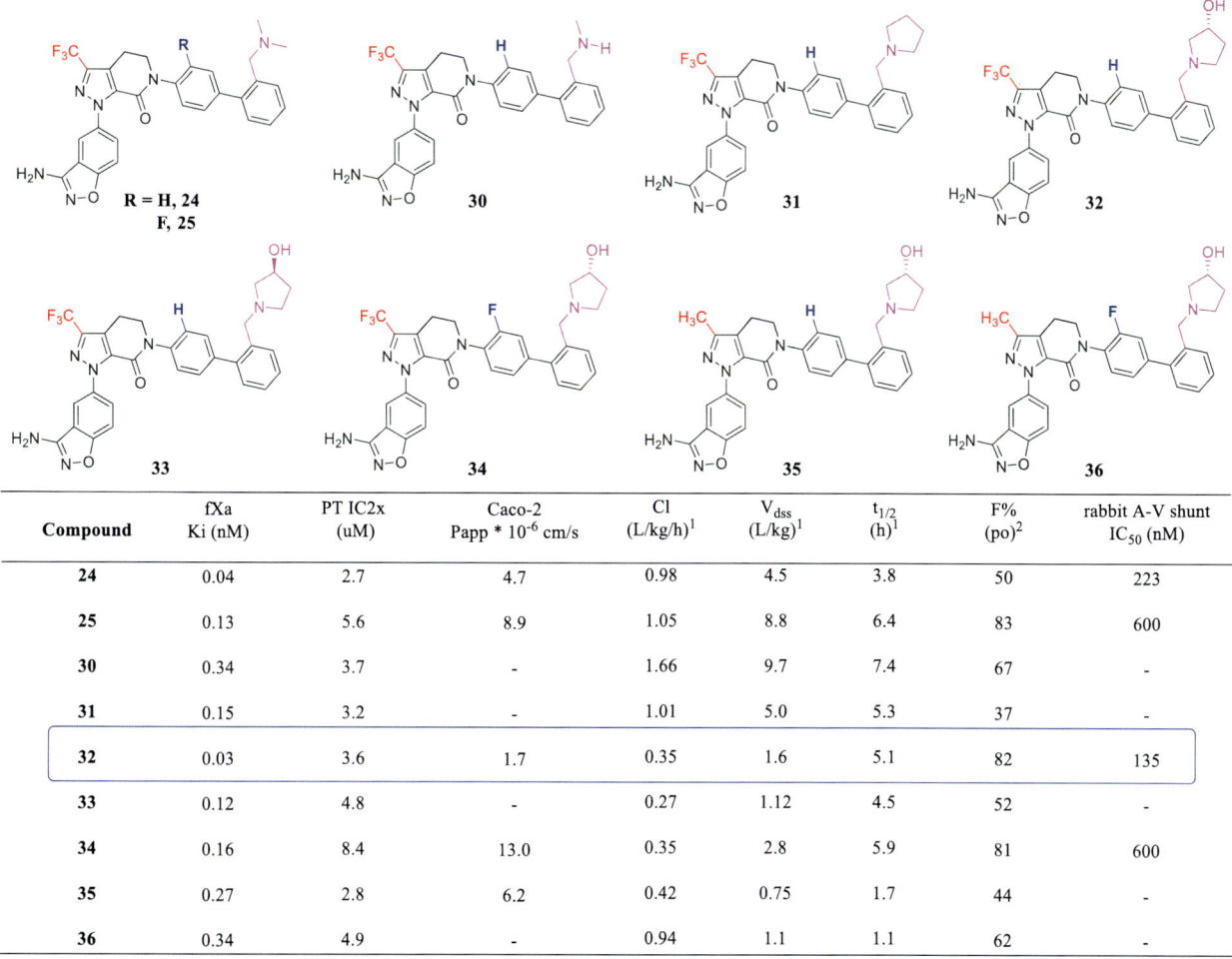

FIGURE 7.15 Compounds optimization of bicyclic series. Compounds were dosed with TFA salt. 1. IV dose of 0.5 mg/kg. 2. Oral dose of 0.2 mg/kg.

significant structure diversity compared with previous aryl substituents. The good FXa binding potency displayed by compound **50** indicates that the configuration of the *N*-methylacetamide substituent is very important for its binding to the active site of FXa. Cyclization of the *N*-methylacetamide substituent in compound **50** led to lactam compounds **51** and **52**, both retained perfect FXa binding potency, but the coagulation efficacy was reduced, which may be due to the increased lipophilicity (*clogP* > 7) and high human PPB rate (PPB > 99%).

Combining the SAR of the P4 substituent (Fig. 7.17) and the SAR of the 3-position substituent on the pyrazole (Fig. 7.16), the trifluoromethyl group at the C3 position of the planar pyrazole ring in compounds **50** and **51** was replaced with the more polar amide substituent in compound **39**, resulting in compounds **53** and **54** (Table 7.6) [20]. Both compounds not only retained sub-digit nanomolar FXa binding potency but also exhibited good anticoagulant efficacy in the PT coagulation assay. PK studies in dogs showed that although compound **53** demonstrated an oral bioavailability of 56%, it had a higher in vivo clearance rate and volume of distribution, as well as a shorter half-life time. In comparison, compound **54** showed a lower in vivo clearance rate and volume of tissue distribution, with better PK properties than those of **BMS-740808** and **razaxaban**. The human serum protein binding of compound **54** was 87%, indicating a relatively higher free concentration. Taking into account all of the above information, scientists finally selected compound **54** (**apixaban**) as the candidate for clinical trial research.

7.3.3 The binding model of apixaban and FXa

Compound **54** binds tightly with FXa to form an inhibitor-enzyme complex (Fig. 7.18) [20]. In the S1 pocket, the para-methoxy group is in the same plane as the benzene ring and does not show specific interactions with the protein residues. The nitrogen atom at the 2-position of the pyrazole ring interacts with Gln192 residue (3.2 Å), the

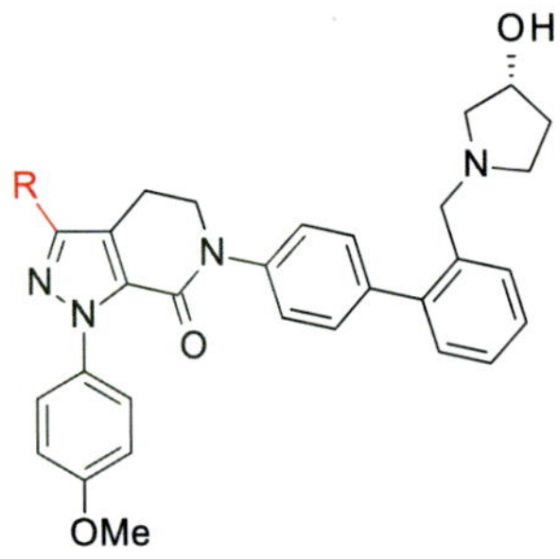

FIGURE 7.16 Exploration of 3-position substituent of pyrazole.

compound	R	fXa Ki (nM)	Thrombin Ki (nM)	PT EC$_{2x}$ (µM)
37	CF$_3$	0.18	330	33.1
38	SO$_2$Me	0.25	180	1.5
39	**CONH$_2$**	**0.07**	**140**	**1.3**
40	CN	0.33	100	2.8
41	CO$_2$Et	3.9	980	6.1
42	COOH	7.6	>20000	25
43	NH$_2$	6.7	9400	4.7
44	NMe$_2$	0.31	1800	NT
45	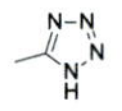 (tetrazole)	0.63	12000	12.4

TABLE 7.5 Pharmacokinetic properties of compound 39 in dogs.

Cl (L/kg/h)[a]	V_{dss} (L/kg)[a]	$t_{1/2}$ (h)[a]	F% (PO)[b]	Caco-2 Papp*10^{-6} cm/s
0.32	1.6	5.6	100	2.3

Note: Compound was dosed as TFA salt.
[a]IV dose of 0.4 mg/kg.
[b]Oral dose of 0.2 mg/kg.

oxygen atom of the bicyclic lactam interacts with the NH of Gly216 (2.9 Å), and the NH in the amide at the pyrazole C$_3$ position interacts with the carbonyl of Glu146 (3.1 Å). The benzamide in the S4 pocket shows an edge-to-face interaction with Trp215 and is positioned between Tyr99 and Phe174, the lactam ring and benzene ring in the P4 substituent adopt an orthogonal conformation to better embed into the S4 pocket. Although the X-ray crystallography study did not show interactions between the oxygen atom in the lactam of P4 and the protein, it did show that it can interact with a water molecule. In summary, compound **54** embeds into the active pocket of the FXa enzyme in a highly complementary manner.

7.3.4 The synthetic routes of apixaban

During the research and development (R&D) process of apixaban and after its launch, chemists developed many synthetic routes. The construction of the bicyclic pyrazole scaffold is the key. This section introduces four related process routes, all of which use compound **55** as a key intermediate. Its synthesis is shown in Fig. 7.19 [20]. 4-methoxyaniline undergoes diazotization in the presence of concentrated hydrochloric acid and sodium nitrite, followed by Japp-Klingemann reaction with ethyl 2-chloroacetoacetate in the presence of sodium acetate, yielding compound **55** (para-methoxyphenyl chlorohydrazone intermediate) in 90% yield.

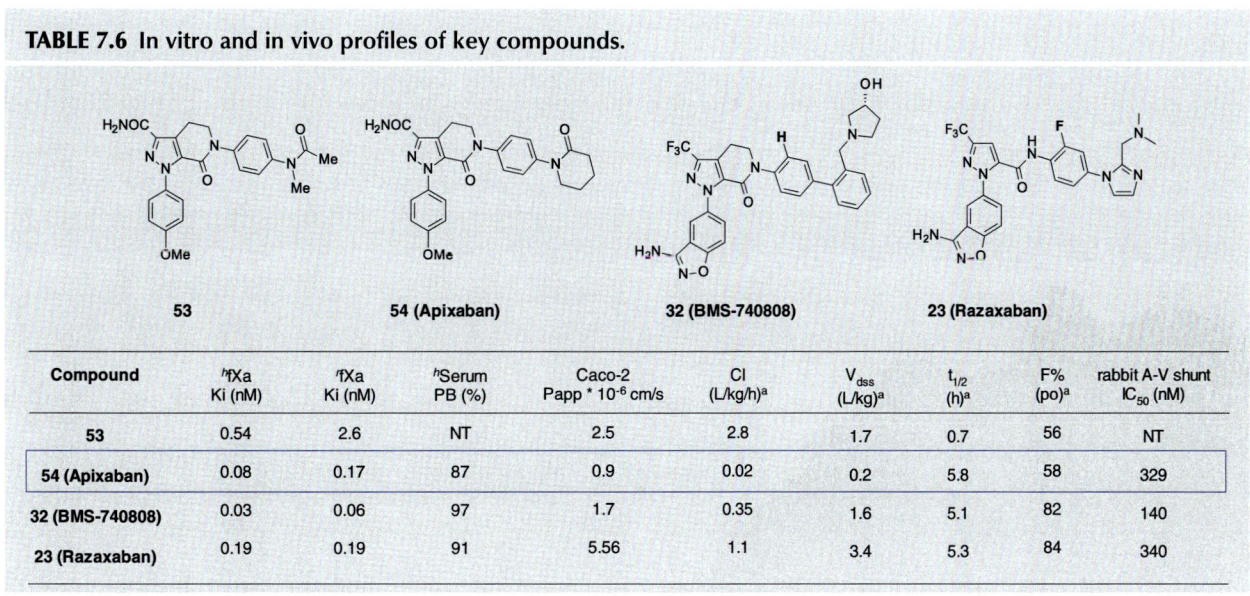

FIGURE 7.17 Investigation of the P4 substituent connected with nitrogen atom.

Compound	R	fXa Ki (nM)	Thrombin Ki (nM)	PT EC2x (μM)
46	NH₂	1600	>6300	NT
47	NHMe	610	>6300	NT
48	NMe₂	6	>13400	40.6
49	NHCOMe	180	>6300	NT
50	N(Me)COMe	0.5	>6300	8.2
51	(piperidinone)	0.23	4400	36
52	(azepanone)	0.47	3300	26

TABLE 7.6 In vitro and in vivo profiles of key compounds.

Compound	^{h}fXa Ki (nM)	^{r}fXa Ki (nM)	^{h}Serum PB (%)	Caco-2 Papp * 10⁻⁶ cm/s	Cl (L/kg/h)^a	V$_{dss}$ (L/kg)^a	t$_{1/2}$ (h)^a	F% (po)^a	rabbit A-V shunt IC$_{50}$ (nM)
53	0.54	2.6	NT	2.5	2.8	1.7	0.7	56	NT
54 (Apixaban)	0.08	0.17	87	0.9	0.02	0.2	5.8	58	329
32 (BMS-740808)	0.03	0.06	97	1.7	0.35	1.6	5.1	82	140
23 (Razaxaban)	0.19	0.19	91	5.56	1.1	3.4	5.3	84	340

^{a} "h" and "r" refer to human and rabbit species respectively. Compounds were dosed in a cassette dosing (PO/IV) N-in-one format. a refers to the cassette dosing (PO/IV) dog pharmacokinetic parameters. PB refers to serum protein binding. "NT" indicates "not tested."

7.3.4.1 Route 1

In the original research synthetic route (Fig. 7.20) [20,42,43], the starting material 4-iodoaniline and 5-bromovaleroyl chloride underwent a condensation reaction, followed by treatment with potassium *tert*-butoxide, and then chlorination with phosphorus pentachloride in refluxing chloroform to obtain the α,α-dichloropiperidone intermediate compound **57**.

156 Medicinal Chemistry and Drug Development

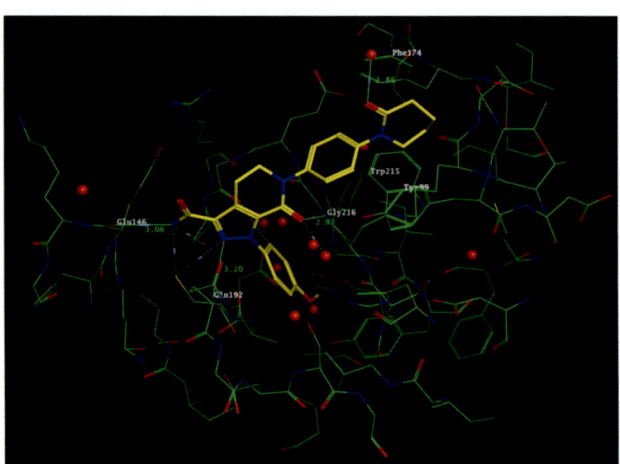

FIGURE 7.18 The binding model of apixaban (compound 54) and FXa.

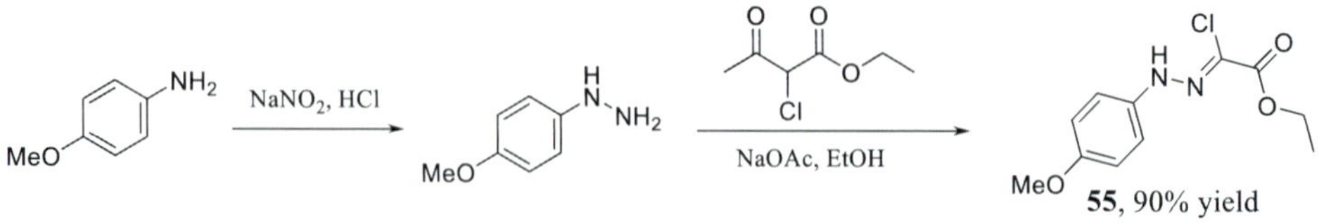

FIGURE 7.19 Synthesis of key intermediate compound 55.

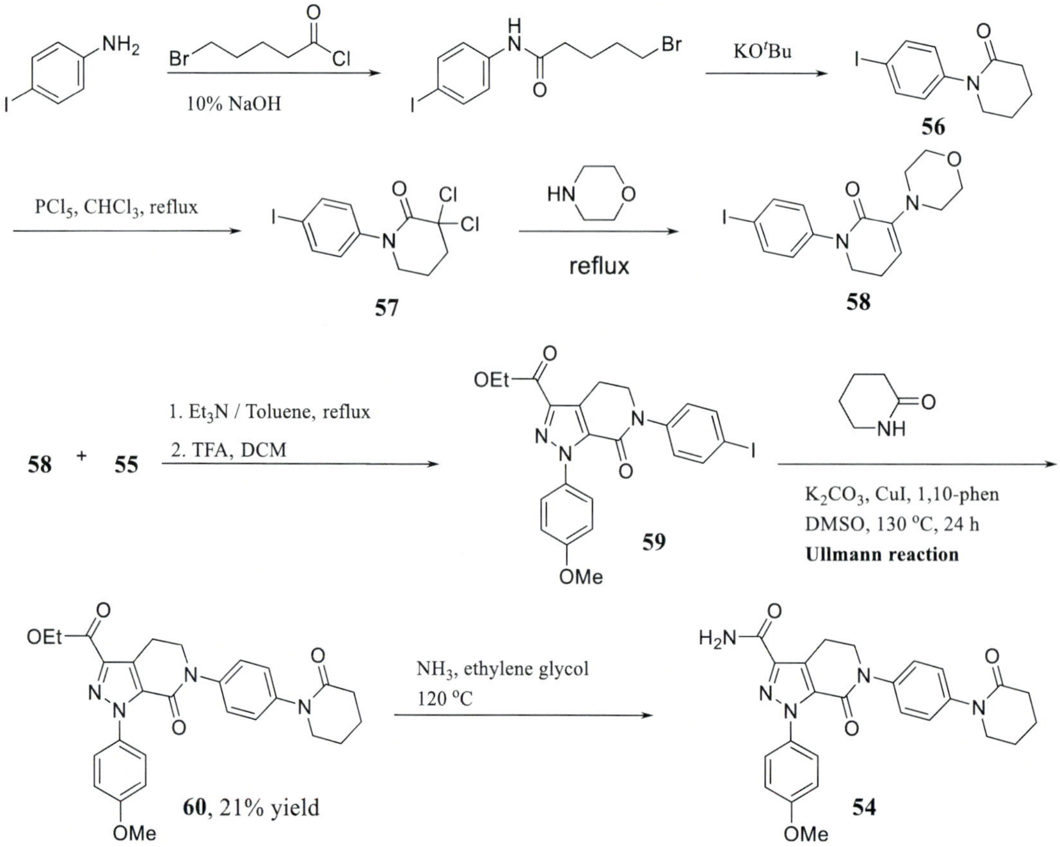

FIGURE 7.20 Synthetic route 1 of apixaban.

Under reflux conditions, compound **57** reacted with excess morpholine to obtain compound **58** with an overall yield of 70%.

Subsequently, compound **58** reacted with compound **55** in the presence of excess triethylamine, the mixture was treated with trifluoroacetic acid in dichloromethane to obtain compound **59** with a yield of 71%. Under conditions similar to the Ullmann reaction, the aryl iodide compound **59** reacted with δ-valerolactam to yield the coupling product **60** with a yield of 21%. Finally, the ester group underwent aminolysis with ammonia in ethylene glycol to ultimately yield the product apixaban.

7.3.4.2 Route 2

In synthetic route 2 (Fig. 7.21) [44], firstly, 2-piperidone underwent an ortho-dichlorination reaction under conditions similar to route 1, followed by elimination and substitution reactions to yield the enamine intermediate **61**. Compound **61** then underwent a consecutive [3 + 2] cycloaddition and elimination reaction with compound **55** to yield compound **62**. Compound **62** reacted with aryl iodide compound **56** under Ullmann reaction conditions to yield the coupling product **63**. Subsequently, the carboxylic acid group in compound **63** reacted with isobutyl chloroformate to obtain a mixed anhydride intermediate. Finally, an aminolysis reaction occurs in the presence of aqueous ammonia to obtain the target product apixaban.

Both route 1 and route 2 required the use of relatively expensive organic iodides, and the Ullmann reaction required the participation of a copper catalyst, which limited the scalability.

7.3.4.3 Route 3

The synthetic route 3 is shown in Fig. 7.22 [45]. Using *p*-nitroaniline and cheaper 5-chlorovaleryl chloride as starting materials, the enamine intermediate **65** was obtained under conditions similar to route 1. Then, using sodium sulfide as

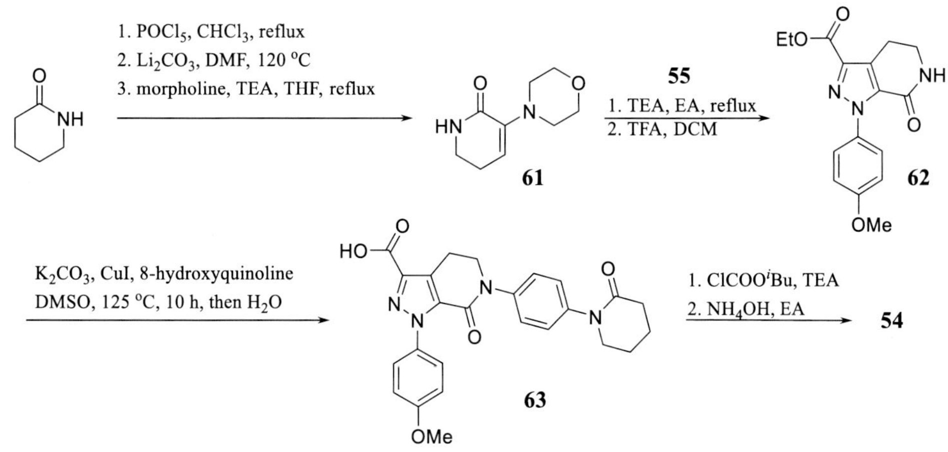

FIGURE 7.21 Synthetic route 2 of apixaban.

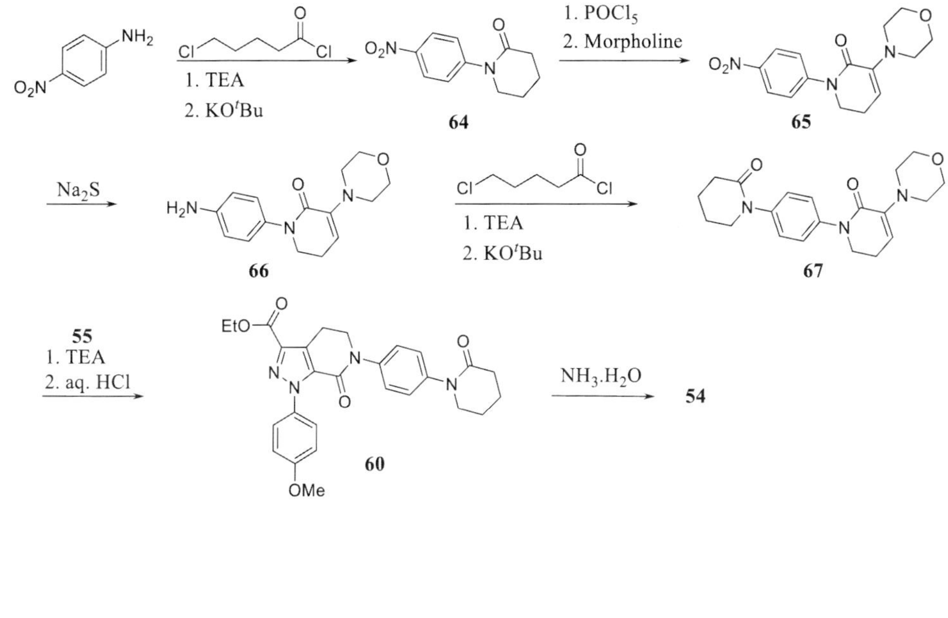

FIGURE 7.22 Synthetic route 3 of apixaban.

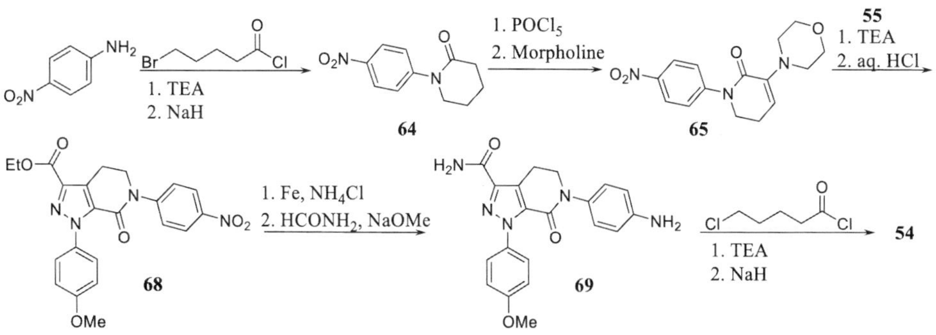

FIGURE 7.23 Synthetic route 4 of apixaban.

a reducing agent, the nitro group in compound **65** was reduced to an amino group to obtain compound **66**. The amino group in compound **66** then underwent a ring-closing reaction with 5-chlorovaleryl chloride to obtain the key intermediate **67**, which contains two δ-valerolactam skeletons. Subsequently, compound **67** and compound **55** underwent consecutive [3 + 2] addition-elimination reactions to obtain compound **60**. In this process, potassium iodide was added as a cocatalyst to improve the reaction yield and shorten the reaction time. Then compound **60** underwent aminolysis in a methanol solution of ammonia to obtain the target product apixaban. The overall yield of this route is 35%, and the use of Ullmann reaction conditions is avoided.

7.3.4.4 Route 4

Synthetic route 4 is shown in Fig. 7.23 [46]. Firstly, compound **65** underwent a consecutive [3 + 2] addition-elimination reaction with compound **55** to construct the bicyclic pyrazole scaffold, resulting in compound **68**. Subsequently, under the action of iron powder as a reducing agent, the nitro group in compound **68** was reduced to an amino group, and then the ester group underwent aminolysis under the conditions of formamide/sodium methoxide to obtain compound **69**. The amino group in compound **69** underwent a ring-closing reaction with 5-chlorovaleryl chloride to obtain the target product apixaban.

In summary, the synthetic route of apixaban mainly includes four key steps: reduction, cyclization, condensation, and amination. The sequence of these four steps and the specific reaction conditions vary slightly among reported literature.

7.4 Clinical indications of apixaban

Apixaban (brand name Eliquis) is a direct, reversible, and highly selective FXa inhibitor. It was firstly approved in the European Union in May 2011 for the prevention of VTE in adult patients undergoing elective hip or knee replacement surgery. In November 2012, the EU further approved it for the prevention of stroke and systemic embolism in adult patients with NVAF. In December 2012, it was approved by the FDA, and in January 2013, it was approved by the former China National Food and Drug Administration to enter the Chinese market for the prevention of VTE in adult patients undergoing elective hip or knee replacement surgery. It was also included in the 2017 edition of the National Medical Insurance Directory. The treatment period varies depending on the condition, some require 3 to 6 months, while others may need a longer treatment period. Apixaban is used to prevent the formation of blood clots and prevent existing clots from expanding, but it cannot dissolve clots that have already formed. Apixaban has the best-in-class clinical trial results in its class, with safety and efficacy exceeding those of similar drugs, significantly reducing the risk of bleeding.

Most of apixaban is excreted in the feces in its original form, with about 25% being metabolized mainly by the CYP3A4 enzyme. The main metabolites in the body are O-demethyl apixaban and hydroxyl apixaban. The total clearance rate of apixaban in the human body is 3.3 L/h, with renal clearance accounting for approximately 27%. There is no need to adjust the dose of apixaban in patients with mild liver dysfunction. Apixaban is not suitable for patients with moderate to severe liver dysfunction and those with renal or hepatic failure.

7.5 Postclass requirements and references

1. Understand the commonly used drugs to prevent blood clots.
2. Understand the coagulation cascade.
3. Understand the specificity and advantages of selective FXa inhibitors.

4. Understand the molecular optimization process of apixaban.
5. Understand the SAR and structure-toxicity relationship of apixaban.
6. Master at least one synthesis route of apixaban.
7. Understand Ullmann reaction.

References

[1] Furie B, Furie BC. Mechanisms of thrombus formation. N Engl J Med 2008;359:938–49.
[2] Mackman N. Triggers, targets and treatments for thrombosis. Nature 2008;451:914–18.
[3] Furie B, Furie BC. Molecular and cellular biology of blood coagulation. N Engl J Med 1992;326:800–6.
[4] Furie B, Furie BC. The molecular basis of blood coagulation. Cell 1988;53:505–18.
[5] Martinelli I, Bucciarelli P, Mannucci PM. Thrombotic risk factors: basic pathophysiology. Crit Care Med 2010;38:S3–9.
[6] Eriksson BI, Borris L, Dahl OE, Haas S, et al. Oral, direct Factor Xa inhibition with BAY 59-7939 for the prevention of venous thromboembolism after total hip replacement. J Thromb Haemost 2006;4:121–8.
[7] Pinto DJ, Smallheer JM, Cheney DL, et al. Factor Xa inhibitors: next-generation antithrombotic agents. J Med Chem 2010;53:6243–74.
[8] Onishi A, St Ange K, Dordick JS, et al. Heparin and anticoagulation. Front Biosci (Landmark Ed) 2016;21:1372–92.
[9] Ansell J, Hirsh J, Hylek E, et al. Pharmacology and management of the vitamin K antagonists: American College of Chest Physicians Evidence-Based Clinical Practice Guidelines (8th Edition). Chest 2008;133:160S–98S.
[10] Yeh CH, Hogg K, Weitz JI. Overview of the new oral anticoagulants: opportunities and challenges. Arterioscler Thromb Vasc Biol 2015;35:1056–65.
[11] Chen A, Stecker E, Warden B. Direct oral anticoagulant use: a practical guide to common clinical challenges. J Am Heart Assoc 2020;9:1–18 e017559.
[12] Baker DE. Formulary drug review: betrixaban. Hosp Pharm 2018;53:29–37.
[13] Bona RD, Hickey AD, Wallace DM. Efficacy and safety of oral anticoagulation in patients with cancer. Thrombosis Haemost 1997;78:137–40.
[14] Girolami A, Ferrari S, Cosi E, et al. Vitamin K-dependent coagulation factors that may be responsible for both bleeding and thrombosis (FII, FVII, and FIX). Clin Appl Thromb Hemost 2018;24:42S–7S.
[15] Dubois EA, Cohen AF. Dabigatran etexilate. Br J Clin Pharmacol 2010;70:14–15.
[16] Hauel NH, Nar H, Priepke H, et al. Structure-based design of novel potent nonpeptide thrombin inhibitors. J Med Chem 2002;45:1757–66.
[17] Roehrig S, Straub A, Pohlmann J, et al. Discovery of the novel antithrombotic agent 5-chloro-N-({(5S)-2-oxo-3-[4-(3-oxomorpholin-4-yl)phenyl]-1,3-oxazolidin-5-yl}methyl)thiophene-2-carboxamide (BAY 59-7939): an oral, direct factor Xa inhibitor. J Med Chem 2005;48:5900–8.
[18] Eriksson BI, Borris LC, Friedman RJ, et al. Rivaroxaban versus enoxaparin for thromboprophylaxis after hip arthroplasty. N Engl J Med 2008;358:2765–75.
[19] Lassen MR, Ageno W, Borris LC, et al. Rivaroxaban versus enoxaparin for thromboprophylaxis after total knee arthroplasty. N Engl J Med 2008;358:2776–86.
[20] Pinto DJ, Orwat MJ, Koch S, et al. Discovery of 1-(4-methoxyphenyl)-7-oxo-6-(4-(2-oxopiperidin-1-yl)phenyl)-4,5,6,7-tetrahydro-1H-pyrazolo[3,4-c]pyridine-3-carboxamide (apixaban, BMS 562247), a highly potent, selective, efficacious, and orally bioavailable inhibitor of blood coagulation factor Xa. J Med Chem 2007;50:5339–56.
[21] Zhu J, Alexander GC, Nazarian S, et al. Trends and variation in oral anticoagulant choice in patients with atrial fibrillation, 2010-2017. Pharmacotherapy 2018;38:907–20.
[22] Nagata T, Nagamochi M, Kobayashi S, et al. Stereoselective synthesis and biological evaluation of 3,4-diaminocyclohexanecarboxylic acid derivatives as factor Xa inhibitors. Bioorg Med Chem Lett 2008;18:4587–92.
[23] Zhang P, Huang W, Wang L, et al. Discovery of betrixaban (PRT054021), N-(5-chloropyridin-2-yl)-2-(4-(N,N-dimethylcarbamimidoyl)benzamido)-5-methoxybenz amide, a highly potent, selective, and orally efficacious factor Xa inhibitor. Bioorg Med Chem Lett 2009;19:2179–85.
[24] FDA approved betrixaban (BEVYXXA, Portola) for the prophylaxis of venous thromboembolism (VTE) in adult patients, n.d. https://www.fda.gov/drugs/resources-information-approved-drugs/fda-approved-betrixaban-bevyxxa-portola-prophylaxis-venous-thromboembolism-vte-adult-patients.
[25] Metharom P, Berndt MC, Baker RI, et al. Current state and novel approaches of antiplatelet therapy. Arterioscler Thromb Vasc Biol 2015;35:1327–38.
[26] Thachil J. Antiplatelet therapy - a summary for the general physicians. Clin Med (Lond) 2016;16:152–60.
[27] Khan IA, Gowda RM. Clinical perspectives and therapeutics of thrombolysis. Int J Cardiol 2003;91:115–27.
[28] Ansell J. Factor Xa or thrombin: is factor Xa a better target? J Thromb Haemost 2007;5(Suppl 1):60–4.
[29] Bates SM, Wettz JI. Coagulation assays. Circulation 2005;112:53–60.
[30] Mann KG, Brummel K, Butenas S. What is all that thrombin for? J Thromb Haemost 2003;1:1504–14.
[31] Quan ML, Wexler RR. The design and synthesis of noncovalent factor Xa inhibitors. Curr Top Med Chem 2001;1:137–49.
[32] Pruitt JR, Pinto DJ, Galemmo Jr RA, et al. Discovery of 1-(2-aminomethylphenyl)-3-trifluoromethyl-N- [3-fluoro-2'-(aminosulfonyl)[1,1'-biphenyl)]-4-yl]-1H-pyrazole-5-carboxyamide (DPC602), a potent, selective, and orally bioavailable factor Xa inhibitor(1). J Med Chem 2003;46:5298–315.
[33] Quan ML, Pruitt JR, Ellis CD, et al. Bisbenzamidine isoxazoline derivatives as factor Xa inhibitors. Bioorg Med Chem Lett 1997;7:2813–18.

[34] Quan ML, Liauw AY, Ellis CD, et al. Design and synthesis of isoxazoline derivatives as factor Xa inhibitors. 1. J Med Chem 1999;42:2752—9.
[35] Quan ML, Ellis CD, Liauw AY, et al. Design and synthesis of isoxazoline derivatives as factor Xa inhibitors. 2. J Med Chem 1999;42:2760—73.
[36] Pruitt JR, Pinto DJ, Estrella MJ, et al. Isoxazolines and isoxazoles as factor Xa inhibitors. Bioorg Med Chem Lett 2000;10:685—9.
[37] Pinto DJ, Orwat MJ, Wang S, et al. Discovery of 1-[3-(aminomethyl)phenyl]-N-3-fluoro-2'-(methylsulfonyl)-[1,1'-biphenyl]-4-yl]-3- (trifluoromethyl)-1H-pyrazole-5-carboxamide (DPC423), a highly potent, selective, and orally bioavailable inhibitor of blood coagulation factor Xa. J Med Chem 2001;44:566—78.
[38] Wong PC, Pinto DJ, Knabb RM. Nonpeptide factor Xa inhibitors: DPC423, a highly potent and orally bioavailable pyrazole antithrombotic agent. Cardiovasc Drug Rev 2002;20:137—52.
[39] Lam PY, Clark CG, Li R, et al. Structure-based design of novel guanidine/benzamidine mimics: potent and orally bioavailable factor Xa inhibitors as novel anticoagulants. J Med Chem 2003;46:4405—18.
[40] Quan ML, Lam PY, Han Q, et al. Discovery of 1-(3'-aminobenzisoxazol-5'-yl)-3-trifluoromethyl-N-[2-fluoro-4-[(2'-dimethylaminomethyl)imidazol-1-yl]phenyl]-1H-pyrazole-5-carboxyamide hydrochloride (razaxaban), a highly potent, selective, and orally bioavailable factor Xa inhibitor. J Med Chem 2005;48:1729—44.
[41] Wong PC, Crain EJ, Watson CA, et al. Razaxaban, a direct factor Xa inhibitor, in combination with aspirin and/or clopidogrel improves low-dose antithrombotic activity without enhancing bleeding liability in rabbits. J Thromb Thrombolysis 2007;24:43—51.
[42] Pinto DJ, Orwat MJ, Quan ML, et al. 1-[3-Aminobenzisoxazol-5'-yl]-3-trifluoromethyl-6-[2'-(3-(R)-hydroxy-N-pyrrolidinyl)methyl-[1,1']-biphen-4-yl]-1,4,5,6-tetrahydropyrazolo-[3,4-c]-pyridin-7-one (BMS-740808) a highly potent, selective, efficacious, and orally bioavailable inhibitor of blood coagulation factor Xa. Bioorg Med Chem Lett 2006;16:4141—7414.
[43] Gant T.G., Shahbaz M. Pyrazole carboxamides inhibitors of factor Xa. WO2010030983, 2010.
[44] Zhou J., Ma P., Li H., et al. Synthesis of 4,5-dihydro-pyrazolo[3,4-c]pyrid-2-ones. WO2003049681, 2003.
[45] Jiang J, Ji Y. Alternate synthesis of apixaban (BMS-562247), an inhibitor of blood coagulation factor Xa. Synth Commun 2013;43:72—9.
[46] Dwivedi S.D., Singh K.K., Tandon N., et al. An improved process for the preparation of apixaban and intermediates thereof. WO2014203275, 2014.

Chapter 8

Development of the anticoagulant drug fondaparinux sodium

Zhongtang Li and Zhongjun Li
State Key Laboratory of Natural and Biomimetic Drugs, School of Pharmaceutical Sciences, Peking University, Beijing, P.R. China

Chapter outline

- 8.1 Thrombotic disorders — 161
  - 8.1.1 Thrombotic disorders and their hazards — 161
  - 8.1.2 Factors and mechanisms of thrombosis formation — 162
  - 8.1.3 Functions of factor Xa — 163
- 8.2 Treatment of thrombotic disorders — 163
  - 8.2.1 Antiplatelet agents, anticoagulants, and thrombolytics — 163
  - 8.2.2 Anticoagulants: the past and present of heparin — 164
  - 8.2.3 Unfractionated heparin — 165
  - 8.2.4 Low-molecular-weight heparin — 166
  - 8.2.5 Ultra-low-molecular-weight heparins — 168
- 8.3 Discovery and history of anticoagulant drug: fondaparinux sodium — 168
  - 8.3.1 Lead compound: discovery of the heparin pentasaccharide sequence — 168
  - 8.3.2 The genesis of fondaparinux sodium: structure-activity relationship studies based on the heparin pentasaccharide sequence — 170
  - 8.3.3 Mechanism of action of fondaparinux sodium — 176
  - 8.3.4 Pharmacokinetics and safety of fondaparinux sodium — 176
- 8.4 Chemical process of fondaparinux sodium — 178
  - 8.4.1 Synthesis challenges of fondaparinux sodium — 178
  - 8.4.2 Chemical synthesis of fondaparinux sodium — 179
  - 8.4.3 Chemo-enzymatic synthesis of fondaparinux sodium — 179
- 8.5 Summary — 182
  - 8.5.1 Development strategy for fondaparinux sodium — 182
  - 8.5.2 Development trends in heparin-like anticoagulants — 183
  - 8.5.3 Development of small-molecule carbohydrate drugs — 183
- References — 183

8.1 Thrombotic disorders

8.1.1 Thrombotic disorders and their hazards

According to the pathological process, thrombotic disorders are typically defined as two classes, including thrombosis and thromboembolism. Thrombosis refers to the physiological or pathological process that forms elements of blood, creating a clot within vessels, causing partial or full obstruction of blood circulation, and finally leading to supply disruption in the affected areas. On the other hand, thromboembolism involves the detachment of thrombuses from their formation site, moving with the bloodstream to obstruct vessels partially or wholly. This obstruction results in ischemia, hypoxia, or even necrosis, as well as congestion and edema in the affected tissues and organs. Therefore, thrombotic diseases refer to arterial, venous, and microvascular thrombosis. When thrombus formation overwhelms hemostatic regulation, an excess of thrombin is generated, which can lead to a hypercoagulable state and eventually cause local thrombotic lesions. The majority of hypercoagulable states are associated with local thrombus formation [1]. Arterial thrombus formation occurs in individuals at high risk for cardiovascular diseases, with coronary artery myocardial infarction and ischemic stroke being the primary outcomes of arteriosclerosis and thrombus formation in coronary arteries [2,3]. Peripheral arterial thrombotic diseases include mesenteric artery embolism and limb arterial embolism, while venous thromboembolism encompasses deep vein thrombosis and its complications, including pulmonary embolism, which represents a serious pathological state [4].

The formation of blood clots in the arterial, venous, and microvascular circulations represents a major contributor to worldwide morbidity and mortality. According to the World Health Organization, deaths resulting from arteriosclerotic thrombotic diseases exceed 25% of all human mortality [5]. Annually, over 12 million people worldwide succumb to cardiovascular diseases. For instance, in the United States, the mortality rate for acute myocardial infarction is 27% in men and even higher at 44% in women. In China, approximately 2 million people die from cardiovascular diseases each year, with deaths from thrombotic diseases accounting for 51% of the global total [2]. Acute arterial embolism is a primary cause of heart disease, with 80% of strokes being associated with it.

8.1.2 Factors and mechanisms of thrombosis formation

The hemostatic system is a vital defense mechanism in host organisms, encompassing platelet aggregation, coagulation, and fibrinolysis, to uphold the integrity of the high-pressure closed circulatory system of mammals following vascular injury. Coagulation comprises both intrinsic and extrinsic coagulation. In the case of extrinsic coagulation, also known as the tissue factor pathway, it is initiated by vascular wall injury, causing extravasation of circulating blood that rapidly results in platelet aggregation at the site of injury. In turn, the membrane glycoproteins of platelets at the injured site specifically bind to a soluble von Willebrand factor, triggering a series of complex reactions, including platelet adhesion, activation, and aggregation [6]. Simultaneously, a transmembrane glycoprotein tissue factor from perivascular cells forms a bimolecular complex with plasma factor VII/VIIa. This complex subsequently activates factors X and IX, leading to the generation of thrombin and the deposition of fibrin, thus facilitating coagulation [7,8].

The multifactorial etiology of thrombus formation signifies that any factor disrupting the balance between coagulation and anticoagulation can induce thrombotic diseases. Such etiology is generally categorized into three types:

1. Coagulation System Abnormalities: Under physiological or pathological conditions, injured tissues release tissue factor III into plasma and form a complex with factor VII and Ca^{2+}. This complex catalyzes factor X to its active forms, i.e., factor Xa (FXa) [9]. FXa, proaccelerin (factor V, FV), Ca^{2+}, and platelet phospholipids together form a prothrombin activator. Subsequently, this activator catalyzes the conversion of prothrombin (factor II, FII) to active thrombin (factor IIa, FIIa). Finally, with the assistance of Ca^{2+}, factor VIII (FVIII), and thrombin, the soluble fibrinogen in the plasma is converted to insoluble fibrin, forming a gel-like clot that traps a large number of blood cells in a cross-linked network [10]. Within health circumstances, an efficient anticoagulation system in the human body, where antithrombin III (AT-III) rapidly serves as an inactivator of the active sites of coagulation factors and prevents the conversion of fibrinogen, ensures blood remains a smooth fluid. Conversely, when the thrombin is generated at an injured site beyond the normal or regular amount, a thrombus will be formed inside the vessel, usually causing occlusion or partial occlusion and supplement disruption to the corresponding tissue area, ultimately leading to local thrombotic lesions. For instance, postsurgery, after trauma, or during tumor tissue breakdown, the human body enters a hypercoagulable state with increased numbers of platelets and coagulation factors that reduce the activity of anticoagulant factors and make thrombus formation more likely in the end.
2. Endothelial Injury: When the vascular endothelium is damaged, endothelial cells undergo degeneration and necrosis, leading to the exposure of underlying collagen fibers, which activates the intrinsic coagulation factor XII. This activation also plays a role in coagulation, leading to thrombus formation [11]. Additionally, damaged endothelial cells can release tissue factors, which activate the extrinsic coagulation pathway. This, combined with the injured vascular intima, promotes platelet aggregation and adherence, making the exposure of collagen fibers more likely. However, concurrent activation of both intrinsic and extrinsic coagulation leads to thrombus formation [12].
3. Hemodynamic Changes: Hemodynamic changes primarily refer to states characterized by reduced blood flow and vortex formation, which promote thrombus formation. Under normal blood flow, red and white blood cells flow in the central axial stream due to density differences, with a platelet layer and an outermost plasma layer surrounding them. Reduced blood flow or the formation of vortices causes platelets to enter the boundary layer, increasing the chances of platelet contact and adhesion to the endothelium. Moreover, the stasis-like conditions enable activated coagulation factors and thrombin to achieve the necessary concentrations for coagulation at the local site, thereby facilitating the coagulation process. Veins are equipped with valvular structures that can impede blood flow and generate vortexes, leading to venous thrombosis occurring four times more frequently than arterial thrombosis, often at the site of valve pockets [13].

Fig. 8.1 summarizes the pathways and key factors involved in the process of thrombus formation.

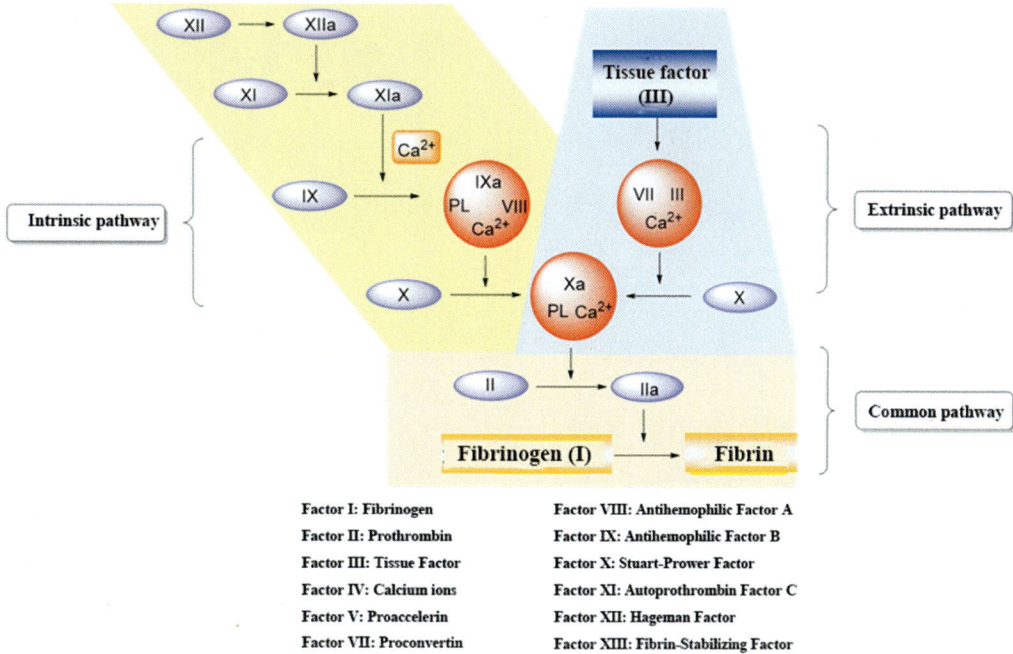

FIGURE 8.1 The coagulation cascade and the involved coagulation factors.

8.1.3 Functions of factor Xa

FXa, located at the convergence of the body's intrinsic and extrinsic coagulation pathways and upstream of thrombin, plays a pivotal role in the coagulation cascade. Inhibiting FXa can simultaneously suppress both the intrinsic and extrinsic coagulation processes. Additionally, due to the amplification effect of biological signals, a single inhibitor molecule of FXa can counteract the physiological effects of 138 thrombin molecules, making FXa inhibition more effective than thrombin inhibition. As a serine protease, FXa functions by cleaving peptide bonds in large protein molecules, resulting in their hydrolysis into smaller proteins. Specifically, FXa hydrolyzes prothrombin downstream, converting it into thrombin, thereby triggering the coagulation process [14].

In 1996, Brandstette et al. elucidated the X-ray diffraction crystal structure of human FXa (Fig. 8.2). Following this, multiple research groups examined the binding modes of active molecules to FXa. As illustrated, S1 serves as the specific binding region of FXa, determining substrate specificity, whereas S4 constitutes the aromatic pocket of FXa, consisting of Phe174, Tyr99, and Trp215 [15].

Currently, the sole marketed glycosidic indirect FXa inhibitor is fondaparinux sodium, which has become the preferred anticoagulant for the prevention and treatment of thromboembolism in orthopedic joint replacement surgery and venous thromboembolic diseases. Fondaparinux sodium induces a conformational change in antithrombin (dissociation constant of 50 nM), significantly amplifying antithrombin's natural neutralizing effect on FXa (approximately 300-fold). This disruption of FXa release ultimately impairs both the intrinsic and extrinsic coagulation pathways, suppressing the production of thrombin and the formation of thrombus (Fig. 8.3) [16].

8.2 Treatment of thrombotic disorders

8.2.1 Antiplatelet agents, anticoagulants, and thrombolytics

Based on the mechanism of action, the medications for treating thrombotic diseases can be briefly categorized into three types: antiplatelet agents, anticoagulants, and thrombolytics. A summary of marketed drugs is provided in Table 8.1 Due to different molecular pathways and targets, these drugs have varying indications, which are not elaborated here.

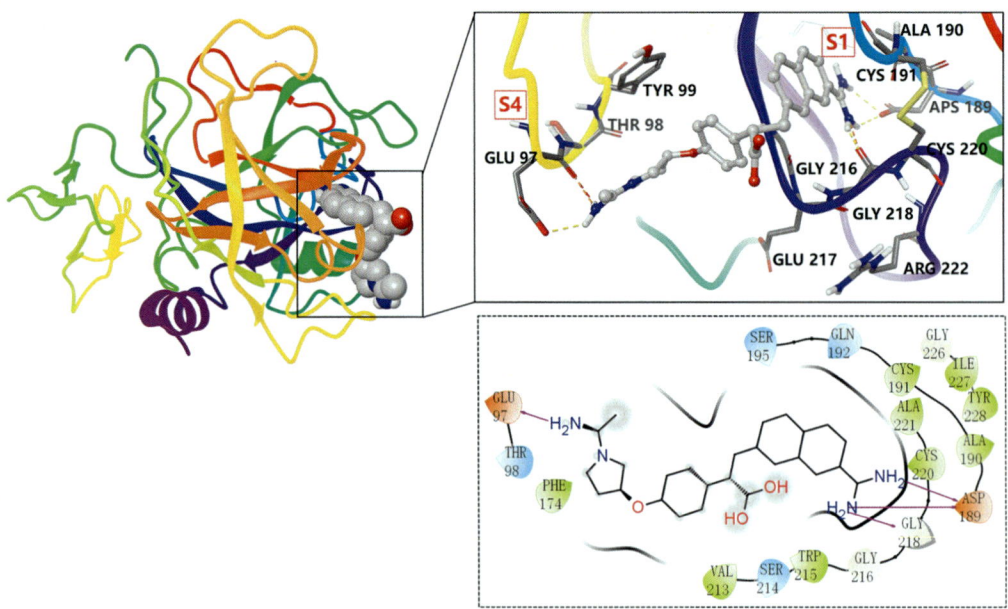

FIGURE 8.2 The active structure of FXa.

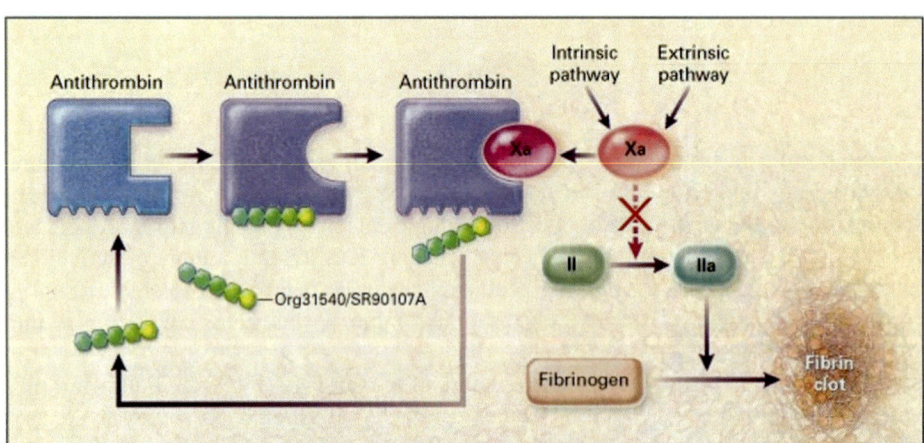

FIGURE 8.3 The mechanism of action of fondaparinux sodium (represented by the five-ball chain structure in the diagram) [16].

8.2.2 Anticoagulants: the past and present of heparin

Natural heparin is found in the mast cells and neutrophils of mammals. It is released into the bloodstream from sites of tissue injury, thereby exerting anticoagulant effects. As early as 1916, McLean, a second-year medical student at Johns Hopkins University, first isolated a lipophilic anticoagulant from canine liver tissue, marking the initial recognition of ordinary heparin in the medical field. As it was derived from animal liver, Mclean's mentor, Professor Howell, named this anticoagulant "heparin" in 1918.

In the 1930s, researchers began exploring the structure and function of heparin. In 1935, Jorpes from the Karolinska Institute first published the molecular structure of heparin. They found that heparin primarily consists of repeating tri-sulfated disaccharides, yet with microscopic heterogeneity due to structural variations (as shown in Fig. 8.4). The amine group of glucosamine can be acetylated, sulfated, or unsubstituted. The 3-position or 6-position of glucosamine can be O-sulfated or not, and the uronic acid can be either L-iduronic acid or D-glucuronic acid, with optional 2-O-sulfation. The average molecular weight is about 15 kDa. Heparin is known as the biomolecule with the highest negative charge density, with each disaccharide unit of heparin containing an average of 2.7 sulfate groups [17].

In May 1935, Vitrum AB, the Swedish company, conducted the first human trials of heparin, thereby validating the safety and efficacy of heparin produced by Connaught. Subsequently, in 1936, the first intravenous heparin product was

TABLE 8.1 Summary of marketed drugs for thrombotic disorders.

Mechanism of action	Signaling pathways and targets	Trade names	Drug categories
Antiplatelet drugs	Thromboxane A2 inhibitors	Aspirin	Small-molecules
	P2Y12 receptor antagonists	Clopidogrel	Small-molecules
		Prasugrel	Small-molecules
		Ticlopidine	Small-molecules
	Platelet IIb/IIIa inhibitors	Abciximab	Monoclonal antibodies
		Tirofiban	Cyclic peptides
		Eptifibatide	Non-peptide Small-molecules
	Phosphodiesterase inhibitors	Cilostazol	Small-molecules
Anticoagulants	Competitive inhibitors of vitamin K	Warfarin	Small-molecules
	Binding with antithrombin III (ATIII) and inhibiting multiple coagulation factors and platelets	Unfractionated Heparin	Macromolecules
	Binding with antithrombin III (ATIII) and inhibiting multiple coagulation factors	Low Molecular Weight Heparins Enoxaparin Nadroparin	Macromolecules
	Binding with antithrombin III (ATIII) and inhibiting factor Xa	Fondaparinux	Small-molecules
	Factor Xa inhibitors	Direct oral anticoagulants: Rivaroxaban Apixaban Edoxaban, Betrixaban	Small-molecules
Thrombolytic drugs	Nonspecific plasminogen activators	Urokinase Streptokinase	Macromolecules
	Specific plasminogen activators	Alteplase Pro-urokinase Reteplase Tenecteplase	Macromolecules

introduced. Connaught Medical Research Laboratories later improved the production process of heparin, facilitating its safe and nontoxic administration *via* intravenous injection in saline solution. Since its clinical application in the 1940s, heparin has been widely used for decades, particularly in various vascular surgeries, owing to its cost-effectiveness and efficacy.

8.2.3 Unfractionated heparin

Unfractionated heparin (UFH), which is commonly used in early clinical settings, is considered the first-generation heparin. Its mechanism of action involves indirect modulation of multiple coagulation factors through AT-III. When UFH binds to AT-III, it induces a conformational change that accelerates the closure of the active centers of coagulation factors and inhibits serine-containing coagulation factors such as factors IIa, IXa, Xa, XIa, and XIIa. Currently, UFH is predominantly used in the clinical treatment of thromboembolic diseases, early management of disseminated intravascular coagulation, and in vitro anticoagulation, characterized by its significant anticoagulant effect, rapid onset of action, and quick neutralization by protamine sulfate.

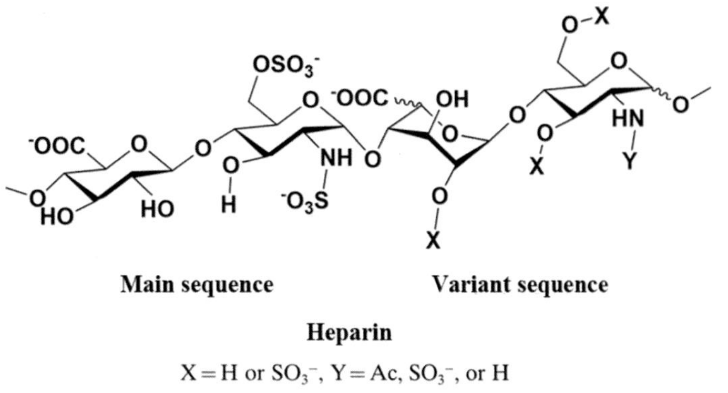

FIGURE 8.4 Representative structure of heparin.

Heparin
X = H or SO$_3^-$, Y = Ac, SO$_3^-$, or H

However, the intrinsic characteristics of UFH also limit its further application and development prospects. One significant limitation is the sourcing of UFH. Over the past few decades, the raw materials for heparin in Western contexts were predominantly extracted from bovine lungs, intestines, or porcine intestinal mucosa. Concerns about the rapid spread of bovine spongiform encephalopathy (mad cow disease) and the risk of potential prion contamination have led to a paradigm shift toward porcine-derived heparin in recent years. Research indicates that porcine-derived heparin is safer and less likely to cause thrombocytopenia compared to bovine sources.

The manufacturing process for UFH is characterized by its rigorous requirements. One of the major concerns during extraction is the potential contamination with other glycosaminoglycans, specifically oversulfated chondroitin sulfate, which exhibits kinin-releasing enzymatic activity and poses a significant risk. Such contamination poses a grave risk to patient health, potentially leading to fatal outcomes. A notable period of severe adverse reactions to heparin occurred globally from late 2007 to early 2008, with the contamination episode in the United States culminating in hundreds of deaths.

The administration of UFH necessitates meticulous dosing surveillance. Its main adverse reactions can be categorized into three types:

1. Osteoporosis: Heparin's interaction with osteoblasts leads to the activation of osteoclasts. Prolonged therapeutic use of heparin can precipitate osteoporosis.
2. Heparin-Induced Thrombocytopenia (HIT): Heparin binds with Platelet Factor 4 (PF4) in the body. Within 5−10 days of heparin therapy, antibodies against the PF4-heparin complex are produced. The Fc segment of these antibodies can bind to platelets, triggering platelet aggregation and the formation of thromboxane, thereby enhancing coagulation. In the presence of a positive feedback mechanism between coagulation and anticoagulation, platelet count decreases, leading to a hypercoagulable state with potentially fatal risks.
3. Potential Hemorrhagic Risks: The heterogeneous structure of UFH results in uncertain dose-response relationships. In 2006, an accidental overdose at an Indianapolis hospital resulted in the deaths of three premature infants, drawing global attention. Hence, stringent monitoring of heparin dosage is imperative in clinical practice to prevent such incidents.

8.2.4 Low-molecular-weight heparin

Currently, the most extensively used in clinical practice is the second generation of heparin products, known as low-molecular-weight heparins (LMWHs). In 1976, Joshon et al. found that LMWHs generate higher anti-FXa activity than UFH, along with a superior selectivity coagulation ratio (anti-Xa/anti-IIa). FXa plays a crucial role at the intersection of intrinsic and extrinsic coagulation pathways, and LMWHs can further reduce thrombin generation. LMWHs exhibit reduced nonspecific binding to endothelial cells and plasma proteins, increased bioavailability, prolonged half-life, decreased risk of bleeding, and superior clinical effectiveness and safety compared to UFH.

LMWHs are produced through controlled chemical or enzymatic degradation of heparin, yielding fragments with a molecular weight range of approximately 4000−6500 Da. The British Pharmacopoeia (BP) mandates an average molecular weight below 8000 Da, with more than 60% of components being less than 8000 Da, and a minimum anti-FXa to anti-FIIa activity ratio of 1.5 [18,19]. Compared to UFH, LMWHs exhibit lower anticoagulant activity and higher antithrombotic activity. They significantly reduce the incidence of adverse bleeding reactions. Additionally, LMWHs are characterized by favorable subcutaneous absorption, high bioavailability, and an extended half-life within the body. The frequency of adverse reactions such as HIT and osteoporosis is considerably lower, making them more convenient for use without the need for special monitoring. Consequently, LMWHs have garnered increasing clinical attention and application in recent years.

The preparation methods for LMWHs are diverse, including acid degradation, alkaline degradation, oxidation, free radical degradation, and enzymatic degradation [20]. These different processes result in variations in molecular weight, distribution, terminal structure, degree of sulfation, pharmacokinetic properties, and anticoagulant activity of LMWHs. These differences might render them noninterchangeable in clinical applications. Currently, over a dozen LMWH products have been developed, and the European Pharmacopoeia and BP have classified several LMWHs based on different processes. Examples include enoxaparin sodium, nadroparin calcium, dalteparin sodium, tinzaparin sodium, and parnaparin sodium. Each LMWH has distinct trade names, manufacturers, and preparation methods, as detailed in Table 8.2. Enoxaparin sodium is a type of LMWH produced from sodium heparin through alkaline β-elimination degradation. It contains numerous undefined oligosaccharides, predominantly characterized by a 4-enepyranosuronic acid structure at the nonreducing end of most oligosaccharide chains and a 15%–25% 1,6-anhydro structure at the reducing end [21]. Nadroparin calcium and dalteparin sodium are both produced *via* sodium nitrite degradation, with structural features, including 2-*O*-*S*-α-L-IdoA at the nonreducing end and a 6-*O*-*S*-2,5-anhydro-D-Man structure at the reducing end. Nadroparin calcium is primarily used in the European market as a calcium salt, while dalteparin sodium, as a sodium salt, is mainly used in the United States. Tinzaparin sodium is prepared through controlled heparinase degradation, while parnaparin sodium is produced *via* a free radical degradation method that preserves the sulfate groups and anticoagulant structures, comprising both odd and even oligosaccharide fragments [21,22].

Compared to UFH, LMWHs are more effective in preventing deep vein thrombosis, offering a better therapeutic window. While increasing the selectivity for FXa, LMWHs still retain the ability to bind with Factor IIa [23], indicating the persistence of bleeding risks and the possibility of HIT. Therefore, rigorous monitoring is still necessary during clinical applications.

TABLE 8.2 Classification of low molecular weight heparins (LMWHs).

Attribute	Daltaparin sodium	Enoxaprin sodium	Nadroparin calcium	Parnaparin sodium	Tinzaparin sodium
Manufacture	Pfizer, USA	Sanofi-Aventis, France	GlaxoSmithKline, UK	Alfa Wassermann, Italy	Leo, Denmark
Production method	Nitrous Acid Degradation	Chemical Degradation β-Elimination Degradation	Nitrous Acid Degradation, Removal of <2000 MW	Peroxide Degradation	Heparinase Degradation β-Elimination Degradation
Reducing end structure	6-*O*-sulfate-2,5-anhydro-mannitol	Sulfated or acetylated glucosamine	6-*O*-sulfate 2, 5-anhydro-mannitol	2-*N*, 6-*O*-disulfate-D-glucosamine	2-*N*, 6-*O*-disulfate-D-glucosamine
Non-reducing end structure	2-*O*-sulfate-α-L-iduronic acid	4-Enepyranosuronic acid	2-*O*-sulfate-α-L-iduronic acid	2-*O*-sulfate-α-L-iduronic acid	4-Enepyranosuronic acid
Average molecular weight	5600~6400	3500~5500	3600~5000	4000~6000	5500~7500
Anti-Factor Xa activity	110~210 IU/mg	90~125 IU/mg	95~130 IU/mg	75~110 IU/mg	70~120 IU/mg
Anti-Xa/IIa factor activity ratio	1.9~3.2	3.3~5.3	2.5~4.0	1.5~3.0	1.5~2.5
Subcutaneous bioavailability	87%	91%	100%	90%	87%
Half-life	2 h	4.1 h	3.7 h	6 h	3~4 h

8.2.5 Ultra-low-molecular-weight heparins

Known as the third generation of heparin products, fondaparinux sodium (Arixtra) is the only clinically approved ultra-low molecular weight heparin (ULMWH) currently available. ULMWHs, also known as small molecule heparins, are chemically synthesized and have shorter molecular chains compared to LMWHs. This shorter chain length reduces the likelihood of HIT. However, ULMWHs are not as widely used in clinical practice as LMWHs. Fondaparinux sodium is a pentasaccharide structure, representing the minimal unit of heparin. It acts as a selective inhibitor of FXa, exerting a potent inhibitory effect on the activity of antithrombin III (AT-III). Compared to LMWHs, fondaparinux has a weaker binding capacity for other plasma proteins. It has a longer half-life and offers better purity and safety since it is nonanimal-sourced. It represents the minimal unit of heparin, a pentasaccharide structure, and serves as a selective inhibitor of FXa, depending on AT-III binding activity. Compared to LMWHs, fondaparinux has a weaker binding capacity for other plasma proteins than LMWHs. Fondaparinux exhibits a sufficiently long half-life relative to LMWHs, and being nonanimal-sourced offers better purity and safety. Although the development of fourth-generation heparin products derived from chemical enzymatic methods or biotechnology is underway, their clinical application is still a long way off. The development of small molecule heparins, exemplified by fondaparinux sodium, remains a primary direction in heparin product research. The next section will provide details on the discovery process for fondaparinux.

8.3 Discovery and history of anticoagulant drug: fondaparinux sodium

8.3.1 Lead compound: discovery of the heparin pentasaccharide sequence

The development of fondaparinux began with the elucidation of the structure of heparin. As mentioned earlier, a significant challenge in developing heparin drugs lies in the heterogeneity of their structure. Initially, the repeating disaccharide units of glucosamine and glucuronic acid were identified. However, for a considerable time, glycochemists struggled to clarify the sugar form of glucuronic acid and the sites of its sulfation. To overcome these challenges, optimized degradation conditions and nuclear magnetic resonance technology were employed. The structure of heparin was further deciphered, ultimately determining the linkage pattern of the heparin sugar backbone, as shown in Fig. 8.5. These findings laid the foundation for further explaining the structure-activity relationship between heparin and its anticoagulant activity.

In the early 20th century, scientists discovered the existence of antithrombin III (AT-III) in plasma, which played a primary role in anticoagulation. Initially, the relationship between the anticoagulant activity of heparin and AT-III was not fully understood. Early perspectives suggested that heparin exerted its anticoagulant activity mainly through highly anionic interactions and binding with plasma proteins. However, this explanation did not account for its dependency on AT-III or the enhanced anticoagulant effects observed when lower molecular-weight heparin molecules bound to AT-III. In 1976, two key discoveries finally unveiled the secret of the anticoagulant action of heparin and its relationship with AT-III. The first discovery was the direct interaction between heparin molecules and AT-III, which was revealed through affinity chromatography studies. The second discovery showed that the strength of the interaction between heparin and AT-III positively correlated with the inhibitory activity against FXa, suggesting that heparin might be an indirect inhibitor of FXa [24–27]. These groundbreaking findings significantly advanced heparin research and led scientists to hypothesize that the binding of AT-III to heparin molecules was achieved by recognizing a specific sequence on the sugar backbone. This raised an important research question: What is the specific structure of the shortest sugar chain sequence in heparin that binds to AT-III?

In the 1970s and 1980s, due to the belated progression of computer simulation and structural biology, glycochemists were constrained to explore the shortest sequence of heparin molecules, binding to AT-III by progressively degrading them. As illustrated in Fig. 8.5, each monosaccharide fragment in the heparin molecule is represented by a letter from A to J. Structure **1** displays the A-J sequence of the heparin molecule, indicating that the heparin sugar chain is mainly composed of 1–4 linked glucuronic acid and glucosamine. Choay et al. [28,29] conducted initial investigations of the shortest effective segment of heparin through degradation methods. They used affinity chromatography to measure the affinity between various-sized fragments and AT-III, discovering that the octasaccharide structure **2** (part A~H) with the disaccharides removed from the reducing end exhibited strong binding to AT-III. In 1980, Lindahl et al. prepared the octasaccharide structure **3** (parts C~J) through nitrous acid degradation by removing the disaccharide at the nonreducing end. This heparin fragment also exhibited a strong binding affinity with AT-III. Further removal of the iduronic acid structure (sugar C) to form a heptasaccharide did not affect the activity. Lindahl et al.'s major contribution was the identification of 3-*O*-sulfate as the key functional group for AT-III binding [30]. Compound **4** (part C~H), a hexasaccharide structure, was prepared by Choay et al. through longer enzymatic degradation of heparin and also demonstrated

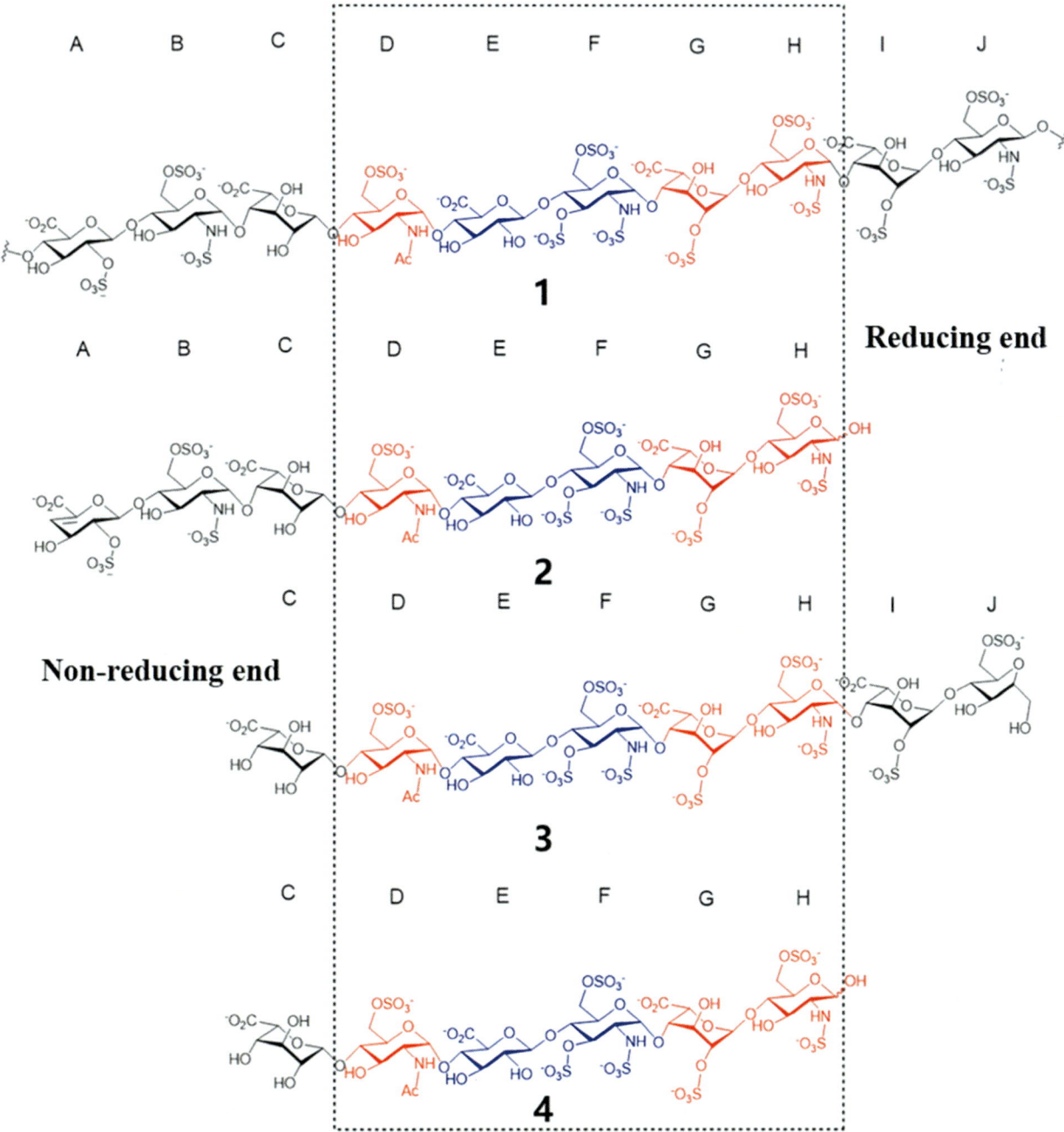

FIGURE 8.5 The minimal effective structural unit of heparin: the pentasaccharide sequence within the dashed box and its sulfation pattern (sites).

high binding activity to AT-III. This finding indicated that the disaccharide-containing parts I and J are not essential for the activity. They concluded that the smallest active segment of heparin is definitely less than or equal to the hexasaccharide. Since it was not feasible to further degrade and study the structure-activity relationship of a pentasaccharide through biological degradation, Choay et al. focused on the chemical synthesis strategy of the pentasaccharide DEFGH, resulting in two tetrasaccharides (DEFG and EFGH). Binding tests with AT-III found that DEFGH still maintained high binding activity, while the two tetrasaccharides showed significantly reduced binding. Through a series of structural simplification studies, it was ultimately determined that the pentasaccharide structure of heparin is the minimal effective structural unit for binding to AT-III and exerting anticoagulant activity (Fig. 8.6). The chemical synthesis method of the pentasaccharide laid the foundation for developing the production process of fondaparinux sodium, which will be discussed in the following section.

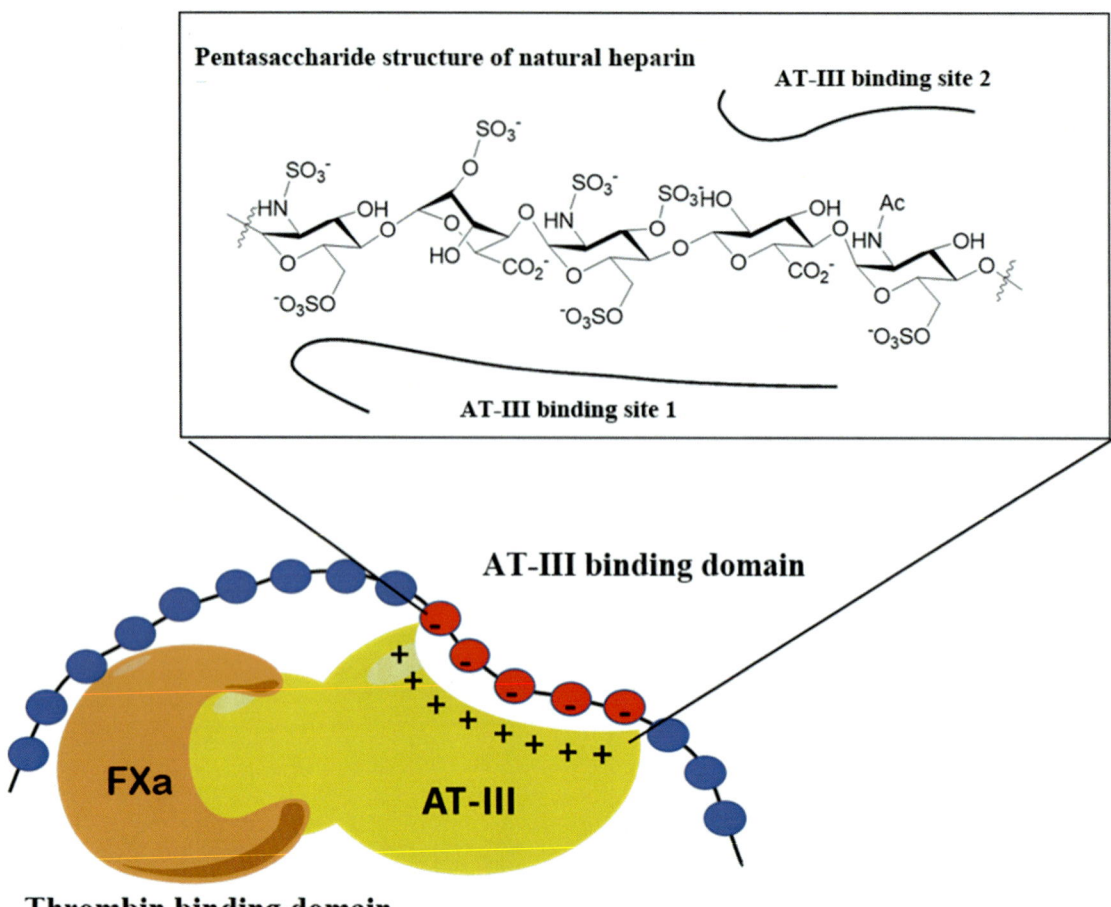

FIGURE 8.6 The binding mode of the pentasaccharide fragment in the heparin sequence with AT-III.

8.3.2 The genesis of fondaparinux sodium: structure-activity relationship studies based on the heparin pentasaccharide sequence

In 1984, Torri et al. pioneered the synthesis of the natural pentasaccharide structure (Compound **1**) through a 75-step chemical synthesis and replaced acetamido groups with sulfamino groups. They demonstrated in vitro that this pentasaccharide inhibits FXa by binding to AT-III, suggesting its potential as a novel anticoagulant drug. However, as shown in Fig. 8.7, compound **1** with a hydroxy group in the hemiacetal form at the reducing end would not be a favorable drug candidate due to the poor stability in the body [31].

The researchers from Sanofi Pharmaceuticals and Organon Pharmaceuticals synthesized a series of pentasaccharide derivatives based on the discovery of the natural pentasaccharide structure. They explored the structure-activity relationship, which was summarized in Fig. 8.8 [23], along with specific details provided in Tables 8.3–8.6. In their study, the researchers performed sulfation modifications on different hydroxyl groups of the heparin pentasaccharide backbone, starting with sulfation of the 3-position and 4-position hydroxyl groups of part D (**7**, **8**, and **12**). However, the results showed that sulfation at these positions did not enhance the anticoagulant activity of the oligosaccharide. Sulfation of the 3-position hydroxyl group on part H (**6**) significantly improved the inhibitory activity against FXa and anticoagulant activity. In contrast, sulfation of the 3-position hydroxyl group on part E (**13**) resulted in a nearly 200-fold decrease in FXa inhibition compared to **6**, also significantly reducing anticoagulant activity. Furthermore, sulfation of the 2-position hydroxyl group of part G played a critical role in FXa inhibition activity, as desulfation (**5** and **7**) almost completely lost FXa inhibitory activity (Table 8.3).

Further studies on the heparin pentasaccharide backbone involved the open-ring structure. They found that opening the rings of parts E (**19**) and G (**15**, **16**, and **18**) almost entirely eliminated the inhibitory effect on FXa (Table 8.4), indicating that disrupting the integrity of the pentasaccharide backbone significantly impacts activity. Other structure-activity relationships are

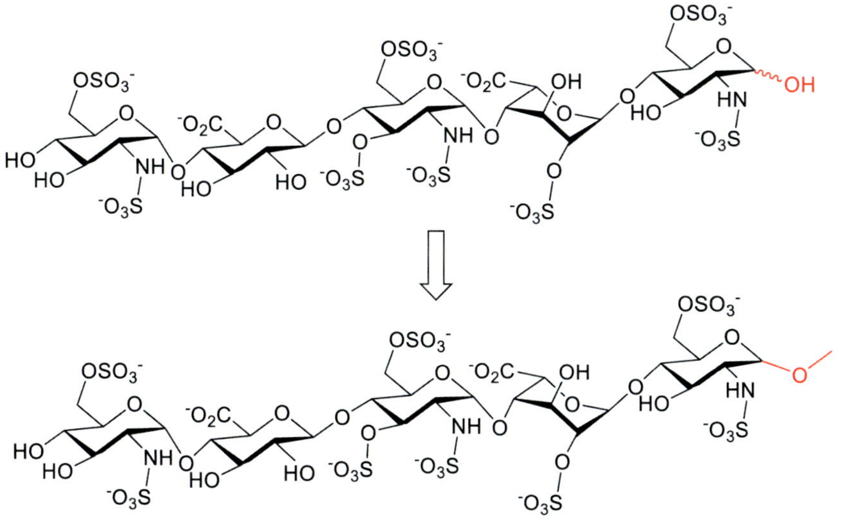

FIGURE 8.7 Conversion of the heparin pentasaccharide binding fragment (**1**) to its stable methyl glycoside product (**2**).

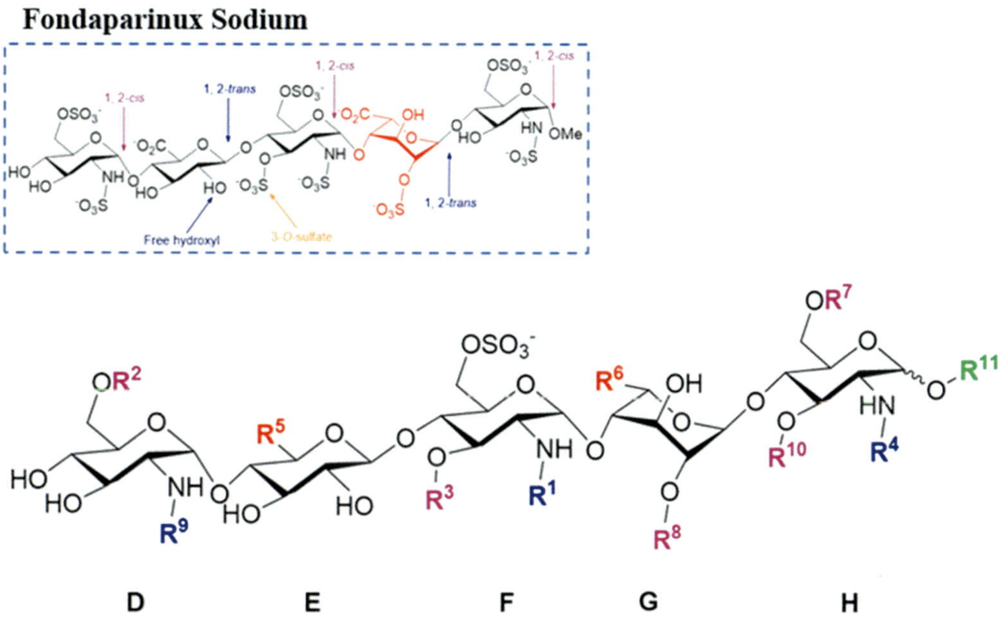

Org31540 / SR90107A

FIGURE 8.8 Structure-activity relationship of fondaparinux sodium.

presented in Table 8.5, including the desulfation or acetylation of the 3-position amine on glucosamine (**22**, **23**, **25**, and **29**), resulting in a significant reduction in activity. Inversion or removal of the carboxyl group at the 5-position of part G's glucuronic acid (**28** and **30**) led to a significant reduction in activity. Methylation of the carboxyl group at the 5-position of part E (**31**) significantly reduced activity. Desulfation of the 6-position hydroxyl group on glucosamine (**20**) or its replacement with a phosphate (**24**) also greatly decreased activity. Replacing sulfamino with *O*-sulfate had little impact on activity (**32**~**34**), and methylation of the 3-position hydroxyl groups on parts D/E/G demonstrated either no effect or a boosting effect on anticoagulant activity (**27**).

The development team replaced all glucosamine units in the pentasaccharide backbone with glucose, creating a new pentasaccharide framework for further structure-activity relationship studies (Table 8.6). By retaining methylation of the reducing end terminus and sulfation of the 2- and 3-positions of parts F and H and derivatizing the hydroxyl groups on the 2- and 3-positions of parts D, E, and F, they found that sulfation and methylation of the hydroxyl groups on part

TABLE 8.3 Structure-activity relationship of methyl glycoside derivatives at different O-sulfate positions.

		K_d (nM)	Axa (u/mg)			K_d (nM)	Axa (u/mg)
2		50	700	9		NA	≈175
3		NA	Inactive	10		NA	SA
4		1560	198	11		NA	SA
5		NA	≈175	12		NA	≈1200
6		1.3	1260	13		218	476
7		NA	≈1200	14		320	700
8		NA	≈1200				

TABLE 8.4 Structure-activity relationship of open-ring methyl glycoside derivatives of sugars E and G.

		K_d (nM)	AXa (u/mg)
15		NA	SA
16		NA	SA
17		NA	Inactive
18		NA	175
19		NA	Inactive

D both improved activities, but methylation had a more significant contribution (**35**). Using longer alkyl chains (four or six carbons) for derivatization significantly increased the inhibitory activity against FXa (**42** and **43**), but the activity decreased with longer chain lengths (**41**). Methylation of the 2-position hydroxyl group on part G also achieved considerable FXa inhibitory activity (**39** and **40**). Methylation or butylation modifications on the 3-position hydroxyl group of parts F and H (**35**, **39**, and **44**) maintained good activity, while other changes reduced it. It is important to note compound **35**, which had significantly higher binding activity to antithrombin III compared to fondaparinux sodium and doubled its inhibitory effect on FXa. In a New Zealand rabbit model, the half-life of compound **35** reached 16.5 hours (compared to 1.6 hours for fondaparinux sodium), indicating its potential for longer-lasting therapeutic effects. This compound, named Idraparinux (SR-34006), entered Phase III clinical trials in 2002 as a candidate treatment for deep vein thrombosis and pulmonary embolism. Unfortunately, due to its longer half-life resulting in a stronger tendency for bleeding, the clinical trials were terminated. The stronger bleeding risk associated with the compound led to concerns about its safety profile, ultimately preventing its further development as a therapeutic option.

In summary, the following conclusions can be drawn from the structure-activity relationship studies of heparin pentasaccharide derivatives:

1. The presence and position of sulfate groups on hydroxyl groups significantly affect the activity of the derivatives. Sulfation at the 6-position of part D (R^2) and 3-position of part F (R^3) is crucial for activating AT-III and enhancing the binding of the compound to the first binding site of AT-III. Sulfation at the 3-position of sugar H (R^{10}) greatly enhances binding to the second site of AT-III and its anticoagulant activity.
2. The sulfamino group structure in parts F and H is essential. Replacing the 2-position sulfamino group (-NH-R^1) on part F with acetyl or hydroxyl groups significantly decreases its anti-FXa activity. Replacing the 2-position sulfamino group (-NH-R^4) on part H with a hydroxyl group reduces activity to only 5% of the original. The 2-position sulfamino group (-NH-R^9) on part D has a smaller impact on activity and can be replaced with a methoxy group in some derivatives (Idraparinux). Additionally, the sulfamino group can be replaced with *O*-sulfate, with a minor impact on activity, as observed in compound **3**.
3. The carboxyl group structure is necessary. When the carboxyl group at the 5-position of sugar E (R^5) is methyl-protected, activity drops to 5% of the original. Removal of the carboxyl group at the 5-position of part G (R^6) also greatly reduces activity, highlighting that negatively charged carboxyl groups play a vital role in activating AT.
4. Replacing sulfate groups with other charged groups yields poor results. For example, replacing the sulfate group at position R^2 of part D with a phosphate group almost completely eliminates activity.

TABLE 8.5 Structure-activity relationship of methyl glycoside derivatives at different O-sulfate positions.

	K_d (nM)	Axa (u/mg)		K_d (nM)	Axa (u/mg)
20	NA	Inactive	28	NA	Inactive
21	NA	Inactive	29	NA	882
22	NA	Inactive	30	NA	Inactive
23	NA	Inactive	31	NA	35
24	NA	Inactive	32	3.0	1302
25	NA	35	33	4.0	1110
26	NA	126	34	NA	819
27	NA	≈1200			

TABLE 8.6 Structure-activity relationship of methyl glycoside derivatives at different O-sulfate and O-alkyl positions.

		K_d (nM)	Axa (u/mg)			K_d (nM)	Axa (u/mg)
35		16	1323	40		28	1318
36		NA	≈1200	41		NA	Inactive
37		NA	≈1200	42		9	910
38		139	1150	43		2	1529
39		13	1611	44		0.3	1080

5. The integrity of the pyranose ring structure is critical. Maintaining carboxyl groups at positions R^5 and R^6 while opening the ring of iduronic acid reduces activity to 25% of the original, and opening the ring of part E almost completely eliminates activity. Hence, the integrity of the pyranose ring structure is crucial for maintaining activity, partly due to its role in dispersing the charge.
6. Epimers show poor activity. Replacing the 1,2-*cis* glycosidic bond between parts D and E with a 1,2-*trans* bond almost completely eliminates activity. Moreover, flipping the carboxyl group of part E downwards results in only 10% of the original activity. Consequently, there are significant limitations in structural modification and optimization related to the replacement of sugar types and the configuration of glycosidic bonds.
7. Methylation does not affect activity. Methylation of the exposed hydroxyl groups on the pentasaccharide structure does not significantly alter its activity but critically impacts the half-life of the compound. However, methylation, at the reducing end ($R^{11} = Me$) significantly increases the compound's plasma stability.

8.3.3 Mechanism of action of fondaparinux sodium

Early research preliminarily verified that DEFGH is the smallest effective structural unit of heparin. Sanofi Pharmaceuticals' research team further elaborated the structure-activity relationship of this pentasaccharide sequence in detail and ultimately chose the methyl glycoside derivative of the heparin pentasaccharide, Org31540/SR90107A (fondaparinux sodium), for further investigation, as shown in Fig. 8.8. In vivo activity studies, fondaparinux sodium was found to enhance the inhibition of FXa by AT-III by 300 times compared to without its presence. Fondaparinux sodium binds to AT-III, inducing a protein conformational change. The formation of a strong fondaparinux sodium-AT-III-FXa ternary complex inhibits the downstream coagulation process induced by FXa. The in vitro binding activity of fondaparinux sodium to AT-III is characterized by a K_d value of about 40 nM, while the measured inhibitory activity of fondaparinux sodium on FXa varied slightly depending on the methods and conditions used. Fondaparinux sodium demonstrates consistent inhibition of FXa across different species, as indicated in Table 8.7, and exhibits high selectivity toward factors IIa, IXa, etc. Scientists also discovered that fondaparinux sodium elevates thrombin levels in platelet-poor plasma but inhibits thrombin generation in platelet-rich plasma. Systematic studies on anticoagulant activity revealed that fondaparinux sodium is particularly effective in the extrinsic coagulation pathway. Its advantage lies in its ability to not affect platelets, thus avoiding inhibition of platelet aggregation, which is typically observed with heparin and low molecular weight heparins.

After thorough research, fondaparinux sodium was confirmed to achieve the desired clinical trial endpoints and received approval for clinical use in the United States and Europe in 2001. Detailed mechanistic studies revealed that the nonreducing trisaccharide sequence, located at the left end of fondaparinux sodium, is responsible for binding to AT-III and forming a complex. This complex alters the conformation of AT-III to selectively inhibit FXa but not Factor IIa. It is important to note that inhibition of IIa requires a longer sugar chain. The reducing disaccharide located at the right end of fondaparinux sodium stabilizes the conformation of activated AT-III, enhancing the stability of the ternary complex (Fig. 8.9).

8.3.4 Pharmacokinetics and safety of fondaparinux sodium

Fondaparinux sodium, which was approved for market in China in 2008 and included in the National Medical Insurance Catalog in 2017, exhibits favorable pharmacokinetic properties and clinical safety compared to UFH and low molecular weight heparins. After subcutaneous administration, sondaparinux sodium is rapidly absorbed with a bioavailability of 100%, and peak plasma concentrations are reached around 2 hours postdosing. The drug predominantly

TABLE 8.7 In vivo activity of fondaparinux sodium.

FXa inhibitory activity (IC_{50} in nM)			Binding affinity for AT-III (K_d in nM)				Thrombin generation (IC_{50} in μM)	
Human	Rabbit	Rat	Human	Rabbit	Baboon	Rat	Extrinsic activation pathway	Intrinsic activation pathway
40 ± 3	45 ± 11	36 ± 12	48 ± 8	132 ± 10	78 ± 2.4	50 ± 2.5	0.3 ± 0.05	2.8 ± 0.4

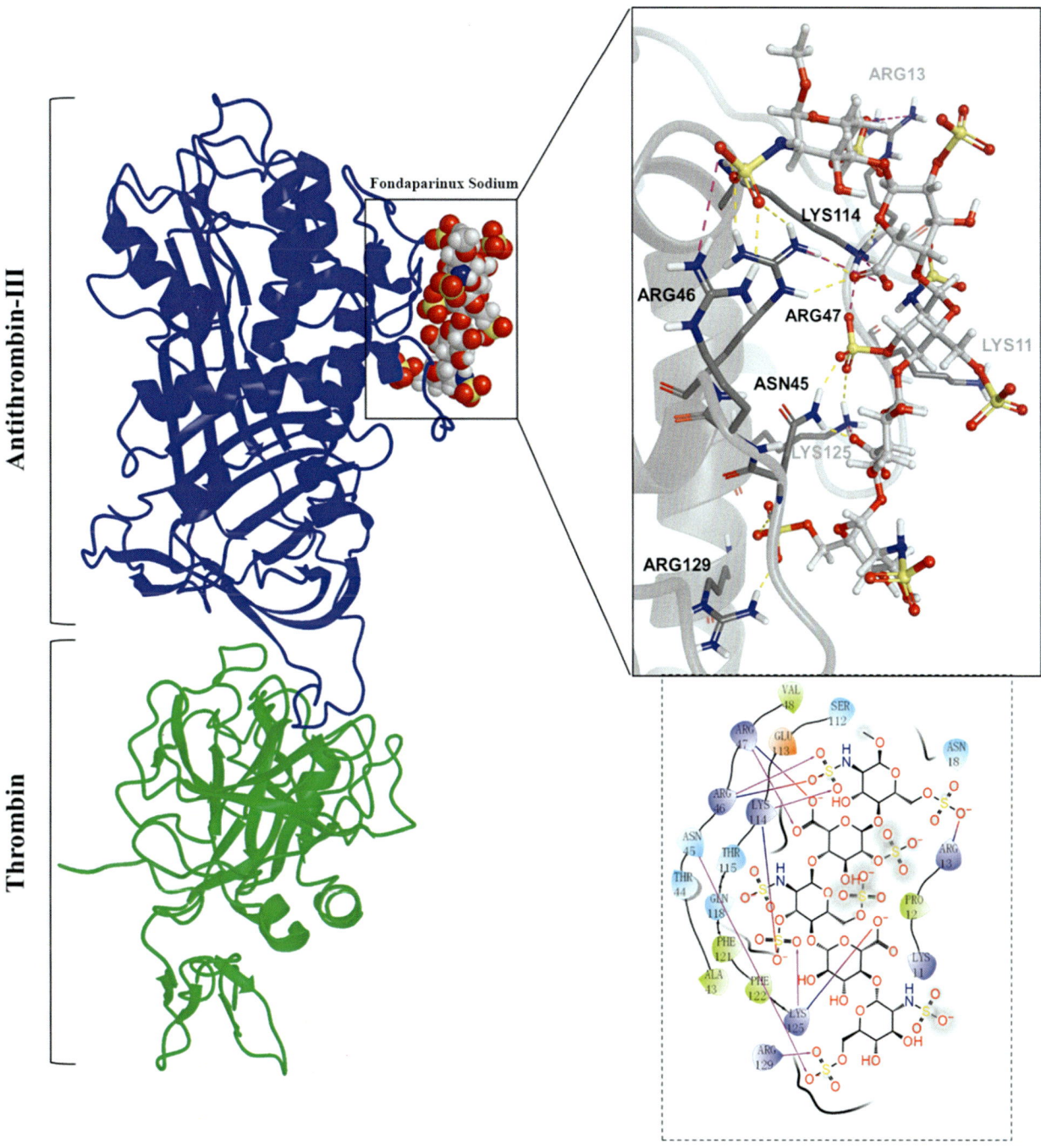

FIGURE 8.9 The binding mode of fondaparinux sodium with AT-III.

distributes in plasma, with a plasma protein binding rate of 97%. Fondaparinux sodium is not metabolized by the liver, and approximately 80% of the drug is excreted unchanged in the urine through renal excretion. The half-life of fondaparinux sodium is 17 hours in young adults and 21 hours in the elderly. It shows good linear pharmacokinetic parameters within a dose range of 2−8 mg [32]. Compared to UFH and low-molecular-weight heparins, fondaparinux sodium demonstrates significant advantages in terms of pharmacokinetics and clinical safety, as shown in Table 8.8.

The metabolic characteristics of fondaparinux sodium result in minimal individual variation in treatment response, ranging from 5.5% to 17%. This characteristic allows for the implementation of fixed dosing regimens, making it easier for healthcare professionals to manage and control bleeding risks. Furthermore, its extended half-life allows once-daily

TABLE 8.8 Comparison of unfractionated heparin, low molecular weight heparin, and fondaparinux sodium.

Type of heparin	Unfractionated heparin	Low molecular weight heparin	Fondaparinux sodium
Source	Bovine lung/porcine intestine	Crude heparin	Synthetic
Sugar chain length	~45 units	~15 units	5 units
Neutralization of DPP4	Strong	Weak	None
Half-life	0.5~2 h	4~7 h	17~21 h
Bioavailability	15%~30%	90%	100%
Platelet activation	Strong	Weak	None
HIT risk	2%~5%	1%~2%	0
Monitoring required	Yes	Yes	No
Neutralizing agent	Protamine	Protamine	Plasma
Bleeding risk	> LMWH	0%~13% bleeding 0%~4% major bleeding	2%~3% minor bleeding 1%~3% major bleeding
Binding to proteins, endothelial cells, and macrophages	High	Low	None
Risk of osteoporosis	High	Low	None
Site of clearance	Reticuloendothelial system/kidney	Reticuloendothelial system/kidney	Kidney
Dose adjustment based on body weigh	Required	Required	Not required

dosing, providing convenience for patients. One significant advantage of fondaparinux sodium is that it is not metabolized by the liver, decreasing the potential for drug-drug interactions. As a short pentasaccharide sequence, fondaparinux sodium does not bind to PF4 proteins, effectively avoiding complications associated with HIT. However, its high rate of renal excretion may pose a significant risk of renal damage, especially in the elderly population. In contrast to UFH and low molecular weight heparins, which can bind to various plasma proteins, macrophages, endothelial cells, and the extracellular matrix, fondaparinux sodium does not bind to endothelial cells or macrophages. This characteristic makes its clinical use more convenient, as it does not require monitoring of coagulation status through tests such as activated partial thromboplastin time.

8.4 Chemical process of fondaparinux sodium

8.4.1 Synthesis challenges of fondaparinux sodium

Compared to conventional small-molecule drugs, fondaparinux sodium possesses a complex structure and is comprised of a charged pentasaccharide. The synthesis route is relatively long and challenging, with key difficulties including:

1. Difficulty in Stereoselective Control: The presence of two 1,2-*cis*-glycosidic bonds (between parts D and E and F and G) in the pentasaccharide makes their synthesis challenging and significantly elevates the complexity of protecting groups for the monosaccharide building blocks, consequently extending the synthesis route.
2. Challenges in Purification and Separation: During glycosylation, a certain proportion of α/β isomers are formed, which complicates the separation process. The deprotection phase presents considerable difficulty in purification due to the high polarity of the products with multiple exposed hydroxyl groups, leading to challenges in purification. Furthermore, the subsequent steps involving catalytic hydrogenation, which utilize palladium-carbon metal catalysts, are hard to purify thoroughly. This complicates the separation process and raises issues for pharmaceutical quality control.

8.4.2 Chemical synthesis of fondaparinux sodium

As one of the small-molecule drugs with the longest synthesis route to date, fondaparinux sodium has remained expensive to produce. Sanofi's mature process for producing Arixtra, which is fondaparinux sodium, involves more than 50 reaction steps, with a total yield of only 0.22%. Different companies employ various synthesis routes for fondaparinux sodium, but the general approach involves synthesizing monosaccharide building blocks through protective group operations, selectively constructing glycosidic bonds, and subsequently deprotecting and sulfating to obtain the target molecule. Here, we selected two representative approaches to introduce.

The first approach is described in a patent published by Reliable Biopharmaceutical in 2012 (US 2012/0116066 A1). The retrosynthetic analysis is depicted in Fig. 8.10. The process begins with readily available and inexpensive materials such as glucal **11**, dehydrated cellobiose **12**, bis-isopropylidene glucose **9**, and methyl glucoside **10**. Various glycosyl building blocks are constructed using these starting materials and then assembled. It is worth noting that the reaction activity of amino sugars is generally low. Therefore, this synthesis route uses 2-azido substituted sugar building blocks, which are reduced to amino groups after the pentasaccharide assembly, followed by sulfation reactions to produce the target molecule. To obtain the fondaparinux sodium pentasaccharide, a fully protected pentasaccharide compound **1** is designed first, which can be synthesized through a single glycosylation from trisaccharide building block **2** and disaccharide building block **3**. Trisaccharide **2** can be obtained from 2-azido-D-glucose building block **7** and azido-substituted dehydrated cellobiose **8** through a single glycosylation. Disaccharide **3**, on the other hand, can be synthesized from iduronic acid building block **5** and 2-azido-D-glucose building block **6** through glycosylation.

This synthesis route involves a total of 56 steps, including three glycosylation reactions, with the majority of steps focusing on the protective group strategy for the sugar building blocks. Starting with fully acetylated glucal **11**, a series of eight reaction steps are performed to yield 2-azido-substituted glucose building block **7**. This compound serves as the trichloroacetimidate glycoside donor. Starting with 1,6-anhydro cellobiose, nine reaction steps lead to the hydroxyl-exposed disaccharide **8** as the following receptor. The trichloroacetimidate glycoside donor **7** and the receptor disaccharide **8** are reacted using TESOTf as a catalyst at $-40°C$ for 2 hours to obtain the target trisaccharide **4**. The subsequent two steps involve opening the dehydrated sugar ring and selective hydrolysis. The trisaccharide **4** is converted to trichloroacetimidate glycoside donor **2** using 1,8-Diazabicyclo[5,4,0]undec-7-ene (DBU) as a catalyst.

Concurrently, starting with bis-isopropylidene glucose **9** as the initial material, thirteen steps were undertaken to obtain iduronic acid building block **5**, which serves as a trichloroacetimidate glycoside donor. Similarly, starting with glucoside **10**, eight steps were carried out to yield the 2-azido-substituted glucose building block **6** as a receptor. The donor and acceptor are mixed at $-20°C$ with boron trifluoride etherate as the catalyst, then raised to room temperature and reacted for 3 hours to produce the β-configured disaccharide building block. Subsequent removal of the Lev protecting group with hydrazine hydrate resulted in the disaccharide building block **3** as an acceptor. Employing TESOTf as the catalyst, the trisaccharide donor **2** and disaccharide donor **3** were reacted at $-30°C$ for two hours, yielding the fully protected pentasaccharide **1**. Deprotection of the fully protected pentasaccharide obtained above led to the target molecule of fondaparinux sodium, which involves acyl deprotection, selective sulfation of hydroxyl groups, catalytic hydrogenation reduction, and sulfamidation, totaling eleven reaction steps.

In 2014, the research team led by Shang-Cheng Hung in Taiwan, adopted a [4 + 1] synthetic strategy, starting from commercially available materials. They completed the synthesis of Arixtra in 22 linear steps with a total yield of 0.63%. The design of orthogonal protective groups significantly shortened the synthesis route. This provides a feasible solution for optimizing the synthesis process of fondaparinux sodium [33], as illustrated in Fig. 8.11.

In summary, the numerous reported chemical synthesis routes for fondaparinux sodium all suffer from common drawbacks: lengthy procedures, cumbersome operations, and low efficiency. Effectively optimizing the synthesis route and enhancing reaction efficiency will significantly promote the widespread use and clinical application of fondaparinux sodium.

8.4.3 Chemo-enzymatic synthesis of fondaparinux sodium

In recent years, significant breakthroughs have been achieved in chemo-enzymatic synthesis and hybrid chemo-enzymatic synthesis. Scientists have endeavored to simplify the synthesis steps of fondaparinux sodium by employing enzymatic methods in conjunction with chemical synthesis.

The enzymes required for the chemo-enzymatic synthesis of fondaparinux sodium can be categorized into two types: glycosyltransferases and glycan-modifying enzymes. Glycosyltransferases can mimic the in vivo synthesis of glycosaminoglycans, with KfiA, KfiC, and PmHSs being the primary enzymes utilized in the synthesis of heparin-like molecules. Glycan-modifying enzymes mainly include sulfotransferases and C_5-epimerases (C_5-*epi*), which are used in the

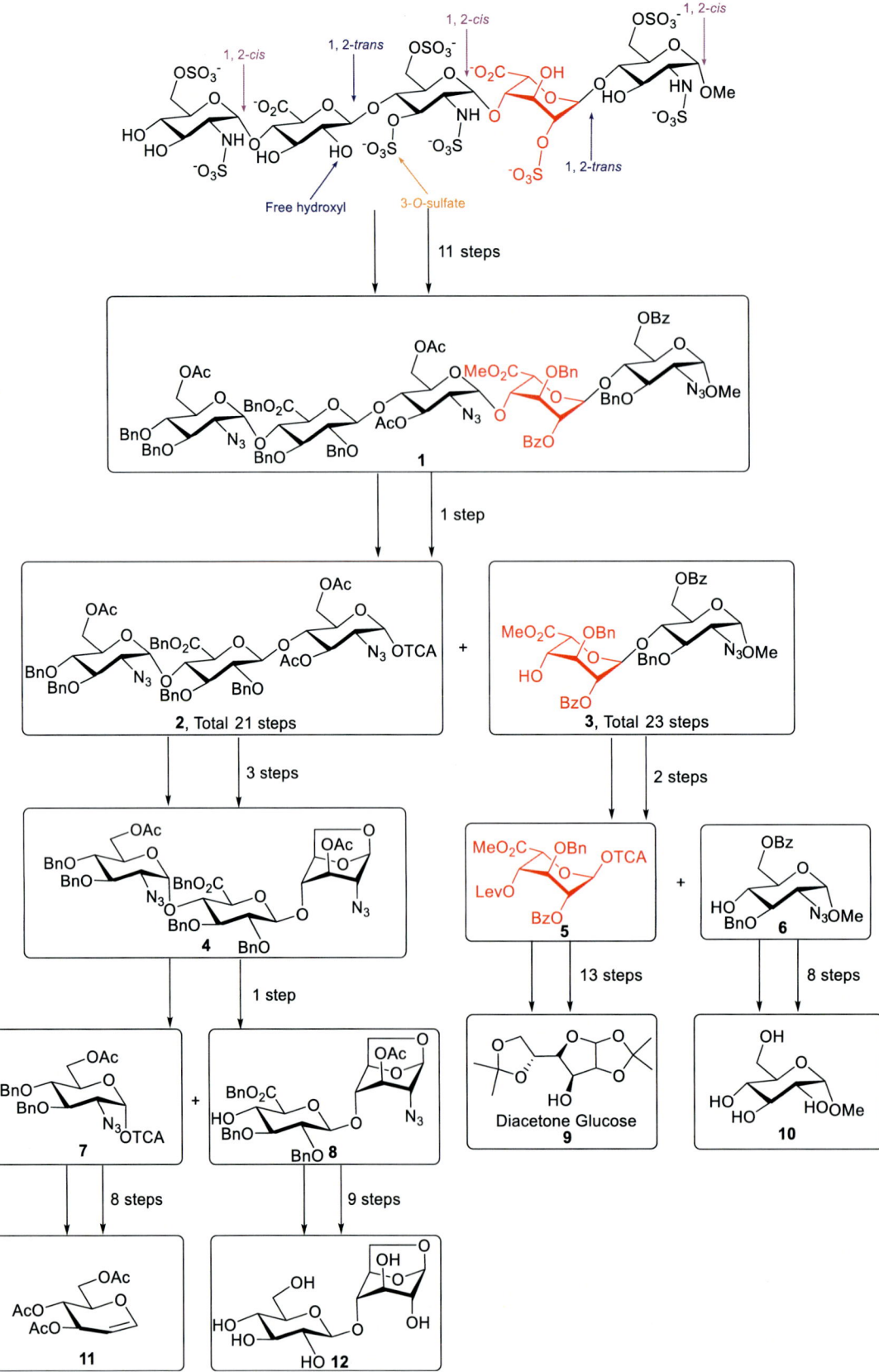

FIGURE 8.10 Retrosynthetic analysis route for fondaparinux sodium (reliable biopharmaceutical, US 2012/0116066 A1).

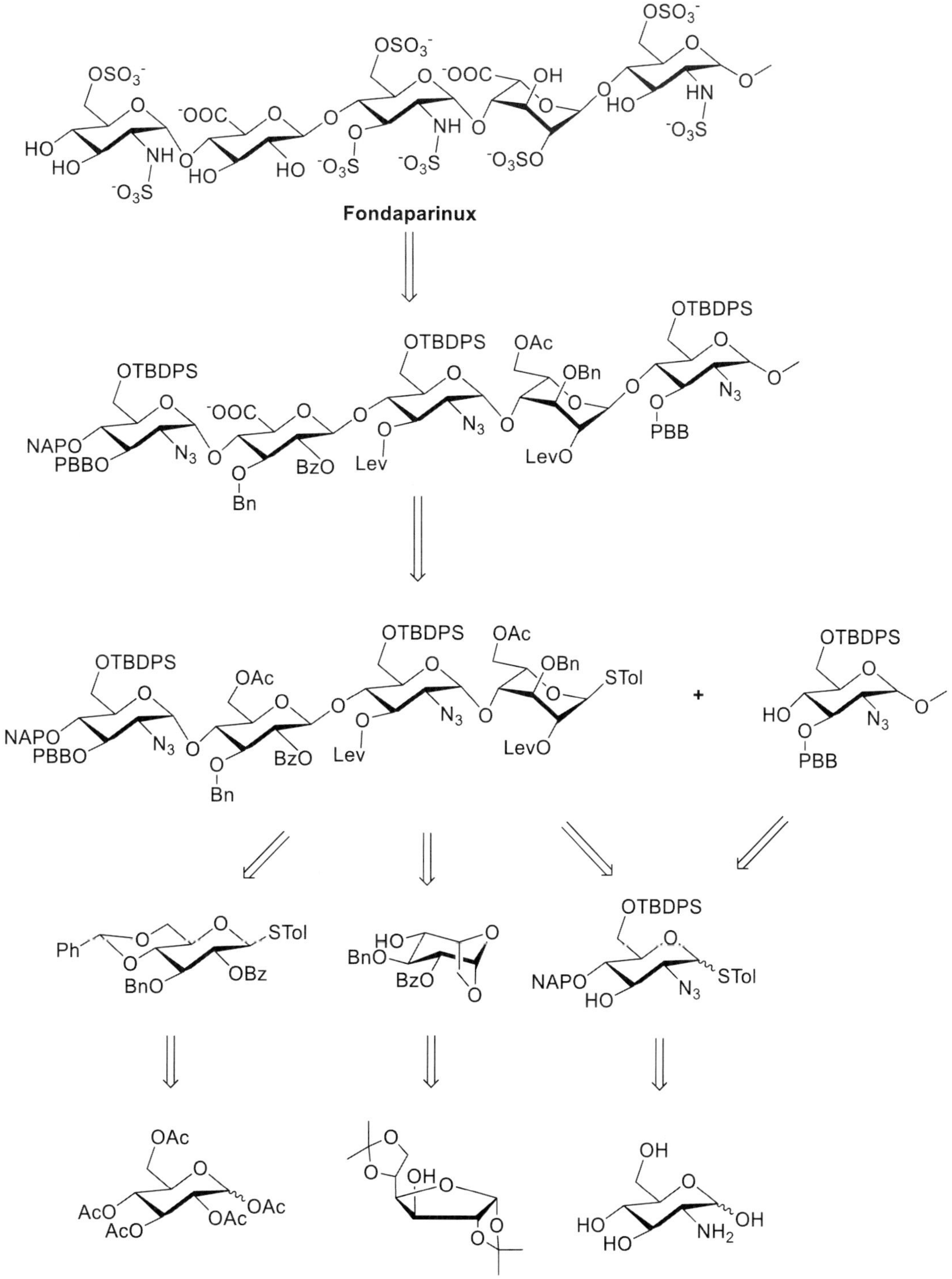

FIGURE 8.11 22-Step linear chemical synthesis and retrosynthetic analysis of fondaparinux sodium.

sulfation process during the synthesis of heparin-like molecules. The natural sulfonate donor 3'-phosphoadenosine-5'-phosphosulfate can be used to modify oligosaccharide segments, exhibiting excellent region-specificity. C_5-*epi* is capable of isomerizing glucuronic acid to iduronic acid, simplifying the operational steps involved. In 2011, the research groups of Linhardt in the USA and Liu Jian collaborated to synthesize two heparin heptasaccharide analogs using chemo-enzymatic methods, as shown in Fig. 8.12. This work achieved yields of 42% in ten steps and 35% in twelve steps [34], respectively, and offered new avenues for the synthesis of small-molecule heparin oligosaccharides.

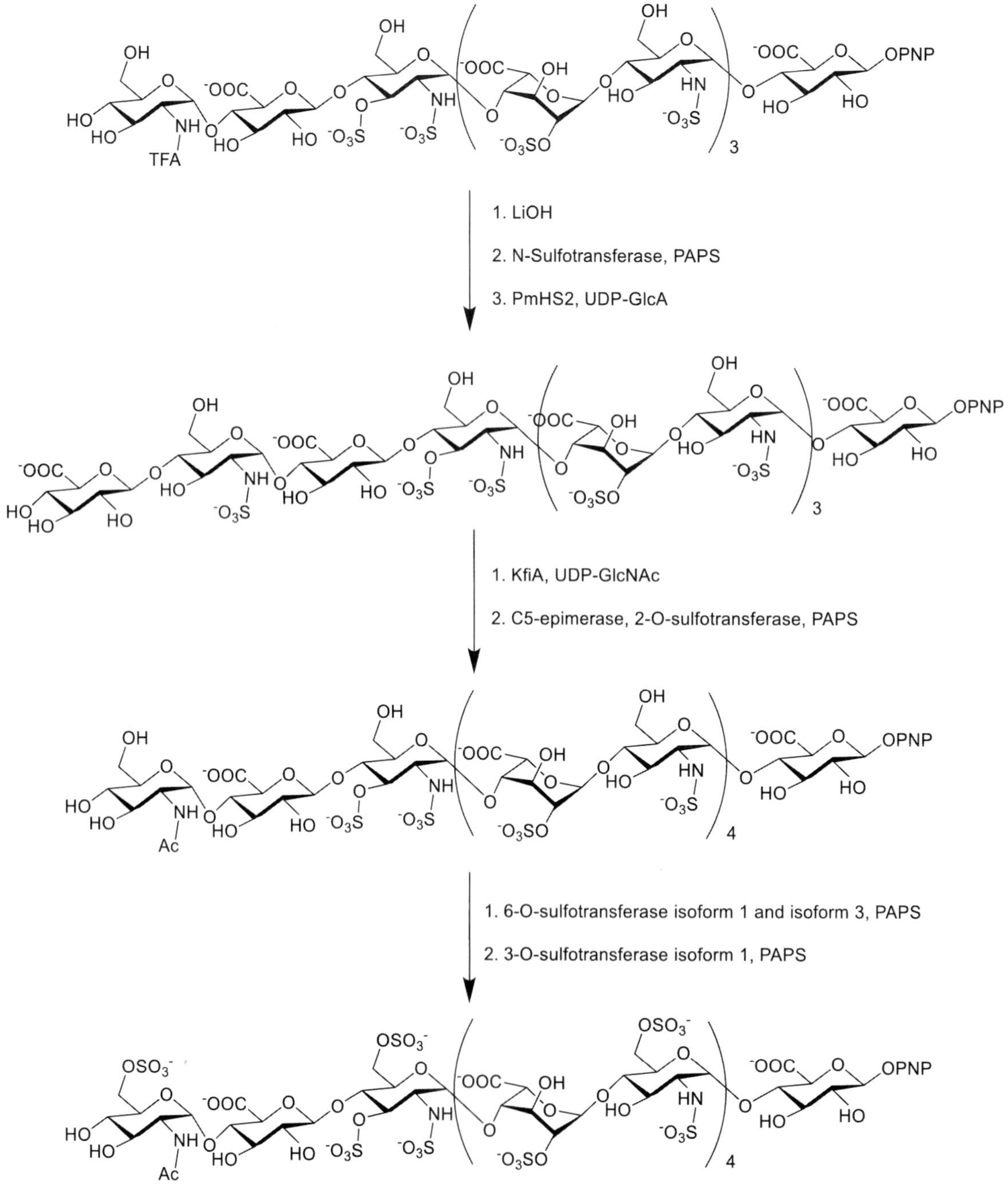

FIGURE 8.12 Chemo-enzymatic synthesis of fondaparinux sodium heptasaccharide derivatives.

8.5 Summary

8.5.1 Development strategy for fondaparinux sodium

Anticoagulant therapy is an essential treatment modality for the prevention and treatment of thromboembolic diseases, and heparin and its derivatives are indispensable anticoagulants on a global scale. Due to the bleeding tendency of UFH as well as potential adverse effects like HIT and osteoporosis, vigilant monitoring is necessary for clinical use. The discovery of fondaparinux sodium aimed to address these issues associated with natural heparin. Its origin lies in the AT-III binding region of natural heparin and its pentasaccharide structure. Research revealed that fondaparinux sodium binds to AT-III to inhibit FXa rather than directly inhibiting thrombin. Based on this mechanism, further studies on the structure-activity relationship of the pentasaccharide structure revealed the impact of sulfation and methylation at different sites on its activity, leading to the development of fondaparinux sodium.

8.5.2 Development trends in heparin-like anticoagulants

To date, four generations of heparin anticoagulants have been developed for anticoagulation. The first generation is UFH (UFH), which is derived from pig intestines, bovine lungs, and bovine intestines. The second generation, known as LMWHs, is produced by controlled chemical or enzymatic degradation of UFH with molecular weights between 3500 and 6000 Da. The third generation, ULMWHs, includes fondaparinux sodium and other low-molecular-weight heparin analogs synthesized chemically. The fourth generation comprises bioengineered low-molecular-weight heparins and heparin analogs prepared from chemical-enzymatic methods.

Chemo-enzymatic synthesis mimics the biological pathway of heparin synthesis, combining chemical and enzymatic synthesis techniques to overcome the bottlenecks faced in chemical synthesis. Enzymatic synthesis enables the construction of stereo-selective and region-selective glycan structures without concern for substituent groups. This approach allows for the rapid generation of oligosaccharide building blocks needed for chemical synthesis. Over the past five years, scientists have developed a series of novel chemical and enzymatic methods for preparing LMWHs, ULMWHs, and bioengineered heparins. These advancements have led to the discovery of safer and more updated heparin products. The successful synthesis of novel heparin derivatives also provided the material foundation for further understanding the structure-activity relationship of heparin oligosaccharides. This knowledge paves the way for developing more ideal heparin products.

8.5.3 Development of small-molecule carbohydrate drugs

Carbohydrate drugs currently have a relatively small representation in the clinical setting compared to their importance in organic matter. The complex and widespread roles of carbohydrate compounds in cells make it challenging to design them as single-target regulatory molecules in drug development. Several obstacles hinder the development of carbohydrate drugs, including strong water solubility, difficulties in crossing the phospholipid bilayer, limited oral administration options, synthetic complexity, and the lack of a uniformly stable source. However, the development of fondaparinux sodium has provided a successful reference for the development of carbohydrate drugs. The process involves starting with the natural carbohydrate molecular framework and conducting in-depth studies on its biological activity and mechanisms. Researchers identify the minimal sugar framework structure through chemical or enzymatic methods to degrade the natural polysaccharide framework and determine the key structural characteristics necessary for biological activity. Subsequent optimization of the structure enhances the pharmaceutical properties of carbohydrate compounds, leading to the discovery of carbohydrate drugs with clinical therapeutic value. Polysaccharides derived from marine sources, microorganisms, and traditional Chinese medicines exhibit significant activities and unique mechanisms of action for various indications. By adopting the research and development approach used for fondaparinux sodium, there is immense potential for discovering carbohydrate-based chemical monomers with high activity and novel mechanisms. This methodology and strategy hold promise for unlocking the vast pharmacological potential inherent in carbohydrate-based therapeutics. They serve as a pivotal instrument in the future exploration and exploitation of carbohydrate drugs.

References

[1] Aird WC. Vascular bed-specific thrombosis. J Thromb Haemost 2007;5(1):283–91 Suppl.
[2] Jackson SP. Arterial thrombosis—insidious, unpredictable and deadly. Nat Med 2011;17(11):1423–36.
[3] Turpie AG, Esmon C. Venous and arterial thrombosis—pathogenesis and the rationale for anticoagulation. Thromb Haemost 2011;105(4):586–96.
[4] Spencer FA, Emery C, Joffe SW, et al. Incidence rates, clinical profile, and outcomes of patients with venous thromboembolism. The Worcester VTE study. J Thromb Thrombol 2009;28(4):401–9.
[5] Hillis LD, Borer J, Braunwald E, et al. High dose intravenous streptokinase for acute myocardial infarction: preliminary results of a multicenter trial. J Am Coll Cardiol 1985;6(5):957–62.
[6] Reininger AJ. VWF attributes – impact on thrombus formation. Thromb Res 2008;122:S9–13.
[7] Mackman N. Role of tissue factor in hemostasis and thrombosis. Blood Cell Mol Dis 2006;36(2):104–7.
[8] Furie B, Furie BC. Mechanisms of thrombus formation. N Engl J Med 2008;359(9):938–49.
[9] Moons A. Tissue factor and coronary artery disease. Cardiovas Res 2002;53(2):313–25.

[10] Lundblad RL, Bradshaw RA, Gabriel D, et al. A review of the therapeutic uses of thrombin. Thromb Haemost 2004;91(5):851−60.
[11] Licari LG, Kovacic JP. Thrombin physiology and pathophysiology. J Vet Emerg Crit Care (San Antonio) 2009;19(1):11−22.
[12] Reininger AJ, Heijnen HF, Schumann H, et al. Mechanism of platelet adhesion to von Willebrand factor and microparticle formation under high shear stress. Blood 2006;107(9):3537−45.
[13] Grotta J, Ackerman R, Correia J, et al. Whole blood viscosity parameters and cerebral blood flow. Stroke 1982;13(3):296−301.
[14] Lin Z, Johnson ME. Proposed cation-π mediated binding by factor Xa: a novel enzymatic mechanism for molecular recognition. FEBS Lett 1995;370(1-2):1−5.
[15] Brandstetter H, Kühne A, Bode W, et al. X-ray structure of active site-inhibited clotting factor Xa. Implications for drug design and substrate recognition. J Biol Chem 1996;271(47):29988−92.
[16] Turpie AG, Gallus AS, Hoek JA, et al. A synthetic pentasaccharide for the prevention of deep-vein thrombosis after total hip replacement. N Engl J Med 2001;344(9):619−25.
[17] Lindahl U, Pejler G. Heparin-like polysaccharides in intra- and extravascular coagulation reactions. Acta Med Scand Suppl 1987;715:139−44.
[18] Fareed J, Jeske W, Hoppensteadt D, et al. Low-molecular-weight heparins: pharmacologic profile and product differentiation. Am J Cardiol 1998;82(5):3L−10L.
[19] Ahsan A, Jeske W, Hoppensteadt D, et al. Molecular profiling and weight determination of heparins and depolymerized heparins. J Pharm Sci 1995;84(6):724−7.
[20] Maddineni J, Walenga JM, Jeske WP, et al. Product individuality of commercially available low-molecular-weight heparins and their generic versions: therapeutic implications. Clin Appl Thromb Hemost 2006;12(3):267−76.
[21] Dogan OT, Polat ZA, Karahan O, et al. Antiangiogenic activities of bemiparin sodium, enoxaparin sodium, nadroparin calcium and tinzaparin sodium. Thromb Res 2011;128(4):e29−32.
[22] Hao C, Sun M, Wang H, et al. Low molecular weight heparins and their clinical applications. Prog Mol Biol Transl Sci 2019;163:21−39.
[23] Herbert JM, Hérault JP, Bernat A, et al. Biochemical and pharmacological properties of SANORG 32701. Comparison with the "synthetic pentasaccharide" (SR 90107/ORG 31540) and standard heparin. Circ Res 1996;79(3):590−600.
[24] Lam LH, Silbert JE, Rosenberg RD. The separation of active and inactive forms of heparin. Biochem Biophys Res Commun 1976;69(2):570−7.
[25] Höök M, Björk I, Hopwood J, Lindahl U, et al. Anticoagulant activity of heparin: separation of high-activity and low-activity heparin species by affinity chromatography on immobilized antithrombin. FEBS Lett 1976;66(1):90−3.
[26] Hopwood J, Höök M, Linker A, Lindahl U. Anticoagulant activity of heparin: isolation of antithrombin-binding sites. FEBS Lett 1976;69(1-2):51−4.
[27] Andersson LO, Barrowcliffe TW, Holmer E, et al. Anticoagulant properties of heparin fractionated by affinity chromatography on matrix-bound antithrombin III and by gel filtration. Thromb Res 1976;9(6):575−83.
[28] Choay J, Lormeau JC, Petitou M, et al. Anti-Xa active heparin oligosaccharides. Thromb Res 1980;18(3-4):573−8.
[29] Casu B, Oreste P, Torri G, et al. The structure of heparin oligosaccharide fragments with high anti-(factor Xa) activity containing the minimal antithrombin III-binding sequence. Chemical and 13C nuclear-magnetic-resonance studies. Biochem J 1981;197(3):599−609.
[30] Thunberg L, Bäckström G, Grundberg H, et al. The molecular size of the antithrombin-binding sequence in heparin. FEBS Lett 1980;117(1-2):203−6.
[31] Sinay P, Jacquinet JC, Petitou M, et al. Total synthesis of a heparin pentasaccharide fragment having high affinity for antithrombin III. Carbohydr Res 1984;132(2):C5−9.
[32] Donat F, Duret JP, Santoni A, et al. The pharmacokinetics of fondaparinux sodium in healthy volunteers. Clin Pharmacokinet 2002;41(Suppl 2):1−9.
[33] Chang CH, Lico LS, Huang TY, et al. Synthesis of the heparin-based anticoagulant drug fondaparinux. Angew Chem Int Ed Engl 2014;53(37):9876−9.
[34] Xu Y, Masuko S, Takieddin M, et al. Chemoenzymatic synthesis of homogeneous ultralow molecular weight heparins. Science 2011;334(6055):498−501.

Chapter 9

Development of the nucleotide antiviral drug sofosbuvir for the hepatitis C virus

Jiamin Zheng[1], Dong Ding[1] and Hong Shen[2]

[1]Department of Medicinal Chemistry, China Innovation Center of Roche (CICoR), Shanghai, P.R. China, [2]China Innovation Center of Roche (CICoR), Shanghai, P.R. China

Chapter outline

9.1 Hepatitis C and hepatitis C virus	185
9.1.1 Hepatitis C: symptoms, causes, and transmission	185
9.1.2 An overview of the epidemiology and genotyping of hepatitis C	186
9.1.3 The discovery of hepatitis C and the development of its therapeutic drugs	186
9.2 Hepatitis C virus biology	187
9.2.1 The structure of the hepatitis C virus	187
9.2.2 The structure of the hepatitis C virus NS5B protein	187
9.3 Discovery of sofosbuvir	189
9.3.1 Mechanism of nucleoside antiviral drugs	189
9.3.2 Structure-activity relationship of the nucleoside scaffold: the birth of PSI-6130	190
9.3.3 Pharmacokinetic study of PSI-6130: design and application of prodrugs	194
9.3.4 The synthesis of sofosbuvir	201
9.4 Clinical studies of sofosbuvir	203
9.4.1 Preclinical studies of sofosbuvir	203
9.4.2 Clinical trial results of sofosbuvir	203
9.4.3 Treatment regimens with sofosbuvir	204
9.5 Summary and outlook	205
9.5.1 Summary	205
9.5.2 Further reading: ProTide technology	206
References	208

9.1 Hepatitis C and hepatitis C virus

9.1.1 Hepatitis C: symptoms, causes, and transmission

Hepatitis C is a liver disease caused by the infection of the hepatitis C virus (HCV) and is one of the leading causes of liver disease-related deaths worldwide. Most individuals with HCV infection initially have no significant symptoms, and 50%−80% of those with acute HCV infection will progress to chronic infection. Of these chronic carriers, 10%−20% will develop cirrhosis, and about 5% will eventually progress to hepatocellular carcinoma (HCC) (Fig. 9.1) [1]. HCV is mainly transmitted through blood, such as through blood transfusions, intravenous drug use, and healthcare-related infections. Due to the implementation of blood donation screening for HCV in western countries since the 1990s, the probability of infection through transfusions and blood products has significantly decreased in these regions, with intravenous drug use and sharing of needles becoming the predominant routes of transmission [2−5]. In some other areas, other routes of exposures, such as contaminated medical injections, nonmedical injections, and blood dialysis, are major factors in HCV infection. For example, in the 1960s and 1970s, Egypt experienced an HCV epidemic due to the reuse of syringes to

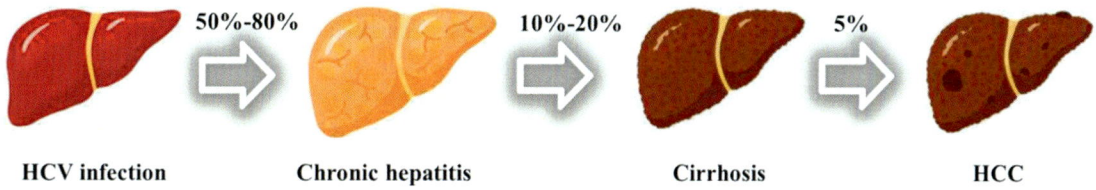

FIGURE 9.1 Stages of HCV infection.

control the schistosomiasis outbreak, given the limited medical resources, resulting in the high prevalence of HCV in Egypt [6]. Additionally, mother-to-child transmission of HCV occurs in less than 5% of cases resulting from this route [7–10]. The likelihood of transmission increases significantly to 19.4% if the mother is coinfected with human immunodeficiency virus (HIV) [11,12]. The role of sexual contact in the transmission of HCV is not conclusive, and it is generally believed that the possibility of HCV transmission through a single heterosexual contact is relatively low [13].

9.1.2 An overview of the epidemiology and genotyping of hepatitis C

Globally, an estimated HCV infection rate of approximately 3%, which translates to around 180 million individuals, have chronic HCV infection, with about 35,000 new infections occurring per year [14–18]. The epidemiology of hepatitis C demonstrates distinct regional disparities, with reported higher incidence rates in Africa, Asia, and Southern Europe [17]. To facilitate the analysis of HCV evolution and distribution, as well as to enable more targeted therapeutic approaches in clinical settings, hepatitis C has been classified into various genotypes, denoted by Arabic numerals. Each genotype further encompasses multiple subtypes, represented by lowercase English letters. To date, a minimum of six HCV genotypes (1–6) have been identified, with the distribution of these genotypes varying geographically. Genotypes 1, 2 and 6 are prevalent in East Asia, with genotype 1 accounting for approximately 44% of the global HCV-infected population, thus representing the most common genotype. Genotype 3 is predominantly found in South Asia, comprising 25% of the global HCV-infected population. Genotype 4, accounting for about 15% of the total HCV-infected population, is commonly observed in North Africa and the Middle East. Genotype 5 is relatively uncommon, representing less than 1% of the total HCV-infected population, and is primarily concentrated in southern Africa [19].

9.1.3 The discovery of hepatitis C and the development of its therapeutic drugs

In the 1970s, Dr. Harvey James Alter and his colleagues at the National Institutes of Health in the United States first discovered hepatitis C. They found that a portion of hepatitis patients tested negative for both hepatitis A and hepatitis B, yet clinically exhibited clear symptoms of hepatitis. They suspected the existence of a third type of hepatitis virus, silently spreading among the population, posing a potential risk to transfusion safety and human health. Dr. Alter named this new type of hepatitis "non-A, non-B hepatitis." However, due to technical limitations in medical research at the time, Dr. Alter and his colleagues were unable to unveil the true nature of this hidden virus for the following 15 years. The emergence of this new type of hepatitis prompted scientists worldwide to actively search for the pathogen. It was not until 1987 that Dr. Michael Houghton's team at Chiron Corporation and Dr. Daniel W. Bradley at the Centers for Disease Control and Prevention isolated ribonucleic acid (RNA) fragments of the new hepatitis virus using molecular cloning technology, marking a new stage in the precise identification of new hepatitis, moving away from the previous method of exclusion of "non-A, non-B" [20]. In 1989, Dr. Houghton's team first reported this new virus and named it HCV [21,22]. The discovery of HCV was a milestone in the history of hepatitis C research. Methods for detecting HCV were quickly established, and screening was carried out in blood banks and blood products, greatly reducing the possibility of HCV transmission through blood transfusion. In recognition of the significant contributions of Dr. Alter and Dr. Houghton in the discovery of HCV, the Lasker Foundation awarded them the Lasker Award in 2000. The two scientists, along with American virologist Dr. Charles M. Rice, were awarded the Nobel Prize in Physiology or Medicine in 2020.

After completing the crucial and arduous step of "discovering the hepatitis C virus", it was anticipated that subsequent research would develop along the lines of other hepatitis treatments, namely, the simultaneous development of vaccines and drugs. However, scientists soon encountered challenges. Due to the genetic diversity of HCV and the relatively weak immune response to its infection, the development of a hepatitis C vaccine has been unsuccessful to this day. The failure of vaccine development prompted scientists to shift their research focus to the development of hepatitis C treatment drugs.

As early as 1989, due to the phased success of interferon alpha (IFNα) in the treatment of hepatitis B, scientists also began clinical research on its treatment of hepatitis C. Clinical trial research found that the sustained virological response rate (SVR) was only 6% for 24 weeks of treatment with IFNα three times a week, and the SVR could be increased to 16% for 48 weeks of continuous treatment, but it was still very low [23,24]. Although IFNα alone did not have a significant anti-HCV effect, scientists quickly found that the combination of IFNα and the broad-spectrum antiviral drug ribavirin (RBV) increased the SVR to 34% for 24 weeks of treatment and further increased to 42% for 48 weeks of treatment [23,24]. Given the effectiveness of this combination, the U.S. Food and Drug Administration (FDA) approved this combination therapy for the treatment of hepatitis C in 1997. However, the biggest drawback of IFNα is its short half-life in the body, requiring multiple doses per week to maintain its efficacy. Later, scientists developed pegylated interferon alpha (PEG-IFNα), a new form of IFNα by cross-linking inactive, nontoxic PEG molecules with IFNα, to delay the clearance of IFNα after injection, extend the drug half-life, and maintain effective blood drug concentration with once-weekly dosing. The monotherapy of PEG-IFNα for 48 weeks, administered once a week, increased the SVR to 39%, and combined with RBV, once-weekly dosing for 48 weeks further increased the SVR to 54%−56% [25−27]. For patients with chronically infected by hepatitis C virus genotypes 2 and 3 the SVR can even reach 76%−82% with 24 weeks of combination therapy [28,29]. The combination of PEG-IFNα and RBV (abbreviated as PR therapy) was the first choice for the treatment of hepatitis C for a long time since it was approved by the FDA in 1998. The combination of PEG-IFNα and RBV has benefited many hepatitis C patients, but because IFNα stimulates the body's immune system to fight the virus rather than acting directly on the virus, it has strict indications, numerous contraindications, serious adverse reactions, and specific routes of administration, all of which limit the broader clinical application of PR therapy [30−32]. In view of this, scientists hope to develop small-molecule drugs that act directly on the virus itself (direct-acting antivirals (DAAs)). After unremitting efforts, anti-HCV small-molecule drug protease inhibitors were born. In 2011, the first generation of HCV protease inhibitors targeting HCV nonstructural protein NS3/4A, boceprevir and telaprevir, were approved by the FDA for use in combination with PR therapy to treat patients with HCV genotype 1 [33]. The first generation of protease inhibitors has several limitations, such as the need to be used in combination with PR. Clinical trial results showed that the adverse reactions caused by the two were significant, and the drug needed to be administered three times a day for a treatment period of up to 48 weeks. Therefore, the development of the second generation of protease inhibitors was quickly planned and launched [20,34]. In November 2013, the FDA approved simeprevir in combination with PR therapy to treat patients with HCV genotype 1. Simeprevir is also an NS3/4A protease inhibitor. Compared with the first generation of NS3/4A protease inhibitors, it only needs to be administered once a day, and the treatment period can be shortened to 24 weeks, with an SVR of up to 80% [35,36]. However, simeprevir also did not solve the problem of needing to be used in combination with PR therapy, and this target protease inhibitor has a low resistance barrier and is prone to resistance [37]. Therefore, scientists turned their attention to another HCV target, the nonstructural protein NS5B. In December 2013, the first NS5B protease inhibitor, sofosbuvir, was approved for marketing. Its great advantage is that it is the first drug for the treatment of hepatitis C that does not need to be combined with IFNα, and the treatment period can be further shortened to 12 weeks. Sofosbuvir showed a high SVR for all types [38−40] (Fig. 9.2).

9.2 Hepatitis C virus biology

9.2.1 The structure of the hepatitis C virus

HCV is a positive single-stranded RNA virus belonging to the *Flaviridae* family, with a diameter of 55−65 nm. Its structure is divided into surface proteins, glycoprotein envelope, nucleocapsid, and the RNA strand (Fig. 9.3). Its RNA is composed of approximately 9600 nucleotides, including one large open reading frame (ORF) and noncoding regions at the 5′ and 3′ ends. The ORF can encode three structural proteins and seven nonstructural proteins. The structural region encodes the virus's core protein (C protein) and envelope proteins (E1 and E2), also known as structural proteins, which are involved in the assembly of the virus; the nonstructural region includes NS2-NS5, which can encode seven nonstructural proteins (Fig. 9.4). These seven nonstructural proteins all play important roles in the viral life cycle [41]. Among them, the NS2 protease, NS3 protease, and NS4 cofactor are related to the posttranslational processing of HCV polyproteins. The NS3/4A protease was one of the earliest targets to be drugged, with several inhibitors of this protease now on the market; the NS5A protein is related to the formation of the replication complex; the NS5B polymerase is the key enzyme catalyzing the synthesis of HCV RNA, and the discovery of sofosbuvir was based on the research targeting this enzyme.

9.2.2 The structure of the hepatitis C virus NS5B protein

The NS5B polymerase is composed of 591 amino acids encoded by 1773 bases [41,42]. The replication of HCV is carried out using single-stranded RNA as a template, catalyzed by the replicase complex involving the NS5B polymerase [43−45]. The NS5B RNA-dependent RNA polymerase (RdRP) has the typical right-hand structure of polymerases, consisting of the thumb domain, finger domain, and palm active site (Fig. 9.5) [46,47]. The function of the thumb domain is to form the catalytic center for the nucleotidyl transfer reaction; the fingers domain mainly interacts with the triphosphate nucleotides required for replication, while the palm domain plays a role in the initiation and extension processes of RNA replication [48]. Within the palm domain, there is a catalytically active motif, Gly317−Asp318−Asp319 (GDD), which is highly conserved across all HCV genotypes [49], and there is no enzyme with similar function to NS5B RdRp expressed in human cells. This means that inhibitors of NS5B RdRp can have the dual advantages of broad-spectrum inhibition across HCV genotypes and high selectivity between HCV and human cells, making the NS5B polymerase an ideal target for anti-HCV drugs.

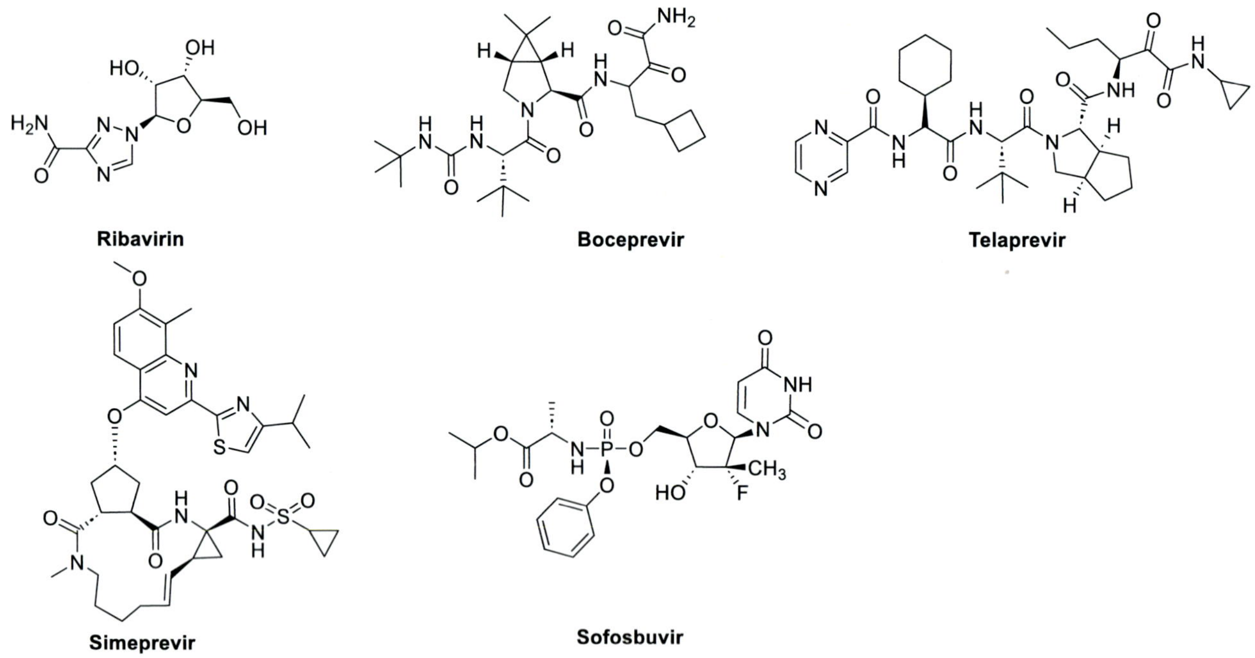

FIGURE 9.2 Structures of representative anti-HCV drugs.

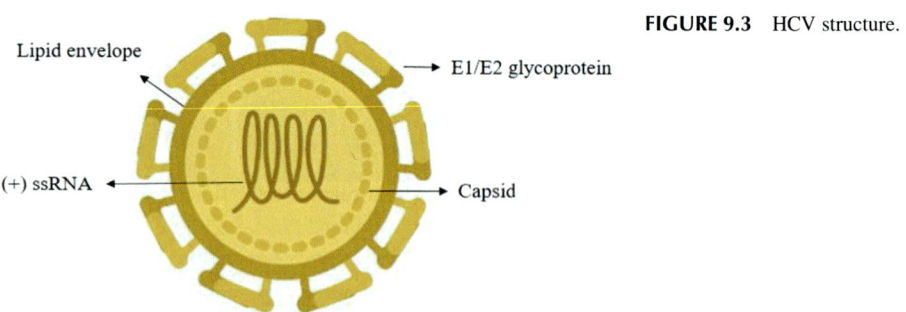

FIGURE 9.3 HCV structure.

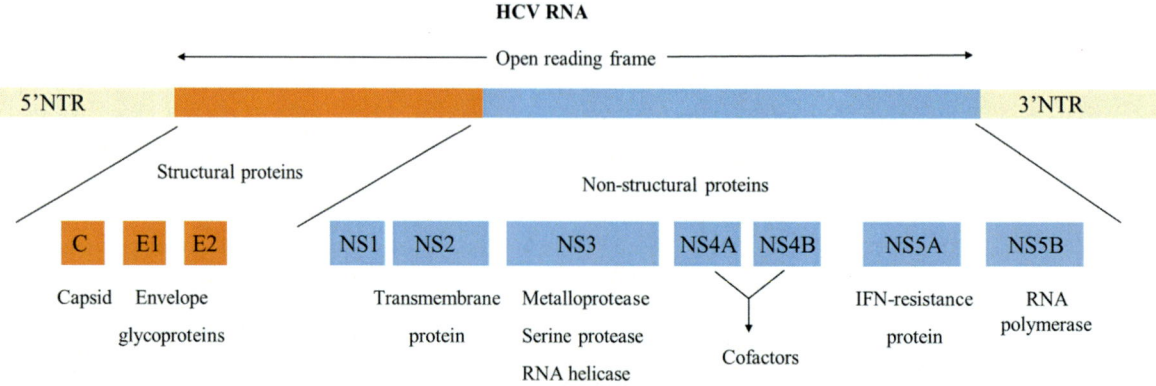

FIGURE 9.4 The composition of RNA and its decoded proteins.

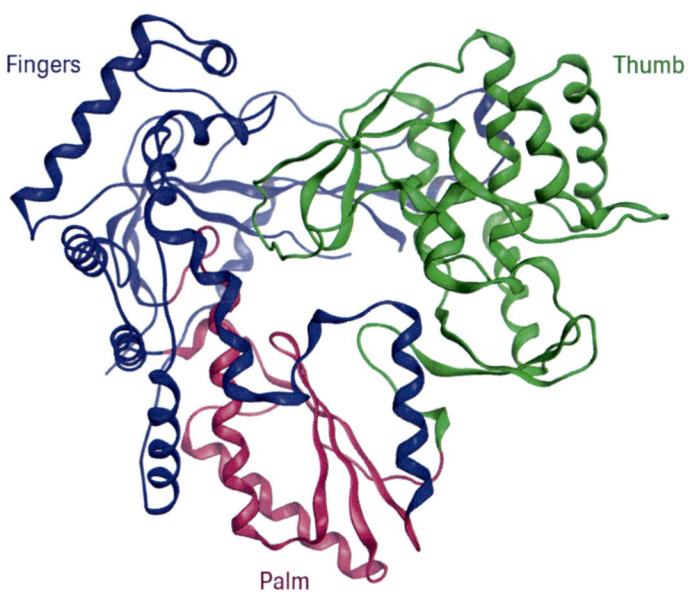

FIGURE 9.5 The X-ray structures of NS5B polymerase. *Adapted from Boyce SE, Tirunagari N, Niedziela-Majka A, et al. Structural and regulatory elements of HCV NS5B polymerase—b-loop and C-terminal tail—are required for activity of allosteric thumb site II inhibitors. PLoS One 9(1): e84808.*

9.3 Discovery of sofosbuvir

9.3.1 Mechanism of nucleoside antiviral drugs

With the HCV NS5B RdRp as the target, scientists began to screen nucleoside analogs that exhibited inhibitory effects on HCV RNA replication. As nucleoside analogs have a rich history in drug development, scientists aim to identify ideal nucleoside analogs that specifically target the desired active site and are capable of deceiving the RNA polymerase during the viral replication process. By substituting nucleoside building blocks for the next generation of RNA synthesis, the molecule subsequently cause RNA synthesis to fail and the virus to lose its ability to replicate, ultimately achieving the goal of treating the disease.

Compared with other nonnucleoside compounds, nucleoside analogs can directly interact with the active site of HCV NS5B RdRp, providing a clear mechanism for the termination of viral RNA replication. They exhibit a broad genotypic coverage (targeting all six genotypes of the virus simultaneously) and a high resistance barrier. However, during the development process, three key issues must be considered: (1) selectivity of the drug molecules toward human DNA and virus RNA polymerases to avoid potential off-target toxicity; (2) metabolic pathways of the molecules and the activity of their metabolites within the body; and (3) optimization of the structure-activity relationship of nucleoside analogs poses significant challenges, deviating from the conventional strategies employed for traditional small molecule optimization.

From a mechanistic standpoint, nucleotide molecules differ from traditional small molecules as they require recognition by different kinases as substrates before binding to the target. They undergo sequential conversions to nucleotide monophosphate and diphosphate and exhibit antiviral activity in the form of the active structure—triphosphate metabolite (NTP). Upon recognition by the polymerase, the triphosphate metabolite binds to the target HCV NS5B RdRp, interrupting the normal elongation of the viral RNA chain (Fig. 9.6). In other words, nucleoside analogs, acting as substitutes for NTP, must be recognized as substrates by three distinct kinases and one polymerase to proceed. Therefore, the inhibitory activity of the viral polymerase depends not only on the efficiency of nucleoside analog phosphorylation but also on the influence of corresponding active metabolites' half-lives within the body.

Before 2000, the development of antiviral drugs against HCV was hindered by the difficulty of replicating the virus in vitro and the lack of suitable in vitro drug screening assays. This problem was eventually addressed when scientists established a cell culture method using Huh7 cells, which allowed for virus replication and cultivation in vitro [50]. Pharmasset, a small pharmaceutical company dedicated to antiviral drug development, utilized an in vitro HCV replicon RNA-containing Huh-7 cell assay to screen nucleoside analogs for their anti-HCV activity. They fortuitously discovered the nucleoside analogs NHC (1), 2′-modified nucleoside analog 2-FdCyd (2), and deoxy-nucleoside analog (3), all of which exhibited potent inhibitory effects on HCV replication in vitro (Fig. 9.7) [51–53].

Further investigations revealed that while the nucleoside triphosphate metabolite of compound **1** showed some antiviral activity, its binding affinity to the NS5B RdRp target was relatively weak, resulting in a lower selective inhibitory

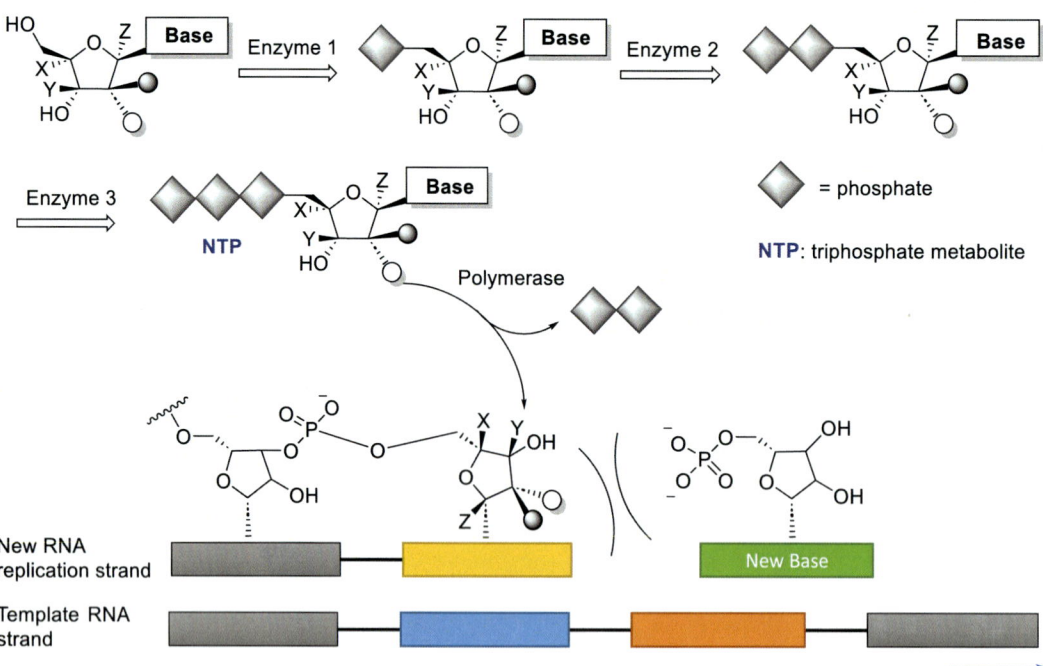

FIGURE 9.6 Mechanism by which nucleotide molecules inhibit viral replication.

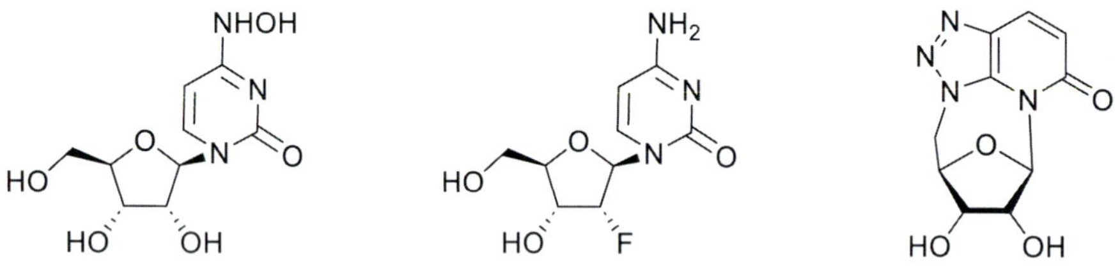

FIGURE 9.7 Pharmasett anti-HCV hit compounds.

effect on HCV. On the other hand, the structurally novel deoxy-nucleoside analog **3** exhibited biological activity that was associated with cytotoxicity concerns. Only the triphosphate metabolite of uridine analog **2** was confirmed to effectively inhibit NS5B polymerase and showed no adverse reactions in short-term animal studies. However, despite the lack of apparent toxicity in vitro and in animal experiments, literature reports suggested the potential risks of host and viral cell selectivity for compound **2**. It inhibited cellular enzyme polymerization, leading to cellular growth arrest, which might contribute to the delayed onset of drug toxicity during long-term administration [50].

Considering these risks, Dr. Clark's team conducted structure-activity relationship studies and optimization on the series of uridine analogs, using compound **2** as the hit compound. Ultimately, they developed a candidate drug molecule, PSI-6130 (Table 9.1), which exhibits high inhibitory activity, selectivity for HCV, and in vivo safety. Here, PSI stands for Pharmasset Small-molecule Inhibitor, while 6130 represents the compound's designation number.

9.3.2 Structure-activity relationship of the nucleoside scaffold: the birth of PSI-6130

Before Pharmasett, numerous pharmaceutical companies and institutions conducted research and development efforts on nucleoside compounds for the treatment of HCV infections. These efforts included base modifications, (deoxy)ribose substitutions, phosphate group preorganization on the ribose, and amino acid-modified prodrugs [54]. Several compounds, exemplified in Fig. 9.8, represented the exploration of nucleoside compounds in the context of anti-HCV activity, including 2′-O-MeC with 2′-α-methoxy substitution instead of a hydroxyl group, NM107 with 2′-β-methyl

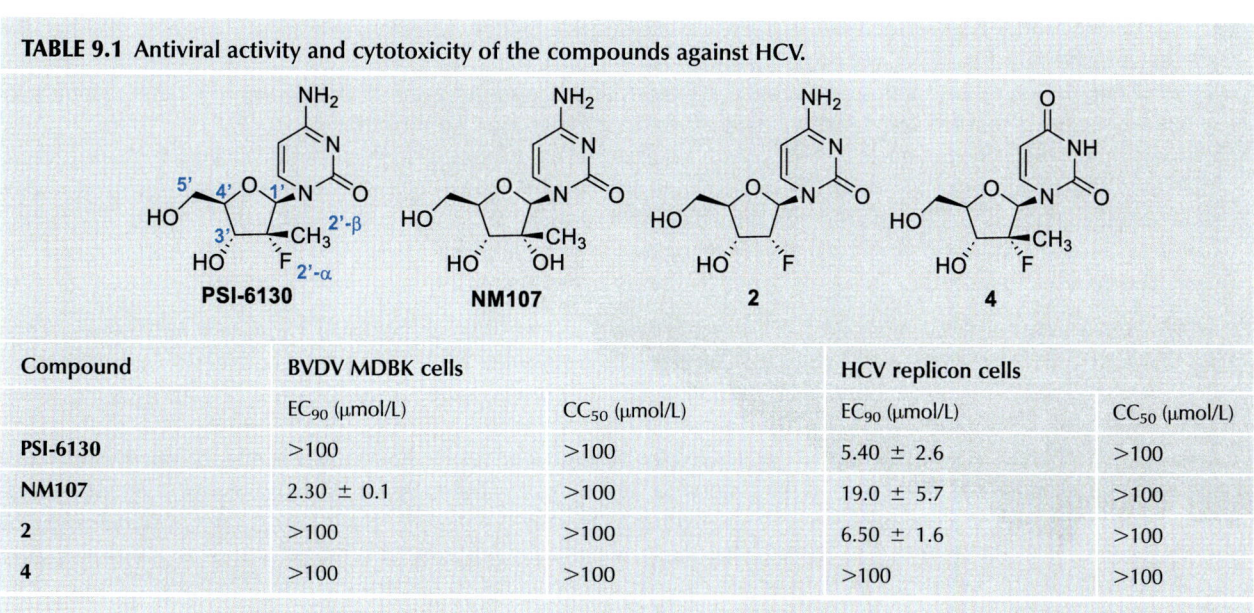

TABLE 9.1 Antiviral activity and cytotoxicity of the compounds against HCV.

Compound	BVDV MDBK cells		HCV replicon cells	
	EC$_{90}$ (μmol/L)	CC$_{50}$ (μmol/L)	EC$_{90}$ (μmol/L)	CC$_{50}$ (μmol/L)
PSI-6130	>100	>100	5.40 ± 2.6	>100
NM107	2.30 ± 0.1	>100	19.0 ± 5.7	>100
2	>100	>100	6.50 ± 1.6	>100
4	>100	>100	>100	>100

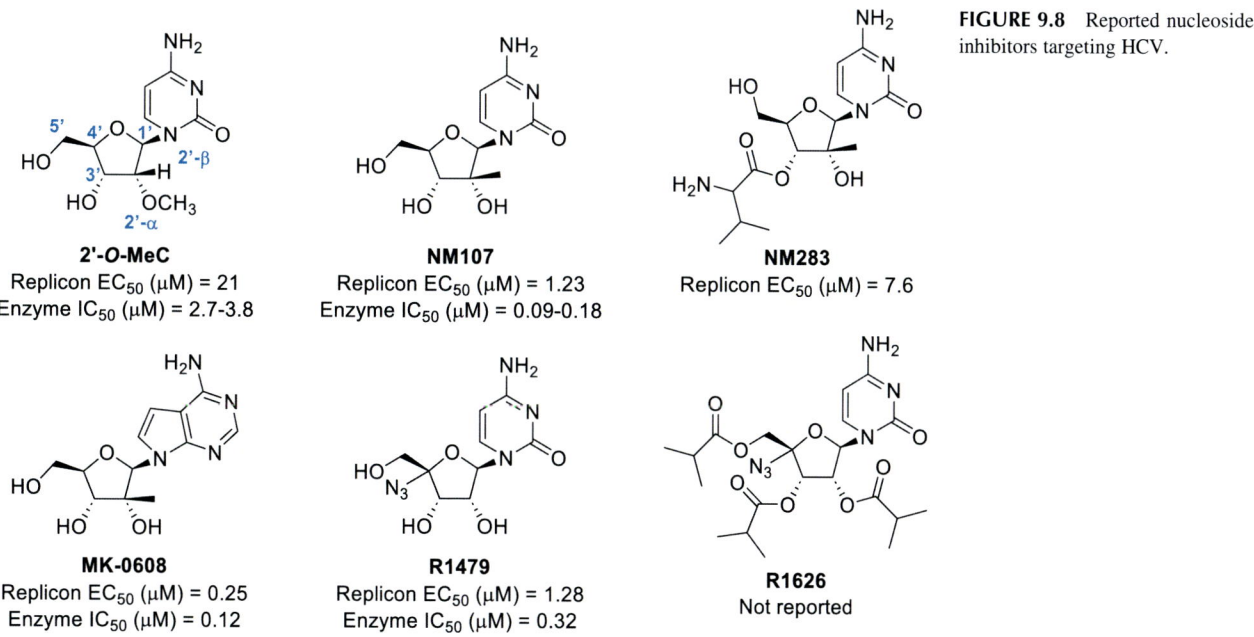

FIGURE 9.8 Reported nucleoside inhibitors targeting HCV.

substitution, R1479 with 4′-azido substitution, and base-modified MK-0608 (Fig. 9.8). The structure-activity relationships of the compounds are illustrated as follows:

1. Research on the 2′-α-position of the nucleoside revealed that after methylation of the 2′-α-hydroxyl group, the triphosphate form of 2′-O-MeC remained a substrate for NS5B polymerase. However, its activity in HCV replicon cell assays was significantly lower compared to other series. Subsequent metabolism studies indicated that this was due to the formation of low-activity triphosphate byproducts during the process of phosphorylation of 2′-O-MeC, thereby reducing its cellular activity.

2. The research on 2′-β-position were extensively explored. In the early stages, nucleoside derivatives were screened using the bovine viral diarrhea virus (BVDV) model as a surrogate assay, which belongs to the same family as HCV. The active structures with a 2′-β-methyl substitution were identified. Subsequent structure-activity relationship studies revealed a limited tolerance for functional groups at the 2′-β-position. Any substitution with bulky groups or changes in chemical configuration, apart from methyl, led to reduced activity. In this series of studies,

Indenix and Novartis codeveloped the first nucleoside NS5B inhibitor, valopicitabine (also known as NM283, the prodrug of NM107; Fig. 9.8), which entered clinical development. However, its clinical development halted at Phase II due to severe gastrointestinal adverse effects. Merck's research team also reported MK-0608, which possesses the same scaffold and improved oral bioavailability through base modifications.

3. Research on the 4′-position of nucleosides revealed that azido-substituted nucleoside analogs maintained high polymerase inhibitory activity and exhibited anti-HCV activity inhibitory activity and exhibit anti-HCV activity. Moreover, studies showed that compound R1479 efficiently underwent phosphorylation metabolism within host cells. However, its prodrug molecule, R1626, exhibited adverse reactions of neutropenia in patients during Phase IIb clinical trials, leading to the discontinuation of the study.

While these endeavors faced hindrances due to a variety of factors, they accumulated experience and knowledge to enable the success of Pharmasset, particularly the research findings on the nucleoside candidate NM107 and its prodrug NM283 (valopicitabine). It was discovered that the introduction of a methyl group at the 2′-β-position enhanced the inhibitory activity against RNA-related viruses, playing a crucial role in subsequent structure-activity relationship studies [55]. Consequently, Dr. Clark's team designed and synthesized the nucleotide molecule PSI-6130, wherein the fluorine atom and methyl group replaced the original moiety at the 2′-position. The fluorine atom in PSI-6130 ribose is similar in electronegativity and size to the oxygen atom and comparable in hydrogen bonding capability to the hydroxyl group. Additionally, the fluorine atom facilitates the formation of stable glycosidic bonds, thereby maintaining comparable in vitro antiviral activity to 2-C-MeCyd (NM107) (Table 9.1). Even more surprisingly, this combination negated the toxic issue of cell growth stagnation observed in BVDV cell experiments with compound **2**, while no cytotoxicity or mitochondrial toxicity was observed in other in vitro cytotoxicity tests [56]. These research findings provided the development team with great encouragement. Dr. Clark and his colleagues continued to optimize the base and ribose portions of the PSI-6130 molecule (Fig. 9.9). They decided to retain the 2′-fluoro-2′-methyl combination unchanged and made modifications to the ribose portion, including altering the hydroxyl group at the 3′-position and introducing substituents at the 4′-position. However, these changes resulted in the loss of inhibitory activity. Moreover, screening of different bases revealed that only cytosine produced sufficient antiviral activity. Subsequently, they maintained cytosine as the compound's base, alongside the unchanged 3′- and 4′-positions, and attempted different substitution combinations at the 2′-α- and 2′-β-positions. However, this direction of exploration did not yield candidate molecules superior to PSI-6130 [57].

Ultimately, the research group identified PSI-6130 as a candidate compound and conducted studies and predictions on its in vivo transformation. The compound was separately incubated with HCV replicon cells and human liver cells to examine its transformation in cellular metabolism at different time points. The experiments not only observed the metabolic products of PSI-6130, including monophosphorylated, diphosphorylated, and triphosphorylated being formed at the 5′-hydroxy position, but also discovered the compound PSI-6206, generated through deamination of PSI-6130, as well as the phosphorylated metabolic products of PSI-6206 [58,59].

The metabolic activation pathway of PSI-6130, as described in Fig. 9.10, involves the catalysis of deoxycytidine kinase (dCK), leading to the formation of cytidine monophosphate, which is further recognized and phosphorylated by the nucleoside monophosphate kinase uridine-cytidine monophosphate kinase (UMP/CMPK) to generate cytidine diphosphate. Finally, under the influence of nucleoside diphosphate kinase, the cytidine diphosphate is converted to the activated form of cytidine triphosphate, which subsequently interacts with the NS5B target to inhibit viral replication. Additionally, PSI-6130 also undergoes binding with cytidine deaminase and oxidative deamination to generate uridine PSI-6206 in liver cells. However, in preliminary structure-activity relationship studies, uridine PSI-6206 showed no activity in HCV replicon assays; further research revealed that this was due to the inability of PSI-6206 to be phosphorylated by dCK, resulting in the molecule's inactivity [58,59]. However, during the metabolism of PSI-6130, its monophosphorylated cytidine can also undergo oxidative deamination driven by deoxycytidine phosphate deaminase, generating PSI-6206-MP, which then undergoes subsequent phosphorylation in liver cells to produce uridine triphosphate. To the researchers' delight, both PSI-6130-TP and PSI-6206-TP exhibited significant inhibitory effects on HCV replication, and the active structure of PSI-6206-TP provided scientists with a new research direction.

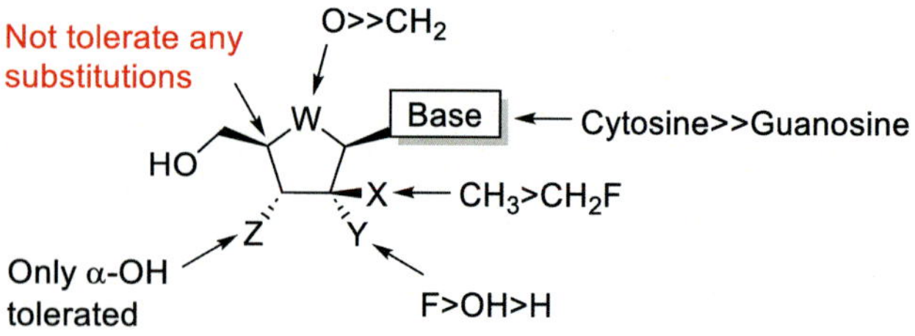

FIGURE 9.9 Structure-activity relationship study of PSI-6130.

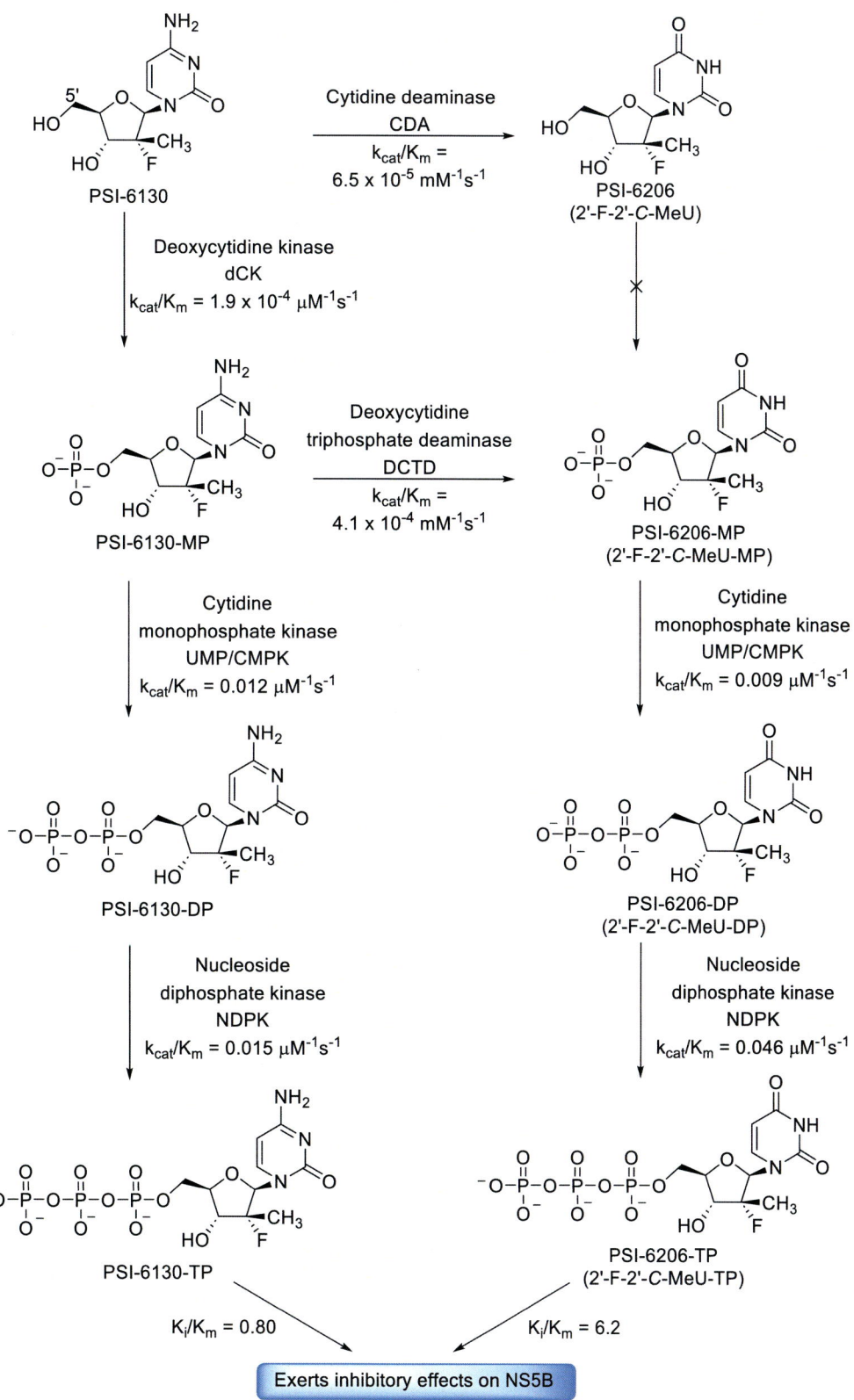

FIGURE 9.10 Metabolic pathways and metabolites of PSI-6130.

Despite the structural similarity between candidate compounds PSI-6130 and NM107, they are quite distinct in terms of antiviral activity, selectivity, toxicity, resistance risks, and intracellular phosphorylation levels. NM107 demonstrates broad-spectrum antiviral activities against multiple viruses [55], while PSI-6130 exhibits high selectivity for inhibiting HCV replication. It has shown no inhibitory effect in activity tests against other viruses such as bovine diarrhea virus (BVDV), Dengue type 2 virus (DV), human immunodeficiency virus (HIV), and hepatitis B virus (HBV), and no significant toxicity findings have been observed in animal experiments and human cell line studies [60]. Furthermore, in resistance experiments, PSI-6130 has demonstrated a low risk, being sensitive only to the S282T mutation in the NS5B polymerase, with a much smaller sensitivity change compared to NM107.

Based on these advantages, Pharmasett moved forward with Phase I clinical trials of PSI-6130 to investigate its safety, tolerability, and pharmacokinetic properties in humans. The results revealed that oral administration of PSI-6130 at doses of 500/1500/3000 mg was well-tolerated with no adverse effects. However, its oral bioavailability was only 25% in humans, and a significant portion of the molecule was metabolized into inactive PSI-6206 in the intestine, hindering the sufficient therapeutic efficacy of PSI-6130. With the development of this compound reaching a deadlock, Dr. Sofia's involvement came at a critical moment and saved the development of PSI-6130. After Dr. Sofia joined Pharmasett, he developed a strong interest in the stagnant development of PSI-6130. He believed that PSI-6130 was a promising drug candidate, and with structural modifications, it could be effectively absorbed and transported to the target site—infected liver cells with HCV. Subsequently, Pharmasett initiated an upgraded development plan for PSI-6130, focusing on prodrug design to develop more superior molecules.

9.3.3 Pharmacokinetic study of PSI-6130: design and application of prodrugs

In the process of drug development, many drug candidates may exhibit excellent biological activities in in vitro testing but fail to achieve the desired therapeutic effects in the human body due to inherent deficiencies in their properties. This is often attributed to inadequate oral bioavailability, metabolic instability, short duration in the blood, poor cell membrane permeability, or a lack of selectivity. To address these issues, researchers will further explore the structure-activity relationship of the molecules with regards to DMPK and safety profiles. When it is proven that structural modifications cannot resolve the challenges, the strategy of prodrug design may become an alternative research direction.

A prodrug is a compound derived from the chemical modification of a drug molecule. It exhibits little or no pharmacological activity in vitro, but upon enzymatic or nonenzymatic conversion in vivo, it releases active metabolites that exert the desired therapeutic effects. The concept of a prodrug was first introduced by Adrien Albert in 1958 in the journal "Nature" to describe the notion of compounds undergoing biotransformation to elicit pharmacological actions [61]. Subsequently, Jarkko Rautio and others further refined the definition of a prodrug to specifically refer to the reversible derivatives of the parent drug molecule that release active moieties capable of achieving the intended pharmacological activity through enzymatic or chemical processes [62].

Prodrugs can be classified into two primary categories based on different principles of parent drug release. The first category is carrier-linked prodrugs, where the parent drug is covalently bonded to a carrier that is removed in vivo through biodegradation or chemical reactions to exert therapeutic effects. Typically, carriers are lipophilic and could be either small molecular entities or macromolecules, such as albumin and antibodies. The second category encompasses bioprecursor prodrugs, which undergo a series of enzymatic transformations within the biological system to alter their molecular structure, thereby generating an active parent drug that manifests its pharmacological action. An exemplary prodrug developed with this rationale is Sulindac, a nonsteroidal antiinflammatory drug [63].

Modification of existing drugs to design prodrugs offers numerous advantages: it can surmount pharmacological barriers; enhance chemical and metabolic stability; improve hydrophilicity or lipophilicity properties; augment the absorption of oral or topical administration; enhance penetration through the blood-brain barrier; extend drug action duration; increase bioavailability; refine tissue distribution of the drug; and elevate target specificity while mitigating adverse reactions [62]. Nowadays, prodrug design has been established as an extensively accepted and effective strategy within the field of medicinal chemistry.

9.3.3.1 The application of conventional prodrug technologies

To address the poor oral bioavailability and metabolic instability of PSI-6130, researchers employed a series of prodrug design strategies for optimization. They sought to enhance the stability of PSI-6130 within the gastrointestinal system and increase systemic absorption, while also delaying the conversion of the compound to inactive metabolic products by chemically modifying the structure of PSI-6130. Guided by this rationale, the research team crafted a series of prodrug entities featuring functional groups like esters, carbamates, and carbonates at the 3′- and/or 5′-hydroxyl positions, as well as the conversion of cytidine's *N4* to urea. These prodrug molecules were first screened in vitro for potency, stability in gastrointestinal fluids, metabolic stability, and membrane permeability. Subsequently, they were evaluated in animal models (rats and monkeys) to determine the efficiency of prodrug conversion and oral bioavailability. The prodrug molecule RG7128 (mericitabine) was identified as optimal, as it lowered the molecule's polarity and enhanced both membrane permeability and absorption through isobutyrate esterification at the 3′- and 5′-hydroxyl positions. Once absorbed, the prodrug underwent first-pass metabolism to release the parent drug (PSI-6130), thereby significantly improving the parent molecule's oral bioavailability, as demonstrated in Table 9.2.

Roche acquired the investigational drug RG7128 from Pharmasett and continued conducting clinical trial research [64–68]. RG7128 demonstrated excellent efficacy and safety in clinical single-dose escalation, multiple-dose escalation, and combination therapy studies with INFα [69,70]. In clinical trials, RG7128 was administered orally twice daily at a dose of 1 g per administration, resulting in a 2.7-log reduction in HCV RNA levels after a 14-day treatment period in patients with genotype 1 HCV infection. Furthermore, RG7128 demonstrated significant efficacy when combined with interferon in the treatment of patients with genotype 2 and 3 HCV, marking a noteworthy achievement in the effective inhibition of the virus with direct antiviral therapy in both genotype 1 and nongenotype 1 HCV patients [71–73]. When RG7128 was coadministered with the NS3/4A protease inhibitor danoprevir, a reduction of 4.9–5.1 logarithmic units was observed in patients with genotype 1 hepatitis C after a 14-day treatment period, offering the first evidence of the possibility of noninterferon-based regimens for the cure of hepatitis C infection [68]. Overall, the clinical data for RG7128 establishes a robust foundation for nucleoside-based therapy for the treatment of hepatitis C. However, it exhibits modest efficacy and has a relatively short half-life in the liver, necessitating high-doses and multiple administrations, thereby limiting its potential as a first-line drug.

9.3.3.2 The design of liver-targeted nucleoside prodrugs

An analysis of the pros and cons of RG7128 led scientists at Pharmasett to continue their research and development of second-generation nucleoside analog drugs. They aimed to retain the unique combination of a 2′-β-fluoro and 2′-α-methyl group and explore compounds with stronger efficacy, a longer half-life, an increased liver-to-plasma ratio, and the potential for low-dose administration. Their attention was attracted by PSI-6206-MP, the uridine metabolite of PSI-6130. The researchers observed that PSI-6206-MP, generated through the activation pathway of PSI-6130, could be metabolized into PSI-6206-TP. It demonstrated not only significant in vitro antiviral activity but also a long half-life of 38 hours. The prolonged half-life of PSI-6206-TP can enhance its accumulation in the body, leading to better viral inhibition compared to PSI-6130-TP. Therefore, PSI-6206-MP shows great potential to become an ideal DAA drug for the inhibition of HCV replication.

As shown in the previous pharmacokinetic studies, the uridine molecule PSI-6206 is not a suitable substrate for kinases and cannot be converted into its monophosphate form, PSI-6206-MP, in the body. Consequently, the team had to face the challenge of delivering PSI-6206-MP directly into hepatocytes. However, due to the presence of unmodified negatively charged and highly polar phosphate groups in the PSI-6206-MP, it faces difficulties in penetrating biological membranes and

TABLE 9.2 Comparative data for PSI-6130 and Prodrug RG7128.

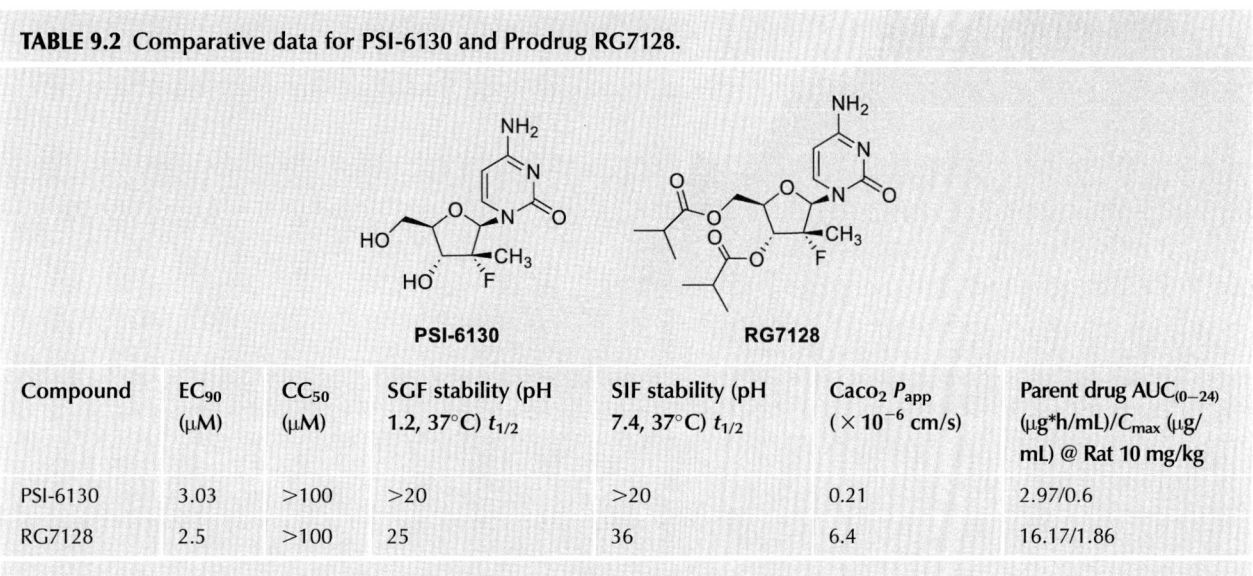

Compound	EC$_{90}$ (μM)	CC$_{50}$ (μM)	SGF stability (pH 1.2, 37°C) $t_{1/2}$	SIF stability (pH 7.4, 37°C) $t_{1/2}$	Caco$_2$ P_{app} (× 10^{-6} cm/s)	Parent drug AUC$_{(0-24)}$ (μg*h/mL)/C$_{max}$ (μg/mL) @ Rat 10 mg/kg
PSI-6130	3.03	>100	>20	>20	0.21	2.97/0.6
RG7128	2.5	>100	25	36	6.4	16.17/1.86

is susceptible to degradation by phosphatases before reaching the liver. Therefore, the phosphate groups in the molecule need to be modified and shielded through an alternative prodrug approach. This approach aims to enhance the molecule's compatibility with biological membranes, prevent premature degradation by phosphatases, and increase its oral bioavailability. Additionally, considering that the liver is the main site of hepatitis C treatment, the prodrug is designed to release the active compound PSI-6206-MP specifically in liver cells under the action of specific enzymes, achieving liver-targeted effects. Clearly, the prodrug design based on PSI-6206-MP is much more complex than the design discussed previously for RG7128. At that time, the concept of nucleoside analog drugs had been widely employed in the development of anticancer and antiviral drugs, leading to significant interest in the study of phosphoryl ester prodrugs. To address the high electronegativity of phosphate groups, medicinal chemists attempted to introduce different protecting groups to decrease the polarity of the drug and enhance its membrane permeability, thereby improving its oral bioavailability. Since the initial simple introduction of alkyl groups to form phosphates, the design of prodrugs for nucleoside-based drugs has been gradually developing and evolving. In 1990, Professor Chris McGuigan and his research group, after many years of investigation, successfully invented a modification method that connected nucleoside phosphates/phosphonate analogs to polar groups *via* phosphodiester and phosphoramidate bonds, aiming to mask the polar groups, decrease molecular polarity, and enhance membrane permeability. This method facilitated the effective release of the active drug in the body through enzymatic hydrolysis in the liver [74].

Therefore, in the process of developing the second generation of antiviral nucleoside drugs against HCV, Dr. Sofia drew inspiration from Professor McGuigan's ProTide prodrug technology using phosphoramidate esters (see Further Reading for details). By incorporating appropriate fragments at the amide and ester linkages of the phosphate group, masking of the phosphate moiety was achieved, aiding in the membrane permeability of the molecule. Upon entering liver cells, the prodrug could be hydrolyzed by esterases, followed by specific recognition and cleavage of the phosphorus-nitrogen bond by phosphoramidases (histidine triad nucleotide-binding protein 1, HNT1). This breakdown allowed for the release of the parent drug within the liver cells, initiating two subsequent phosphorylation steps to convert it into active triphosphorylated uridine (Fig. 9.11A). Throughout this process, apart from ensuring the successful release of the phosphate moieties during the hepatic first-pass effect, considerations also had to be given to the tolerability and sufficient absorption of the prodrug molecule in the gastrointestinal tract and blood transport environment. Evidently, these multiple factors mutually influence one another, thereby increasing the complexity of molecular design and prediction.

To identify the optimal molecular combinations, the research and development team conducted in-depth and extensive structure-activity relationship studies. Compound screening was performed through the in vitro and in vivo compound

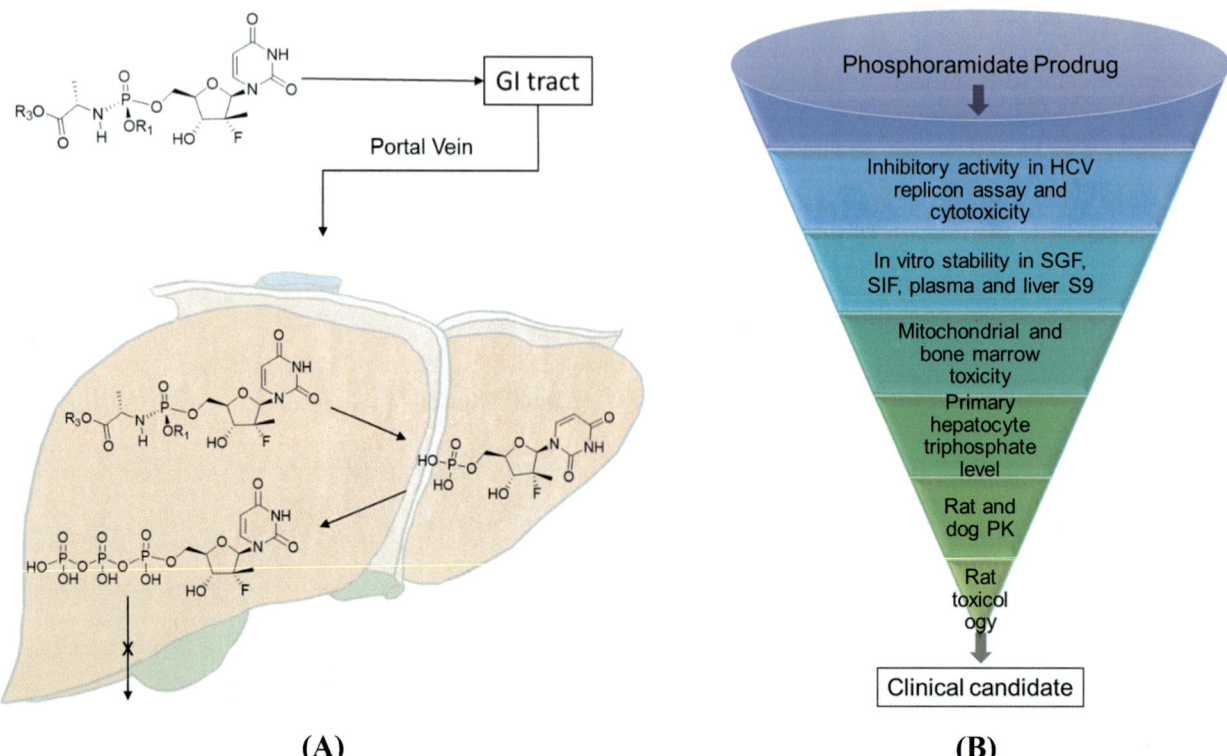

FIGURE 9.11 Design and screening cascade of liver-targeted nucleoside prodrugs. (A) Liver-targeted prodrug strategy, (B) Screening cascade of nucleoside prodrugs.

evaluation processes illustrated in Fig. 9.11B. In vitro tests encompassed the assessment of the activity against whole-cell HCV replicon, toxicity in different cell lines, stability in the gastrointestinal system, and stability against enzymes in plasma and liver microsomes, as well as the level of in vitro conversion into triphosphorylated nucleoside by key prodrug molecules in human liver cells. This screening cascade enabled the identification of compounds with submicromolar-level whole-cell viral inhibition activity in the absence of cytotoxicity, stability in the gastrointestinal system and plasma, exclusive hydrolysis by specific enzymes within liver cells, and rapid triphosphorylation, making them ideal candidates. Moreover, by indirectly evaluating the concentration of triphosphorylated nucleosides in the liver after oral administration of the drug, the assessment of in vivo activity was accomplished, thereby addressing the challenges and time constraints associated with comparing molecular in vivo activity using animal models. Additionally, early screening also included testing for mitochondrial toxicity and bone marrow toxicity to avoid similar toxic issues exhibited by many nucleoside-based drugs.

9.3.3.3 Structure-activity relationship of liver-targeting prodrug molecule PSI-7851

The research team initially synthesized the relatively simple phosphoramidate prodrug PSI-7672 (Fig. 9.12), which exhibited comparable inhibitory activity to PSI-6130 in cellular assays of HCV replication [57]. This result boosted confidence in the successful design of phosphoramidate prodrugs, prompting the team to further investigate the structure-activity relationship of this series. In the design of phosphoramidate prodrugs, there are three variable groups within the structure (Fig. 9.12): (1) R_1, which forms an ester bond with phosphate. The bond is hydrolyzed upon entry into liver cells. Therefore, consideration must be given to the absence of significant hepatotoxicity in the resulting alcohol or phenol after its removal. (2) R_2, a side chain substitute of α-amino acids, affects the stability of the phosphoramidate bond in the prodrug molecule before liver entry and its ability to undergo hydrolysis upon entry into the liver. (3) R_3, an amino acid ester group, which can be modified to modulate the physicochemical properties of the molecule.

First, as shown in Table 9.3, compounds **5** to **9** were designed with the R_1 and R_2 groups of PSI-7672 fixed while varying the carboxylic ester group R_3. The derivatives were evaluated by in vitro testing for their inhibitory activity (EC_{90}) against NS5B polymerase and their ability to inhibit normal cell rRNA synthesis (inhibition%) at a concentration of 50 μmol/L. The results revealed that when linear or branched alkyl chains and cyclic substituents such as cyclohexane and benzyl groups were attached at the R_3 position, the molecules maintained submicromolar activity. However, the benzoic ester exhibited a decrease in antiviral activity. Although the data showed that increasing steric hindrance of the substituent could further enhance the molecule's antiviral activity, larger R_3 groups also resulted in cytotoxicity toward rRNA synthesis. For example, compound **7**, despite having a potent EC_{90} at 0.06 μmol/L, showed an increase in cell toxicity from 0% inhibition for PSI-7672 to 93.8%. Balancing the antiviral activity and cytotoxicity, methyl and isopropyl became favorable choices for the R_3 carboxylic ester. Subsequently, with the R_2 and R_3 groups fixed as methyl, variations were made to the phosphate ester at the R_1 position. The results, as shown in Table 9.3 (compounds **10–14**), demonstrated the significance of an aromatic ring at the phosphate ester position for inhibiting viral replication. Halogens and a naphthalene ring on the aromatic ring further increased activity but also resulted in cytotoxicity.

Following the optimization of R_1 and R_3, with the R_3 being fixed as the methyl group, the compounds with different natural amino acid side chains at the R_2 position were evaluated. The results shown in Table 9.4 indicate that the R_2 position can only tolerate relatively small substituent groups, such as methyl (**10**), ethyl (**16**), and gem-methyl (**18**), while larger substituents like isopropyl in comound **17** and cyclopropyl in compound **19** resulted in a complete loss of antiviral activity in the in vitro HCV replicon assay. Additionally, compound **20**, the enantiomer of PSI-7672, showed a complete loss of inhibitory activity against viral replication. Therefore, the selection range for the R_2 group is limited, and the optimal choice is the *S*-configuration methyl group—the natural alanine.

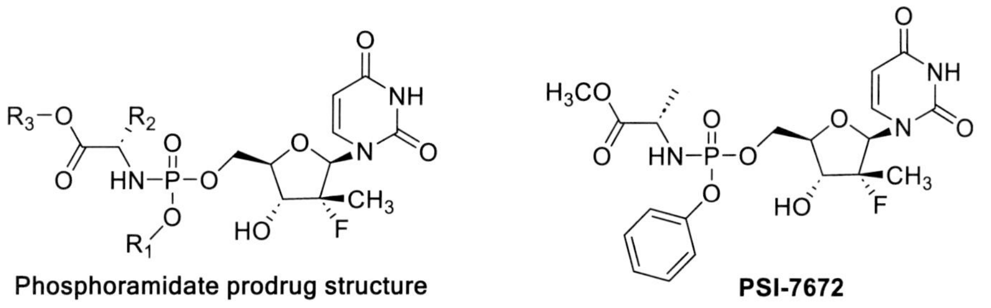

FIGURE 9.12 Structure of the phosphoramidate prodrug.

Phosphoramidate prodrug structure

PSI-7672

TABLE 9.3 Effect of R₁ and R₃ on the inhibitory activity and cytotoxicity.

Compound	R₁	R₃	EC₉₀ cloneA (μmol/L)	Inhibition% of rRNA synthesis @ 50 μmol/L
PSI-7672	Ph	Me	0.91	0
5	Ph	i-Pr	0.52	25.9
6	Ph	c-Hex	0.25	61
7	Ph	2-Bu	0.06	93.8
8	Ph	Ph	18.5	0
9	Ph	Bn	0.13	74.3
10	4-F-Ph	Me	0.69	16.8
11	4-Cl-Ph	Me	0.58	62.8
12	3,4-Cl-Ph	Me	0.45	63.7
13	1-Napth	Me	0.09	95.4
14	Et	Me	>50	16.8

TABLE 9.4 Effect of R₁ and R₂ on the inhibitory activity and cytotoxicity

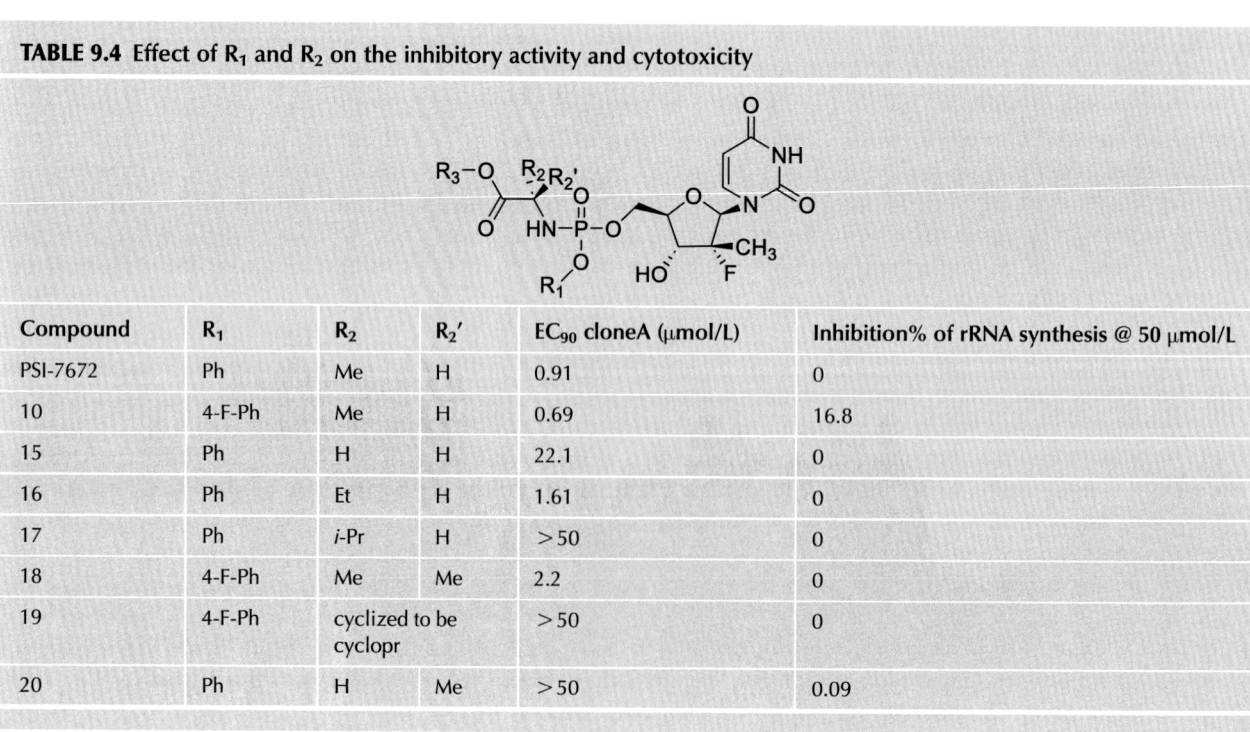

Compound	R₁	R₂	R₂'	EC₉₀ cloneA (μmol/L)	Inhibition% of rRNA synthesis @ 50 μmol/L
PSI-7672	Ph	Me	H	0.91	0
10	4-F-Ph	Me	H	0.69	16.8
15	Ph	H	H	22.1	0
16	Ph	Et	H	1.61	0
17	Ph	i-Pr	H	>50	0
18	4-F-Ph	Me	Me	2.2	0
19	4-F-Ph	cyclized to be cyclopr		>50	0
20	Ph	H	Me	>50	0.09

After the structure-activity relationship studies on the substituents at R₁, R₂, and R₃ positions, the research team selected seven compounds with R₃ as isopropyl or methyl and R₁ as either unsubstituted or halogen-substituted phenyl groups. These compounds exhibited favorable selectivity, inhibitory activity, and structural diversity and were chosen for further in vitro evaluations, including stability in simulated gastric fluid and simulated intestinal fluid, as well as plasma stability, to ensure the stability of the drug molecules during distribution in the body. Subsequently, the stability of the molecules in human S9 enzymes was tested to estimate the rate of release of the prodrug into hepatocytes, where it is converted into the active parent drug structure.

As shown in Table 9.5, all seven tested nucleoside molecules tolerate gastric and intestinal fluids (with a half-life exceeding 15 hours), remain stable in plasma, and rapidly undergo cleavage of the prodrug phosphate ester group within

TABLE 9.5 Biological activity, stability, and PK properties of phosphoramidate prodrugs.

Compound	R_1	R_3	EC_{90} cloneA (µM)	% Inhib @50 µM	In vitro stability		Pharmacokinetic data in rat			
					SGF^a/SIF^b (h)	Human plasma^c/ human S9^d (h)	C_{max} (ng/g)	T_{max} (h)	$AUC_{(0-t)}$ (ng*h/g)	$AUC_{(inf)}$ (ng*h/g)
PSI-7672	Ph	Me	0.91	0	15.5/>20	16.7/0.18	1985	6	14206	18 968
5	Ph	i-Pr	0.52	25.9	22/>24	>24/0.57	1934	4	16796	18 080
6	Ph	c-Hex	0.25	61.1	17/>20	>24/1.4	557	2	6487	8 831
21	4-F-Ph	Et	0.76	55.3	17/>20	>8/0.23	291	4	4191	5 423
22	4-F-Ph	i-Pr	0.77	0	>20/>20	>24/0.42	519	6	6140	7 375
23	4-F-Ph	c-Hex	0.04	52.1	20/>20	>24/0.18	716	4	8937	9 888
24	4-Cl-Ph	i-Pr	0.42	0	>20/>20	>24/0.35	339	1	5143	8 468

^{a}SGF: simulated gastric fluid, pH 1.2, 50 µg/mL concentration, 37°C, 20 h.
^{b}SIF: simulated intestinal fluid, pH 7.5, 50 µg/mL concentration, 37°C, 20 h.
^{c}100 µM, 37°C, 24 h.
^{d}100 µM concentration, 37°C, 24 h, pH 7.4.

hepatocytes to release the active parent compound PSI-6206-MP. These characteristics fulfill the requirements for the prodrug to exert its effects on the body. Although the final activated molecular structure formed by these prodrugs is the same, different modifying groups can influence their drug metabolism behavior, resulting in variations in absorption rate, hepatocyte permeability rate, and conversion to the triphosphate form. Consequently, the in vitro data cannot accurately predict the effects of the drug molecules in vivo.

To validate the clinical efficacy of the molecules against HCV, researchers conducted tests on the concentration of uridine triphosphate generated within hepatocytes after oral absorption of the drug molecules. Pharmasset administered the seven lead compounds orally to rats (at a dose of 50 mg/kg), and measured the maximum concentration (C_{max}) and area under the concentration-time curve (AUC) of the prodrug in plasma. After 4 days of dosing, the dissection was performed to measure the concentration of the active triphosphate structure in the rat liver. As presented in Table 9.6, the data indicated the successful oral absorption of the prodrug, hepatocyte uptake, active parent drug conversion, and ultimately the conversion into the active triphosphate nucleotides, thus achieving the desired prodrug liver-targeting effect. Among these seven compounds, PSI-7672, **5**, and **23** exhibited the highest drug exposure levels in rats.

Pharmacokinetic studies of these three compounds in dogs and monkeys revealed that compound **5** achieved plasma exposure levels 15-fold higher than PSI-7672 and 110-fold higher than compound **23** in dogs. In monkeys, compound **5** had 3-fold higher plasma exposure levels than PSI-7672. Results from liver samples also demonstrated that compound **5** exhibited higher concentrations of the active triphosphate structure in the liver compared to the other two compounds. In in vitro experiments using rat, dog, monkey, and human hepatocyte cultures, all three compounds showed higher levels of conversion to uridine triphosphate than the traditional prodrug molecule RG7128. Compound **5** exhibited a favorable conversion rate, with its triphosphate concentration in human hepatocytes surpassing that of PSI-7672 and **23** by three fold.

In terms of the safety evaluation, in vitro experiments conducted on mitochondria and bone marrow cells showed that only the compound with cyclohexyl-substituted carboxylic ester exhibited bone marrow toxicity (red progenitor cells $IC_{50} = 37 \pm 5\ \mu M$, myeloid progenitor cells $IC_{50} = 30 \pm 5\ \mu M$). In other acute toxicity tests conducted in animals, none of the three compounds showed any toxicity findings, even at high doses (> 1800 mg/kg). Taking into consideration the evaluations of activity, pharmacokinetic data, levels of prodrug conversion to active uridine triphosphate, and safety aspects, compound **5** was ultimately designated as the clinical candidate drug and named PSI-7851.

In-depth investigations were conducted on the metabolism of PSI-7851 in animal models (Fig. 9.13) [64]. The results demonstrated that during the metabolism process, the ester moiety of the prodrug PSI-7851 was primarily hydrolyzed by cathepsin A and carboxylesterase 1, leading to the generation of a carboxylic acid with a negative charge under physiological pH conditions. Subsequently, the oxygen anion of the carboxyl group attacks the phosphorus atom, resulting in the departure of the phenol moiety and the formation of an unstable five-membered cyclic acid anhydride. After the ring

TABLE 9.6 Pharmacokinetic data of phosphoramidate prodrugs in dog and monkey at a dose of 50 mg/kg.

Compound			PSI-7672	5	23
Dog	Day 3 plasma sampling	C_{max} (ng/mL)	317	6 179	36
		T_{max} (h)	1	0.5	0.25
		AUC $_{(inf)}$ (ng h/mL)	420	6 903	62
		AUC $_{(0-t)}$ (ng h/mL)	418	6 894	54
	Day 4 liver sampling	Prodrug (ng/g liver)	5.24	612	8.72
		NTP (ng/g liver)	4 960	10 560	476
Monkey	Day 3 plasma sampling	C_{max} (ng/mL)	19	33	1.8
		T_{max} (h)	0.25	1	6
		AUC $_{(inf)}$ (ng h/mL)	34	170	NA
		AUC $_{(0-t)}$ (ng h/mL)	27	86	NA
	Day 4 liver sampling	Prodrug (ng/g liver)	4.66	177	13
		NTP (ng/g liver)	26	57	NA

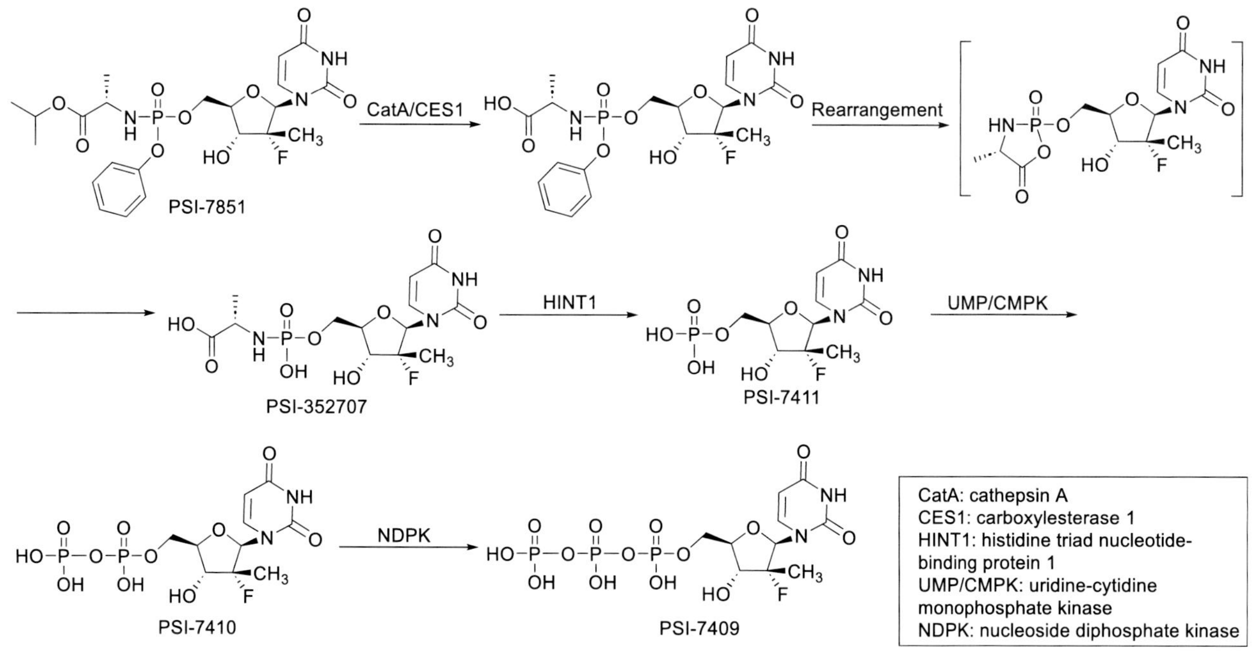

FIGURE 9.13 Metabolic pathway of phosphoramidate prodrug PSI-7851.

opening of the cyclic intermediate, the phosphoryl amine metabolite PSI-352707 is formed. The phosphorus-nitrogen bond is then cleaved by the phosphoramidase (histidine triad nucleotide-binding protein 1, HINT1), generating the monophosphate nucleoside PSI-7411 (also known as PSI-6206-MP), which ultimately undergoes successful conversion into the active triphosphate nucleoside PSI-7409 (also known as PSI-6206-TP) within the liver. In this metabolic pathway, all enzymes are liver-associated, thereby achieving the desired liver-targeting objectives.

After the completion of investigational new drug studies on PSI-7851, it successfully progressed into Phase I clinical trials to evaluate its safety and pharmacokinetic properties in humans. Daily oral administration of PSI-7851 at a dose of 800 mg did not elicit any adverse effects. The pharmacokinetic data obtained in humans were consistent with preclinical animal experiment results, demonstrating rapid hepatic absorption and low plasma concentrations, indicative of liver targeting. In a multiple-dose escalation study conducted in patients with genotype 1 hepatitis C, oral administration of PSI-7851 at doses ranging from 50 to 400 mg per day resulted in a reduction of HCV RNA levels by 0.49–1.98 log units, with no observed viral mutations or development of resistance. These findings confirm the success of the liver-targeting prodrug strategy and demonstrate the clinical efficacy of PSI-7851 in anti-HCV treatment.

9.3.3.4 Characterization of the active diastereomer: PSI-7977

PSI-7851, selected as a clinical candidate compound, is actually a pair of 1:1 diastereomers of phosphoramidate. It possesses a chiral center at the phosphorus atom, and the mixture exhibits the characteristics of an amorphous solid with a relatively low melting point (66°C–75°C). During the preclinical development process, to expedite the demonstration of the feasibility of the novel liver-targeting prodrug strategy, the team did not separate the diastereomeric pair. Once the efficacy of PSI-7851 was established, researchers separated the diastereomers using chiral high performance liquid chromatograpy (HPLC), resulting in the isolation of two individual stereoisomers: PSI-7976 and PSI-7977 (Table 9.7). These two molecules exhibited more than a 10-fold difference in HCV replicon activity in vitro. Subsequently, the crystal structure of the highly active compound PSI-7977 was determined through single-crystal X-ray diffraction, confirming its *Sp* configuration. This molecule was eventually advanced into clinical application and became the first approved nucleoside analog drug for HCV, known as sofosbuvir.

9.3.4 The synthesis of sofosbuvir

During the early development of sofosbuvir, synthetic chemists utilized D-glyceraldehyde as a starting material to develop the chiral synthesis of the nucleoside molecule PSI-6206 (Fragment A). Subsequently, PSI-6206 was transformed into the phosphoramidate prodrug PSI-7851. Then, by means of recrystallization, the active isomer PSI-7977 was selectively prepared with high efficiency. However, as clinical research progressed, there was a significant increase

TABLE 9.7 Comparison of PSI-7851 diastereoisomers.

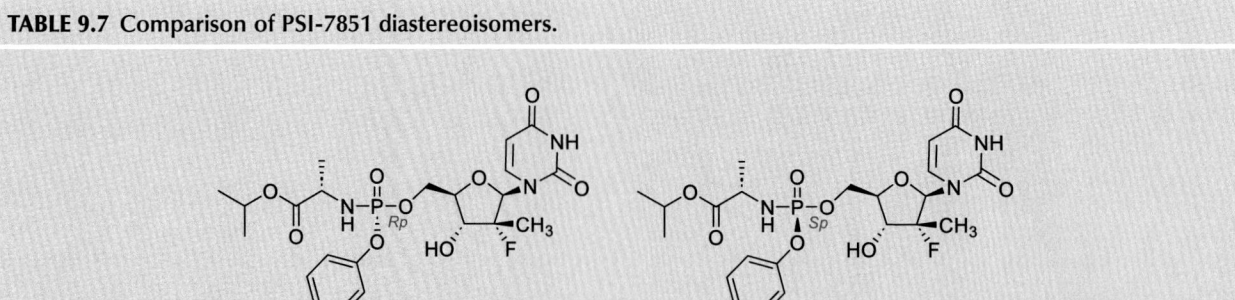

Compound	cloneA: EC_{90} (μM)		S282/WT	ET-lunet: EC_{90} (μM)		S282/WT
	WT	S282T	E_{90} ratio	WT	S282T	E_{90} ratio
PSI-7976	7.50 ± 3.0	>100	>13	3.3 ± 1.4	1.3 ± 0.3	0.4
PSI-7977	0.42 ± 0.23	7.80 ± 5.3	18.6	0.23 ± 0.15	0.11 ± 0.039	0.5

FIGURE 9.14 The synthetic route towards Fragment A.

in the demand for this drug, necessitating further optimization of the synthetic process [64]. The optimized synthetic route consists of the linkage between Fragment A and Fragment B (Fig. 9.14). The synthesis of Fragment A begins with the starting material (R)-2,2-dimethyl-1,3-dioxane-4-carboxaldehyde (A1), which undergoes a Wittig reaction to generate the olefin intermediate A2. Subsequent dihydroxylation is employed to yield the *cis*-diol compound A3. A3 reacts with thionyl chloride in an ice-water bath to form a cyclic sulfite compound, which is further oxidized by

2,2,6,6-tetramethylpiperidine 1-oxyl radical (TEMPO) catalysis to produce the cyclic sulfate compound A4. Without purification, A4 undergoes fluorination using tetraethylammonium fluoride, followed by hydrolysis in a solution of hydrochloric acid and dioxane to generate intermediate A5. A6 is then obtained through condensation and cyclization in concentrated hydrochloric acid, forming a five-membered lactone compound. A7 is obtained through benzoylation of A6, which is subsequently reduced by Red-Al to form a hemiacetal intermediate. Without purification, the intermediate reacts with thionyl chloride to yield the chlorinated intermediate A8, which undergoes nucleophilic substitution with N_4-benzoylcytosine to yield A9. A9 is hydrolyzed with acetic acid to remove the amino group, resulting in the formation of a benzoyl-protected nucleoside intermediate. The benzoyl group is then removed using an aqueous solution of ammonium methanol, leading to intermediate A (Fig. 9.14). The single enantiomer of Fragment B can be obtained from diphenylphosphoryl chloride as the starting material, which reacts with L-alanine isopropyl ester hydrochloride and pentafluorophenol (Fig. 9.15). Intermediate B, upon reaction with intermediate A using the t-butylmagnesium chloride reagent, yields the final product, sofosbuvir (Fig. 9.16).

9.4 Clinical studies of sofosbuvir

9.4.1 Preclinical studies of sofosbuvir

In preclinical studies, sofosbuvir demonstrated high inhibitory activity against viral replication in HCV RdRp activity assays. It exhibited potent activity with an EC_{90} of 0.42 μM in genotype 1b replicon assays and demonstrated broad-genotype inhibitory activity against HCV strains of genotypes 1–6. Furthermore, when evaluating the combination effects of sofosbuvir with other antiviral agents against HCV, including IFNα, other types of DAAs such as NS5A inhibitors, NS3/4A protease inhibitors, and nonnucleoside NS5B inhibitors, cumulative effects or synergistic actions were observed. On the other hand, in preclinical pharmacological studies and safety evaluations of sofosbuvir, no safety issues commonly associated with other nucleoside drugs were observed. In vitro safety assessments of sofosbuvir, even at doses several times higher than the effective dose, did not result in any cytotoxicity, mitochondrial toxicity, or myelotoxicity. Sofosbuvir is neither a substrate nor an inducer of human DNA and RNA polymerases or mitochondrial polymerases. Studies on drug-drug interactions have shown that sofosbuvir and its major uridine metabolites are not substrates or inducers of CYP450 enzymes, but they are substrates of P-glycoprotein (P-gp) and breast cancer resistance protein (BCRP). In genetic toxicity, embryotoxicity, and reproductive toxicity experiments conducted on rats, no toxic effects of sofosbuvir were observed. Consequently, sofosbuvir was successfully advanced to clinical trial research.

9.4.2 Clinical trial results of sofosbuvir

To evaluate the efficacy of sofosbuvir in clinical settings, Pharmasett designed a clinical study called ATOMIC to investigate the treatment response of sofosbuvir in combination with pegylated IFNα and RBV in patients infected with

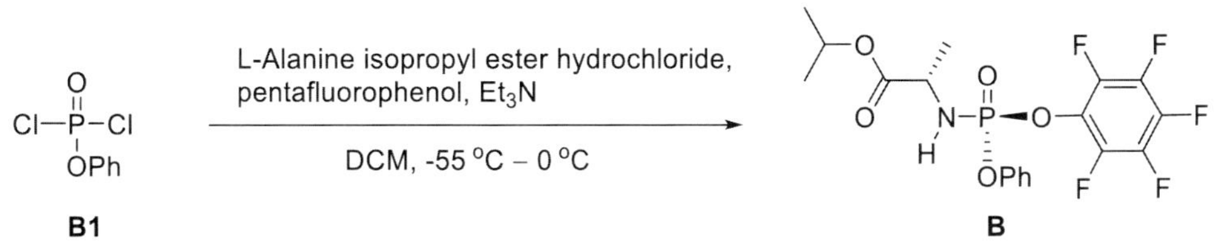

FIGURE 9.15 The synthetic route towards Fragment B.

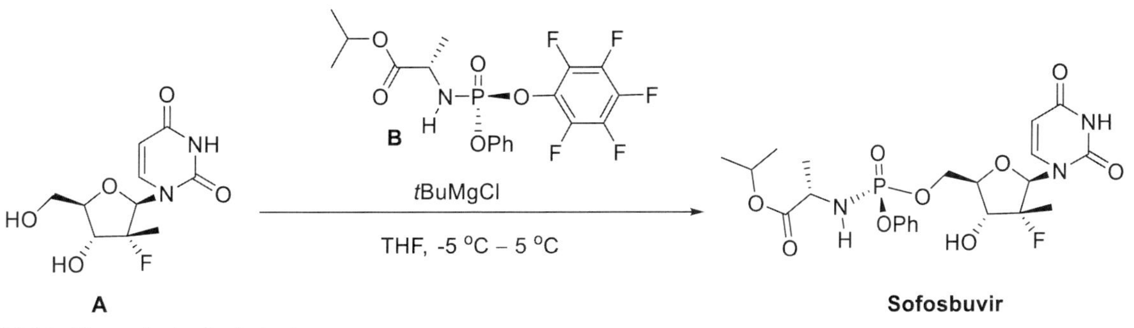

FIGURE 9.16 The synthesis of sofosbuvir.

genotype 1 HCV. In the combination regimen, sofosbuvir was administered orally at doses of 100, 200, and 400 mg per day for 28 days. Experimental data demonstrated that the sofosbuvir combination group achieved a reduction of the HCV RNA levels in plasma by 5 log units, which was significantly better than the placebo and PR combination group (reduction of 2.8 log units). Moreover, compared to the lower rapid virologic response rate of 21% in the control group, the sofosbuvir combination group achieved high response rates ranging from 88% to 94%, with sustained virologic response rates of 76% after a 24-week follow-up period. No significant adverse effects were observed during the treatment period with sofosbuvir, and the most reported drug-related adverse reactions were fatigue and nausea, which were consistent with the expected safety profile during RBV and pegylated IFNα treatment [75].

Afterward, Pharmasett conducted a crucial ELECTRON clinical trial to assess the feasibility of sofosbuvir monotherapy. Before the ELECTRON, the treatment regimen of sofosbuvir in combination with RBV for genotype 1 HCV-infected patients, even with an extended treatment duration of 24 weeks, showed lower efficacy compared to the triple therapy of sofosbuvir/RBV/IFNα. The Electron study focused on individuals with chronic genotype 2 or 3 HCV infections. The trial evaluated three treatment options: sofosbuvir monotherapy, sofosbuvir/RBV combination therapy, and sofosbuvir/RBV/IFNα triple therapy for 12 weeks. The efficacy of the three treatment regimens was assessed at 12 and 24 weeks after treatment discontinuation. Results showed that the combination of sofosbuvir and RBV exhibited comparable efficacy to the combination with IFNα. For naïve or previously IFN treated genotype 2 HCV-infected patients, the SVR rate for sofosbuvir/RBV treatment for 12 weeks reached 92%. For genotype 3 HCV-infected patients, the efficacy of sofosbuvir/RBV was lower than that for genotype 2, but after extending the treatment duration to 24 weeks, the SVR rate could reach 86% [76]. In the clinical trial process mentioned above, sofosbuvir did not exhibit the common resistance issue observed with nucleoside therapies. The S282T polymerase mutation reported in the early stages of the experiment did not occur during the clinical trial [77]. These encouraging clinical data finally demonstrated the possibility of interferon-free treatment for HCV and opened the revolutionary path for anti-HCV therapy (Fig. 9.17).

9.4.3 Treatment regimens with sofosbuvir

After the ELECTRON trial, clinical studies were conducted with sofosbuvir targeting different viral genotypes, diverse ethnicities, treatment-naïve individuals, patients who had previously received interferon-based regimens, and with compensated liver disease (such as cirrhosis). These studies consistently demonstrated the effectiveness of sofosbuvir. Due to variations in response rates among different patient populations and different genotypes of HCV infection, treatment regimens and durations may vary slightly. Table 9.8 presents the treatment regimens recommended in the 2015 European guidelines for hepatitis C, which include sofosbuvir.

Due to the tremendous potential demonstrated by sofosbuvir in clinical research, Gilead Sciences promptly seized the opportunity and acquired Pharmasett in November 2011, making sofosbuvir their flagship drug. On December 6, 2013, the combination regimen of sofosbuvir and ledipasvir was officially approved by the FDA for the treatment of genotype 1–4 hepatitis C patients. The remarkable advancement with this approval was the elimination of the need for interferon in the treatment regimen. In commemoration of Dr. Sofia's significant contributions during the development process, the

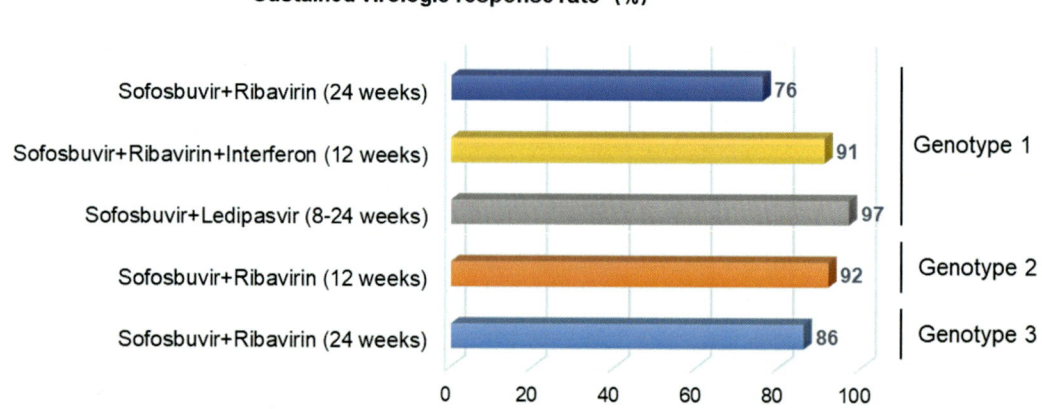

FIGURE 9.17 Clinical results of sofosbuvir. *From ELETRON, PHOTON, NEUTRINO, ION, FISSION, POSITRON, FUSION, and VALENCE studies.*

TABLE 9.8 EMA suggested treatment regimens containing sofosbuvir for different genotypes.

Patient population	Recommended treatment plan
All genotypes of HCV-infected patients	Sofosbuvir + Pegylated Interferon + Ribavirin (12 weeks)
Genotypes 1/4/5/6 of HCV-infected patients with intolerance or contraindications to Interferon	Non-cirrhotic: Sofosbuvir + Daclatasvir (12 weeks)
	Cirrhotic: Sofosbuvir + Daclatasvir + Ribavirin (12–24 weeks)
Genotypes 1/4 of HCV-infected patients with intolerance or contraindications to Interferon	Non-cirrhotic: Sofosbuvir + Simeprevir (12 weeks)
	Cirrhotic: Sofosbuvir + Simeprevir (24 weeks) or Sofosbuvir + Simeprevir + Ribavirin (12 weeks)
Genotypes 2 of HCV-infected patients	Noncirrhotic: Sofosbuvir + Ribavirin (12 weeks)
	Cirrhotic or treatment-experienced: Sofosbuvir + Ribavirin (16–20 weeks) or Sofosbuvir + Daclatasvir (12 weeks)
Genotypes 3 of HCV-infected patients	Noncirrhotic: Sofosbuvir + Ribavirin (24 weeks) or Sofosbuvir + Daclatasvir (12 weeks)
	Cirrhotic: Sofosbuvir + Daclatasvir + Ribavirin (24 weeks)

molecule was named sofosbuvir, derived from his surname, and marketed under the trade name Sovaldi. Dr. Sofia also shared the 2016 Lasker-DeBakey Clinical Medical Research Award for this groundbreaking contribution.

Subsequently, Gilead developed a series of combination therapies for chronic hepatitis C based on sofosbuvir. It was discovered that the coadministration of sofosbuvir with the NS5A inhibitor ledipasvir or daclatasvir could effectively treat patients infected with genotype 1 HCV, which posed higher treatment challenges. A treatment duration of 8–12 weeks achieved a remarkable SVR rate of 95%–100%. In October 2014, the fixed-dose combination of sofosbuvir and ledipasvir, known as Harvoni, received official approval from the FDA for the treatment of genotype 1 chronic hepatitis C. The coadministration of sofosbuvir and daclatasvir was also approved in 2015. In recent years, with the successful introduction of more DAA drugs, sofosbuvir has overcome the need for interferon and/or RBV, which often have significant side effects. Instead, sofosbuvir is used in combination with next-generation DAAs. This approach undoubtedly enhances both the efficacy and safety of treatment, offering HCV patients greater benefits.

9.5 Summary and outlook

9.5.1 Summary

In 2016, the World Health Organization set forth the overarching goal of "eliminating viral hepatitis by 2030." However, according to the 2017 report, it is estimated that in 2015, there were still 71 million people worldwide living with chronic hepatitis C. Due to the vast population size, the actual number of infections in China has also reached tens of millions. In the fundamental eradication of hepatitis C, DAA therapies, with sofosbuvir as a representative, undoubtedly make a significant contribution. The introduction of sofosbuvir has shattered the impasse in the field of hepatitis C treatment, characterized by the lack of vaccines, the lack of specific drugs, and the inability to achieve a cure. The 12-week cure has brought immense relief to a vast number of hepatitis C patients. As the first drug approved for an all-oral treatment regimen for hepatitis C patients, its global sales reached a staggering 10.28 billion dollars in the first year after its launch. For patients with specific genotypes of hepatitis C, sofosbuvir treatment can eliminate the reliance on interferon, while demonstrating outstanding efficacy with minimal side effects, greatly improving patients' quality of life. It can be considered a new era in the treatment of hepatitis C. Furthermore, considering the risk of hepatitis C progressing to cirrhosis and liver cancer, sofosbuvir can also be viewed, to some extent, as a preventive drug for liver cancer.

Sofosbuvir is the first drug to be launched that targets HCV NS5B polymerase. HCV NS5B RNA-dependent RNA polymerase is crucial for HCV and is present in all genotypes. When the drug binds to this target, it can effectively halt the replication of viral RNA and generate pan-genotypic efficacy, making it an excellent solution for eliminating HCV. However, the design and development of inhibitors that bind to this target are not easy. Scientists have conducted numerous experimental designs and accumulated experience to identify key nucleotide structures with high activity, remarkable selectivity, and sufficient safety. After confirming the clinical efficacy of the parent nucleoside, the research and development team encountered issues related to drug metabolism and absorption during clinical trials. Based on the concept of metabolic activation, researchers applied a prodrug strategy to construct the chemical structure of sofosbuvir. Throughout the tumultuous development process, scientists skillfully addressed issues such as the design of in vitro and in vivo experiments, the conversion of parent drugs to prodrugs, the stability of prodrugs, and their targeting properties. Ultimately, they successfully developed the "game-changer" sofosbuvir.

9.5.2 Further reading: ProTide technology

Nucleoside-based drugs are widely used in various fields, such as antitumor and antiviral therapies. After entering the cells, nucleoside-based drugs need to undergo three phosphorylation steps by enzymes to generate the biologically active triphosphate form, which is responsible for their therapeutic effects. Among these steps, monophosphorylation is the rate-determining step. Therefore, in the development of nucleoside-based drugs, it is common to directly introduce a monophosphate or phosphate ester group to bypass the first rate-limiting step. However, early phosphate or phosphate ester derivatives often possess high polarity, which leads to difficulties in membrane penetration and poor metabolic stability of the phosphorous-oxygen bond. To address these challenges, prodrug strategies have been extensively explored and utilized.

ProTide technology is one of the most prominent prodrug strategies in nucleoside-based drug research. The term "ProTide" is derived from "prodrug" and "nucleotide," representing the combination of a prodrug and nucleotide technology. It was initially developed by Professor Chris McGuigan and his research group at Cardiff University in the 1990s. During their work on the synthesis of azidothymidine (AZT) phosphoramidate using chlorophosphate esters, they observed that the phosphate derivatives of AZT exhibited enhanced anti-HIV activity in certain cases compared to the parent nucleoside. Additionally, the cellular activity of the substituted phosphoramidate was found to be ten times higher ($EC_{50} = 10$ μM vs $EC_{50} = 100$ μM) than that of AZT. Based on these findings, they patented a structure consisting of an aromatic substituent and an amino acid ester, which protected the phosphate group of the nucleoside in the form of a phosphoramidate. This prodrug technology effectively shields the polarity of the phosphate group, allowing efficient cellular transport of the nucleoside prodrug molecule. Subsequently, upon enzymatic action inside the cell, the phosphate form of the parent drug structure is released [74,78].

The development of ProTide technology has undergone more than 20 years of research and development and can be traced back to the late 1980s, when six major categories were identified (Table 9.9) [79]. In the field of anti-HIV research, scientists initially employed alkyl and halogenated alkyl esters to mask the phosphate group, rendering the drug molecules neutral under physiological pH conditions and facilitating absorption. This strategy indeed enhanced the stability of the phosphate group in the body. However, the resulting alkyl phosphates were too stable, leading to a slow release of the parent drug and compromising the bioactivity of the prodrug molecule. Subsequently, inspired by studies demonstrating the ability of HIV protease to cleave phosphate ester bonds, alkoxymethyl and halogenated alkoxymethyl phosphoramidates were introduced into the design of nucleoside monophosphate prodrugs. Explorations in this direction revealed that the amino acid side chains masking the phosphate group were crucial for molecular activity, with the α-amino acids demonstrating superior activity compared to β- and γ-types of amino acids, thus laying the foundation for the subsequent maturation of ProTide technology. However, the phosphate prodrug molecules derived from alkoxymethyl and halogenated alkoxymethyl phosphoramidates still fell short of the desired anti-HIV activity. As a result, phosphoramidate and lactate derivatives were attempted as modifications for the phosphate group. Although these modifications aided in membrane permeability, they failed to achieve the same level of bioactivity as the parent nucleosides. It was not until the emergence of diaryl phosphates that a phosphorus prodrug molecule in the nucleoside prodrug technology demonstrated superior activity to the parent drug structure. Building upon previous research, Professor McGuigan's team successfully developed the ProTide technology by combining the aryloxy group with the amino acid side chain of phosphoramidate.

As a versatile technology, the widespread adoption of ProTide technology has significantly advanced the development of nucleoside-based drugs. Representative examples of ProTide nucleoside drugs include tenofovir alafenamide for anti-HIV/hepatitis B therapy and sofosbuvir for anti-hepatitis C therapy. Furthermore, Gilead's newly developed drug for COVID-19 in 2020 also utilizes a similar prodrug technology. In recent years, the application of ProTide technology has expanded to nonnucleotide-based drugs as well. Examples include glucosamine monophosphate for the treatment of osteoarthritis, anticancer small molecule monophosphates, panthotenate kinase-dependent neurodegenerative disease drugs, S1P receptor modulators, 6-PGDH inhibitors, and tyrosine phosphate mimetics [80]. Experimental data for these molecules have demonstrated improved stability and oral bioavailability compared to the parent drugs. Considering the potential of ProTide technology to enhance the pharmacokinetic properties of compounds with suboptimal performance, it is undoubtedly a tremendous opportunity to benefit patients. We anticipate that more drugs will be optimized with ProTide technology in the future (Fig. 9.18).

TABLE 9.9 The development of ProTide technology.

Number	Class	Phosphate masking group
1	Alkyl and haloalkyl phosphate ester	$\xi\text{-O-P(=O)(OR}_1\text{)OR}_2$; R_1/R_2 = Me, Et, Pr, -CH$_2$CCl$_3$, -CH$_2$CF$_3$
2	Alkoxyl and haloalkoxy phosphoramidate	Three structures shown. Left: R_1 = Me, Et, Pr, Bu, Hex; R_2 = H, Me, Bn, -CH(CH$_3$)$_2$, -CH$_2$CH(CH$_3$)$_2$, -CH(CH$_3$)CH$_2$CH$_3$. Middle: n = 1–6. Right: R = H, Me, iPr; X = H, F, Cl
3	Phosphordiamidate	R = H, Me, iPr, -CH$_2$Ph, -CH$_2$CO$_2$CH$_3$
4	Lactyl-derived systems	R_1 = Me, nPr, nC$_{12}$H$_{25}$, R_2 = H, Me, R_3 = Me, Et
5	Diaryl phosphates	Ar = Ph, p-X-Ph
6	Aryloxy phosphoramidates	R_1 = H, Me, -CH$_2$iPr, -CH$_2$Ph...; R_2 = Me, Et, iPr, tBu, Bn...

Source: Adapted from Mehellou Y, Rattan HS, Balzarini J. The ProTide prodrug technology: from the concept to the clinic. J Med Chem, 2018, 61(6): 2211–2226.

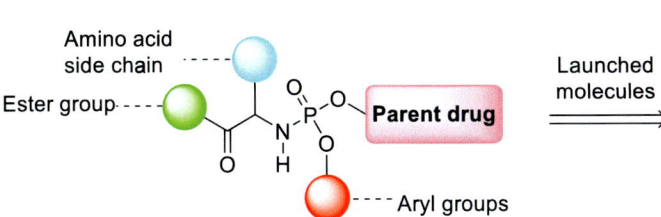

Tenofovir alafenamide
for treatment of chronic hepatitis B and HIV infection

Remedesivir
Broad-spectrum antiviral drugs for treating COVID-19

FIGURE 9.18 The application of ProTide technology.

References

[1] Stanaway JD, Flaxman AD, Naghavi M, et al. The global burden of viral hepatitis from 1990 to 2013: findings from the global burden of disease study 2013. Lancet 2016;388(10049):1081–8.

[2] Dalgard O, Egeland A, Ervik R, et al. Risk factors for hepatitis C among injecting drug users in Oslo. Tidsskr Nor Laegeforen 2009;129(2):101–4.

[3] Mann AG, Ramsay ME, Brant LJ, et al. Diagnoses of, and deaths from, severe liver disease due to hepatitis C in England between 2000 and 2005 estimated using multiple data sources. Epidemiol Infect 2009;137(4):513–18.

[4] Razavi H, Waked I, Sarrazin C, et al. The present and future disease burden of hepatitis C virus (HCV) infection with today's treatment paradigm. J Viral Hepat 2014;21(s1):34–59.

[5] Duberg A, Janzon R, Bäck E, et al. The epidemiology of hepatitis C virus infection in Sweden. Euro Surveill 2008;13(21):18882–6.

[6] Arafa N, Hoseiny ME, Rekacewicz C, et al. Changing pattern of hepatitis C virus spread in rural areas of Egypt. J Hepatol 2005;43(3):418–24.

[7] Compagnone A, Catenazzi P, Riccardi R, et al. Mother-to-child transmission of hepatitis C virus. Minerva Pediatr 2019;71(2):174–80.

[8] Delgado-Borrego A, Smith L, Jonas MM, et al. Expected and actual case ascertainment and treatment rates for children infected with hepatitis C in Florida and the United States: epidemiologic evidence from statewide and nationwide surveys. J Pediatr 2012;161(5):915–21.

[9] Kuncio DE, Newbern EC, Johnson CC, et al. Failure to test and identify perinatally infected children born to hepatitis C virus-infected women. Clin Infect Dis 2016;62(8):980–5.

[10] Pott Junior H, Theodoro M, de Almeida Vespoli J, et al. Mother-to-child transmission of hepatitis C virus. Eur J Obstet Gynecol Reprod Biol 2018;224:125–30.

[11] Domínguez-Rodríguez S, Prieto L, Fernández McPhee C, et al. Perinatal HCV transmission rate in HIV/HCV coinfected women with access to ART in Madrid, Spain. PLoS One 2020;15(4):e0230109.

[12] Marine-Barjoan E, Berrebi A, Giordanengo V, et al. HCV/HIV co-infection, HCV viral load and mode of delivery: risk factors for mother-to-child transmission of hepatitis C virus? AIDS 2007;21(13):1811–15.

[13] Tohme RA, Holmberg SD. Is sexual contact a major mode of hepatitis C virus transmission? Hepatology 2010;52(4):1497–505.

[14] Global Burden Of Hepatitis C working group. Global burden of disease (GBD) for hepatitis C. J Clin Pharmacol 2004;44(1):20–29.

[15] Lavanchy D. The threat to public health of hepatitis C. Res Virol 1997;148(2):143–5.

[16] Lavanchy D. Hepatitis C: public health strategies. J Hepatol 1999;31(s1):146–51.

[17] Lavanchy D. The global burden of hepatitis C. Liver Int 2009;29(s1):74–81.

[18] Lavanchy D. Evolving epidemiology of hepatitis C virus. Clin Microbiol Infect 2011;17(2):107–15.

[19] Polaris observatory hcv collaborators. Global prevalence and genotype distribution of hepatitis C virus infection in 2015: a modelling study. Lancet Gastroenterol Hepatol 2017;2(3):161–76.

[20] Pawlotsky J-M, Feld JJ, Zeuzem S, et al. From non-A, non-B hepatitis to hepatitis C virus cure. J Hepatol 2015;62(1s):S87–99.

[21] Choo QL, Kuo G, Weiner AJ, et al. Isolation of a cDNA clone derived from a blood-borne non-A, non-B viral hepatitis genome. Science 1989;244(4902):359–62.

[22] Kuo G, Choo QL, Alter HJ, et al. An assay for circulating antibodies to a major etiologic virus of human non-A, non-B hepatitis. Science 1989;244(4902):362–4.

[23] McHutchison JG, Gordon SC, Schiff ER, et al. Interferon alfa-2b alone or in combination with ribavirin as initial treatment for chronic hepatitis C. Hepatitis Interventional Therapy Group. N Engl J Med 1998;339(21):1485–92.

[24] Poynard T, Marcellin P, Lee SS, et al. Randomised trial of interferon α2b plus ribavirin for 48 weeks or for 24 weeks versus interferon α2b plus placebo for 48 weeks for treatment of chronic infection with hepatitis C virus. International hepatitis interventional therapy group (IHIT). Lancet 1998;352(9138):1426–32.

[25] Heathcote EJ, Shiffman ML, Cooksley WG, et al. Peginterferon alfa-2a in patients with chronic hepatitis C and cirrhosis. N Engl J Med 2000;343(23):1673–80.

[26] Lindsay KL, Trepo C, Heintges T, et al. A randomized, double-blind trial comparing pegylated interferon alfa-2b to interferon alfa-2b as initial treatment for chronic hepatitis C. Hepatology 2001;34(2):395–403.

[27] Reddy KR, Wright TL, Pockros PJ, et al. Efficacy and safety of pegylated (40-kd) interferon alpha-2a compared with interferon alpha-2a in noncirrhotic patients with chronic hepatitis C. Hepatology 2001;33(2):433–8.

[28] Manns MP, McHutchison JG, Gordon SC, et al. Peginterferon alfa-2b plus ribavirin compared with interferon alfa-2b plus ribavirin for initial treatment of chronic hepatitis C: a randomised trial. Lancet 2001;358(9286):958–65.

[29] Fried MW, Shiffman ML, Reddy KR, et al. Peginterferon alfa-2a plus ribavirin for chronic hepatitis C virus infection. N Engl J Med 2002;347(13):975–82.

[30] Beilharz MW, Cummins MJ, Bennett AL, et al. Oromucosal administration of interferon to humans. Pharmaceuticals (Basel) 2010;3(2):323–44.

[31] Ebinuma H, Saito H, Tada S, et al. Disadvantages of peginterferon and ribavirin treatment in older patients with chronic hepatitis C: an analysis using the propensity score. Hepatol Int 2012;6(4):744–52.

[32] Manns MP, Wedemeyer H, Cornberg M. Treating viral hepatitis C: efficacy, side effects, and complications. Gut 2006;55(9):1350–9.

[33] Wilby KJ, Partovi N, Ford J-AE, et al. Review of boceprevir and telaprevir for the treatment of chronic hepatitis C. Can J Gastroenterol 2012;26(4):205–10.

[34] Park C, Jiang S, Lawson KA. Efficacy and safety of telaprevir and boceprevir in patients with hepatitis C genotype 1: a meta-analysis. J Clin Pharm Ther 2014;39(1):14—24.

[35] Jacobson IM, Dore GJ, Foster GR, et al. Simeprevir with pegylated interferon alfa 2a plus ribavirin in treatment-naive patients with chronic hepatitis C virus genotype 1 infection (QUEST-1): a phase 3, randomised, double-blind, placebo-controlled trial. Lancet 2014;384 (9941):403—13.

[36] Manns M, Marcellin P, Poordad F, et al. Simeprevir with pegylated interferon alfa 2a or 2b plus ribavirin in treatment-naive patients with chronic hepatitis C virus genotype 1 infection (QUEST-2): a randomised, double-blind, placebo-controlled phase 3 trial. Lancet 2014;384 (9941):414—26.

[37] Romano KP, Ali A, Royer WE, et al. Drug resistance against HCV NS3/4A inhibitors is defined by the balance of substrate recognition versus inhibitor binding. Proc Natl Acad Sci U S A 2010;107(49):20986—91.

[38] Jacobson IM, Gordon SC, Kowdley KV, et al. Sofosbuvir for hepatitis C genotype 2 or 3 in patients without treatment options. N Engl J Med 2013;368(20):1867—77.

[39] Lawitz E, Mangia A, Wyles D, et al. Sofosbuvir for previously untreated chronic hepatitis C infection. N Engl J Med 2013;368(20):1878—87.

[40] Lawitz E, Poordad F, Brainard DM, et al. Sofosbuvir with peginterferon-ribavirin for 12 weeks in previously treated patients with hepatitis C genotype 2 or 3 and cirrhosis. Hepatology 2015;61(3):769—75.

[41] Bartenschlager R, Lohmann V, Penin F. The molecular and structural basis of advanced antiviral therapy for hepatitis C virus infection. Nat Rev Microbiol 2013;11(7):482—96.

[42] Gehring S, Gregory SH, Wintermeyer P, et al. Generation of immune responses against hepatitis C virus by dendritic cells containing NS5 protein-coated microparticles. Clin Vaccine Immunol 2009;16(2):163—71.

[43] Biswal BK, Cherney MM, Wang M, et al. Crystal structures of the RNA-dependent RNA polymerase genotype 2a of hepatitis C virus reveal two conformations and suggest mechanisms of inhibition by non-nucleoside inhibitors. J Biol Chem 2005;280(18):18202—10.

[44] Jin Z, Leveque V, Ma H, et al. Assembly, purification, and pre-steady-state kinetic analysis of active RNA-dependent RNA polymerase elongation complex. J Biol Chem 2012;287(13):10674—83.

[45] Rigat K, Wang Y, Hudyma TW, et al. Ligand-induced changes in hepatitis C virus NS5B polymerase structure. Antiviral Res 2010;88 (2):197—206.

[46] Boyce SE, Tirunagari N, Niedziela-Majka A, et al. Structural and regulatory elements of HCV NS5B polymerase-b-loop and C-terminal tail—are required for activity of allosteric thumb site II inhibitors. PLoS One 9(1):e84808.

[47] Bressanelli S, Tomei L, Roussel A, et al. Crystal structure of the RNA-dependent RNA polymerase of hepatitis C virus. Proc Natl Acad Sci U S A 1999;96(23):13034—9.

[48] Lesburg CA, Cable MB, Ferrari E, et al. Crystal structure of the RNA-dependent RNA polymerase from hepatitis C virus reveals a fully encircled active site. Nat Struct Biol 1999;6(10):937—43.

[49] Poch O, Sauvaget i, Delarue M, et al. Identification of four conserved motifs among the RNA-dependent polymerase encoding elements. EMBO J 1989;8(12):3867—74.

[50] Stuyver LJ, McBrayer TR, Tharnish PM, et al. Dynamics of subgenomic hepatitis C virus replicon RNA levels in Huh-7 cells after exposure to nucleoside antimetabolites. J Virol 2003;77(19):10689—94.

[51] Stuyver LJ, Whitaker T, McBrayer TR, et al. Ribonucleoside analogue that blocks replication of bovine viral diarrhea and hepatitis C viruses in culture. Antimicrob Agents Chemother 2003;47(1):244—54.

[52] Chun B-K, Wang P, Hassan A, et al. Synthesis of 5′,9-anhydro-3-(beta-D-ribofuranosyl)xanthine, and 3,5′-anhydro-xanthosine as potential anti-hepatitis C virus agents. Tetrahedron Lett 2005;46(16):2825—7.

[53] Chun B-K, Wang P, Hassan A, et al. Synthesis and biological activity of 5′,9-anhydro-3-purine-isonucleosides as potential anti-hepatitis C virus agents. Nucleos Nucleot Nucl 2007;26(1):83—97.

[54] Furman PA, Lam AM, Murakami E. Nucleoside analog inhibitors of hepatitis C viral replication: recent advances, challenges and trends. Future Med Chem 2009;1(8):1429—52.

[55] Pierra C, Amador A, Benzaria S, et al. Synthesis and pharmacokinetics of valopicitabine (NM283), an efficient prodrug of the potent anti-HCV agent 2′-C-methylcytidine. J Med Chem 2006;49(22):6614—20.

[56] Clark JL, Hollecker L, Mason JC, et al. Design, synthesis, and antiviral activity of 2′-deoxy-2′-fluoro-2′-methylcytidine, a potent inhibitor of hepatitis C virus replication. J Med Chem 2005;48(17):5504—8.

[57] Sofia MJ, Bao D, Chang W, et al. Discovery of a β-D-2′-deoxy-2′-α-fluoro-2′-β-C-methyluridine nucleotide prodrug (PSI-7977) for the treatment of hepatitis C virus. J Med Chem 2010;53(19):7202—18.

[58] Murakami E, Niu CR, Bao HY, et al. The mechanism of action of beta-D-2′-deoxy-2′-fluoro-2′-C-methylcytidine involves a second metabolic pathway leading to beta-D-2′-deoxy-2-fluoro-2′-C-methyluridine 5′-triphosphate, a potent inhibitor of the hepatitis C virus RNA-dependent RNA polymerase. Antimicrob Agents Chemother 2008;52(2):458—64.

[59] Ma H, Jiang WR, Robledo N, et al. Characterization of the metabolic activation of hepatitis C virus nucleoside inhibitor beta-D-2′-deoxy-2′-fluoro-2′-C-methylcytidine (PSI-6130) and identification of a novel active 5′-triphosphate species. J Biol Chem 2007;282(41):29812—20.

[60] Stuyver LJ, McBrayer TR, Tharnish PM, et al. Inhibition of hepatitis C replicon RNA synthesis by beta-D-2′-deoxy-2′-fluoro-2′-C-methylcytidine: a specific inhibitor of hepatitis C virus replication. Antivir Chem Chemother 2006;17(2):79—87.

[61] Albert A. Chemical aspects of selective toxicity. Nature 1958;182(4633):421—2.

[62] Rautio J, Kumpulainen H, Heimbach T, Oliyai R, et al. Prodrugs: design and clinical applications. Nat Rev Drug Discov 2008;7(3):255—70.

[63] Shen T-Y. Discovery of sulindac, a reversible prodrug, as a second-generation indomethacin. The search for anti-inflammatory drugs: case histories from concepts to clinic. Boston, MA: Birkhäuser Boston; 1995. p. 105–28.

[64] Sofia M.A. Sofosbuvir: the discovery of a curative therapy for the treatment of hepatitis C virus. Successful drug discovery. Wiley-VCH Verlag GmbH & Co. KGaA: Weinheim, Germany: 163-188.

[65] Guedj J, Dahari H, Shudo E, et al. Hepatitis C viral kinetics with the nucleoside polymerase inhibitor mericitabine (RG7128). Hepatology 2012;55(4):1030–7.

[66] Wedemeyer H, Jensen D, Herring R, et al. PROPEL: a randomized trial of mericitabine plus peginterferon alpha-2a/ribavirin therapy in treatment-naive HCV genotype 1/4 patients. Hepatology 2013;58(2):524–37.

[67] Wedemeyer H, Forns X, Hézode C, et al. Mericitabine and either boceprevir or telaprevir in combination with peginterferon alfa-2a plus ribavirin for patients with chronic hepatitis C genotype 1 infection and prior null response: the randomized DYNAMO 1 and DYNAMO 2 studies. PLoS One 2016;11(1):e0145409.

[68] Gane EJ, Roberts SK, Stedman CAM, et al. Oral combination therapy with a nucleoside polymerase inhibitor (RG7128) and danoprevir for chronic hepatitis C genotype 1 infection (INFORM-1): a randomised, double-blind, placebo-controlled, dose-escalation trial. Lancet 2010;376 (9751):1467–75.

[69] Lalezari J, Gane E, Rodriguez-Torres M, et al. Potent antiviral activity of the HCV nucleoside polymerase inhibitor R7128 with peg-IFN and ribavirin: interim results of R7128 500mg BID for 28 days. J Hepatol 2008;48:S29.

[70] Rodriguez-Torres M, Lalezari J, Gane EJ, et al. Potent antiviral response to the HCV nucleoside polymerase inhibitor R7128 for 28 days with peg-IFN and ribavirin: subanalysis by race/ethnicity, weight and HCV genotype. Hepatology 2008;48(4):1160a.

[71] Le Pogam S, Seshaadri A, Ewing A, et al. RG7128 alone or in combination with pegylated interferon-alpha2a and ribavirin prevents hepatitis C virus (HCV) replication and selection of resistant variants in HCV-infected patients. J Infect Dis 2010;202(10):1510–19.

[72] Gane EJ, Rodriguez-Torres M, Nelson DR, et al. Antiviral activity of the HCV nucleoside polymerase inhibitor R7128 in HCV genotype 2 and 3 prior non-responders: interim results of R7128 1500mg BID with peg-IFN and ribavirin for 28 days. Hepatology 2008;48(4):1024a.

[73] Gane EJ, Rodriguez-Torres M, Nelson DE, et al. Sustained virologic response (SVR) following RG7128 1500mg BID/peg-IFN/RBN for 28 days in HCV genotype 2/3 prior non-responders. J Hepatol 2010;52:S16.

[74] Mcguigan C, Pathirana RN, Mahmood N, et al. Aryl phosphate derivatives of AZT inhibit HIV replication in cells where the nucleoside is poorly active. Bioorg Med Chem Lett 1992;2(7):701–4.

[75] Rodriguez-Torres M, Lawitz E, Kowdley KV, et al. Sofosbuvir (GS-7977) plus peginterferon/ribavirin in treatment-naive patients with HCV genotype 1: a randomized, 28-day, dose-ranging trial. J Hepatol 2013;58(4):663–8.

[76] Gane EJ, Stedman CA, Hyland RH, et al. Nucleotide polymerase inhibitor sofosbuvir plus ribavirin for hepatitis C. New Engl J Med 2013;368 (1):34–44.

[77] Lam AM, Espiritu C, Bansal S, et al. Genotype and subtype profiling of PSI-7977 as a nucleotide inhibitor of hepatitis C virus. Antimicrob Agents Chemother 2012;56(6):3359–68.

[78] Cahard D, McGuigan C, Balzarini J. Aryloxy phosphoramidate triesters as pro-tides. Mini Rev Med Chem 2004;4(4):371–81.

[79] Mehellou Y, Rattan HS, Balzarini J. The ProTide prodrug technology: from the concept to the clinic. J Med Chem 2018;61(6):2211–26.

[80] Alanazi AS, James E, Mehellou Y. The ProTide prodrug technology: where next? ACS Med Chem Lett 2019;10(1):2–5.

Chapter 10

The first HIV-1 integrase inhibitor, raltegravir

Xiaoqing Wang[1], Xiaowen Wei[2] and Hong Shen[3]

[1]Roche Innovation Center Shanghai, Shanghai, P.R. China, [2]WuXi AppTec, Shanghai, P.R. China, [3]China Innovation Center of Roche (CICoR), Shanghai, P.R. China

Chapter outline

10.1 AIDS and HIV 211	10.3.4 Optimization of dihydroxy pyrimidine lead compound 226
10.1.1 Discovery, transmission, and current status of AIDS 211	10.3.5 Clinical investigation of raltegravir 232
10.1.2 Structure and replication of HIV 212	10.4 Research on the synthetic process of raltegravir 234
10.2 Anti-HIV drugs 213	10.4.1 Synthetic route in medicinal chemistry 234
10.2.1 Classification of anti-HIV drugs 213	10.4.2 Optimization of the first-generation synthetic process 234
10.2.2 Drug resistance to HIV 214	10.4.3 Optimization of the second-generation synthetic process 236
10.3 The discovery journey of raltegravir 215	10.5 Summary and knowledge expansion 239
10.3.1 Structure and mechanism of action of HIV-1 integrase 215	10.5.1 Summary of the discovery journey of raltegravir 239
10.3.2 Discovery and optimization of hit compounds 216	10.5.2 Knowledge expansion 241
10.3.3 Optimization of 1,6-naphthyridine lead compound 221	References 242

10.1 AIDS and HIV

10.1.1 Discovery, transmission, and current status of AIDS

Acquired immunodeficiency syndrome (AIDS), also known as human immunodeficiency syndrome, was first reported in 1981 [1] and rapidly emerged as a highly lethal communicable disease on a global scale. In 1983, scientists successfully isolated the human immunodeficiency virus (HIV) [2], confirming its role as the culprit behind AIDS. HIV primarily attacks CD4 T-lymphocytes within the human body, causing a significant decline in their numbers and subsequently resulting in varying degrees of immune system dysfunction. Untreated HIV-infected individuals are prone to developing severe opportunistic infections and malignant tumors in the advanced stages of the disease, ultimately leading to patient mortality.

The transmission of AIDS primarily occurs through three main pathways:

1. Sexual transmission: Sexual contact is the chief mode of HIV transmission. Unsafe sexual practices, both homosexual and heterosexual, can transmit HIV to sexual partners through seminal fluid or vaginal secretions. Therefore, the use of barrier methods, such as condoms, can greatly reduce the transmission of AIDS.
2. Bloodborne transmission: AIDS can be transmitted through blood, including the transfusion of HIV-infected blood or blood products, the sharing of injection needles for intravenous drug use, and invasive procedures that do not adhere to safety regulations, such as tattooing and eyeliner tattooing. Choosing reputable healthcare facilities and refraining from substance abuse can effectively prevent the spread of AIDS.
3. Mother-to-child transmission: HIV-infected mothers can transmit the virus to their offspring during pregnancy, childbirth, or breastfeeding. Medications can intervene to reduce the risk of mother-to-child transmission.

The AIDS epidemic once sparked profound societal panic. However, with the continuous discovery of anti-HIV drugs, AIDS has transformed from a fatal disease into a manageable chronic condition. While current medical interventions do not offer a complete cure, proper medication adherence enables individuals with AIDS to achieve lifespans and quality of life comparable to those without the disease. As of 2019, there were approximately 38 million people worldwide living with HIV. In the same year, there were 1.7 million new HIV infections globally, marking a downward trend in new infections for the past 20 years. The number of AIDS-related deaths also decreased from 17 million in 2004 to 6.9 million in 2019. These improvements underscore the significant impact of increased awareness of prevention strategies and advancements in anti-HIV therapy. However, regional disparities persist in the prevalence of AIDS, with Eastern and Southern Africa being the most severely affected regions, housing approximately 54% of global HIV carriers [3,4].

10.1.2 Structure and replication of HIV

HIV is a lentivirus, a type of retrovirus, consisting of two subtypes: HIV-1 and HIV-2 [5]. These subtypes can both impair the immune function of the human body, but they only share approximately 55% of their genetic sequence [6]. Approximately 95% of HIV carriers are infected with the HIV-1 subtype, while HIV-2 is predominantly found in a small number of individuals in West Africa and exhibits significantly lower transmission capacity compared to HIV-1. Similar to other lentiviruses, HIV has a relatively long latency period, typically ranging from 6 to 10 years.

HIV is generally spherical in shape (Fig. 10.1), with a radius of approximately 120 nm, only about 1/60th the size of a red blood cell [7]. The virus is enveloped, and the membrane is covered with numerous envelope proteins (spikes) that are responsible for host cell recognition. The envelope proteins consist of three glycoproteins (gp120) that assemble together to form a cap, which is connected to the viral membrane by three other glycoproteins (gp41) [8]. Inside the membrane is the matrix protein, which surrounds the viral core and various enzymes to ensure the integrity of the virus. The viral core is ellipsoidal and consists of tightly connected arrangements of around 2000 identical proteins. Within the core, there are two identical single-stranded RNA molecules that encode the virus's nine genes. The RNA is tightly associated with the nucleocapsid. Additionally, various enzymes required for viral replication, such as reverse transcriptase (RT), integrase, RNase, etc., are also encapsulated within the core.

The replication cycle of the virus encompasses four stages: fusion and entry, replication, release, and maturation (Fig. 10.2).

1. Fusion and entry [9,10]: In the human body, immune cells such as CD4 T-lymphocytes possess a receptor known as CD4, which aids in immune cell recognition of antigens. CD4 also functions as the receptor for HIV. Initially, HIV utilizes the envelope protein gp120 to recognize and bind to the CD4 receptor on the surface of immune cells. Subsequently, there is a conformational change in gp120, enabling it to bind to coreceptors on the immune cell surface, such as CCR5 or CXCR4. This interaction allows the distal end of gp41 to insert into the host cell membrane, leading to protein folding and fusion of the viral membrane with the host cell membrane. Finally, the virus's capsid encapsulates RNA and various enzymes as it enters the host cell.

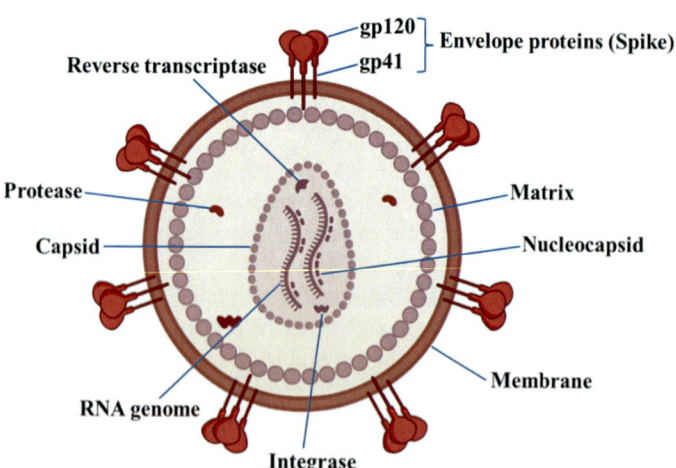

FIGURE 10.1 The structure of HIV.

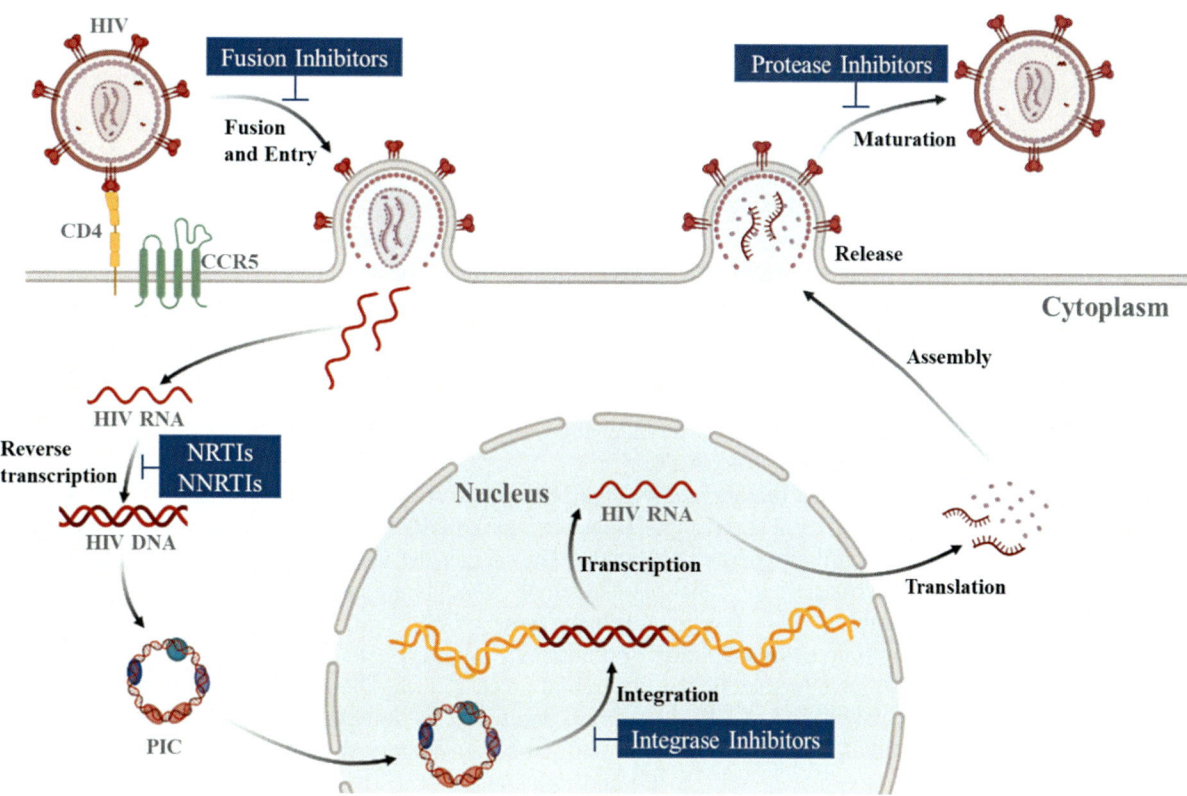

FIGURE 10.2 The replication cycle of HIV.

2. Replication [11]: Upon entering the host cell, HIV first sheds its capsid. Subsequently, under the action of RT, the single-stranded RNA dissociates from the attached nucleocapsid and undergoes reverse transcription to synthesize complementary DNA. However, this process of reverse transcription is prone to errors, which is a major contributing factor to the emergence of HIV drug resistance. RT also possesses the activity of ribonuclease (RNase), which simultaneously degrades the viral RNA during the formation of complementary DNA. Subsequently, RT acts as a DNA polymerase, utilizing the complementary DNA to synthesize a sense DNA strand, ultimately forming a double-stranded DNA. The newly formed viral DNA then interacts with HIV integrase, forming a preintegration complex (PIC), which enters the nucleus of the host cell. With the assistance of HIV integrase, the viral DNA becomes integrated into the host DNA. Transcription ensues, generating new RNA that is released into the cytoplasm. A portion of this RNA is processed into messenger RNA (mRNA) through trimming and subsequently translated to produce viral proteins. Another portion of the RNA serves as newly synthesized viral RNA, which, together with these viral proteins, reassembles into new HIV particles.
3. Release: The newly formed viral RNA and viral proteins initially accumulate at the inner side of the host cell membrane, following which gp41 integrates gp120 into the cell membrane. Subsequently, the viral RNA and viral proteins, enveloped by the cell membrane, are released into the extracellular space.
4. Maturation: The newly released viruses are not yet matured. The polyproteins within them are cleaved into various functional proteins, such as matrix protein, capsid protein, and nucleocapsid, by the action of protease. Subsequently, these functional proteins further assemble to form mature HIV particles. Mature HIV particles can then infect the next host cell and initiate a new replication cycle.

10.2 Anti-HIV drugs

10.2.1 Classification of anti-HIV drugs

In 1987, the FDA approved the first anti-HIV drug, zidovudine (AZT), only 6 years after the discovery of the first case of AIDS. Over the next three decades, the FDA has approved more than 50 anti-HIV drugs. These drugs can be broadly classified into the following five categories based on their mechanisms of action.

1. Fusion Inhibitors: Fusion inhibitors act at the initial step of the virus replication cycle, the fusion and entry stage. They function by inhibiting the recognition or fusion of HIV with host cells, thereby preventing HIV from infecting host cells. Currently, clinically used fusion inhibitors include maraviroc (MVC) and enfuvirtide (ENF). MVC targets the coreceptor CCR5 on the surface of CD4 T-lymphocytes, blocking the recognition between the virus and host cells. ENF, on the other hand, acts on the distal end of the viral surface protein gp41, inducing conformational changes that prevent its insertion into the cell membrane, thereby inhibiting the fusion of the virus with host cells.
2. Nucleoside Reverse Transcriptase Inhibitors (NRTIs): NRTIs act on the reverse transcription process during the viral replication stage. HIV, being an RNA virus, can only integrate into the host cell's DNA after successful reverse transcription into DNA by its RT, thereby completing its replication process. As RT is absent in the healthy human body, it becomes a highly selective target for antiviral drugs. NRTIs are nucleoside analogs that can replace normal nucleosides and participate in DNA synthesis during the virus's reverse transcription. However, due to the absence of a 3′-OH group in their structure, once NRTIs are incorporated into the DNA chain, they inhibit (terminate) subsequent DNA synthesis, thereby suppressing viral reverse transcription. Currently, clinically used drugs of this class include abacavir (ABC), lamivudine (3TC), emtricitabine (FTC), tenofovir (TDF), and the first anti-HIV drug, AZT.
3. Nonnucleoside Reverse Transcriptase Inhibitors (NNRTIs): Similar to NRTIs, NNRTIs also act on the reverse transcription process during the viral replication stage. However, unlike NRTIs, these inhibitors do not belong to the nucleoside analog class based on their chemical structure. They target the allosteric site of RT, preventing it from performing its normal reverse transcription function. Therefore, NNRTIs are considered noncompetitive inhibitors. Currently, clinically used drugs of this class include nevirapine (NVP), efavirenz (EFV), and etravirine (ETR), among others. It is important to note that these drugs do not have inhibitory effects on HIV-2.
4. Integrase Inhibitors: Integrase inhibitors act on the integration process during the viral replication stage. These drugs function by binding to the catalytic site of HIV-1 integrase, inhibiting the integration of viral DNA into host DNA, thus suppressing viral replication and proliferation. In 2007, the FDA approved the first HIV-1 integrase inhibitor, raltegravir (RAL). Subsequently, elvitegravir (EVG) and dolutegravir (DTG) were approved by the FDA in 2012 and 2013, respectively.
5. Protease Inhibitors (PIs): PIs act on the maturation stage of the virus. Under the influence of these drugs, the protease enzyme is unable to cleave the polyproteins within newly formed viruses into various functional proteins, such as matrix protein and capsid protein, thereby impeding viral maturation. Consequently, immature HIV particles are rendered noninfectious. As of 2018, the FDA has approved over 10 HIV PIs. Among them, darunavir (DRV) and atazanavir (ATV) are currently recommended as first-line therapies [12].

10.2.2 Drug resistance to HIV

The approval of the first anti-HIV drug, AZT, brought a glimmer of hope to AIDS patients. However, it was soon discovered that after a certain period of treatment, the viral levels in patients whose symptoms had been temporarily controlled would rise again, and the previously used drugs would no longer be effective.

Within the human body, HIV replicates at a remarkably fast pace, with infected individuals producing an average of 10.3×10^9 viruses per day. The lifecycle of each virus, from generation to infecting another cell and producing new viruses, takes an average of only 2.6 days [13]. During the replication process, errors often occur during the reverse transcription of RNA into DNA. As HIV lacks proofreading enzymes, it undergoes mutations at a rapid rate. Although some mutations are disadvantageous to the virus itself, such as decreasing its infectivity, others reflect the superiority of natural selection, allowing the mutated HIV to resist previously encountered antiviral drugs, thus developing drug resistance.

Although several NRTIs have been approved and introduced to the market in the subsequent years, the rapid development of HIV drug resistance has hindered the effectiveness of AIDS treatment. This is especially true as multidrug-resistant HIV mutations have emerged, prompting scientists to continue developing anti-HIV drugs with different mechanisms of action and devising new treatment strategies. Against this backdrop, cocktail therapy, also known as cocktail treatment, emerged in 1996 [14]. Clinical practitioners at the time discovered that when patients simultaneously received three to four different anti-HIV drugs, HIV levels in their bodies rapidly decreased to undetectable limits. It was postulated that even if HIV developed mutations and acquired resistance to a particular drug during treatment, the concomitant use of other medications could still inhibit the replication of the mutated virus. Consequently, cocktail therapy was established as the standard treatment for AIDS [12]. Clinical research data indicates that cocktail therapy typically consists of a combination of three distinct drugs with at least two different mechanisms of action, requiring long-term adherence to medication by patients. Nonadherence to the prescribed drug regimen significantly increases the risk of viral drug resistance. However, the concurrent administration of multiple drugs also increases the risk of side effects and places a financial burden on patients, subsequently decreasing medication adherence.

Combining 3–4 different medications in specific proportions into a single tablet not only yields excellent therapeutic results but also greatly simplifies the medication regimen, effectively improving patient adherence. Presently, the market's top-selling drugs, Triumeq (ABC/3TC/DTG) and Stribild (EVG/FTC/TDF), consist of an integrase inhibitor combined with two NRTIs (Stribild also contains a CYP3A4 inhibitor).

As mentioned previously, integrase inhibitors play a pivotal role in the therapeutic approach of HIV cocktail therapy. This chapter will primarily delve into the discovery journey of the first integrase inhibitor, RAL, in subsequent sections.

10.3 The discovery journey of raltegravir

10.3.1 Structure and mechanism of action of HIV-1 integrase

The HIV-1 integrase is a 32 kDa protein (Fig. 10.3), comprising three structural domains: the N-terminal domain [15], the catalytic core domain (CCD) [16], and the C-terminal domain [17]. Within the CCD, the amino acid residues D64, D116, and E152 form the catalytic triad, constituting the active site of the HIV-1 integrase. In living organisms, the integrase exists as a dimer or other oligomeric forms [18], and the interactions between subunits exhibit a highly dynamic nature [19]. Each monomer on the dimeric CCD interface features four α-helical structures (α1, α3, α5, and α6) and one β-folded structure (β3). Strong hydrophobic and electrostatic interactions exist between α1 and α5′, as well as α1′ and α5, critically stabilizing the dimeric structure [16].

As previously mentioned, the primary function of HIV-1 integrase is to catalyze the integration of viral and host DNA, whereby only the viral DNA integrated into the host DNA can be successfully transcribed into viral RNA and ultimately translated into viral proteins. The catalytic process of integrase can be divided into three key steps: assembly of the PIC, 3′ end processing (3′-P), and strand transfer (ST) [20–22].

1. Assembly of the PIC: Initially, the ends of the viral DNA chain bind to the catalytic sites of the dimeric integrase, forming a stable PIC. In addition to integrase and viral DNA, this complex comprises components such as the matrix, RT, nucleocapsid, and viral proteins [23–25]. These constituents play vital roles in the transfer and functionality of the complex. Additionally, the complex contains certain host cell proteins [26] that activate integrase, regulate integration processes, promote intermolecular integration, and suppress self-integration, among other functions.

2. 3′ End Processing: The 3′-P takes place in the cytoplasm of the host cell. The 3′ end of the viral DNA, synthesized by RT, is composed of four nucleotides: cytosine, adenine, guanine, thymine (CAGT). During this process, the guanine, thymine (GT) units at the 3′ ends of both viral DNA strands are cleaved by integrase, exposing the cytosine, adenine (CA) units at the ends of the chains. This cleaving step not only facilitates the subsequent binding of the host DNA but also provides spatial accommodation. After the excision of the GT units, integrase and viral DNA remain in the form of the PIC as they enter the nucleus of the host cell, initiating the next step, ST (Fig. 10.4).

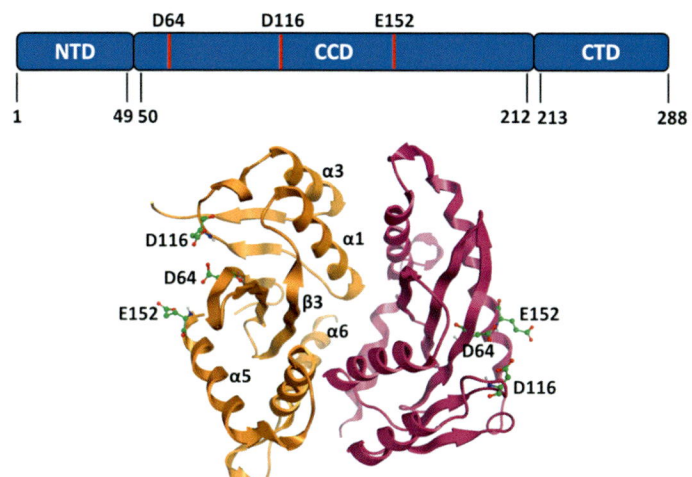

FIGURE 10.3 Protein sequence diagram of HIV-1 integrase and tertiary structure of the catalytic core domain.

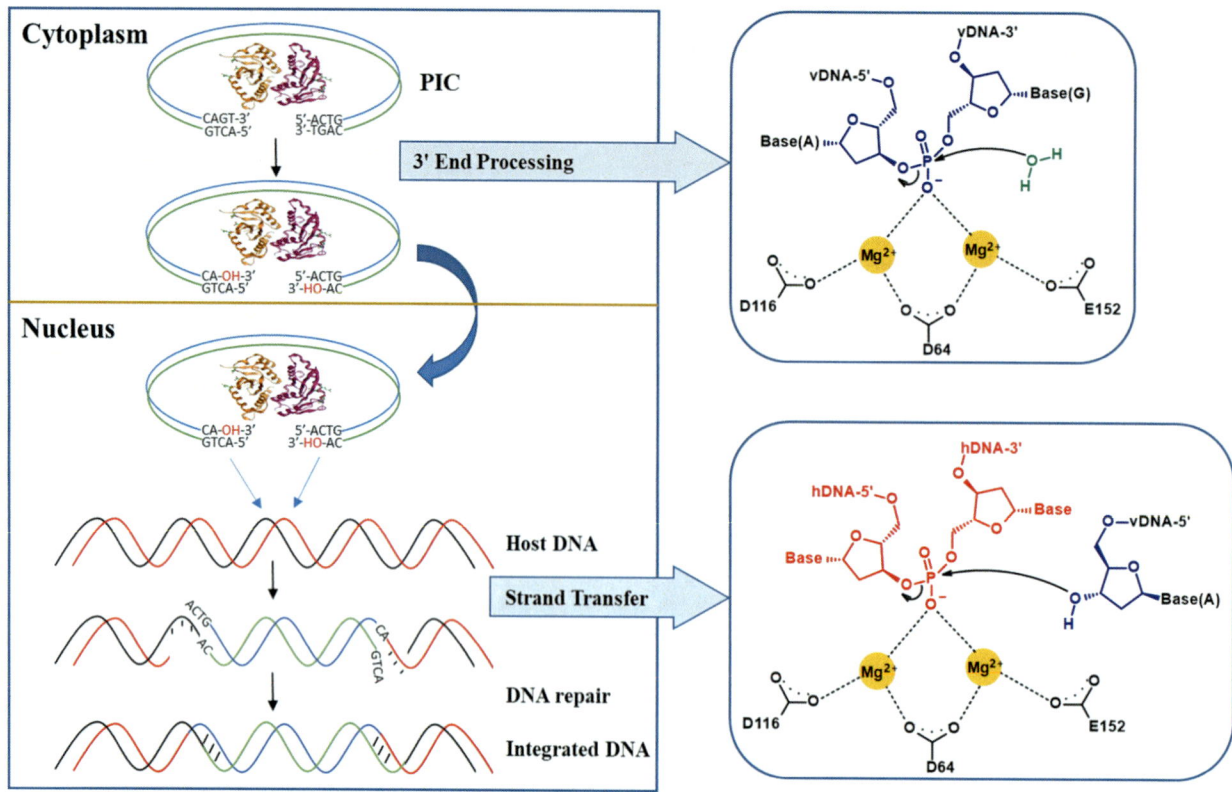

FIGURE 10.4 Integration process of viral DNA and host DNA catalyzed by HIV-1 integrase.

3. Strand Transfer: During the ST process, the host DNA initially binds to the catalytic site of integrase, followed by the joining of the viral DNA's 3′ end with the complementary strand of the host DNA. Lastly, facilitated by the host cell polymerase, the viral DNA's 5′ end undergoes cleavage and connects with the other complementary strand of the host DNA, completing the entirety of the ST process (Fig. 10.4).

The hydrolysis of nucleotides during the 3′-P and the subsequent ST process involves a bivalent magnesium ion-mediated phosphodiester hydrolysis and ester exchange process, respectively (Fig. 10.4). At the catalytic site of integrase, two bivalent magnesium ions interact with the catalytic triad (D64, D116, and E152) and the phosphoryl group of the DNA, enhancing the stability of the PIC and activating the phosphoryl group, making it more susceptible to attack by nucleophiles. During the 3′-P, the nucleophile is mainly water, leading to the hydrolysis of the phosphodiester bond between the A and G at the 3′ end of the viral DNA. On the other hand, during the ST process, the nucleophile is the CA-3′-OH of the viral DNA, causing an ester exchange reaction in the phosphodiester bond of the host DNA, thereby linking the viral DNA to the host DNA [20]. Therefore, from the perspective of drug design, it is possible to develop a small molecule compound that inhibits the interaction between magnesium ions and viral DNA or host DNA, thereby preventing ester hydrolysis during the 3′-P or ester exchange during the ST process, achieving the goal of inhibiting the action of integrase.

10.3.2 Discovery and optimization of hit compounds

Due to the crucial role of HIV-1 integrase in the replication of the virus and the absence of integrase in the human body, it serves as a selective target for anti-HIV drugs. The research on integrase inhibitors began in the 1990s, with early molecular studies including peptides [27], nucleosides, oligonucleotides [28], and polyhydroxy aromatic compounds. Some of these small molecule inhibitors are derived from natural products [29–32], while others are designed through medicinal chemistry approaches [33–35]. The biological activity screening models primarily rely on purified or recombinant HIV-1 integrase as the basis, (Fig. 10.5, left), along with viral DNA, host DNA, and the compounds being simultaneously added to the test system. Therefore, even if a compound exhibits the desired bioactivity, it is

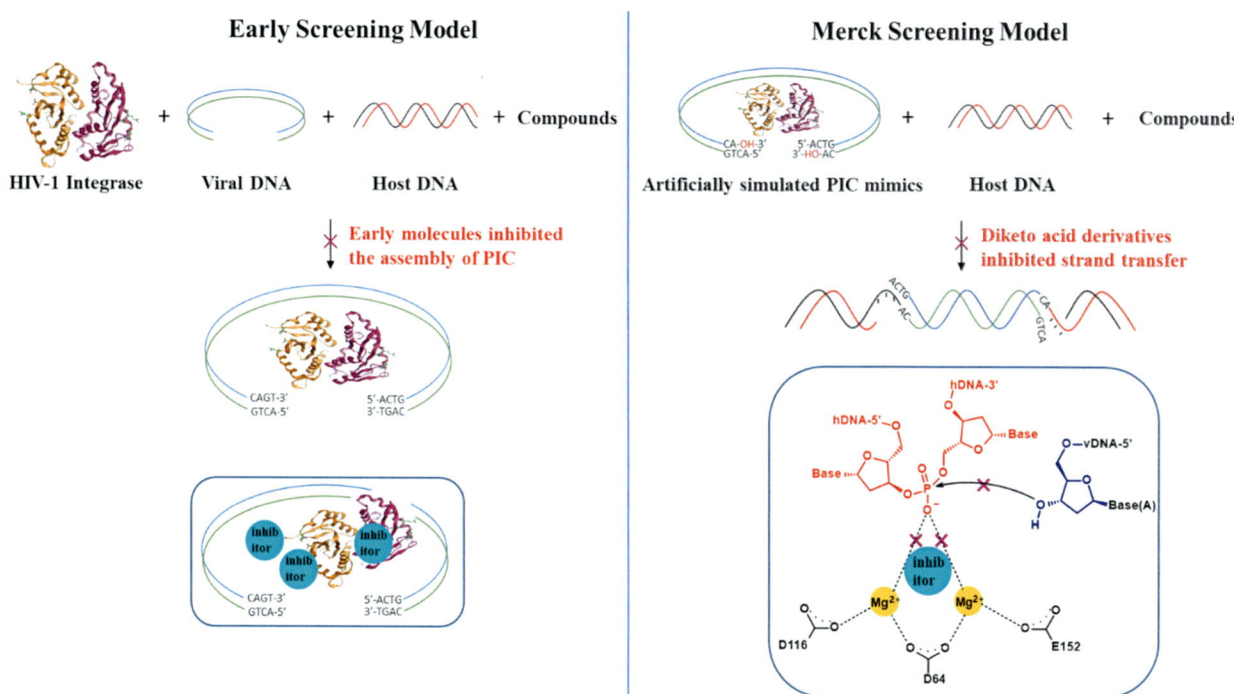

FIGURE 10.5 Early screening model and Merck screening model for HIV-1 integrase inhibitors.

challenging to quickly discern at which specific step of the integration process the active compound inhibits. Retrospective studies have shown that these early discoveries of so-called HIV-1 integrase inhibitors merely affect the assembly process of the PIC [36–38]. Since the assembly of the PIC is a prerequisite for integrase to exert its catalytic function, these early molecules, although seemingly inhibitory to the catalytic process of integrase, fail to demonstrate the expected inhibitory effects when evaluated using preassembled PICs or at the cellular level. In fact, the compound libraries screened in the early stages did not contain molecules that truly inhibited the ST step, thereby contributing to the unsuccessful identification of active molecules at the cellular level at that time.

To discover small molecules that can effectively inhibit the catalytic process of HIV-1 integrase, researchers at Merck Laboratories in Pennsylvania, United States, utilized a unique bioactivity screening model based on the biochemical mechanism of integrase [39]. In this model (Fig. 10.5, right), recombinant HIV-1 integrase was combined with specific HIV-1 oligonucleotides, followed by 3'-P, thereby creating a mimic of the postprocessed PIC. This mimic was then used for bioactivity screening, allowing for the identification of active compounds with ST inhibitory capabilities. Using this model, Merck scientists focused on screening their own proprietary library of influenza virus nucleic acid endonuclease inhibitors (as the structure and function of influenza virus nucleic acid endonuclease are similar to HIV-1 integrase). They discovered a class of diketo acid derivatives that exhibited activity in inhibiting ST. These compounds demonstrated a good correlation with the activity measured using preassembled PICs isolated from infected cells, confirming that these artificially simulated complex mimics can properly execute the functions of the PIC. Taking the hit compounds L-731988 and L-708906 (Fig. 10.6) as examples, the measured inhibitory activity against ST (ST IC_{50}) in this model was 50 and 100 nM, respectively. The IC_{50} values obtained using preassembled PICs isolated from infected cells were 80 and 150 nM, respectively. These two compounds were reported to be the most potent inhibitors of HIV-1 integrase at that time. In cellular level functional tests, scientists used MT4 human T-lymphocyte cells infected with HIV-1 virus and cultured in medium containing 10% fetal bovine serum (FBS). Both compounds also exhibited antiviral activity, with IC_{95} values (FBS IC_{95}) of 9.6 and 17.7 μM, respectively. They were also the earliest reported compounds to demonstrate HIV-1 integrase inhibitory activity in cellular assays. Further investigations revealed that these compounds had no inhibitory effect on viral fusion and entry, reverse transcription, PIC assembly, or 3'-P. Interestingly, these two compounds could induce mutations in HIV-1, resulting in the generation of new mutants, with the mutations occurring near the catalytic triad D64-D116-E152 of integrase (L-731988 induced T66I and S153Y mutations; L-708906 induced T66I and M154I mutations). These experimental results indirectly confirmed that these two compounds inhibit the ST process by binding to the catalytic site of integrase.

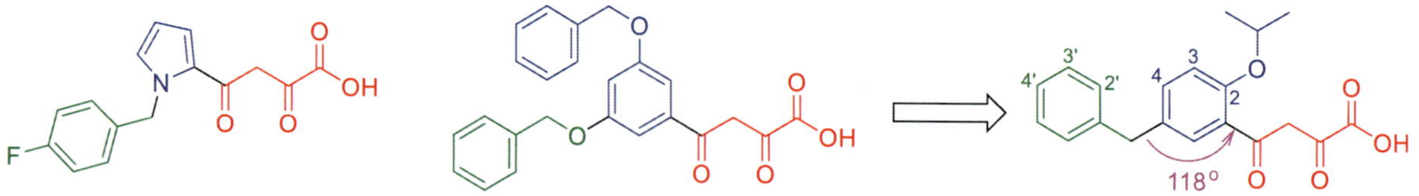

FIGURE 10.6 SAR of diketo acid derivatives.

	L-731988	L-708906	1
ST IC$_{50}$ (nM):	50	100	<100
FBS IC$_{95}$ (nM):	9 600	17 700	100

From a structural perspective, hit compounds are composed of three parts (Fig. 10.6): the diketo acid moiety on the right side (highlighted in red), the central (blue) and left (green) aromatic rings. Scientists conducted structure-activity relationship (SAR) studies on these three parts [40], and the results revealed the following:

1. The diketo acid structure on the right side is the pharmacophore of these compounds, playing a critical role in maintaining their activity. The 1,3-diketo acid structure can effectively mimic the phosphoryl group in DNA, suggesting that these compounds likely exert their inhibitory effects by chelating with the metal ions in the integrase through the 1,3-diketo acid structure (Fig. 10.7).
2. The central aromatic ring acts as a linker between the left and right parts. A 5-membered (L-731988) or 6-membered (L-708906) aromatic ring both exhibit some degree of activity, but the optimal angle between the two opposing parts is 118 degrees, indicating that a meta-substituted benzene ring has the best activity. The activity can be further enhanced by substituting the 2-position of the benzene ring with an alkoxyl group, with the 2-isopropoxy group showing the highest activity.
3. The benzene ring of the left benzyl group can be replaced by other aromatic heterocycles, but the activity is generally reduced. The benzene ring can also be substituted by smaller halogen atoms or methyl groups.

After careful SAR studies, it was discovered that compound 1 (Fig. 10.6) exhibited optimal ST inhibitory activity (ST IC$_{50}$ < 100 nM) and antiviral activity at the cellular level (FBS IC$_{95}$ = 100 nM), surpassing the cellular inhibitory activity of L-731988 by nearly 100-fold. Furthermore, compound 1 showed no cytotoxicity at 50 μM, indicating a higher therapeutic index (therapeutic index = EC$_{50}$/CC$_{50}$, calculated by dividing the antiviral activity EC$_{50}$ by the compound's cytotoxicity CC$_{50}$ at the cellular level). However, the diketo acid structure of such compounds has a tendency to bind with glutathione in the human body, undergo decarboxylation reactions in alkaline environments, and exhibit poor cellular permeability, posing challenges for further development of diketo acid-based compounds. Despite these limitations, this class of compounds remained the only confirmed inhibitors of ST at the time, leaving the project team with no alternative options. Therefore, based on an understanding of the pharmacophore, the team focused on designing alternative structures or bioisosteres to replace the diketo acid moiety.

In the diketo acid structure, the carboxyl group plays a significant role and possesses both proton acidity and Lewis basicity. However, at that time, researchers were uncertain about which characteristic of the carboxyl group influenced the inhibition of integrase activity. Therefore, medicinal chemists replaced the carboxyl group with the basic pyridine, resulting in compound 3, which displayed ST inhibitory activity and antiviral activity at the cellular level (Fig. 10.8). When the pyridine was replaced with a benzene ring or when the nitrogen atom in the pyridine ring was shifted to the 3-position, the activity was completely lost. These findings suggested that the carboxyl group in the diketo acid serves as a Lewis base, and this role could be substituted by the basicity exhibited by the nitrogen atom in the aromatic heterocycle. Further SAR studies revealed that introducing an aromatic heterocycle through a methylene at the 3-position of the central aromatic ring could enhance the activity. Similar to the aromatic heterocycle, a 5-membered cyclic sulfonamide also increased the antiviral activity at the cellular level (compound 4), with its IC$_{95}$ value being half of the previous diketo acid compound 2 in medium containing 10% FBS.

At this juncture, Shionogi & Co., Ltd. in Japan and the National Institutes of Health (NIH) in the United States adopted the soaking approach, leading to the first elucidation of the crystal structure of the CCD of HIV-1 integrase in complex with small molecule inhibitors [41]. The small molecule, 5-CITEP, also features a diaryl diketone structure (Fig. 10.9), wherein the molecule utilizes tetrazole as a substituent for the carboxyl group. Although 5-CITEP possesses a certain degree of ST inhibitory activity (ST IC$_{50}$ = 2.1 μM), it does not exhibit antiviral activity at the cellular level (IC$_{95}$ > 50 μM). In the crystal structure of the complex, two small molecules occupy the catalytic site of integrase in a dimeric form, with each molecule adopting an approximate planar conformation. Contrary to the earlier speculation of

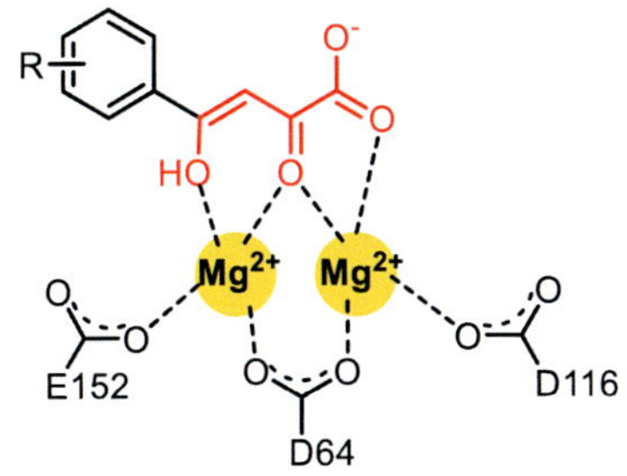

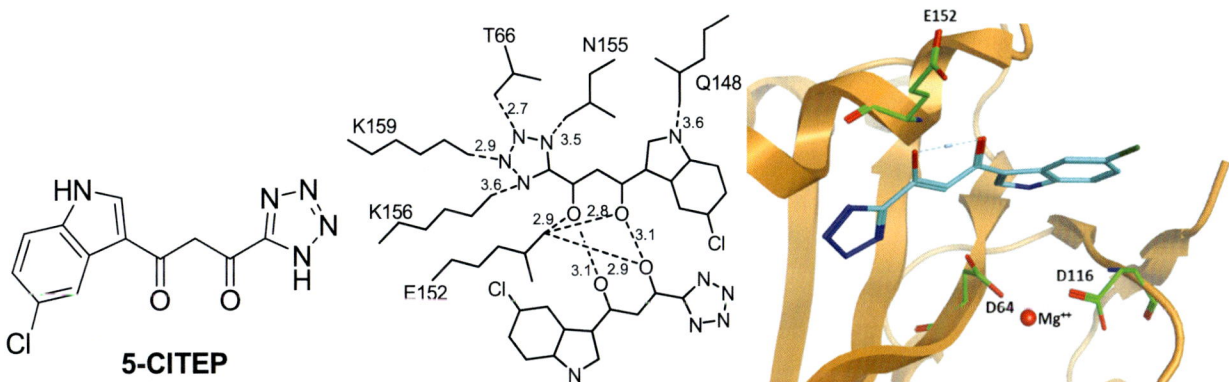

FIGURE 10.7 Proposed binding mode of diketo acid derivatives with HIV-1 integrase.

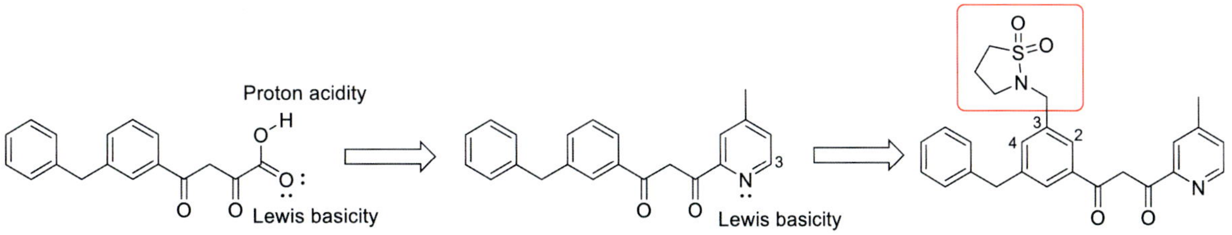

FIGURE 10.8 Design and optimization of diaryl diketone derivatives.

FIGURE 10.9 Molecular structure of 5-CITEP and its crystal structure in complex with the catalytic core domain of HIV-1 integrase.

Merck scientists, the small molecules do not interact with metal ions, but rather form hydrogen bonds solely with the E152 residue of the catalytic triad. In fact, this co-crystal structure was obtained under artificially designed in vitro experimental conditions and does not reflect the true physiological conditions. Subsequent research findings confirmed that this crystal structure did not substantially contribute to the development of RAL. Fortunately, based on the results of SAR studies, Merck scientists persevered with their own conjectures, and the outcome of this article did not alter their optimization direction. Ultimately, they successfully discovered the first HIV-1 integrase inhibitor, RAL. This fact strongly emphasizes the importance for researchers to maintain a vigilant scientific critical thinking mindset during the drug discovery process. This applies not only to their own experimental results but also to the reported findings in the literature.

During medicinal chemistry research, it is common to employ cyclization strategies or introduce intramolecular hydrogen bonds to constrain the conformation of compounds to precisely match the conformation required for binding with proteins. This approach often leads to a significant enhancement of the compound's biological activity. Hence, starting from compound 3, scientists have fused the diketone motif with the pyridine on the right side by introducing a benzene ring, yielding compound 5 (Fig. 10.10), thereby fixing the conformation of the pyridine and diketone moiety. However, the activity of this compound was diminished [42]. It is postulated that there is steric repulsion between the

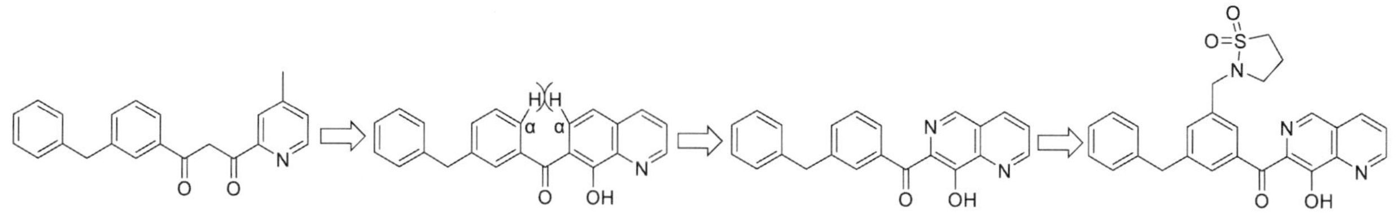

220 Medicinal Chemistry and Drug Development

	3	5	6	7
ST IC$_{50}$ (nM):	200	370	40	10
FBS IC$_{95}$ (nM):	5 000	5 000	6 200	390

FIGURE 10.10 Evolution of diaryl diketone compounds to 1,6-naphthyridine compounds.

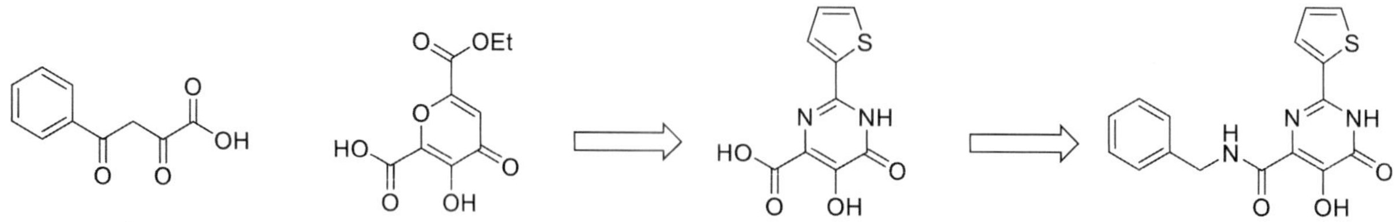

FIGURE 10.11 Hit compounds of HCV polymerase inhibitor and their evolution to dihydroxypyrimidine compounds.

α-H atoms on both sides of the carbonyl group, causing the central benzene ring to deviate from coplanarity with the quinoline ring. Consequently, the conformation of compound 5 does not fully align with the desired planar conformation for molecular-protein binding, resulting in reduced activity. To achieve a more planar conformation, scientists introduced a nitrogen atom at one of the α-positions of the carbonyl group, resulting in compound 6, which indeed exhibited a significantly improved ST inhibitory activity, four times higher than that of compound 3. Building upon previous SAR findings, the introduction of a cyclic sulfonamide at the 3-position of the central benzene ring led to further enhancements in both ST inhibitory activity and antiviral activity at the cellular level, as observed in compound 7.

While Merck's research center in Pennsylvania, USA, was studying HIV-1 integrase inhibitors, their research center in Rome, Italy, was conducting research on hepatitis C virus (HCV) polymerase inhibitors. Both enzymes share significant structural and functional similarities, with a catalytic triad and chelation of two metal ions. Researchers in Rome identified two lead compounds, 8 and 9 (Fig. 10.11), with HCV polymerase inhibitory activity through high-throughput screening [43,44]. Particularly, compound 8 also possessed a diketo acid motif. Consequently, scientists from both research centers decided to collaborate on these projects and sent the synthesized molecules to each other's laboratories for activity testing. This decision greatly facilitated the research process of HIV-1 integrase inhibitors.

Although compound 9 possesses a novel scaffold, it is also unstable and prone to decarboxylation under acidic conditions. Therefore, medicinal chemists began searching for bioisosteres that preserve the carboxyl, hydroxyl, and carbonyl moieties that may participate in metal ion chelation. Compound 10, derived from the structural modification of compound 9, exhibits HCV polymerase inhibitory activity and demonstrates notable stability under both acidic and alkaline environments. Additionally, it does not undergo any covalent binding with proteins and exhibits improved drug-like properties. However, at the cellular level, compound 10 shows weak anti-HCV activity, possibly due to the presence of a carboxyl group and a highly acidic phenolic hydroxyl group in its molecular structure. Both groups exist as oxygen anions under physiological conditions, leading to excessive polarity of the molecule and poor cell permeability. In an effort to enhance cell permeability, medicinal chemists explored several bioisosteres of carboxylic acids, including amides and esters. Unfortunately, none of these attempts yielded compounds with higher HCV polymerase inhibitory activity. However, when these compounds were tested for their inhibition of HIV-1 integrase activity, amide compound 11 exhibited potent ST inhibitory activity with an IC$_{50}$ value of 80 nM [45].

Although the scaffold of compound 11 differs from the previously discovered classes of HIV-1 integrase inhibitors, comparing the structures of these various series of molecules reveals that they all contain a common core structure with 1,3,4-trisubstituted heteroatoms (highlighted in red in Fig. 10.12). This structure represents the pharmacophore of HIV-1 integrase inhibitors. By overlaying the core structures of compounds 6 and 11, it becomes apparent that the benzylamine moiety in compound 11 aligns with the benzyl-substituted phenyl group in compound 6 (highlighted in blue). Leveraging the synthetic convenience of the amide bond, researchers incorporated an amide

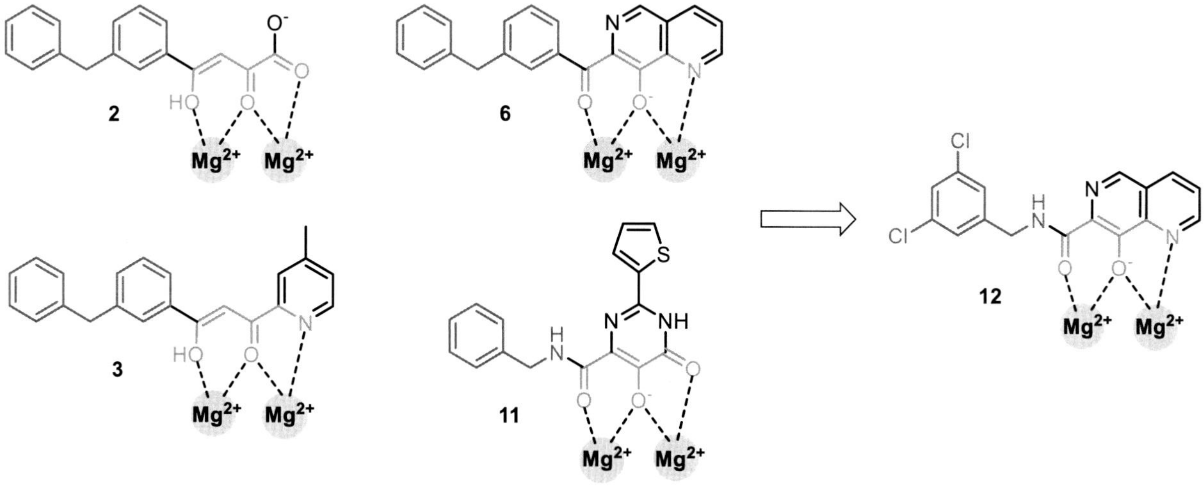

FIGURE 10.12 HIV-1 integrase inhibitors with diverse scaffolds and their proposed binding modes.

structure into compound 6, resulting in compound 12 with a novel scaffold (the introduction of two chlorine atoms enhances activity). Compound 12 still exhibits good ST inhibitory activity (IC_{50} = 90 nM) and antiviral activity at the cellular level (FBS IC_{95} = 1.2 μM) [46].

Compounds 11 and 12 exhibit favorable ST inhibitory activity and possess drug-like properties. Furthermore, they do not exhibit inhibitory activity against human DNA polymerases α, β, and γ, showcasing good selectivity. As a result, the project team identified these two compounds as lead compounds and proceeded with further optimization of the dihydroxypyrimidine compounds represented by compound 11 and the 1,6-naphthyridine compounds represented by compound 12.

10.3.3 Optimization of 1,6-naphthyridine lead compound

The two classes of lead compounds represented by 11 and 12 share a similar amide structure on the left side, indicating that the SAR on the left side are likely to be analogous. Considering synthetic convenience, medicinal chemists synthesized over 200 amide compounds with different amine fragments based on the dihydroxypyrimidine compound 11 [47]. The resulting SAR are as follows (Table 10.1):

1. The presence of an NH group is essential.
2. Substituents on nitrogen must contain a benzene ring.
3. There should be at least one sp^3 carbon atom between the benzene ring and the nitrogen atom.
4. Substitution of the CH_2 between the benzene ring and nitrogen decreases activity.
5. 4-Fluoro substitution on the benzene ring is optimal.

Similarly, for the 1,6-naphthyridine compound 12, similar SAR were observed. Amide compound formed by 4-fluoro substituted benzylamine (Table 10.3, compound 23) exhibited the most potent ST inhibitory activity with an IC_{50} value of 33 nM.

Upon comparing the structures of the two lead compounds, it is evident that apart from the difference in skeletal framework, the 5-position of the 1,6-naphthyridine lacks a thiophene moiety. Consequently, while optimizing the amine fragments in the amide group, medicinal chemists also explored the 5-position of the 1,6-naphthyridine (Table 10.2). Introducing a thiophene at the 5-position (compound 20) maintained the ST inhibitory activity (data undisclosed) but exhibited a decrease in antiviral activity at the cellular level [46]. However, introducing a piperazine at the 5-position (compound 21) further enhanced the activity, particularly in terms of its antiviral activity at the cellular level. During the synthesis of compound 21, a byproduct 22 was inadvertently generated due to the use of dimethylformamide (DMF) as a solvent. As medicinal chemistry is an empirical science, successful medicinal chemists must possess the ability to acknowledge every possibility or opportunity. Therefore, instead of disregarding this byproduct, they also tested its activity. Surprisingly, compound 22 exhibited even better activity with an antiviral activity at the cellular level of 156 nM. Subsequent research further revealed that introducing various functional groups at the 5-position maintained

TABLE 10.1 SAR of amine fragments in amide group.

Compound	R	R_1	ST IC_{50} (nM)
11	CH_2Ph	H	85
13	CH_2Ph	Me	530
14	Ph	H	1000
15	CH_2CH_2Ph	H	20
16	CH_2-cyclohexyl	H	>1000
17	4-Pyridine	H	>1000
18	$CH(CH_3)Ph$	H	200
19	$(4-F)PhCH_2$	H	10

TABLE 10.2 SAR of the 5-position of 1,6-naphthyridine compounds.

Compound	R	ST IC_{50} (nM)	FBS IC_{95} (nM)	NHS IC_{95} (nM)
12	H	90	1250	nd
20	2-thienyl	/	2500	>50,000
21	piperazinyl	70	467	1250
22	4-formylpiperazinyl	21	156	625

good antiviral activity, suggesting that this position may not directly interact with the protein but rather exist in a solvent exposed area. Therefore, modifying the functional groups at this position can fine-tune the physicochemical properties of the entire molecule without significantly affecting the compound's activity.

The cellular antiviral screening models used in the aforementioned studies employed culture media supplemented with 10% FBS. Therefore, the cellular antiviral activity was expressed as FBS IC_{95} in the previous sections. In this model, compounds generally exhibit limited binding to FBS, and mostly exist in a free form, resulting in strong inhibitory activity. However, under physiological conditions in the human body, small molecules often bind to plasma proteins, leading to a decrease in the free concentration of the compounds. It can be envisioned that the antiviral activity values obtained from screening using cost-effective FBS media may sometimes not accurately reflect the compounds' antiviral activity in the human body. To bridge this gap and make the in vitro cellular screening model more physiologically relevant, the research team developed a third screening model, utilizing 50% normal human serum (NHS) instead of 10% FBS to evaluate the cellular antiviral activity. In the following sections, the IC_{95} values obtained under the condition of adding 50% NHS will be denoted as NHS IC_{95}. It should be noted that compound 22 was the first compound discovered with an NHS IC_{95} value less than 1.0 μM.

The three different screening models can reflect the activity of compounds from three different perspectives:

1. Enzyme-based ST inhibition assay can reflect the direct inhibitory activity of compounds on the enzyme and is suitable for high-throughput screening.
2. The cell-based screening model using culture media supplemented with 10% FBS can demonstrate the cellular antiviral activity of compounds and indirectly reflect their membrane permeability. Additionally, this model is cost-effective.
3. The cell-based screening model with the addition of 50% NHS provides a closer representation of the antiviral activity under physiological conditions in the human body. The higher the binding affinity of the compound to human plasma proteins, the lower the percentage of free small molecules, resulting in larger differences in cellular antiviral activity between NHS and FBS conditions.

Taking into consideration the SAR obtained from studying the amine fragments in the amide group, the introduction of the most effective 4-fluorobenzylamine moiety into the 1,6-naphthyridine series also demonstrated good anti-HIV activity (Table 10.3). Compound 24 showed an FBS IC_{95} value of 16 nM, but its NHS IC_{95} value was only 1875 nM, indicating a higher plasma protein binding (PPB = 98.2%) for this compound. Therefore, reducing the plasma protein binding of the compound became the next important optimization direction. It has been reported in the literature [48] that introducing functional groups such as methylated glycine, β-alanine, or acetyl amide within the molecule can lower its binding affinity to human plasma proteins. Hence, researchers introduced similar functional groups at the 5-position of the 1,6-naphthyridine, resulting in compound 25. Although compound 25 showed a roughly 10-fold decrease in FBS IC_{95} compared to compound 24, its NHS IC_{95} value significantly improved [49]. Unfortunately, compound 25 exhibited high plasma clearance (CL = 150 mL/min/kg) in rats, approximately 2.5 times the rat liver blood flow (60 mL/min/kg). Further investigations revealed that compound 25 was primarily metabolized through glucuronidation of the hydroxyl group at the 8-position of the 1,6-naphthyridine ring. Scientists speculated that the nitrogen atom at the 5-position possessed an electron-donating conjugation effect, increasing the nucleophilicity of the hydroxyl group at the 8-position. Thus, reducing the electron density of the naphthyridine ring might potentially decrease the rate of glucuronidation at the 8-position. In the literature [50], it has been reported that acetylation of the amino group in para-position to a phenolic hydroxyl group could reduce the rate of phenolic glucuronidation. Therefore, compound 26 was further synthesized, resulting in a significant decrease in its plasma clearance in rats, as it is only 1.8 mL/min/kg. Although compound 26 exhibited an FBS IC_{95} value similar to compound 25, its plasma protein binding was higher (95.6% vs 83.3%), leading to a slight reduction in its cellular activity under NHS conditions.

To incorporate the characteristics of both lower plasma protein binding in compound 25 and lower plasma clearance in compound 26 into a single molecule, medicinal chemists integrated two substituents and designed compound 27. This compound not only exhibited good antiviral activity under NHS conditions (NHS IC_{95} = 250 nM) but also had lower plasma clearance in rats, with a clearance of 5.6 mL/min/kg upon intravenous administration of 2 mg/kg. Additionally, when administered orally at a dose of 10 mg/kg, compound 27 demonstrated a high oral bioavailability (F%) of 71%. The average blood concentration over 24 hours was approximately 600 nM, surpassing twice the concentration required to inhibit 95% of viral proliferation under NHS conditions (NHS IC_{95}).

Compound 27 not only inhibits the replication of HIV-1 but also exhibits good inhibitory activity against simian immunodeficiency virus (SIV). When evaluated using 50% monkey serum instead of 10% FBS, the cellular antiviral activity of compound 27 against SIV yielded an IC_{95} value of 350 nM. In pharmacokinetic studies conducted in rhesus macaques, oral administration of 10 mg/kg of compound 27 demonstrated favorable oral bioavailability (60%) and a long half-life (5 hours). In in vivo antiviral activity experiments, rhesus macaques infected with SIV were treated with oral doses of 10 mg/kg of compound 27 twice daily, starting from day 10 of infection. The results showed sustained inhibitory effects of compound 27 on SIV in the animal's

TABLE 10.3 SAR and SPR (structure-property relationship) of the 5-position of 1,6-naphthyridine compounds.

Compound	R	ST IC$_{50}$ (nM)	FBS IC$_{95}$ (nM)	NHS IC$_{95}$ (nM)	PPB (%)	Rat CL (mL/min/kg)
23	H	33	1250	6000	99.2	NA
24	*N-formyl piperazine*	30	16	1875	98.2	NA
25	*N,N-dimethyl glycinamide with N-methyl*	58	156	234	83.3	150.0
26	*N-methyl-N-acetyl*	25	125	612	95.6	1.8
27	*N-methyl-N-(N,N-dimethyloxamoyl)*	40	103	250	93.2	5.6

body over a period of 4 weeks. Subsequently, the dosing regimen was adjusted to once daily at a dose of 20 mg/kg, maintaining the experiment for 87 days, during which compound 27 consistently exhibited good antiviral effects.

These experimental results provided the first in vivo evidence that HIV-1 integrase inhibitors can suppress the replication of HIV-1, significantly boosting the confidence of the project team members in the development of HIV-1 integrase inhibitor drugs. However, another experiment revealed that the duration of sustained reduction in viral load in rhesus macaques treated with compound 27 decreased when the treatment was initiated after 87 days of infection. Moreover, as the viral RNA load in the animal's body increased, the efficacy of compound 27 decreased, prompting the scientists to search for compounds with even more ideal activity to enhance the anti-HIV effect.

Based on a profound understanding of the SAR at the 5-position of the 1,6-naphthyridine, medicinal chemists decided to further explore this position. Halogen atoms in organic chemistry, especially iodine and bromine, are good leaving groups and are often used as intermediates for the synthesis of derivatives due to their ease of preparation. Common reactions include aromatic nucleophilic substitution and metal-catalyzed coupling reactions, which enable the convenient introduction of various types of substituents. Employing this organic chemistry strategy, by replacing the acetyl group in compound 26 with a methylsulfonyl group, compound 28 exhibited further improved activity (Table 10.4).

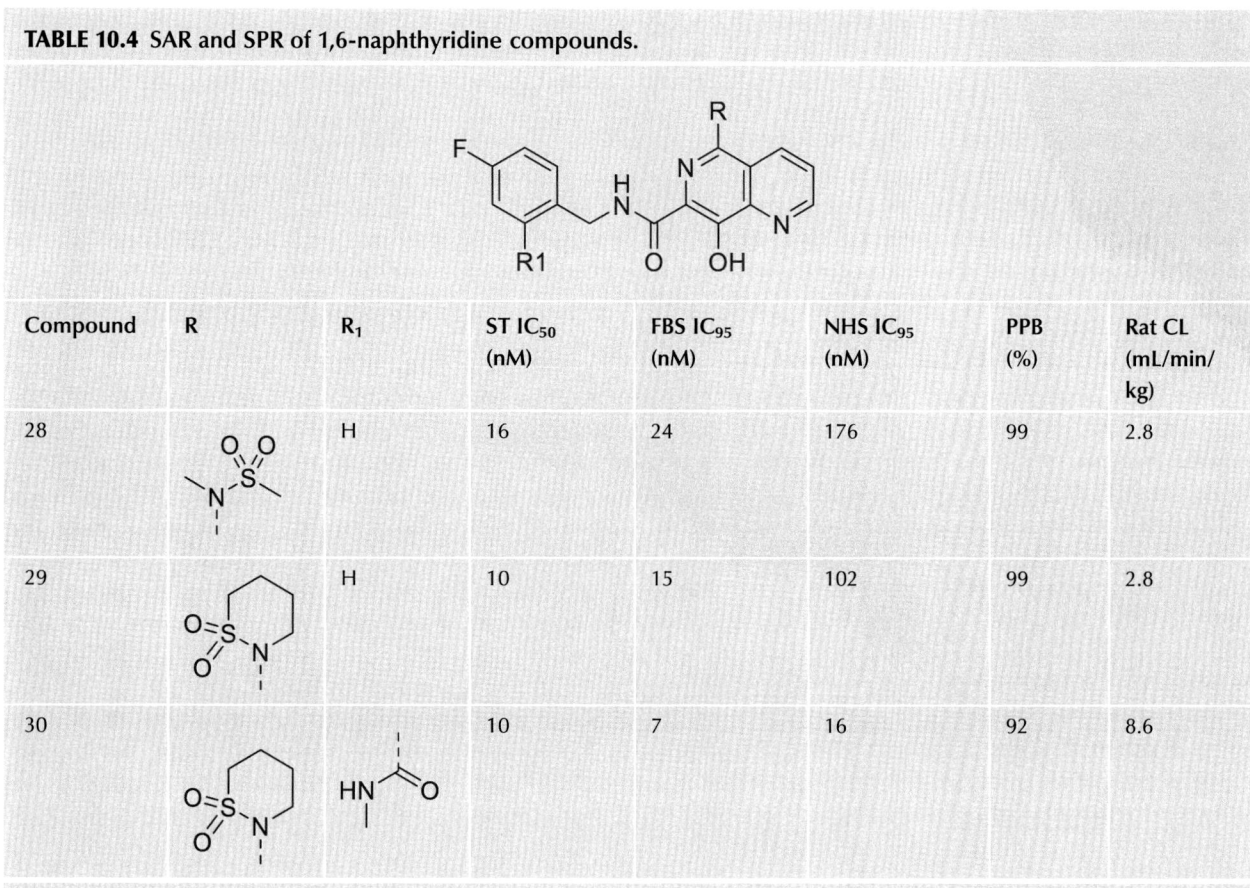

TABLE 10.4 SAR and SPR of 1,6-naphthyridine compounds.

Compound	R	R_1	ST IC_{50} (nM)	FBS IC_{95} (nM)	NHS IC_{95} (nM)	PPB (%)	Rat CL (mL/min/kg)
28	(dimethylsulfamoyl)	H	16	24	176	99	2.8
29	(cyclic sulfonamide)	H	10	15	102	99	2.8
30	(cyclic sulfonamide)	NHC(O)N(Me)	10	7	16	92	8.6

Although its plasma protein binding remained high at 99%, the cellular antiviral activity under NHS conditions was more than two times higher compared to compound 26. Compound 29, a cyclized sulfonamide, exhibited even better activity with cellular activity under NHS conditions of 102 nM, more than doubling that of compound 27. Evidently, this was mainly attributed to a significant improvement in the cellular antiviral activity under FBS conditions (IC_{95} = 15 nM). Subsequent studies on the cocrystal structures of the complexes revealed that the threonine residue (T66) in the integrase was located near the sulfonamide group of this small molecule, which could move freely and interact with various groups. Compounds capable of binding to T66, including compounds 28 and 29, showed increased activity.

Compound 29 exhibits excellent pharmacokinetic properties [51], with low clearance of 2.8, 2.0, and 6.6 mL/min/kg in rats, dogs, and monkeys, respectively. The oral bioavailability is 41%, 24%, and 51% for each respective species. Furthermore, the subsequent animal toxicology studies support the potential of this compound for clinical trials, aiming to demonstrate the therapeutic effects of integrase inhibitors in AIDS patients. As anticipated, the results of the clinical proof-of-concept trial in HIV-1 infected patients showed a remarkable average reduction of over 50-fold in viral RNA load after oral administration of compound 29 at a dosage of 400 mg twice daily. This milestone achievement confirms for the first time in a clinical setting the effectiveness of integrase inhibitors in countering HIV-1.

The positive clinical outcomes have provided immense encouragement and confidence to the entire project team. They strongly believe that by further enhancing the compound's activity, improving its pharmacokinetic properties, and ensuring sufficient tolerability and safety over the course of treatment, humanity can develop a novel class of anti-HIV drugs that target the unique mechanism of action exhibited by integrase inhibitors.

In the ongoing battle against AIDS, it has been two decades since humanity embarked on this fight. Scientists have come to a profound realization that inhibiting viral mutations is crucial in achieving optimal clinical outcomes. The most effective approach to minimize the emergence of viral resistance lies in maximizing the antiviral activity of compounds, ensuring that the minimum blood drug concentration within the human body reaches levels sufficient to suppress viral replication and proliferation (approximately two to three times the NHS IC_{95} of the drug).

Although compound 29 has displayed excellent ST inhibition activity and cellular antiviral activity, its high plasma protein binding (99%) results in a sixfold reduction in cellular activity under NHS conditions compared to FBS conditions. During the earlier investigation of SAR of the amine fragment in the amide group, it was found that introducing polar groups such as amide at the 2-position of the phenyl ring could decrease the molecule's log$P$ value, thereby reducing plasma protein binding, while maintaining the activity essentially unchanged. Hence, medicinal chemists introduced an N-methylformamide group at the 2-position of the phenyl ring of compound 29, resulting in compound 30 (Table 10.4). The plasma protein binding of compound 30 was lowered to 92%. It exhibited a noticeable improvement in cellular activity under NHS conditions, with an NHS IC_{95} value of 16 nM, only onefold lower than its cellular activity under FBS conditions. The pharmacokinetic properties of compound 30 were similar to compound 29 [52], with clearance of 8.6, 2.8, and 18.3 mL/min/kg in rats, dogs, and monkeys, respectively. The oral bioavailability was 45%, 65%, and 23% for each respective species.

Compound 30 also exhibits excellent activity against HIV-1 mutants. Fig. 10.13 illustrates the inhibitory capabilities of compounds 29 and 30 against site-directed mutants of HIV-1. These mutants were induced through continuous passage of the virus in cell culture media containing diketo acid compounds L-731988 and L-708906 or compound 29, with the mutation sites located near the catalytic site of the integrase enzyme. Compound 29 showed weak inhibitory activity against F121Y and N155S mutants (with IC_{50} values 4 times and 12 times higher than the wild-type virus, respectively), whereas compound 30 maintained relatively good inhibitory activity (with IC_{50} values 2 times and 4 times higher than the wild-type virus, respectively) [52]. This indicates that compound 30 has a better ability to suppress the development of HIV-1 resistance. Consequently, compound 30 becomes the second clinical candidate compound following compound 29. The inhibitory capabilities of compounds 29 and 30 against HIV-1 resistant mutants have once again inspired the project team members, and the scientists believe they can identify drug candidate compounds that exhibit high inhibitory activity against HIV-1 mutants within the patients' bodies.

Unfortunately, in the long-term safety study conducted in experimental dogs concurrently with clinical trials, compound 29 exhibited severe hepatotoxicity due to the inhibition of copper ion secretion. Although this adverse effect was not observed in rats, Merck & Co. made the decision to suspend further clinical trial research on 1,6-naphthyridine compounds, including compound 30.

10.3.4 Optimization of dihydroxy pyrimidine lead compound

While optimization of 1,6-naphthyridine compounds was being conducted at Merck's research center in Pennsylvania, their research center in Rome also focused on optimizing dihydroxy pyrimidine compounds. As mentioned earlier, medicinal chemists initially conducted SAR studies on the amine fragment of the amide group (Table 10.1) and discovered that compound 19, substituted with 4-fluorobenzylamine, exhibited the best ST inhibition activity. However, this compound did not demonstrate the desired antiviral activity in cellular assays, possibly due to its poor solubility, low membrane permeability, and high plasma protein binding. Comparing the scaffold structures of these two lead compounds reveals that, during the binding of ligands to HIV-1 integrase, the 2-position of pyrimidine and the 5-position of

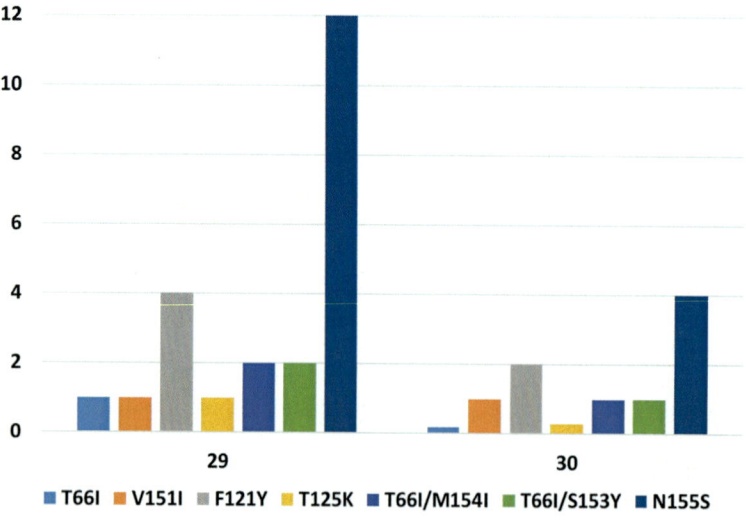

FIGURE 10.13 The inhibitory efficacy of compounds 29 and 30 against site-directed mutants of HIV-1. The vertical axis represents the fold change in IC_{50} values between the compounds' inhibitory activity against site-directed mutants of HIV-1 and the wild-type HIV-1 in a single host cell infection experiment.

naphthyridine occupy the same location in the solvent-exposed area of the binding pocket. Therefore, following the same optimization strategy as for the 1,6-naphthyridine compounds, medicinal chemists focused on structural optimization of the 2-position of the pyrimidine ring (Table 10.5). They initially removed the thiazole structure, resulting in compound 31, which also exhibited good ST inhibition activity ($IC_{50} = 60$ nM), but did not demonstrate antiviral activity at the cellular level. After introducing a benzyl group at the 2-position, compound 32 showed similar ST inhibition activity to compound 31. However, due to an increased log$P$, its membrane permeability was improved, resulting in some activity in cellular assay under FBS conditions. Because the hydroxyl group at the 5-position of the pyrimidine ring possesses a certain acidity and can lose a hydrogen ion to form an oxygen anion under physiological conditions, medicinal chemists introduced a tertiary amine at the benzyl position of compound 32, giving rise to compound 33. Although its ST inhibition activity was somewhat reduced, its cellular activity under FBS conditions significantly increased. This compound became the first in the series to exhibit cellular activity below 1.0 μM. However, due to a plasma protein binding exceeding 99.9% [53], the compound did not show antiviral activity under NHS conditions.

There is a strong correlation between plasma protein binding and the log$P$ value of a molecule. Decreasing the log$P$ value of a molecule helps reduce its plasma protein binding. Based on compound 33, medicinal chemists employed two strategies to lower the molecule's log$P$ value. The first strategy involved directly removing the phenyl ring from the 2-position substituent, while the second strategy involved substituting the 2-position with a nitrogen-containing cycloalkyl group (Fig. 10.14) [53].

Firstly, by substituting the phenyl ring with a methyl group, compound 34 was obtained, exhibiting a slight improvement in both ST inhibition activity and cellular activity under FBS conditions (Table 10.6). However, due to a significant decrease in plasma protein binding, the cellular activity under NHS conditions also showed a noticeable improvement, with an NHS IC_{95} value of 500 nM. To simplify the molecule and remove its chiral center, chemists further removed the methyl group (compound 35) or introduced a gem-dimethyl (compound 36). Compound 35 completely lost its cellular activity, while compound 36 showed further improvement in cellular activity under NHS conditions (NHS $IC_{95} = 110$ nM), which was only twice the value of the FBS IC_{95}, primarily attributed to a further decrease in plasma protein binding.

TABLE 10.5 SAR of the 2-position of dihydroxy pyrimidine compounds.

Compound	R	ST IC$_{50}$ (nM)	FBS IC$_{95}$ (nM)	NHS IC$_{95}$ (nM)	PPB (%)
19	thiophene	10	>10,000	>10,000	/
31	H	60	>10,000	>10,000	/
32	benzyl	50	5800	>10,000	/
33	α-(dimethylamino)benzyl	200	300	>10,000	>99.9

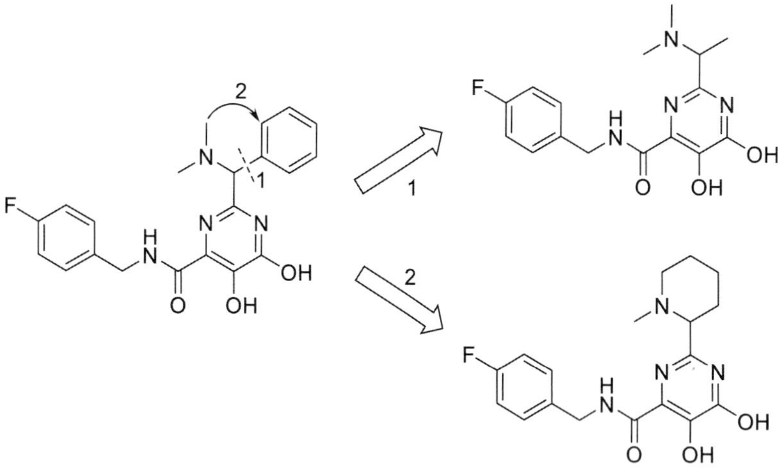

228 Medicinal Chemistry and Drug Development

FIGURE 10.14 Two strategies for reducing the log*P* value of a molecule.

TABLE 10.6 SAR and SPR of the 2-position of dihydroxy pyrimidine compounds.

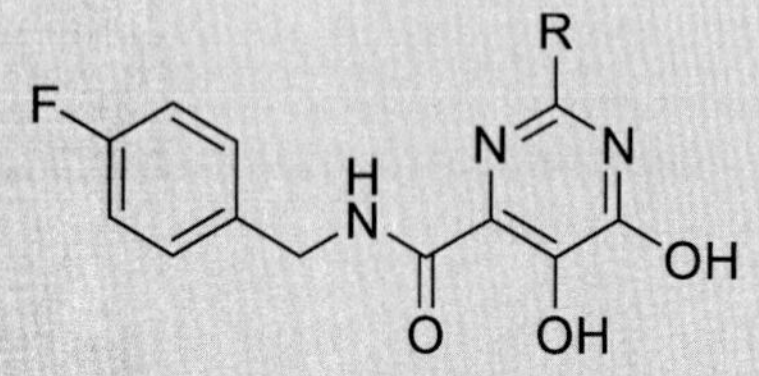

Compound	R	ST IC$_{50}$ (nM)	FBS IC$_{95}$ (nM)	NHS IC$_{95}$ (nM)	PPB (%)
34	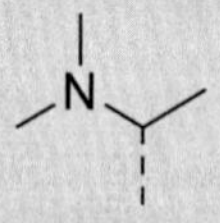 –CH(CH$_3$)N(CH$_3$)$_2$	80	125	500	92.5
35	–CH$_2$N(CH$_3$)$_2$	200	>1000	>1000	/
36	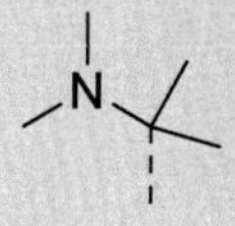 –C(CH$_3$)$_2$N(CH$_3$)$_2$	50	50	110	88.7
37	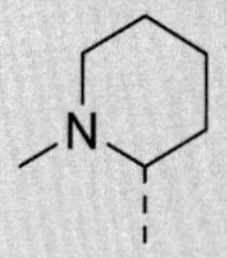 N-methylpiperidin-2-yl	200	150	400	94.8
38	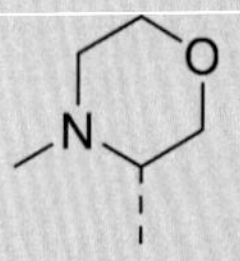 N-methylmorpholin-3-yl	27	30	240	96.7

Compound 36 demonstrated low clearance in rats, dogs, and monkeys, with values of 16, 2, and 15 mL/min/kg, respectively, and oral bioavailability of 28%, 100%, and 61%, respectively. In the selectivity test, compound 36 did not exhibit inhibitory effects on human DNA polymerase α, β, and γ but showed toxicity in rodents at high doses, leading to its discontinuation.

In the second strategy, the removal of the phenyl ring and cyclization of the alkylamine led to the formation of compound 37. This strategy also lowered the plasma protein binding, resulting in a less than threefold discrepancy in cellular activity IC_{95} values observed under both conditions. However, if the position of nitrogen was shifted from ortho to meta or para, or if the methyl group on nitrogen was removed, the activity was greatly reduced. Substituting N-methylpiperidine with N-methylmorpholine (compound 38) further improved the activity, with cellular activities under FBS and NHS conditions being 30 and 240 nM, respectively.

In the project of HCV polymerase inhibitors mentioned earlier, it was discovered that the N-methyl pyrimidone compounds, obtained by single methylation of the dihydroxy pyrimidine compounds, maintained or further improved their activity and pharmacokinetic properties. This finding was also applied in the research of HIV-1 integrase inhibitors. Based on compounds 37 and 38, medicinal chemists synthesized compounds 39 and 40, respectively (Table 10.7). The plasma protein binding of both compounds significantly decreased to 48% and 70%, respectively. Compound 39 exhibited weaker cellular activity compared to compound 37, but compound 40 showed higher cellular activity under NHS conditions (NHS IC_{95} = 100 nM) than compound 38. Chiral separation of compound 40 resulted in two enantiomers, 41 and 42, both of which displayed similar ST inhibition activity, further demonstrating that the substituent at the 2-position does not directly interact with the protein. However, compound 41 exhibited higher antiviral activity at the cellular level, with IC_{95} values of 40 and 65 nM under the respective conditions. Furthermore, compound 41 demonstrated excellent pharmacokinetic properties, with low clearance in rats, dogs, and monkeys—9, 2.2, and 14 mL/min/kg, respectively—and oral bioavailability of 56%, 69%, and 73%, respectively. Compound 41 also showed no inhibitory effects on human DNA polymerases α, β, and γ (IC_{50} > 10 μM). As another preclinical candidate compound, various in vitro toxicity studies were conducted. Unfortunately, compound 41 tested positive in the mutagenicity (Ames) assay, leading scientists to once again face disappointment in their pursuit of a clinically viable HIV-1 integrase inhibitor.

Based on the benefits of N-methyl pyrimidone in terms of compound activity and pharmacokinetic properties, medicinal chemists also carried out N-methylation of the dihydroxy pyrimidine in compound 36, yielding compound 43 (Table 10.8). However, this compound exhibited weaker ST inhibition activity and antiviral activity at the cellular level compared to compound 36. At this point, they recalled the use of an oxamide (compound 27) in the 1,6-naphthyridine series and introduced it into the N-methyl pyrimidone series, resulting in compound 44. Fortunately, compound 44 displayed excellent ST inhibition activity (IC_{50} = 10 nM) as well as antiviral activity at the cellular level [54], with IC_{95} values under FBS and NHS conditions being close to each other, at 45 and 74 nM, respectively. Meanwhile, they also attempted some other similar derivatives such as acetamide, sulfonamide, urea, and sulfonylurea, but none of them exhibited activity comparable to compound 44.

TABLE 10.7 SAR and SPR of the 2-position of N-methyl pyrimidone compounds.

Compound	X	ST IC_{50} (nM)	FBS IC_{95} (nM)	NHS IC_{95} (nM)	PPB (%)
39	CH_2 (±)	210	840	1100	48
40	O (±)	60	65	100	70
41	O (+)	20	40	65	81
42	O (−)	25	90	190	/

TABLE 10.8 SAR and SPR of the 2-position of N-methyl pyrimidone compounds.

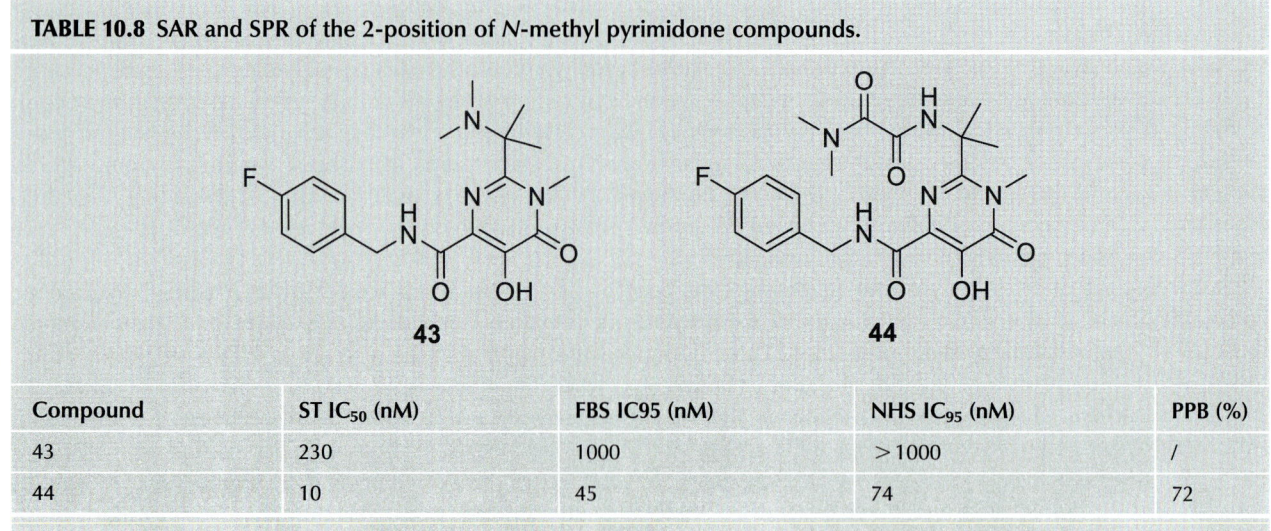

Compound	ST IC$_{50}$ (nM)	FBS IC95 (nM)	NHS IC$_{95}$ (nM)	PPB (%)
43	230	1000	>1000	/
44	10	45	74	72

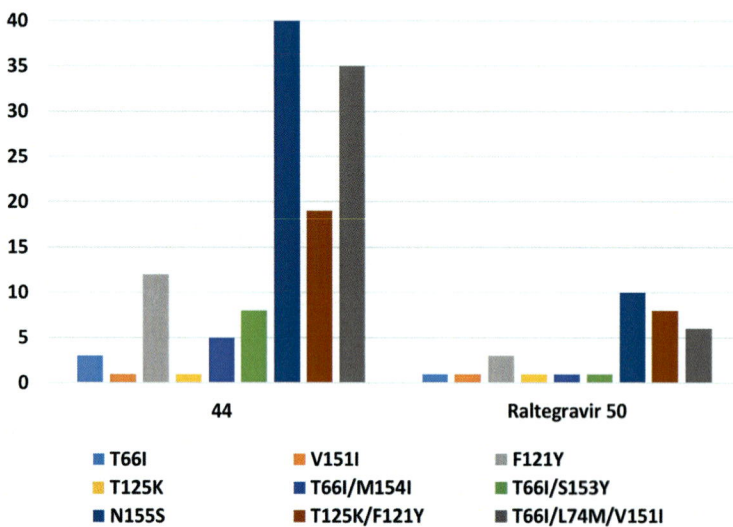

FIGURE 10.15 The inhibitory efficacy of compounds 44 and raltegravir against site-directed mutants of HIV-1. The vertical axis represents the fold change in IC$_{50}$ values between the compounds' inhibitory activity against site-directed mutants of HIV-1 and the wild-type HIV-1 in a single host cell infection experiment.

Compound 44 also exhibited favorable pharmacokinetic properties, with clearance of 21, 8, and 20 mL/min/kg in rats, dogs, and monkeys, respectively, and oral bioavailability of 36%, 93%, and 24%, respectively. Similar to previous compounds, the primary metabolic pathway for 44 involved glucuronidation of the hydroxyl group at the 5-position of the pyrimidone. Compound 44 also did not exert inhibitory effects on human DNA polymerases α, β, and γ and showed no significant inhibition activity (IC$_{50}$ > 10 μM) on 150 unrelated off-targets, including enzymes, ion channels, and receptors, indicating good selectivity. Promisingly, compound 44 demonstrated good safety in animal toxicity studies, with no observed adverse effects or mutagenicity. Therefore, compound 44 was selected as a clinical candidate, and phase I clinical trials were initiated.

During the safety evaluation of compound 44, scientists also investigated its inhibitory ability against various HIV-1 mutants. Unfortunately, the compound exhibited weaker inhibitory activity against the single point mutants F121Y and N155S, with IC$_{50}$ values of 12-fold and 40-fold higher than the wild-type virus, respectively (Fig. 10.15). As a result of these findings, Merck & Co. had to once again pause the clinical trial on compound 44 and continue their search for more promising clinical candidate compounds.

Medicinal chemists continued to optimize the 2-position of N-methyl pyrimidone [54] and attempted to replace the oxamide with heteroaromatic rings while ensuring that heteroatoms on the aromatic ring are positioned similarly to those on the oxamide (Table 10.9). The objective was to maintain the activity of compound 44 while altering the

TABLE 10.9 SAR of the 2-position of N-methyl pyrimidone compounds.

Compound	R	ST IC$_{50}$ (nM)	FBS IC$_{95}$ (nM)	NHS IC$_{95}$ (nM)
45	2-pyridyl	20	125	1000
46	pyridazinyl	15	62	500
47	pyrimidinyl	7	20	50
48	oxazolyl	7	500	500
49	imidazolyl	6	250	250
50	methyl-oxadiazolyl	15	19	31
51	methyl-triazolyl	4	250	1000
52	isopropyl-oxadiazolyl	7	20	160

molecular physicochemical properties to improve drug-likeness. When using a six-membered heteroaromatic ring, such as 2-pyridyl (compound 45), the ST inhibition activity could be maintained, but the cellular activity under NHS conditions significantly decreased. Pyridyl, substituted in other positions, led to a further reduction in activity. Introducing an additional nitrogen atom on the pyridyl ring resulted in compounds 46 and 47, which showed improved activity compared to 45, particularly compound 47, with cellular activity under NHS conditions reaching 50 nM. For five-membered heteroaromatic rings, better activity was observed when there were two or three heteroatoms (compounds 48–52). Additionally, the presence of a heteroatom at the 2-position shows superior activity compared to a carbon atom. Among all these compounds, the methyloxadiazole-substituted compound 50 demonstrated the highest antiviral activity at the cellular level, with activity of 19 and 31 nM under FBS and NHS conditions, respectively, and a plasma protein binding of 82%. The more polar triazole compound 51 exhibited better ST activity but lower cellular activity. By increasing lipophilicity and replacing the methyl group with isopropyl in compound 50 (compound 52), a significant difference in cellular activity under the two conditions was observed, primarily due to the increased plasma protein binding caused by the higher lipophilicity of the molecule.

Compound 50 exhibited IC_{50} values threefold and 10-fold higher than the wild-type virus for the single point mutants F121Y and N155S, respectively [54], indicating a significant improvement compared to compound 44. Additionally, compound 50 demonstrated favorable selectivity in vitro, as it did not inhibit human DNA polymerases α, β, and γ and showed no significant inhibitory activity on 150 unrelated off-targets. In vitro safety evaluation experiments revealed that compound 50 did not exhibit potent inhibition against human Ether-a-go-go Related Gene (hERG) and showed negative results in the Ames mutagenicity assay. Furthermore, compound 50 did not bind to glutathione and did not form irreversible covalent bonds with proteins.

Compound 50 demonstrated similar plasma protein binding in rats, dogs, monkeys, and humans, with the fractions of unbound compounds in plasma being 26.6%, 29.1%, 15.4%, and 17.2% respectively. In vitro metabolism studies using liver microsomes and hepatocytes showed that the primary metabolic pathway of compound 50 involved glucuronidation of the hydroxyl group at the 5-position of the pyrimidone. The metabolic rates in rat, dog, monkey, and human liver microsomes were found to be 34, 2, 36, and 9 μL/min/kg, respectively. Pharmacokinetic data in vivo (Table 10.10) revealed that compound 50 exhibited a moderate volume of distribution (0.9–2 L/kg) in rats, dogs, and monkeys; moderate clearance in rats (39 mL/min/kg) and monkeys (18 mL/min/kg); and low clearance in dogs (6 mL/min/kg). When administered orally as the free form, compound 50 demonstrated moderate oral bioavailability in rats and dogs (approximately 40%) but poor bioavailability in monkeys (<10%). However, when administered orally as the sodium or potassium salt, the drug plasma exposure, area under the concentration-time curve (AUC), in rats and dogs was significantly higher compared to the free form, and the AUC increased proportionally with the dose, indicating dose-dependent effects. Plasma concentrations of the drug in dogs at 12 hours after oral administration of the potassium salt at doses of 2 and 10 mg/kg were 160 and 350 nM, respectively, which were considerably higher than the IC_{95} value for antiviral activity at the cellular level under NHS conditions (31 nM). Based on the analysis of all in vitro and in vivo metabolism data and the anti-HIV activity of compound 50, its pharmacokinetic profile in humans was predicted to closely resemble that in dogs, with twice-daily dosing being the most appropriate regimen.

Additionally, compound 50 dose not exhibit inhibitory activity against UGT1A1 or major cytochrome P450 enzymes, such as CYP1A2, 2C9, 2D6, and 3A4. It also does not display time-dependent inhibition of CYP3A4. Therefore, the probability of potential drug-drug interactions mediated by compound 50 is extremely low, making it suitable for multidrug regimens in the treatment of AIDS.

To evaluate the toxicity of compound 50 on cardiovascular, respiratory, and central nervous systems, toxicologists conducted toxicity experiments in dogs and rats. At the highest administered doses (a single dose of 45 mg/kg in dogs and a single dose of 120 mg/kg in rats), compound 50 did not exhibit any toxicity. Furthermore, they performed single-dose and multiple-dose toxicity studies in mice, rats, rabbits, and dogs to investigate various toxicities, including mutagenicity, carcinogenicity, and reproductive toxicity. No toxic side effects were observed in any of these studies.

Considering the excellent antiviral activity against HIV-1 and favorable absorption, distribution, metabolism, excretion and toxicity (ADME/T) properties of compound 50, Merck conducted comprehensive clinical trials. Finally, on October 12, 2007, it was approved by the FDA for use in combination with other HIV RT inhibitors to treat adult HIV-1 positive patients who had been previously treated with other drugs. It was named RAL (brand name: Isentress, Fig. 10.16).

10.3.5 Clinical investigation of raltegravir

The Phase 1 clinical trial of RAL primarily investigated the pharmacokinetic properties of the compound in healthy individuals after single and multiple doses [55,56]. Consistent with preclinical predictions, raltegravir exhibited

TABLE 10.10 Pharmacokinetic parameters of compound 50.

Species	IV dose (mg/kg)	CL (mL/min/kg)	$T_{1/2}$ (h)	V_d (L/kg)	Oral F (%)			AUC (μM*h)		
					Na^+	K^+	OH	Na^+	K^+	OH
Rat	3	39	2	2	nd	45	37	$1.4_{(3)}$	$1.3_{(3)}$	$1.0_{(3)}$
Dog	1	6	11	0.9	nd	69–85	45	nd	$11_{(2)}$–$45_{(10)}$	$7_{(2)}$–$21_{(10)}$
Monkey	1	18	4	1.2	nd	nd	8	nd	nd	$1.8_{(10)}$

The values in parentheses represent the oral dosages administered (in mg/kg).

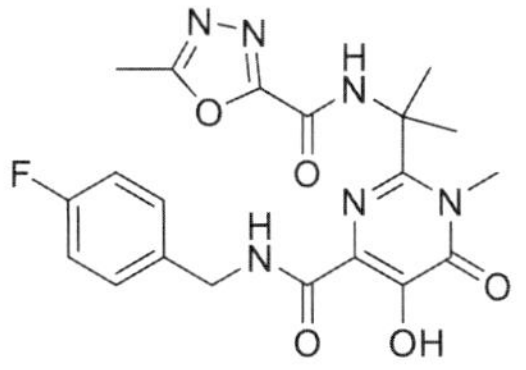

FIGURE 10.16 The chemical structure of raltegravir.

pharmacokinetic characteristics in humans that were most similar to those observed in dogs. After oral administration of 200 mg of the drug to healthy subjects, the half-life ranged from 7 to 12 hours, with a 12-hour blood concentration (C_{trough}) of 94 nM, significantly higher than the NHS IC_{95} value (31 nM). Therefore, RAL is suitable for twice-daily dosing. In multiple-dose studies, within a range of oral dosages from 100 to 1600 mg, both AUC and maximum blood concentration of the compound increased proportionally with the dosage. The blood concentration at 12 hours postdose also increased proportionally with dosage within the range of 100–800 mg. Steady-state plasma concentrations were achieved after 2 days of dosing when administered twice daily. Additionally, the results indicated that food intake did not have a clinically significant impact on the pharmacokinetic properties of RAL, and no dose adjustment was required for patients with renal or hepatic impairment.

The study on the drug–drug interactions of RAL was conducted in HIV-1-negative individuals [55]. RAL is neither a substrate nor an inducer or inhibitor of P450 enzymes, thus there are no P450 enzyme-related drug–drug interactions associated with this compound. RAL is a substrate of P-glycoprotein (P-gp) but not an inhibitor of P-gp. Currently, there is no data indicating that the pharmacokinetics of RAL in the human body are affected by other P-gp inducers or inhibitors. RAL is primarily metabolized through glucuronidation catalyzed by UGT1A1. Therefore, the drug–drug interactions associated with RAL mainly revolve around the induction or inhibition of UGT1A1. For example, coadministration of rifampin (an inducer of UGT1A1) can lead to decreased blood concentrations of RAL, while coadministration of ATV (an inhibitor of UGT1A1) can result in increased blood concentrations of RAL.

The Phase 2 clinical trials of RAL consisted of a concept validation study of monotherapy in treatment-naïve HIV-1-positive patients and a dose-ranging study of combination therapy, as well as a dose-ranging study in previously treated HIV-1-positive patients. In the concept validation study [57], treatment-naïve HIV-1-positive patients were selected to assess the efficacy and safety of RAL given as monotherapy for 10 days. The results showed a significant reduction in HIV-1 RNA levels in all dose groups (100, 200, 400, 600 mg twice daily) compared to the placebo group, with no significant difference observed between the different dose groups. In the first dose-ranging study of combination therapy [58], treatment-naïve HIV-1 positive patients were again selected. Some patients received RAL (100, 200, 400, and 600 mg twice daily) in combination with tenofovir and lamivudine, while others received efavirenz in combination with tenofovir and lamivudine. After 24 weeks of treatment, 85%–92% of patients in all treatment groups achieved HIV-1 RNA levels below the detection limit. Within both treatment groups, a similar proportion of patients maintained HIV-1 RNA levels below 50 copies/mL for over 48 weeks. However, patients receiving RAL achieved a faster reduction in HIV-1 RNA levels to below 50 copies/mL compared to those receiving efavirenz (80% vs 70% at week 16). This clinical study confirms the significant efficacy of RAL as monotherapy or in combination therapy for treatment-naïve HIV-1-positive patients, offering a novel alternative treatment option for patients intolerant to standard therapy.

In the second dose-ranging study of combination therapy [59], patients who had previously received treatment and developed resistance to multiple drugs (at least one nonnucleoside RT inhibitor, one nucleoside RT inhibitor, and one protease inhibitor) were selected. In addition to optimized background therapy, various doses of RAL (200, 400, and 600 mg, twice daily) or placebo were administered orally. After 2 weeks of treatment, all three doses of RAL demonstrated approximately a 100-fold reduction in HIV-1 RNA levels in patients, which was sustained for 24 weeks. The proportion of patients achieving HIV-1 RNA levels below 50 copies/mL was significantly higher compared to the placebo group. Alongside the reduction in HIV-1 RNA levels, there was a corresponding increase in CD4 T-lymphocyte count. Patients receiving different doses of RAL exhibited a similar incidence of adverse effects compared to the placebo group, and no dose-related side effects were observed. In summary, this trial demonstrated that RAL can provide rapid and sustained treatment for advanced HIV-1-positive patients who have developed resistance to at least three kinds of drugs. Based on the results of these two Phase 2 clinical trials and experimental research on drug–drug interactions, Merck decided to proceed with Phase 3 clinical trials using a dosage of 400 mg twice daily, without the need for dose adjustment in combination therapy.

The Phase 3 clinical trials of RAL enrolled patients who had previously received treatment and developed resistance to multiple drugs in HIV-1-positive individuals [60]. RAL (400 mg twice daily) was added to the patients' optimized background therapy to evaluate its safety and efficacy. The trial results demonstrated that adding RAL to the optimized background therapy had superior therapeutic effects in terms of HIV-1 suppression and immune function restoration compared to adding a placebo. At week 16, the proportions of patients achieving HIV-1 RNA levels below 400 copies/mL were 77.5% and 41.9% in the RAL group and placebo group, respectively. The proportions achieving HIV-1 RNA levels below 50 copies/mL were 61.8% and 34.7% in the respective groups. By week 48, the proportions achieving HIV-1 RNA levels below 50 copies/mL reached 62.1% and 32.9%, respectively. Adverse events related to medication occurred at a similar frequency in both the RAL and placebo groups, primarily including diarrhea, headache, nausea, and fever.

The above Phase 2 and Phase 3 clinical trial results served as the primary basis for FDA approval of RAL. In addition to these trials, Merck & Co. conducted several other clinical trials to broaden the patient population for its clinical application.

For instance, in another Phase 3 clinical trial [61], treatment-naïve HIV-1 positive patients were enrolled to compare the efficacy of RAL and efavirenz in combination with tenofovir and emtricitabine. The trial results demonstrated that at week 48, 86.1% of patients in the RAL group and 81.9% of patients in the efavirenz group achieved a reduction in HIV-1 RNA levels to below 50 copies/mL. Additionally, the time required for patients in the RAL group to reach HIV-1 RNA levels below 50 copies/mL was shorter compared to the efavirenz group. The proportion of patients experiencing drug-related adverse effects in the RAL group was 44%, significantly lower than the 77% observed in the efavirenz group. The proportion of both groups experiencing drug-related serious adverse effects was less than 2%. Therefore, based on the RAL-based combination therapy, it exhibits excellent efficacy against HIV-1, and the efficacy at week 48 is equivalent to or better than that of efavirenz. Based on these Phase 3 clinical trial results, the FDA expanded the clinical indication for RAL on July 8, 2009, approving its use in combination with other HIV RT inhibitors for initial treatment in adult HIV-1 positive patients. In the same year, in December, the U.S. Department of Health and Human Services modified the guidelines for anti-HIV therapy, incorporating RAL-based combination therapy as a preferred option for initial treatment in adult HIV-1-positive patients. Subsequently, the FDA approved the expansion of the RAL population to include children aged 2–18 years and newborns in 2011 and 2017, respectively.

10.4 Research on the synthetic process of raltegravir

The synthesis of RAL has undergone several generations of optimization, from its early laboratory synthesis to its final commercial production [62]. Although the overall synthetic route has not changed significantly, optimization of reaction conditions has increased the overall yield from 3% to 35%, significantly reducing production costs and the discharge of wastewater and organic reagents.

10.4.1 Synthetic route in medicinal chemistry

The earliest synthetic route is illustrated in Fig. 10.17. Starting from cyanohydrin 53, amino nitrile 54 is obtained via the Strecker reaction. Intermediate 55 is formed by protecting the amino group with carbobenzoxy (Cbz), followed by the nucleophilic addition of hydroxylamine to yield amino oxime 56. The overall yield for these three steps is 37%. Subsequently, intermediate 56 undergoes a Michael addition with dimethyl 2-butynedioate to yield adduct 57 in two configurations. Under high temperature, a rearrangement of intermediate 57 occurs, leading to the formation of the key intermediate, multiply-substituted pyrimidine ring 58, in a two-step process with a yield of 41%. After successful construction of the pyrimidine ring, selective protection of the hydroxyl group, N-methylation, and hydrogenation to remove the Cbz protecting group yield intermediate 61. The amino group of intermediate 61 is then subjected to amide formation with acyl chloride 67 to give 62. Finally, through amide formation with 4-fluorobenzylamine and concomitant removal of the benzoyl group yield RAL in a single step.

The synthesis of the oxadiazole fragment begins with the commercially available starting material, methyl tetrazole 63, which undergoes an acylation reaction with ethyl oxalyl monochloride to form intermediate 64. Subsequently, a rearrangement occurs at 70°C, leading to the elimination of one molecule of nitrogen and the subsequent hydrolysis by potassium hydroxide, resulting in the formation of methyl oxadiazole potassium formate. Finally, intermediate 66 is quantitatively converted to acyl chloride 67 in the presence of oxalyl chloride.

10.4.2 Optimization of the first-generation synthetic process

Process chemists have conducted an analysis of the entire synthetic route and identified some areas for improvement. While the starting materials and reagents are readily available and cost-effective, and the construction of key intermediate 58 is highly efficient and atom economical, there are low yields observed in the Strecker reaction, rearrangement of 57, N-methylation, and the final step of amide formation. Furthermore, the route involves multiple uses of solvents such as chloroform, dichloromethane, and dioxane, which are environmentally unfriendly and pose potential toxicity risks to humans. Based on these considerations, the process chemists have implemented the following optimizations in the synthetic process.

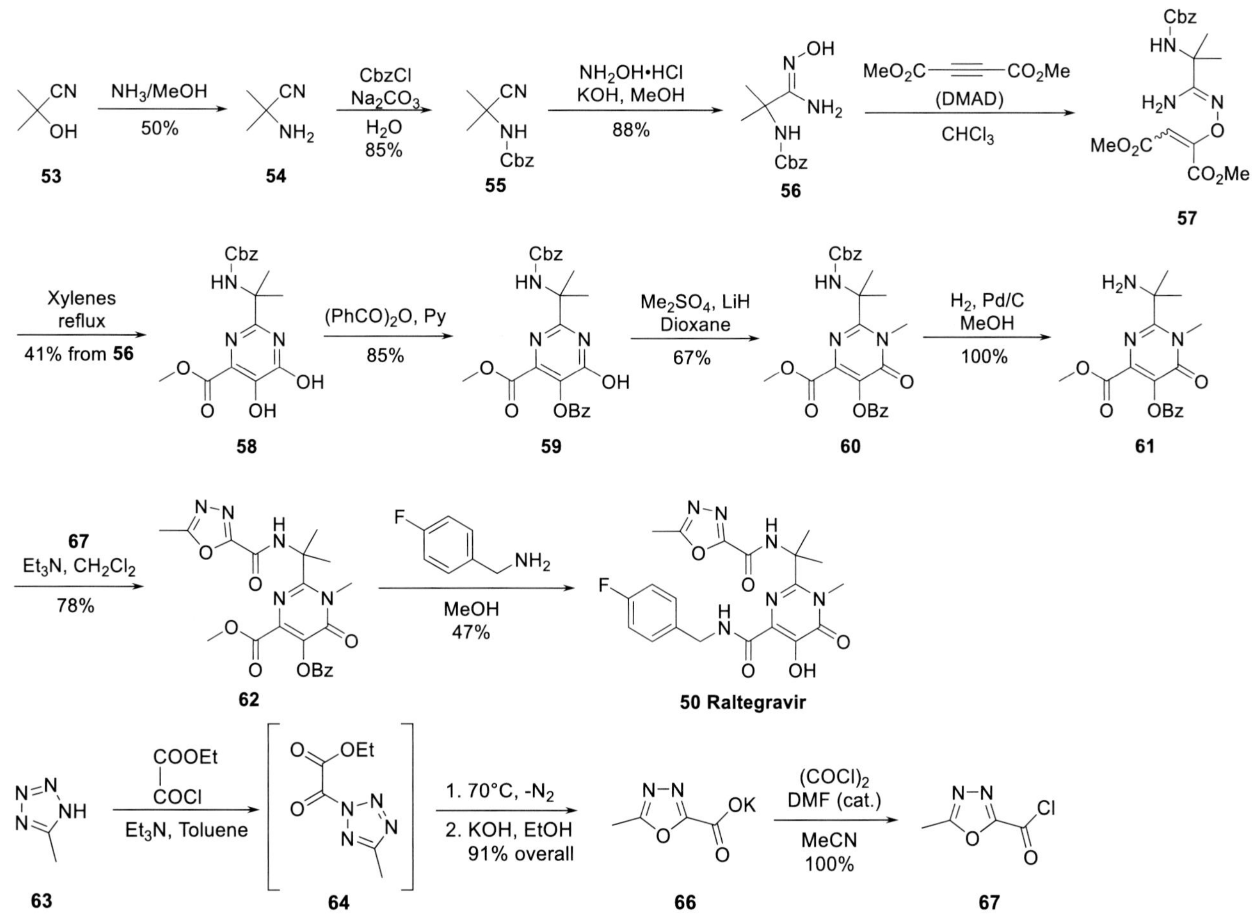

FIGURE 10.17 Medicinal chemistry synthetic route of raltegravir.

By replacing the ammonia methanol solution with liquid ammonia, the yield of the Strecker reaction was increased to 99%. Simple optimizations of the subsequent Cbz protection and hydroxylamine addition to the cyano group have resulted in an overall yield improvement of the first three steps, increasing the total yield for the synthesis of 56 from the previous 37% to 81% (Fig. 10.18).

To avoid the use of the highly toxic solvent chloroform, process chemists investigated the Michael addition reaction between intermediate 56 and dimethyl 2-butynedioate and found that the solvent had a significant influence on the cis-trans selectivity of the reaction product. Polar aprotic solvents, such as DMF and dimethyl sulfoxide (DMSO), favored the formation of the E-isomer, while protic solvents, such as methanol, favored the formation of the Z-isomer. The chemists separated the Z- and E-isomers and subjected them to rearrangement reactions. It was found that the Z-isomer could be converted to 58 with a yield of 72% at 125°C, while the E-isomer required a temperature of 135°C for rearrangement with a yield of only 48%. Because neither the Z- nor E-isomers underwent isomerization under common conditions for double bond isomerization (e.g., heating in the presence of catalytic amounts of acid, base, iodine, or trialkyl phosphine), methanol was ultimately chosen as the solvent for the Michael addition reaction to maximize the formation of the Z-isomer. The solvent was then switched to xylene and heated at 125°C for 2 hours, followed by a temperature increase to 135°C and further heating for 4 hours, to ensure the maximum conversion of both isomers to 58. Finally, by recrystallization, the rearranged product 58 was obtained with an overall yield of 54% (Fig. 10.19).

In the medicinal chemistry synthesis route, it is necessary to protect the phenolic hydroxy group before methylation. In order to minimize the use of protective groups, process chemists investigated the direct methylation reaction of 58. Unexpectedly, under the same reaction conditions, only the desired product 68 and the side product 69, resulting from oxygen methylation, were obtained in a ratio of 7:3, without any phenolic hydroxy methylation side products (70–72) (Fig. 10.20). To avoid the use of environmentally unfriendly dioxane and lithium hydride, as well as to improve the selectivity and yield of the reaction, process chemists conducted a detailed investigation on this reaction. It was found that the addition of magnesium salt could

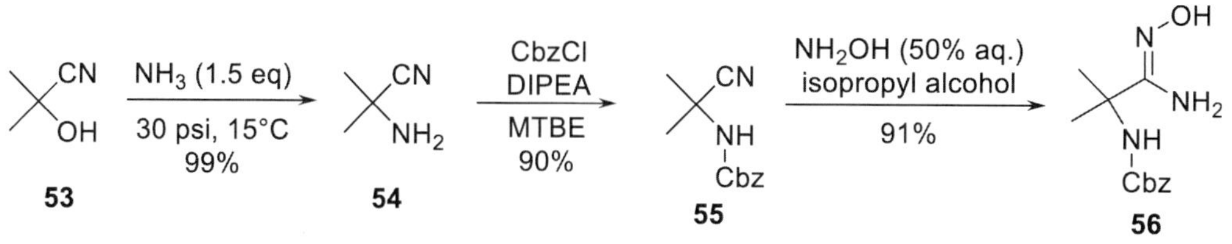

FIGURE 10.18 Synthetic process of intermediate 56.

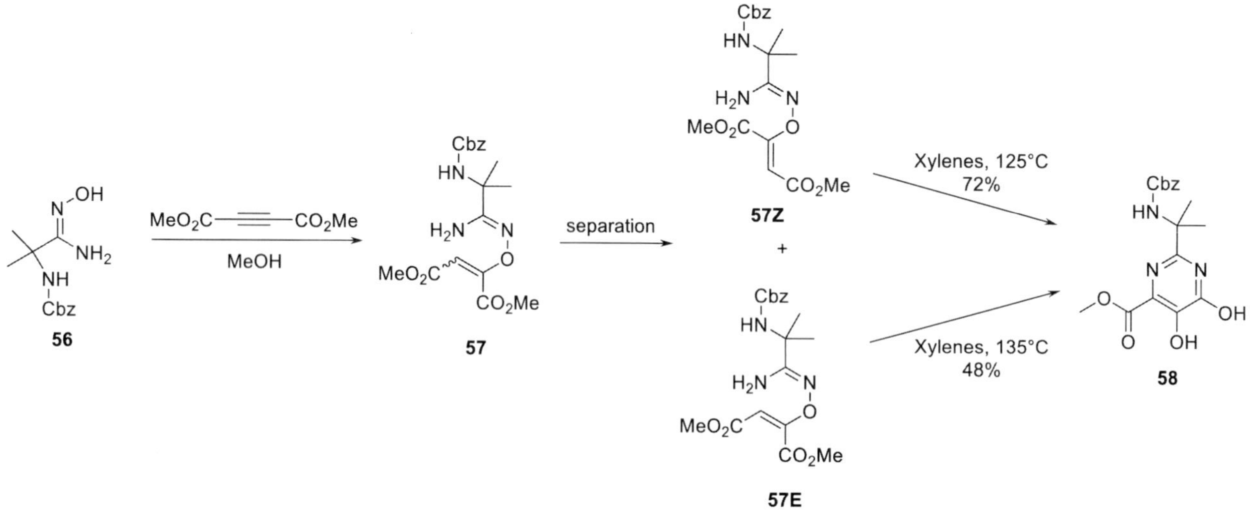

FIGURE 10.19 Research on the synthetic process of intermediate 58.

enhance the selectivity of the reaction, and it was proposed that magnesium salt could act as a Lewis acid to coordinate with the phenolic hydroxy group and amide oxygen (Fig. 10.21), thereby impeding the oxygen methylation reaction. Ultimately, using iodomethane as the methylation reagent, Mg(OMe)$_2$ as the base, and dimethyl sulfoxide as the solvent at 60°C, complete conversion of 58 was achieved with a selectivity of 78:22 for the mixture of 68 and 69. Through recrystallization, intermediate 68 can be obtained with a yield of 70% and a purity of >99%.

In the medicinal chemistry synthesis route, the oxadiazole fragment is initially introduced, followed by the introduction of the 4-fluorobenzylamine fragment. However, the yields of these two steps are only 37%. To improve the reaction yields, process chemists reversed the order of these two steps during process optimization. Initially, intermediate 68 undergoes amide formation with a 2.2 equivalent of 4-fluorobenzylamine in ethanol, resulting in intermediate 75 with a yield of 90%. Subsequently, the Cbz protecting group is hydrogenated and removed using palladium on a carbon catalyst. Due to the requirement of 1 equivalent of methanesulfonic acid in this reaction, neutralization with sodium hydroxide is necessary after the reaction to achieve a yield of 99% for intermediate 76, which contains a crystalline water molecule. Surprisingly, this water molecule is highly stable and cannot be removed by conventional drying methods, leading to an impact on the subsequent amide formation reaction. Therefore, process chemists employ a coboiling method with tetrahydrofuran to remove the crystalline water before the final amide formation reaction. Under the conditions of *N*-methylmorpholine as the base and tetrahydrofuran as the solvent, intermediate 76 reacts with acyl chloride 67 through amide formation, yielding the desired product RAL in a 10:1 ratio with side product 78. By adding an aqueous methylamine solution to the reaction mixture, 78 can be hydrolyzed completely to RAL. By further neutralization with hydrochloric acid, RAL is obtained with the phenolic hydroxy group in its free state, with a yield of 88%. Finally, the RAL solution is treated with potassium ethoxide, resulting in the crystalline RAL potassium salt with a yield of 93% and a purity of 99.5% (Fig. 10.22).

10.4.3 Optimization of the second-generation synthetic process

Although the first-generation synthetic process has made significant improvements compared to the initial medicinal chemistry synthetic route—such as the yield of critical intermediate 58 was increased from 15% to 44%, and the overall yield from intermediate 58 to the final RAL potassium salt was increased from 20% to 51%—process chemists believed that there is still room

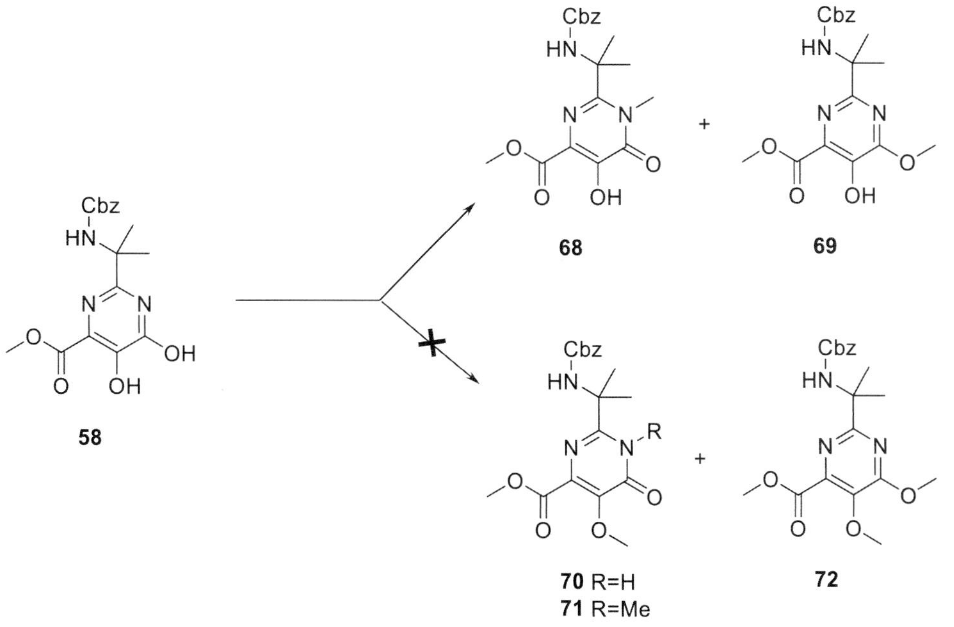

FIGURE 10.20 Selectivity in methylation reaction.

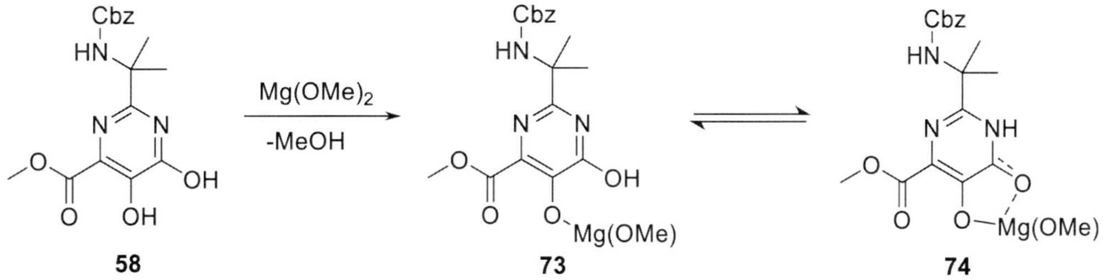

FIGURE 10.21 Coordination of magnesium salt with intermediate 58.

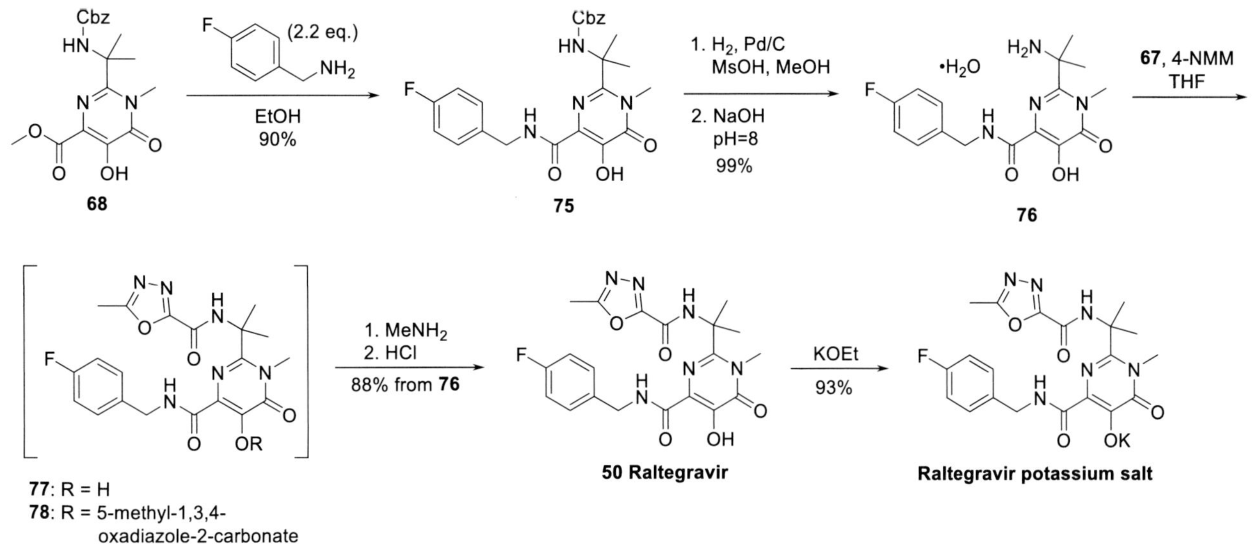

FIGURE 10.22 First-generation synthetic process of raltegravir potassium salt from intermediate 68.

77: R = H
78: R = 5-methyl-1,3,4-oxadiazole-2-carbonate

for further optimization for the ultimate purpose of commercial production. Through further analysis of the first-generation synthetic process, process chemists have deemed the synthesis of intermediate 58 to be already concise and efficient. Therefore, the focus of optimization for the second-generation synthetic process lies in the synthetic process from intermediate 58 to the final product.

The first-generation synthetic process still has shortcomings including low selectivity in the methylation reaction of nitrogen (70% yield), high solvent consumption, and significant discharge of waste solvents. Previous research experience has shown that achieving complete regioselectivity through kinetics is nearly impossible. Therefore, process chemists are hopeful that 100% nitrogen methylation can be achieved through a cyclic reaction involving demethylation and remethylation of compound 69 in the synthetic process. However, compound 69 decomposed under various attempted conditions, possibly due to the instability of its ester group under harsh demethylation conditions. Consequently, the researchers decided to adjust the reaction sequence, initiating the reaction between compound 58 and 4-fluorobenzylamine, yielding amide 79 with a yield of 99% (Fig. 10.23). Through optimization of experimental conditions, the amount of 4-fluorobenzylamine can be reduced from the previous 2.2 equivalents to 1.2 equivalents.

Upon obtaining 79, using the previous methylation reaction conditions did not result in any change in selectivity (78:22). However, by heating the reaction to 65°C for 4 hours, the selectivity can be increased to 80:20. Further prolonging the reaction time to 20 hours allows for the production of the nitrogen-methylated product 75 with a selectivity of 99:1 (Fig. 10.24). Through careful examination of the reaction conditions, process chemists discovered that increasing the reaction temperature, substrate concentration, and reagent amount all contribute to higher proportions of nitrogen-methylated products. Taking into account factors such as reagent cost, availability, toxicity, safety, and ease of operation, process chemists ultimately selected magnesium hydroxide as the base, Me$_3$S(O)I as the methylation reagent, and NMP as the solvent. Under these conditions, the reaction is carried out at 100°C for 6 hours, yielding intermediate

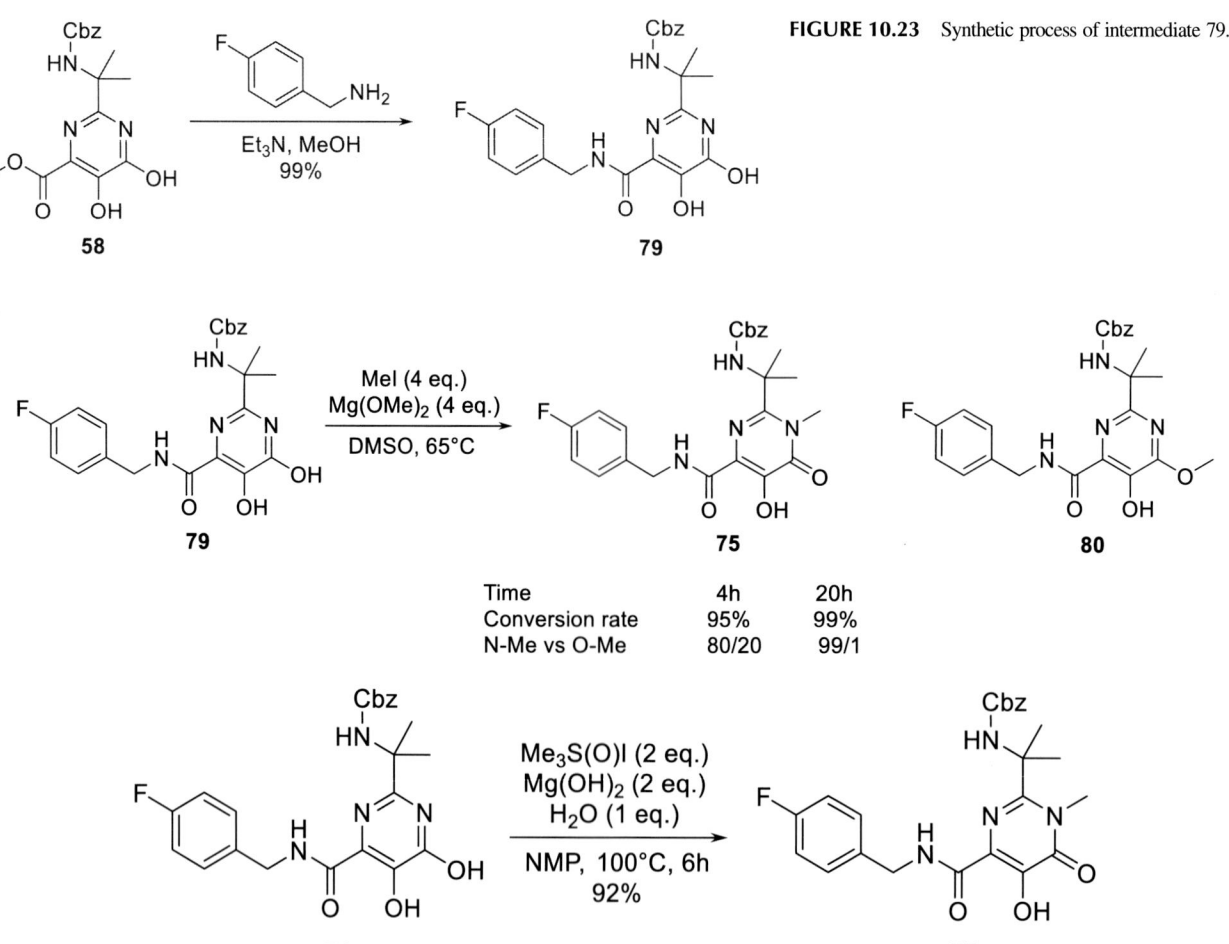

FIGURE 10.23 Synthetic process of intermediate 79.

FIGURE 10.24 The research on the nitrogen methylation reaction of intermediate 79.

75 with a 92% yield. The addition of 1 equivalent of water promotes the complete conversion of oxygen-methylated products to nitrogen-methylated products.

In the first-generation synthetic process, the amide formation reaction between 76 and 67 inevitably generates the byproduct 78 through diacylation. Therefore, it requires the use of 2.2 equivalents of acyl chloride 67 to improve the yield. To reduce the consumption of the expensive starting material 67 and achieve higher yields, process chemists attempted to protect the phenolic hydroxyl group. Considering the cost-effectiveness, efficiency in the introduction and removal of the protecting group, stability, and ease of storage of the intermediate, the t-butyl acyl group was ultimately selected as the protecting group. By optimizing the reaction conditions, the overall yield of the two-step process involving t-butyl acyl chloride protection of the phenolic hydroxyl group and palladium-catalyzed hydrogenation of the Cbz protecting group reached 98%. The obtained intermediate 82, unlike the unprotected intermediate 76 in the first-generation synthetic process, exhibits low hygroscopicity. Therefore, before the final amide formation reaction, complex water removal operations, as in the case of 76, are no longer required for 82. This significantly improves the synthesis efficiency while reducing solvent consumption. Finally, the amino group of intermediate 82 reacts with 1.15 equivalents of acyl chloride 67 to form the amide. Deprotection of the t-butyl ester in potassium hydroxide solution yields RAL. The overall yield of the two-step reaction reaches 97%, not only further enhancing the yield but also significantly reducing the consumption of 67 (Fig. 10.25).

Compared to the first-generation synthetic process, the second-generation synthetic process has significantly increased the overall yield of RAL potassium salt from intermediate 58, from 51% to 81%, while concurrently reducing the discharge of organic solvents and wastewater by 65%.

10.5 Summary and knowledge expansion

10.5.1 Summary of the discovery journey of raltegravir

RAL stands as the inaugural HIV-1 integrase inhibitor to attain commercial approval. The successful discovery of RAL underwent several crucial milestones (Fig. 10.26). Firstly, the discovery of two hit compounds marked a significant achievement. Scientists at Merck utilized their unique bioactivity screening model and an exclusive library of influenza virus endonuclease inhibitor molecules to successfully screen and identify the diketo acid compound L-731988. Through an investigation of the SAR pertaining to this hit compound, the pharmacophore was determined to be a core structure substituted with 1,3,4-triheteroatoms. By preserving this pharmacophore, further optimization of the scaffold led to the discovery of 1,6-naphthyridine compounds with improved drug-like properties, eventually resulting in the lead compound 12. Additionally, through a profound understanding of multiple target mechanisms, Merck scientists were able to perceptively

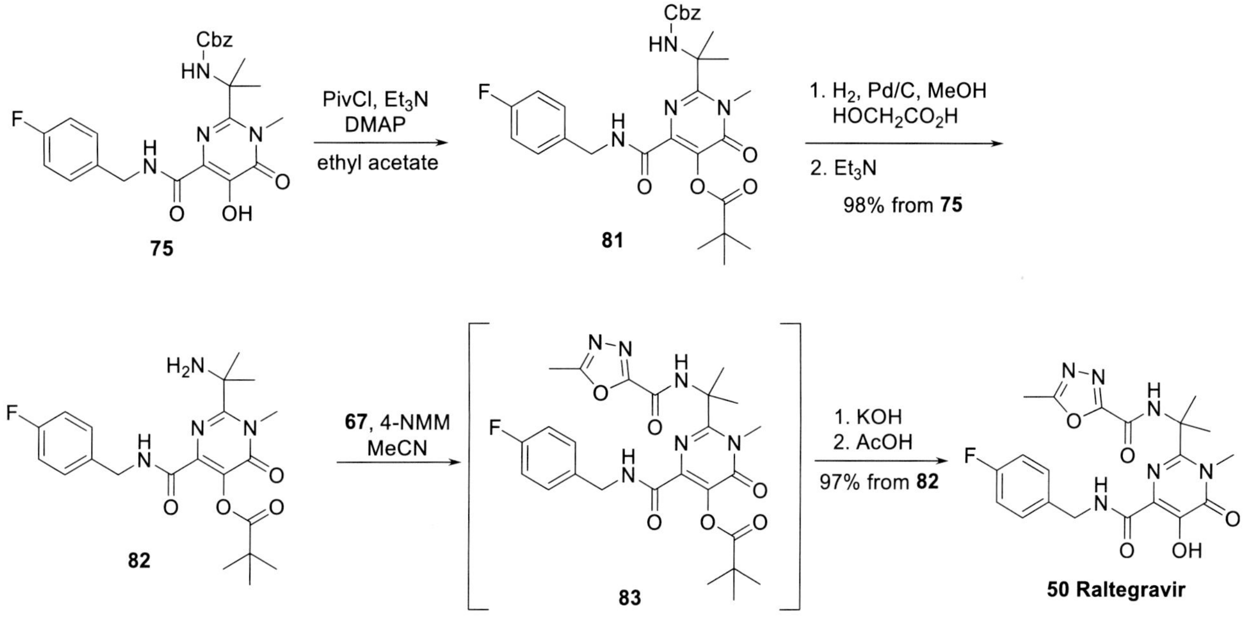

FIGURE 10.25 Second-generation synthetic process of raltegravir from intermediate 75.

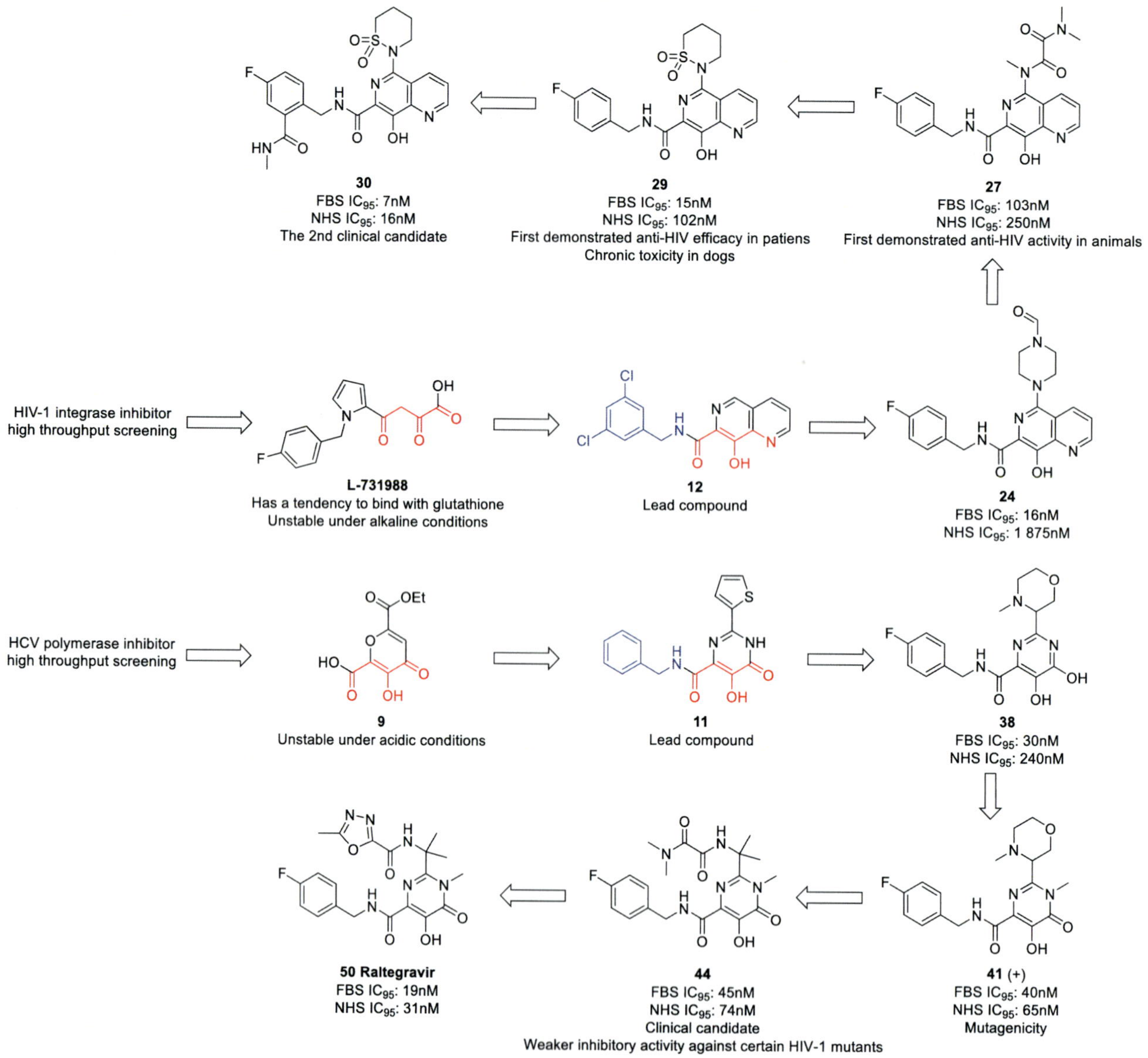

240 Medicinal Chemistry and Drug Development

FIGURE 10.26 The discovery journey of raltegravir.

link the HIV-1 integrase inhibitor project with the HCV polymerase inhibitor project, leading to the discovery of another hit compound, 9. Thus, combining insights into the SAR of 1,6-naphthyridine compounds with scaffold optimization of 9, another lead compound, 11, was obtained.

During the optimization process of the two lead compounds (11 and 12), the medicinal chemists first investigated the amine group of the amide for ease of synthesis and determined 4-F benzylamine as the optimal moiety. Subsequently, they meticulously optimized the solvent-exposed area of the binding pocket for both series, specifically the 5-position of 1,6-naphthyridine and the 2-position of N-methyl pyrimidone (dihydroxypyrimidine). For the 1,6-naphthyridine series, the introduction of a formylpiperazine at the 5-position (compound 24) improved the activity. However, due to high plasma protein binding, significant discrepancies in inhibitory activity were observed in cell experiments with the addition of FBS and NHS. By introducing an oxamide group at the 5-position (compound 27), the plasma protein binding was significantly reduced, narrowing the differences in cell activity under the two experimental conditions. Furthermore, the reduced nucleophilicity of the hydroxyl group at the 8-position lowered the rate of glucuronidation metabolism, improving the pharmacokinetic properties of the compound. This compound (27) demonstrated anti-HIV activity in animals for the first time. Further optimization by replacing the oxamide group at the 5-position with a sulfonamide group resulted in the enhanced activity of compound 29, which became the first compound to enter clinical trial. Its anti-HIV efficacy was confirmed in HIV-1-infected patients. Through further optimization of the amine group of the amide, compound 30 further reduced plasma protein binding. However, due to certain toxicities revealed in long-term safety evaluations in dogs for similar compound 29, Merck halted further clinical trials on the 1,6-naphthyridine compounds 29 and 30.

For the dihydroxypyrimidine series, the activity of compound 38 was noticeably enhanced by introducing N-methylmorpholine at the 2-position. Similarly, drawing from the experience of the HCV polymerase inhibitor project, the methylation of dihydroxypyrimidine resulted in compound 41, which significantly reduced plasma protein binding, improved cell activity under NHS conditions, and exhibited excellent pharmacokinetic properties. However, due to positive results in mutagenicity experiments, the compound had to be abandoned. By introducing an oxamide group similar to compound 27 at the 2-position, the first clinical candidate compound 44 in this series was obtained. Nonetheless, due to the compound's weaker inhibitory activity against certain HIV-1 mutants, Merck halted further clinical trials on compound 44. Through continued exploration of the 2-position, the medicinal chemists ultimately discovered that methyl oxadiazole formamide could serve as a substituent for the oxamide group, resulting in compound 50. Compound 50 not only further enhanced cell activity but also exhibited improved inhibitory potency against various HIV-1 mutants. Furthermore, it demonstrated favorable ADME/T properties, and clinical trials confirmed the safety and efficacy of this compound. Ultimately, compound 50 became the first successfully commercialized HIV-1 integrase inhibitor.

The research and development process of RAL can be briefly summarized as follows, aiming to provide inspiration for fellow students:

1. Through a profound understanding of HIV biology, a unique bioactivity screening model was established. Emphasis was placed on screening the company's proprietary library of influenza virus endonuclease inhibitor molecules, leading to the identification of diketo acid compounds with integrase inhibitory activity. The pharmacophore of 1,3-diketo acid effectively mimicked the phosphoryl group in DNA. However, these compounds had poor cell permeability, stability, and a tendency to bind with glutathione.
2. By comprehensively understanding the pharmacophore of the diketo acid compounds, innovative structural scaffolds of 1,6-naphthyridine and dihydroxypyrimidine were successfully designed to overcome the limitations of the original compound. These new scaffolds exhibited improved drug-like properties.
3. Precise optimization of the 5-position of 1,6-naphthyridine and the 2-position of dihydroxypyrimidine (N-methyl pyrimidone) (both located in the solvent-exposed area of the binding pocket) not only enhanced the compounds' potency but also reduced plasma protein binding, improved metabolic stability, and enhanced pharmacokinetic properties. This optimization improved safety, inhibitory potential against clinical HIV-1 mutant strains, and drug-like characteristics.
4. Crucially, cohesive team collaboration, critical thinking, a meticulous scientific attitude, and an innovative spirit are indispensable for the successful discovery of RAL.

Several years later, the main inventors of RAL, Summa, and Egbertson, along with their colleagues, provided a comprehensive account of the entire research and development process of RAL in two books published by John Wiley & Sons, Inc. [46,63]. Interested readers are encouraged to further explore these valuable resources.

10.5.2 Knowledge expansion

In 2007, scientists at Pfizer established a computational model [64] to predict the drug-likeness of various targets, with HIV-1 integrase being considered the "least druggable" target. Interestingly, in the same year, the HIV-1 integrase inhibitor RAL was approved by the FDA. The erroneous conclusion drawn by Pfizer's scientists was due to their reported model only considering the protein structure information of HIV-1 integrase, in which they did not identify any pockets capable of binding small molecules. However, they failed to consider that conformational changes occur when HIV-1 integrase binds to viral DNA, resulting in the formation of a small molecule binding pocket, which is precisely the site of action for integrase inhibitors like RAL. This conclusion was validated in the crystal structures (Fig. 10.27) [65] of prototype foamy virus integrase (which bears a striking resemblance to HIV-1 integrase in structure and function) bound to viral DNA and RAL. Additionally, it confirmed the binding mode proposed earlier by Merck scientists, involving chelation of the small molecule with two magnesium ions in the integrase.

Furthermore, upon binding of viral DNA with integrase, the 3′-P occurs immediately, whereby the GT unit is swiftly excised by the integrase. This elucidates why RAL does not inhibit the 3′-P. Once the 3′-P has taken place, during the transition of the PIC from the cytoplasm to the nucleus, RAL has ample time to bind with it, thereby inhibiting subsequent ST processes.

The successful discovery of RAL serves as a reminder for us to maintain a vigilant scientific critical mindset throughout the process of scientific research. Even in the face of authoritative reports, we should approach them with

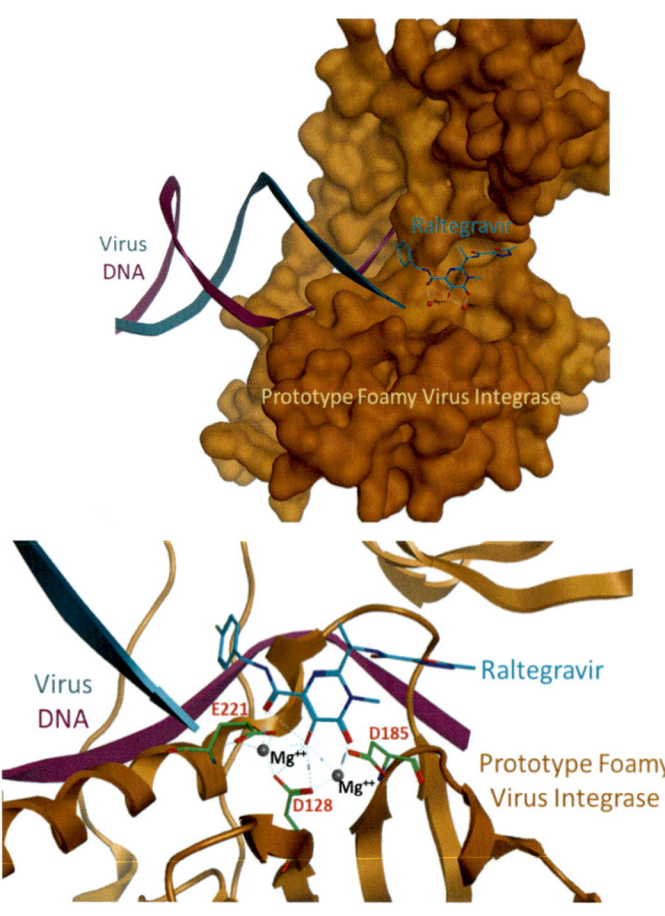

FIGURE 10.27 The crystal structure of the prototype foamy virus integrase complexed with viral DNA and raltegravir.

cautious skepticism. The notions of "undruggability" or "druggability" pertaining to targets should be approached with utmost caution to avoid missing the discovery of a new class of drugs or veering in the wrong direction.

References

[1] Gottlieb MS, Schroff R, Schanker HM, et al. Pneumocystis-carinii pneumonia and mucosal candidiasis in previously healthy homosexual men - evidence of a new acquired cellular immunodeficiency. N Engl J Med 1981;305(24):1425–31.

[2] Barresinoussi F, Chermann JC, Rey F, et al. Isolation of a T-lymphotropic retrovirus from a patient at risk for acquired immune-deficiency syndrome (AIDS). Science 1983;220(4599):868–71.

[3] UNAIDS[EB/OL], [2021-03-10], http://www.unaids.org.

[4] UNAIDS DATA 2020[EB/OL], [2021-03-10], http://old.aidsdatahub.org/sites/default/files/publication/UNAIDS_2020_aids-data-book_1.pdf.

[5] Wikipedia: HIV[EB/OL], [2021-03-10], https://en.wikipedia.org/wiki/HIV.

[6] Motomura K, Chen JB, Hu WS. Genetic recombination between human immunodeficiency virus type 1 (HIV-1) and HIV-2, two distinct human lentiviruses. J Virol 2008;82(4):1923–33.

[7] Harvey RA, Champe PC, Fisher BD. Microbiology. Lippincott Williams & Wilkins; 2006.

[8] Chan DC, Fass D, Berger JM, et al. Core structure of gp41 from the HIV envelope glycoprotein. Cell 1997;89(2):263–73.

[9] Chan DC, Kim PS. HIV entry and its inhibition. Cell 1998;93(5):681–4.

[10] Wyatt R, Sodroski J. The HIV-1 envelope glycoproteins: fusogens, antigens, and immunogens. Science 1998;280(5371):1884–8.

[11] Zheng YH, Lovsin N, Peterlin BMA. Newly identified host factors modulate HIV replication. Immunol Lett 2005;97(2):225–34.

[12] Guidelines for the Use of Antiretroviral Agents in Adults and Adolescents with HIV[EB/OL]. Department of Health and Human Services, 2019 [2020-04-12], http://www.aidsinfo.nih.gov/ContentFiles/AdultandAdolescentGL.pdf.

[13] Perelson AS, Neumann AU, Markowitz M, et al. HIV-1 dynamics in vivo: virion clearance rate, infected cell life-span, and viral generation time. Science 1996;271(5255):1582–6.

[14] Hammer SM, Squires KE, Hughes MD, et al. A controlled trial of two nucleoside analogues plus indinavir in persons with human immunodeficiency virus infection and CD4 cell counts of 200 per cubic millimeter or less. N Engl J Med 1997;337(11):725–33.

[15] Cai ML, Huang Y, Caffrey M, et al. Solution structure of the His12 —> Cys mutant of the N-terminal zinc binding domain of HIV-1 integrase complexed to cadmium. Protein Sci 1998;7(12):2669—74.

[16] Goldgur Y, Dyda F, Hickman AB, et al. Three new structures of the core domain of HIV-1 integrase: an active site that binds magnesium. Proc Natl Acad Sci USA 1998;95(16):9150—4.

[17] Lodi PJ, Ernst JA, Kuszewski J, et al. Solution structure of the DNA binding domain of HIV-1 integrase. Biochemistry 1995;34(31):9826—33.

[18] Passos DO, Li M, Yang RB, et al. Cryo-EM structures and atomic model of the HIV-1 strand transfer complex intasome. Science 2017;355 (6320):89—92.

[19] Mckee CJ, Kessl JJ, Shkriabai N, et al. Dynamic modulation of HIV-1 integrase structure and function by cellular lens epithelium-derived growth factor (LEDGF) protein. J Biol Chem 2008;283(46):31802—12.

[20] Engelman A, Mizuuchi K, Craigie R. HIV-1 DNA integration - mechanism of viral-DNA cleavage and DNA strand transfer. Cell 1991;67 (6):1211—21.

[21] Lee GE, Mauro E, Parissi V, et al. Structural insights on retroviral DNA integration: learning from foamy viruses. Viruses 2019;11(9):770.

[22] Wielens J, Crosby IT, Chalmers DK. A three-dimensional model of the human immunodeficiency virus type 1 integration complex. J Comput Aid Mol Des 2005;19(5):301—17.

[23] Miller MD, Farnet CM, Bushman FD. Human immunodeficiency virus type 1 preintegration complexes: studies of organization and composition. J Virol 1997;71(7):5382—90.

[24] Farnet CM, Haseltine WA. Determination of viral-proteins present in the human-immunodeficiency-virus type-1 preintegration complex. J Virol 1991;65(4):1910—15.

[25] Bukrinsky MI, Sharova N, Mcdonald TL, et al. Association of integrase, matrix, and reverse-transcriptase antigens of human-immunodeficiency-virus type-1 with viral nucleic-acids following acute infection. Proc Natl Acad Sci USA 1993;90(13):6125—9.

[26] Turlure F, Devroe E, Silver PA, et al. Human cell proteins and human immunodeficiency virus DNA integration. Front Biosci-Landmrk 2004;9:3187—208.

[27] Maurin C, Bailly F, Cotelle P. Structure-activity relationships of HIV-1 integrase inhibitors-enzyme-ligand interactions. Curr Med Chem 2003;10(18):1795—810.

[28] Jing N, Xu X. Rational drug design of DNA oligonucleotides as HIV inhibitors. Curr Drug Targets Infect Disord 2001;1(2):79—90.

[29] Fesen MR, Kohn KW, Leteurtre F, et al. Inhibitors of human-immunodeficiency-virus integrase. Proc Natl Acad Sci USA 1993;90 (6):2399—403.

[30] Mazumder A, Gazit A, Levitzki A, et al. Effects of tyrphostins, protein-kinase inhibitors, on human-immunodeficiency-virus type-1 integrase. Biochemistry 1995;34(46):15111—22.

[31] Fesen MR, Pommier Y, Leteurtre F, et al. Inhibition of HIV-1 integrase by flavones, caffeic acid phenethyl ester (Cape) and related-compounds. Biochem Pharmacol 1994;48(3):595—608.

[32] Lin ZW, Neamati N, Zhao H, et al. Chicoric acid analogues as HIV-1 integrase inhibitors. J Med Chem 1999;42(8):1401—14.

[33] Artico M, Di Santo R, Costi R, et al. Geometrically and conformationally restrained cinnamoyl compounds as inhibitors of HIV-1 integrase: synthesis, biological evaluation, and molecular modeling. J Med Chem 1998;41(21):3948—60.

[34] Di Santo R, Costi R, Artico M, et al. HIV-1 integrase inhibitors that block HIV-1 replication in infected cells. Planning synthetic derivatives from natural products. Pure Appl Chem 2003;75(2-3):195—206.

[35] Costi R, Di Santo R, Artico M, et al. 2,6-bis(3,4,5-trihydroxybenzylydene) derivatives of cyclohexanone: novel potent HIV-1 integrase inhibitors that prevent HIV-1 multiplication in cell-based assays. Bioorg Med Chem 2004;12(1):199—215.

[36] Hazuda DJ, Felock PJ, Hastings JC, et al. Differential divalent cation requirements uncouple the assembly and catalytic reactions of human immunodeficiency virus type 1 integrase. J Virol 1997;71(9):7005—11.

[37] Hazuda D, Felock PJ, Hastings JC, et al. Discovery and analysis of inhibitors of the human immunodeficiency integrase. Drug Des Discov 1997;15(1):17—24.

[38] Neamati N, Hong HX, Owen JM, et al. Salicylhydrazine-containing inhibitors of HIV-1 integrase: implication for a selective chelation in the integrase active site. J Med Chem 1998;41(17):3202—9.

[39] Hazuda DJ, Felock P, Witmer M, et al. Inhibitors of strand transfer that prevent integration and inhibit HIV-1 replication in cells. Science 2000;287(5453):646—50.

[40] Wai JS, Egbertson MS, Payne LS, et al. 4-aryl-2,4-dioxobutanoic acid inhibitors of HIV-1 integrase and viral replication in cells. J Med Chem 2000;43(26):4923—6.

[41] Goldgur Y, Craigie R, Cohen GH, et al. Structure of the HIV-1 integrase catalytic domain complexed with an inhibitor: a platform for antiviral drug design. Proc Natl Acad Sci USA 1999;96(23):13040—3.

[42] Zhuang LC, Wai JS, Embrey MW, et al. Design and synthesis of 8-hydroxy-[1,6]naphthyridines as novel inhibitors of HIV-1 integrase in vitro and in infected cells. J Med Chem 2003;46(4):453—6.

[43] Pace P, Nizi E, Pacini B, et al. The monoethyl ester of meconic acid is an active site inhibitor of HCVNS5B RNA-dependent RNA polymerase. Bioorg Med Chem Lett 2004;14(12):3257—61.

[44] Summa V, Petrocchi A, Pace P, et al. Discovery of alpha, gamma-diketo acids as potent selective and reversible inhibitors of hepatitis C virus NS5b RNA-dependent RNA polymerase. J Med Chem 2004;47(1):14—17.

[45] Pace P, Di Francesco ME, Gardelli C, et al. Dihydroxypyrimidine-4-carboxamides as novel potent and selective HIV integrase inhibitors. J Med Chem 2007;50(9):2225—39.

[46] Neamati. N. HIV-1 integrase: mechanism and inhibitor design. John Wiley & Sons, Inc; 2011.
[47] Petrocchi A, Koch U, Matassa VG, et al. From dihydroxypyrimidine carboxylic acids to carboxamide HIV-1 integrase inhibitors: SAR around the amide moiety. Bioorg Med Chem Lett 2007;17(2):350—3.
[48] Chapman RG, Ostuni E, Takayama S, et al. Surveying for surfaces that resist the adsorption of proteins. J Am Chem Soc 2000;122 (34):8303—4.
[49] Guare JP, Wai JS, Gomez RP, et al. A series of 5-aminosubstituted 4-fluorobenzyl-8-hydroxy-[1,6]naphthyridine-7-carboxamide HIV-1 integrase inhibitors. Bioorg Med Chem Lett 2006;16(11):2900—4.
[50] Mulder GJ, Van Doorn AB. A rapid NAD + -linked assay for microsomal uridine diphosphate glucuronyltransferase of rat liver and some observations on substrate specificity of the enzyme. Biochem J 1975;151(1):131—40.
[51] Hazuda DJ, Anthony NJ, Gomez RP, et al. A naphthyridine carboxamide provides evidence for discordant resistance between mechanistically identical inhibitors of HIV-1 integrase. Proc Natl Acad Sci USA 2004;101(31):11233—8.
[52] Egbertson MS, Moritz HM, Melamed JY, et al. A potent and orally active HIV-1 integrase inhibitor. Bioorg Med Chem Lett 2007;17 (5):1392—8.
[53] Summa V, Petrocchi A, Matassa VG, et al. 4,5-dihydroxypyrimidine carboxamides and N-alkyl-5-hydroxypyrimidinone carboxamides are potent, selective HIV integrase inhibitors with good pharmacokinetic profiles in preclinical species. J Med Chem 2006;49(23):6646—9.
[54] Summa V, Petrocchi A, Bonelli F, et al. Discovery of raltegravir, a potent, selective orally bioavailable HIV-integrase inhibitor for the treatment of HIV-AIDS infection. J Med Chem 2008;51(18):5843—55.
[55] Cocohoba J, Dong BJ. Raltegravir: the first HIV integrase inhibitor. Clin Ther 2008;30(10):1747—65.
[56] Iwamoto M, Wenning LA, Petry AS, et al. Safety, tolerability, and pharmacokinetics of raltegravir after single and multiple doses in healthy subjects. Clin Pharmacol Ther 2008;83(2):293—9.
[57] Markowitz M, Morales-Ramirez JO, Nguyen BY, et al. Antiretroviral activity, pharmacokinetics, and tolerability of MK-0518, a novel inhibitor of HIV-1 integrase, dosed as monotherapy for 10 days in treatment-naive HIV-1-infected individuals. Jaids-J Acq Imm Def 2006;43 (5):509—15.
[58] Markowitz M, Nguyen BY, Gotuzzo E, et al. Rapid and durable antiretroviral effect of the HIV-1 integrase inhibitor raltegravir as part of combination therapy in treatment-naive patients with HIV-1 infection - results of a 48-week controlled study. Jaids-J Acq Imm Def 2007;46 (2):125—33.
[59] Grinsztejn B, Nguyen BY, Katlama C, et al. Safety and efficacy of the HIV-1 integrase inhibitor raltegravir (MK-0518) in treatment-experienced patients with multidrug-resistant virus: a phase II randomised controlled trial. Lancet 2007;369(9569):1261—9.
[60] Steigbigel RT, Cooper DA, Kumar PN, et al. Raltegravir with optimized background therapy for resistant HIV-1 infection. N Engl J Med 2008;359(4):339—54.
[61] Lennox JL, Dejesus E, Lazzarin A, et al. Safety and efficacy of raltegravir-based versus efavirenz-based combination therapy in treatment-naive patients with HIV-1 infection: a multicentre, double-blind randomised controlled trial. Lancet 2009;374(9692):796—806.
[62] Humphrey GR, Pye PJ, Zhong YL, et al. Development of a second-generation, highly efficient manufacturing route for the HIV integrase inhibitor raltegravir potassium. Org Process Res Dev 2011;15(1):73—83.
[63] Kazmierski WM. Antiviral drugs: from basic discovery through clinical trials. John Wiley & Sons, Inc; 2011.
[64] Cheng AC, Coleman RG, Smyth KT, et al. Structure-based maximal affinity model predicts small-molecule druggability. Nat Biotechnol 2007;25(1):71—5.
[65] Hare S, Gupta SS, Valkov E, et al. Retroviral intasome assembly and inhibition of DNA strand transfer. Nature 2010;464(7286):232—6.

Chapter 11

Discovery and development of the human immunodeficiency virus protease inhibitor Saquinavir

Daoyuan Chen[1,2] and Xianzhang Bu[2]

[1]School of Bioengineering, Zhuhai Campus of Zunyi University, Zhuhai, Guangdong, P.R. China, [2]School of Pharmaceutical Sciences, Sun Yat-Sen University, Guangzhou, P.R. China

Chapter outline

11.1 Overview of virus	245
11.1.1 Virus structure and its biological functions	245
11.1.2 Classification and nomenclature of viruses	246
11.1.3 Viral infection and pathogenic properties	246
11.1.4 The human antiviral warfare	247
11.2 Human immunodeficiency virus and acquired immunodeficiency syndrome	247
11.2.1 HIV and AIDS	247
11.2.2 Structure of HIV	248
11.2.3 Mechanisms of HIV infection and HIV life cycle	248
11.3 HIV protease and inhibitor saquinavir	249
11.3.1 Structural characteristics of HIV proteases	249
11.3.2 The design of HIV protease inhibitors	250
11.3.3 Design and discovery of saquinavir	251
11.3.4 Pharmacokinetic properties and deficiencies of saquinavir	253
11.4 Further development of Saquinavir	254
11.4.1 Enhancement of pharmacokinetic properties	254
11.4.2 The discovery of the Darunavir	256
11.5 Anti-HIV/AIDS drugs and novel treatment strategies	260
11.5.1 Classification of anti-HIV/AIDS drugs	260
11.5.2 New strategies for HIV/AIDS prevention and treatment	261
References	263

11.1 Overview of virus

11.1.1 Virus structure and its biological functions

A virus is an infectious nucleic acid entity that parasitically replicates within host cells at the molecular level. It belongs to a category of minute noncellular microorganisms. The fundamental architecture of a virus consists of nucleic acid encapsulated within a proteinaceous capsid often adorned with additional layers such as envelopes derived from host cell membranes.

The nucleic acid resides centrally within the virus, often denoted as the viral core. The viral core typically consists solely of DNA or RNA, approximately containing 300–400 kilobases (kb). These base sequences make up the viral genome, carrying the entirety of the virus's genetic information, which in turn determines its biological functions such as infectivity, replication, heredity, and variation.

The capsid is a protein coat formed by the assembly of a specific number of capsomeres following certain arrangement rules. Its primary roles are to protect the viral core and facilitate infection. Capsomeres, the substructural units that compose the capsid, are typically folded into ordered patterns by proteins encoded by the viral genome and are thereby classified as viral structural proteins. Different virus particles exhibit varying numbers and arrangements of capsomeres, which dictate their morphological structures. Based on the arrangement of capsomeres, viral capsids can exhibit helical symmetry (e.g., tobacco mosaic virus), icosahedral symmetry (e.g., poliovirus), or complex symmetry (e.g., bacteriophage T-series). The capsid envelops the viral core, forming a nucleocapsid. The simplest viral particles consist solely of a nucleocapsid, exemplified by naked viruses like the poliovirus.

Some viruses also possess additional auxiliary structures, such as an envelope, enzymes, and fibers. The envelope is a membrane or membrane-like structure that surrounds the viral capsid, consisting of lipid bilayers, proteins, and polysaccharides. Among these components, proteins and polysaccharides combine to form glycoprotein subunits, which are embedded in the lipid structure and exhibit spike-like protrusions known as "spike proteins." These spike proteins are critical for determining viral specificity and high antigenicity. Located between the envelope and the capsid is a matrix composed of matrix proteins, which not only provide support to the envelope but also maintain the viral structure. The envelope is generated during the budding and release process of progeny viruses from host cells. Due to its high homology with the host cell membrane, enveloped viruses can even evade the host's immune defenses. The enveloped virus nucleocapsid also contains functional proteins such as RNA polymerase, reverse transcriptase, proteases, and others, which play important roles in the viral life cycle. Fibers, on the other hand, are found only in adenoviruses and consist of linear polymer peptides and spherical terminal proteins. They are located at various protruding regions on the surface of the capsid. These fibers can attach to host cells and are associated with their pathogenic effects.

Mature and fully infectious viral particles are referred to as virions. These virions are considered nanoscale microorganisms, typically measuring around 100 nm in size. Some larger virions, such as the vaccinia virus, can reach up to 300 nm, while smaller ones like the poliovirus are only about 20 nm in size. Viruses exhibit various morphologies, including sphericity, filamentous structures, bullet-shaped forms, and brick-shaped configurations.

11.1.2 Classification and nomenclature of viruses

Based on the chemical nature of nucleic acids, viruses are broadly categorized into DNA viruses and RNA viruses. Further classification is based on the composition of nucleic acid chains, distinguishing between double-stranded viruses and single-stranded viruses. Single-stranded RNA viruses can be further divided into + ssRNA viruses and −ssRNA viruses. + ssRNA can directly serve as mRNA for protein translation, while −ssRNA requires the synthesis of a complementary positive-sense chain with mRNA functionality. In addition to these, there is a special type of single-stranded RNA virus that first synthesizes a double-stranded DNA through the action of reverse transcriptase. This DNA is then integrated into the host cell genome to complete the subsequent viral replication process. These viruses are known as retroviruses.

Virus nomenclature is determined by the International Committee on Taxonomy of Viruses (ICTV). According to the naming and writing conventions set by the ICTV, viruses are typically named based on their unique characteristics, using italicized uppercase letters to denote the taxonomic units such as order, family, subfamily, genus, and species. The Tenth Report on Virus Classification and Nomenclature, published by the ICTV in 2017, reveals that there are currently 8 orders, 122 families, 35 subfamilies, 735 genera, and 4404 species of classified viruses. Additionally, there are 80 families that cannot be assigned to known viral orders. The ICTV also terms subviral agents as entities that are smaller and structurally simpler than typical viruses. These agents lack complete viral structures but are capable of infecting both animals and plants.

11.1.3 Viral infection and pathogenic properties

Viruses are composed of simple chemical structures and lack any characteristics of life. Purified viruses can even be crystallized. Due to the absence of cellular structures such as ribosomes, transfer RNA, and protein synthesis enzyme systems, viruses lack the ability for independent growth, reproduction, and metabolism. Instead, they rely on parasitizing specific host cells. In some cases, viral nucleic acids can integrate into the host cell's DNA, allowing for proliferation and exhibiting genetic and mutational characteristics. Thus, viruses possess attributes of both biological macromolecules and organisms.

Viruses can spread through various means, including the respiratory and digestive tracts, contact, and bodily fluids. The processes of viral infection and replication primarily involve attachment, fusion, replication, amplification, maturation, and release. When infecting a host with normal immune function, viruses may not exhibit significant clinical symptoms, which is referred to as a latent infection. However, when the immune function of the host is compromised, the extensive replication and proliferation of the virus can not only damage cells—leading to cell lysis, death, functional transformation, chromosomal aberrations, and other consequences—but also induce immune responses in the host, resulting in immune-mediated pathological damage and significant clinical symptoms, known as an overt infection.

Clinically, overt infections can be further classified as acute or chronic infections. Acute infections have a short incubation period and rapid onset, with recovery possible within a few days after treatment. On the other hand, chronic infections refer to persistent viral infections within the body, with an incubation period that can last for more than a decade. Clinical symptoms may be mild or even asymptomatic, but the infection remains transmissible, as seen in cases such as hepatitis B and AIDS caused by the corresponding viruses.

11.1.4 The human antiviral warfare

Throughout history, due to a lack of scientific understanding of viruses, humanity has been virtually powerless in the face of virulent infectious diseases, paying an exceedingly devastating price. Events such as the Black Death in medieval Europe, the 1918 Spanish flu pandemic, and the centuries-long scourge of smallpox have all resulted in millions of deaths within a short period. However, with the advancements in modern science, our comprehension of viruses has deepened, and conquering viral infections has become a genuine possibility. After arduous and remarkable efforts, the World Health Organization (WHO) declared the global eradication of smallpox in 1979, marking a significant milestone in human history's fight against viral infectious diseases.

Nevertheless, the struggle between humans and viruses is an ongoing battle, and the prevention and treatment of viral infections remain an arduous task. Diseases such as AIDS (1981), severe acute respiratory syndrome (2003), Ebola hemorrhagic fever (2014), and the sudden outbreak of the novel coronavirus pneumonia in late 2019 have posed severe challenges to humanity. The broad scope of transmission, rapid spread, and significant societal impact caused by viral infectious diseases not only affect health and endanger lives but also become critical social issues that affect national stability and development. Effectively preventing and controlling these diseases has become a focal point and a hot topic in the field of global public health.

11.2 Human immunodeficiency virus and acquired immunodeficiency syndrome

11.2.1 HIV and AIDS

On the 5th of June, 1981, the Centers for Disease Control and Prevention in the United States documented an unusual series of case reports in the "Morbidity and Mortality Weekly Report," detailing conditions observed in five homosexual males. These patients exhibited symptoms such as persistent high fevers and severe immunodeficiency, along with Pneumocystis pneumonia and oral candidiasis infections, with no efficacy from symptomatic treatments. Tragically, two of the patients succumbed to their ailments [1]. The disease was then named AIDS in 1982 by the CDC, a term that has since become widely recognized around the world.

AIDS rapidly proliferated across the globe, earning it the designation of "the plague of the century." According to reports by the WHO, as of the year 2020, there were approximately 37.7 million individuals living with AIDS worldwide, with an annual increase of about 1.5 million new infections and around 680,000 deaths attributed to AIDS-related complications. Africa has been particularly hard-hit by the epidemic, with infection rates in some countries reaching up to 30% of the total population. In China, the prevalence of AIDS remains relatively low overall, yet certain regions are experiencing a surge in cases [2]. The effective prevention and control of AIDS remains a universal challenge.

In the wake of the AIDS epidemic, pinpointing the causative pathogen became a critical focus in the fight against the disease. In 1983, a team led by Luc Montagnier at the Pasteur Institute in France isolated a novel retrovirus from the lymph nodes of an early AIDS patient, which they named lymphadenopathy associated virus (LAV) [3]. In early 1984, a team led by Robert Gallo in the United States isolated a virus from the peripheral blood mononuclear cells of AIDS patients, which was named human T-cell lymphotropic virus type III (HTLV-III) [4]. Shortly thereafter, a team from the University of California, led by Levy, isolated the AIDS-related virus (ARV) from the peripheral blood lymphocytes of AIDS patients, marking the first instance of the virus being linked to AIDS through its nomenclature [5]. Subsequent research confirmed that these three strains of the virus were members of the same retrovirus family and were the pathogens responsible for AIDS. These discoveries highlighted the global effort in identifying the pathogen responsible for AIDS. In 1986, the ICTV unified the nomenclature of LAV/HTLV-III/ARV under the designation human immunodeficiency virus (HIV) [6].

HIV belongs to the genus Lentivirus within the family of retroviruses. There are two main subtypes of the virus: HIV-1 and HIV-2 [7]. HIV-1 is found worldwide and is more virulent, making it the primary cause of the global AIDS epidemic. Most research focuses on this subtype due to its widespread prevalence and severe impact on human health. HIV-1 is known for its rapid progression to AIDS in untreated individuals, leading to a higher mortality rate. Conversely, HIV-2 is primarily found in West Africa. It is less virulent and less transmissible than HIV-1, leading to a slower progression of AIDS [7,8]. Due to its geographical concentration and lower virulence, HIV-2 has not spread as extensively as HIV-1 and thus has a smaller impact on global health. However, for individuals infected with HIV-2, the disease can still lead to serious health issues and necessitates medical treatment.

HIV is transmitted through sexual contact, blood exposure (including needle sharing or transfusions), and from mother to child during pregnancy, childbirth, or breastfeeding. To date, the virus has caused over 30 million deaths worldwide, making it one of the most devastating infectious diseases in human history. Recognizing the urgent need for public awareness and prevention measures, the WHO designated December 1st as World AIDS Day in 1988. This day is observed annually to raise awareness about the disease, commemorate those who have died from AIDS-related illnesses, and mobilize efforts to address the epidemic.

11.2.2 Structure of HIV

HIV particles are spherical in shape with a diameter ranging from 100 to 120 nm and are characterized by an enveloped morphology. As shown in Fig. 11.1, the envelope's surface is studded with protrusions formed by the glycoprotein gp120 and gp41, which are present as trimers and serve as the principal binding sites for the interaction between HIV and the CD4 receptors on host cells. Within the virus is a spherical matrix composed of the p17 protein and a conical capsid constructed of the capsid protein p24. Encased within the capsid are the nucleocapsid protein p7, the RNA genome, and enzymes vital for viral replication, including reverse transcriptase, integrase, protease, and various regulatory proteins [9].

The genome of HIV consists of two identical positive-sense RNA single strands, with a total length of approximately 9.8 kb. It encompasses three structural genes (*gag, env, and pol*), two regulatory genes (*tat and vif*), and four accessory genes (*vpr, vpu/vpx, nef, and rev*) [10,11]. The *gag* gene is responsible for encoding the core proteins, while the *pol* encodes the reverse transcriptase, integrase, and protease necessary for HIV replication. The *env* encodes the viral membrane protein, which acts as the primary antigen for HIV immunological diagnostics.

11.2.3 Mechanisms of HIV infection and HIV life cycle

HIV infects host cells by relying on the cell surface CD4 receptor, which is crucial for the selective infection of CD4-positive host cells such as T-lymphocytes, monocytes, and dendritic cells. The process of infection includes key stages such as attachment and fusion, entry into the nucleus, reverse transcription and genome integration, transcription and translation, assembly and release, and maturation [7,12].

Attachment and Fusion: During infection, the HIV viral envelope glycoprotein gp120, with the assistance of the host cell surface coreceptor CCR5 (or CXCR4), binds to the host cell surface CD4 molecule, forming a gp120/CD4/CCR5 (or CXCR4) trimeric complex. At the same time, gp120 undergoes a conformational change, exposing the transmembrane protein gp41. The exposed gp41, utilizing its own hydrophobic properties, induces fusion of the viral envelope with the host cell membrane, thus facilitating the entry of the viral capsid into the host cell.

Reverse Transcription and Integration: The viral capsid releases the RNA genome and enzymes, and under the action of reverse transcriptase, the RNA is reverse transcribed into previral DNA. The previral DNA forms a complex with integrase, enters the host cell nucleus, and integrates into the chromosome.

Transcription and Translation: The previrus utilizes the host expression system for transcription and translation, synthesizing Env protein and Gag and Gag-Pol polyproteins. The Env protein is cleaved by host cell proteases in the endoplasmic reticulum into glycoproteins gp120 and gp41 and is transported to the cell membrane.

Assembly and Release: Gag, Gag-Pol polyproteins, and replicated RNA genome assemble to form viral particles, acquiring the envelope protein through budding.

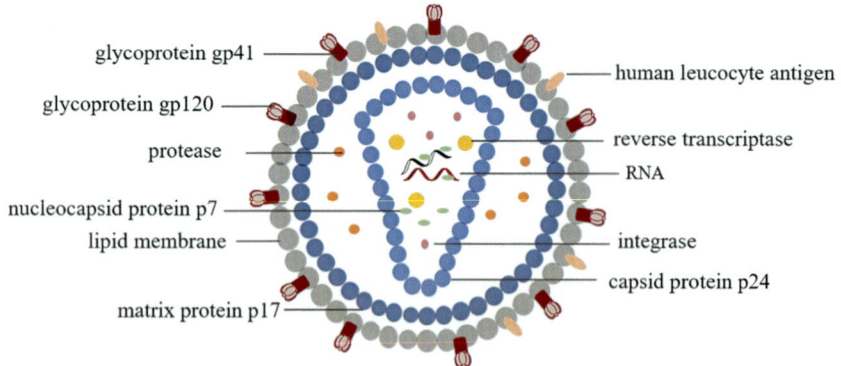

FIGURE 11.1 Structural model of HIV.

Maturation: Under the processing of HIV protease, Gag and Gag-Pol polyproteins are cleaved into structural proteins such as p24, p17, p7, and p6, as well as enzymes like reverse transcriptase, integrase, and protease within the viral particle. This ultimately leads to the formation of mature infectious progeny viruses, thereby initiating a new replication cycle.

Throughout the lengthy process of evolution, organisms have developed both innate immunity and adaptive immunity to combat external pathogen attacks. Among these, a series of immune cells, exemplified by human CD4 + T lymphocytes, play a vital role in adaptive immunity, responsible for eradicating pathogens within infected host cells. HIV primarily invades human CD4 + T lymphocytes and, through its replication, compromises the immune system. This acquired immunodeficiency resulting from such acquired factors is known as AIDS. Patients with compromised immune systems are susceptible to opportunistic infections or malignant tumors, ultimately leading to fatality.

11.3 HIV protease and inhibitor saquinavir

11.3.1 Structural characteristics of HIV proteases

HIV protease contains a conserved -Asp-Thr-Gly-sequence, which is characteristic of the aspartic protease family and indicates its membership within this family. During the replication cycle of HIV, HIV protease cleaves the precursor Gag and Gag-Pol polyproteins encoded by the virus, generating core structural proteins such as p24 and p17, as well as functional proteins such as reverse transcriptase and integrase. This process is crucial for the maturation of progeny viruses. Inhibiting HIV protease can disrupt the maturation of the virus, thus preventing the production of infectious viral particles. Consequently, HIV protease has become one of the key targets for anti-HIV therapy [13].

HIV-1 protease, as revealed by protein crystallography studies, is composed of two identical peptide chains, each containing 99 amino acid residues, and exhibits a twofold rotational symmetry axis (C2 axis) [14,15]. The active site of the protease is located between the two peptide chains and consists of two β-hairpin structures and two segments of aspartyl-serine-glycine (-Asp25-Thr26-Gly27-), where the Asp25/Asp25' residues regulate catalytic activity by transferring hydrogen atoms to activate water molecules, thereby facilitating the attack of water molecules on peptide bonds. The active site is capped by two "flap" structures, and as substrates bind or are released, the dimer adopts a closed or open conformation [13,16]. Additionally, Gly27/Gly27' can form hydrogen bonds with substrates to stabilize the substrate at the top of the flap region, in coordination with Ile50/Gly50' (Fig. 11.2A).

During the precision-driven process of drug design and refinement, researchers frequently utilize standardized nomenclature to delineate the locational relationship between substrates and proteins. Focused around the peptide bond at the substrate's cleavage site, the flanking amino acid residue side chains are denoted as the P1 and P1' regions, corresponding to the protease's S1 and S1' pockets. Progressing laterally from the cleavage site, these are sequentially identified as P2, P3, and P2', P3', etc., with the matching receptor areas labeled as S2, S3, S2', S3', and so on (refer to Figs. 11.2B and 11.3) [17].

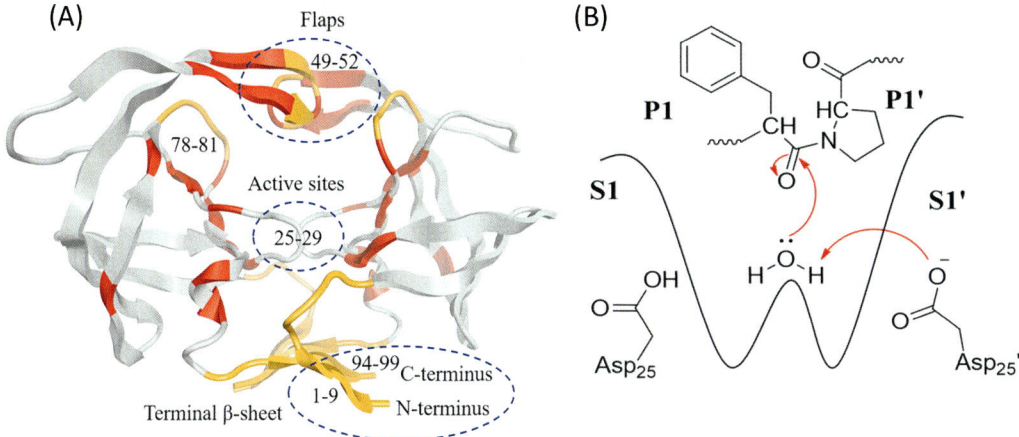

FIGURE 11.2 (A) Structural diagram of HIV-1 protease. Yellow represents the relatively conserved sequence and red indicates the mutation-prone region; (B) Catalytic center.

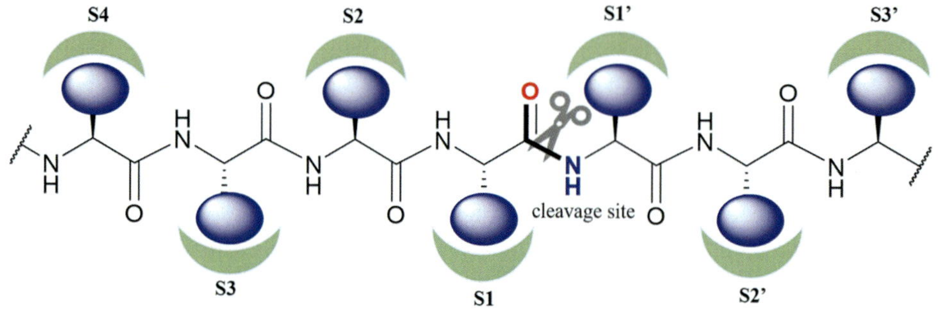

FIGURE 11.3 General binding model of enzyme and substrate.

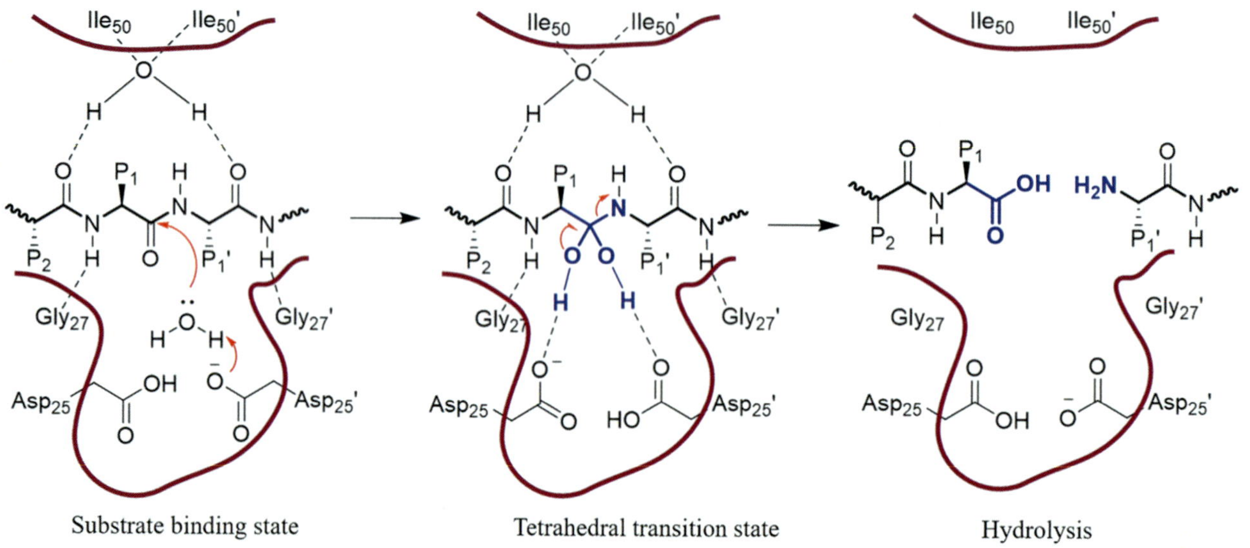

FIGURE 11.4 Schematic diagram of the hydrolysis mechanism of HIV protease based on the tetrahedral transition state model.

11.3.2 The design of HIV protease inhibitors

Developing highly selective HIV PIs to reduce their effects on endogenous human aspartic proteases is crucial in minimizing drug side effects. Mammalian aspartic proteases such as pepsin primarily cleave at the Leu (P1)-Val/Ala (P1′) sites. In contrast, HIV protease targets over 10 asymmetric and nonhomologous cleavage sites in the cleavage of Gag and Gag-Pol polyproteins, with the Tyr/Phe (P1)-Pro (P1′) site being extremely rare among other members of the aspartic protease family. This rarity presents an opportunity for the design of selective HIV PIs that specifically target the Tyr/Phe-Pro site [18–20].

It is generally believed that the hydrolysis catalyzed by aspartic protease is a part of acid-base catalysis, relying on the involvement of a water molecule. The two Asp residues at the active site have different dissociation states, with the negatively charged Asp residue first obtaining a proton from a water molecule. The activated water then attacks the carbonyl carbon atom at the cleavage site, changing the carbon atom from sp2 to sp3 hybridization; simultaneously, another Asp residue loses a proton to the substrate intermediate, forming a tetrahedral transition state with a gem-diol structure through proton transfer, followed by the generation of free amino and carboxyl groups, releasing the hydrolyzed shortened peptide product and then starting a new reaction cycle. Despite the fact that the precise roles or mechanisms of Asp25/25′ residues' protonation states, the relative positions of acidic protons, and the cap structure in the catalytic process of HIV protease have not been completely elucidated, researchers generally agree that HIV protease adheres to the common catalytic hydrolysis mechanism of the aspartic protease family. This recognition has significantly guided the early development of inhibitors for HIV protease (Fig. 11.4) [13,17].

The theory of transition-state mimicry in drug design suggests that due to the influence of multiple hydrogen bonds, the transition state exhibits markedly greater enzymatic affinity compared to both the substrate and the resultant product. Therefore, if stable compounds with spatial structure, hydrophobicity, or electronegativity similar to the transition state can be designed, it may be possible to obtain highly active and selective enzyme inhibitors. Because the gem-diol structure in the sp³ hybridized state of the transition state is unstable, further optimization and substitution of the gem-diol structure are required, using electron-withdrawing groups or other strategies. A common method is to first remove a hydroxyl group and simultaneously replace the -NH- in the original amide bond with -CH$_2$- through electron-withdrawing substitution, achieving a stable hydroxyethyl core structure (Fig. 11.5). So far, the development of peptide bond transition state analogs for aspartic protease hydrolysis has led to the use of various electron-withdrawing groups such as hydroxyethyl, phosphonate, hydrazine, and hydroxyethylamine, resulting in several successful drug design examples [17].

11.3.3 Design and discovery of saquinavir

11.3.3.1 From dipeptide Phe-Pro to the lead compound 3

In the process of drug design and optimization, achieving a detailed structure-activity relationship (SAR) is particularly important. Based on the existing SAR, further structural optimization of lead compounds to obtain higher-activity candidate drugs is the main focus of medicinal chemistry, spanning the entire drug development process. In 1990, researchers began with the protease cleavage site, using the inactive dipeptide Phe (P1)-Pro (P1′) as the basic structure (1, Fig. 11.6). The free amine and carboxyl groups were protected using benzyl carbonyl and tert-butyl groups, respectively. Additionally, hydroxyethylamine was used to replace the peptide bond based on transition state characteristics, resulting in a pseudo-dipeptide compound 2 that mimics the transition state of the hydrolysis process. Compound 2 exhibited a half-maximal inhibitory concentration (IC$_{50}$) of 6500 nM against HIV-1 protease activity [18], indicating a relatively weak level of activity.

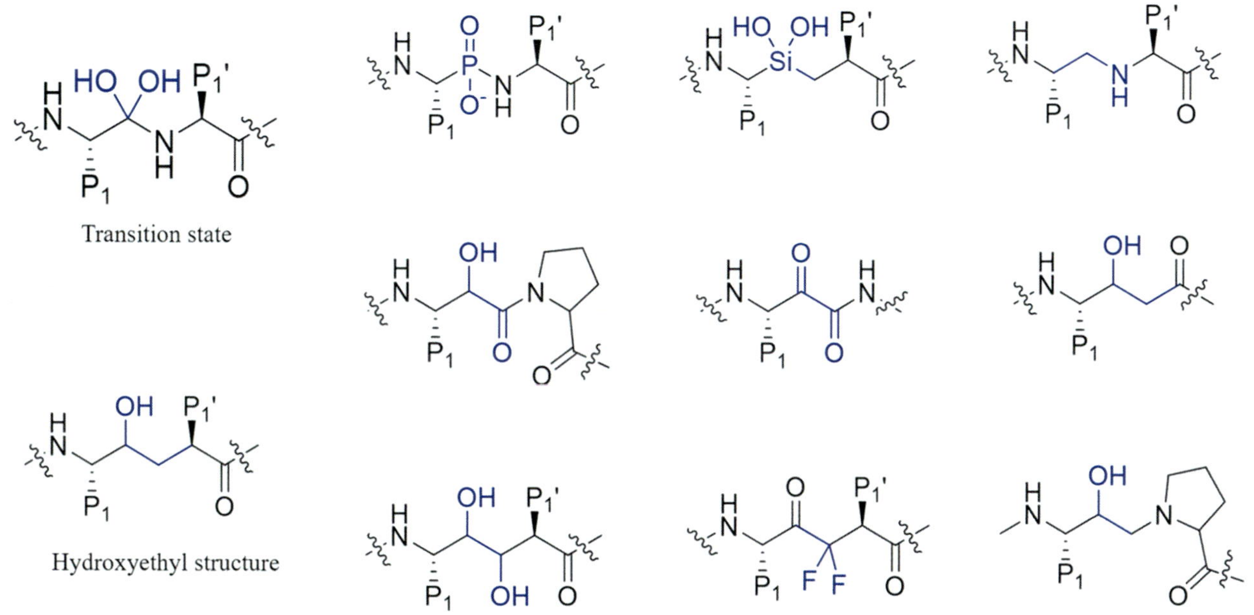

FIGURE 11.5 Representative analogs based on tetrahedral transition state strategy used for designing protease inhibitors.

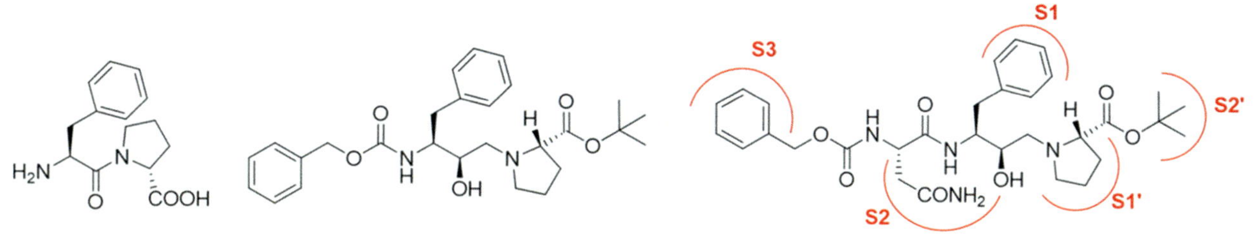

FIGURE 11.6 Structural and activity characteristics of Phe-Pro-based peptidomimetics.

Similarly, by simulating the substrate Leu165-Ile169 pentapeptide sequence Leu-Asn-Phe-Pro-Ile, where the Phe-Pro segment was replaced and an additional Asn residue was introduced at the N-terminus of compound 1, compound 3 was obtained with an IC$_{50}$ value of 140 nM, representing a more than 40-fold increase in activity (Fig. 11.6). It was also observed that extending an additional Leu at the N-terminus or an additional Ile at the C-terminus of compound 3, or simultaneously extending both termini, did not significantly improve the activity. Due to possessing the minimal molecular framework required for high enzyme inhibitory activity, compound 3 has become the lead structure for subsequent systematic structural optimization [18].

11.3.3.2 Optimization of the lead compound 3

The research team conducted an optimization design for the spatial volume and electrostatic strength of the end and side chain groups of lead compound 3 and obtained the following SAR through activity screening and evaluation (Fig. 11.7) [18,21].

N-terminus hydrophobicity enhancement: The substitution of the benzyl group at the N-terminus (P3 region) of lead compound 3 to the more hydrophobic 2-naphthyl group (4) resulted in an enhancement of activity (IC$_{50}$ = 53 nM). This suggests the possible presence of a large hydrophobic pocket in the S3 region of the protease, and the presence of a larger hydrophobic group in the P3 region is conducive to enhancing enzyme inhibitory activity. Furthermore, the replacement of the 2-naphthyl group with 2-quinoline resulted in a further enhancement of the activity of compound 5 to an IC$_{50}$ of 23 nM, indicating the potential involvement of the nitrogen atom in the binding process.

C-terminus stability considerations: The hydrophobic tert-butyl group in the structure of lead compound 3 is an essential pharmacophore, and no superior substituents have been identified in the study. Substitution of the tert-butoxy group with a tert-butylamine group resulted in a slight decrease in enzyme inhibitory activity to an IC$_{50}$ of 210 nM. However, the conversion of the ester bond to the chemically more stable amide bond is advantageous for enhancing the *in vivo* stability of the drug, thereby possessing better drug potential. Subsequent structural optimization also largely retained this key feature.

P1′ region ring expansion: Expanding the P1′ region of compound 6 from the proline residue tetrahydropyrrole framework to a piperidine ring, resulting in a significant improvement in the activity of compound 7 (IC$_{50}$ = 18 nM). Further cyclization to the decahydroisoquinoline structure in compound 8 led to a further

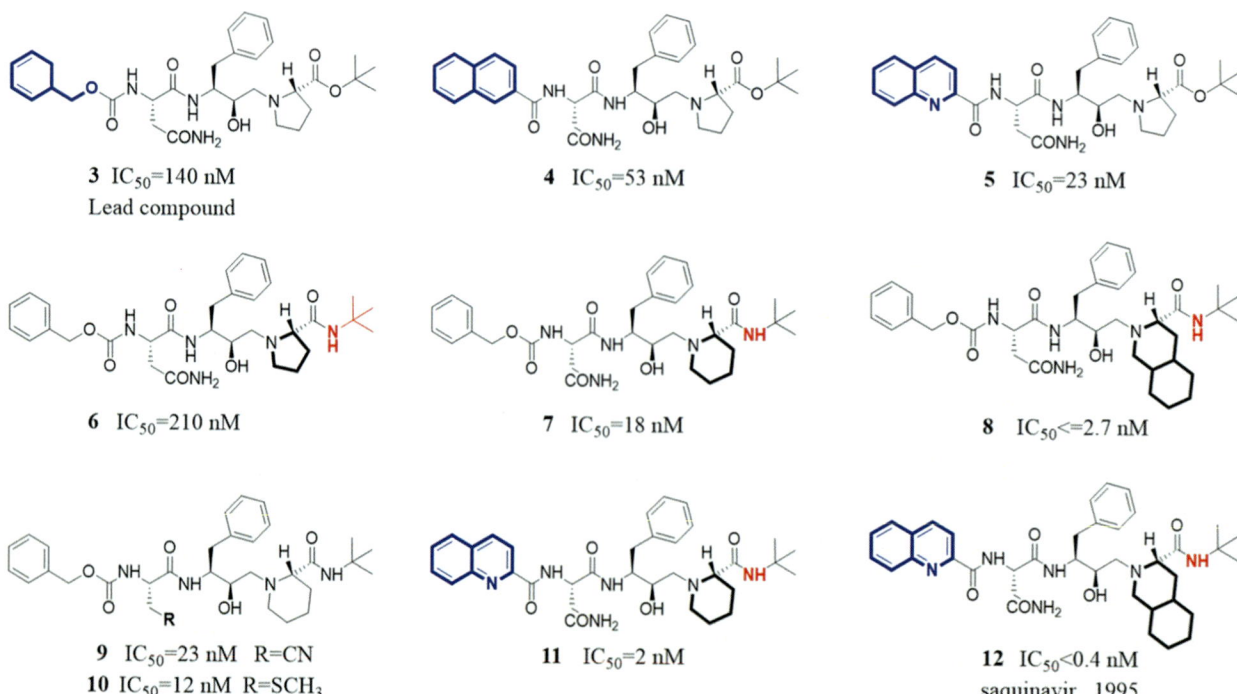

FIGURE 11.7 Derivative structures and activity characteristics based on the lead structure **3**.

enhancement of activity. This indicates that increasing the volume and hydrophobicity of the P1′ region ring framework is advantageous for binding to the protease S1′ region, thereby enhancing inhibitory activity.

The significance of aspartyl amide residue: The Asn residue in the P2 region of lead compound 3 mimics the substrate protein Leu165-Ile169 peptide sequence, while the P2 region of the other two Tyr/Phe-Pro cleavage sites of the substrate protein also contains Asn residues. This suggests that the Asn residue may be closely involved in the binding of the substrate to the HIV protease and is crucial for maintaining the activity of the compound. Furthermore, researchers did not find any superior natural amino acid residues that could significantly enhance the activity. However, when Asn was replaced with the nonnatural β-cyanoalanine (9) or S-methylcysteine (10), both effectively maintained the enzyme inhibitory activity of compound 7. This information provides new clues for the derivatization of the P2 region.

11.3.3.3 Discovery of the Saquinavir

Based on the aforementioned SAR study, researchers opted to maintain the Asn residue in the P2 region and the benzyl moiety in the P1 region of compound 3, while substituting the P3 region with a 2-quinoline moiety and the P1′ region with a piperidine ring, leading to the discovery of compound 11 with an IC_{50} value of 2 nM. Furthermore, it was observed that the activity of the S enantiomer of 11 significantly decreased (IC_{50} = 470 nM), indicating the chiral selectivity of the catalytic active site of the HIV protease. Subsequent adjustment of the P1′ piperidine ring to a decahydroisoquinoline resulted in the highly active compound 12 (Ro 31−8959). Compound 12 exhibited an IC_{50} value of less than 0.4 nM, representing a more than 16,000-fold increase in activity compared to the initial lead compound 2 (Fig. 11.7).

Compound **12** exhibits antiviral activity against infected cells with an EC_{50} value of 2 nM, while its IC_{50} values for *in vitro* proliferation inhibition toxicity in different host cell lines range from 5 to 100 μM, resulting in a high therapeutic index of 2500−50,000. It demonstrates excellent selectivity for the HIV protease, as at 10 μM (thousands of times the effective inhibitory concentration), no more than 50% inhibition was observed for aspartic proteases such as pepsin, cathepsin D, and cathepsin E. Furthermore, it showed no significant inhibitory effect on representative serine, cysteine, or metalloproteases. Compound 12 was ultimately named saquinavir and was approved by the FDA in 1995 as the first marketed HIV PI.

The study shows that saquinavir can form a wide-ranging interaction network with HIV-1 protease upon binding. The hydroxyl group of hydroxyethylamine forms hydrogen bonds with the active center Asp25/Asp25′. The P1′ decahydroisoquinoline group predominantly occupies the protease S1′ pocket, creating favorable hydrophobic interactions with the top flap region. The top Ile50/Ile50′ is mediated by water molecules, forming a hydrogen bond network with the inhibitor's structure. The P2′ tert-butylamine group tightly fits into the S2′ region but does not induce polar effects. The P1 benzyl moiety and the P3 quinoline group effectively fill the hydrophobic cavities of S1 and S3, while the P2 Asn amide group forms a stable hydrogen bond system with the Asp29-Asp30 amide backbone and the side-chain carboxyl group (Fig. 11.8) [22].

11.3.4 Pharmacokinetic properties and deficiencies of saquinavir

Saquinavir was initially approved in hard capsule formulation and used in combination with nucleoside drugs such as zidovudine or zalcitabine to treat HIV-1-infected adults. This combination therapy has been shown to be more effective in increasing CD4 + cell count and reducing the incidence of AIDS-related complications and mortality compared to the use of zidovudine or zalcitabine alone. For adults and adolescents aged 16 and above, the FDA-approved standard treatment dosage is 1000 mg of saquinavir and 100 mg of ritonavir twice daily, with the initial dose halved for the first 7 days of treatment for new patients.

Pharmacokinetic Challenges:

Solubility Issues: Saquinavir has poor water solubility, less than 0.01 mg/mL in phosphate buffer at pH 7.4. To improve solubility, it is formulated as a methanesulfonate salt in clinical settings.

Bioavailability and Metabolism: Saquinavir exhibits high plasma protein binding (up to 98%) and undergoes significant first-pass elimination, resulting in a short half-life of only 1−2 hours. It is primarily metabolized by the P450 3A4 enzyme in the liver into an inactive form, with most of it excreted through the biliary route and less than 3% eliminated via the kidneys [23]. The absolute oral bioavailability of 600 mg of saquinavir, when taken by healthy volunteers 30 minutes after a meal, is about 4%, which drops significantly when taken on an empty stomach. The peptidic character of saquinavir and the extensive first-pass liver metabolism are key factors contributing to its low bioavailability.

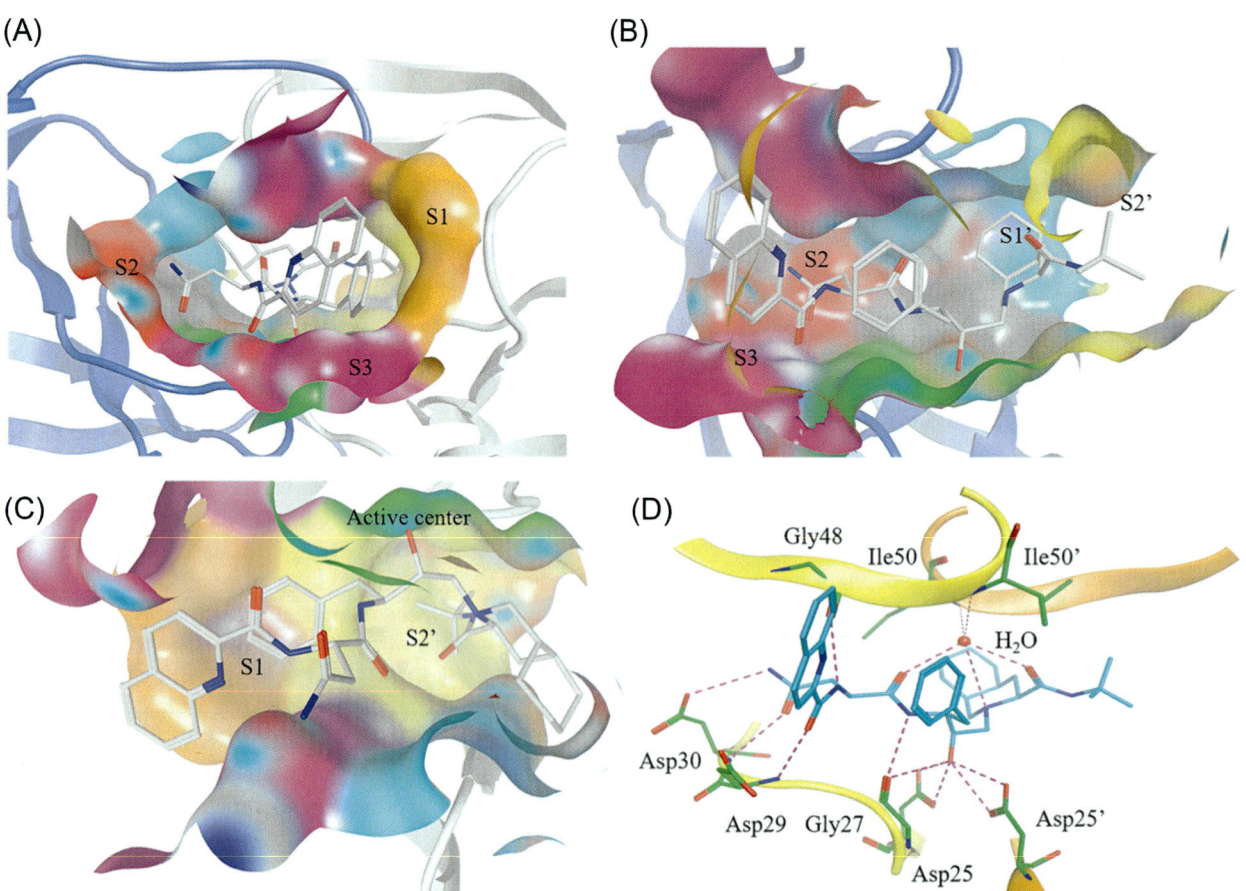

FIGURE 11.8 Schematic diagram of the interaction between saquinavir and HIV-1 protease. (A)–(D) represent side view, front view, back view, and interaction network, respectively.

In 1997, the soft capsule formulation of saquinavir, known as Fortovase, was introduced with an improved oral bioavailability of 13% compared to the hard capsule. Initially, it was expected to replace the hard capsule formulation. However, subsequent studies indicated that the combination of ritonavir with the hard capsule form of saquinavir resulted in higher blood drug concentrations and better drug tolerability. Consequently, Fortovase was discontinued in 2006.

Adverse Effects:

Common Side Effects: The most common adverse effects are relatively mild, including diarrhea (4%), abdominal pain (1%), and nausea (2%).

Metabolic Disturbances: Prolonged use of saquinavir can lead to disturbances in lipid metabolism, a typical adverse effect of HIV PIs. This includes hypertriglyceridemia, hypercholesterolemia, and insulin resistance, which may manifest clinically as facial and peripheral fat wasting, as well as abnormal fat accumulation in the abdomen, back, and chest areas [24].

Cardiac Risks: Recent findings suggest that the combination of saquinavir and ritonavir therapy may increase the risk of abnormal heart rhythms, necessitating cautious use in patients with ischemic heart disease, cardiomyopathy, and related conditions.

11.4 Further development of Saquinavir

11.4.1 Enhancement of pharmacokinetic properties

In 1993, in an effort to combat HIV/AIDS, Merck & Co., Inc. collaborated with over a dozen pharmaceutical companies to engage in cross-company cooperation and resource sharing. Following the release of saquinavir, subsequent medications with high structural similarity, such as indinavir and nelfinavir, were successively introduced, thereby forming the first generation of the HIV PI family (Fig. 11.9). Concurrently, ritonavir, developed by Abbott (divested by Abbott

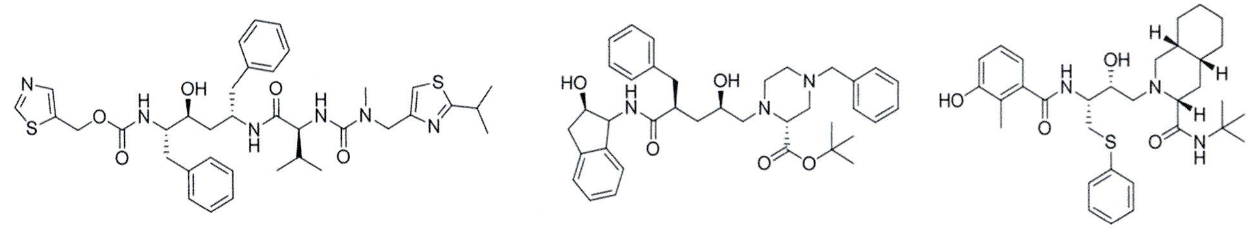

ritonavir
1996

indinavir
1996

nelfinavir
1997

FIGURE 11.9 First-generation HIV protease inhibitors following saquinavir.

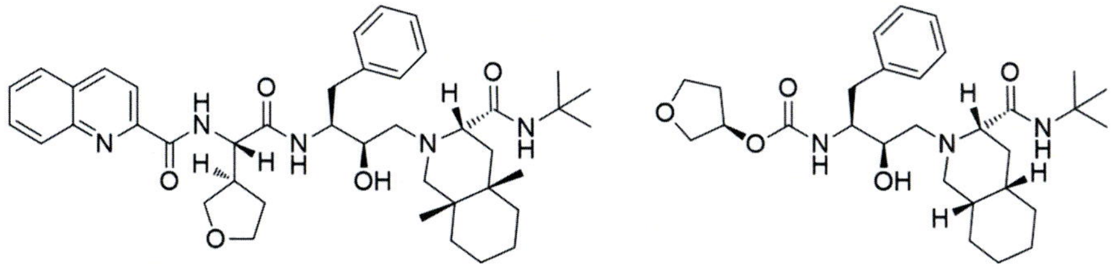

13 IC$_{50}$=0.054 nM

14 IC$_{50}$=132 nM

FIGURE 11.10 Molecular structures of compounds **13** and **14**.

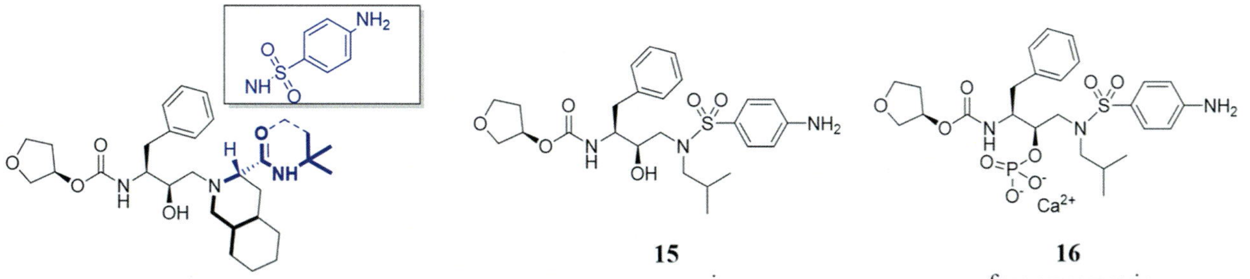

14

15
amprenavir
1999

16
fosanmprenavir
2003

FIGURE 11.11 Molecular structures of compounds **14–16**.

Laboratories as AbbVie), was primarily designed to target the C2 symmetry feature of the HIV protease. Due to the poor bioavailability and suboptimal metabolic performance of saquinavir, researchers undertook targeted structural modifications to eliminate peptidomimetic features and reduce its molecular weight, leading to the development of amprenavir, which exhibited improved metabolic performance.

In the preceding discussion, the importance of the P2 region Asn as an essential active group is underscored by its ability to form hydrogen bonds with the NH of the protease Asp29-Asp30 backbone. However, compounds 9 and 10 also maintain high inhibitory activity, demonstrating the feasibility of substituting Asn with nonnatural amino acids. Ghosh et al. discovered that by replacing the Asn residue with a rigid 3-tetrahydrofuran (THF) glycine residue, the THF group can also form hydrogen bonds with the backbone NH, leading to a significant enhancement in the activity of compound 13, with an IC$_{50}$ of only 0.054 nM [25]. However, its peptidomimetic features and molecular weight remained largely unchanged. The removal of the quinoline acylamide in the P3 region resulted in compound 14, which, despite a significant reduction in activity to an IC$_{50}$ of 132 nM due to the loss of binding with the S3 region, exhibited a markedly reduced backbone, indicating potential for optimization and modification (Fig. 11.10) [26].

The Vertex team simplified the decahydroisoquinoline scaffold of compound 14 in the P1′ region to an isobutyl and innovatively introduced a phenylsulfonyl group in the P2′ region, which is more prevalent in clinical drugs than the t-butylamino group. The phenylsulfonyl group plays a role in regulating the acid-base properties and solubility of the drug, providing multiple hydrogen bond acceptors. Structurally, the phenylsulfonyl group bears some resemblance to the t-butylamine fragment in the P2′ region (Fig. 11.11). Through this design, the resulting compound 15 (VX-478) simplifies the basic scaffold structure of saquinavir (MW = 505.63), reduces its peptidomimetic features, and eliminates the three chiral carbon atoms in the original P1' region, thereby significantly reducing the synthetic difficulty [27]. The enzyme inhibitory activity of 15 (K_i, the drug concentration corresponding to 50% of the HIV protease bound by the drug) is 1.6 nM. In the cell experiments with virus-infected cells, the drug concentration corresponding to 50% antiviral effect (EC_{50}) is 15 nM, comparable to the activity of saquinavir (K_i and EC_{50} values determined in the same group are 1.4 and 18 nM, respectively) [28]. **15** was named amprenavir and was approved for marketing in the United States in 1999.

Amprenavir, like saquinavir, binds within the catalytic activity cavity of the HIV protease and engages in extensive interactions with the surrounding amino acid residues in the S1/S1', S2/S2' regions, as depicted in Fig. 11.12 [27]. Notably, the oxygen atom of the sulfonyl group in its structure can mediate hydrogen bonding with the "flaps" Ile50 backbone NH of the HIV protease through water molecules, while the amino group in the benzene ring forms a hydrogen bond with Asp30 (Fig. 11.12). This characteristic has inspired the subsequent design and discovery of scaffold-targeted antiretroviral inhibitors [27].

Due to the introduction of furan and para-aminobenzenesulfonamide, amprenavir's solubility has significantly improved compared to saquinavir. This enhancement allows for more versatile dosing options, including capsule formulations and an oral solution (150 mg/10 mL), which facilitates improved medication compliance, particularly in pediatric populations with infections. A notable metabolic advantage of amprenavir is its significantly extended half-life in the human body, lasting between 7.1 and 10.6 hours [29], surpassing all similar inhibitors on the market prior to its introduction. Even at present, only darunavir, with a half-life of 15 hours and derived from further optimization of amprenavir, has comprehensively surpassed it.

Furthermore, amprenavir is rapidly absorbed, reaching peak plasma concentrations approximately 2 hours after administration in adult HIV-infected individuals. However, due to the lack of intravenous formulations for human use, its absolute bioavailability has yet to be determined. Bioequivalence studies have indicated that the oral solution of amprenavir has a bioavailability of less than 14% compared to the capsule formulation, with significant individual variability. Therefore, simple dose conversion based on formulation interchange is not advisable [29]. Similar to saquinavir, amprenavir is primarily metabolized by hepatic cytochrome P450 3A4, with approximately 75% of metabolites excreted in feces and 14% in urine. The urinary metabolites include the parent compound and 10 metabolites, all of which are present at levels below the limit of detection.

In 2003, fosamprenavir, the prodrug of amprenavir, was introduced. Fosamprenavir further enhances patient medication compliance and reduces medication dosage. Upon cellular entry, it is converted into amprenavir by phosphatase enzymes, thereby exerting its effect. Just two tablets of fosamprenavir per day are sufficient to maintain the therapeutic effect of 16 amprenavir tablets per day.

11.4.2 The discovery of the Darunavir

The first-generation PIs, represented by saquinavir, have played a crucial role in early HIV infection and AIDS treatment. However, due to the lack of proofreading activity in HIV reverse transcriptase, leading to a high base mismatch rate, combined with the influence of drug evolution pressure and other factors, the issue of drug resistance caused by HIV mutations has become increasingly severe [30].

Mutations in the HIV protease can be classified into primary and secondary mutations. Primary mutations occur in the active center residues of the protease, mainly involving positions 25–32, 47–53, or 80–84, directly affecting substrate

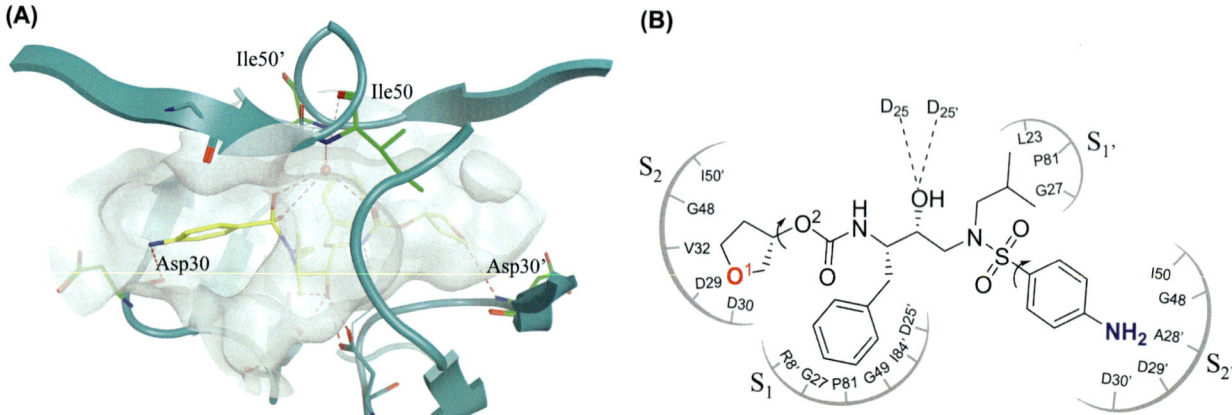

FIGURE 11.12 Schematic representation of the binding mode of amprenavir with HIV-1 protease. (A) Amprenavir (in yellow) bound to the active site cavity of HIV protease (in cyan) (PDB code: 1HPV), with its sulfonamide moiety interacting with the backbone residues Asp30' and Ile50 shown in green; (B) Binding region of amprenavir with the active site cavity of HIV protease.

binding. Secondary mutations occur at other sites and are believed to compensate for the decreased natural substrate binding ability caused by primary protease mutations. Dozens of HIV protease resistance mutation types have been identified, significantly reducing the efficacy of inhibitors (Table 11.1) [31]. Although optimizing lead compound structures based on the nature of key residues in the target protein or the characteristic cavities formed by them—considering spatial volume, hydrophobicity, and electrostatic features—is an effective approach in drug design, this residue side chain-targeted design strategy cannot overcome the challenge of drug resistance in the face of highly mutable HIV.

11.4.2.1 From side-chain targeting to backbone targeting

Researchers observed that when comparing the crystal structures of wild-type and mutant HIV protease in complex with saquinavir, the protease's active center backbone only underwent a slight distortion. Additionally, after mutation, saquinavir primarily lost its hydrogen bond with the side chain of Asp30 in the protease. However, its interaction with the protease's main chain, including the hydrogen bonds formed with the main chain of Asp29, Asp30, and Val (mutation)/Gly (wild-type) at position 48, is still preserved (Fig. 11.13) [32].

During the study of the substrate recognition mechanism, researchers also observed that, compared to the wild-type mode of action, the D25N mutant HIV-1 protease retains most of its backbone hydrogen bonds and water molecules when

TABLE 11.1 The inhibitory activity of Saquinavir against mutant HIV protease.

Virus	Mutation sites	IC_{50}/nM			
		SQV	RTV	IDV	NFV
1	L10I	17	15	30	32
2	L10I, K14R, L33I, M36I, M46I, F53L, K55R, I62V, L63P, A71V, G73S, V82A, L90M, I93L	230	>1000	>1000	>1000
3	L10I, Ll15V, K20R, M36I, M46L, I54V, K55R, I62V, L63P, K71Q, V82A, L89M	100	>1000	500	310
4	L10I, V11I, T12E, I15V, L19I, R41K, M46L, L63P, A71T, V82A, L90M	59	>1000	500	170
5	L10I, K14R, R41K, M46L, L54V, L63P, A71V, V82A, L90M, I93L	250	>1000	>1000	>1000
6	L10V, K20R, L33F, M36I, M46I, I50V, I54V, D60E, L63P, A71V, V82A, L90M	>1000	>1000	>1000	>1000
7	L10I, M46L, K55R, I62V, L63P, I72L, G73C, V77I, I84V, L90M	>1000	>1000	>1000	>1000
8	L10F, D30N, K45I, A71V, T74S	20	57	260	>1000

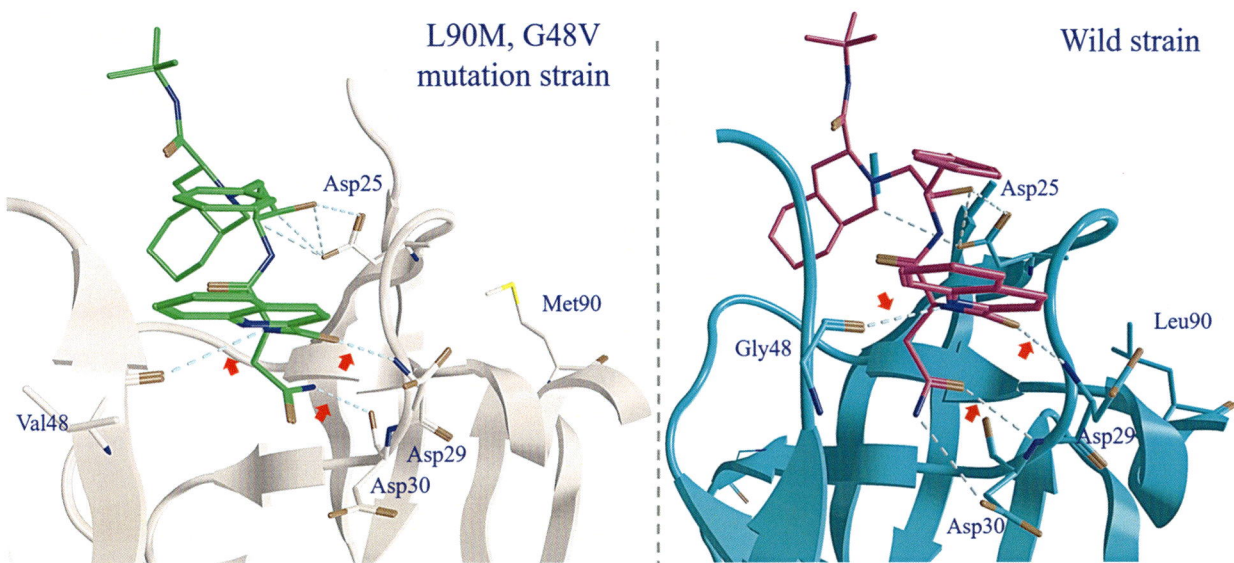

FIGURE 11.13 Interaction of the G48V/L90M mutant type (brown, PDB code: 1FB7) and wild type (blue, PDB code: 1HXB) HIV-1 protease with saquinavir. The image displays a single side of the HIV protease, with saquinavir represented in green for the mutant strain and purple for the wild-type strain. A red arrow indicates the hydrogen bonds formed between saquinavir and the main chain of the protease.

binding to the substrate, while the side-chain hydrogen bonds show differences [33]. These characteristics have inspired Ghosh and his collaborators to propose a backbone-targeted strategy for designing antiretroviral PIs, namely, the design of small molecule inhibitors that can form extensive hydrogen bond interactions with the protein backbone [34]. Even if the HIV protease mutates, the inhibitor can still maintain its characteristic interaction with the backbone, thus demonstrating the potential to overcome HIV protease resistance. With the successful launch of the first antiretroviral-resistant inhibitor, darunavir, the backbone-targeted antiretroviral strategy is gradually gaining recognition.

11.4.2.2 From amprenavir to darunavir

In the optimization design of darunavir, Ghosh et al. found that the introduction of THF residues in the P2 region could maintain the hydrogen bond interaction between the Asn residue and the Asp29-Asp30 backbone NH, thereby eliminating the P3 region and obtaining a significantly simplified structure, 14 (Fig. 11.14). To further enhance the backbone binding ability and compensate for the loss of hydrophobic quinoline ring function, Ghosh expanded the single THF structure to a double tetrahydrofuran (Bis-THF) structure. Compound 17 exhibited increased activity with an IC_{50} of 1.8 nM. It was also observed that the position of the epoxide atom had a significant impact on the activity (18, 19) [35]. Bis-THF is an important structural unit of the natural product ginkgolide and possesses rich biological activity, particularly antiviral activity [36]. The introduction of this structure may contribute to the enhancement of the compound's pharmacological properties. It is worth noting that, given the potential of Bis-THF to enhance backbone activity, pharmaceutical giants such as AbbVie and GlaxoSmithKline have incorporated it into their respective inhibitor structures.

As previously mentioned, amprenavir was obtained by simplifying the decahydroisoquinoline ring and introducing a sulfonamide moiety based on compound 14. The introduction of the sulfonamide moiety not only allows for the adjustment of the drug's acidity and solubility and improvement of metabolic performance but also holds significant importance in promoting the interaction between the inhibitor and the protease backbone (Fig. 11.12). The successful market launch of amprenavir inspired the Ghosh team to introduce the sulfonamide group into compound 17 to further enhance its interaction with the protease backbone. Building on this concept, the Ghosh team designed and discovered the highly potent TMC-114 and TMC-126, both of which have enzyme inhibition constants in the picomolar range, surpassing all previously marketed HIV PIs (Fig. 11.14) [34].

The molecular structure of TMC-114 is highly similar to that of amprenavir, and their functional characteristics are also similar. However, TMC-114 is capable of forming more hydrogen bonds with the protein backbone. Whether it is the wild-type or mutant strain, TMC-114, in addition to forming hydrogen bonds with the flap Ile50 mediated by water molecules, can form a total of four sets of hydrogen bonds with the protease Asp29, Asp30, and Asp30' main chain backbones, involving both the bis- THF and sulfonamide moieties (Fig. 11.15). In contrast, amprenavir and other marketed inhibitors can form at most two sets of hydrogen bonds. Furthermore, the conformation of TMC-114 matches well with the active cavity, and all of these features are crucial for its high activity and ability to resist mutant proteases [34].

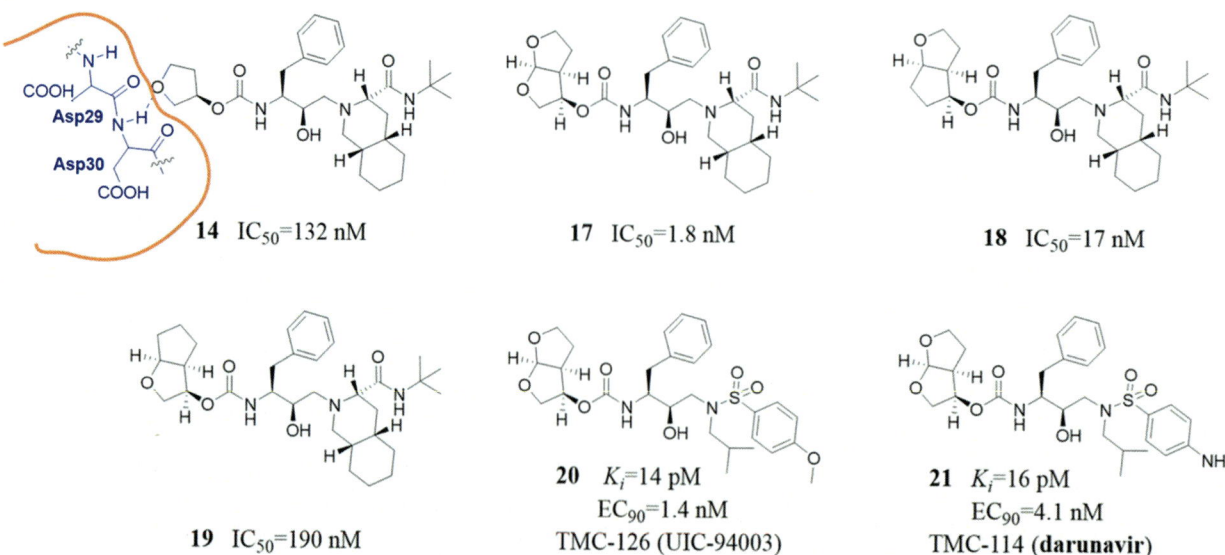

FIGURE 11.14 Molecular structures derived from **14**. The EC90 value represents the lowest drug concentration corresponding to a 90% antiviral effect in cell-based experiments infected with the virus.

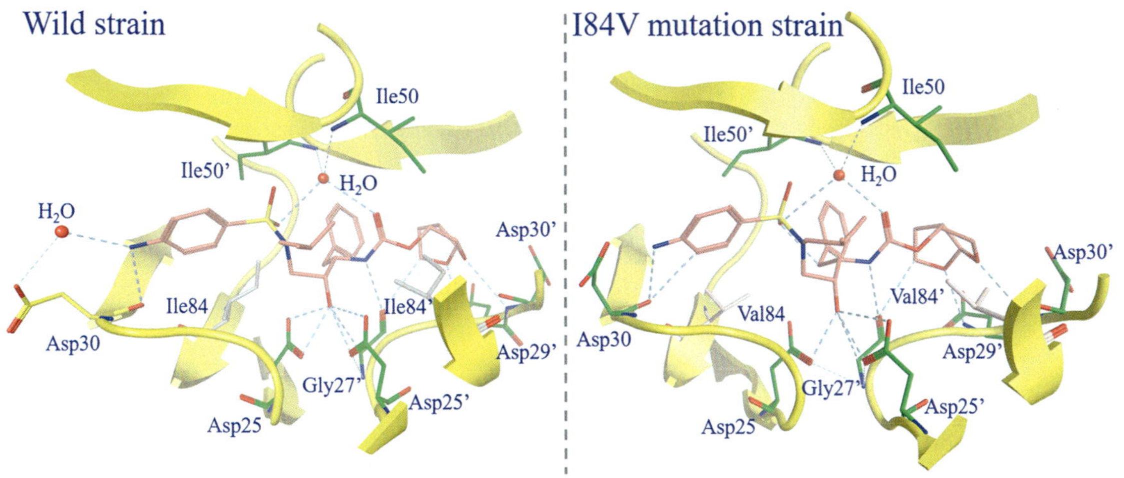

FIGURE 11.15 Interaction of the wild type (left, PDB code: 2IEN) and I84V mutant type (right, PDB code: 2IEO) HIV-1 protease with the TMC-114 complex. The HIV protease is shown in yellow, while TMC-114 is represented in dark brown. Amino acid residues involved in key interactions are depicted in green, and the mutated amino acid residues are shown in gray.

In drug sensitivity experiments, TMC-126 exhibited more than 10 times stronger antiviral activity than that of first-generation inhibitors such as saquinavir, while TMC-114 showed a range of 6–13 times [37]. Clinical testing with multidrug-resistant isolates demonstrated that the efficacy of TMC-114 (21) and TMC-126 (20) was only marginally diminished in a few resistant strains, with a reduction of 7 to 10-fold, but retaining high antiviral activity within the 10 nM IC50 value range. In contrast, the first-generation inhibitors typically exhibited a substantial decrease ranging from several to tens of times [37]. TMC-114 and TMC-126 have demonstrated outstanding resistance to resistance, providing preliminary validation for the skeleton-targeted resistance design concept.

Due to significant shortcomings in the development of resistance strains, stability, and metabolic kinetics, TMC-126 has hindered its further pharmaceutical development. In contrast, TMC-114, with its combination of high activity and excellent drug metabolic properties, was eventually named darunavir. In June 2006, it was approved by the FDA for the treatment of HIV-infected adults with treatment-resistant HIV, becoming the first and currently the only PI used to treat drug-resistant HIV. Today, the use of darunavir has expanded to include all AIDS patients, including children, and is commonly used in clinical practice in combination with low-dose ritonavir to enhance efficacy.

11.4.2.3 Pharmacokinetic properties of darunavir

Resistance Profile: One of the critical parameters in evaluating antiretroviral drugs is their ability to inhibit the emergence of drug-resistant strains. The resistance profile of darunavir, compared to other PIs such as TMC-126, amprenavir, and ritonavir, shows significant advantages. In studies involving MT-4-LTR-EGFP cells infected with wild-type HIV strains, TMC-126 led to mutations at known protease-resistant sites within 100 days, resulting in a drastic 100-fold reduction in drug sensitivity. This sensitivity continued to decrease over time. In contrast, darunavir exhibited a much slower rate of resistance development; even after one year, the reduction in drug sensitivity was only about 20-fold, substantially less than that observed with TMC-126 and other tested inhibitors [38]. Notably, the resistance induced by darunavir did not result in the emergence of clinically resistant strains, maintaining sensitivity to other PIs.

Metabolic Stability: Darunavir also demonstrates superior metabolic stability. When tested on liver microsomes from various species, including rats, dogs, and humans, the prototype components of darunavir accounted for 92%, 80%, and 85% respectively. This performance is on par with other marketed PIs like amprenavir and indinavir. In comparison, TMC-126 showed significantly lower values of 25%, 11%, and 56%, respectively, indicating weaker metabolic stability [38]. From a structural perspective, the P2′ functional groups of the two compounds exhibit only subtle differences, with the presence of an amino group and a methoxy group. This suggests that in the framework of such PIs, the amino group may contribute more to metabolic stability than the methoxy group.

Oral Bioavailability: The oral bioavailability of darunavir is another area where it excels. Animal studies focused on oral absorption demonstrated that darunavir, administered at a dose of 80 mg/kg in a PEG-400 solution, achieved significantly higher peak plasma concentrations (C_{max}) and area under the concentration-time curve (AUC_{last}) compared to TMC-126, with nearly a 20-fold difference [38]. Further clinical studies have shown that the absolute oral bioavailability of a single 600 mg dose of darunavir reached 37%, which significantly increased to 82% when coadministered with a low dose of ritonavir [39]. This excellent metabolic profile has been crucial in the successful market launch and widespread acceptance of darunavir as an effective treatment for HIV.

From saquinavir to amprenavir and then to darunavir, the antiviral activity has continuously strengthened, and the pharmacokinetic properties such as half-life have been continuously improved, making it a classic example of structure-based drug design and discovery. The timely approval of amprenavir and darunavir has continued to save the lives of numerous AIDS patients. However, the challenge of viral resistance has not been completely resolved, and there remains room for improvement in the antiviral activity of drugs. The structural redesign of darunavir remains highly active. To date, researchers have developed over ten new classes of structures by introducing aromatic heterocycles, crown ether rings, and other functional groups (Fig. 11.16), progressing toward more efficient and broad-spectrum antiresistance activity [30,40–49].

11.5 Anti-HIV/AIDS drugs and novel treatment strategies

11.5.1 Classification of anti-HIV/AIDS drugs

In theory, intervening in any process of the HIV infection and replication cycle will impact the virus's replication and proliferation, leading to antiviral effects. Therefore, the key enzymes or receptors involved in various stages of virus replication and proliferation may become targets for drug design and are commonly used as the primary basis for classifying antiretroviral drugs.

In 1987, the first nucleoside reverse transcriptase inhibitor (NRTI), zidovudine (AZT), was approved for the treatment of HIV infection, AIDS, and AIDS-related syndrome, marking the beginning of antiretroviral therapy. Since then, more than 30 antiretroviral drugs and multiple combination formulations have been approved for market use. These drugs are mainly classified into six categories based on their structural characteristics and antiviral mechanisms (Table 11.2): (1) nucleoside reverse transcriptase inhibitors (NRTIs), (2) nonnucleoside reverse transcriptase inhibitors (NNRTIs), (3) integrase strand transfer inhibitors (INSTIs), (4) PIs, (5) fusion inhibitors (FIs), and (6) CCR5 receptor antagonists [50]. Due to the close interconnection of HIV with host cell attachment, coreceptor binding, and fusion, FIs and CCR5 receptor antagonists are often referred to as entry inhibitors (EIs).

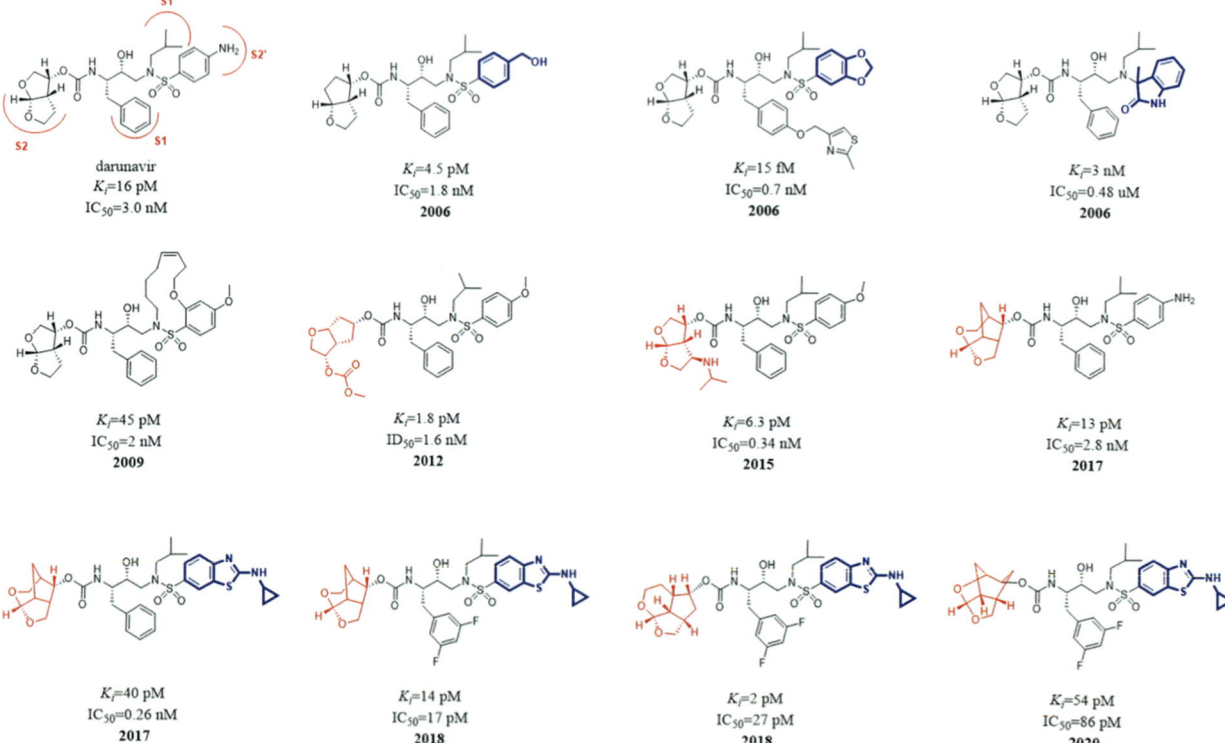

FIGURE 11.16 Further optimization design based on the structure of Darunavir.

TABLE 11.2 Classification of major anti-HIV/AIDS drugs [51].

Classification	Generic name/ abbreviation	Company Abbreviation	Approval year	Generic name/ abbreviation	Company Abbreviation	Approval year
NRTIs	Zidovudine/AZT	GSK	1987	Abacavir/ABC	GSK	1998
	Didanosine/DDI	BMS	1991	Tenofovir/PMPA	GILEAD	2001
	Stavudine/dT4	BMS	1994	Emtricitabine/FTC	GILEAD	2003
	lamivudine/3-TC	GSK	1995	Tenofovir Alafenamide/TAF	GILEAD	2016
NNRTIs	Nevirapine/NVP	BI	1996	Etravirine/ETR	JANSSEN	2008
	Delavirdine/DLV	GSK	1997	Rilpivirine/DPV	JANSSEN	2011
	Efavirenz/EFV	BMS	1998	Doravirine/DOR	MSD	2018
PIs	Saquinavir/SQV	Roche	1995	Fosamprenavir/FPV	GSK	2003
	Indinavir/IDV	MSD	1996	Amprenavir/APV	GSK	2003
	Ritonavir/RTV	ABBVIE	1996	Atazanavir/ATV	BMS	2003
	Nelfinavir/NFV	Pfizer	1997	Tipranavir/TPV	BI	2005
	Lopinavir/LPV	ABBVIE	2000	Darunavir/DRV	JANSSEN	2006
FIs	Enfuvirtide/ENF	Roche	2003	Albuvirtide/ABT	Frontier Biotech.	2018
INSTIs	Raltegravir Potassium/RAL	MSD	2007	Dolutegravir Sodium/DTG	GSK	2013
	Elvitegravir	GILEAD	2007	Bictegravir/BIC	GILEAD	2018
CCR5 Receptor Antagonists	Maraviroc/MVC	GSK	2007			

TABLE 11.3 Recommendations on first- and second-line antiretroviral regimens [52].

Treatment	Clinical features	Preferred regimen	Alternative regimen
First-line	Initial detection	TDF + 3TC (or FTC) + DTG	TDF + 3TC (or FTC) + EFV
Second-line	EFV/NVP resistance	Two core NRTIs + DTG	Two core NRTIs + ATV/r (or LPV/r or DRV/r)
	DTG resistance	Two core NRTIs + ATV/r (or LPV/r)	Two core NRTIs + DRV/r

11.5.2 New strategies for HIV/AIDS prevention and treatment

11.5.2.1 Highly active antiretroviral therapy

With the rapid emergence of HIV drug resistance, the efficacy of AIDS drugs has sharply declined. In 1995, Professor David D. Ho discovered that the structure and function of HIV proteins undergo continuous variation during host cell proliferation while existing drugs act on the characteristics of the virus prior to mutation. Based on this understanding, Professor Ho proposed the concept of HAART, widely known as cocktail therapy. The core of HAART is based on the concurrent use of three or more highly effective drugs with different antiviral mechanisms to overcome the problem of drug resistance and maximize the inhibition of viral replication, thereby controlling the progression of AIDS.

Currently, the combination therapy regimen has matured, and the WHO has updated its recommendations on first- and second-line antiretroviral regimens in July 2019 (Table 11.3). In China, the government has made relevant adjustments to the first-line and second-line regimens based on the WHO guideline (Table 11.4) and has implemented "Four Frees and One Care" AIDS policy for AIDS patients.

TABLE 11.4 National free AIDS antiviral drug treatment guidelines (4th edition).

Population	First-line regimen	Preferred second-line regimen
Adults and adolescents	AZT/d4T + 3TC + NVP/EFV	TDF + 3TC + LPV/r
	TDF + 3TC + EFV (or NVP)	AZT + 3TC + LPV/rAZT + TDF + 3TC + LPV/r (Co-infection of HIV/HBV)

The combination therapy has profoundly altered the AIDS treatment landscape, greatly extending the incubation period for those infected with HIV, lowering both the incidence and mortality of AIDS and successfully turning AIDS from a once deadly disease into a manageable chronic condition that requires ongoing medication. Patients who consistently adhere to their medication regimen can lead lives similar to those of healthy individuals. However, combination therapy also has apparent limitations. While it is highly effective for early-stage AIDS patients, its therapeutic effects are relatively limited for patients in the advanced stages, where irreversible damage to the immune system has already occurred.

11.5.2.2 Developments in HIV prevention and treatment strategies

HAART cannot completely eradicate HIV, as it can conceal itself within host cells at extremely low viral loads, forming viral reservoirs. Even brief interruptions in medication may lead to disease rebound, necessitating lifelong treatment for patients. However, long-term drug exposure is also prone to causing serious adverse reactions and exacerbating issues such as viral resistance. Therefore, the development of new mechanistic approaches to AIDS therapy is of significant importance [53].

Vaccines were once considered an ideal approach to combat AIDS. However, due to factors such as the highly glycosylated nature of the HIV envelope protein, its strong variability, and its ability to integrate into the host genome, progress in the development of HIV vaccines has been slow. At the end of 2007, the highly anticipated adenovirus type 5 vaccine suffered a clinical failure. Not only did this virus fail to prevent HIV infection or reduce viral load in patients, but it also resulted in a higher HIV infection rate in the vaccinated group. This study was prematurely terminated, marking a significant setback in the development of second-generation HIV vaccines aimed at reducing viral load through the induction of T-cell immunity. In 2009, a novel canarypox virus-gp120 protein combination vaccine developed by the Thailand Ministry of Public Health and other institutions was reported to provide a 31.2% protective effect for the vaccinated population. In the vaccine group (8197 healthy volunteers), 51 individuals were infected, while in the control group (8197 healthy volunteers), 74 individuals were infected. Despite the relatively limited protective effect, statistical results indicate the feasibility of HIV infection prevention through vaccination.

With the rapid advancement of molecular biology technologies such as RNA interference and gene editing, new therapeutic strategies for AIDS have gradually gained attention. These novel treatment approaches, including antisense drugs, RNA decoys, nucleases, and gene editing, have certain representative drug candidates enter the phase II clinical trial research stage [53,54]. Whether used as a standalone or adjunct therapy, these new treatment modalities demonstrate promising prospects for development.

11.5.2.3 The dawn of humanity's conquest of AIDS?

The auxiliary receptor CCR5 plays a crucial role in promoting the fusion process of HIV with host cells and is considered one of the effective targets for anti-HIV therapy. In addition to CCR5 receptor antagonists, another strategy for treating AIDS involves mutating the CCR5 receptor and reducing the affinity between HIV and host cell membranes to block the fusion process. In 1995, Timothy Brown was infected with AIDS, but his condition was controlled after receiving antiretroviral therapy. However, in 2006, he also developed acute myeloid leukemia. His attending physician, Gero Hütter, hoped to use a bone marrow transplant with a CCR5 gene-deficient match to simultaneously treat leukemia and AIDS. In 2007, after receiving the bone marrow transplant, Timothy Brown not only cured his leukemia but also miraculously cleared the HIV virus from his body. The successful cure of the "Berlin patient" offered a glimmer of hope for humanity in conquering AIDS. Although Timothy Brown passed away at the end of September 2020 due to a relapse of leukemia, he has been immortalized as the world's first person to be cured of AIDS [55].

In 2016, similar to the "Berlin patient," the "London patient" Adam Castillejo, who was concurrently suffering from AIDS and Hodgkin's lymphoma, interrupted antiviral therapy 16 months after receiving a CCR5-Δ32 genotype bone marrow transplant. Subsequently, for 18 months, HIV was also not detected in his body [56]. In 2020, the treatment team published their findings in Lancet HIV, confirming the "London patient" as the second globally cured AIDS patient [57].

The successful cure of the "Berlin patient" and the "London patient" has inspired millions of AIDS patients and reignited hope among scientists to conquer AIDS using the CCR5 target. However, considering that both patients had nonreplaceable malignant blood diseases, as well as the high medical costs and significant treatment risks, the applicability of bone marrow transplant schemes remains relatively limited. For ordinary AIDS patients, cocktail therapy remains the optimal option.

References

[1] Centers for Disease Control. Pneumocystis pneumonia—Los Angeles. MMWR Morb Mortal Wkly Rep 1981;30(21):250—2.
[2] Wang N, Zhong P. Molecular epidemiology of HIV in China:1985-2015. Chin J Epidemiol 2015;36(6):541—6.
[3] Barré-Sinoussi F, Chermann JC, Rey F, et al. Isolation of a T-lymphotropic retrovirus from a patient at risk for acquired immune deficiency syndrome. Science 1983;220(4599):868—71.
[4] Gallo RC, Salahuddin SZ, Popovic M, et al. Frequent detection and isolation of cytopathic retroviruses (HTLV-III) from patients with AIDS and at risk for AIDS. Science 1984;224(4648):500—3.
[5] Levy JA, Hoffman AD, Kramer SM, et al. Isolation of lymphocytopathic retroviruses from San Francisco patients with AIDS. Science 1984;225(4664):840—2.
[6] Brown F. Human immunodeficiency virus. Science 1986;232(4757):1486.
[7] Maartens G, Celum C, Lewin SR. HIV infection: epidemiology, pathogenesis, treatment, and prevention. Lancet 2014;384(9939):258—71.
[8] Sharp PM, Hahn BH. Origins of HIV and the AIDS pandemic. Cold Spring Harb Perspect Med 2011;1(1):a006841.
[9] Turner BG, Summers MF. Structural biology of HIV. J Mol Biol 1999;285(1):1—32.
[10] Gallo R, Wong-Staal F, Montagnier L, et al. HIV/HTLV gene nomenclature. Nature 1988;333(6173):504.
[11] Levy JA. Human Immunodeficiency Viruses and the Pathogenesis of AIDS. JAMA 1989;261(20):2997—3006.
[12] Engelman A, Cherepanov P. The structural biology of HIV-1: mechanistic and therapeutic insights. Nat Rev Microbiol 2012;10(4):279—90.
[13] Brik A, Wong CH. HIV-1 protease: mechanism and drug discovery. Org Biomol Chem 2003;1(1):5—14.
[14] Wlodawer A, Miller M, Jaskolski M, et al. Conserved folding in retroviral proteases: crystal structure of a synthetic HIV-1 protease. Science 1989;245(4918):616—21.
[15] Yang Zh H, Bai XG, Wang JX et al. Recent advance in research and development of HIV-1 protease inhibitors. Chin J New Drugs 2014; 23 (19): 2246—55.
[16] Louis JM, Aniana A, Weber IT, et al. Inhibition of autoprocessing of natural variants and multidrug resistant mutant precursors of HIV-1 protease by clinical inhibitors. Proc Natl Acad Sci U S A 2011;108(22):9072—7.
[17] Voshavar C. Protease inhibitors for the treatment of HIV/AIDS: recent advances and future challenges. Curr Top Med Chem 2019;19 (18):1571 98.
[18] Roberts NA, Martin JA, Kinchington D, et al. Rational design of peptide-based HIV proteinase inhibitors. Science 1990;248(4953):358—61.
[19] Roberts NA, Craig JC, Duncan IB. HIV proteinase inhibitors. Biochem Soc Trans 1992;20(2):513—16.
[20] Martin JA. Recent advances in the design of HIV proteinase inhibitors. Antivir Res 1992;17(4):265—78.
[21] Guo ZR. Structure-based drug design of protease inhibitors saquinavir, amprenavir and darunavir. Acta Pharm Sin 2017;52(5):832—6.
[22] Krohn A, Redshaw S, Ritchie JC, et al. Novel binding mode of highly potent HIV-proteinase inhibitors incorporating the (R)-hydroxyethylamine isostere. J Med Chem 1991;34(11):3340—2.
[23] Bao YL (translator). Clinical pharmacology and drug effects of saquinavir. J Int Pharm Res 1999;26(1):17—20.
[24] Bucher HC, Young J, Battegay M. Protease inhibitor-sparing simplified maintenance therapy: a need for perspective. J Antimicrob Chemother 2004;54(2):303—5.
[25] Thompson WJ, Ghosh AK, Holloway MK, et al. 3'-Tetrahydrofuranylglycine as a novel, unnatural amino acid surrogate for asparagine in the design of inhibitors of the HIV protease. J Am Chem Soc 1993;115(2):801—3.
[26] Ghosh AK, Thompson WJ, McKee SP, et al. 3-Tetrahydrofuran and pyran urethanes as high-affinity P2-ligands for HIV-1 protease inhibitors. J Med Chem 1993;36(2):292—4.
[27] Kim EE, Baker CT, Dwyer MD, et al. Crystal structure of HIV-1 protease in complex with VX-478, a potent and orally bioavailable inhibitor of the enzyme. J Am Chem Soc 1995;117:1181—2.
[28] Ghosh AK, Kincaid JF, Cho W, et al. Potent HIV protease inhibitors incorporating high-affinity P2-ligands and (R)-(hydroxyethylamino)sulfonamide isostere. Bioorg Med Chem Lett 1998;8(6):687—90.
[29] Sadler BM, Stein DS. Clinical pharmacology and pharmacokinetics of amprenavir. Ann Pharmacother 2002;36(1):102—18.
[30] Ghosh AK, Osswald HL, Prato G. Recent progress in the development of HIV-1 protease inhibitors for the treatment of HIV/AIDS. J Med Chem 2016;59(11):5172—208.
[31] Hao GF, Yang GF. Progress in the New Generation Nonpeptide Sulfonamide Anti-HIV Protease Inhibitor Darunavir. Chin J Org Chem 2008;28 (9):1545—52.

[32] Hong L, Zhang XC, Hartsuck JA, et al. Crystal structure of an in vivo HIV-1 protease mutant in complex with saquinavir: insights into the mechanisms of drug resistance. Protein Sci 2000;9(10):1898−904.

[33] Prabu-Jeyabalan M, Nalivaika E, Schiffer CA. Substrate shape determines specificity of recognition for HIV-1 protease: analysis of crystal structures of six substrate complexes. Structure 2002;10(3):369−81.

[34] Ghosh AK, Chapsal BD, Weber IT, et al. Design of HIV protease inhibitors targeting protein backbone: an effective strategy for combating drug resistance. Acc Chem Res 2008;41(1):78−86.

[35] Ghosh AK, Kincaid JF, Walters DE, et al. Nonpeptidal P2 ligands for HIV protease inhibitors: structure-based design, synthesis, and biological evaluation. J Med Chem 1996;39(17):3278−90.

[36] Nakanishi K. The ginkgolides. Pure Appl Chem 1967;14(1):89−113.

[37] Ghosh AK, Ramu Sridhar P, Kumaragurubaran N, et al. Bis-tetrahydrofuran: a privileged ligand for darunavir and a new generation of hiv protease inhibitors that combat drug resistance. ChemMedChem 2006;1(9):939−50.

[38] Surleraux DL, Tahri A, Verschueren WG, et al. Discovery and selection of TMC114, a next generation HIV-1 protease inhibitor. J Med Chem 2005;48(6):1813−22.

[39] Rittweger M, Arasteh K. Clinical pharmacokinetics of darunavir. Clin Pharmacokinet 2007;46(9):739−56.

[40] Ghosh AK, Schiltz G, Perali RS, et al. Design and synthesis of novel HIV-1 protease inhibitors incorporating oxyindoles as the P2'-ligands. Bioorg Med Chem Lett 2006;16(7):1869−73.

[41] Ghosh AK, Sridhar PR, Leshchenko S, et al. Structure-based design of novel HIV-1 protease inhibitors to combat drug resistance. J Med Chem 2006;49(17):5252−61.

[42] Wang YF, Tie Y, Boross PI, et al. Potent new antiviral compound shows similar inhibition and structural interactions with drug resistant mutants and wild type HIV-1 protease. J Med Chem 2007;50(18):4509−15.

[43] Ghosh AK, Kulkarni S, Anderson DD, et al. Design, synthesis, protein-ligand X-ray structure, and biological evaluation of a series of novel macrocyclic human immunodeficiency virus-1 protease inhibitors to combat drug resistance. J Med Chem 2009;52(23):7689−705.

[44] Ghosh AK, Chapsal BD, Steffey M, et al. Substituent effects on P2-cyclopentyltetrahydrofuranyl urethanes: design, synthesis, and X-ray studies of potent HIV-1 protease inhibitors. Bioorg Med Chem Lett 2012;22(6):2308−11.

[45] Ghosh AK, Martyr CD, Osswald HL, et al. Design of HIV-1 protease inhibitors with amino-bis-tetrahydrofuran derivatives as P2-ligands to enhance backbone-binding interactions: synthesis, biological evaluation, and protein-ligand X-ray studies. J Med Chem 2015;58(17):6994−7006.

[46] Ghosh AK, Rao KV, Nyalapatla PR, et al. Design and development of highly potent HIV-1 protease inhibitors with a crown-like oxotricyclic core as the P2-ligand to combat multidrug-resistant HIV variants. J Med Chem 2017;60(10):4267−78.

[47] Ghosh AK, Nyalapatla PR, Kovela S, et al. Design and synthesis of highly potent HIV-1 protease inhibitors containing tricyclic fused ring systems as novel P2 ligands: structure-activity studies, biological and X-ray structural analysis. J Med Chem 2018;61(10):4561−77.

[48] Ghosh AK, Rao KV, Nyalapatla PR, et al. Design of highly potent, dual-acting and central-nervous-system-penetrating HIV-1 protease inhibitors with excellent potency against multidrug-resistant HIV-1 variants. ChemMedChem 2018;13(8):803−15.

[49] Ghosh AK, Kovela S, Osswald HL, et al. Structure-based design of highly potent HIV-1 protease inhibitors containing new tricyclic ring P2-ligands: design, synthesis, biological, and X-ray structural studies. J Med Chem 2020;63(9):4867−79.

[50] Reeves JD, Piefer AJ. Emerging drug targets for antiretroviral therapy. Drugs 2005;65(13):174766.

[51] Ma QS, Wang Zh P, Li JL, et al. Anti-aids Drugs: Status Quo and Challenges. J Liaocheng Univ Nat Sci Ed 2020;33(01):70−8.

[52] World Health Organization, Update of recommendations on first- and second-line antiretroviral regimens, 2019.

[53] Yao Ch, Zhu PP, Xie D. Advances in antiretroviral therapy and drug development for AIDS. Progress in Pharm Sci 2018;42(2):84−98.

[54] Zheng H. Advances in research on HIV-1 gene therapy. Progress in Pharm Sci 2018;42(2):122−128.

[55] Hütter G. The cure of Timothy Brown. How is his condition now and has this case been repeated? MMW Fortschr Med 2018;160(Suppl 2):27−30.

[56] Gupta RK, Abdul-Jawad S, McCoy LE, et al. HIV-1 remission following CCR5Delta32/Delta32 haematopoietic stem-cell transplantation. Nature 2019;568(7751):244−8.

[57] Gupta RK, Peppa D, Hill AL, et al. Evidence for HIV-1 cure after CCR5Δ32/Δ32 allogeneic haemopoietic stem-cell transplantation 30 months post analytical treatment interruption: a case report. Lancet HIV 2020;7(5):340−7.

Chapter 12

Baloxavir: an antiinfluenza drug with a novel mechanism of action

Peng Zhan, Kai Tang and Xinyong Liu
Department of Medicinal Chemistry, School of Pharmaceutical Sciences, Shandong University, Jinan, Shandong, P.R. China

Chapter outline

12.1 Influenza virus	**265**
12.1.1 Transmission and status quo of influenza virus	265
12.1.2 Structure, function, and classification of influenza viruses	265
12.1.3 Life cycle of influenza virus	266
12.2 Antiinfluenza drugs	**268**
12.2.1 M2 ion channel blockers	268
12.2.2 Neuraminidase inhibitors	268
12.2.3 Broad-spectrum antiviral drugs	268
12.2.4 Influenza virus inhibitors targeting the polymerase complex	269
12.3 Development of baloxavir	**270**
12.3.1 The structure and function of endonuclease	270
12.3.2 Discovery of baloxavir	271
12.3.3 Synthesis of baloxavir	279
12.3.4 Clinical study of baloxavir	283
12.3.5 Inspiration from the study of baloxavir	284
References	**285**

12.1 Influenza virus

12.1.1 Transmission and status quo of influenza virus

Influenza, also known as the flu, is an acute respiratory tract illness caused by the influenza virus infection. The most notable epidemiological characteristics of influenza include sudden outbreaks, rapid spread, and varying degrees of epidemics. Influenza can be mainly categorized into two types, including seasonal influenza and pandemic influenza. Seasonal influenza, which recurs annually, encompasses a wide range of strains that necessitate vigilant monitoring and prediction by researchers to develop updated vaccines for the predicted viral variants. The pandemic influenza is a highly pathogenic strain of influenza that occurs sporadically, and its viral strains can rapidly disseminate among individuals, resulting in high morbidity and mortality. Each outbreak of pandemic influenza could cause a huge economic and social burden to human beings, such as the 1918–1920 H1N1 subtype "Spanish flu," the 1957–1958 H2N2 subtype "Asian flu," the 1968–1969 H3N2 subtype "Asian flu," the 1977–1978 H1N1 subtype "Hong Kong flu," the 2009 H1N1 subtype influenza outbreak in Mexico, the 2013 H7N9 subtype influenza first reported in China, and the 2019–2020 US influenza outbreak (Table 12.1). The World Health Organization reports an annual mortality of 290–650,000 individuals due to respiratory diseases caused by influenza. Even in the United States, which boasts a highly advanced healthcare system, the annual incidence of influenza infection among the population ranges from 5% to 20%, resulting in over 200,000 hospitalizations and more than 36,000 fatalities [1–6].

12.1.2 Structure, function, and classification of influenza viruses

The influenza virus belongs to the Orthomyxoviridae family and is characterized by its segmented single-stranded negative-strand ribonucleic acid (RNA) structure. They typically exist in two distinct forms: spherical and filamentous [7]. The spatial structure of influenza viruses can be categorized into three components, progressing from the innermost to the outermost: the core (materials storing viral genetic information and various enzymes related to replication), matrix protein (M1, the scaffold of the viral shell), and envelope (phospholipid bilayer) (Fig. 12.1A). Due to the absence of

TABLE 12.1 Typical influenza pandemic events [1–5].

Name of influenza occurrence time	Toxic strain lethality rate	Epidemic severity (PSI)
Spanish flu 1918–1920	H1N1 2%	5
Asian flu 1957–1958	H2N2 0.13%	2
Hong Kong flu 1977–1978	H1N1 <0.1%	2
Influenza A (H1N1) 2009–2010	H1N1 0.03%	–
US influenza 2019–2020	B/Victoria <0.11%	2
	H1N1pdm09	

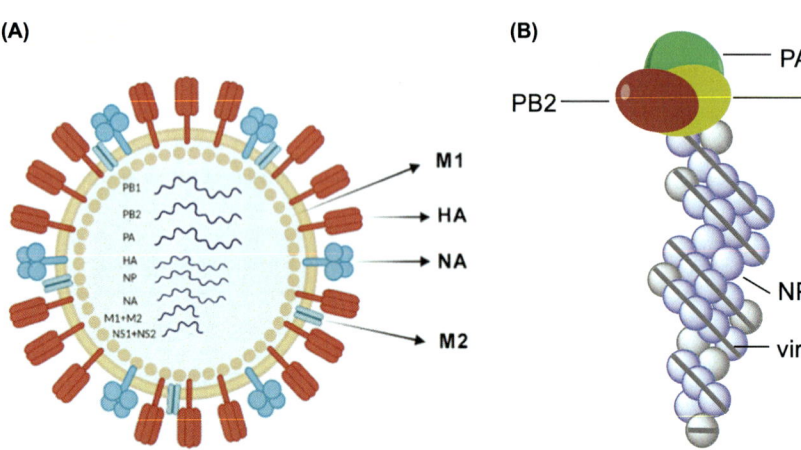

FIGURE 12.1 The structure of the influenza virus: (A) A diagram of the structural pattern of influenza virus particles; (B) vRNP complex structure [8]. *vRNP*, Viral RNA ribonucleoprotein.

proofreading capabilities in the RNA polymerase utilized during influenza virus replication, an error arises approximately every 10,000 nucleotides, leading to a heightened frequency of RNA mutations. Moreover, concurrent infection by different subtypes and genotypes of influenza viruses can potentially induce gene rearrangement, leading to substantial alterations in the viral genome. According to the different antigen determinants of viral nucleoprotein (NP) and M1, influenza viruses can be divided into four types: A, B, C, and D [9]. The primary differentiating factor lies in the varying host range of infection. Influenza A viruses have the broadest host range, infecting humans, pigs, horses, and birds. They are highly prone to mutation and recombination, which leads to susceptibility in human populations and seasonal epidemics. Consequently, they pose the greatest threat to human health [10]. For example, the 2009 pandemic influenza A (H1N1) virus is a result of genetic recombination between avian, swine, and human strains. Influenza B viruses primarily infect humans and pigs, while influenza C viruses exclusively infect only humans, and a new class of influenza viruses known as type D influenza has been recently identified in cattle and pigs but predominantly circulates among humans and other mammals.

Influenza A viruses consist of eight distinct RNA fragments that encode a minimum of 12 functional proteins, such as nonstructural protein 1 (NS1) and nuclear export protein (NEP) encoded by the NS fragment. Additionally, it encodes receptor-binding proteins such as hemagglutinin (HA), neuraminidase (NA), NP, polymerase acidic protein (PA), polymerase basic protein 1 (PB1), and polymerase basic protein 2 (PB2) (Fig. 12.1B) [8,11–13]. According to the protein structure and gene characteristics of surface antigen HA and NA, influenza A viruses can be further divided into multiple subtypes, each subtype is named based on the combination of different subtypes of NA and HA, such as H1N1, H3N2, and H5N1. So far, there are 18 subtypes of HA (H1~H18) and 11 subtypes of NA (N1~N11). The functions of these proteins are shown in Table 12.2:

12.1.3 Life cycle of influenza virus

The replication process of the influenza virus can be broadly categorized into eight distinct stages, namely attachment, endocytosis, fusion, replication, translation, assembly, budding, and release. The specific steps are shown in Fig. 12.2:

TABLE 12.2 Genome-encoded proteins of influenza A virus and their functions [13].

Protein	Function
Hemagglutinin (HA)	Binding to host receptors; Promotes fusion of viral envelope with cell membrane
Neuraminidase (NA)	Promote the release of progeny viruses; Prevent the aggregation of released viruses
Matrix protein (M1)	Interacts with the genome and nuclear export factors to assist in viral assembly
Proton channel protein (M2)	Control the pH in Golgi apparatus during HA synthesis and virion dehulling
Nucleoprotein (NP)	Expression of nucleocapsid and virus synthesis
Polymerase acidic protein (PA)	"Capture" the 5′ cap structure of the mRNA of the host cell
Polymerase basic protein 1 (PB1)	Binds to the viral promoter and is responsible for the synthesis of mRNA strands
Polymerase basic protein 2 (PB2)	Recognize and bind to the cap-like structure of the host cell's mRNA
Nonstructural protein 1 (NS1)	Posttranscriptional RNA control; Inhibition of nuclear factor-KB activation and interferon-α/-mediated antiviral action
Nuclear export protein (NEP)	Nuclear export of viral RNA; Viral assembly

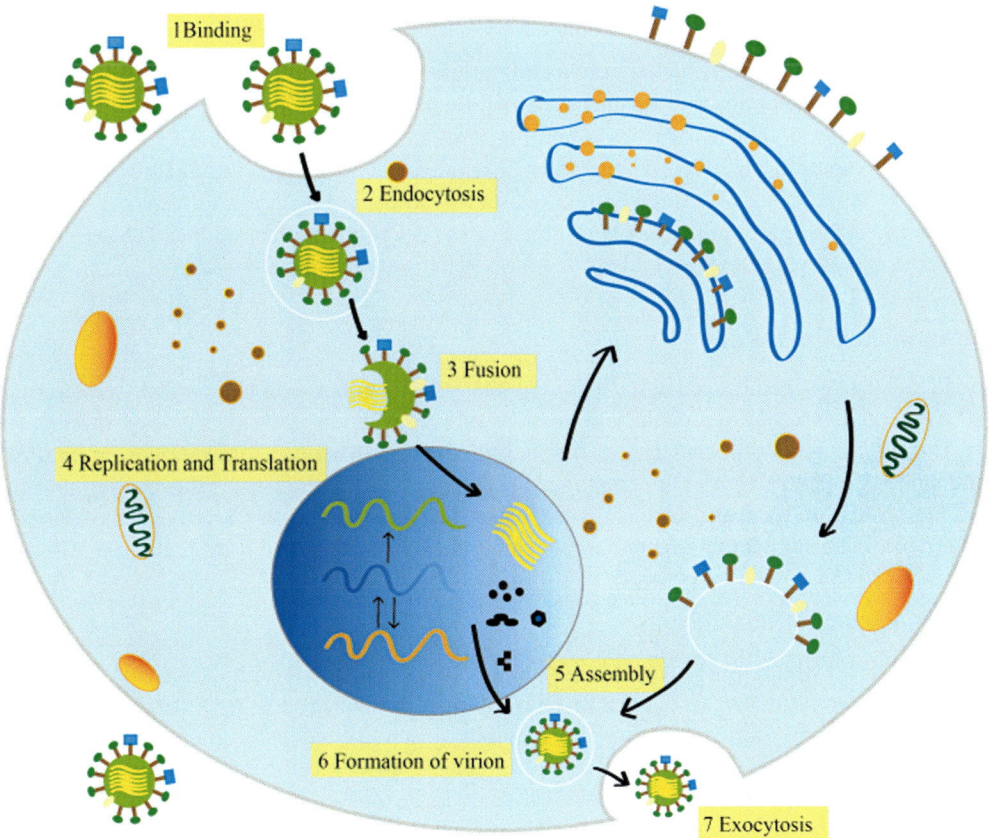

FIGURE 12.2 The life cycle of influenza virus [14].

(1) The influenza virus binds to the sialic acid receptor on the host cell surface through its HA, facilitating adherence of the virus to the host cell surface; (2) Endocytic vesicles (endosomes) are formed and enter the cytoplasm through endocytosis; (3) The low pH environment within the endosome promotes fusion between the viral membrane and cellular vesicle membrane, leading to H^+ influx through M2 ion channels. This reduces the internal pH of the virus, resulting in the shedding of the M1 protein and the release of viral RNA ribonucleoprotein (vRNP) particles composed of NP, PA,

PB1, and PB2. Subsequently, vRNP is transported into the host nucleus by recognition of nuclear localization sequences on NP; (4) Within the host nucleus, viral polymerase initiates the synthesis of viral mRNA by cleaving the 5′-cap RNA fragment from host mRNA. Subsequently, it proceeds with transcription and replication of viral RNA while concurrently inhibiting transcription and replication processes in host cells; (5) The viral mRNA is transported to the cytoplasm and synthesizes various functional proteins of the virus on ribosomes; (6) The assembly of viral particles is accomplished through the regulation facilitated by packaging signals, resulting in the formation of new progeny virus particles; (7) The new progeny virus particles sprout on the host cell membrane; and (8) The NA on the surface of the viral particles cleaves the viral HA and sialic acid residues present on the host cell surface, subsequently facilitating the release of new virus particles [9,14].

12.2 Antiinfluenza drugs

Influenza vaccination is an effective measure for preventing influenza and reducing the risk of severe complications in vaccinated individuals. However, due to the limitations of the seasonal influenza vaccine, antiinfluenza drugs are still the main measures for the prevention and treatment of influenza [15,16]. Current drugs for the treatment of influenza mainly include M2 ion channel blockers (amantadine and rimantadine); NA inhibitors (oseltamivir, zanamivir, peramivir, and laninamivir); RNA polymerase inhibitors (baloxavir); and broad-spectrum antiviral drugs (favipiravir, arbidol hydrochloride, and nitazoxanide). While these drugs play a significant role in combating influenza viruses, they still have some notable shortcomings [17].

12.2.1 M2 ion channel blockers

Before the 1990s, amantadine drugs, including amantadine released in 1966 (**1**) and rimantadine released in 1987 (**2**), were the primary choice for preventing and treating type A influenza. Amantadine specifically targets type A influenza viruses by blocking the M2 ion channel, thereby inhibiting virus uncoating and preventing viral RNA release into the host cytoplasm. This mechanism effectively disrupts the early stages of viral replication. However, prolonged usage of amantadine drugs has resulted in widespread drug resistance among almost all influenza virus strains [18, 19]. Consequently, since the 2004–2005 influenza season, the Food and Drug Administration (FDA) no longer recommends the use of amantadine derivatives but instead advocates for NA inhibitors (Fig. 12.3) [20].

12.2.2 Neuraminidase inhibitors

Mature virus particles attach to the host cell surface through the interaction between HA on their surface and HA receptors on the host cell membrane. NA plays a crucial role in catalyzing the hydrolysis of the glycosylation between sialic acid on the host cell surface and influenza virus HA, facilitating the release of mature viruses from infected cells for further infection. Neuraminidase inhibitors (NAIs) are employed as therapeutic agents against influenza by impeding this process [21]. Currently, four NAIs are available in the market (Table 12.3): oseltamivir (**3**, trade name: Tamiflu), zanamivir (**4**, trade name: Relenza), laninamivir phosphate (**5**, trade name: Inavir), and peramivir (**6**, trade name: Rapiacta) [22].

12.2.3 Broad-spectrum antiviral drugs

The nucleoside compound favipiravir (**7**) is a prodrug that undergoes conversion into its active triphosphate form within the human body. This active form acts as a competitive inhibitor of influenza virus polymerase, directly impeding viral replication and transcription. Favipiravir demonstrates inhibitory activity against certain oseltamivir-resistant H275Y mutant strains, with EC_{50} values ranging from 0.5 to 6 μM. Initially approved for influenza treatment in Japan in 2014, this drug has subsequently obtained approval for clinical trials in Europe and the United States, currently progressing through phase III [28].

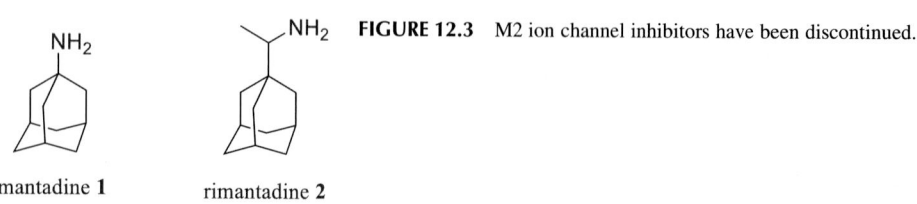

FIGURE 12.3 M2 ion channel inhibitors have been discontinued.

amantadine **1**   rimantadine **2**

TABLE 12.3 Marketed neuraminidase inhibitors [22–27].

Inhibitors	The primary role of influenza virus types	Route of administration	Drug characteristics
oseltamivir (3)	Suppress influenza A and B viruses; The most commonly used treatment and prevention for childhood influenza	Take orally	Ninety percent of circulating virus strains show resistance to it
zanamivir (4)	For the treatment of influenza A and B	Oral inhalation or nasal drip administration	Low oral bioavailability (<5%); It is more effective than oseltamivir, and adverse reactions are less common than oseltamivir
laninamivir phosphate (5)	For the treatment of influenza A and B	Nasal delivery	After a single nasal administration, the drug is retained in the lungs for a long time with long-lasting activity
peramivir (6)	It can be used to treat patients who are unable to inhale or take oral drugs or who are not sensitive to oseltamivir or zanamivir	Intravenous injection	It can bind to the active site of neuraminidase and has the characteristics of rapid onset and long duration

Arbidol hydrochloride (**8**) prevents the fusion of the virus with host cells by targeting the virus HA, while the therapeutic effect is limited by its antiviral activity and drug resistance. Currently, it is exclusively available in Russia and China [29].

Thiazole compound nitazoxanide (**9**) is originally an antiparasitic drug that also exhibits efficacy in treating influenza virus infection. Its mechanism involves inhibiting the glycosylation of HA after translation, thereby affecting the maturation of viral HA. The drug is effective for both type A and type B influenza and is currently undergoing the phase III clinical trial stage in the United States (Fig. 12.4) [30, 31].

12.2.4 Influenza virus inhibitors targeting the polymerase complex

In recent years, significant advancements have been achieved in the field of structural biology of influenza virus polymerase complexes, thereby facilitating the progress of market and clinical research on certain compounds. For example,

favipiravir(**7**)   arbidol hydrochloride(**8**)   nitazoxanide(**9**)

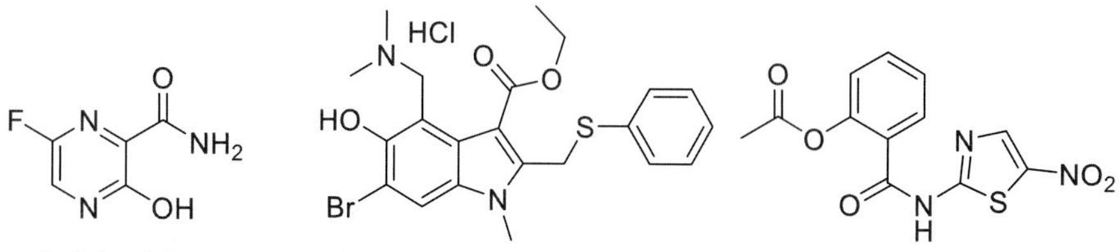

FIGURE 12.4 Broad-spectrum antiviral drugs.

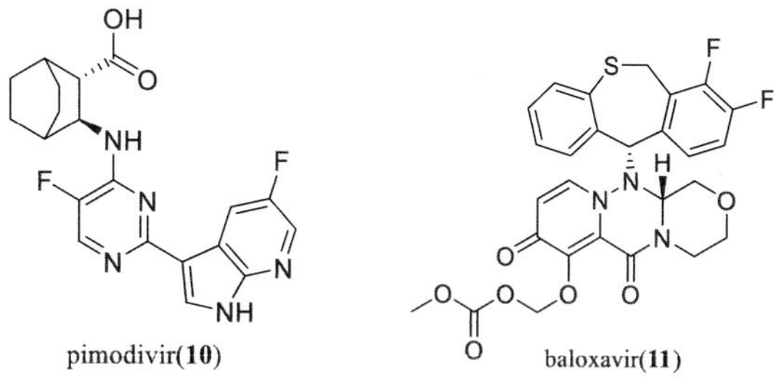

pimodivir(**10**)   baloxavir(**11**)

FIGURE 12.5 Antiinfluenza virus inhibitors targeting polymerase.

PB2 polymerase-targeted pimodivir (**10**) impedes viral gene transcription by obstructing the binding of the polymerase to the host-side RNA's 7-methyl-GTP cap structure. Due to distinct structural disparities in the PB2 cap-binding domain among various influenza types, pimodivir exclusively exhibits efficacy against the type A influenza virus [32]. Nevertheless, outcomes from phase III clinical trials revealed that pimodivir did not demonstrate superior effectiveness compared to existing drugs. Consequently, Janssen Pharmaceuticals eventually terminated its development as an anti-type A influenza medication [33].

Baloxavir marboxil (**11**, Xofluza) is a novel PA inhibitor that targets the initiation stage of mRNA synthesis to inhibit influenza virus replication [34]. The development history, mechanism of action, and clinical trial results of baloxavir are summarized below (Fig. 12.5).

12.3 Development of baloxavir

12.3.1 The structure and function of endonuclease

Influenza viruses are segmented, single-stranded negative-strand RNA viruses. Both type A and type B influenza viruses possess eight RNA sequences encoding proteins, while type C influenza viruses have seven RNA sequences. Unlike plus-strand RNA viruses, each gene sequence of influenza viruses is reversely complementary to its mRNA. The negative-strand genome of the virus is encapsulated by viral proteins, including NP and the RNA-dependent RNA polymerase complex. The complex consists of three protein subunits, PA, PB1, and PB2, which play a crucial role in the virus's life cycle by directly facilitating replication and transcription of viral RNA [35]. Additionally involved in the viral replication process, the PA subunit of the polymerase also exhibits endonuclease and protease activities while participating in viral RNA (vRNA) transcription and assembly of viral particles. Due to their small genome size, influenza viruses rely on host cell translation systems for protein synthesis. Therefore, the mRNA of influenza viruses requires both 5′ cap (CAP) structure and 3′-poly (A) tail structure that can be recognized by host cell translation machinery. However, intrinsic influenza virus mRNA lacks a 5′ cap structure; hence, endonuclease PA seizes this cap structure from the 5′ terminus of host cell mRNA as primers for viral genome transcription—a process known as "CAP-snatching" (Fig. 12.6). "CAP-snatching" represents a pivotal step in influenza virus replication without any analogous mechanism or corresponding enzyme present within host cells. Consequently, inhibitors targeting PA endonuclease can selectively impede the specific transcription process of the influenza virus without affecting normal cellular function—rendering it an ideal target for antiinfluenza drug development [36,38–40]. For instance, by inhibiting the activity of endonuclease PA, baloxavir effectively suppresses viral mRNA synthesis.

PA subunits are divided into the *C*-terminal domain (PA$_C$) and *N*-terminal domain (PA$_N$), which are connected by a long and flexible peptide chain (Fig. 12.7A). PA$_C$ is primarily responsible for combining with the PB1 subunit to form a complex and transporting it into the nucleus, while PA$_N$ mainly provides primers for viral genome transcription. Among them, PA$_N$ contains a domain composed of α-helix and β-fold, where 7 α-helices surround 5 reverse β-folds to form a curved surface that includes an active pocket capable of binding divalent metal cations. Studies have identified

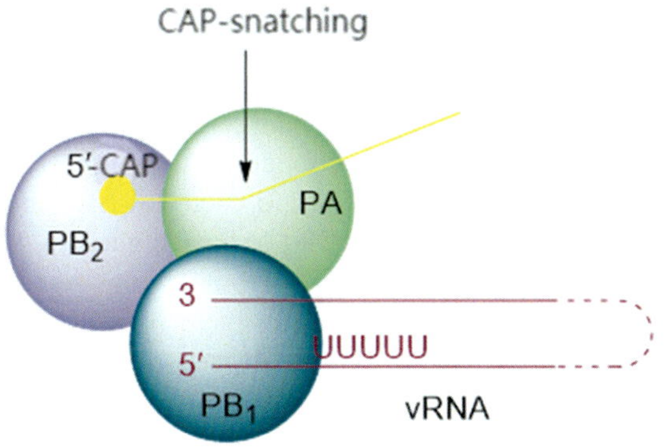

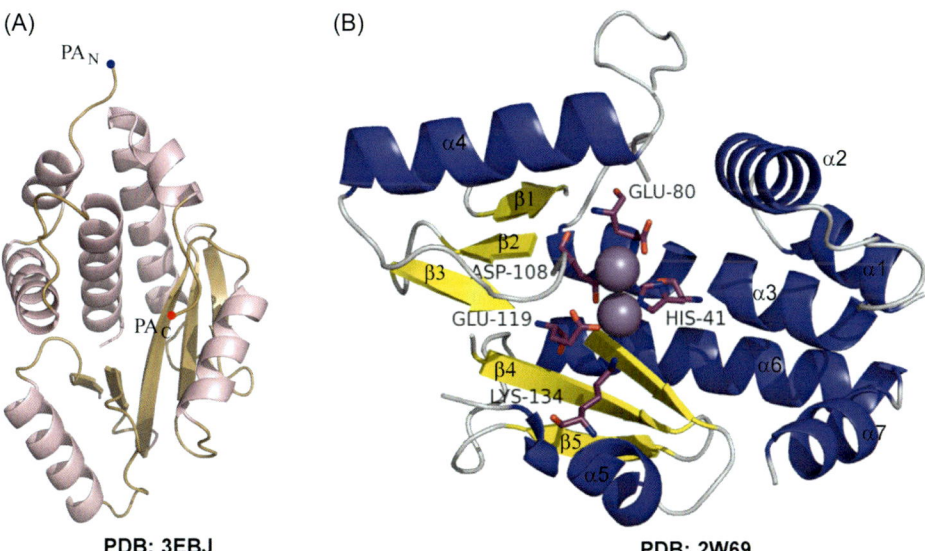

FIGURE 12.6 Graphic illustration of the "CAP-snatching" process [36,37].

FIGURE 12.7 Crystal structure of PA and structure of PA$_N$ [39,41]. *PA*, Polymerase acidic protein; PA$_N$, *N*-terminal domain.

this active site as a negatively charged pocket consisting of histidine (His41), conservative lysine (Lys134), and three acidic amino acid residues (Glu80, Asp108, and Glu119) (Fig. 12.7B). The endonuclease activity of this site requires the activation of divalent metal cations (Mg^{2+} or Mn^{2+}) [39, 42]. Notably, PA$_N$ exhibits an affinity for Mn^{2+} that is approximately 500~600 times higher than that for Mg^{2+}. Interestingly, the binding between PA$_N$ and Mn^{2+} is exothermic whereas it is endothermic with Mg^{2+}. The majority of PA inhibitors that have been researched contain a metal ion chelating group as well as peripheral substituents that interact with the active site. The active site has a variety of large hydrophobic structure fragments within the cavity, providing opportunities for designing inhibitors targeting PA's endonuclease domain [41].

12.3.2 Discovery of baloxavir

Baloxavir marboxil, an oral drug jointly developed by Shionogi Pharmaceutical Company and Roche Pharmaceutical Company of Switzerland, is marketed under the trade name Xofluza. It was first approved for the treatment of influenza A and B in Japan on February 24, 2018, and subsequently received approval from the U.S. FDA on October 25, 2018. The development of the first generation of PA inhibitors lacked structural biology guidance and exhibited weak antiviral activity [43]. In 2009, researchers determined the crystallographic structure of PA and identified the active site of viral endonuclease in its N-terminal domain (Fig. 12.7A) [38]. Furthermore, they discovered that the catalytic domain of PA nucleic acid endonuclease is located at its N-terminal, requiring bimetallic ions (Mg^{2+} or Mn^{2+}) for activity. This finding provided a theoretical basis for studying PA inhibitors based on metal ion chelation mechanisms [44]. Based on highly active metal-binding pharmacophores, guided by coordination chemistry and structure-based drug design, researchers have found many PA inhibitors in recent years. The inhibitors typically comprise two components: one is the metal-binding group (MBG) that can be coordinated with divalent metal ions (Mn^{2+} or Mg^{2+}), which plays a leading role in the binding of nucleic acid endonuclease; the other is the large hydrophobic group that can occupy the PA_N to enhance the affinity and selectivity toward PA [45]. The MBG of baloxavir was generated through a relocation strategy employing the "privileged structure" concept based on the bimetallic pharmacophore model observed in HIV integrase inhibitor dolutegravir (**12**) (Fig. 12.8). The privileged structure refers to the core scaffold chemical structure found across various drug molecules. Molecules possessing privileged scaffolds are considered to possess higher drugability. Therefore, medicinal chemists often adopt effective strategies such as "structural reuse" based on target similarity, "activity redevelopment" utilizing fragments from privileged structures, and "functional reassessment" considering target heteromorphism during the lead compound discovery process. The baloxavir lead compound herein was designed based on target similarity [46]. Dolutegravir (**12**) is a bimetallic chelating model targeting the catalytic active site of integrase. Through multiple rounds of modification, it has been transformed into an analog of carbamyl pyridone, possessing a metal chelating group capable of binding to the active site of HIV integrase via two divalent metal ions (Fig. 12.8A). Given the similarity in metal coordination between PA nucleic acid endonuclease and HIV integrase (the carbamyl pyridone scaffold of dolutegravir can form coordination bonds with two Mn^{2+} in the active site of PA endonuclease, Fig. 12.8B), researchers naturally sought to incorporate the metal chelating scaffold (red part) from **12** into the design of PA inhibitors while modifying its advantageous scaffold with various substituents targeting pockets 2, 3, and 4. On the one hand, the metal chelation of pocket 1 is guaranteed (the 2,4-difluorobenzylamine of dolutegravir has a certain deviation in the binding of the scaffold with metal ions due to its large volume); on the other hand, occupying other pockets can enhance the activity and selectivity of the compound. Consequently, Shionogi Pharmaceutical Company of Japan conducted a systematic investigation on structure-activity relationships based on highly potent matrix structure **13a** (Table 12.4), ultimately yielding valuable baloxavir acid derivative **13** [47–49] (Fig. 12.8).

The specific process is as follows: In the initial structural modification (Table 12.4), the compound with C1-benzyl substitution significantly enhances the inhibitory activity against the enzyme (**14b**). Furthermore, when the C1-position is replaced by an N heteroatom, the compound with N1-benzyl substitution (**14d**) also exhibits a significant

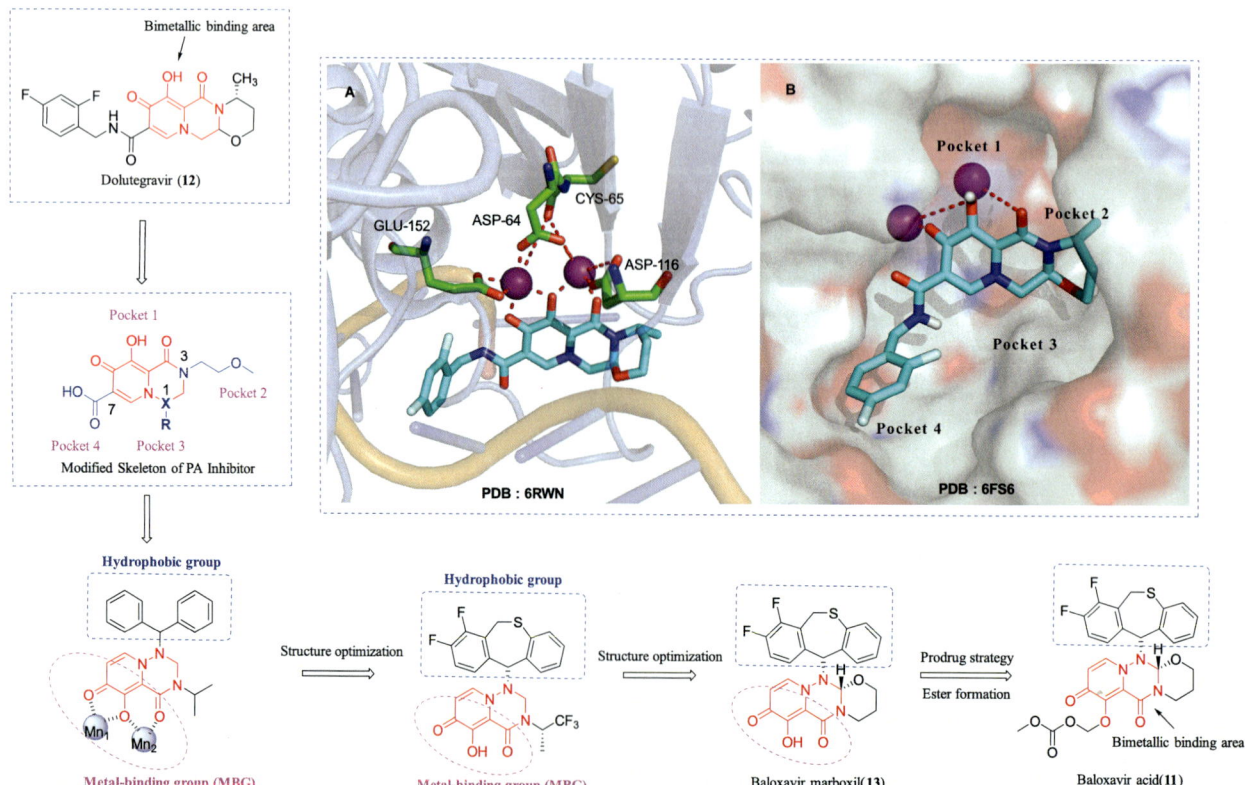

FIGURE 12.8 Structure of dolutegravir (**12**) and discovery of baloxavir (**11**). (A) Pattern of interaction between dolutegravir and HIV integrase; (B) The docking model of dolutegravir and PA endonuclease. *PA*, Polymerase acidic protein.

TABLE 12.4 Early structure-activity relationships of baloxavir.

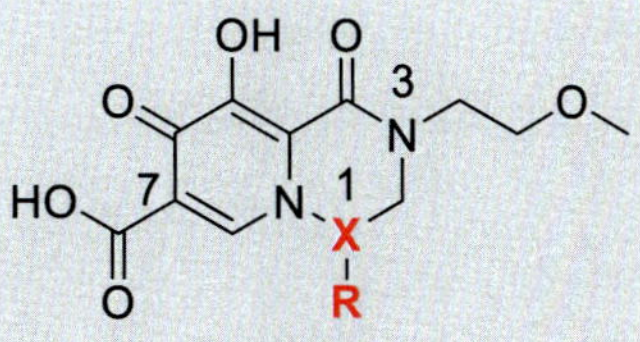

14a-14j

Compound number	X	R	Cap-dependent endonuclease (CEN) IC$_{50}$^{a} (μM)	Cytopathic effect (CPE) EC$_{50}$^{b} (μM)
14a	CH	H	68.6	N.D.
14b	CH(S)	Bn	0.241	>50
14c	CH(R)	Bn	27.4	>50
14d	N	p-F-Bn	0.419	>25
14e	CH(S)	Ph	27.8	>50
14f	CH(S)	Phenethyl	1.35	N.D.
14g	CH(S)	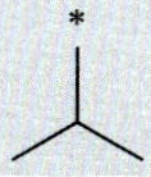 isobutyl*	2.99	N.D.
14h	CH(S)	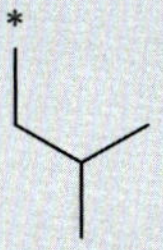 isopentyl*	9.31	N.D.
14i	CH(S)	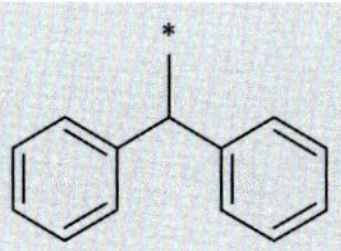 benzhydryl*	0.0478	0.293
14j	N	benzhydryl*	0.116	1.47

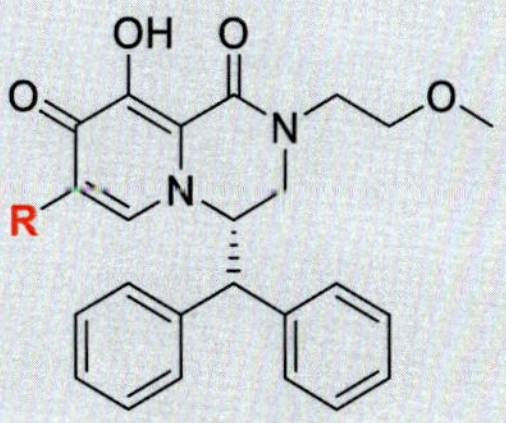

15a-15g

Compound Number	R	CEN IC$_{50}$^{a}(μM)	CPE EC$_{50}$^{b}(μM)
15a	COOEt	0.298	2.53
15b	CONHMe	1.59	7.11
15c	NH$_2$	0.358	3.86
15d	OMe	0.110	1.68
15e	Me	0.281	2.47
15f	Cl	0.114	0.541
15g	H	0.115	0.134

(Continued)

TABLE 12.4 (Continued)

16a–16g

Compound Number	X	R	CEN IC$_{50}$[a] (nM)	CPE EC$_{50}$[b] (nM)	Met. Stab. microsome[c] (%)	iv CL[d] (mL/min/kg)
16a	CH(S)	*–CH$_2$CH$_2$–O–CH$_3$	115	134	79.7	42.2
16b		Me	80.4	144	79.9	31.6
16c		i-Pr	239	57.5	78.7	25.3
16d	N	*–CH$_2$CH$_2$–O–CH$_3$	103	75.2	83.4	47.4
16e		Me	164	81.6	92.1	18.8
16f		i-Pr	286	81.6	86.0	10.9
16g		*–CH$_2$-furyl	588	478	50.6	42.6

*The attachment point of the substituent to the parent ring.
[a] CEN (Cap-dependent endonuclease) inhibitory activity was determined according to previously reported methods.
[b] The Madin–Darby bovine kidney (MDBK) cells were infected with influenza A virus (diluted A/WSN/33 at 50 TCID$_{50}$ per well in a 96-well plate) and incubated with the test compound for 72 h at 37°C in a CO$_2$ incubator, using the concentration of EC$_{50}$ required for 50% cell survival of the test compound.
[c] Liver microsomal stability was determined by calculating the percentage of compounds retained after incubating them with rat liver microsomes at a concentration of 2 μM for 30 minutes at 37°C
[d] Rat clearance was measured through LC/MS/MS analysis following administration of a single intravenous dose.

improvement in activity. However, it is noteworthy that the highest enzyme inhibitory activity is observed for the S configuration substitution compound **14i** of C1-diphenyl, which demonstrates three orders of magnitude increase in activity compared to **14a**. Despite this remarkable enhancement, its IC$_{50}$ value remains near 50 nM, which is unsatisfactory for medicinal chemists. To further optimize this compound, various modifications were implemented at the carboxylic acid group located at position C7 of **14i**. These modifications included ethyl esterification, formamide incorporation, and amino group introduction, as well as methyl and methoxy substitutions (**15a∼15g**). Unfortunately, none of these derivatives exhibited superior activity compared to **14i**. Efforts to remove substituents from position C7 also failed to yield desired results. Medicinal chemists then turned their attention to the study of the structure-activity relationships of the N-3 position and found that although the substitution derivative of this position did not further improve the in vitro enzyme inhibition activity, the hydrophobic substituents reduced the venous clearance rate of rats and improved the stability of rat liver microsomes in vitro. The most noteworthy derivative among these was **16f** [50].

After obtaining information on the N-3 position, medicinal chemists redirected their focus toward optimizing the diphenylmethyl group at the C-1 position. They initially optimized the two benzene rings through various alkylation, halogenation, and addition of electron-donor groups and electron-withdrawing groups (as shown in Table 12.5). As a result, compound **17g** with dichloride substitution exhibited an IC$_{50}$ value of 37 nM. Of course, medicinal chemists also introduced various polar groups to the benzene ring; however, the activities of compounds obtained were all diminished to varying extents, likely due to the reduced permeability of these compounds across the cell membrane caused by the presence of polar groups. Interestingly, the two chlorine atoms exhibited higher activity at the ortho-position (**17g**) of the C3-substituted methylene group compared to the meta position (**17h**), as well as surpassing the activity of the ortho-mono-chlorine atom substituted **17c**.

Considering the potential benefits of the molecule's rigid structure in mimicking the hydrophobic pocket in the active site of PA, medicinal chemists confirmed the molecular structure, such as the scaffold of annulene (**17k**), and incorporated easily synthesized polar molecules **17l** and **17m** into the completely hydrophobic fragment. Among them,

TABLE 12.5 Structure-activity relationship analysis of baloxavir after scaffold determination.

Compound number	R₁	CEN IC$_{50}$a (nM)	CPE EC$_{50}$b (nM)
16f	diphenylmethyl	286	81.6
17a	(2-methylphenyl)(phenyl)methyl	142	73.4
17b	(3-methylphenyl)(phenyl)methyl	276	219
17c	(2-chlorophenyl)(phenyl)methyl	210	77.8
17d	(3-chlorophenyl)(phenyl)methyl	101	75.9
17e	(4-chlorophenyl)(phenyl)methyl	291	94.0
17f	bis(4-methylphenyl)methyl	394	440
17g	bis(2-chlorophenyl)methyl	37.0	48.2
17h	bis(3-chlorophenyl)methyl	230	65.8
17i	bis(3-methoxyphenyl)methyl	1310	589

(Continued)

276 Medicinal Chemistry and Drug Development

TABLE 12.5 (Continued)

Compound	Structure	CEN IC$_{50}$ (nM)	CPE EC$_{50}$ (nM)
17j	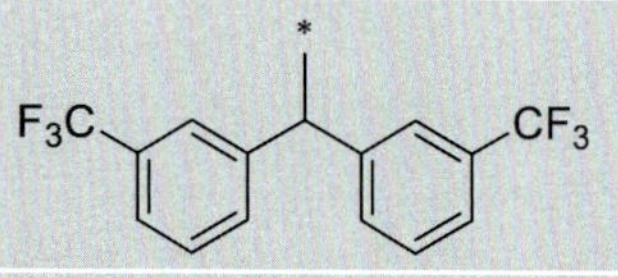 1-(3-CF$_3$-phenyl)-1-(3-CF$_3$-phenyl)ethyl	456	386
17k	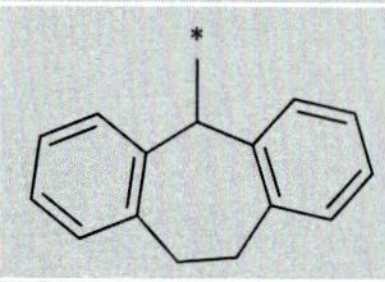 10,11-dihydro-5H-dibenzo[a,d]cycloheptene	60.1	20.1
17l	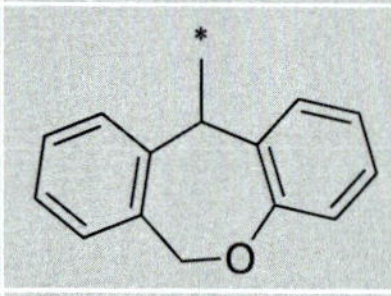 dibenz[b,f]oxepine	264	71.0
17m	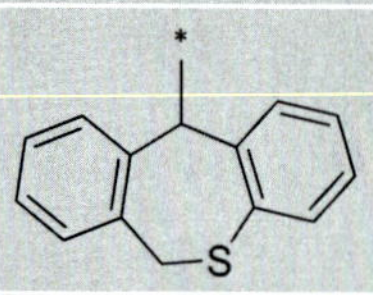 dibenz[b,f]thiepine	61.9	16.9

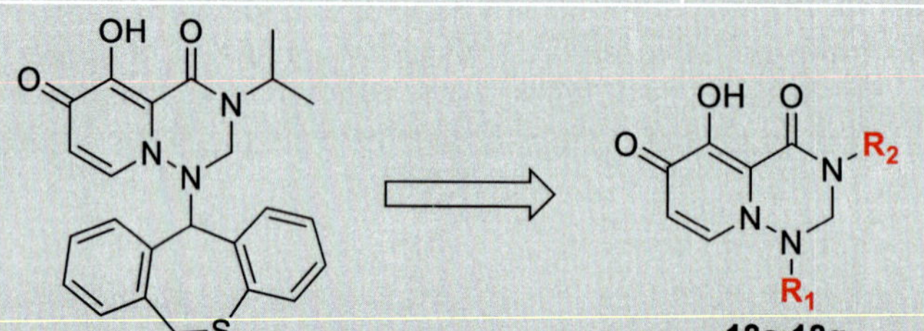

Compounds 18a–18g share a common R$_1$ (dibenz[b,f]thiepin-10(11H)-yl) with R$_2$ varied:

Compound number	R$_1$	R$_2$	CEN IC$_{50}$[a] (nM)	CPE EC$_{50}$[b] (nM)	Met. Stab. microsome[c] (%)	iv Cl[d] (mL/min/kg)
17m	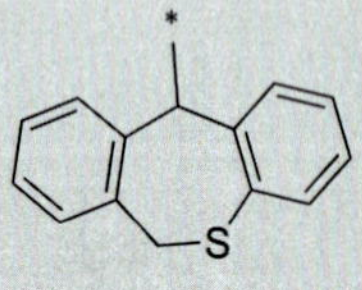 dibenz[b,f]thiepine	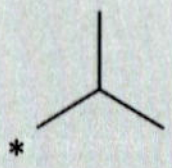 isobutyl	61.9	16.9	72.6	32.7
18a		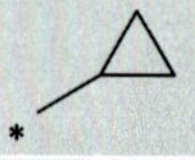 cyclopropylmethyl	35.0	13.7	73.7	46.0
18b		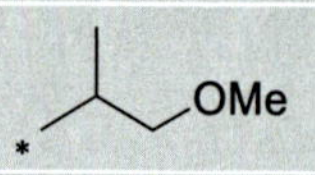 CH$_2$CH(CH$_3$)OMe	57.9	20.7	58.6	49.1
18c		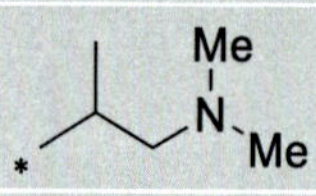 CH$_2$CH(Me)NMe$_2$	151	84.1	76.4	98.7
18d		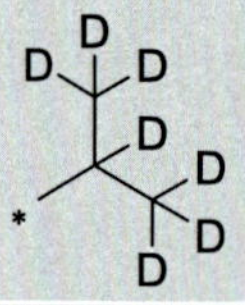 d$_7$-isobutyl	43.4	11.7	74.4	39.1
18e		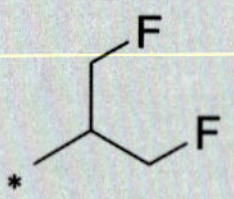 CH$_2$CHFCH$_2$F	113	27.5	84.9	33.5

(Continued)

TABLE 12.5 (Continued)

Compound	Structure		CEN IC50	CPE EC50	Met. Stab.	iv Cl
(R)-18f	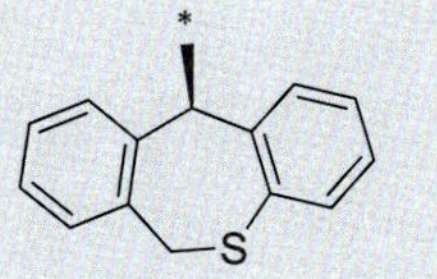 [dibenzothiepine structure]	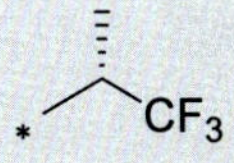 CF3 group	1890	131	NT	NT
(S)-18f	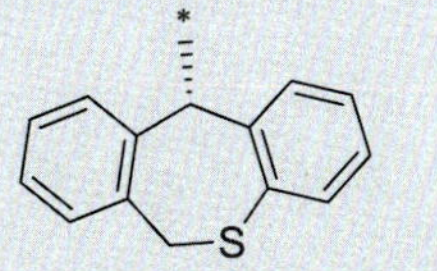 [dibenzothiepine structure]		49.7	4.69	98.1	15.8
(R)-18g	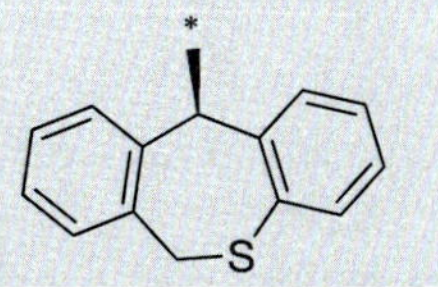 [dibenzothiepine structure]	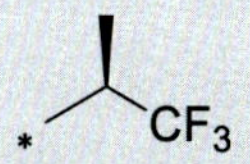 CF3 group	285	21.7	NT	NT
(S)-18g	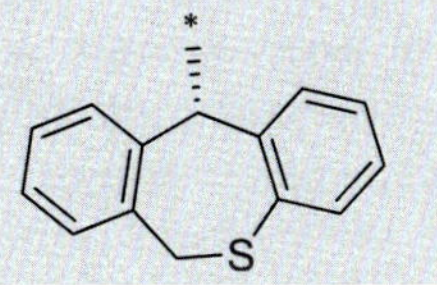 [dibenzothiepine structure]		112	18.6	79.8	NT

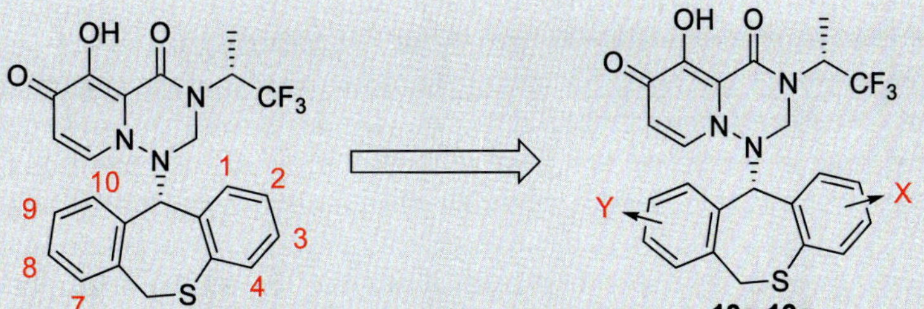

19a-19q

Compound number	X or Y	CEN IC$_{50}$[a] (nM)	CPE EC$_{50}$[b] (nM)	Met. Stab. microsome[c] (%)	iv Cl[d] (mL/min/kg)
(S)-18f	H	49.7	4.69	98.1	15.8
19a	1-F	37.1	15.1	97.4	9.09
19b	2-F	39.2	8.16	103	15.4
19c	3-F	48.2	14.3	93.9	13.4
19d	4-F	66.4	3.41	95.6	10.3
19e	7-F	12.5	3.85	91.8	8.37
19f	8-F	12.3	3.54	95.3	11.6
19g	9-F	44.3	4.68	98.9	21.3
19h	10-F	31.8	3.75	102	18.0
19i	7,8-F,F	5.57	4.28	81.1	11.0
19j	1-Cl	76.2	18.8	85.4	10.2
19k	2-Cl	24.9	70.8	NT	NT
19l	3-Cl	62.1	21.2	101	12.2
19m	4-Cl	23.2	13.5	92.3	6.78
19n	7-Cl	30.0	3.04	102	7.36

(Continued)

TABLE 12.5 (Continued)

19o	8-Cl	6.99	10.5	96.1	5.70
19p	9-Cl	16.6	4.21	94.1	12.4
19q	10-Cl	9.95	3.52	93.3	19.6

*The attachment point of the substituent to the parent ring.
[a]CEN (Cap-dependent endonuclease) inhibitory activity was determined according to previously reported methods.
[b]The Madin–Darby bovine kidney (MDBK) cells were infected with influenza A virus (diluted A/WSN/33 at 50 $TCID_{50}$ per well in a 96-well plate) and incubated with the test compound for 72 h at 37°C in a CO_2 incubator, using the concentration of EC_{50} required for 50% cell survival of the test compound.
[c]Liver microsomal stability was determined by calculating the percentage of compounds retained after incubating them with rat liver microsomes at a concentration of 2 μM for 30 minutes at 37°C.
[d]Rat clearance was measured through LC/Ms/MS analysis following administration of a single intravenous dose.

both **17k** and **17m** exhibited comparable enzyme inhibition activity to the lead compound **14i** in vitro. Since then, the basic scaffold of baloxavir has been officially formed!

Thirdly, medicinal chemists turned to the derivation of the N-3 substituent with the concern of improving metabolic stability and reducing clearance of the molecule in vivo. The above introduction of isopropyl substituted **16f** naturally prompted pharmacologists to consider cyclopropyl substitution (**18a**), as well as various polar groups based on isopropyl groups, halogenated groups, and even deuterated groups. However, the compounds obtained did not yield the desired results. Interestingly, it was found that the CF_3-substituted compound (**S**)-**18f** exhibited more ideal results. Its IC_{50} value was measured at 49.7 nM, with 98% of the compounds demonstrating metabolic stability in vitro and a clearance rate of only 15.8 mL/min/kg. Interestingly, the activity of its stereoisomer (**R**)-**18f** was lost, indicating that the stereostructure of the small molecule was crucial for binding to the active site of the target enzyme.

At this point, medicinal chemists anticipated reducing the enzyme inhibition activity in vitro of the lead compound to the nanomolar concentration level. (Note: modern antiviral molecules are generally optimized to this level to increase the effective inhibition of virus concentration in plasma, reduce the chance of virus mutation in response to drug pressure, and minimize potential side effects). Researchers proceeded to conduct various halogenation derivatives of the thiofazine scaffold of (**S**)-**18f**, with a specific focus on the impact of substitutions involving fluorine and chlorine atoms. It could be seen that the inhibitory activity of cap-dependent endonuclease (CEN) was further improved when the F atom was introduced at the 7′- and 8′-positions. Additionally, the inhibitory activity in vitro of the compound below 10 nM was observed upon introducing chlorine atoms at the 8′- and 10′-positions, indicating the presence of a small lipophilic pocket adjacent to the CEN binding site that could accommodate both fluorine and chlorine atoms. Among them, compounds **19i** and **19q** exhibited potent inhibitory activity against CEN and demonstrated antiviral efficacy in the single-digit nanomolar range. Additionally, during the investigation of pharmacokinetic properties, it was observed that **19i** exhibited a lower venous clearance rate compared to **19q** (**19i**: 11.0 mL/min/kg vs. **19q**: 19.6 mL/min/kg).

In a mouse model inoculated with A/WSN/33 influenza virus (100 tissue culture infectious dose $(TCID)_{50}$/mouse), **19i** or oseltamivir phosphate was orally administered twice (BID) on day 5 postinfection. Twenty-four hours after the first dose, pharmacologists quantified viral titers (log $TCID_{50}$/mL) in mouse lung tissue using Madin–Darby canine kidney cells. When **19i** was administered at 0.4 mg/kg bis in die (BID), compared with the clinical equivalent dose of oseltamivir phosphate (5 mg/kg BID), the viral load in the lung of mice was reduced by one-tenth. Increasing the dose of **19i** to 10 mg/kg BID reduced the pulmonary viral load to approximately one-thirtieth of the level observed after oseltamivir phosphate administration (Fig. 12.9) [51]. By further optimizing **19i**, medicinal chemists successfully identified baloxavir acid (**13**); unfortunately, a detailed optimization process was not provided by the authors and requires further investigation. However, comparing the structure of **19i** and **13**, it can be found that the change of N-3 position substituent deserved additional explanation: the replacement of methyl ethyl ether substituent (**16d**) with isopropyl (**16f**) resulted in a decrease in venous clearance rate in rats and enhanced stability of rat liver microsomes in vitro. This suggested that N-alkyl substitution served as a common metabolic site (Table 12.4). The replacement of the isopropyl group by the trifluoromethyl isopropyl group ((**S**)-**18f**) was also aimed to further improve the metabolic stability of the isopropyl group (the methyl group or tertiary carbon of isopropyl group was also a common metabolic site), but the introduction of trifluoromethyl group was likely to greatly improve the lipid solubility of the molecule. Therefore, medicinal chemists used the method of intramolecular cyclization to introduce oxygen atoms to obtain **13**. The low oral bioavailability of baloxavir acid **13** prompted medicinal chemists to favor the "prodrug strategy." Introducing ester bonds is a commonly employed approach for prodrugs. This mechanism involves the hydrolysis of drug molecules' ester bonds by various human carboxylesterases present in plasma, cells, and different tissues, leading to the release of active drug molecules. Baloxavir **11** is a dimethyl carbonate ester of **13**, with one end attached to the acidic hydroxyl group of **13** (Fig. 12.8). The dimethyl ester bond is susceptible to hydrolysis catalyzed by carboxylesterase, leading to the formation

FIGURE 12.9 Pulmonary viral inhibition by **19i** was observed in a mouse model infected with A/WSN/33 influenza virus [51].

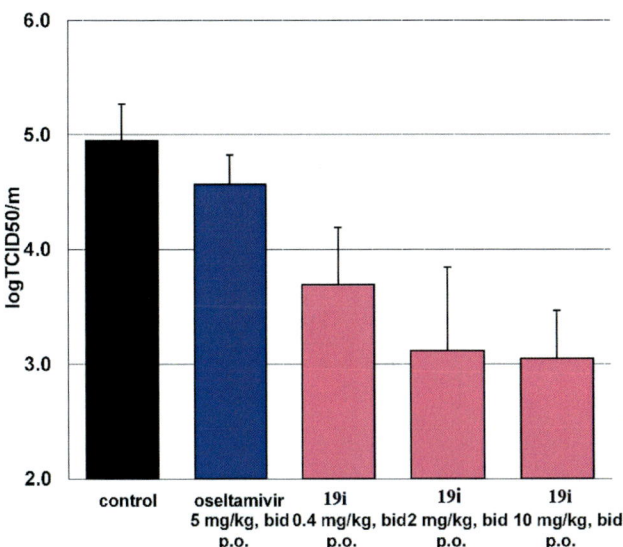

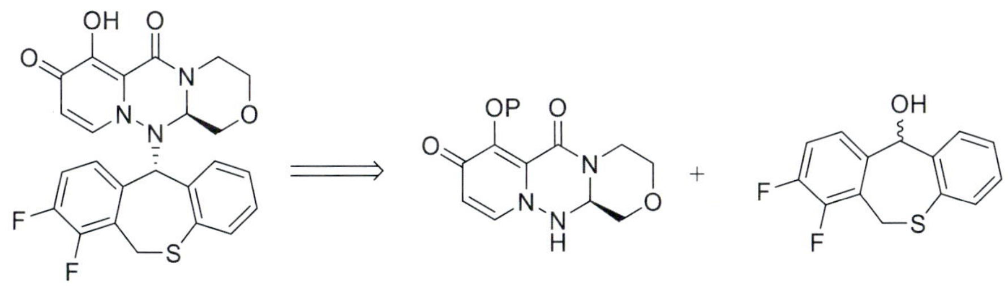

FIGURE 12.10 Inverse synthesis analysis of baloxavir.

of an unstable hydroxymethyl ester that spontaneously decomposes, releasing one molecule of formaldehyde and one molecule of baloxavir acid. The oral bioavailability of baloxavir **11** ($F = 18.4\%$) is 2.5 times higher than that of baloxavir acid **13** ($F = 7.1\%$) [52].

12.3.3 Synthesis of baloxavir

The baloxavir consists primarily of two fragments (A and B) (Fig. 12.10), each containing a chiral center. Fragments A and B can be transformed into the desired compounds through coupling and deprotection reactions [53], with three main synthesis routes available:

Route 1: Fragment **A** was synthesized in 10 steps. Lactam **20** was used as starting material, protected by allyl chloroformate (alloc), then reduced by the carbonyl group, and reacted with methanol to obtain methoxy ether **23**. The carboxylic acid of another starting material, **24**, was esterified and underwent an exchange reaction with butyl *tert*-butyl hydrazine carboxylate (Boc-NHNH$_2$) to form pyridinone **26**, which was deprotected with anhydrous hydrochloric acid to obtain **27**. After the substitution reaction of intermediate **23** with **27** to obtain compound **28** and subsequent catalytic hydrogenation for deprotecting the group, the ammonolysis reaction of molecular lactonide was conducted to yield closed-loop product **29**. Subsequently, (R)-tetrahydrofuran-2-carboxylic acid was introduced through an acylation reaction to afford diastereomers **29A** and **29B**, which were further recrystallized using ethanol to isolate pure compound **29A**. Finally, the tetrahydrofuran-2-formyl group was removed to obtain fragment **A** (Fig. 12.11).

3, 4-difluorobenzoic acid **30** was used as raw material and reacted with N,N-dimethylformamide (DMF) by strong alkali LDA treatment to introduce an aldehyde group at the o-position of its carboxylic acid and undergo intramolecular hemiacetal reaction with carboxylic acid to form compound **31**. **31** reacted with thiophenol to give thioacetal **32**. **32** underwent hydroreduction catalyzed by Lewis acid (AlCl$_3$), followed by Friedel−Crafts in polyphosphate to form cyclic thioether **34**, which was then reduced with sodium borohydride to give racemic sulfide **B**. Finally, the catalytic coupling

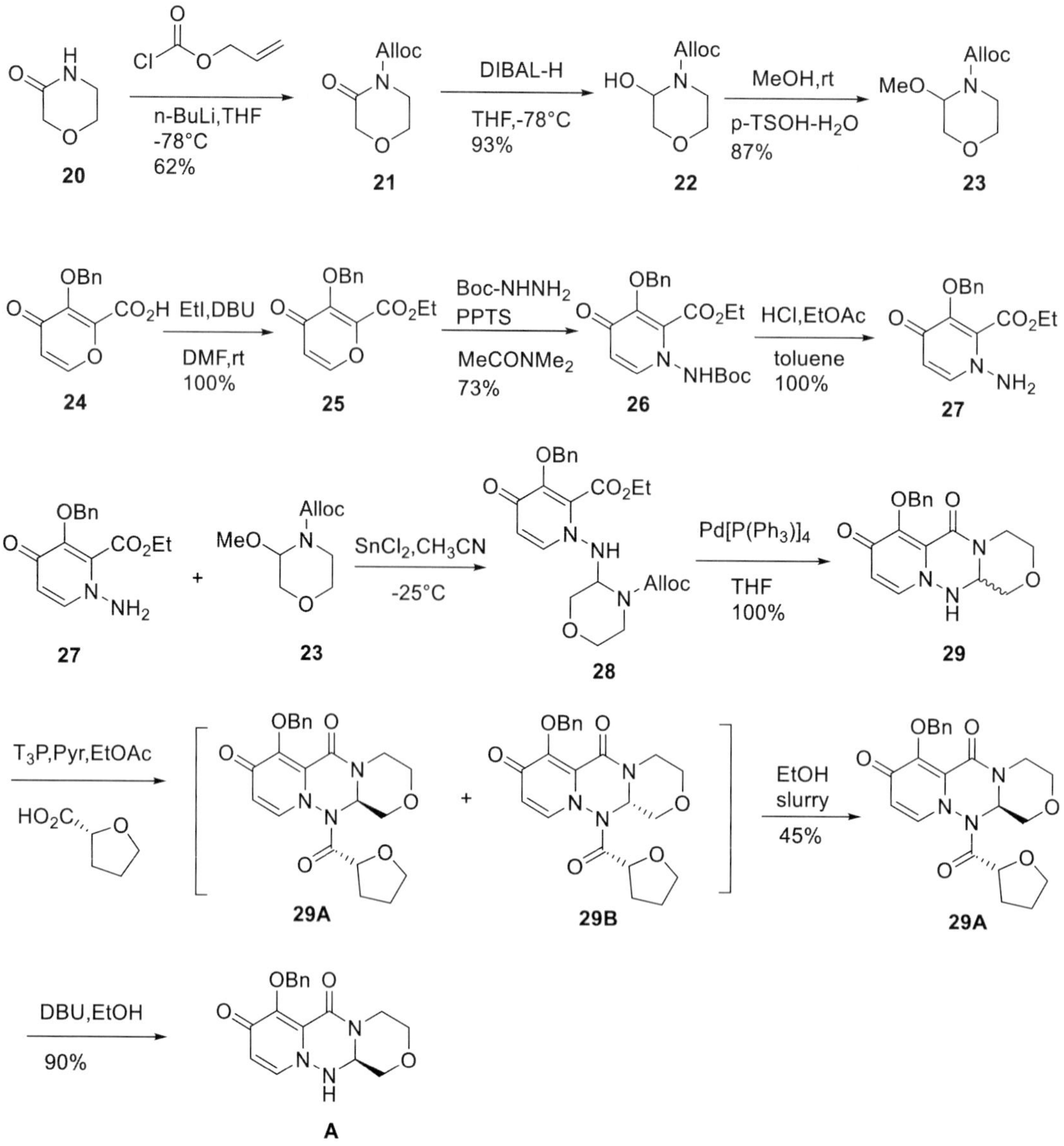

FIGURE 12.11 Synthesis of fragment **A**.

and debenzylization of fragments **A** and **B** ultimately led to the formation of baloxavir acid 13 with S configuration with a high yield of 93% (Fig. 12.12) [52].

The main problems of this route include (1) the long reaction time and the necessity to obtain the pure enantiomers by synthesizing covalent diastereomers in low yields; (2) limited coupling efficiency and inadequate diastereomeric selectivity between the two major fragments **A** and **B**.

Route 2: Synthetic fragment **A** was shortened from 10 steps to 8 steps. The primary alcohol 36 was first alkylated and then deprotected with hydrazine hydrate to obtain a primary amine 38 with a hemiacetal at one end. The compound 39 obtained by amidation reaction of compounds 26 and 38 was treated with MeCN aqueous solution of MeSO$_3$H to obtain tricyclic amine 29. Like the first-generation route, 29 was subjected to acylation reaction, recrystallization to obtain **29A**, and then amide reduction to obtain fragment **A** (Fig. 12.13). Different from route 1, before the combination of fragment **A** and fragment **B**, compound 41 was obtained by protecting fragment **A** with n-hexyl and then reacting with fragment **B**. Finally, baloxavir acid 13 was obtained in 91% yield by deprotection (Fig. 12.14). The use of n-hexyl-protected fragment **A** in this route greatly improved the selectivity of diastereoisomers and the yield [54,55].

Route Three: The separation (**29–29A**) yield of diastereoisomers in the first two routes was 45%. In this route, the required asymmetric center was set by using a chiral directing group to avoid the low-yield separation of

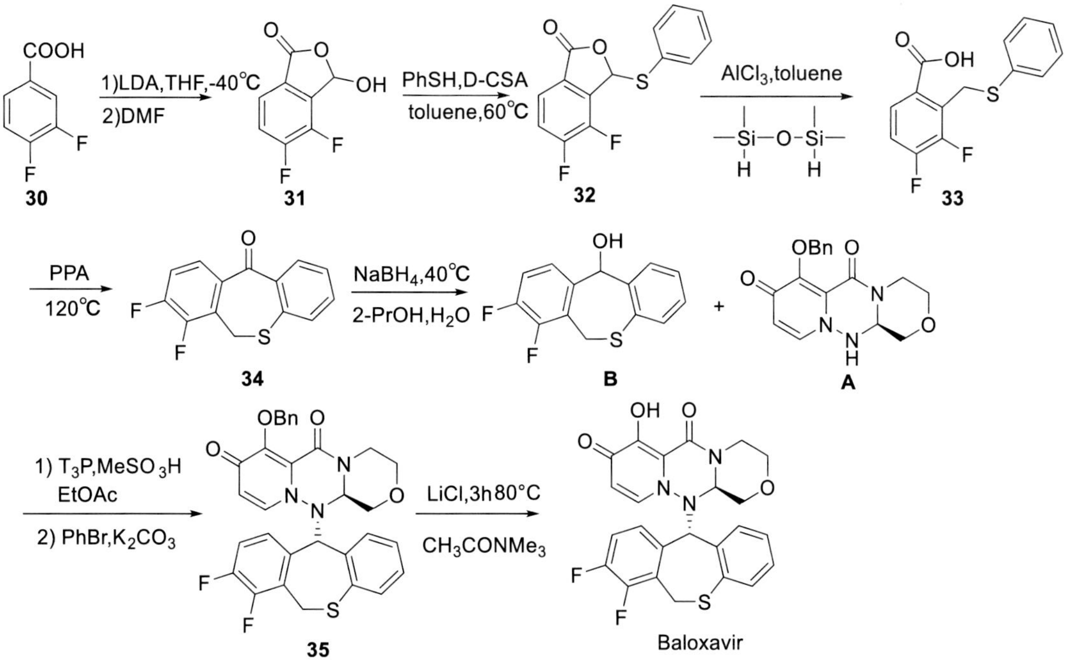

FIGURE 12.12 Synthesis of baloxavir (fragment **A** + fragment **B**).

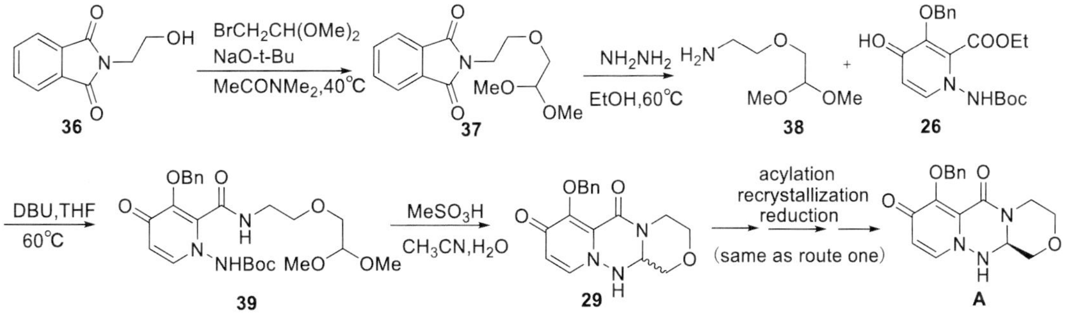

FIGURE 12.13 Synthesis of fragment **A**.

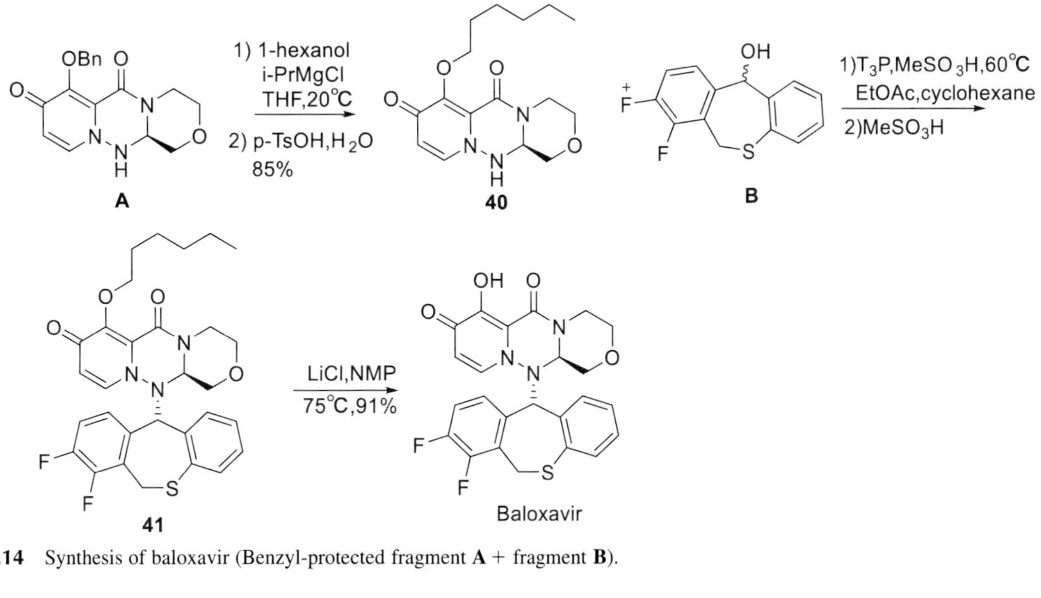

FIGURE 12.14 Synthesis of baloxavir (Benzyl-protected fragment **A** + fragment **B**).

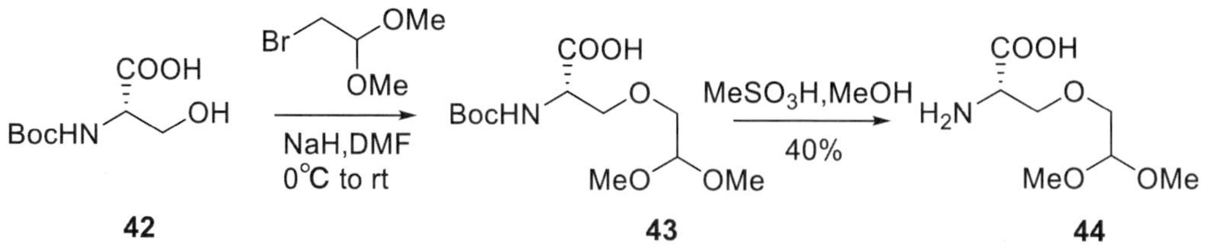

FIGURE 12.15 Preparation of chiral fragment **44**.

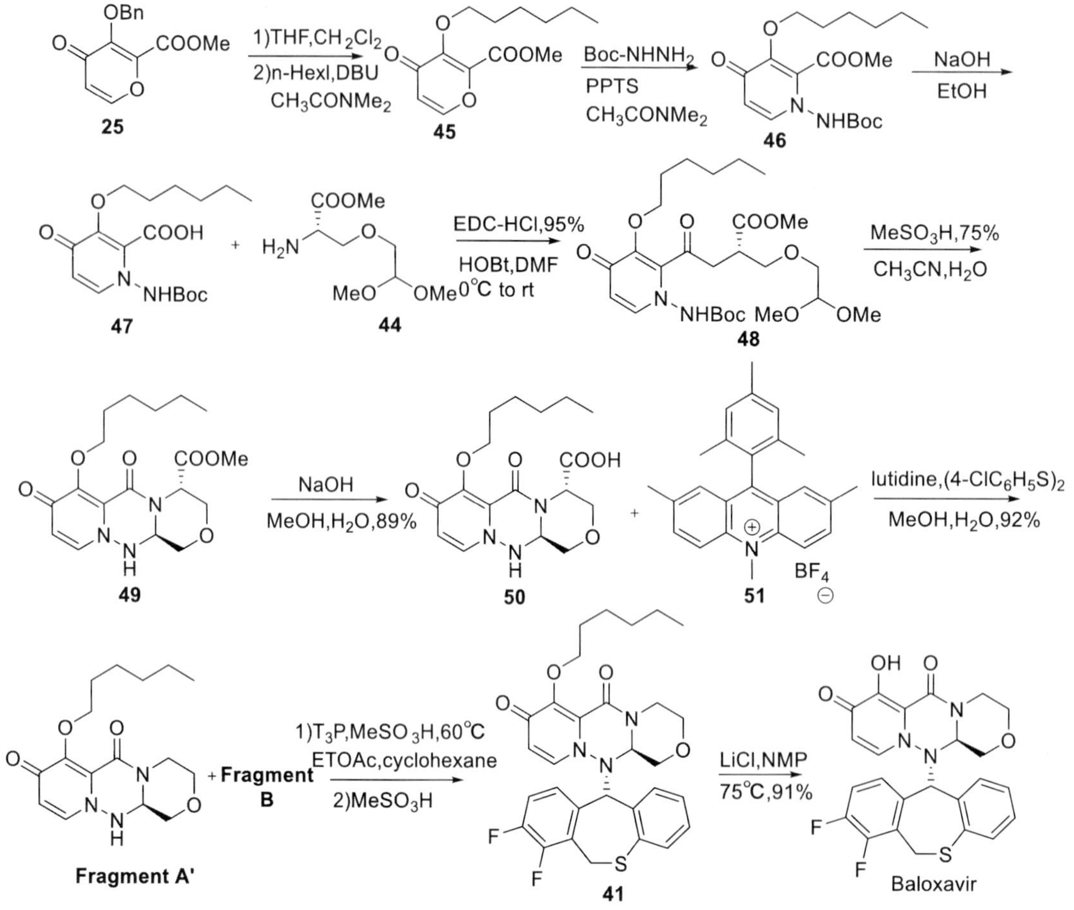

FIGURE 12.16 Preparation of fragment **A′** and synthesis of baloxavir.

diastereoisomers. The route also avoided the switching of late protective groups by introducing n-hexyl protective groups earlier. A total of 10 steps were required for the synthesis of fragment **A′**. Although there were two more steps than Route 2, the yield was still about twice that of Route 2 due to the avoidance of the diastereoisomeric separation step.

Using Boc-protected serine **42** as the starting material, a chiral fragment **44** (Fig. 12.15) was obtained by etherification and esterification (simultaneous removal of the Boc group). The preparation of fragment **A′** started from benzyl-protected pyranone **25**, which was debenzylated by TFA, and then alkylated with n-hexyl iodide (the protecting group was switched to n-hexyl in two steps) to obtain intermediate **45**. **45** was reacted with Boc-NHNH$_2$ and then saponified to obtain **47**. The chiral fragment **44** was coupled with **47** to obtain **48**, and the tricyclic product **49** (diastereoisomeric ratio of 20:1) was obtained after treatment with acetonitrile/aqueous solution of MeSO$_3$H, which avoided diastereoisomeric separation. Finally, compound **50** was obtained by ester hydrolysis. Finally, **50** and **51** were decarboxylated in the alkaline solution of methanol to obtain fragment **A′**, and fragment **A′** was condensed with fragment **B** to obtain baloxavir acid **13** (yield 91%) (Fig. 12.16) [56].

12.3.4 Clinical study of baloxavir

12.3.4.1 Pharmacological action of baloxavir

Baloxavir exhibited significant antiviral activity against influenza A and B viruses and clinical isolates, including the NA-H274Y mutant strain, and showed synergistic antiviral activity with NA inhibitors such as oseltamivir and zanamivir [57].

In a mouse model inoculated with clinical isolates of influenza A or B virus (including oseltamivir-resistant H5N1 and H7N9 virus strains), baloxavir treatment alone or in combination with oseltamivir significantly reduced mortality in mice compared with an equal dose of oseltamivir (5 mg/kg twice daily for 5 days). In addition, the baloxavir group exhibited a significant reduction in virus titer within 24 hours after administration. The efficacy of baloxavir was evident in a mouse model even when administration was delayed 24—96 hours after inoculation with a lethal dose of influenza A virus. However, in the tolerance test in vitro of influenza A and B virus strains, it was found that mutant strains with I38T amino acid mutation in the PA active site (the binding target of baloxavir) were 100-fold less sensitive to baloxavir than wild strains [58].

12.3.4.2 Pharmacokinetics study

Absorption and distribution: As a small molecule prodrug, baloxavir could be rapidly converted to its active metabolite **13** after oral administration, which could reach its maximum plasma concentration (C_{max}) in about 4 hours with an apparent volume of distribution of 1180 L. C_{max} could be reduced by 48% if taken with food, area under the curve decreased by 36%, and the binding rate of **13** to plasma protein in vitro was 92.9%—93.9%.

Metabolism and elimination: **13** was mainly metabolized by UGT1A3 to form a glucuronic acid conjugate and then metabolized by CYP3A to form sulfoxide. Baloxavir was mainly eliminated by bile excretion. Radioactive marker detection showed that about 80% of the drug was excreted through feces after administration, and a small amount (about 15%) was excreted from urine. The half-life was 79.1 hours and the clearance rate was 10.3 L/h. In addition, population pharmacokinetic studies showed that age, gender, and mild or moderate liver and kidney injury had no significant effect on the pharmacokinetics of baloxavir, and the effect of severe liver and kidney injury on the pharmacokinetics of baloxavir was not clear.

12.3.4.3 Drug administration

Baloxavir should ideally be administered within 48 hours of symptom onset. A single dose was taken orally once and should not be taken with dairy products, calcium-fortified beverages, multivalent cations with laxatives, antacids, or oral supplements. It needed to be administered according to body weight, as shown in Table 12.6 [59,60].

Phase II clinical trial: The phase II trial was a double-blind, placebo-controlled, dose-ranging, randomized controlled trial. Researchers assessed the efficacy of baloxavir in 400 patients who were randomly assigned to receive single doses of 10, 20, or 40 mg of baloxavir or placebo. The findings demonstrated that the duration of influenza symptoms was significantly shorter (49.5—54.2 vs 77.7 hours) and the duration of fever was significantly reduced (28.9—33.4 vs 45.3 hours) in the baloxavir group compared to the placebo group, while each dosage level of baloxavir exhibited a significant reduction in viral load within the body [60].

12.3.4.4 Phase III clinical trial

CAPSTONE-1 was a global, multicenter, randomized, double-blind, placebo-controlled phase III study. Researchers used this method to evaluate the efficacy and safety of baloxavir. A total of 1436 influenza patients without other complications were included in the trial. Patients aged 20—64 years were randomly divided into three groups according to the weight ratio of 2: 2: 1. According to body weight, they received a single oral dose of 40 or 80 mg of baloxavir, twice a day, along

TABLE 12.6 Baloxavir for adults and adolescents 12 years of age and older [56].

Weight of the patient	Recommended oral dose
40~80 kg	A single dose of 40 mg
≧80 kg	A single dose of 80 mg

with 75 mg of oseltamivir or placebo for a total of five days. Patients aged 12–19 years were randomly divided into two groups according to the weight ratio of 2: 1 and received a single oral administration of baloxavir or placebo (only on the first day). The results showed that in adolescents (38.6 hours) and adults (25.6 hours), the median time of symptom relief in the baloxavir group was shorter than that in the placebo group. Compared with patients who began to receive drug treatment within 24 hours after the onset of symptoms (32.8 hours) and those who began to receive drug treatment after 24 hours (13.3 hours), the difference in symptom relief time between the baloxavir group and the placebo group was significant. Compared with the oseltamivir group, the median time of symptom relief was similar in the baloxavir group (53.5 hours) and the oseltamivir group (53.8 hours), but the viral load in the baloxavir group decreased faster. PA 138T/M mutation was also detected in 9.7% (usually on day 5 or later) of the 370 baloxavir subjects, and these subjects experienced longer remission of influenza symptoms than those who did not detect the mutation [61].

CAPSTONE-2 was a phase III, multicenter, randomized, double-blind study to evaluate the efficacy of a single oral dose of baloxavir versus placebo and oseltamivir in patients aged 12 years or older with high-risk factors for influenza complications. The results showed that in the high-risk group of severe complications of influenza, the duration of influenza symptoms was significantly shorter in the baloxavir group than in the placebo-control group (median time was 73.2 vs. 102.3 hours). In the analysis of influenza virus subtypes, the time to improvement of influenza symptoms (TTIIS) of influenza A/H3N2 and influenza B viruses was significantly shorter in the baloxavir group than in the placebo group (median time was 75.4 vs. 100.4 hours, and 74.6 vs 100.6 hours, respectively). Additionally, the virus titer was significantly reduced (48.0 vs. 96.0 hours). Compared with the oseltamivir group, significant differences were observed in the duration of symptoms and the time of viral replication reduction (74.6 vs. 101.6 hours; 48.0 vs. 96.0 hours). Compared with the placebo-control group (29.7%) and the oseltamivir group (28.0%), the total incidence of adverse reactions reported in the baloxavir treatment group was lower (25.1%). In addition, baloxavir was well tolerated, patients with high-risk influenza recovered faster, and the risk of complications was reduced. It usually takes 72 hours for oseltamivir to take effect, while baloxavir only needs a single oral dose, which could kill the virus in only 24 hours, greatly improving patient compliance [62].

12.3.4.5 Adverse reactions

In CAPSTONE-1, a single dose of baloxavir was well tolerated against influenza A or B in 12-year-old adults and children. The results showed that 20.7% of baloxavir recipients, 24.6% of placebo recipients, and 24.8% of oseltamivir recipients had adverse reactions, suggesting that patients had certain psychological implications. However, compared with oseltamivir recipients (8.4%), patients taking baloxavir (4.4%, $P = 0.009$) had significantly fewer adverse reactions. The incidence of adverse reactions in clinical trials in adults and children was 5.4% ($n = 910$). The most common adverse reactions are diarrhea, followed by headache and nausea [60].

12.3.5 Inspiration from the study of baloxavir

The drug design strategy in this chapter is different from the methods in other chapters. The development of structural biology played a decisive role in the design and discovery of active molecules in this chapter. Through the study of structural biology, researchers understood the structure of the functional domain of endonucleases and the basic components of nuclear endonuclease active molecules, including groups that could coordinate with divalent metal ions and large-volume hydrophobic groups that could occupy PA_N. Therefore, it was a good starting point to select bimetallic pharmacophores for simulation from HIV integrase inhibitors. Another feature of this chapter was the optimization strategy of "privileged scaffold refining." Combining the two strategies organically, it was obvious that time and cost were saved in the discovery of drug-active molecules and some time was shortened in the optimization stage. The focus was on the use of "privileged scaffold" molecules may greatly improve the probability of drug-like molecules. Therefore, the use of "privileged scaffold refining" has the following advantages: by modifying the core scaffold of existing active drugs or lead compounds, the number of new structural compound libraries can be rapidly expanded and the synthesis efficiency can be improved; the candidate drugs with good druggability and high safety can be developed. The key pharmacophore model in the molecule can predict the possible binding mode between the ligand and the target, etc. [63].

As a novel endonuclease PA inhibitor, baloxavir has already shown satisfactory results in clinical studies. Baloxavir showed at least two advantages over other available antiinfluenza drugs. First, baloxavir can be administered orally in a single dose, which is convenient to use and can suppress the virus within 24 hours, greatly improving patient compliance; Secondly, baloxavir can overcome the resistance of influenza virus to NA inhibitors.

Although the introduction of baloxavir provides a new drug treatment option for patients with influenza, the emergence of baloxavir-resistant strains soon becomes an urgent problem to be solved. PA I38T mutation was found in 1.5% (5/323) of pH1N1 and 9.5% (32/337) of H3N2 virus in 2018−2019. The frequency of PA I38T mutation was higher in the influenza A/H3N2 virus than in the influenza B virus or pH1N1 virus. Most worrisome is the possibility of human-to-human transmission of PA I38T mutant H3N2 influenza virus [64]. It can be expected that with the extension of clinical use, the frequency of PA/I38T mutant virus strains may continue to increase, and the reduced susceptibility of mutant strains to baloxavir will affect the clinical efficacy of baloxavir.

References

[1] Xiu SY, Zhang J, Ju H, et al. Progress on IFV drug targets and small molecule inhibitors. Acta Pharm Sin 2020;55(04):611−26.
[2] Lee VJ, Ho ZJM, Goh EH, et al. Advances in measuring influenza burden of disease. Influ Other Respir Viruses 2018;12(1):3−9.
[3] Fan VY, Jamison DT, Summers LH. Pandemic risk: how large are the expected losses? B World Health Organ 2018;96(2):129−34.
[4] Wang XY, Chai CL, Li FD, et al. Epidemiology of human infections with avian influenza A (H7N9) virus in the two waves before and after October 2013 in Zhejiang province, China. Epidemiol Infect 2015;143(9):1839−45.
[5] U.S. flu season: preliminary burden estimates[EB/OL]. [2020-10-1], https://www.cdc.gov/flu/about/burden/preliminary-in-season-estimates.htm.
[6] Thompson CM, Petiot E, Lennaertz A, et al. Analytical technologies for influenza virus-like particle candidate vaccines: challenges and emerging approaches. Virol J 2013;10:141.
[7] Badham MD, Rossman JS. Filamentous influenza viruses. Curr Clin Microbiol Rep 2016;3(3):155−61.
[8] Yuan S, Wen L, Zhou J. Inhibitors of influenza A virus polymerase. ACS Infect Dis 2018;4(3):218−23.
[9] Cheng CK, Tsai CH, Shie JJ, et al. From neuraminidase inhibitors to conjugates: a step towards better anti-influenza drugs? Future Med Chem 2014;6(7):757−74.
[10] Taubenberger JK, Morens DM. The pathology of influenza virus infections. Annu Rev Pathol Mech Dis 2008;3:499−522.
[11] Watanabe T, Watanabe S, Kawaoka Y. Cellular networks involved in the influenza virus life cycle. Cell Host Microbe 2010;7(6):427−39.
[12] Zhang J, Pekosz A, Lamb RA. Influenza virus assembly and lipid raft microdomains: a role for the cytoplasmic tails of the spike glycoproteins. J Virol 2000;74(10):4634−44.
[13] Das K, Aramini JM, Ma LC, et al. Structures of influenza A proteins and insights into antiviral drug targets. Nat Struct Mol Biol 2010;17(5):530−8.
[14] Niu YH, Cao XP, Ye XS. Advances in influenza virus sialidase inhibitors. Prog Chem 2007;Z1:420−30.
[15] Treanor JJ. Prospects for broadly protective influenza vaccines. Am J Prev Med 2015;49(6 Suppl 4):S355−63.
[16] Beard KR, Brendish NJ, Clark TW. Treatment of influenza with neuraminidase inhibitors. Curr Opin Infect Dis 2018;31(6):514−19.
[17] Yang J, Huang Y, Liu S. Investigational antiviral therapies for the treatment of influenza. Expert Opin Investig Drugs 2019;28(5):481−8.
[18] Ison MG. Antiviral treatments. Clin Chest Med 2017;38(1):139−53.
[19] Dong G, Peng C, Luo J, et al. Adamantane-resistant influenza a viruses in the world (1902−2013): frequency and distribution of M2 gene mutations. PLoS One 2015;10(3):e0119115.
[20] Principi N, Camilloni B, Alunno A, et al. Drugs for influenza treatment: is there significant news? Front Med (Lausanne) 2019;6:109.
[21] Gong J, Xu W, Zhang J. Structure and functions of influenza virus neuraminidase. Curr Med Chem 2007;14(1):113−22.
[22] Chamni S, De-Eknamkul W. Recent progress and challenges in the discovery of new neuraminidase inhibitors. Expert Opin Ther Pat 2013;23(4):409−23.
[23] Esposito S, Principi N. Oseltamivir for influenza infection in children: risks and benefits. Expert Rev Respir Med 2016;10(1):79−87.
[24] Esposito S, Molteni CG, Colombo C, et al. Oseltamivir-induced resistant pandemic A/H1N1 influenza virus in a child with cystic fibrosis and Pseudomonas aeruginosa infection. J Clin Virol 2010;48(1):62−5.
[25] Shie JJ, Fang JM. Development of effective anti-influenza drugs: congeners and conjugates—a review. J Biomed Sci 2019;26(1):1−20.
[26] Ikematsu H, Kawai N. Laninamivir octanoate: a new long-acting neuraminidase inhibitor for the treatment of influenza. Expert Rev Anti Infect Ther 2011;9(10):851−7.
[27] Birnkrant D, Cox E. The emergency use authorization of peramivir for treatment of 2009 H1N1 influenza. N Engl J Med 2009;361(23):2204−7.
[28] Tarbet EB, Maekawa M, Furuta Y, et al. Combinations of favipiravir and peramivir for the treatment of pandemic influenza A/California/04/2009 (H1N1) virus infections in mice. Antivir Res 2012;94(1):103−10.
[29] Kadam RU, Wilson IA. Structural basis of influenza virus fusion inhibition by the antiviral drug Arbidol. Proc Natl Acad Sci USA 2017;114(2):206−14.
[30] Rossignol JF, La Frazia S, Chiappa L, et al. Thiazolides, a new class of anti-influenza molecules targeting viral hemagglutinin at the post-translational level. J Biol Chem 2009;284(43):29798−808.
[31] Behzadi MA, Leyva-Grado VH. Overview of current therapeutics and novel candidates against influenza, respiratory syncytial virus, and middle east respiratory syndrome coronavirus infections. Front Microbiol 2019;10:1327.
[32] Zhang J, Hu Y, Musharrafieh R, et al. Focusing on the influenza virus polymerase complex: recent progress in drug discovery and assay development. Curr Med Chem 2019;26(13):2243−63.

[33] Janssen Pharmaceutical. Janssen to stop clinical development of pimodivir for influenza[EB/OL]. [2020-09-03], https://www.clinicaltrialsarena.com/news/janssen-pimodivir-development.
[34] Heo YA. Baloxavir: first global approval. Drugs 2018;78(6):693−7.
[35] Loregian A, Mercorelli B, Nannetti G, et al. Antiviral strategies against influenza virus: towards new therapeutic approaches. Cell Mol Life Sci 2014;71(19):3659−83.
[36] Mifsud EJ, Hayden FG, Hurt AC. Antivirals targeting the polymerase complex of influenza viruses. Antivir Res 2019;169:104545.
[37] Shaw ML. The next wave of influenza drugs. ACS Infect Dis 2017;3(10):691−4.
[38] Dias A, Bouvier D, Crépin T, et al. The cap-snatching endonuclease of influenza virus polymerase resides in the PA subunit. Nature 2009;458 (7240):914−18.
[39] Liu YF, Lou ZY, Bartlam M, et al. Structure-function studies of the influenza virus RNA polymerase PA subunit. Sci China C Life Sci 2009;52 (5):450−8.
[40] Te Velthuis AJ, Fodor E. Influenza virus RNA polymerase: insights into the mechanisms of viral RNA synthesis. Nat Rev Microbiol 2016;14 (8):479−93.
[41] Crépin T, Dias A, Palencia A, et al. Mutational and metal binding analysis of the endonuclease domain of the influenza virus polymerase PA subunit. J Virol 2010;84(18):9096−104.
[42] Yuan P, Bartlam M, Lou Z, et al. Crystal structure of an avian influenza polymerase PA_N reveals an endonuclease active site. Nature 2009;458 (7240):909−13.
[43] Yang T. Baloxavir marboxil: the first cap-dependent endonuclease inhibitor for the treatment of influenza. Ann Pharmacother 2019;53(7):754−9.
[44] Credille CV, Morrison CN, Stokes RW, et al. SAR exploration of tight-binding inhibitors of influenza virus PA endonuclease. J Med Chem 2019;62(21):9438−49.
[45] Ju H, Zhan P, Liu X. Designing influenza polymerase acidic endonuclease inhibitors via 'privileged scaffold' re-evolution/refining strategy. Future Med Chem 2019;265−8.
[46] Wu G, Zhao T, Kang D, et al. Overview of recent strategic advances in medicinal chemistry. J Med Chem 2019;62(21):9375−414.
[47] Johns BA, Kawasuji T, Weatherhead JG, et al. Carbamoyl pyridone HIV-1 integrase inhibitors 3. A diastereomeric approach to chiral nonracemic tricyclic ring systems and the discovery of dolutegravir (S/GSK1349572) and (S/GSK1265744). J Med Chem 2013;56(14):5901−16.
[48] Omoto S, Speranzini V, Hashimoto T, et al. Characterization of influenza virus variants induced by treatment with the endonuclease inhibitor baloxavir marboxil. Sci Rep 2018;8(1):9633 −9633.
[49] Wang L, Sarafianos SG, Wang Z. Cutting into the substrate dominance: pharmacophore and structure-based approaches toward inhibiting human immunodeficiency virus reverse transcriptase-associated ribonuclease H. Acc Chem Res 2020;53(1):218−30.
[50] Miyagawa M, Akiyama T, Taoda Y, et al. Synthesis and SAR study of carbamoyl pyridone bicycle derivatives as potent inhibitors of influenza cap-dependent endonuclease. J Med Chem 2019;62(17):8101−14.
[51] Taoda Y, Miyagawa M, Akiyama T, et al. Dihydrodibenzothiepine: promising hydrophobic pharmacophore in the influenza cap-dependent endonuclease inhibitor. Bioorg Med Chem Lett 2020;30(22):127547.
[52] Kawai M, Tomita K, Akiyama T, et al. Substituted polycyclic pyridone derivatives and prodrugs thereof. U.S. Patent Application 16/221,733. 2019-4-18.
[53] Hughes DL. Review of the patent literature: synthesis and final forms of antiviral drugs tecovirimat and baloxavir marboxil. Org Process Res Dev 2019;23(7):1298−307.
[54] Sumino Y., Okamoto K., Masui M., et al. Method of producing pyrone and pyridone derivatives. U.S. Patent 8,865,907. 2014-10-21.
[55] Brands KM, Davies AJ. Crystallization-induced diastereomer transformations. Chem Rev 2006;106(7):2711−33.
[56] Cassani C, Bergonzini G, Wallentin CJ. Photocatalytic decarboxylative reduction of carboxylic acids and its application in asymmetric synthesis. Org Lett 2014;16(16):4228−31.
[57] O'Hanlon R, Shaw ML. Baloxavir marboxil: the new influenza drug on the market. Curr Opin Virol 2019;35:14−18.
[58] Fukao K., Ando Y., Noshi T., et al. Delayed oral dosing of S-033188, a novel inhibitor of influenza virus cap-dependent endonuclease, exhibited significant reduction of viral titer and prolonged survival in mice infected with influenza A virus. *Abstract presented at the 27th European Congress of Clinical Microbiology and Infectious Diseases.* 2017, pp. 22−25.
[59] Hayden FG, Sugaya N, Hirotsu N, et al. Baloxavir marboxil for uncomplicated influenza in adults and adolescents. N Engl J Med 2018;379 (10):913−23.
[60] Ng KE. Xofluza (Baloxavir Marboxil) for the treatment of acute uncomplicated influenza. P T 2019;44(1):9−11.
[61] Beigel JH, Hayden FG. Influenza therapeutics in clinical practice—challenges and recent advances. Cold Spring Harb Perspect Med 2020;10 (4):a038463.
[62] Ison MG, Portsmouth S, Yoshida Y, et al. LB16. Phase 3 trial of Baloxavir Marboxil in high-risk influenza patients (CAPSTONE-2 study). Open forum infectious diseases. Oxf Univ Press 2018;5:S764.
[63] Da Fonseca MA, Casamassimo P. Old drugs, new uses. Pediatr Dent 2011;33(1):67−74.
[64] Takashita E, Ichikawa M, Morita H, et al. Human-to-human transmission of influenza A (H3N2) virus with reduced susceptibility to baloxavir. Emerg Infect Dis 2019;25(11):2108−11.

Chapter 13

Paclitaxel: a natural antitumor agent

Yi Dong[1], Yao Ma[1] and Gang Liu[2]
[1]*Institute of Materia Medica, Chinese Academy of Medical Science, Beijing, P.R. China,* [2]*School of Pharmaceutical Sciences, Tsinghua University, Beijing, P.R. China*

Chapter outline

13.1 Discovery and development of taxol 287
   13.1.1 Discovery of paclitaxel 287
   13.1.2 The antitumor action of mechanism 288
   13.1.3 The clinical research on paclitaxel 288
   13.1.4 The application limitations of injectable paclitaxel 289
   13.1.5 Other commercially available taxanes for anticancer therapy 292
   13.1.6 Other taxane-based drug candidates that have been studied in clinical trials 293
   13.1.7 The method of obtaining natural paclitaxel 296

13.2 The pharmaceutical chemistry of paclitaxel 297
   13.2.1 The total synthesis of paclitaxel 297
   13.2.2 The semisynthesis of paclitaxel 300
   13.2.3 Study on the structure-activity relationship of paclitaxel 302
13.3 Design strategy for paclitaxel prodrugs 310
   13.3.1 A prodrug utilizing hydrophilic small molecule moieties as carriers 310
13.4 Summary and outlook 320
References 321

13.1 Discovery and development of taxol

Cancer, also known as malignant tumor, possesses characteristics such as uncontrolled proliferation, infiltration, and metastasis. Since the mid-20th century, cancer has progressively emerged as major disease posing a significant threat to human health and well-being, second to cardiovascular disorders. To conquer the formidable challenge of cancer, the pursuit and development of safe and effective anticancer drugs with novel mechanisms of action have become a continuous endeavor worldwide. Throughout the history of human efforts against cancer, the invention and utilization of chemotherapy drugs hold paramount significance as groundbreaking milestones. From the 1950s to the 1980s, the National Cancer Institute (NCI), a subsidiary of the National Institute of Health in the United States, conducted a high throughput screening program for extensive identification of the extracts from more than 35,000 plant species worldwide, with the aim of discovering new naturally occurring molecules (or components) with anticancer activities. Paclitaxel, also known as taxol, is one of the most successful natural molecules. Paclitaxel, whose trade name is taxol, is a white powder (melting point, 213°C–216°C) with a molecular composition of $C_{47}H_{51}NO_{14}$ and a relative molecular mass of 853.33. It is a diterpenoid alkaloid natural compound isolated from the bark of the Pacific yew tree. Clinically, paclitaxel has been widely used in the treatment of ovarian cancer, breast cancer, nonsmall cell lung cancer, and melanoma, among other types of cancer. Currently, it is commonly used in combination with platinum-based drugs, particularly in conjunction with novel immune checkpoint antitumor medications, such as PD-1 or PD-L1 antibodies, which are emerging as a new trend in cancer treatment. The development of paclitaxel, including its discovery, studies on its anticancer action mechanisms, chemical synthesis (including process chemistry), formulation development, and determination of clinical therapeutic indications, has undergone a research and development process spanning over 30 years.

13.1.1 Discovery of paclitaxel

Taxus, commonly known as the Pacific yew, is a valuable medicine plant belonging to the gymnosperms, scattered mainly in the northern hemisphere. In 1962, Dr. Barclay, an American botanist, conducted the extraction and activity evaluation of Taxus brevifolia Nutt in Washington state. He found that the component labeled NSC670549 exhibited significant cytotoxicity against KB tumor cells. In 1966, Drs. Wall and Wani from the North Carolina Triangle Institute followed a screening approach called activity-guided components isolation and successfully isolated approximately 500 mg of an antitumor active ingredient, coded as K172, from about 12 kg of air-dried Taxus brevifolia Nutt bark, with an isolated yield of 0.004%. This ingredient was further purified in 1967, finally resulting in the product of white crystals and was named Taxol by Dr. Wall, which means a class of alcohol compounds derived from the Taxus. "Tax" is from the Taxus, and the suffix "-ol" represents alcohol. At that moment, it was known that the compound involved a hydroxyl group. On the 153rd meeting of the American Chemical Society held in Miami in the same year, Dr. Wall presented a report detailing the extraction of Taxol, highlighting its extensive antitumor activities. In 1971, Dr. McPhail, a crystallographer from Duke University, employed magnetic resonance and single-crystal X-ray diffraction techniques to definitively determine the chemical structure of Taxol (Fig. 13.1). The core structure of Taxol consists of a tricyclic carbon framework with a 6/8/6 ring system, along with a heterocyclic tetrahydrofuran ring and a side chain involving hydroxyl and amide groups derived from phenylalanine. The entire molecule consists of 11 chiral carbon atoms as well as several functional groups, that is, benzene rings and acetoxy groups, contributing to its highly complex chemical structure [1]. The determination of the structure of paclitaxel enables researchers to intuitively understand this natural antitumor star molecule.

13.1.2 The antitumor action of mechanism

In 1979, Dr. Susan B. Horwitz, a molecular pharmacologist at the Albert Einstein College of Medicine in the United States, first elucidated the unique antitumor mechanism of paclitaxel. It functionalizes by promoting the polymerization of microtubules while simultaneously inhibiting the normal physiological depolymerization of microtubules in cells, leading to cell mitosis arrest at the G2 and M phases. During cell mitosis, if microtubules fail to form the spindle apparatus and spindle fibers, it will prevent the mitosis and proliferation of tumor cells, thereby exerting cytotoxic or growth-inhibitory effects on tumor cells [2–5].

13.1.3 The clinical research on paclitaxel

In 1977, NCI considered paclitaxel as a drug candidate and initiated preclinical studies, which were finalized in 1982. In 1983, NCI formally applied to the Food and Drug Administration (FDA) for Phase I clinical investigation, which was approved 1 year later with ovarian cancer as the designated indication. Phase II clinical trials were started in 1985, and the results of Phase II clinical investigation were published in 1988 by the FDA for advanced-stage ovarian cancer treated with paclitaxel. The report disclosed a response rate of 30%, indicating that at least 3 out of every 10 patients with advanced-stage ovarian cancer experienced tumor shrinkage or no disease progression after treatment with paclitaxel. In 1989, Bristol-Myers Squibb (BMS), a global pharmaceutical company, licensed a paclitaxel drug development project and provided 17 kg of pure paclitaxel, which led to the continuation of the Phase III clinical investigation in 1990.

In 1992, BMS submitted a new drug application for paclitaxel to the FDA. Six months later, injectable paclitaxel received official approval for the second-line treatment of advanced-stage ovarian cancer. As a result, BMS obtained a 10-year patent right for the production, research, and commercialization of paclitaxel. Subsequently, paclitaxel received approvals for the treatment of breast cancer (1994), Kaposi's sarcoma associated with AIDS (1997), first-line therapy in combination with cisplatin for ovarian cancer (1998), first-line therapy for non-small cell lung cancer (1999), and combination therapy with other chemotherapy agents for the treatment of breast cancer, including early-stage breast cancer with positive lymph nodes (2000) and so on.

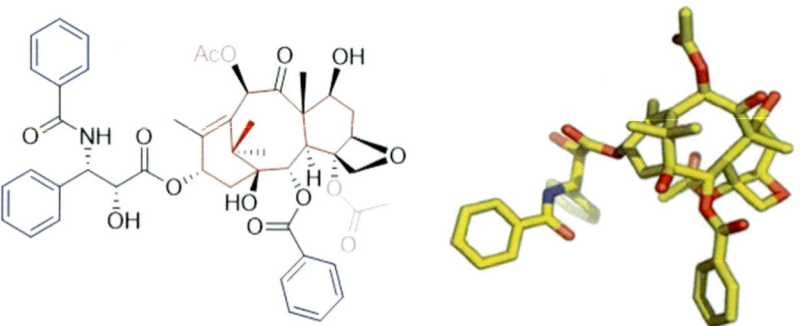

FIGURE 13.1 (A) Chemical structure of paclitaxel; (B) Single-crystal structure of paclitaxel.

13.1.4 The application limitations of injectable paclitaxel

Currently, injectable paclitaxel is widely employed for treating various cancer types such as breast cancer, lung cancer, ovarian cancer, esophageal cancer, and prostate cancer. However, its extensive application is limited by concerns related to its tolerability, drug resistance, low monotherapy response rate, and formulation issues.

13.1.4.1 Dose tolerance issues (adverse effects)

Paclitaxel exhibits dose-dependent adverse effects, including the hematopoietic, cardiovascular, respiratory, and nervous systems. The observed adverse effects are closely linked to the administration regimen of paclitaxel. Therefore, determining the appropriate dosage and route of administration is crucial for ensuring its clinical treatment efficacy. Initially, paclitaxel was administered via a 24-hour intravenous infusion. More recently, the preferred approach, the optimal medication, involves a 3-hour intravenous infusion and adjunctive preventive treatment, such as the pretreatment with dexamethasone, to mitigate allergic side effects.

13.1.4.1.1 Myelosuppression

A high dose of paclitaxel can induce significant myelosuppression. The clinical signs and symptoms are characterized by a decrease in neutrophil count, which exhibits dose-dependent effects. When the dose reaches 275 mg/m^2, 80% of patients experienced varying degrees of myelosuppression, with most cases being severe. Patients undergoing radiation therapy are at an even higher risk of developing myelosuppression. Long-term infusion of paclitaxel can also lead to a significant decrease in white blood cell count, and this effect is time-dependent. Shortening the infusion time or simultaneous treatment with granulocyte colony-stimulating factor can mitigate the incidence of myelosuppression. In instances of severe myelosuppression, intravenous administration of red blood cells or a reduction in the dosage of paclitaxel may be necessary.

13.1.4.1.2 Hypersensitivity reactions

Hypersensitivity reactions are commonly observed adverse reactions during the administration of paclitaxel injection, often occurring during the first or second infusion. The main factors causing hypersensitivity reactions are the polyoxyethylene castor oil and anhydrous ethanol present in the paclitaxel injection. These reactions manifest primarily as skin rash, hypotension, asthma, difficulty breathing, and bronchospasm.

13.1.4.1.3 Neurotoxicity

Neurotoxicity is the main adverse effect of paclitaxel, leading to toxic reactions in the motor nerves, central nervous system, peripheral nervous system, muscles, etc. This neurotoxicity poses a significant limitation on the clinical use of paclitaxel dosage. Typically, when the dose exceeds 200 mg/m^2, most patients experience varying degrees of neurotoxicity. The incidence and severity of paclitaxel-induced neurotoxicity are closely associated with its dosage, with higher doses leading to a greater likelihood of peripheral neuropathy. Moreover, there is evidence of dose accumulation contributing to the impact on neurotoxicity.

Furthermore, paclitaxel can cause cardiovascular toxicity, often accompanied by adverse effects such as abnormal heart rate, hypertension, and venous thrombosis during infusion, which are not dose-dependent. It can also induce mild to moderate gastrointestinal symptoms, including nausea and vomiting, likely because of its stimulating effect on the emetic center. Additionally, paclitaxel can cause muscle and joint pain to a certain extent, with the intensity of pain increasing with higher doses. Moreover, a small proportion of patients may experience hepatotoxicity, mainly characterized by elevated alkaline phosphatase, serum transaminases, and aspartate aminotransferase levels. For the majority of patients, hair loss occurs when the dose of paclitaxel exceeds 200 mg/m^2.

13.1.4.2 Resistance issue

As a frontline antitumor drug, paclitaxel has shown significant potential and promising prospects since its integration into clinical practice. However, the emergence of tumor cell resistance, combined with the increasing occurrence of cross-resistance phenomena, has to some extent limited its clinical application. Comprehensive investigations into the mechanisms of paclitaxel resistance have revealed a complex process with numerous contributing factors. Among them, the overexpression of the P-glycoprotein (P-gp) gene, encoded by MDR1, is widely recognized as a primary cause. Moreover, substantial research in recent years has indicated that abnormal expression of β-III tubulin represents an additional mechanism of paclitaxel resistance.

13.1.4.2.1 Multiple drug resistance

Multiple drug resistance (MDR) refers to the phenomenon in which tumor cells exist or develop a lack of response to various chemotherapy drugs. P-gp, a 170 kDa membrane protein encoded by the MDR gene, serves as an ATP-dependent transmembrane transporter. Functioning as an energy-dependent drug efflux pump, P-gp is widely distributed in tissues such as the gastrointestinal tract. Upon binding to chemotherapy drugs, it immediately releases ATP to pump the intracellular drugs out of the cell, preventing the drugs from reaching an effective concentration within the cell. This, in turn, reduces or completely negates the drugs' cytotoxic effects, resulting in resistance. The high hydrophobicity of paclitaxel and its strong affinity for P-gp are the main reasons for the development of resistance in cells.

13.1.4.2.2 β-Tubulin isoforms

The microtubule system is a vital part of the cellular cytoskeleton and is involved in numerous cellular functions. Microtubules are dynamic structures composed of α- and β-tubulin heterodimers and serve as important targets for various anticancer drugs, including paclitaxel. Research has demonstrated a close link between mutations in β-tubulin, affecting microtubule assembly and drug binding, and paclitaxel resistance. Abnormal expression of β-III tubulin, in particular, has been found to play a significant role in tumor invasion and chemotherapy resistance in clinical settings [6]. In a study by Panda, cells expressing different subtypes of β-tubulin showed that cells with high expression of β-III tubulin (TUBB3) exhibited significantly higher dynamic activity of microtubules. This increased dynamic property regulated microtubule polymerization, allowing the microtubules to maintain sufficient dynamic behavior for cell mitosis even in the presence of paclitaxel, thereby leading to resistance [7]. This resistance mechanism has been further confirmed in nonsmall cell lung cancer [8,9], breast cancer [10], and ovarian cancer [11], all of which exhibit chemotherapy resistance to paclitaxel.

Furthermore, paclitaxel resistance is also associated with β-tubulin-related proteins, with the tau protein being the most abundant microtubule-associated protein. In normal brain tissue, the tau protein binds to microtubule proteins in neural cells, facilitating their polymerization into microtubules. Studies have revealed that at appropriate concentrations, tau protein primarily binds to the exterior of microtubules, synergistically enhancing microtubule polymerization in conjunction with internally bound paclitaxel. However, when tau protein is overexpressed, it binds to both the interior and exterior surfaces of microtubules. The tau protein bound to the interior competes with paclitaxel for the same binding sites, reducing paclitaxel's binding affinity to microtubules, diminishing its capacity to promote microtubule polymerization, and ultimately leading to paclitaxel resistance.

13.1.4.2.3 Chemotherapy resistance induced by the tumor microenvironment

The occurrence, growth, and metastasis of tumors are closely related to the microenvironment in which tumor cells exist. This microenvironment can also contribute to chemotherapy resistance. Subsequently, as discussed in the third section, the design of paclitaxel prodrugs, leveraging the characteristics of the tumor microenvironment, such as hypoxic and inflammatory conditions, to develop novel drug candidates aimed at sensitizing chemotherapy. Readers are encouraged to explore how the tumor microenvironment impacts chemotherapy resistance by delving into the following sections.

13.1.4.3 The response rate to monotherapy is limited (combination therapy)

When paclitaxel is administered as a standalone treatment, concerns such as suboptimal targeting, poor tolerability, and a higher incidence of adverse reactions can lead to reduced treatment efficacy. On average, patients experience relapse and metastasis within 24–42 months after treatment. Consequently, clinicians often utilize combined drug regimens to enhance therapeutic effectiveness, mitigate toxicity and adverse reactions, improve drug tolerance, and promote patient adherence. For example, the combination of paclitaxel and carboplatin is the most common clinical chemotherapy regimen used for breast cancer, ovarian cancer, nonsmall cell lung cancer, and other types of cancer. The main adverse reaction associated with this regimen is myelosuppression. Additionally, ongoing clinical trials explore (or directly implement) the utilization of paclitaxel in combination with immunotherapeutic agents and targeted drugs, which have demonstrated clinical efficacy. For instance, gemcitabine, a second-line chemotherapy drug that interacts with DNA, exhibits a monotherapy response rate of only 15%–20% in the treatment of ovarian cancer. However, when combined with paclitaxel, it demonstrates improved tolerability in cancer patients previously exposed to high-dose chemotherapy. This combination therapy is commonly employed as a treatment option for patients resistant to platinum-based therapies, leading to a significant extension in patient survival. Irinotecan, an inhibitor of topoisomerase I and an analog of camptothecin, represents another effective regimen when combined with paclitaxel and carboplatin for treating advanced ovarian cancer. The combination of paclitaxel, cisplatin, and ifosfamide is currently recognized as a widely accepted treatment approach for advanced ovarian cancer.

13.1.4.4 Issues about dosage form

13.1.4.4.1 Paclitaxel injection (conventional dosage form)

It has a complex chemical structure and multiple hydrophobic groups, which contribute to its highly hydrophobic nature. It has a solubility in water of less than 0.01 mg/mL and is practically insoluble. Therefore, the traditional formulation of paclitaxel (paclitaxel injection) requires it to be dissolved in a mixed solvent of polyoxyethylene castor oil and anhydrous ethanol in a volume ratio of 1:1 that improves its water solubility. This dosage form has a certain impact on the safety and efficacy of paclitaxel in clinical use: [12] (1) polyoxyethylene castor oil is a nonionic surfactant that, when degraded in the human body, can stimulate the release of histamine, leading to severe allergic and neurotoxic reactions; (2) polyoxyethylene castor oil can delay nerve conduction and cause peripheral nerve damage; (3) polyoxyethylene castor oil can also adhere to the surface of paclitaxel molecules, affecting their diffusion into tissues and thereby reducing the anticancer effect; (4) anhydrous ethanol can suppress the central nervous system and cause red blood cell degeneration or hemolysis through the human red blood cell membrane. On the other hand, although paclitaxel exhibits significant anticancer effects, its therapeutic selectivity is poor, as it lacks sufficient discrimination between normal cells and tumor cells, leading to pronounced adverse effects. To alleviate the adverse effects caused by the cosolvent, pretreatment with antihistamines or corticosteroids is necessary before paclitaxel administration. However, the accumulation of these drugs in the body can also have varying negative effects on chemotherapy.

13.1.4.4.2 Paclitaxel liposomes

To address the limitations, various new formulations of paclitaxel have been developed in recent years, aiming to improve water solubility, increase tumor tissue distribution, decrease the dose, and alleviate the multiple adverse effects associated with traditional paclitaxel injections. Among them, liposomal paclitaxel was approved by the center for drug evaluation of China involving encapsulated paclitaxel within lipid particles that have a phospholipid outer membrane. Liposomes composed of phospholipids, which are amphiphilic substances, possess the properties of being carriers for both lipophilic and hydrophilic drugs. By embedding paclitaxel within the liposomes (lipid layer) with an aqueous exterior, the "water solubility" of paclitaxel is increased without the need for the addition of polyoxyethylene castor oil as a cosolvent. This avoids the various adverse effects caused by the polyoxyethylene castor oil formulation. Liposomes are lipid particles with a cell-like structure that can fuse with cell membranes, facilitating the efficient delivery of paclitaxel into the interior of cells. As a result, the dosage and toxicity of paclitaxel can be further reduced, leading to an improved therapeutic index. Relevant research data has shown that the maximum tolerated dose of paclitaxel liposomes in mice via intravenous injection can reach 200 mg/kg, while the maximum tolerated dose of conventional paclitaxel injection is only 30 mg/kg [13]. The first paclitaxel liposome injection product (brand name: Lipusu) in China was approved and launched in 2003. It is used as a first-line chemotherapy for malignant tumors such as breast cancer and nonsmall cell lung cancer.

The application issues faced by paclitaxel liposomes include the following concerns, (1) poor stability, short shelf life, and high-level storage condition requirements; (2) high production costs and relatively expensive prices; (3) potential accumulation in the liver, leading to hepatotoxicity; (4) the commonly used clinical dose ranges from 135 to 175 mg/m^2, with no significant improvement in the actual human tolerability threshold.

13.1.4.4.3 Albumin-bound paclitaxel (abraxane)

Abraxane, an albumin-bound paclitaxel formulation, completely eliminates the associated toxicity of polyoxyethylated castor oil. It not only improves drug absorption and release kinetics but also exhibits superior tumor cell targeting, demonstrating advantages in clinical settings. Abraxane is a novel nanosized paclitaxel formulation that utilizes endogenous human serum albumin as a carrier. It is prepared as particles with a diameter of 130 nm, which interact with the albumin receptor Gp60 on cell membranes, thereby activating caveolin-1 protein for drug transport. Caveolin-1, a glycoprotein located on the cell membrane, directly participates in transmembrane drug transport, effectively delivering albumin-bound paclitaxel into tumor cells [14]. Furthermore, tumors often exhibit a rich secretion of the acidic protein SPARC (secreted protein acidic and rich in cysteine), which attracts and adheres to albumin, leading to the accumulation of the drug in tumor tissues and increased the local drug concentration of albumin-bound paclitaxel, thereby improving its tumor-killing capabilities [15].

Albumin-bound paclitaxel, created through high-pressure homogenization, is a nanosized colloidal suspension composed of paclitaxel and human serum albumin. It is the most successful formulation of albumin-bound paclitaxel in recent years. By directly utilizing the suspension formed by injecting the nanosized paclitaxel into saline, the need for pretreatment steps to prevent allergies, as required with traditional paclitaxel injections, can be avoided. In 2005, albumin-bound paclitaxel was first approved in the United States for the treatment of breast cancer. In 2012, it received further approval as a first-line treatment for metastatic nonsmall-cell lung cancer patients who are ineligible for curative or chemotherapy treatments. In 2013, it was approved in combination with gemcitabine as a first-line treatment for metastatic pancreatic cancer.

Phase I clinical trials of albumin-bound paclitaxel determined its maximum tolerated dose to be 300 mg/m^2, higher than that of traditional paclitaxel injections (175 mg/m^2), with a standard infusion time of 30 minutes, shorter than that of traditional paclitaxel (3 hours). When administered without prior corticosteroid or antihistamine prophylaxis, the dose range of albumin-bound paclitaxel is 135–373 mg/m^2, with a dosing interval of once every 3 weeks. No significant hypersensitivity reactions were observed during administration or on the day of administration. Dose-limiting toxicities include myelosuppression, peripheral sensory neuropathy, and mucositis, with the majority of toxic reactions being grade 1 or 2. The hematological toxicity of the drug is mild, grade 1 or 2, and does not accumulate in the blood [16]. Phase II clinical trials evaluated the efficacy and toxicity of albumin-bound paclitaxel in the treatment of metastatic breast cancer. Compared to traditional paclitaxel injections, albumin-bound paclitaxel allows for higher dose administration without the use of premedication with antiallergic drugs, resulting in increased antitumor efficacy and improved safety. It demonstrates favorable efficacy in advanced breast cancer patients, regardless of prior chemotherapy treatment. The toxicity reactions of albumin-bound paclitaxel are significantly reduced compared to traditional paclitaxel injections [17]. A randomized Phase III clinical trial compared the efficacy of albumin-bound paclitaxel (administered at 260 mg/m^2 over 30 minutes every 3 weeks) with that of traditional paclitaxel injections (175 mg/m^2). In terms of overall objective response rate, albumin-bound paclitaxel showed a significant improvement over paclitaxel injections [18].

In general, albumin-bound paclitaxel offered a higher dose than that of traditional paclitaxel injection, and the drug tolerance was greatly improved, but the neutropenia was much lower than that of traditional paclitaxel injection. Unfortunately, higher doses of albumin-bound paclitaxel can still cause some degree of neurotoxicity, which is generally mitigated clinically by discontinuing treatment or reducing the dose. Of course, albumin-bound paclitaxel has no obvious allergic reaction, reflecting its advantages in clinical application.

The combination therapy of albumin-bound paclitaxel, especially in combination with cytotoxic drugs and molecular targeted therapies, has made significant progress. Clinical trials and studies related to ovarian cancer have shown that the combination of carboplatin and albumin-bound paclitaxel has outstanding therapeutic effects, greatly reducing the incidence of chemotherapy-related adverse reactions and minimizing severe hypersensitivity reactions [19]. In clinics, albumin-bound paclitaxel is commonly used in combination with carboplatin, pemetrexed, erlotinib, and other drugs for the treatment of nonsmall cell lung cancer. This not only significantly improves the overall response rate but also results in a low incidence of neuropathy and a notable reduction in drug-related adverse reactions [20].

13.1.4.4.4 Alternative formulations

To achieve lower dosage, reduced toxicity, and minimal adverse reactions, the formulation of paclitaxel is continuously evolving toward water solubility, targeted delivery, sustained release, and oral formulations. In recent years, several promising new formulations of paclitaxel have emerged, such as polymer micelles [21], emulsions [22], and cyclodextrin complexes [23], which hold great potential for further development. An oral formulation of paclitaxel has been submitted to the FDA as a new drug and is awaiting approval for clinical use [24].

13.1.5 Other commercially available taxanes for anticancer therapy

13.1.5.1 Docetaxel

Docetaxel (Fig. 13.2) is a 3′-*tert*-butoxycarbonyl amide derivative and 10-deacetylated analog of paclitaxel, developed by the French company Rhône-Poulenc Rorer. It is obtained through semisynthetic methods using 10-baccatin III extracted from the leaves of the taxus baccate. Docetaxel is currently the most successful modification of paclitaxel. It was approved by the FDA in 1996 for the treatment of breast cancer, colon cancer, lung cancer, and other cancers. Its antitumor mechanism is similar to that of paclitaxel, but it exhibits significantly better efficacy while also having more pronounced adverse effects.

Unlike paclitaxel, the docetaxel currently used in clinical practice is still in the form of a conventional injection. Although docetaxel injection in polymeric micelles has been approved for market in South Korea, there is no significant improvement in its effectiveness and safety compared to the conventional formulation. Currently, several companies both domestically and internationally are striving for improved formulations of docetaxel, aiming for "safer, more convenient,

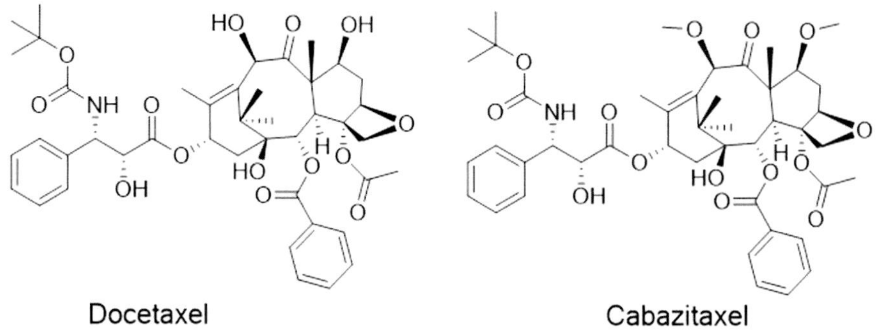

FIGURE 13.2 Other commercially available taxane-based antineoplastic drugs.

and more effective" options. These include injectable micellar nanoparticles, injectable liposomes, injectable albumin-bound formulations, and oral formulations, among others, all of which are in the clinical investigation stage. Among them, ModraDoc006/r, an oral tablet formulation of docetaxel developed by Modra, stands out in terms of its antitumor activity, safety, and convenience, demonstrating clinical advantages unmatched by other formulations. ModraDoc006/r has a dual inhibitory effect on P-gp and CYP3A4, which reduces the efflux of docetaxel from tumor cells and hepatic metabolism, leading to increased exposure of docetaxel within tumor cells and enhanced antitumor efficacy. Compared to other oral formulations of paclitaxel and docetaxel, although the efficacy of ModraDoc006/r is equivalent to that of intravenous docetaxel, its safety profile is higher, with almost no occurrences of severe neutropenia adverse reaction and peripheral neurotoxicity, which could potentially improve patient compliance [25,26].

13.1.5.2 Cabazitaxel

Cabazitaxel (Fig. 13.2) is a 7,10-dihydroxymethyl derivative of docetaxel developed by Sanofi-Aventis. In 2010, it received FDA approval for its use in combination with prednisone for the treatment of hormone-refractory metastatic prostate cancer in patients previously treated with docetaxel [27,28]. Docetaxel has a high affinity for P-gp, making it prone to resistance. However, one advantage of cabazitaxel is its lower affinity for P-gp. It is the first effective taxane-based chemotherapy drug for prostate cancer that has failed to respond to docetaxel treatment.

13.1.6 Other taxane-based drug candidates that have been studied in clinical trials

13.1.6.1 Larotaxel (RPR-109881A)

Larotaxel, a paclitaxel analog that is modified at the 7,8-positions with a cyclopropane ring and at the 10-position with hydroxyethyl acylation (Fig. 13.3), exhibits a mechanism of action similar to that of docetaxel. It possesses a broad spectrum of antitumor activity, particularly against docetaxel-resistant P388 leukemia and tumor cells with high expression of MDR1, demonstrating significant cytotoxic effects [29]. Larotaxel has the ability to penetrate the blood-brain barrier [30] and has shown superior intracranial antitumor efficacy in a nude mouse U251 glioma model [31]. Results from Phase I clinical trials indicate that the main dose-limiting toxicities of larotaxel include neutropenia and diarrhea, with doses below 45 mg/m^2 demonstrating good tolerability [32]. Phase II clinical trials have been designed to evaluate the use of larotaxel as a monotherapy and in combination with other cytotoxic drugs for the treatment of breast cancer, bladder cancer, and pancreatic cancer; however, the final trial results have not been disclosed [33,34].

13.1.6.2 Milataxel (MAC-321)

Milataxel (Fig. 13.4) is a modified derivative of docetaxel, with a furan group substitution at the 3′-position and acetylation at the 7-position. It shares a similar mechanism of action with docetaxel, exerting its antitumor effects by arresting cell division in the G2-M phase of the cell cycle and promoting microtubule protein polymerization. This novel taxane agent, Milataxel, demonstrates significant antitumor activity against various human cancer cell lines that are resistant to paclitaxel or docetaxel, indicating its potential as a modified taxane compound [35]. In phase I clinical trials conducted for advanced solid tumors, both oral and intravenous administration were evaluated to determine the maximum tolerated dose and dose-limiting toxicity of Milataxel, aiming to establish the dosage and optimal dosing regimen for phase II trials [36]. In a phase II clinical trial specifically targeting platinum-refractory nonsmall cell lung cancer, the weekly intravenous administration of 35 mg/m^2 milataxel exhibited sustained responsiveness and tolerability [37]. However, there is currently no available data regarding further results from phase III clinical trials.

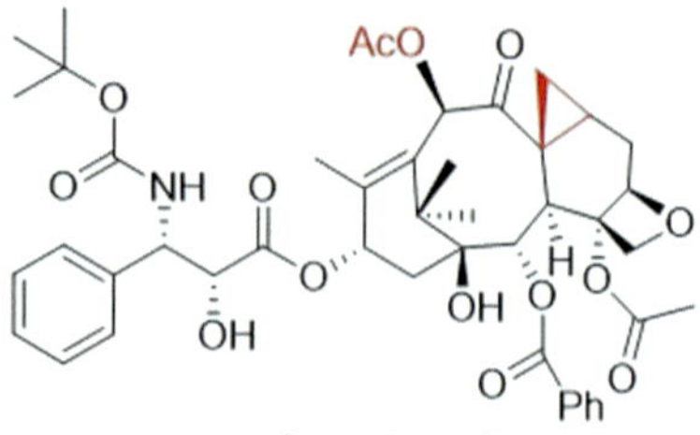

FIGURE 13.3 The structural representation of larotaxel.

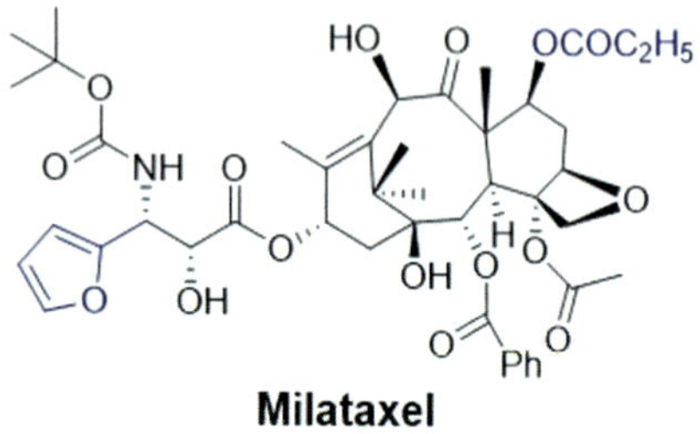

FIGURE 13.4 The structural representation of milataxel.

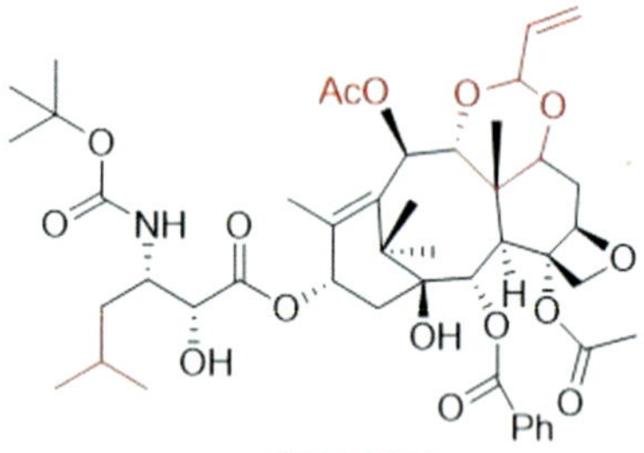

FIGURE 13.5 The structural representation of TPI-287.

13.1.6.3 TPI-287

TPI-287 (Fig. 13.5) is a third-generation taxane derivative with significant modifications to the structure of docetaxel. These modifications include the introduction of an isobutyl group at the 3′-position, aldehyde semiacetalization at the 7,9-positions, and acetylation at the 10-position hydroxyl group. These alterations enable TPI-287 to overcome resistance mediated by MDR1 and mutant microtubule proteins. TPI-287 exhibits excellent oral bioavailability and demonstrates higher antitumor activity compared to paclitaxel. It can evade inactivation and efflux through multiple resistance pathways, allowing effective penetration across the blood-brain barrier and reducing brain metastasis of breast cancer cells [38]. In the nude mice U251 glioblastoma model, TPI-287 has shown significant intracranial tumor inhibition [39]. Clinical Phase I trial results of TPI-287 in combination with temozolomide for the treatment of refractory or recurrent neuroblastoma or medulloblastoma have demonstrated good tolerability at a dose of 125 mg/m^2 [40].

13.1.6.4 TL-310

TL-310 (Fig. 13.6) is a taxane derivative with modifications that include a furan group at the 3′-position and an isobutoxycarbonylamino group, as well as a cyclopropylmethyl group, at the 10-position hydroxyl group. At the nanomolar concentration level, TL-310 exhibits significant cytotoxic activity against various human tumor cell lines. Its activity surpasses that of paclitaxel and it can overcome paclitaxel resistance caused by overexpression of P-gp and mutations in specific microtubule proteins [41]. Oral administration of TL-310 demonstrates remarkable antitumor efficacy, comparable to that of intravenous administration of paclitaxel or docetaxel [42], and even superior in certain tumor models. TL-310 also exhibits favorable safety characteristics, which are crucial assurances for its successful progression into clinical trial research stages [41].

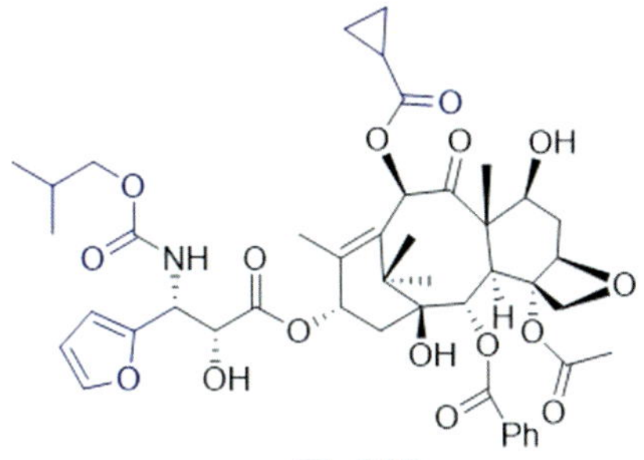

FIGURE 13.6 The structural representation of TL-310.

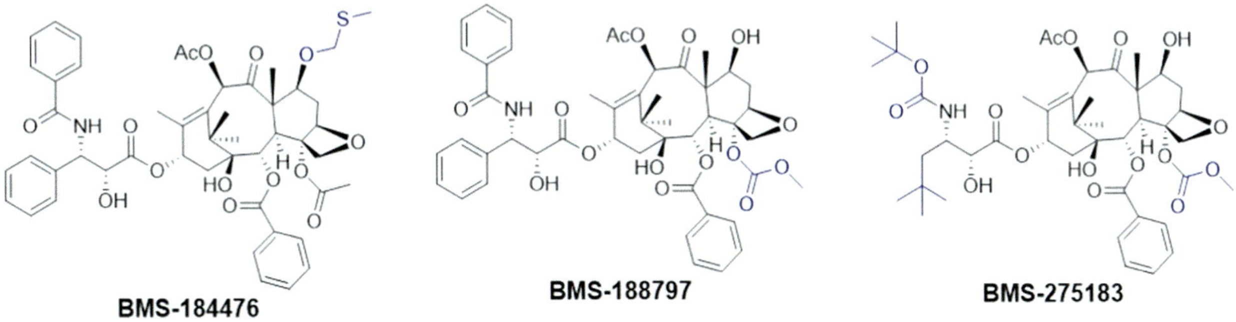

FIGURE 13.7 Bristol-Myers Squibb's class of clinical drugs.

13.1.6.5 BMS series taxane drugs

BMS has developed several taxane analogs, three of which have moved onto clinical investigation as drug candidates, including BMS-184476, BMS-188797, and BMS-275183 (Fig. 13.7).

BMS-184476 is a representative derivative of paclitaxel with a 7-position methylthiomethyl ether, which earns better solubility than paclitaxel derivatives [43]. The modification of the 7-hydroxythiomethyl ether significantly increases the drug's solubility in aqueous cosolvents, reducing the required amount of polyoxyethylene castor oil and minimizing the use of antiallergy drugs and adverse effects caused by polyoxyethylene castor oil [44]. BMS-184476 exhibits significant antitumor activity, surpassing paclitaxel in efficacy and partially overcoming paclitaxel resistance. It is the most extensively studied drug candidate in the BMS series of taxane compounds [45–48]. BMS-188797, designed as a paclitaxel analog derived from paclitaxel, differs from paclitaxel only in the substitution of the hydroxy group at the C_4-position with a methoxycarbonyl group. BMS-188797 does not show significant improvement in water solubility compared to paclitaxel [49] but demonstrates superior antitumor effects over paclitaxel in various paclitaxel-resistant tumor models [50]. BMS-275183 has a greater structural difference from paclitaxel and is an analog of BMS-188797 with a tert-butyl-substituted phenyl group at the 3′-position. It exhibits significant inhibitory activity against tumors with P-gp overexpression and microtubule protein mutations [51]. Due to its low affinity for P-gp, BMS-275183 has better oral bioavailability compared to paclitaxel, with oral administration showing comparable efficacy to intravenous injection [52,53].

13.1.6.6 Ortataxel (BAY-59–8862; IDN-5109)

Ortataxel (Fig. 13.8) is a derivative of paclitaxel that has been modified at the 3′-position with isobutyl and tert-butoxycarbonylamino groups, and at the $C_{1,14}$-positions with hydroxy carbonate esterification [54]. It has the ability to overcome resistance in cell lines expressing the MDR phenotype [55]. Ortataxel exhibits more pronounced advantages over paclitaxel in terms of antitumor activity, adverse effects, and tolerability. Ortataxel exhibits favorable oral bioavailability. In a murine model of MNB-PTX1 ovarian cancer resistant to paclitaxel, oral administration at a dose of 120 mg/kg showed comparable efficacy to intravenous injection at a dose of 60 mg/kg [56]. Additionally, ortataxel shows significantly stronger inhibitory activity against hormone-refractory prostate cancer cells compared to paclitaxel [57].

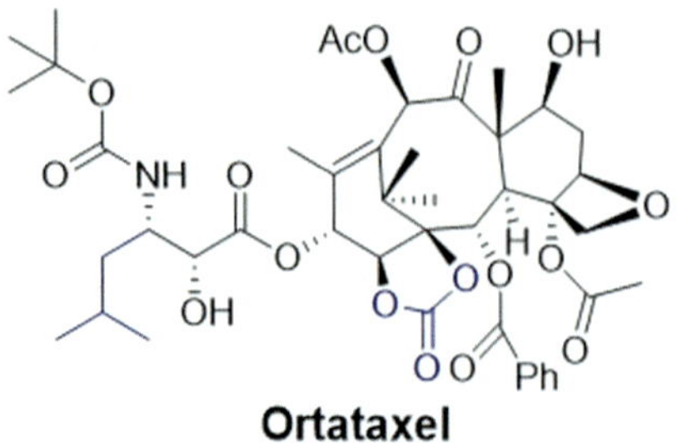

FIGURE 13.8 Structure of ortataxel.

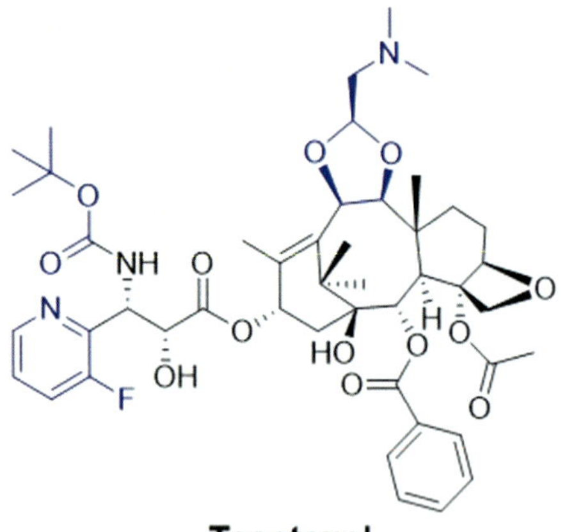

FIGURE 13.9 Structure of tesetaxel.

13.1.6.7 Tesetaxel (DJ-927)

Tesetaxel is a novel orally available taxane anticancer medication (Fig. 13.9). In comparison to other clinically investigating taxanes, it exhibits significant structural differences from paclitaxel. These variances include modifications at the 3′-position with 2-(3-fluoropyridyl) and *tert*-butoxycarbonyl groups, hydroxylation at the C_7-position, and alkylation at the $C_{9,10}$-position with diethylaminomethyl. Tesetaxel exhibits notable advantages compared to paclitaxel and docetaxel, such as improved water solubility, longer half-life, enhanced bioavailability, and resistance to P-gp efflux [58,59]. It demonstrates stronger activity against P-gp-mediated multidrug-resistant tumor cells than paclitaxel and docetaxel [60] (Table 13.1). Unfortunately, the development of this long-acting oral taxane agent was ultimately terminated due to safety concerns. In August 2020, odonate announced the results of Phase III clinical trials of tesetaxel in the treatment of HR + /HER2- metastatic breast cancer. Compared to the single-agent capecitabine group, the combination therapy group with tesetaxel showed higher incidence rates of grade 3 or higher neutropenia (71.2% vs. 8.3%), febrile neutropenia (12.8% vs. 1.2%), leukopenia (10.1% vs. 0.9%), and neuropathy (5.9% vs. 0.9%) as adverse events.

13.1.7 The method of obtaining natural paclitaxel

13.1.7.1 Extracting directly from the bark of the taxus tree

During the initial discovery of natural paclitaxel, scientists primarily obtained it through extraction from the bark of Taxus trees. However, the yield of paclitaxel in the bark is extremely low, approximately 0.004%. It requires about 13,000 kg of Taxus bark to extract 1 kg of paclitaxel. Based on this estimation, the extraction and isolation of 100 kg of paclitaxel would necessitate the felling of millions of Taxus trees. Due to the scarcity of Taxus tree resources and their slow growth rate, it takes hundreds of years for a Taxus tree with a trunk diameter of approximately 20 cm to mature. With the continuous increase in clinical demand for paclitaxel, it is evident that the extraction of paclitaxel through natural means is no longer able to meet human needs.

13.1.7.2 Semisynthesis and total synthesis

In the 1990s, numerous research groups worldwide embarked on exploratory studies for the total synthesis of paclitaxel, aiming to obtain an adequate supply of this natural product through chemical means. However, despite significant progress in

TABLE 13.1 Comparative characteristics of paclitaxel, docetaxel, and tesetaxel.

	Paclitaxel	Docetaxel	Tesetaxel
Subjected to extrusion by P-gp	Yes	Yes	No
Oral bioavailability in preclinical studies (%)	8	18	56
Solubility (μg/mL)	0.3	0.5	41,600
Drug half-life (h)	11	11	193

the artificial total synthesis of paclitaxel, challenges such as lengthy synthesis routes and low yields hindered the achievement of large-scale production of natural paclitaxel. Consequently, chemical semisynthesis emerged as the primary method for obtaining sufficient amounts of paclitaxel. Researchers utilized a crucial intermediate, known as 10-deacetylbaccatin III (10-DAB), which contains the 6/8/6 tricyclic structure of paclitaxel, extracted from the leaves and branches of the yew tree. By employing appropriate protective group strategies and a few simple steps, the coupling of the paclitaxel side chain with the core structure was achieved, leading to the efficient synthesis of paclitaxel. The semisynthesis route offered several advantages, including the renewable nature of yew tree resources, a shorter synthesis pathway, and higher yields, ultimately realizing the industrial-scale production of paclitaxel [61].

In addition to semisynthesis, other approaches have been explored, such as genetic engineering [62], microbial transformation [63], and microbial fermentation [64]. However, none of these methods have reached industrial-level production due to the inhibitory effect of paclitaxel on microbial growth when it reaches a certain concentration.

13.1.7.3 Milestones in the development of paclitaxel

Table 13.2 provides a comprehensive summary of the major historical events in the development of paclitaxel. This journey began in 1962 but is summarized in this book only until 1999.

13.2 The pharmaceutical chemistry of paclitaxel

As previously mentioned, the inherent limitations of the first-generation paclitaxel are primarily characterized by limited natural sources, poor water solubility, and MDR. These factors have attracted attention to the total synthesis, semisynthesis, and exploration of structure-activity relationships (SAR) surrounding its antitumor activity.

13.2.1 The total synthesis of paclitaxel

The content of paclitaxel in the bark of yew trees is only 0.069% (nonyield data). Even if all of it is extracted, obtaining 1 kg of paclitaxel would require at least 10,000 kg of yew tree bark, which corresponds to 2000–3000 yew trees. However, the average dose for treating a cancer patient typically requires 3–12 yew trees. Therefore, at the end of the 20th century, the total synthesis of paclitaxel gained widespread attention in the field of organic synthesis. There were approximately dozens of leading research groups worldwide engaged in the study of its total synthesis. In 1994, the research groups of Nicolaou and Holton simultaneously announced their respective total synthesis routes for paclitaxel to the world. Subsequently, Danishefsky, Wende, and others also reported distinctly different total synthesis methods for paclitaxel. This chapter focuses on several classic total synthesis strategies, combining the retrosynthetic analysis of paclitaxel.

13.2.1.1 Analysis of the structure and synthetic strategies of paclitaxel

From a holistic perspective, paclitaxel consists of a benzoyl ester side chain and a tetracyclic core (rings A, B, and C are carbon rings, while ring D is a heterocyclic oxygen-containing tetrahydropyran ring), encompassing a total of eleven chiral centers (Fig. 13.10). Due to the intricate nature of the tetracyclic core structure, the primary challenge in the total synthesis of paclitaxel lies in this aspect. Traditional strategies for the synthesis of the tricyclic carbon rings mainly involve two approaches: (1) linear synthesis strategy, sequentially constructing the tricyclic rings ABC from A to C or from C to A; (2) convergent synthesis strategy, building the tricyclic rings ABC by converging A and C through a synthesis approach. Finally, the total synthesis of paclitaxel is accomplished through the Ojima coupling reaction between baccatin III and β-lactam, ultimately achieving the desired compound.

298 Medicinal Chemistry and Drug Development

TABLE 13.2 Major historical milestones in the development of paclitaxel and docetaxel injection.

Years	Historical events
1962	The collection of Taxus brevifolia occurred in Washington, United States
1966	A pure form of paclitaxel was isolated
1971	The structural determination of paclitaxel was established (the utilization of X-ray diffraction and magnetic resonance techniques)
1977	Preclinical studies on paclitaxel were initiated
1979	The mechanism of action of paclitaxel has been elucidated (promotion of microtubule protein polymerization)
1983–84	The United States has initiated Phase I clinical trial investigations
1985–86	Initiation of Phase II clinical trial investigations (ovarian cancer)
1988–90	Achieving industrial-scale semisynthetic production of paclitaxel
1990	Initiation of Phase III clinical trial investigations
1992	Approved as second-line therapy for advanced ovarian cancer
1994	Approved treatment for breast cancer
1995	The European regulatory authorities have granted approval for the use of docetaxel injection (docetaxel) in the treatment of breast cancer and nonsmall cell lung cancer
1997	Approved for Kaposi's sarcoma associated with AIDS:
1998	Approved as first-line treatment for ovarian cancer
1999	Approved for first-line treatment of nonsmall cell lung cancer in combination with cisplatin
2005	Albumin-bound paclitaxel injection (Abraxane) has received approval for the treatment of breast cancer, nonsmall cell lung cancer, and pancreatic cancer
2017	China has approved a Phase I clinical trial study of Conmutaxel injection and Salutaxel injection

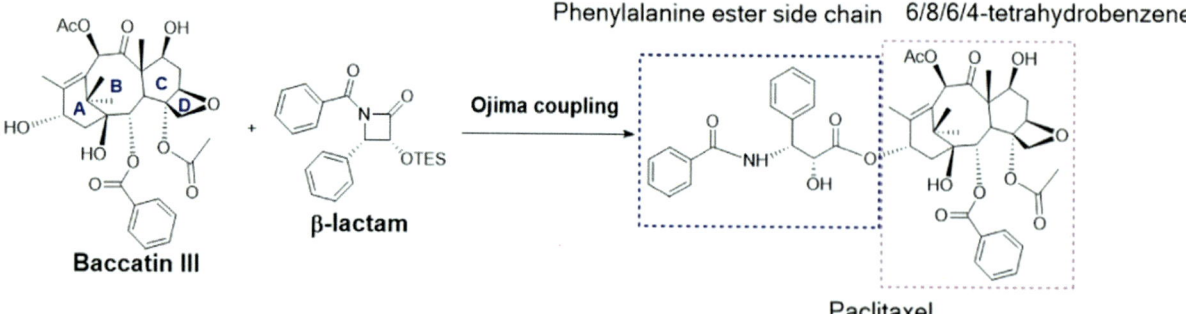

FIGURE 13.10 Synthesis strategy of paclitaxel.

13.2.1.2 The Nicolaou total synthesis route (1994)

The paclitaxel total synthesis was accomplished by the Nicolaou research group in the United States through an efficient convergent synthetic route [65,66]. The Diels–Alder key reaction was employed to construct the intermediate for the A-ring (compound 3) and the intermediate for the C-ring (compound 6) separately. The coupling of compound 3 and compound 6 resulted in the formation of the A/C-ring intermediate (compound 7). Through a series of reactions, the B-ring was then constructed via McMurry cyclization, leading to the formation of the tricyclic ABC core (compound 9). Subsequently, the oxygen-containing D-ring was built upon this core, yielding the crucial intermediate, baccatin III. Finally, the connection of the side chain was accomplished through a reaction with β-lactam, thereby completing the total synthesis of paclitaxel (Fig. 13.11).

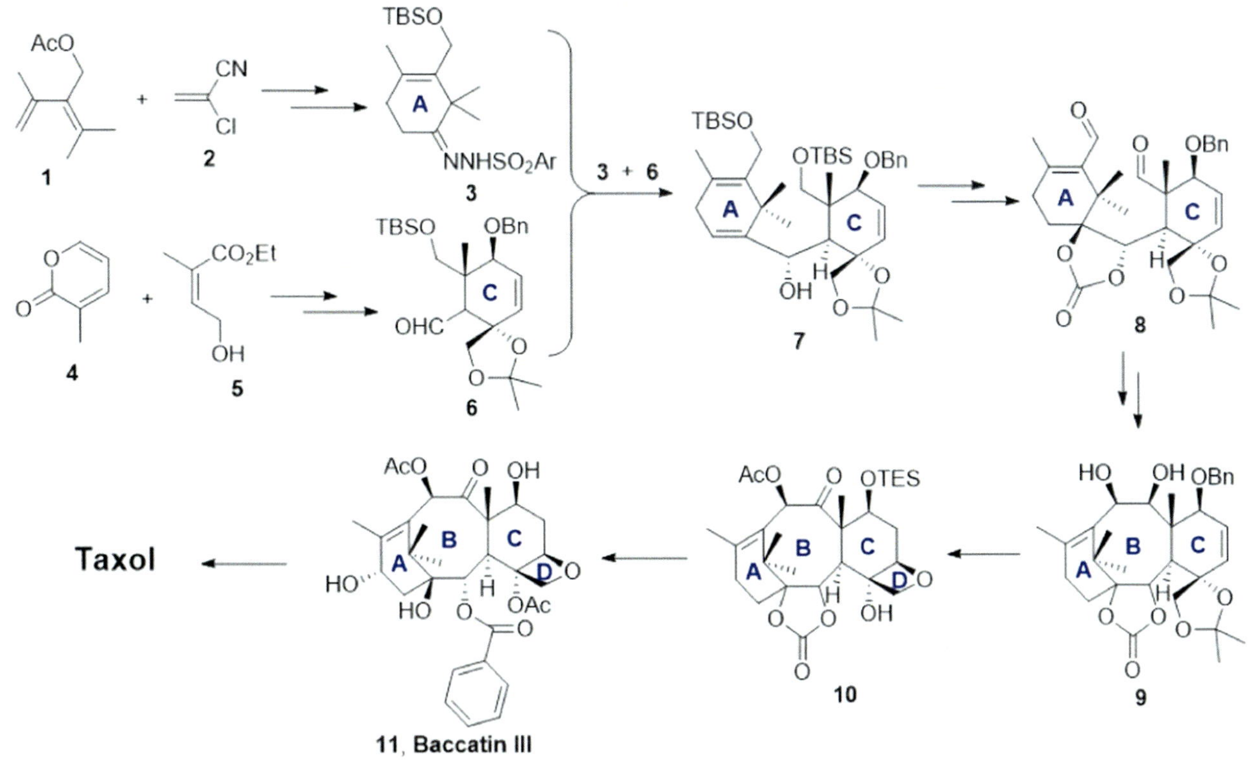

FIGURE 13.11 The Nicolaou total synthesis route.

13.2.1.3 The Holton total synthesis route (1994)

The Holton research group reported a distinct linear synthesis route for the total synthesis of paclitaxel, almost simultaneously with the Nicolaou research group [67–69]. They utilized commercially available taxadiene oxide (compound 12) as the starting material, which contains 15 carbon atoms of the A and B rings of paclitaxel. Through a protective group strategy, oxidation and rearrangement reactions led to the formation of compound 13, followed by epoxy alcohol cleavage to obtain the A/B ring intermediate (compound 14). In the structure of the A/B ring intermediate, a five-membered lactone compound 15 was further constructed, and the ABC tricyclic system compound 16 was synthesized through Dieckmann cyclization. By derivatization of functional groups on the C ring structure, the D ring was formed, resulting in the ABCD core intermediate (compound 17). Subsequently, the crucial intermediate, a baccatin III analog (compound 18), was synthesized. Finally, the connection of the side chain was achieved through a reaction with β-lactam, completing the total synthesis of paclitaxel (Fig. 13.12).

13.2.1.4 The Danishefsky total synthesis route (1990)

The synthetic strategy chosen by the Danishefsky research group is also a convergent approach [70]. On one hand, starting from Wieland–Miescher ketone 19, they initially constructed a CD bicyclic system containing an oxygen heterocycle (compound 21). On the other hand, using 1,3-cyclohexanedione (compound 22) as a starting material, they built an A-ring intermediate (compound 24). Compound 24 was then further combined with compound 21 to form an ACD system intermediate (compound 25). Through oxidation and intramolecular Heck reaction, the ABCD tetracyclic system (compound 27) was obtained. Further oxidation reactions led to the formation of a key intermediate resembling baccatin III. Finally, the connection of the side chain was achieved through a reaction with β-lactam, completing the total synthesis of paclitaxel (Fig. 13.13).

In addition to the aforementioned strategy, there are numerous other total synthesis methods for paclitaxel. For instance, Wender utilized verbenone (an oxidized product of the natural compound pinene, containing the A-ring domain of paclitaxel) as a starting material to achieve the total synthesis of paclitaxel in 37 steps [71,72]. Kuwajima, on the other hand, embarked on the total synthesis of paclitaxel from simple starting materials such as propionaldehyde, completing the synthesis in 47 steps [73,74]. Mukaiyama employed D-serine as a starting material and accomplished

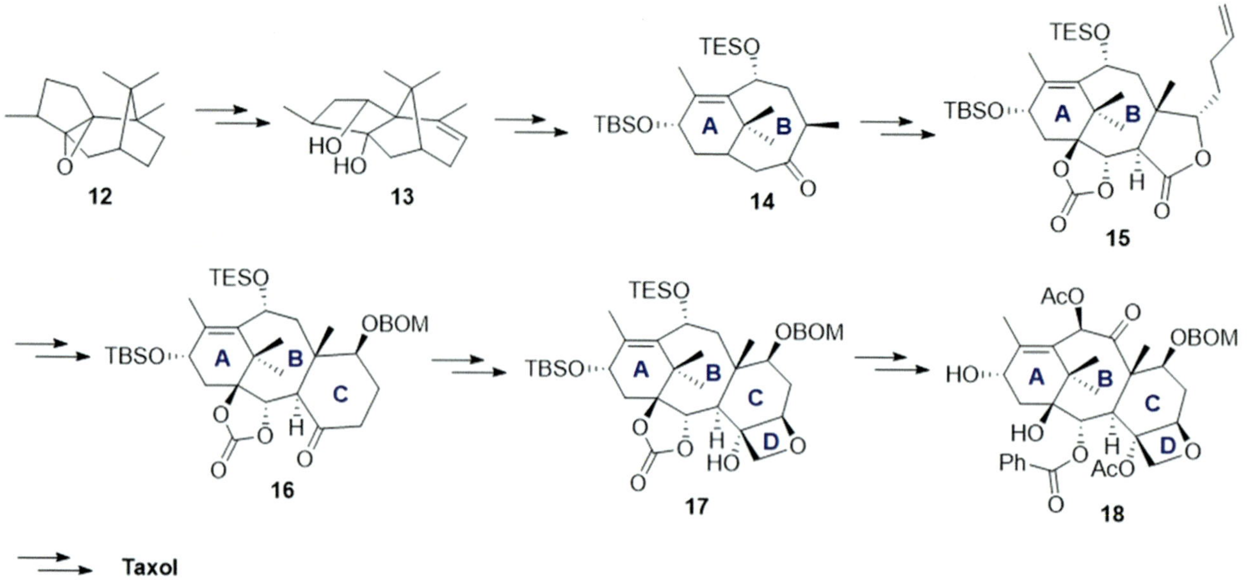

300 Medicinal Chemistry and Drug Development

FIGURE 13.12 The Holton total synthesis route.

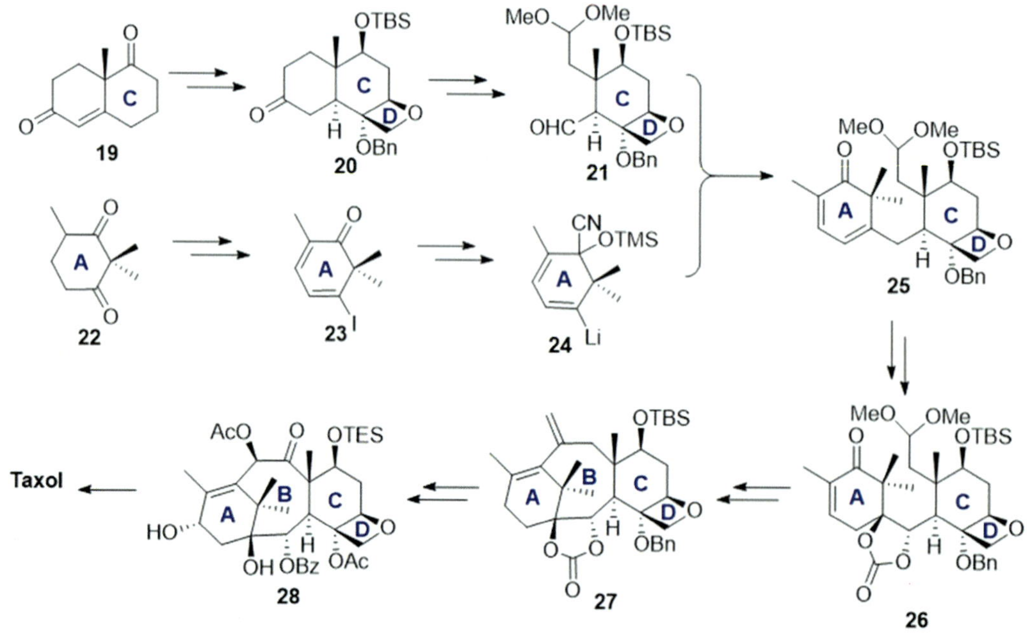

FIGURE 13.13 The Danishefsky total synthesis route.

the total synthesis of paclitaxel through a 38-step reaction sequence [75]. Since the first report on the total synthesis of paclitaxel in 1991, scientists have been diligently searching for more efficient methods to further refine the artificial synthetic approaches for paclitaxel, leading to the emergence of numerous innovative and ingenious total synthesis strategies for this compound over the past three decades.

13.2.2 The semisynthesis of paclitaxel

Since the isolation of key tetracyclic precursor, 10-DAB, and baccatin III from the leaves of yew trees, the synthesis of paclitaxel has been simplified. The abundance of 10-DAB and baccatin III in the leaves of yew trees, coupled with the simplicity of their extraction, has proven advantageous. Furthermore, the regenerative nature of the leaves ensures that large-scale collection does not deplete the yew tree population. The advancements in semisynthesis techniques have significantly reduced the synthetic steps involved in paclitaxel production, laying a solid foundation for its industrial synthesis.

13.2.2.1 The semisynthetic strategy starting from 10-deacetylbaccatin III

13.2.2.1.1 Potier semisynthesis route (1988)

Leveraging the differential reactivity of the hydroxyl groups in the structure of 10-DAB (7-OH > 10-OH > 13-OH), the research group led by Potier employed pyridine as the reaction solvent. They sequentially protected the 7-hydroxyl group with triethylchlorosilane (TES) and the 10-hydroxyl group with acetyl groups [76]. By coupling with 2-hydroxy-3-benzamido-phenylpropionic acid protected with ethoxyethyl groups, they introduced the side chain at the 13-hydroxyl position to obtain the precursor of paclitaxel. The removal of the protecting groups at the 7-position and 2′-hydroxyl group using hydrochloric acid completed the semisynthesis of paclitaxel. This method, starting from 10-DAB, achieves the chemical synthesis of paclitaxel in only four steps, significantly enhancing synthesis efficiency and reducing the cost of industrial production compared to the multistep total synthesis methods. However, this method has the drawback of using pyridine as a reaction medium, which has an unpleasant odor and can lead to air pollution. Therefore, it requires adequate ventilation conditions during industrial production. Additionally, the large quantity, high price, and relatively high cost of TES used in the synthesis process should be considered (Fig. 13.14).

13.2.2.1.2 Holton semisynthesis route (1988)

Similar to Potier's synthetic strategy, Professor Holton utilized imidazole and LHMDS as bases, replacing the odorous pyridine [77]. This enabled selective TES protection at the 7-position hydroxyl and acetylation at the 10-position hydroxyl. By employing a β-lactam protected with a 2-hydroxyl group as the side chain donor, 2′- and 7′-hydroxyl-protected paclitaxel derivatives were obtained. Subsequent deprotection under acidic conditions yielded paclitaxel with an overall yield of up to 80%. Following FDA approval, Shiquibao Company officially employed Holton's patent to produce paclitaxel through a semisynthetic approach (Fig. 13.15).

13.2.2.2 The semisynthetic strategy involving baccatin III as the starting material

13.2.2.2.1 The semisynthetic route proposed by commercon in 1992

The Commercon research group utilized baccatin III as the starting material, employing trichloroacetyl protection of the hydroxyl group at the 7th position [78]. By utilizing (4S,5R)-N-Boc-2,2-dimethyl-4-phenyl-5-imidazolylcarboxylic acid

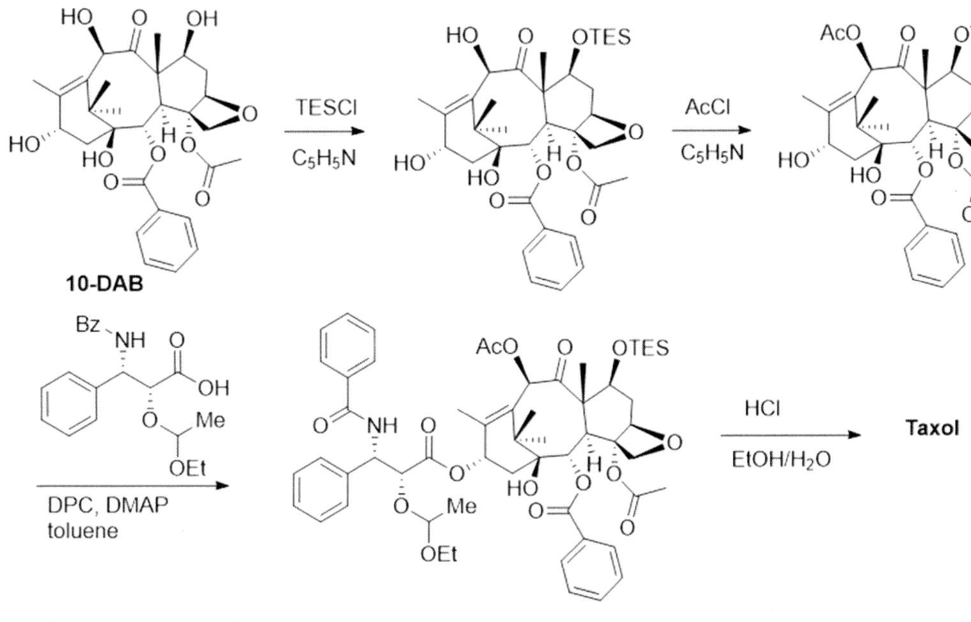

FIGURE 13.14 The Potier semisynthesis route.

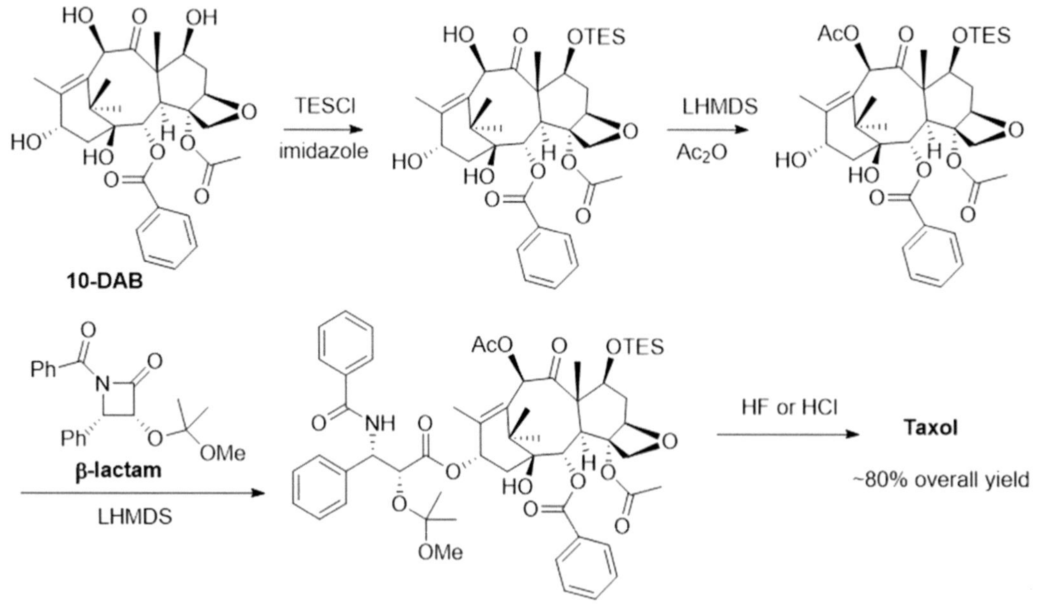

FIGURE 13.15 Holton's semisynthetic route.

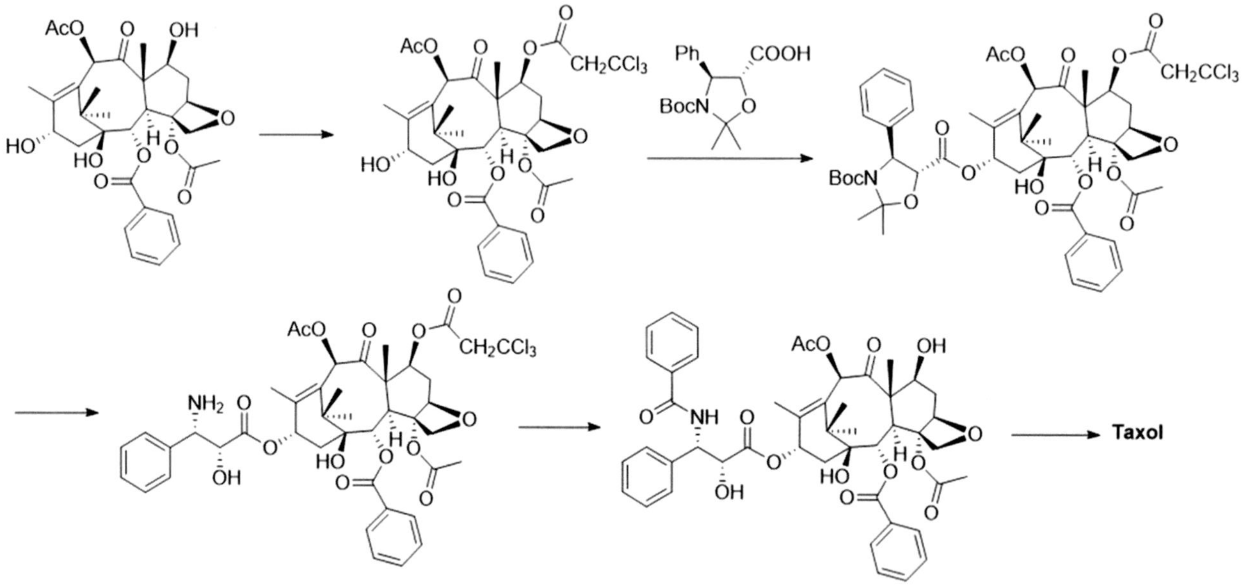

FIGURE 13.16 Commercon's semisynthetic route.

for condensation with the hydroxyl group at the 13th position, a 3′-amino-free derivative of paclitaxel was obtained. Benzoylation and subsequent hydrolysis yielded paclitaxel. This approach not only substituted the expensive triethylsilyl chloride with chloroacetic-(β-trichloroethyl) ester but also designed a five-membered ring side-chain donor at the 2nd position of the phenyl group, which facilitated the condensation reaction with the core structure and improved the condensation yield (Fig. 13.16).

13.2.3 Study on the structure-activity relationship of paclitaxel

On the basis of the increasingly mature total synthesis techniques for paclitaxel, significant efforts have been devoted to the exploration of structural modifications, aiming to elucidate the structure-activity relationship between its intricate structure and anticancer activity. The objective is to identify crucial functional groups and structural motifs essential for its activity, with the ultimate goal of designing and synthesizing paclitaxel analogs that exhibit simpler structures, greater pharmacological potency, and reduced side effects. In this chapter, we focus on the structural modification strategies for paclitaxel's benzoyl side chain and the 6/8/6/4 tetracyclic bacatin III motif (Fig. 13.17), presenting the research findings on the structure-activity relationship in detail through both the "position-based" and "fragment-based" approaches.

13.2.3.1 The structure-activity relationship of the C_1- and C_2-positions in bacatin III

Compared to the natural product paclitaxel, the removal of the hydroxyl group at the C_1-position of bacatin III (replaced with a hydrogen atom) and the subsequent acetylation of the C_9-position in derivative 29 have shown a two- to threefold decrease in microtubule polymerization promotion and cytotoxic activity, indicating that the hydroxyl group at the C_1-position is beneficial but not a critical factor for activity [79] (Fig. 13.18).

The removal of the benzoyloxy group at the C_2-position (compound 30) [80] or its relocation to the C_1-position (compound 31) [81] abolishes the activity. When the phenyl group is replaced with a cyclohexyl group of the same carbon number (compound 32), the microtubule assembly activity decreases by 130-fold compared to paclitaxel [82]. These results demonstrate that the benzoyloxy group at the C_2-position is an essential active group. Furthermore, the absolute configuration at the C_2-position is also essential for activity. For example, the derivative obtained by reversing the configuration of the benzoyloxy group at the C_2-position (compound 33) shows no cytotoxicity against HCT116 colon cancer cells and no significant promotion of microtubule protein assembly [83].

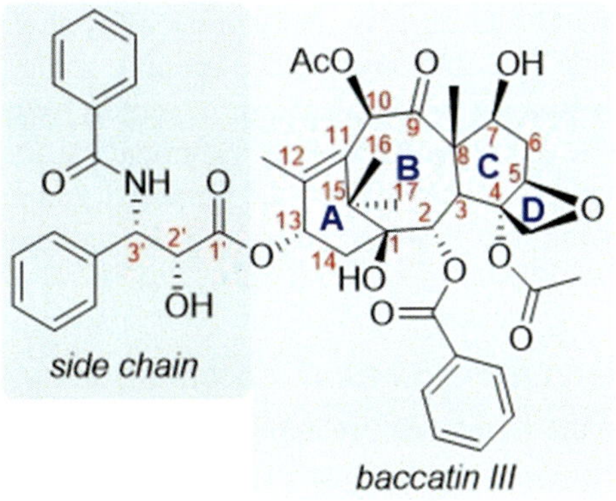

FIGURE 13.17 The structural composition of paclitaxel.

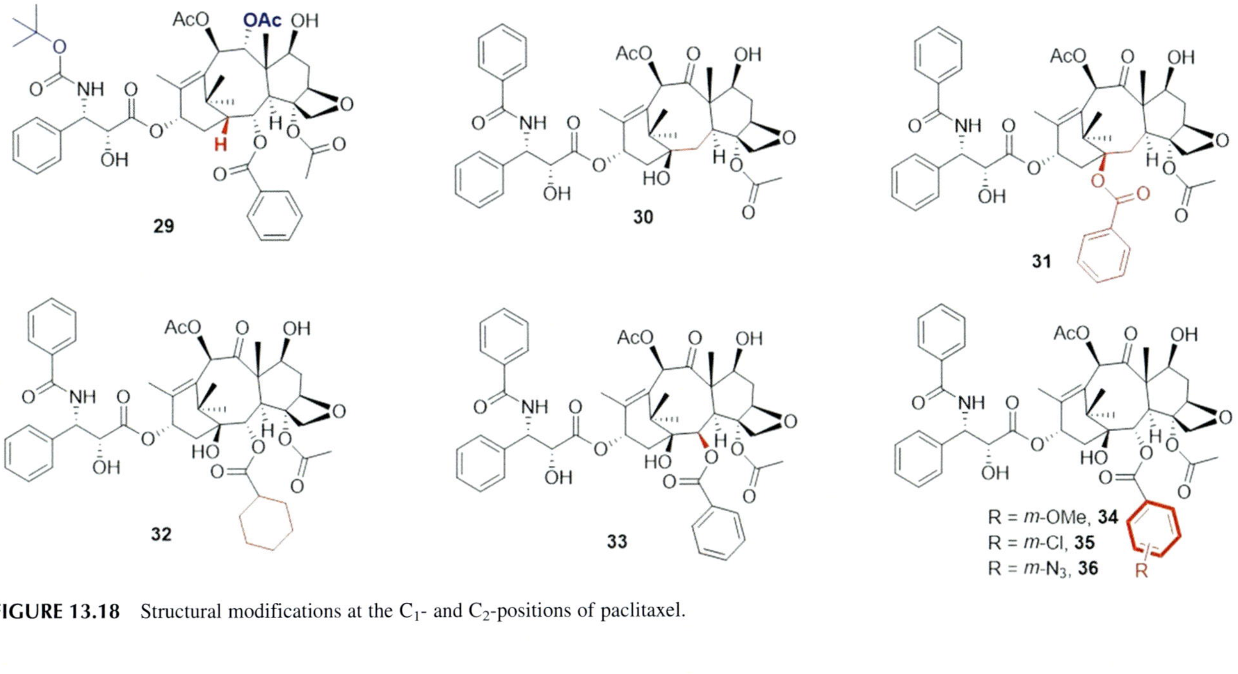

FIGURE 13.18 Structural modifications at the C_1- and C_2-positions of paclitaxel.

The experimental results indicate that the substituents on the phenyl ring of the C_2-position benzoyloxy group have a significant impact on the activity. When ortho-substituents such as N_3, CN, OMe, and Cl are introduced, both the microtubule assembly activity and cytotoxicity are markedly reduced. Conversely, when these substituents are introduced at the metaposition, the microtubule assembly activity and cytotoxicity are significantly increased. For instance, the metamethoxy and metadiazonium derivatives exhibit three times the cytotoxicity against HL60 human leukemia cells compared to paclitaxel, while the metamethoxy and metachloro derivatives demonstrate antitumor activity against P388 mouse leukemia cells that is 800 and 700 times greater than paclitaxel, respectively. When a chlorine atom is introduced at the para-position, the activity is slightly decreased compared to paclitaxel. From the above results, it can be observed that the effects of ortho, meta, and para substituents on the activity of paclitaxel derivatives are distinctly different, with the order of effectiveness being meta > ortho > para [84].

Overall, small substituents at the metaposition can enhance the assembly ability of microtubule proteins, while substituents at the para-position generally lead to a decrease in activity. The structure-activity relationship for alkyl and halogen substituents is relatively clear, with the order of effectiveness being methyl > ethyl > propyl and bromine > chlorine > fluorine > iodine [85] (Fig. 13.19).

13.2.3.2 The relationship between structure and activity at the C_4 position

The compound 37 obtained by replacing the C_4-acetyl group with cyclopropionyl exhibits higher cytotoxicity against HCT116 human colon cancer cells compared to paclitaxel (Fig. 13.19). When the acetyl group is replaced with isopropionyl (compound 38), the assembly ability of microtubule proteins and cytotoxicity against B16 melanoma cells are slightly lower than paclitaxel [86]. A significant decrease in cytotoxicity is observed when the acetyl group is replaced with the benzoyl group (compound 39) [87]. Removal of the C_4-acetoxy group (compound 40) [88] or removal of the acetyl group (compound 41) [89] leads to a significant decrease in activity. When the acetyl group is replaced with a methoxycarbonyl group (compound 42), its antitumor activity is stronger than paclitaxel [90]. These results indicate that the C_4-ester group is essential. Studies have shown that the C_4-acetyl group structure is the most significant factor influencing the conformation of the A-ring and plays a crucial role in maintaining the diterpene conformation in paclitaxel and its derivatives [91].

13.2.3.3 The relationship between the structural modifications at the C_7- to C_{10}-positions

After removing the hydroxyl group at the C_7-position (compound 43), the cytotoxicity against leukemia cell lines is higher compared to paclitaxel, and the toxicity against human colon cancer HCT116 cell line can also reach a similar level as paclitaxel (Fig. 13.20). Similarly, when the C_7-hydroxyl group is replaced with fluorine (compound 44), it

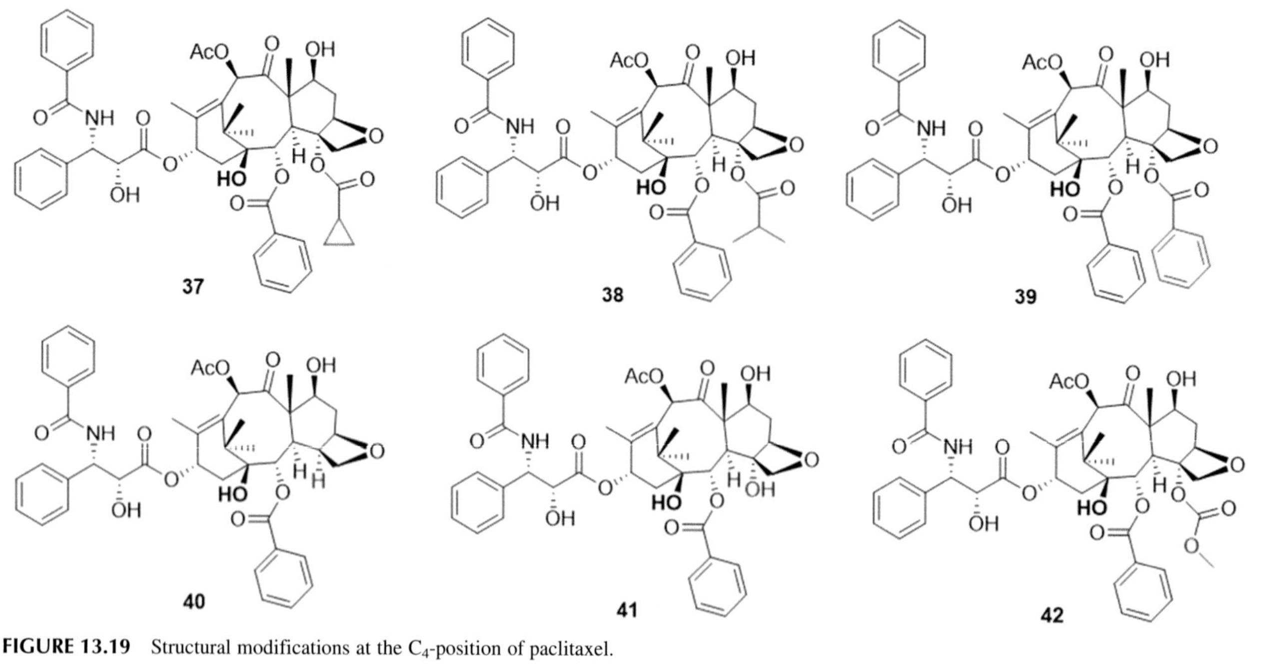

FIGURE 13.19 Structural modifications at the C_4-position of paclitaxel.

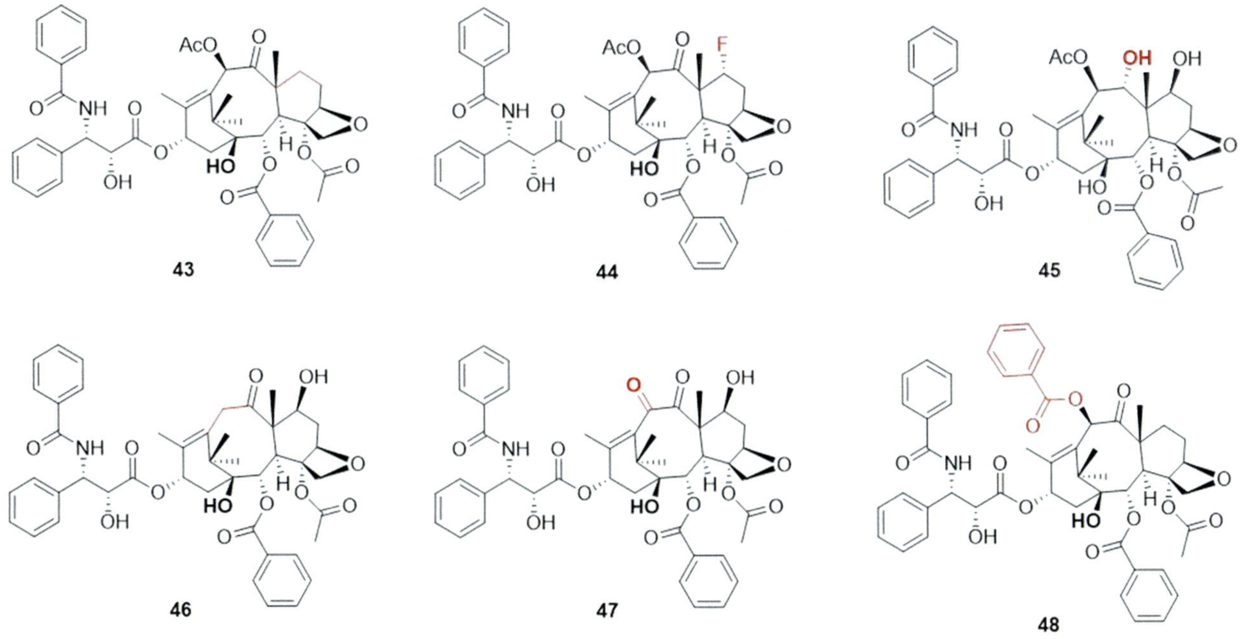

FIGURE 13.20 Structural modifications at positions C$_7$-to C$_{10}$-of paclitaxel.

exhibits a comparable ability to bind to polymerized microtubules and similar cytotoxicity to paclitaxel, indicating that the C$_7$-hydroxyl group is not an essential active moiety [92,93]. After reducing the carbonyl group at the C$_9$-position to a hydroxyl group (compound 45), the activity is slightly enhanced. The derivative with the acetyl group removed at the C$_{10}$-position (compound 46) shows comparable antitumor activity to paclitaxel [94]. However, the activity is significantly reduced when replaced with a carbonyl group (compound 47) [95]. The derivative with C$_{10}$-benzoyloxy and C$_7$-dehydroxy substitution (compound 48) exhibits activity equivalent to paclitaxel [96].

13.2.3.4 The relationship between the structure and effectiveness of the C$_{13}$-side chain

The derivative Bacatin III (compound 49), obtained by removing the entire side chain, exhibits no antitumor activity. However, the derivative of Bacatin III (compound 50), with a substituted diazo group at the metaposition of the phenyl ring at the C$_2$-position, can still inhibit human cancer cell proliferation at nanomolar concentrations, despite lacking a side chain. This finding provides valuable insights for the study of simplified taxane derivatives [97]. When the ester structural unit of the side chain is replaced with an amide, the activity is lost [98] (compound 51). Overall, the ester-based side chain is essential for activity (Fig. 13.21).

Compound 52, obtained by hydroxyacylation at the C$_2'$-position, exhibits diminished in vitro activity and significantly loses its microtubule-stabilizing effect. However, its impact on activity in vivo is minimal, indicating that the acylated ester derivatives decompose and release paclitaxel in the presence of esterases [99]. This also suggests that the ester modification at the C$_2'$-position holds promise as an important approach for developing paclitaxel prodrugs. The C$_2'$-methylated paclitaxel analog (Compound 53) demonstrates stronger in vitro cytotoxicity against HCT116 human colon cancer cells compared to paclitaxel. This could be attributed to the introduction of the methyl group, which potentially reduces the rotational freedom of the C$_2'$-C$_3'$ single bond or enhances the hydrophobic binding between the methyl group and the tubulin-binding site [100]. Furthermore, paclitaxel derivatives with restricted side-chain conformations (Compound 54) can still maintain their antitumor activity (Fig. 13.22) [101].

The removal of the phenyl ring at the C$_3'$-position (Compound 55) results in a significant decrease in microtubule polymerization-promoting activity [102]. However, it can be substituted with individual alkenyl groups. For example, when the phenyl group at the C$_3'$-position is replaced by 2-methylpropenyl (Compound 56), it exhibits highly potent antitumor activity against B16 melanoma in nude mice [103]. The presence of the C$_3'$-acylamino group is also essential for activity, as the removal of the acyl group (57) significantly reduces the activity. However, the phenyl group on the amide is not necessary for activity and can be replaced by alkoxy groups. For instance, the derivative (Compound 58) with a tert-butoxy group replacing the phenyl group demonstrates higher activity than paclitaxel [104]. When the C$_3'$-phenyl group is substituted with

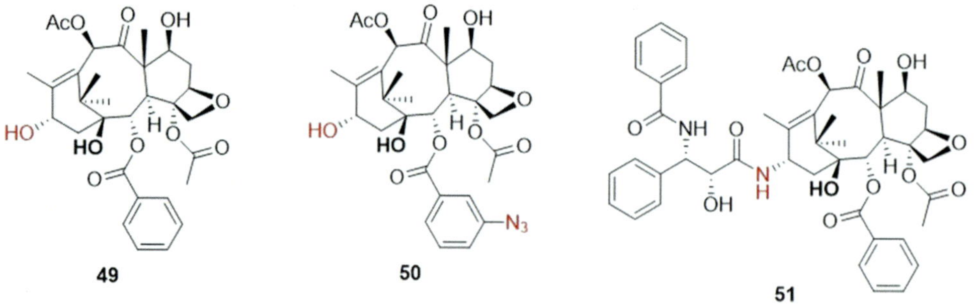

FIGURE 13.21 Structural modification at the C_{13}-position of taxol.

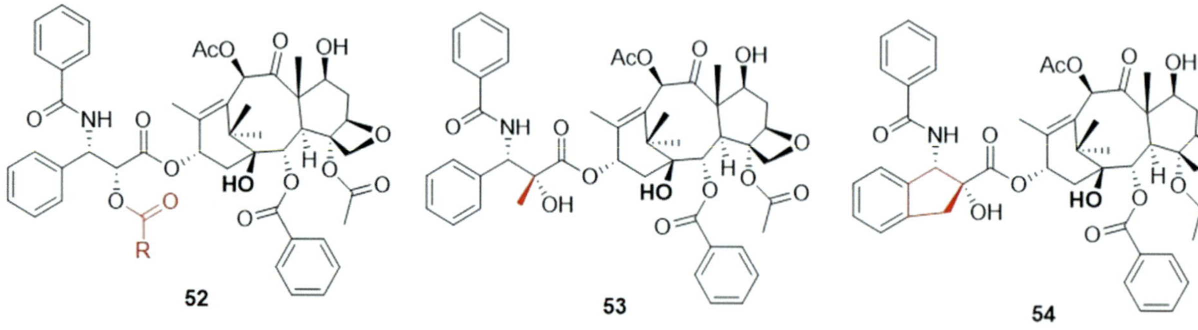

FIGURE 13.22 Structural modification at the C_2'-position of paclitaxel.

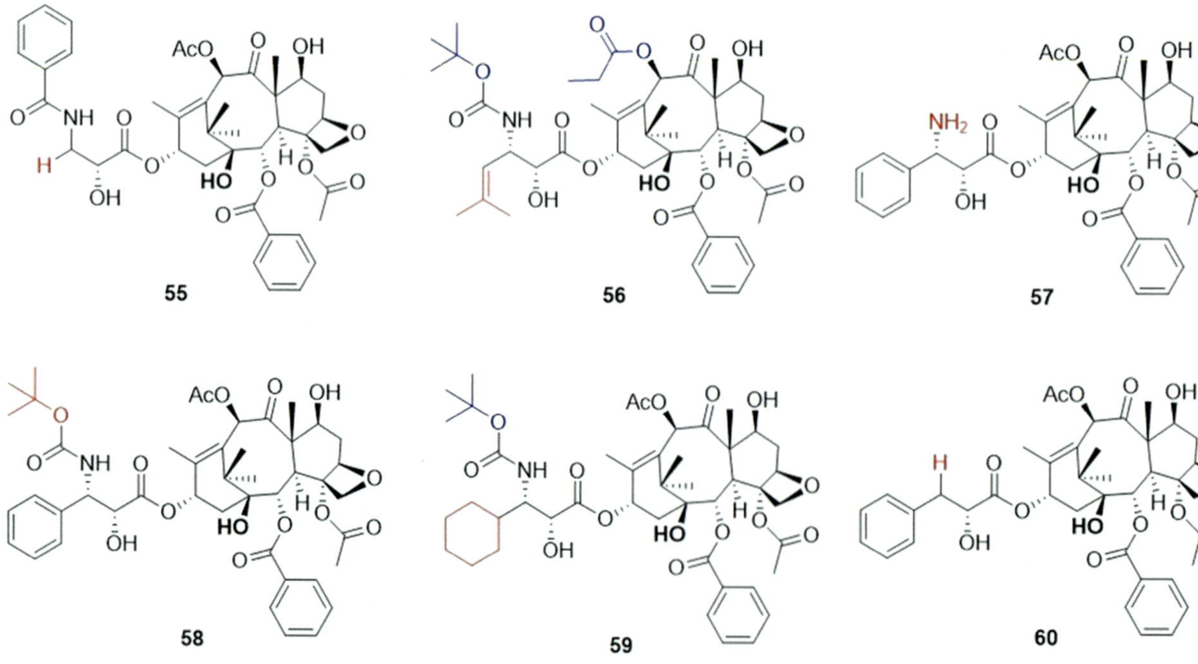

FIGURE 13.23 Structural modification at the C_3'-position of paclitaxel.

an equally sized hydrophobic group, such as cyclohexyl (Compound 59), the activity is maintained [105]. The removal of the C_3'-phenylcarbamoyl group (Compound 60) leads to a four- to fivefold decrease in activity [106]. The removal of either the C_2'-hydroxyl or C_3'-amino group has little impact on activity, but their simultaneous removal or interchange results in a more than 10-fold decrease in activity. Furthermore, the configuration of C_2' and C_3' is closely related to activity. The (2′S,3′S) and (2′R,3′R) diastereomers exhibit activity comparable to the natural product paclitaxel with the (2′R,3′S) configuration, while the activity of the (2′S,3′R) diastereomer is weaker than paclitaxel (Fig. 13.23).

13.2.3.5 Structure-activity relationship based on ring A

The C=C double bond in ring A is oxidized to form an epoxyethane structure, while the derivative (Compound 61) with the removal of the acetoxy group at C_{10} of paclitaxel exhibits higher activity in promoting microtubule polymerization compared to paclitaxel, but lower cytotoxicity against B16 melanoma cells [107]. When ring A is reduced to a five-membered carbon ring and ring B is replaced with an equivalent-sized eight-membered lactone ring, the resulting derivative (Compound 62) shows comparable ability to promote microtubule protein polymerization as paclitaxel but does not exhibit significant cytotoxicity against HCT116 cell line. However, the derivatives (Compound 63) and (Compound 64) obtained by reducing ring A and ring B to five-membered and seven-membered rings, respectively, show significantly lower activity in promoting microtubule protein polymerization compared to paclitaxel [108]. Opening of ring A leads to a simplified ester derivative (Compound 65) with reduced cytotoxicity, but it can maintain comparable antitumor activity to paclitaxel. The amide derivative (Compound 66) loses its antitumor activity, while the methylated amide derivative (Compound 67) exhibits antitumor activity comparable to paclitaxel [109,110]. When ring A is reduced from cyclohexene to cyclopentene (Compound 68), although it shows microtubule depolymerization activity comparable to paclitaxel, its inhibitory activity against KB cells is completely lost, indicating the importance of the 6/8/6 tricyclic structure for maintaining activity [111]. The derivative (Compound 69), with ring D replaced by a four-membered carbon ring and ring A and ring B reduced to five-membered and seven-membered rings, respectively, exhibits weaker cytotoxicity than paclitaxel but maintains activity in inhibiting microtubule polymerization comparable to that of paclitaxel (Fig. 13.24) [112].

13.2.3.6 Structure-activity relationship based on ring C

The reduction of ring C to a five-membered ring (Compound 70) [113] or its opening (Compound 71) resulted in a decrease in the antitumor activity. However, the open-ring derivative with modified side chains (Compound 72) was still able to retain the antitumor activity of paclitaxel [114]. These findings have provided a solid foundation for the study of simplified paclitaxel-like antitumor molecules after ring opening (Fig. 13.25).

13.2.3.7 Structural-functional relationship based on ring D

Research has demonstrated that the D ring plays a crucial role in stabilizing the conformation of paclitaxel and facilitating microtubule assembly [115]. When the oxygen atom in the D ring is replaced with a nitrogen atom (compound 73), the activity in promoting microtubule protein assembly significantly decreases [116]. Derivatives with a C_4-substituted methoxycarbonyl group exhibit enhanced microtubule protein assembly activity and cytotoxicity compared to paclitaxel.

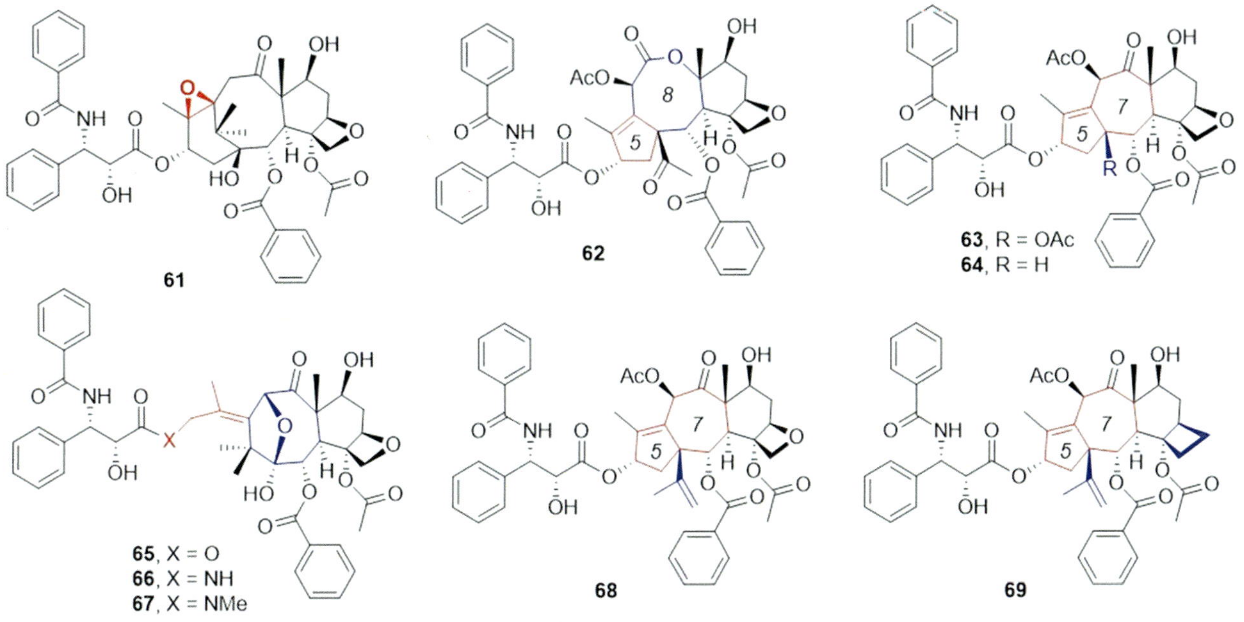

FIGURE 13.24 Structure modification based on ring A.

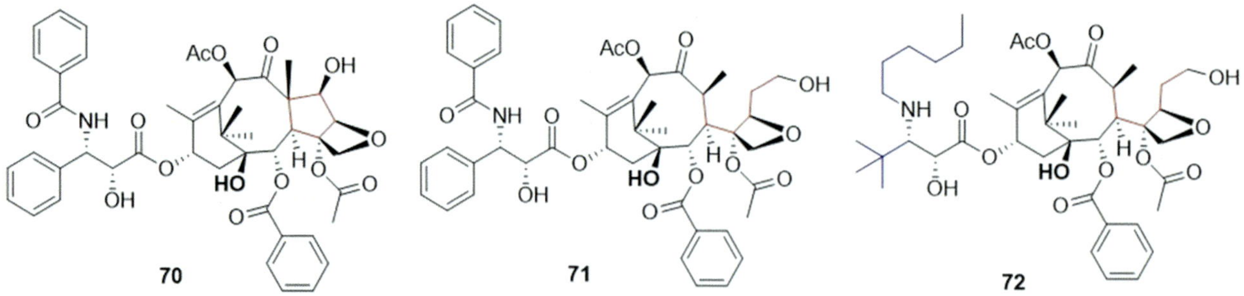

FIGURE 13.25 Structural modifications based on ring C.

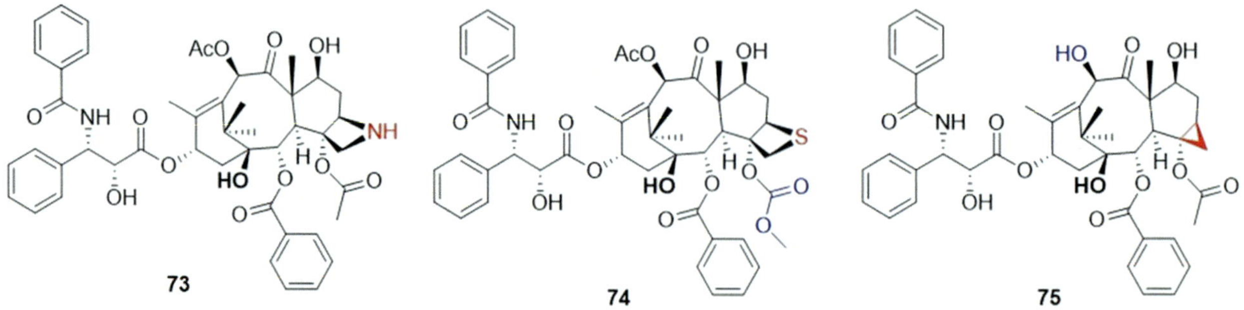

FIGURE 13.26 Structural modifications based on ring D.

However, when the oxygen atom in the D ring is replaced with a sulfur atom (compound 74), both the activity in promoting microtubule protein assembly and cytotoxicity noticeably decrease, indicating that the oxygen atom in the tetrahydropyran D ring is indispensable for activity. Nevertheless, by removing the oxygen atom and replacing it with a tricyclic carbon ring in the C_{10}-deacetylated derivative (compound 75), the microtubule assembly activity remains comparable to that of paclitaxel, suggesting that the tetrahydropyran D ring is not essential for activity (Fig. 13.26) [117].

Compounds 76 and 77, as open-ring derivatives of the D ring, exhibit no cytotoxicity and microtubule assembly activity [91,118]. The open-ring derivatives of the D ring lack the ability to promote microtubule protein assembly and demonstrate cytotoxicity. This could be attributed to the altered spatial conformation of the C_4-acetyl group upon removal of the D ring, which hinders its optimal interaction with the substrate protein. From a spatial perspective, the D ring likely plays a role in stabilizing the C ring, allowing the acetyl oxygen group at the C_4-position to assume a more favorable binding position with the microtubule protein. Electronically, the D-ring could conceivably exploit the hydrogen bond acceptor capacity of its oxygen atom to partake in and affect the polymerization of tubulin proteins via hydrogen bonding interactions (Fig. 13.27).

When the D ring is removed and the C_5/C_6-positions are substituted with a C=C double bond, it can still stabilize microtubule proteins similar to paclitaxel (compound 78). This indicates that the entire D ring may not be essential for activity, as long as the appropriate spatial conformation is maintained. The simplification or removal of the D ring provides a new approach to the design and synthesis of simplified paclitaxel derivatives [119]. The C_4-position methyl or methylene group plays a crucial role in the conformation of the C ring, and the derivative lacking this group (compound 79) shows a significant decrease in activity (Fig. 13.28) [120].

13.2.3.8 Summary of the structure-activity relationship of paclitaxel

As shown in Fig. 13.29, the hydroxyl groups at the C_1- and C_7-positions have minimal impact on the activity. The acyloxy group at the C_2-position is an essential active moiety, while partial substitution with the benzoyl group enhances the activity. Removal of the acyloxy group at the C_4-position leads to a decrease in activity, indicating that the acetyl group is not an essential active moiety. The oxygen heterocycle at the C_5- and C_6-positions is a necessary requirement for activity, as the activity diminishes upon ring opening. Reduction of the carbonyl group at the C_9-position to a hydroxyl group slightly enhances the activity, while removal of the acetyl group at the C_{10}-position

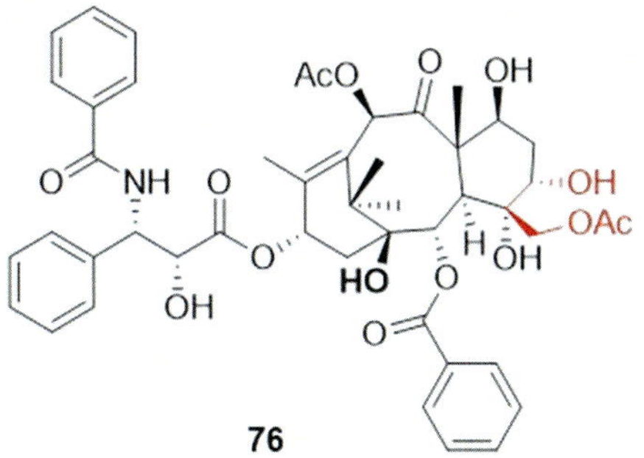

FIGURE 13.27 Open-ring modification of ring D.

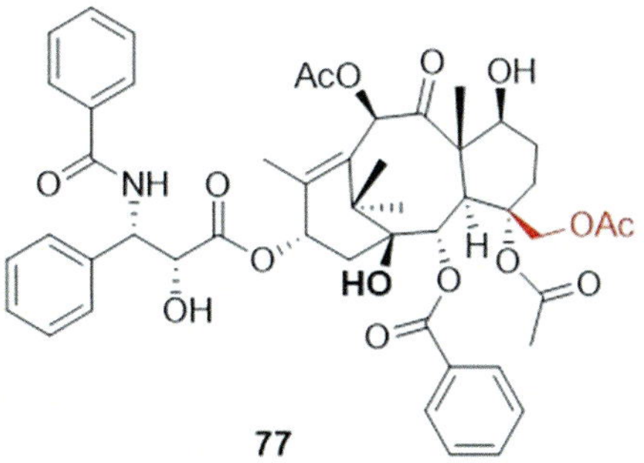

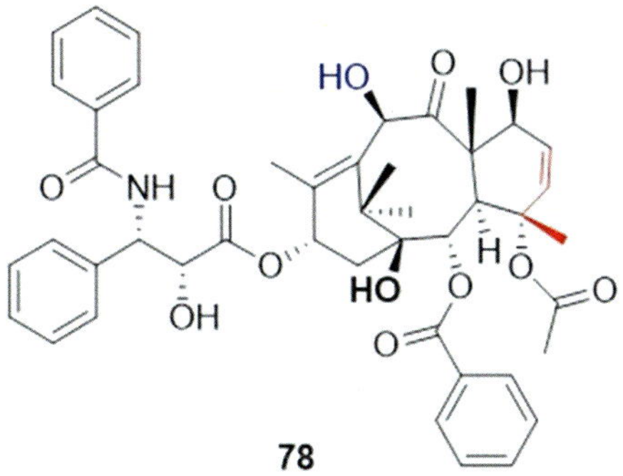

FIGURE 13.28 Structural modification removing ring D.

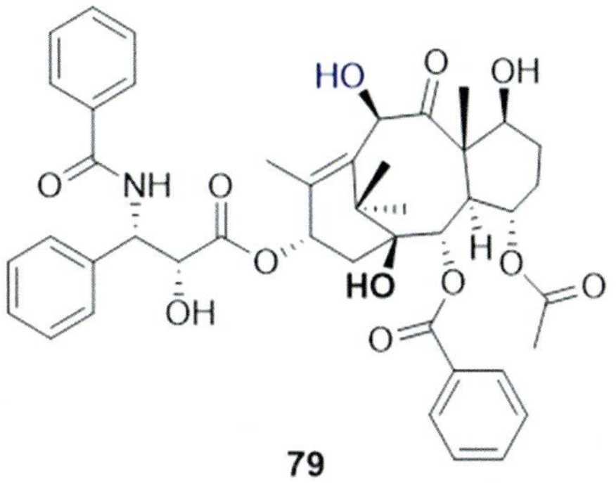

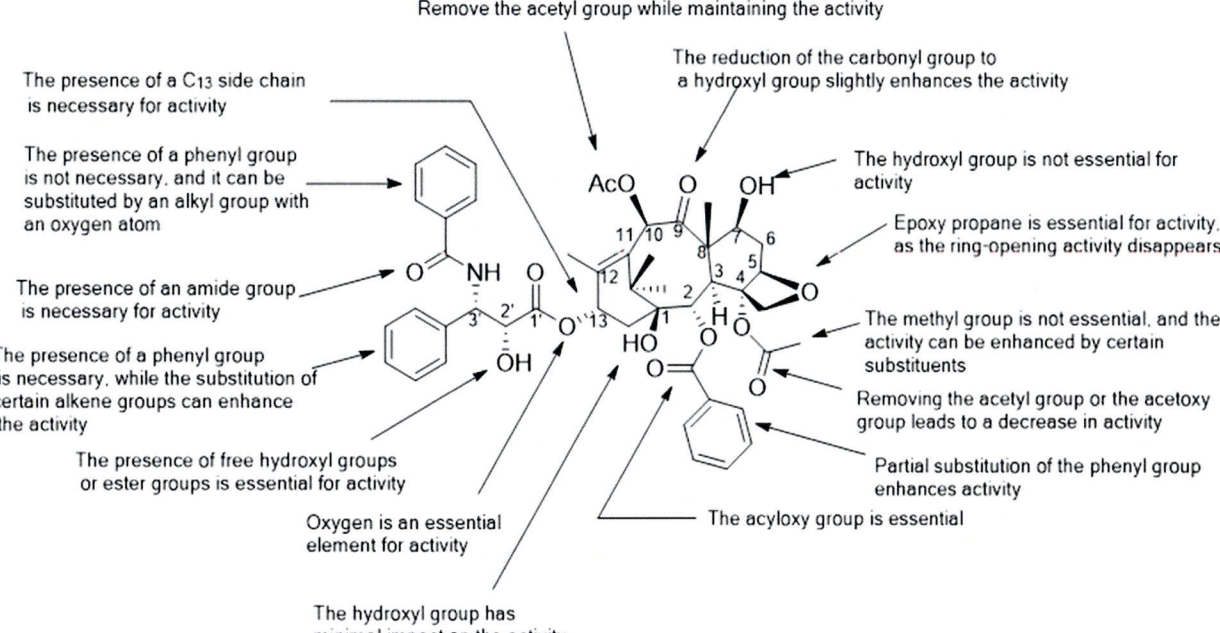

FIGURE 13.29 The structure-activity relationship of paclitaxel.

maintains the activity to a large extent. Multiple positions in the C_{13} side chain of paclitaxel obviously influence the activity. The presence of a free hydroxyl or ester group at the C_2'-position is an essential requirement for activity and the C_2'-hydroxyl group serves as a major modification site in the prodrug strategy of paclitaxel. The phenyl group and amide group at the C_3'-position are essential active moieties, and the amide group can be partially replaced with alkoxyl groups.

13.3 Design strategy for paclitaxel prodrugs

The use of prodrug strategies in the design of paclitaxel analogs has been shown to significantly improve the drug's solubility (or lipophilicity), targeting specificity, and stability. The main methods for designing and obtaining paclitaxel prodrugs typically involve the preparation of esters at the C_2'-OH and C_7-OH positions of paclitaxel (with C_2'-OH and C_7-OH being the primary modification sites). The structure-activity relationship of paclitaxel, as summarized in Fig. 13.29, reveals that the C_2'-OH group is an essential pharmacophore, and its derivatization eliminates the cytotoxic activity. This suggests that prodrugs derived from the C_2'-OH position of paclitaxel need to be effectively converted into free paclitaxel to exert their anticancer effects. Studies have demonstrated that ester prodrugs derived from the C_2'-OH group of paclitaxel can be enzymatically hydrolyzed in vivo to release the active parent drug, paclitaxel. On the other hand, prodrugs based on modification of the C_7-OH position of paclitaxel exhibit enhanced structure stability. Therefore, the C_2'-OH position is considered the preferred site for designing paclitaxel prodrugs.

13.3.1 A prodrug utilizing hydrophilic small molecule moieties as carriers

Introducing hydrophilic moieties at the C_2'-OH position is employed to enhance the water solubility of paclitaxel. As depicted in Fig. 13.30, the paclitaxel derivative 80, bearing an amino methyl sulfonic acid salt moiety at the C_2'-OH position, exhibits favorable water solubility and demonstrates comparable antitumor activity to paclitaxel in rat models [121]. Another classical prodrug design strategy involves the modification of the C_2'-OH position to obtain paclitaxel phosphate ester sodium salt (compound 81). This prodrug rapidly distributes along the intestinal wall and undergoes enzymatic hydrolysis by hepatic phosphatases, releasing the parent drug. However, it exhibits a slightly reduced activity compared to paclitaxel, possibly due to extensive plasma protein binding, leading to incomplete conversion of the prodrug by phosphatase hydrolysis to release the active drug and consequently displaying inferior biological activity [122]. On the other hand, the paclitaxel malate complex compound 82, derived from modification at the C_2'-OH position, demonstrates a half-life of 4 hours in plasma, indicating higher stability. It exhibits equivalent inhibitory activity against human breast cancer cell lines MCF-7 and EVSA-T as paclitaxel and displays superior activity in a mouse P388 leukemia tumor model [123].

13.3.1.1 Prodrugs of paclitaxel utilizing water-soluble polymers as carriers

Tumor tissues exhibit high permeability to polymers and can prolong drug efficacy. In light of this characteristic, it is possible to utilize certain polymers as carriers in prodrug design.

13.3.1.2 Polyethylene glycol—paclitaxel conjugates

PEG possesses remarkable hydrophilicity, and when conjugated with drugs, it can render the drugs highly water-soluble and easily cleared by renal metabolism. Compound 83 represents the conjugation between the C_2'-hydroxyl group of paclitaxel and PEG, exhibiting good water solubility. Its activity in vitro is comparable to paclitaxel, while its inhibitory activity against P388 nonleukemic white blood cells is slightly lower than that of paclitaxel [124]. Compound 84 is a paclitaxel prodrug linked with an amino acid PEG as a linker. It not only possesses excellent water solubility but also exhibits stronger in vitro activity compared to paclitaxel. Furthermore, its activity in vivo is fair with paclitaxel, while reducing adverse reactions (Fig. 13.31) [125].

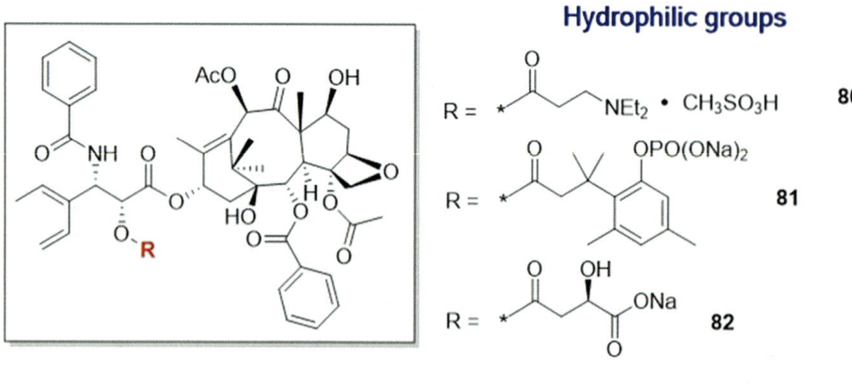

FIGURE 13.30 Prodrugs utilizing hydrophilic small molecular moieties as carriers.

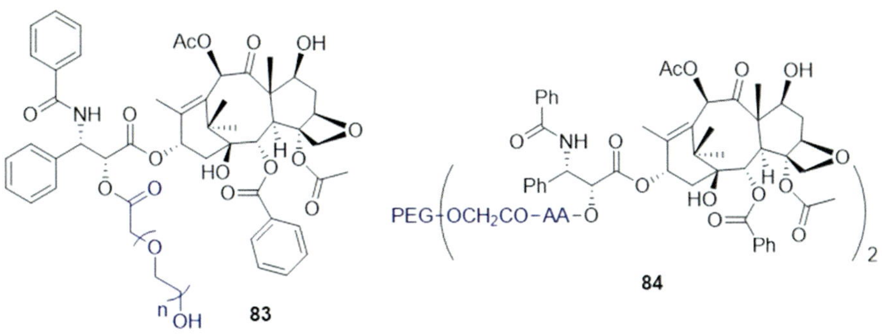

FIGURE 13.31 PEG-paclitaxel conjugate prodrug.

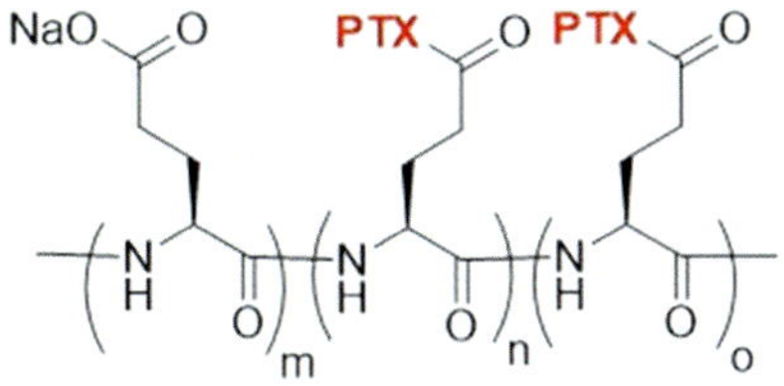

FIGURE 13.32 PLGA-paclitaxel conjugate prodrug (PTX = paclitaxel or taxol).

13.3.1.3 Poly L-glutamic acid–paclitaxel conjugate

PLGA is a water-soluble conjugate carrier that degrades into nontoxic L-glutamic acid in the body. The prodrug obtained by conjugating L-glutamic acid with paclitaxel at the C_7-OH position (Compound 85) exhibits a remarkable aqueous solubility of up to 100 g/L. This water-soluble paclitaxel prodrug demonstrates significant antitumor activity in vivo and low toxicity compared to traditional paclitaxel. It completely inhibits tumor growth in the Oca-1 ovarian cancer cell line at a dose of 160 mg/kg. In comparison to paclitaxel, PLGA-paclitaxel exhibits a longer half-life in plasma and greater tumor uptake. Apart from selectively delivering the paclitaxel drug to the tumor site, PLGA-paclitaxel also exerts unique pharmacological effects, resulting in significant antitumor efficacy [126]. Polyglutamic acid-paclitaxel 86 (Xyotax, CT-2103) is a prodrug that conjugates paclitaxel at the C_2'-OH position with PGA [127]. It has been used for the treatment of nonsmall cell lung cancer, ovarian cancer, and breast cancer. However, its phase II clinical trial investigations were terminated due to its neurotoxicity and hypersensitivity reactions (Fig. 13.32) [128,129].

13.3.1.4 Peptide-paclitaxel conjugate

The compound referred to as paclitide is a peptide-drug conjugate (PDC) formed by the ester bond between paclitaxel and a peptide at the C_2'-OH position. This conjugate exhibits specific immunomodulatory properties, as described in the subsequent text, pertaining to the prodrug portion of paclitaxel with immunomodulatory function.

13.3.1.5 Prodrugs designed for targeted tissue delivery

13.3.1.5.1 Enzymes or transport proteins overexpressed in tumor tissue as target

The enzymes or transport proteins overexpressed in target cells are specific targets that enable targeted actions through enzymatic degradation or transport processes in tumor tissues. Currently, identified specific targets include glucose transporter and plasmin. Compound 87 is a paclitaxel-glucose derivative designed with a butanedioyl linker at the C_2'-OH position, which can be transported by overexpressed glucose transporters as a prodrug. Studies have shown that compound 87 not only exhibits good water solubility but also demonstrates activity against human breast cancer cell line MCF-7 comparable to paclitaxel. Moreover, it exhibits strong targeting properties and minimal cytotoxicity to normal RPTEC cells (paclitaxel exhibits high cytotoxicity to RPTEC cells). Plasmin, overexpressed on the surface of cancer cells, is involved in a series of physiological activities of cancer cells, such as extracellular matrix degradation activation, tumor growth, and angiogenesis [130]. Compound 88 is a prodrug targeting plasmin, designed as a tripeptide conjugate with a carbonate-protected amino benzyl ester linker at the paclitaxel C_2'-OH position. The enzyme-sensitive linker can be cleaved by plasmin, leading to the controlled release of the parent drug paclitaxel. The enzymatic process is depicted in Fig. 13.33. However, in terms of inhibitory activity, its effectiveness against tumor strains is weaker than paclitaxel, possibly due to incomplete activation of plasmin [131].

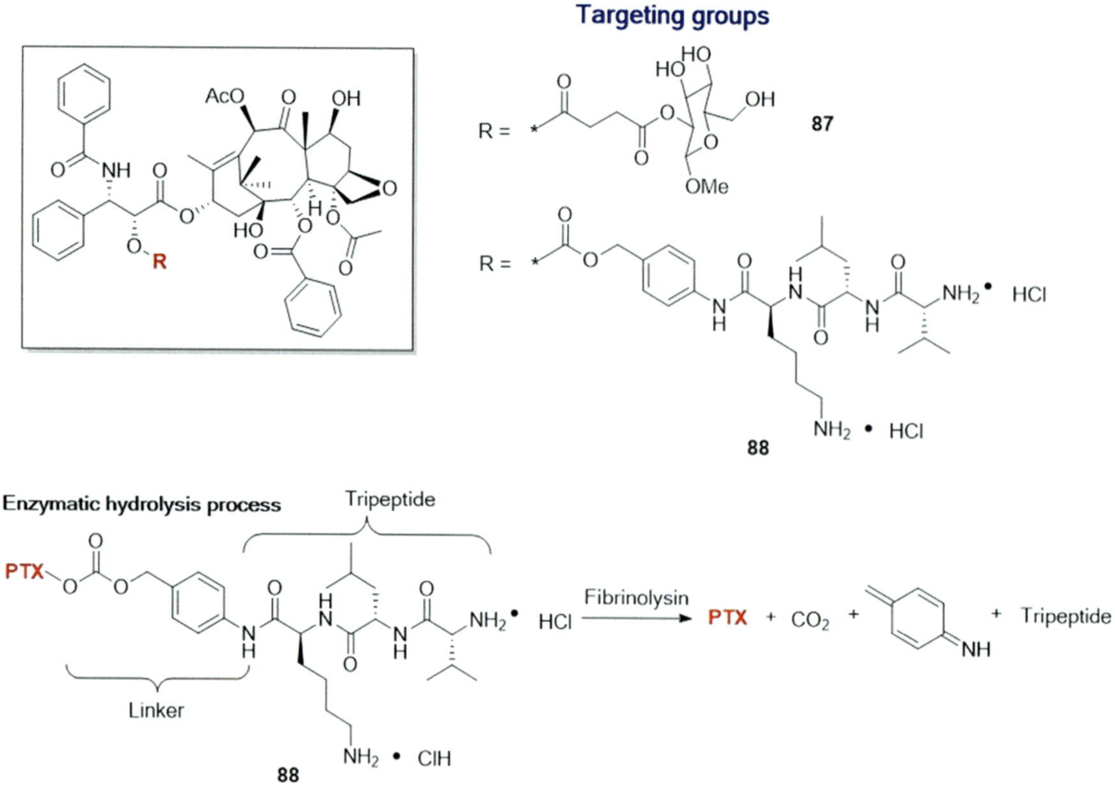

312 Medicinal Chemistry and Drug Development

FIGURE 13.33 Targeting prodrugs for enzymes or transport proteins overexpressed in tumor tissues (PTX = paclitaxel or taxol).

13.3.1.6 Targeting the hypoxic microenvironment of cancer cells

Cancer cells possess a highly active metabolism, requiring a significant amount of oxygen and energy throughout their physiological processes. As a result, most tumor cells exist in a hypoxic environment. Therefore, the hypoxic condition of tumors can serve as a target for prodrug design. Building upon this design concept, Damen et al. developed a prodrug (Compound 89) by coupling paclitaxel C_2'-OH, in the form of a carbonate ester, with a nitro-stilbene moiety (Fig. 13.34). The aim was to activate the nitro group using the intracellular reductase in the hypoxic tumor environment, leading to the release of paclitaxel through a 1,8-elimination electron cascade reaction. Unfortunately, this prodrug failed to achieve effective activation within the hypoxic physiological environment of the tumor. However, successful liberation of paclitaxel was observed through chemical reduction of the nitro group in vitro, demonstrating the feasibility of this design. Thus, the search for a suitable nitro group structural unit remains crucial for the efficacy of such prodrugs [132].

13.3.1.7 Targeting cancer cells overexpressing receptors

A fraction of cancer cells often exhibit overexpression of certain membrane receptors. This characteristic can be utilized as a strategy for prodrug design. By appropriately linking paclitaxel with a membrane receptor-ligand at the C_2'-OH position, targeted delivery of paclitaxel can be achieved. The cyclic peptide RGD, composed of arginine, glycine, and aspartic acid, has been found to inhibit the activity of the Rv integrin protein, inducing apoptosis in endothelial cells, inhibiting angiogenesis, and increasing endothelial cell monolayer permeability. Chen et al. used succinyl as a linking chain to conjugate paclitaxel with the bicyclic peptide RGD at the C_2'-OH position, resulting in a prodrug targeting integrin (compound 90) (Fig. 13.35). This prodrug can specifically recognize the cell adhesion molecule αvβ3 integrin, enabling targeted delivery of paclitaxel, reducing its toxicity, and enhancing its selective cytotoxicity against cancer cells [133].

13.3.1.8 Paclitaxel–unsaturated fatty acid conjugates

Multiple PUFAs, such as docosahexaenoic acid (DHA) and α-linolenic acid (LNA), have been proven to effectively suppress the expression of oncogenic proteins, inhibit tumor angiogenesis, and demonstrate excellent cytotoxic effects against various cancer cells, including breast cancer and gastric cancer. Through an ester bond linkage with DHA at the

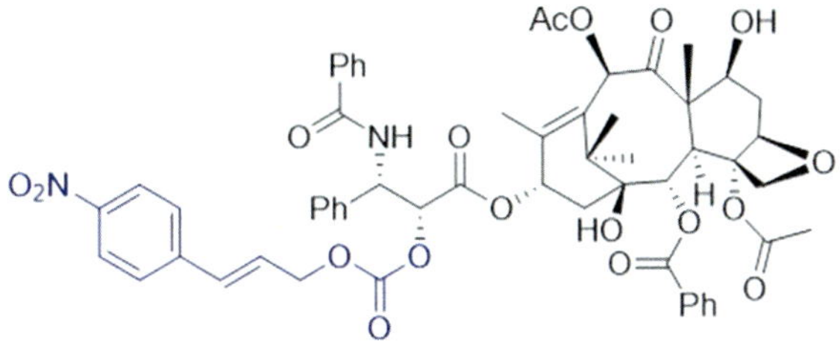

FIGURE 13.34 Prodrug targeting hypoxic cancer cells.

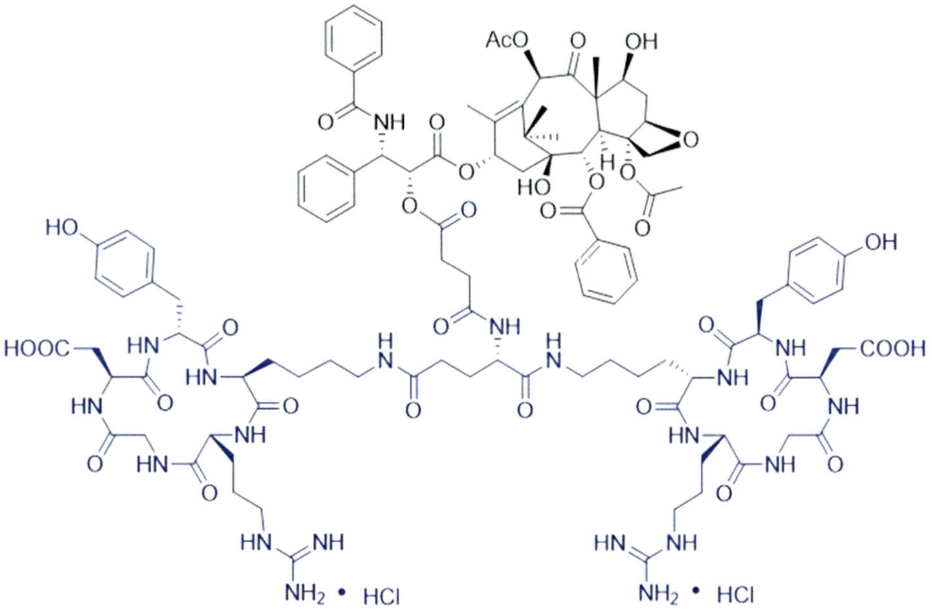

FIGURE 13.35 Targeting prodrugs overexpressed in cancer cells.

C_2'-OH position of paclitaxel, a conjugate (compound 91) (Fig. 13.36) can prolong the duration of action on tumor cells, significantly increase the concentration of paclitaxel at the site of tumor cells, and exhibit superior targeting ability and antitumor activity compared to paclitaxel [134].

13.3.1.9 Paclitaxel prodrug targeting the inflammatory microenvironment of tumors

Pattern recognition receptors (PRRs) are a type of recognition molecules expressed on the surface or intracellularly in innate immune cells, which play an important role in regulating chemotherapy resistance mediated by the inflammatory microenvironment of tumors. Among them, nucleotide-binding oligomerization domain 1/2 (NOD1/2) are important PRRs in the human body. Activated NOD1/2 can initiate downstream signaling pathways, including NF-κB, MAPKs (RIP2K, JNK, p38, ERK), and interferon regulatory factors (IRF3 and IRF7). Activation of NF-κB and MAPK pathways can result in the production of inflammatory cytokines such as TNF-α, IL-6, and IL-8. These cytokines can foster the construction of an inflammatory microenvironment in tumors and induce chemotherapy resistance, thereby facilitating tumor growth and metastasis. Based on the literature and assumptions described, the authors of this chapter have, for the first time, conjugated the natural exogenous ligand (muramyl dipeptide, MDP) of NOD2 with paclitaxel at its C_2'-OH position using succinic anhydride, resulting in the MDP-Taxol conjugate (2'-O-MTC-01). The team hopes to discover a new drug candidate that can simultaneously inhibit tumor growth and metastasis [135]. As shown in Fig. 13.37, (1) The literature reports that in addition to serving as a microtubule stabilizer, paclitaxel can mimic the action of lipopolysaccharide (LPS) on Toll-like receptor 4 (TLR4) in immune cells and activate downstream inflammatory signaling pathways such as the NF-

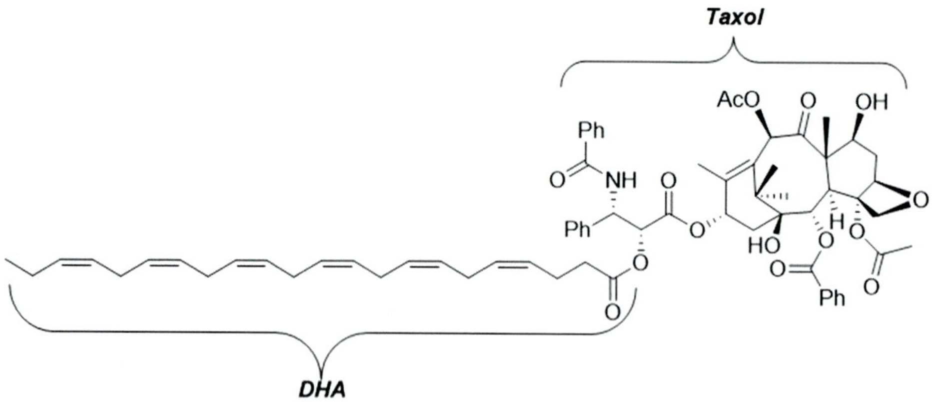

314 Medicinal Chemistry and Drug Development

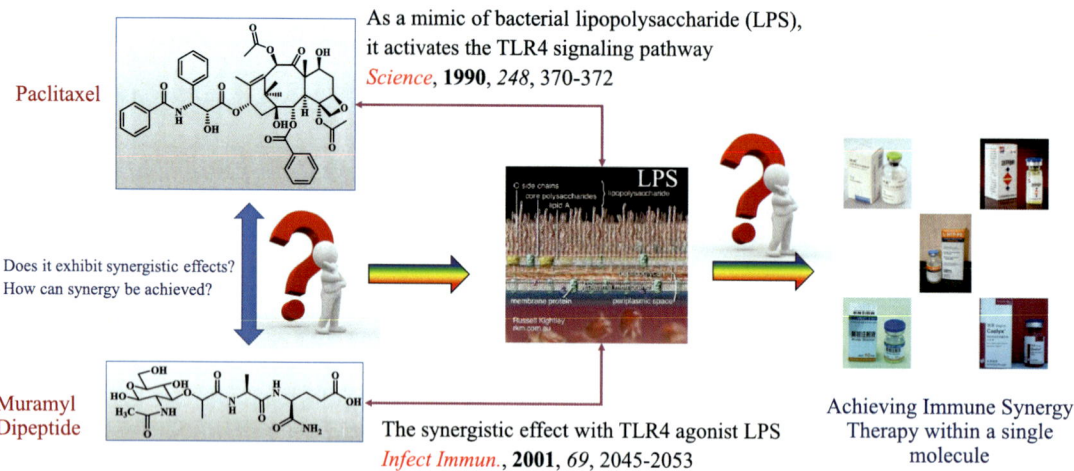

FIGURE 13.36 Paclitaxel—PUFA conjugate prodrug.

FIGURE 13.37 The rationale for designing a conjugate of paclitaxel with MDP.

κB pathway; [136] (2) When MDP activates immune cells, such as macrophages, through PRR NOD2, it can intensely synergistically interact with LPS when TLR4 is simultaneously activated, significantly enhancing the inflammatory response in infected individuals; [137] (3) This synergistic inflammatory response may suppress tumor metastasis by generating a large amount of tumor necrosis factor TNF-α (which was an incorrect assumption at that time!); (4) The strong hydrophilicity of MDP can improve the hydrophilicity of the conjugated paclitaxel molecule, facilitating modifications to the formulation of paclitaxel; (5). Conversely, the strong hydrophobicity of paclitaxel can balance the strong hydrophilicity, which aids in the easy excretion of MDP in urine, resulting in both paclitaxel and MDP possessing suitable physicochemical properties, thereby enhancing their druggability. Consequently, this type of PDC is likely to have dual functions: antitumor (paclitaxel) and antitumor metastasis (NOD2 signaling pathway agonist), thus addressing the critical clinical unmet need for preventing tumor metastasis while inhibiting tumor growth.

Based on this, Dr. Xuqin Li employed solid-phase synthesis methods to design and synthesize three compounds depicted in Fig. 13.38. These compounds individually were conjugated to the C_2'-, C_3'-, and C_7-positions of paclitaxel with MDP, marking the first successful implementation of molecular conjugation [135]. Excitingly, compound 2′-O-MTC-01 exhibited significant synergistic stimulation of murine macrophages, leading to highly elevated levels of TNF-α and IL-12 secretion compared to the individual use of equimolar doses of paclitaxel, MDP, or their mixture (Table 13.3). This synergistic effect did not occur in the mixture of the two components, suggesting that the conjugation of paclitaxel effectively enhanced the cell membrane permeability of MDP.

The results of this study validated the initial hypothesis on a cell level; however, the data indicated that 2′-O-MTC-01 only inhibited tumor growth in mice but did not suppress tumor metastasis. Despite this outcome, the study continued, and two decisions made by the authors in this chapter were deemed crucial and correct. Firstly, the development of

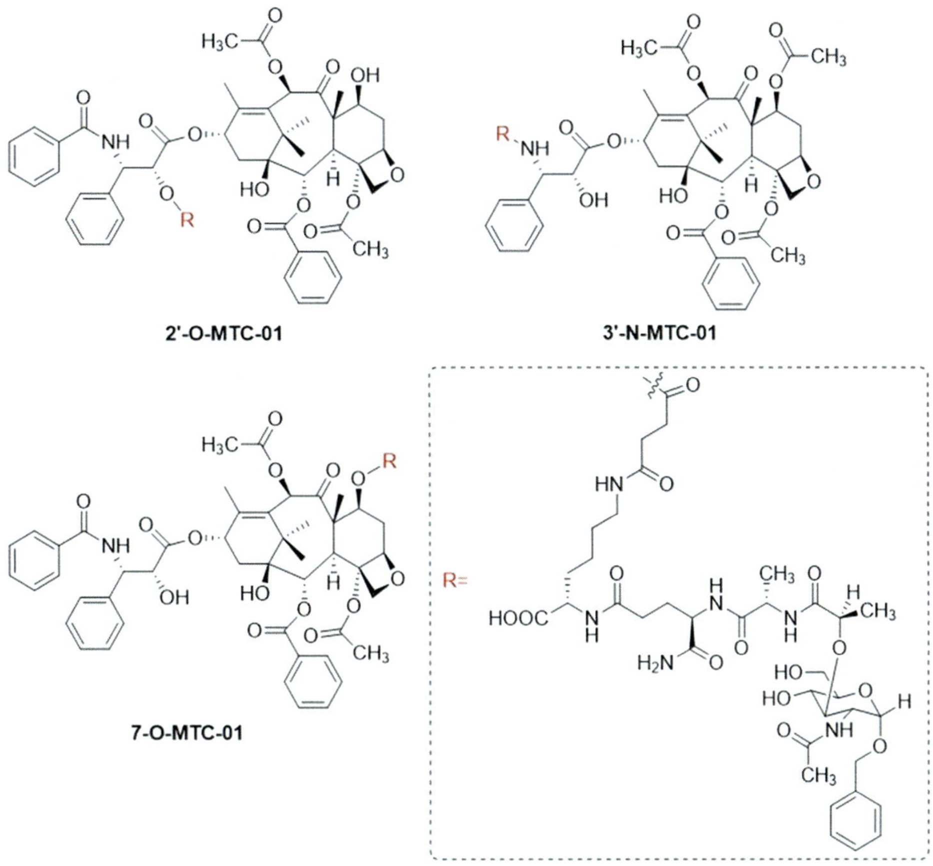

FIGURE 13.38 The first-generation conjugate of paclitaxel with MDP synthesized with the solid-phase synthesis method.

TABLE 13.3 Influence of compound 2'-*O*-MTC-01 on the secretion of inflammatory cytokines by murine macrophages.

Compound		TNF-α (pg/mL)	IL-12 (pg/mL)	MHC II (positivity rate %)	CD54 (positivity rate %)
Control group		10.8 ± 1.1	262 ± 2	2.95 ± 0.03%	0.79 ± 0.003%
Paclitaxel (5.0 μmol/L)		30.7 ± 2.4*	530 ± 33*	4.50 ± 0.02*%	3.27 ± 0.06*%
MDP (5.0 μmol/L)		40.2 ± 2.9*	486 ± 22*	3.64 ± 0.04*%	2.73 ± 0.02*%
MDP (5.0 μmol/L) + Paclitaxel (5.0 μmol/L)		91.0 ± 3.2	676 ± 49*	4.89 ± 0.02*%	3.6 ± 0.05*%
2'-*O*-MTC-01	10.0 μmol/L	664.8 ± 4.4*	1790 ± 64*	4.58 ± 0.48*	4.57 ± 0.02*
	5.0 μmol/L	537.0 ± 5.3*,**	1592 ± 73*,**	5.51 ± 0.03*,**	4.57 ± 0.01*,**
	1.0 μmol/L	245.5 ± 3.1*	900 ± 80*	4.58 ± 0.02*	4.13 ± 0.02*
	0.1 μmol/L	87.9 ± 4.3*	356 ± 56*	4.01 ± 0.02*	3.13 ± 0.02*

*$P < 0.01$; compared to the combination of MDP and paclitaxel, **$P < 0.01$.

solid-phase synthesis methods enabled the rapid synthesis of sufficient quantity and quality of such covalent compounds. This fulfilled the need for a large number of compounds required for rapid screening in vitro and test in vivo. It also provided an opportunity to replace the sugar-based fragments of MDP with other organic fragments, thus constructing a related chemical library. The results obtained from this decision not only challenged the existing understanding of the SAR between MDP's chemical structure and function, specifically the notion that the amino sugar fragment is the core fragment maintaining its activity, but also laid the foundation for the discovery of NOD1/2 antagonists. The establishment of an appropriate and efficient animal screening model was another crucial decision made by the researchers. This model directly involved animal experiments with the most meaningful phenotypic relevance for screening. Undoubtedly, the rapid animal screening that was achieved imposed high demands on the convenience of synthesizing complex conjugated compounds, as well as the workload, accuracy, and reproducibility of animal experiments. As a result, researchers deeply value animal experimental tests as they represent crucial preclinical data, inspiring drug developers and guiding research direction. Similar outcomes have been observed in multiple cases throughout this book.

Fig. 13.39 illustrates the early-stage construction and screening process of a chemical library containing conjugated compounds of paclitaxel and MDP. Dr. Xuqin Li constructed the chemical library, and Dr. Yao Ma developed and executed the animal screening model. They both made outstanding contributions to this project.

Regarding the structural optimization of N-acetylglucosamine around MDP, researchers subsequently found that the compound MTC-220, also known as Conmutaxel, derived from N-acetylglucosamine with a substituted acyl group of para-chlorocinnamoyl, exhibited dual inhibition of tumor growth and metastasis [138]. Conmutaxel can effectively deliver the prototype drug (MTC-220) to tumor tissues, followed by the release of paclitaxel from the prodrug via esterases in the blood, thus improving the distribution of paclitaxel in the tumor tissue. Moreover, Conmutaxel antagonizes the NOD2 signaling pathway activated by paclitaxel chemotherapy, effectively reversing chemotherapy resistance caused by the remodeling tumor inflammatory microenvironment. Ultimately, this enhances paclitaxel's antitumor efficacy and inhibits tumor metastasis, as illustrated in Fig. 13.40. Furthermore, a conjugate of docetaxel and MDP derivatives (trade name, Salutaxel, Fig. 13.41) has been found to enhance docetaxel's effectiveness against 4T1 triple-negative breast cancer in mice by antagonizing the NOD1 signaling pathway activated by docetaxel chemotherapy [139]. Moreover, considering all these factors, researchers have progressed Salutaxel to the clinical investigations, which is currently ongoing in Phase Ib. Current data is promising to move onto Phase II.

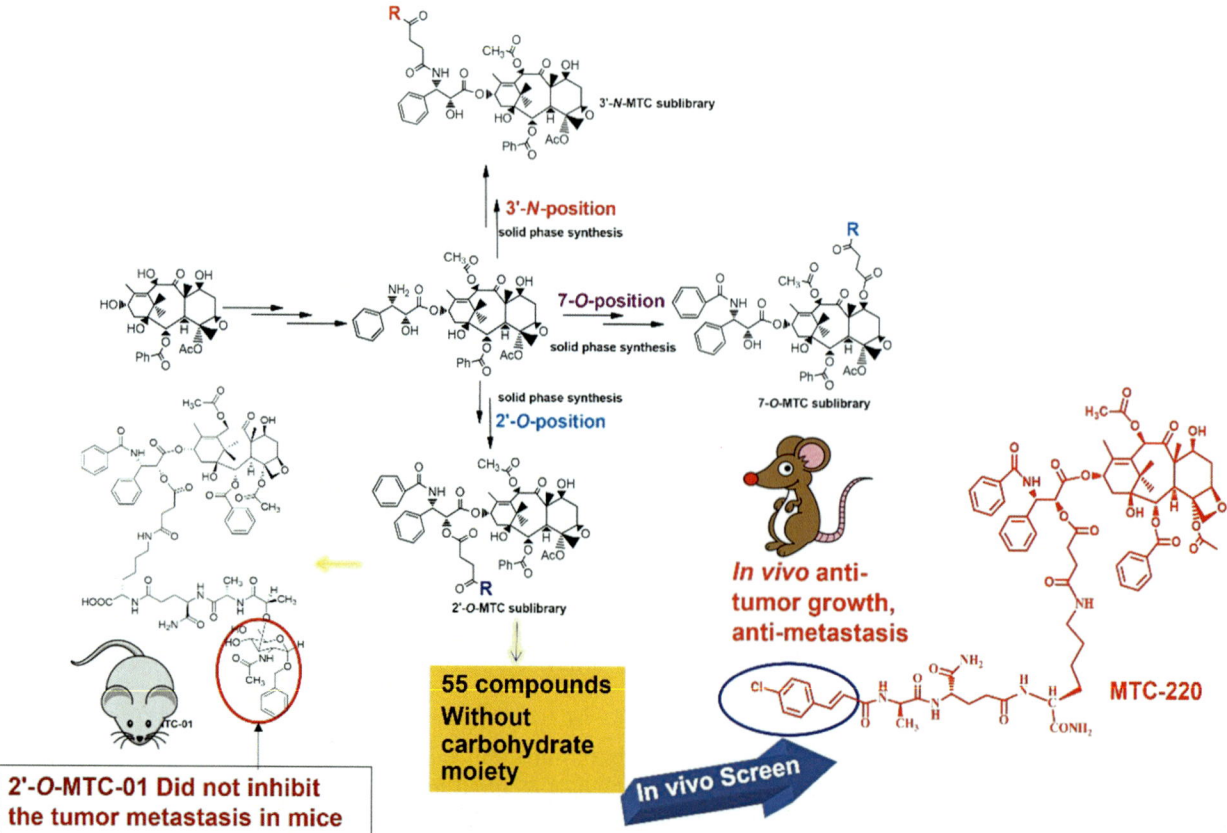

FIGURE 13.39 The chemical library constructed with paclitaxel and MDP\covalent compounds, incorporating modifications at the 2'-O, 3'-N, and 7-O positions of paclitaxel.

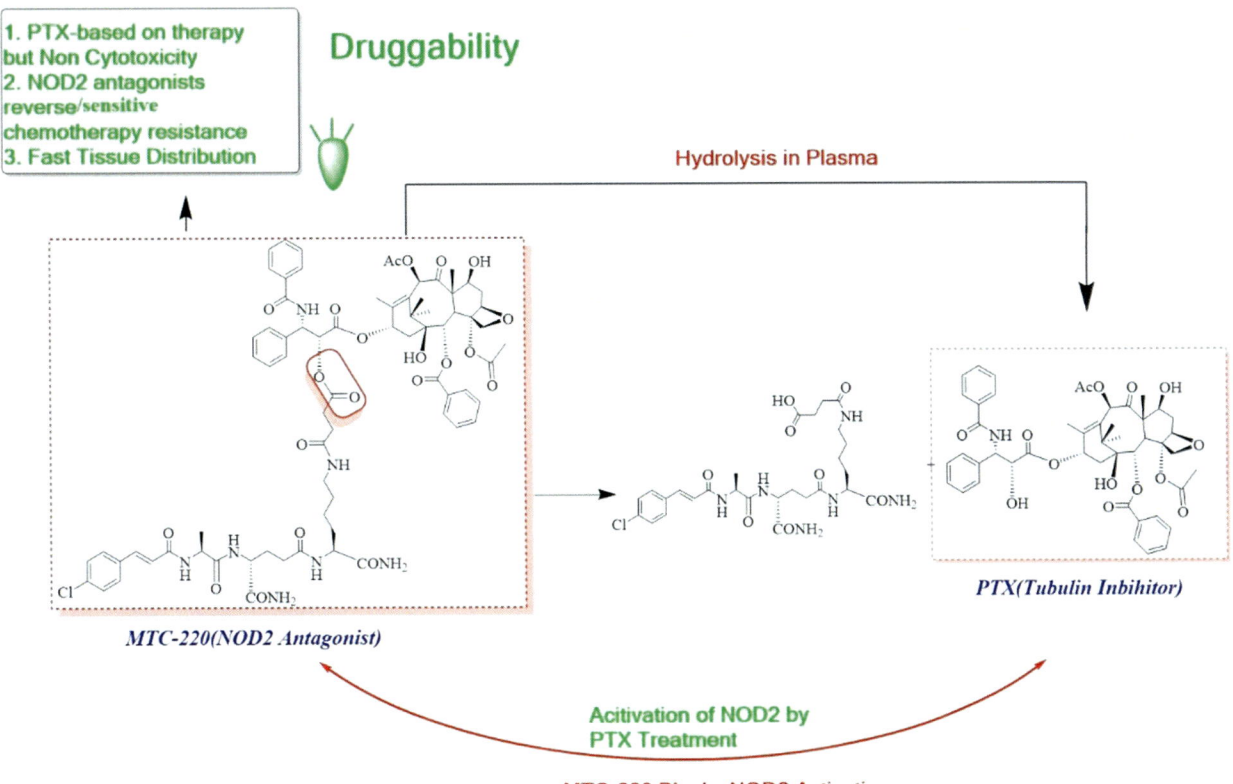

FIGURE 13.40 Schematic illustration of the mechanism of action of Conmutaxel as a prodrug molecule for anticancer activity and inhibition of tumor metastasis.

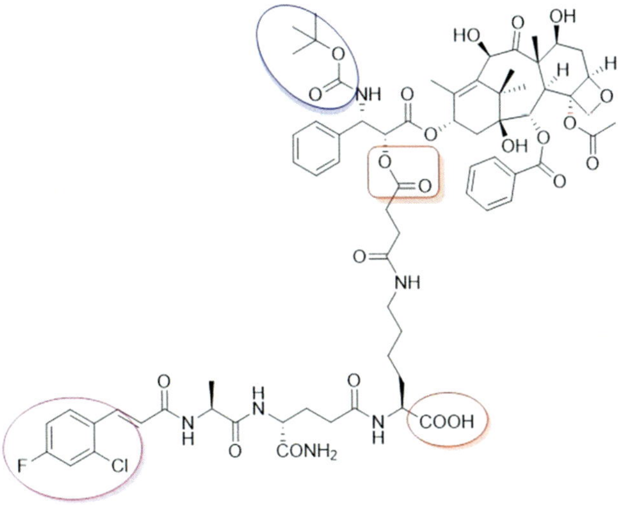

FIGURE 13.41 Molecular structure of docetaxel.

At the moment, the reader may pose the following question: Does Conmutaxel antagonize NOD2 through its prototype molecule or through the released peptide molecule or paclitaxel itself after hydrolysis occurs antagonizing the chemotherapy-activated NOD2 inflammatory signaling pathway? The best approach to addressing this question is to synthesize a nonhydrolyzable prodrug molecule and conduct in vitro and in vivo experiments by coadministering it with paclitaxel. Therefore, Dr. Yi Dong, an expert in organic chemical synthesis, has successfully accomplished the vinylation reaction of the C_2'-hydroxyl group of paclitaxel for the first time and obtained the molecule DY-16−43 (Fig. 13.42), which is connected to the C_2'-hydroxyl group

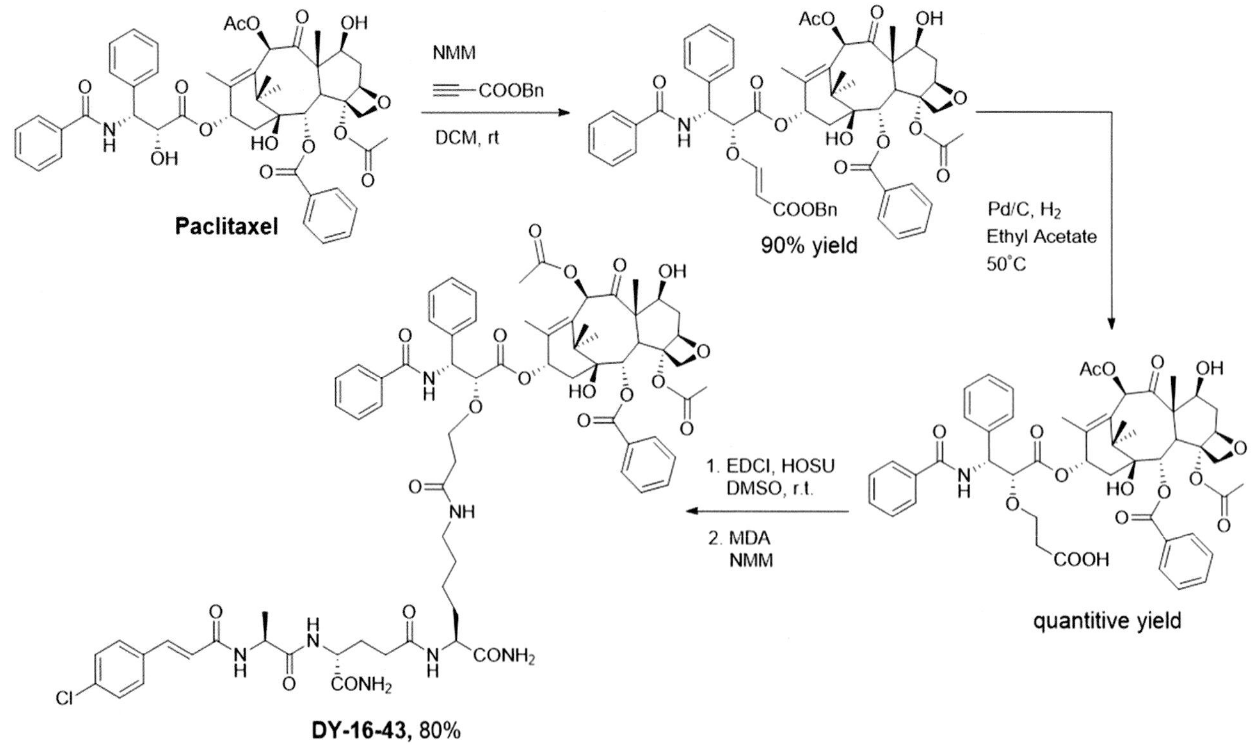

FIGURE 13.42 Synthesis of nonhydrolyzable paclitaxel and MDP conjugate (DY-16−43).

of paclitaxel through an ether linkage using a simple chemical method. This molecule cannot be hydrolyzed by esterases in animal blood, thereby maintaining its complete prototype conjugation structure by coadministering it with paclitaxel. Fig. 13.43 illustrates the antagonistic effect of DY-16−43 on the NOD2 inflammatory signaling pathway, rather than peptides or paclitaxel, significantly enhancing the antitumor growth and metastasis inhibition of paclitaxel [140]. The findings unequivocally demonstrate that NOD2 in macrophages can be activated by damage-associated molecular patterns (DAMPs) produced during paclitaxel chemotherapy. This activation leads to chemotherapy resistance and facilitates tumor metastasis. Simultaneously antagonizing the NOD2 signaling pathway during chemotherapy can improve the therapeutic efficacy against cancer and inhibit tumor metastasis [140]. The verification of this point is greatly supported by the exceptional organic chemical synthesis expertise of the researcher, Dr. Yi Dong.

Fig. 13.43A demonstrates that DY-16−43, rather than MDP derivatives, antagonizes the signal transduction activation of NOD2 in vitro. In Fig. 13.43B, DY-16−43 is shown to antagonize the NOD2 signal transduction activation in 293/hNOD2 cells, exhibiting a clear inhibition of the phosphorylation of RIP2 (p-RIP2). Fig. 13.43C indicates that DY-16-43 significantly enhances the anticancer effect of paclitaxel in mice. Furthermore, Fig. 13.43D illustrates that DY-16-43 noticeably enhances the antitumor metastasis effect of paclitaxel.

Optimally, compared to current paclitaxel formulations (including albumin-bound paclitaxel) or docetaxel injection, Conmutaxel [138] or Salutaxel [139] demonstrates their advantages, including:

1. *Tolerance*: Safety evaluations have shown that Conmutaxel or Salutaxel significantly reduces relative adverse effects, allowing for short-term multiple administrations. This may overcome the limitations of administering paclitaxel or docetaxel injections only once or twice a month.
2. *Adverse Effects Caused by Solvents*: The improved physicochemical properties of the molecules eliminate the need for surfactant polysorbate castor oil in the formulation, significantly decreasing the risks of allergies and hemolysis when administrating in patients.
3. *Target-related Adverse Effects*: Conmutaxel and Salutaxel are primarily distributed and eliminated as prototype drugs. Structure-activity relationship studies reveal that the prototype drugs (with a 2′-position appendage) do not exhibit cytotoxicity; however, they are effectively metabolized into paclitaxel or docetaxel in tumor tissues rich in blood vessels. This process significantly enhances the distribution of both drugs within tumor tissues while minimizing the release of paclitaxel or docetaxel in the bone marrow and normal tissues, thereby significantly reducing neurotoxicity and bone marrow suppression associated with taxanes.

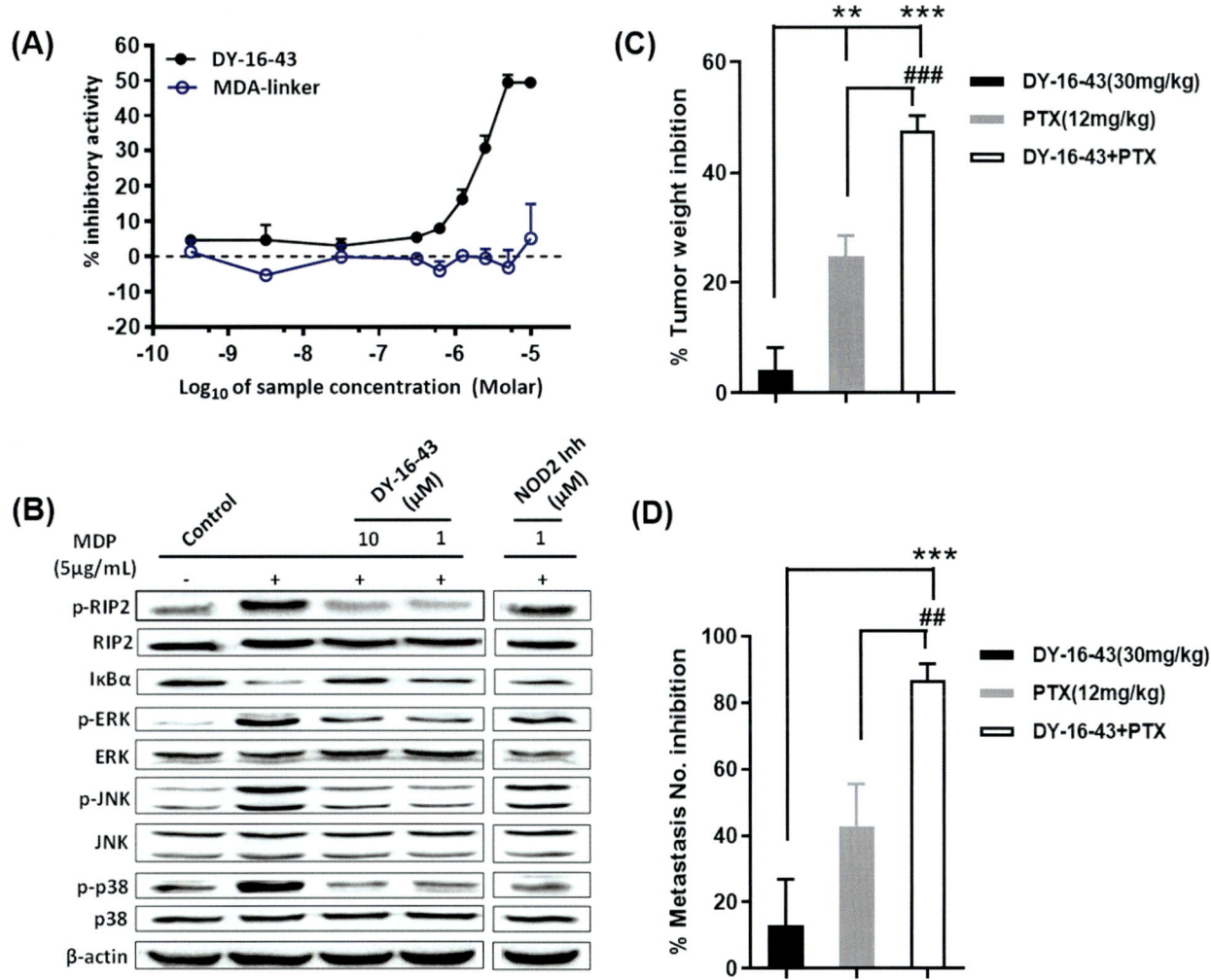

FIGURE 13.43 DY-16-43 antagonizes the chemotherapy-activated NOD2 signaling pathway and inhibits tumor metastasis. (A) Inhibitory response of MDP (5 μg/mL) induced NOD2 activation by DY-16-43 and MDA-linker in HEK-Blue hNOD2 cells. (B) 16-43 inhibits NOD2-mediated NF-B and MAPK signaling in 293/hNOD2 cells. (C, D) 16-43 sensitized the PTX treatment of Lewis lung carcinoma in mice. (C) Tumor weight inhibition rate. (D) Lung metastasis number inhibition rate. Data are shown as the mean ± SEM (n = 10): (**) $p < 0.01$, (***) $p < 0.001$ vs the 16-43 group; (##) $p < 0.01$, (###) $p < 0.001$ vs the PTX group.

4. *Drug Resistance and Metastasis Issues*: Research has shown that chemotherapy can trigger the NF-κB and MAPKs inflammatory signaling pathways through PRRs NOD1/2. Conmutaxel prototype antagonizes the NOD2 signaling pathway, while the Salutaxel prototype antagonizes the NOD1 signaling pathway. Both drugs effectively modulate the tumor inflammatory microenvironment, reversing chemotherapy resistance, significantly enhancing the therapeutic effects of paclitaxel or docetaxel, and inhibiting tumor metastasis.
5. *Tumor Recurrence*: Conmutaxel or Salutaxel may be considered for further combined clinical use with novel immune checkpoint inhibitors, resulting in enhanced efficacy and reduction or postponement of cancer recurrence.
6. *Formulation*: Conmutaxel or Salutaxel are lyophilized powders that can be stored and transported at room temperature, with a long shelf life, avoiding the issues associated with cold chain transportation of taxanes.

The authors of this chapter are currently conducting clinical investigations of Salutaxel. The volunteer selection and enrollment for each dose group in the Phase Ia trial (dose escalation study) have been successfully completed. Phase Ib (dose-expansion study) trials are underway, with a recommended dose of 175 mg/m^2. Research findings demonstrate that intravenous administration of Salutaxel exhibits pharmacokinetic characteristics consistent with animal studies, effectively releasing more docetaxel. Out of the 22 patients with advanced solid tumors who completed tumor assessment, 11 achieved stable disease (SD) and one patient experienced a 26% reduction in tumor size.

Notably, all patients who received a dose of 175 mg/m² demonstrated favorable therapeutic efficacy by achieving SD. We anticipate that Salutaxel will further enhance its effectiveness in benefiting cancer patients, significantly improving patient compliance.

13.4 Summary and outlook

Thanks to the large-scale screening of chemotherapy drugs that began in the 1950s, the NCI in the United States discovered the molecule of natural paclitaxel by establishing high-throughput drug screening assays using various tumor human cancer cells. The first generation of injectable paclitaxel, which was introduced to the market, underwent a 30-year journey during which various challenges were addressed. These challenges included structural identification (chemistry), target identification (biology), formulation issues (pharmacy), industrial synthesis (source), clinical administration routes and methods (such as 3-hour intravenous infusion to achieve tolerable Cmax levels in the bloodstream), clinical safety evaluations, and the balance between patient benefits (medicine). Additionally, the use of combination therapy to enhance treatment efficacy has also been explored. Paclitaxel remains a first-line treatment for many cancer indications till now.

Due to the prominent therapeutic efficacy and notable adverse reactions associated with taxane drugs, various improvements have been continuously pursued, including formulation enhancement, structural modifications, prodrug strategies, and more recently dual-function strategies. Through the content of this chapter, the author not only endeavors to present a comprehensive account of paclitaxel itself to the readers but also aims to showcase the latest advancements in improving taxane drugs, driven by unresolved clinical needs, and to acknowledge the endless pursuit of drug development. Specifically, from the cases presented in this chapter, we not only learn about the structural modifications of traditional or classical natural product drug chemistry but also about the research strategies for Conmutaxel and Salutaxel, which are discussed at the end of the chapter. Researchers have gained several experiences or insights into the development process of Conmutaxel and Salutaxel. (1) The starting point of the hypothesis is crucial. When considering hypotheses, researchers should fully consider clinical unresolved problems or unmet needs that are likely to persist in the long term and propose hypotheses based on existing knowledge to meet the characteristics of the lengthy drug development cycle. For example, metastasis is still the main cause of death in cancer patients. Conmutaxel and Salutaxel, which have been studied for over 20 years, still have great development value because they potentially prevent cancer metastasis and recurrence while inhibiting tumor growth. At this point, readers might question why, despite the article introducing many new molecules of taxanes with activity advantages obtained through structure-activity relationship studies, these have not been developed into drugs, including orally administered taxane molecules? Obviously, these molecules are all based on the microtubule protein target, and while they improve activity, they often come with established on-target adverse effects. The therapeutic window of the drugs has not been significantly improved, in other words, patients do not benefit significantly, and therefore, there is no meaningful continuation of their development. (2) In certain environments or knowledge contexts, reasonable assumptions may not necessarily be correct. For instance, initially, the researchers obtained the shared substructure molecule 2′-O-MTC-01, which was capable of inhibiting tumor growth in animals but did not inhibit tumor metastasis. The researchers devised a unique solid-phase synthesis method that not only fulfilled the requirements for constructing a chemical library of such shared substructures but also ensured an ample supply of compounds (including both the quantity and quality of synthesized compounds) for direct screening in animal models. It was eventually demonstrated that only through this meticulous and labor-intensive extreme phenotype screening approach could Conmutaxel and Salutaxel be discovered. (3) As for the third fundamental question of why activating NOD1/2 cannot inhibit tumor metastasis, when the initial hypothesis was proposed in 2000, there had been limited substantial progress in international research on the tumor and inflammatory microenvironment. Consequently, the researchers only considered the TNF-α factor, presuming that an elevation in TNF-α secretion levels would be sufficient to suppress tumor metastasis. However, they were unaware that inflammation (microenvironment) constitutes the 7th major characteristic of tumors, and they were also unaware of the DAMPs generated by chemotherapy, which can reshape the tumor microenvironment and lead to chemotherapy resistance. At that time, the available knowledge indicated that the response rate of metastatic breast cancer to single-agent paclitaxel therapy was approximately 25%, primarily due to limitations in the dose tolerance of taxane drugs. Later, through the synthesis of appropriate noncleavable docetaxel analog (DY-16−43) and studies conducted using animal models with intact immune function, the initial hypothesis was proven wrong. However, fortunately, the deviation from the intended outcome was not significant. It was found that the research should be focused on antagonists of NOD1/2 rather than the initial choice of agonists. (4) The unique metabolic mechanism of the docetaxel analog in vivo ensured the activation of NOD2 signaling during chemotherapy while simultaneously being antagonized by the prototype molecule. This combination conferred the desired therapeutic effect in animal models and demonstrated significant superiority over albumin-bound paclitaxel (data not shown), along with enhanced safety. Clearly, to validate this point, it was imperative to leverage the researchers' exceptional organic chemistry synthesis skills. Under the premise of preserving the delicate structure of paclitaxel, which is highly sensitive to various organic reaction conditions, the noncleavable docetaxel analog, DY-16−43, was successfully prepared.

Chemical medications will continue to dominate the market and find extensive applications in the future due to their advantages in convenience, low cost, and high patient compliance. Therefore, the authors of this chapter maintain a confident outlook on the development and prospects of anticancer chemotherapy drugs. It must be emphasized once again that drug development should focus on unresolved or unmet clinical need issues, and researchers need to possess the qualities and capabilities to persistently discover and address these challenges. It is believed that the development of successors to taxane-based drugs will not cease. Future advancements will strive to maximize their anticancer activity while minimizing the various adverse effects they may cause, significantly attenuating cancer metastasis and recurrence.

References

[1] Wani MC, Taylor HL, Wall ME, et al. Plant antitumor agents. VI. The isolation and structure of taxol, a novel antileukemic and antitumor agent from *Taxus brevifolia*. J Am Chem Soc 1971;93(9):2325−7.

[2] Schiff PB, Fan J, Horwitz SB. Promotion of microtubule assembly in vitro by taxol. Nature 1979;277(5698):665−7.

[3] Parness J, Horwitz SB. Taxol binds to polymerized tubulin in vitro. J Cell Biol 1981;91(2):479−87.

[4] Manfredi JJ, Parness J, Horwitz SB. Taxol binds to cellular microtubules. J Cell Biol 1982;94(3):688−96.

[5] Schiff PB, Horwitz SB. Taxol stabilizes microtubules in mouse fibroblast cells. Proc Natl Acad Sci USA 1980;77(3):1561−5.

[6] Kavallaris M. Microtubules and resistance to tubulin-binding agents. Nat Rev Cancer 2010;10(3):194−204.

[7] Panda D, Miller HP, Banerjee A, et al. Microtubule dynamics in vitro are regulated by the tubulin isotype composition. Proc Natl Acad Sci USA 1994;91(24):11358−62.

[8] Azuma K, Sasada T, Kawahara A, et al. Expression of ERCC1 and class III beta-tubulin in non-small cell lung cancer patients treated with carboplatin and paclitaxel. Lung Cancer 2009;64(3):326−33.

[9] Sève P, Reiman T, Dumontet C. The role of βIII tubulin in predicting chemoresistance in non-small cell lung cancer. Lung Cancer 2010;67(2):136−43.

[10] Hasegawa S, Miyoshi Y, Egawa C, et al. Prediction of response to docetaxel by quantitative analysis of class I and III β-tubulin isotype mRNA expression in human breast cancers. Clin Cancer Res 2003;9(8):2992−7.

[11] Hetland TE, Hellesylt E, Flørenes VA, et al. Class III β-tubulin expression in advanced-stage serous ovarian carcinoma effusions is associated with poor survival and primary chemoresistance. Hum Pathol 2011;42(7):1019−26.

[12] Gelderblom H, Verweij J, Nooter K, et al. Cremophor EL: the drawbacks and advantages of vehicle selection for drug formulation. Eur J Cancer 2001;37(13):1590−8.

[13] Cabanes A, Briggs KE, Gokhale PC, et al. Comparative in vivo studies with paclitaxel and liposome-encapsulated paclitaxel. Int J Oncol 1998;12(5):1035−40.

[14] Aapro MS, Minckwitz GV. Molecular basis for the development of novel taxanes in the treatment of metastatic breast cancer. Eur J Cancer Suppl 2008;6(10):3−11.

[15] Desai N, Trieu V, Damascelli B, et al. SPARC expression correlates with tumor response to albumin-bound paclitaxel in head and neck cancer patients. Transl Oncol 2009;2(2):59−64.

[16] Ibrahim NK, Deasi N, Legha S, et al. Phase I and pharmacokinetic study of ABI-007, a Cremophor-free, protein-stabilized, nanoparticle formulation of paclitaxel. Clin Cancer Res 2002;8(5):1038−44.

[17] Ibrahim NK, Samuels B, Page R, et al. Multicenter Phase II trial of ABI-007, an albumin-bound paclitaxel, in women with metastatic breast cancer. J Clin Oncol 2005;23(25):6019−26.

[18] Gradishar WJ, Tjulandin S, Davidson N, et al. Phase III trial of nanoparticle albumin-bound paclitaxel compared with polyethylated castor oil-based paclitaxel in women with breast cancer. J Clin Oncol 2005;23(31):7794−803.

[19] Parisi A, Palluzzi E, Cortellini A, et al. First-line carboplatin/nab-paclitaxel in advanced ovarian cancer patients, after hypersensitivity reaction to solvent-based taxanes: a single-institution experience. Clin Transl Oncol 2019;22(1):158−62.

[20] Socinski MA, Bondarenko I, Karaseva NA, et al. Weekly nab-paclitaxel in combination with carboplatin versus solvent-based paclitaxel plus carboplatin as first-line therapy in patients with advanced non-small-cell lung cancer: final results of a phase III trial. J Clin Oncol 2012;30(17):2055−62.

[21] Gong C, Xie Y, Wu Q, et al. Improving anti-tumor activity with polymeric micelles entrapping paclitaxel in pulmonary carcinoma. Nanoscale 2012;4(19):6004−17.

[22] Lundberg BB, Risovic V, Ramaswamy M, et al. A lipophilic paclitaxel derivative incorporated in a lipid emulsion for parenteral administration. J Control Release 2003;86(1):93−100.

[23] Yu SL, Zhang YJ, Wang X, et al. Synthesis of paclitaxel conjugated β-cyclodextrin polyrotaxane and its antitumor activity. Angew Chem Int Ed 2013;52(28):7272−7.

[24] https://ir.athenex.com/news-releases/news-release-details/athenex-announces-oral-paclitaxel-and-encequidar-had.

[25] De Weger VA, Sturman FE, Koolen SLW, et al. A phase I dose escalation study of once-weekly oral administration of Docetaxel as ModraDoc001 capsule or ModraDoc006 tablet in combination with Ritonavir. Clin Cancer Res 2019;25(18):5466–74.

[26] Vermunt MAC, De Veger VA, Janssen JM, et al. Effect of food on the pharmacokinetics of the oral docetaxel tablet formulation ModraDoco06 combined with Ritonavir (ModraDoco06/r) in patients with advanced solid tumors. Drugs R&D 2021;21:103–11.

[27] De Bono JS, Oudard S, Ozguroglu M, et al. Prednisone plus cabazitaxel or mitoxantrone for metastatic castration-resistant prostate cancer progressing after docetaxel treatment: a randomized open-label trial. Lancet 2010;376(9747):1147–54.

[28] Paller CJ, Aantonarakis ES. Cabazitaxel: a novel second line treatment for metastatic castration-resistant prostate cancer. Drug Des Devel Ther 2011;5:117–24.

[29] Gelmon KA, Latreille J, Tolcher A, et al. Phase I dose-finding study of a new taxane, RPR 109881A, administered as a one-hour intravenous infusion days 1 and 8 to patients with advanced solid tumors. J Clin Oncol 2000;18(24):4098–108.

[30] Bissery MC. Preclinical evaluation of new toxoids. Curr Pharm Des 2001;7(13):1251–7.

[31] Bissery MC, Vrignaud P, Combeau C, et al. Preclinical evaluation of XRP9881A, a new toxoid. Cancer Res 2004;64(7_Supplement):1253.

[32] Kurata T, Shimada Y, Tamura T, et al. Phase I and pharmacokinetic study of a new toxoid, RPR 109881A, given as a 1-hour intravenous infusion in patients with advanced solid tumors. J Clin Oncol 2000;18(17):3164–71.

[33] Dieras V, Valero V, Limentani S, et al. Multicenter, non-randomized Phase II study with RPR109881 in taxane-exposed metastatic breast cancer (MBC) patients (pts): final results. J Clin Oncol 2005;23(16_suppl):565.

[34] Zatloukal P, Gervais R, Vansteenkiste J, et al. Randomized multicenter phase II study of larotaxel (XRP9881) in combination with cisplatin or gemcitabine as first-line chemotherapy in nonirradiable stage IIIB or stage III non-small cell lung cancer. J Thorax Oncol 2008;3(8):894–901.

[35] Sampath D, Discafani CM, Loganzo F, et al. MAC-321, a novel taxane with greater efficacy than paclitaxel and docetaxel in vitro and in vivo. Mol Cancer Ther 2003;2(9):873–84.

[36] Lockhart AC, Bukowski R, Rothenberg ML, et al. Phase I trial of oral MAC-321 in subjects with advanced malignant solid tumors. Cancer Chemother Pharmacol 2007;60:203–9.

[37] Mekhail T, Serwatowski P, Dudek A, et al. A Phase II study of intravenous (III) milataxel (M) for the treatment of non-small cell lung cancer (NSCLC) refractory to platinum-based therapy. J Clin Oncol 2006;24(18_suppl):7098.

[38] Helson L, Ferrara J, Jones M, et al. NBT-287, a third generation taxane analog, and paclitaxel resistance due to MDR-1 and mutant tubulin. J Clin Oncol 2004;22(14_suppl):3114.

[39] Hwang JJ, Marshall JL, Ahmed T, et al. A phase I study of TPI287: a third generation taxane administered weekly in patients with advanced cancer. J Clin Oncol 2007;25(18_Suppl):2575.

[40] Modiano MR, Plezia P, Baram J, et al. A Phase I study of TPI 287, a third generation taxane, administered every 21 days in patients with advanced cancer. Proc Am Soc Clin Oncol 2007;25(18):2569.

[41] Glasspool RM, Boddy AV, Evans TR, et al. A Phase I study of a novel taxane, TL310, orally administered every week in patients (pts) with advanced solid tumors. Proc Am Soc Clin Oncol 2007;25(18):2544.

[42] Longley RE, Clement C, Metts L, et al. In vivo efficacy of TL-310; a new, orally active taxane analog. Cancer Res 2006;66(8_Supplement):120.

[43] Altstadt TJ, Fairchild CR, Golik J, et al. Synthesis and antitumor activity of novel C-7 paclitaxel ethers: discovery of BMS-184476. J Med Chem 2001;44(26):4577–83.

[44] Hidalgo M, Aylesworth C, Hammond LA, et al. Phase I and pharmacokinetic study of BMS-184476, a taxane with greater potency and solubility than paclitaxel. J Clin Oncol 2001;19(9):2493–503.

[45] Camps C, Felip E, Sanchez JM, et al. Phase II trial of the novel taxane BMS-184476 as second-line in non-small-cell lung cancer. Ann Oncol 2005;16(4):597–601.

[46] Plummer R, Ghielmini M, Calvert P, et al. Phase I and pharmacokinetic study of the new taxane analog BMS-184476 given weekly in patients with advanced malignancies. Clin Cancer Res 2002;8(9):2788–97.

[47] Sun W, Stevenson JP, Gallagher ML, et al. Phase I and pharmacokinetic trial of the novel taxane BMS-184476 administered as a 1-hour intravenous infusion in combination with cisplatin every 21 days. Clin Cancer Res 2003;9(14):5221–7.

[48] Sessa C, Perotti A, Salvatorelli E, et al. Phase IB and pharmacological study of the novel taxane BMS-184476 in combination with doxorubicin. Eur J Cancer 2004;40(4):563–70.

[49] Garrett CR, Fishmann MN, Rago RR, et al. Phase I study of a novel taxane BMS-188797 in adult patients with solid malignancies. Clin Cancer Res 2005;11(9):3335–41.

[50] Advani R, Fisher GA, Lum BL, et al. Phase I and pharmacokinetic study of BMS-188797, a new taxane analog, administered on a weekly schedule in patients with advanced malignancies. Clin Cancer Res 2003;9(14):5187–94.

[51] Mastalerz H, Cook D, Fairchild CR, et al. The discovery of BMS-275183: an orally efficacious novel taxane. Bioorg Med Chem 2003;11(30):4315–23.

[52] Rose WC, Long BH, Fairchild CR, et al. Preclinical pharmacology of Bms-275183, an orally active taxane. Clin Cancer Res 2001;7(7):2016–21.

[53] Broker LE, De Vos FY, Van Groeningen CJ, et al. Phase I trial with BMS-275183, a novel oral taxane with promising antitumor activity. Clin Cancer Res 2006;12(6):1760–7.

[54] Ojima I, Park YH, Sun CM, et al. Structure-activity relationships of new taxoids derived from 14 beta-hydroxy-10-deacetylbaccatin III. J Med Chem 1994;37(10):1408–10.
[55] Distefano M, Scambia G, Ferlini C, et al. Anti-proliferative activity of a new class of taxanes (14beta-hydroxy-10-deacetylbaccatin III derivatives) on multidrug-resistance-positive human cancer cells. Int J Cancer 1997;72(6):844–50.
[56] Nicoletti MI, Colombo T, Rossi C, et al. IDN5109, a taxane with oral bioavailability and potent antitumor activity. Cancer Res 2000;60 (4):842–6.
[57] Cassinelli G, Lanzi C, Supino R, et al. Cellular bases of the antitumor activity of the novel taxane IDN 5109 (BAY59-8862) on hormone-refractory prostate cancer. Clin Cancer Res 2002;8(8):2647–54.
[58] Moore MR, Jones C, Harker G, et al. Phase II trial of DJ-927, an oral tubulin depolymerization inhibitor, in the treatment of metastatic colorectal cancer. J Clin Oncol 2006;24(18_suppl):3591.
[59] Szczesna A, Milanowski E, Juhász E, et al. A Phase II study of DJ-927 administered orally once every three weeks as second line therapy to subjects with locally advanced or metastatic non-small cell lung cancer (NSCLC) after failure of platinum-based non-taxane regimen. J Clin Oncol 2006;24(18_suppl):17006.
[60] Shionoya M, Jimbo T, Kitagawa M, et al. DJ-927, a novel oral taxane, overcomes P-glycoprotein-mediated multidrug resistance in vitro and in vivo. Cancer Sci 2003;94(5):459–66.
[61] Stone R. Surprise! A fungus factory for taxol. Science 1993;260(5105):154–5.
[62] Han KH. Genetic transformation of mature Taxus: an approach to genetically control the in vitro production of the anticancer drug. Plant Sci 1994;95(2):187–96.
[63] Zhang JZ, Zhang LH, Wang XH, et al. Microbial transformation of 10-deacetyl-7-epitaxol and 1-β-hydroxybaccatin I by fungi from the inner bark of Taxus yunnanensis. J Nat Prod 1998;61(4):497–500.
[64] Strobel GA, Yang XS, Sears J, et al. Taxol from pestalotiopsis microspore, an endophytic fungus of *Taxuus wallachiana*. Microbiology 1996;142(Pt 2):435–40.
[65] Nicolaou KC, Yang Z, Liu JJ, et al. Total synthesis of taxol. Nature 1994;367(6464):630–4.
[66] Nicolaou KC, Nantermet PG, Ueno H, et al. Total synthesis of taxol. J Am Chem Soc 1995;117(2):624–59.
[67] Holton RA, Juo RR, Kim HB, et al. A synthesis of taxusin. J Am Chem Soc 1988;110(19):6558–60.
[68] Holton RA, Somoza C, Kim HB, et al. First total synthesis of taxol. 1. Functionalization of the B ring. J Am Chem Soc 1994;116(4):1597–8.
[69] Holton RA, Kim HB, Somoza C, et al. First total synthesis of taxol. 2. Completion of C and D rings. J Am Chem Soc 1994;116(4):1599–600.
[70] Danishefsky SJ, Masters JJ, Young WB, et al. Total synthesis of baccatin III and taxol. J Am Chem Soc 1996;118(12):2843–59.
[71] Wender PA, Badham NF, Conway SP, et al. The pinene path to taxanes. 5. Stereocontrolled synthesis of a versatile taxane precursor. J Am Chem Soc 1997;119(11):2755–6.
[72] Wender PA, Badham NF, Conway SP, et al. The pinene path to taxanes. 6. A concise stereocontrolled synthesis of taxol. J Am Chem Soc 1997;119(11):2757–8.
[73] Morihira K, Hara R, Kawahara S, et al. Enantioselective total synthesis of taxol. J Am Chem Soc 1998;120(49):12980–1.
[74] Kusama H, Hara R, Kawahara S, et al. Enantioselective total synthesis of taxol. J Am Chem Soc 2000;122(16):3811–20.
[75] Mukaiyama T, Shiina I, Iwadare H, et al. Asymmetric total synthesis of taxol. Chem Eur J 1999;5(1):121–61.
[76] Denis JN, Greene AE, Guenard D, et al. Highly efficient, practical approach to natural taxol. J Am Chem Soc 1988;110(17):5917–19.
[77] Holton, R.A. Eur. Pat. Appl. EP 1990, 400971.
[78] Commercon A, Bérnard D, Bernard F, et al. Improved protection and esterification of a precursor of the taxotere® and taxol side chains. Tetrahedron Lett 1992;33(36):5185–8.
[79] Kingston D, Chordia MD, Jagtap PG, et al. Synthesis and biological evaluation of 1-deoxypaclitaxel analogues. J Org Chem 1999;64 (6):1814–22.
[80] Chen S, Wei J, Farina V. Taxol structure-activity relationships: synthesis and biological evaluation of 2-deoxytaxol. Tetrahedron Lett 1993;34 (20):3205–6.
[81] Chaudhary AG, Chordia MD, Kingston DG. A novel benzoyl group migration: synthesis and biological evaluation of 1-benzoyl-2des(benzoyloxy)paclitaxel. J Org Chem 1995;60(10):3260–2.
[82] Chen H, Farina V, Wei J, et al. Structure-activity relationships of Taxol: synthesis and biological evaluation of C2 Taxol analogs. Bioorg Med Chem Lett 1994;4(3):479–82.
[83] Chordia MD, Kingston DG. Synthesis and biological evaluation of 2-*epi*-paclitaxel. J Org Chem 1996;61(2):799–801.
[84] Chaudhary AG, Gharpure MM, Rimoldi JM, et al. Unexpectedly facile hydrolysis of the 2-benzoate group of taxol and syntheses of analogs with increased activities. J Am Chem Soc 1994;116(9):4097–8.
[85] Kingston DGI, Chaudhary AG, Chordia MD, et al. Synthesis and biological evaluation of 2-acyl analogues of paclitaxel (taxol). J Med Chem 1998;41(19):3715–26.
[86] Georg GI, Ali SM, Boge TC, et al. Selective C-2 and C-4 deacylation and acylation of Taxol: the first synthesis of a C-4 substituted Taxol analogue. Tetrahedron Lett 1994;35(48):8931–4.
[87] Chen S, Kadow JF, Farina V. First syntheses of novel paclitaxel (Taxol) analogs modified at the C4-position. J Org Chem 1994;59 (21):6156–8.
[88] Chordia MD, Chaudhary AG, Kingston DGI. Synthesis and biological evaluation of 4-deacetoxypaclitaxel. Tetrahedron Lett 1994;35 (37):6843–6.

[89] Neidigh KA, Gharpure MM, Rimoldi JM, et al. Synthesis and biological evaluation of 4-deacetoxypaclitaxel. Tetrahedron Lett 1994;35 (37):6839–42.

[90] Chen S, Wei J, Long B, et al. Novel C-4 paclitaxel (taxol®) analogs: potent antitumor agents. Bioorg Med Chem Lett 1995;5(22):2741–6.

[91] Barboni L, Datta A, Dutta D, et al. Novel d-seco paclitaxel analogues: synthesis, biological evaluation, and model testing. J Org Chem 2001;66 (10):3321–9.

[92] Chaudhary AG, Rimoldi JM, Kingston DGI. Modified taxols. 10. Preparation of 7-deoxytaxol, a highly bioactive taxol derivative, and interconversion of taxol and 7-epi-taxol. J Org Chem 1993;58(15):3798–9.

[93] Chen S, Huang S, Kant J, et al. Synthesis of 7-deoxy- and 7,10-dideoxytaxol via radical intermediates. J Org Chem 1993;58(19):5028–9.

[94] Chen S, Fairchild C, Mamber SW, et al. Taxol structure-activity relationships: synthesis and biological evaluation of 10-deoxytaxol. J Org Chem 1993;58(11):2927–8.

[95] Kingston DGI. The chemistry of taxol. Pharmacol Ther 1991;52(1):1–34.

[96] Cheng Q, Oritani T, Horiguchi T. The synthesis and biological activity of 9- and 2'-cAMP 7-deoxypaclitaxel analogues from 5-cinnamoyltriacetyltaxicin-I. Tetrahedron 2000;56(12):1667–79.

[97] He L, Jagtap PG, Kingston DGI, et al. A common pharmacophore for taxol and the epothilones based on the biological activity of a taxane molecule lacking a C-13 side chain. Biochemistry 2000;39(14):3972–8.

[98] Chen S, Farina V, Vyas DM, et al. Synthesis and biological evaluation of C-13 amide-linked paclitaxel (taxol) analogs. J Org Chem 1996;61 (6):2065–70.

[99] Mellado W, Magri NF, Kingston DGI, et al. Preparation and biological activity of taxol acetates. Biochem Biophys Res Commun 1984;124(2):329–36.

[100] Kant J, Schwartz WS, Fairchild C, et al. Diastereoselective addition of Grignard reagents to azetidine-2,3-dione: synthesis of novel taxol® analogues. Tetrahedron Lett 1996;37(36):6495–8.

[101] Barboni L, Lambertucci C, Ballini R, et al. Synthesis of a conformationally restricted analogue of paclitaxel. Tetrahedron Lett 1998;39 (39):7177–80.

[102] Swindell CS, Krauss NE, Horwitz SB, et al. Biologically active taxol analogs with deleted A-ring side chain substituents and variable C-2' configurations. J Med Chem 1991;34(3):1176–84.

[103] Ojima I, Slater JC, Michaud E, et al. Syntheses and structure-activity relationships of the second-generation antitumor toxoids: exceptional activity against drug-resistant cancer cells. J Med Chem 1996;39(20):3889–96.

[104] Gueritte-Voegelein F, Guenard D, Lavelle F, et al. Relationships between the structure of taxol analogs and their antimitotic activity. J Med Chem 1991;34(3):992–8.

[105] Ojima I, Duclos O, Zucco M, et al. Synthesis and structure-activity relationships of new antitumor toxoids. Effects of cyclohexyl substitution at the C-3' and/or C-2 of taxotere (docetaxel). J Med Chem 1994;37(16):2602–8.

[106] Botta M, Armaroli S, Castagnolo D, et al. Synthesis and biological evaluation of new toxoids derived from 2-deacetoxytaxinine. Bioorg Med Chem Lett 2007;17(6):1579–83.

[107] Harriman GCB, Jalluri RK, Granewald GL, et al. The chemistry of the taxane diterpene: stereoselective synthesis of 10-deacetoxy-11,12-epoxypaclitaxel. Tetrahedron Lett 1995;36(49):8909–12.

[108] Yuan H, Kingston DGI, Long BH, et al. Synthesis and biological evaluation of C-1 and ring modified A-norpaclitaxels. Tetrahedron 1999;55 (30):9089–100.

[109] Ojima I, Kuduk SD, Chakrakravarty S, et al. A novel approach to the study of solution structures and dynamic behavior of paclitaxel and docetaxel using fluorine-containing analogs as probes. J Am Chem Soc 1997;119(24):5519–27.

[110] Ojima I, Lin S, Chakravarty S, et al. Syntheses and structure-activity relationships of nover nor-seco taxoids. J Org Chem 1998;63 (5):1637–45.

[111] Samaranayake G, Magri NF, Jitrangsri C, et al. Modified taxols. 5. Reaction of taxol with electrophilic reagents and preparation of a rearranged taxol derivative with tubulin assembly activity. J Org Chem 1991;56(17):5114–19.

[112] Kingston DGI. Studies on the chemistry of taxol®. Pure Appl Chem 1998;70(2):331–4.

[113] Liang X, Kingston DGI, Long BH, et al. Paclitaxel analogs modified in ring C: synthesis and biological evaluation. Tetrahedron 1997;53 (10):3441–56.

[114] Appemdino G, Danieli B, Jakupovic J, et al. Synthesis and evaluation of C-seco paclitaxel analogues. Tetrahedron Lett 1997;38(24):4273–6.

[115] Wang M, Cornett B, Nettles J, et al. The oxetane ring in taxol. J Org Chem 2000;65(4):1059–68.

[116] Marder-Karsenti R, Dubois J, Bricard L, et al. Synthesis and biological evaluation of D-ring-modified taxanes: 5(20)-azadocetaxel analogs. J Org Chem 1997;62(19):6631–7.

[117] Dubois J, Thoret S, Guéritte F, et al. Synthesis of 5(20)deoxydocetaxel, a new active docetaxel analogue. Tetrahedron Lett 2000;41 (18):3331–4.

[118] Gunatilaka AAL, Ramdayal FD, Sarragiotto MH, et al. Synthesis and biological evaluation of novel paclitaxel (Taxol) D-ring modified analogues. J Org Chem 1999;64(8):2694–703.

[119] Barboni L, Giarlo G, Ricciutelli M, et al. Synthesis, modeling, and anti-tubulin activity of a D-seco paclitaxel analogue. Org Lett 2004;6 (4):461–4.

[120] Deka V, Dunois J, Thoret S, et al. Deletion of the oxetane ring in docetaxel analogues: synthesis and biological evaluation. Org Lett 2003;5 (26):5031–4.

[121] Mathew AE, Mejillano MR, Nath JP, et al. Synthesis and evaluation of some water-soluble prodrugs and derivatives of taxol with antitumor activity. J Med Chem 1992;35(1):145−51.
[122] Ueda Y, Mikkilineni AB, Knipe JO, et al. Novel water soluble phosphate prodrugs of taxol possessing in vivo antitumor activity. Bioorg Med Chem Lett 1993;3(8):1761−6.
[123] Damen EWP, Wiegerinck PHG, Braamer L, et al. Paclitaxel esters of malic acid as prodrugs with improved water solubility. Bioorg Med Chem 2000;8(2):427−32.
[124] Greenwald RB, Gilbert CW, Pendri A, et al. Drug delivery systems: water soluble taxol 2'-poly(ethylene glycol) ester prodrugs—Design and in vivo effectiveness. J Med Chem 1996;39(2):424−31.
[125] Feng X, Yuan Y, Wu J. Synthesis and evaluation of water-soluble paclitaxel prodrugs. Bioorg Med Chem Lett 2002;12(22):3301−3.
[126] Li C, Yu DF, Newman RA, et al. Complete regression of well-established tumors using a novel water-soluble poly(L-glutamic acid)-paclitaxel conjugate. Cancer Res 1998;58(11):2404−9.
[127] Singer JW, Baker B, De Vries P, et al. Poly-(L)-glutamic acid-paclitaxel (CT-2103) [Xyotax], a biodegradable polymeric drug conjugate: characterization, preclinical pharmacology, and preliminary clinical data. Adv Exp Med Biol 2003;519:81−99.
[128] Sabbatini P, Aghajanian C, Dizon D, et al. Phase II study of CT-2103 in patients with recurrent epithelial ovarian, fallopian tube, or primary peritoneal carcinoma. J Clin Oncol 2004;22(22):4523−31.
[129] Richards DA, Richards P, Bodkin D, et al. Efficacy and safety of paclitaxel poliglumex as first-line chemotherapy in patients at high risk with advanced-stage non-small-cell lung cancer: results of a Phase II study. Clin Lung Cancer 2005;7(3):215−20.
[130] Lin Y, Tungpradit R, Sinchaikul S, et al. Targeting the delivery of glycan-based paclitaxel prodrugs to cancer cell via glucose transporters. J Med Chem 2008;51(23):7428−41.
[131] De Groot FMH, Van Berkom LWA, Scheeren HW. Synthesis and biological evaluation of 2'-carbamate-linked and 2'-carbonate-linked prodrugs of paclitaxel: selective activation by the tumor-associated protease plasmin. J Med Chem 2000;43(16):3093−102.
[132] Damen EWP, Nevalainen TJ, Van Den Bergh TJM, et al. Synthesis of novel paclitaxel prodrugs designed for bioreductive activation in hypoxic tumour tissue. Bioorg Med Chem 2002;10(1):71−7.
[133] Chen X, Plasencia C, Hou Y, et al. Synthesis and biological evaluation of dimeric RGD peptide-paclitaxel conjugate as a model for integrin-targeted drug delivery. J Med Chem 2005;48(4):1098−106.
[134] Sparreboom AW, Verweij AC, Zabelina J, et al. Disposition of docosahexaenoic acid-paclitaxel, a novel taxane, in blood: in vitro and clinical pharmacokinetic studies. Clin Cancer Res 2003;9(1):51−159.
[135] Li X, Yu J, Xu S, et al. Chemical conjugation of muramyl dipeptide and paclitaxel to explore the combination of immunotherapy and chemotherapy for cancer. Glycoconjugate J 2008;25(5):415−25.
[136] Ding AH, Porteu F, Sanchez E, et al. Shared actions of endotoxin and taxol on TNF receptors and TNF release. Science 1990;248 (4953):370−2.
[137] Yang S, Tamai R, Akashi S, et al. Synergistic effect of muramyldipeptide with lipopolysaccharide or lipoteichoic acid to induce inflammatory cytokines in human monocytic cells in culture. Infect Immun 2001;69(4):2045−53.
[138] Ma Y, Zhao N, Liu G. Conjugated (MTC-220) of muramyl dipeptide analogue and paclitaxel prevents both tumor growth and metastasis in mice. J Med Chem 2011;54(8):2767−77.
[139] Wen X, Zheng P, Ma Y, et al. Salutaxel, a conjugate of docetaxel and a muramyl dipeptide (MDP) analogue, acts as multifunctional prodrug that inhibits tumor growth and metastasis. J Med Chem 2018;61(4):1519−40
[140] Dong Y, Wang S, Wang C, et al. Antagonizing NOD2 signaling with conjugates of paclitaxel and muramyl dipeptide derivatives sensitizes paclitaxel therapy and significantly prevents tumor metastasis. J Med Chem 2017;60(3):1219−24.

Chapter 14

Antitumor drug eribulin

Yefeng Tang[1], Tianwen Sun[2] and Hai Shang[3]
[1]School of Pharmaceutical Sciences, Tsinghua University, Beijing, P.R. China, [2]Jiangsu Simcere Pharmaceutical Co., Ltd., Nanjing, Jiangsu, P.R. China, [3]Institute of Medicinal Plant Development, Chinese Academy of Medical Sciences and Peking Union Medical College, Beijing, P.R. China

Chapter outline

14.1 Introduction	327
14.2 Antitumor mechanism of eribulin	328
14.2.1 Structure and function of microtubules	328
14.2.2 Tubulin inhibitors	329
14.2.3 The mechanism of action of eribulin	329
14.3 The development process of eribulin	330
14.3.1 Discovery and chemical synthesis of antitumor natural product halichondrin B	330
14.3.2 Study on the structure-activity relationship of halichondrin B - discovery process of eribulin	333
14.3.3 Study on the process chemistry of eribulin	336
14.4 Pharmacological characteristics of eribulin	342
14.4.1 Pharmacodynamics of eribulin	342
14.4.2 Pharmacokinetics and toxicology of eribulin	343
14.5 Clinical research and safety evaluation of eribulin	343
14.5.1 Clinical research of eribulin	343
14.5.2 Adverse effects of eribulin	344
14.6 Conclusion	345
References	346

14.1 Introduction

Cancer is a serious disease that poses a significant threat to human health and safety. According to the statistics from the International Agency for Research on Cancer in 2020 [1], there were more than 19 million new cancer cases worldwide in 2019, resulting in nearly 10 million deaths. Indeed, cancer has become the first or second leading cause of mortality among individuals under 70 years old. Additionally, among the 36 types of cancer included in the statistics, breast cancer, lung cancer, and colorectal cancer are the top three with the highest incidence rates.

Antitumor drugs are effective weapons to fight against cancer. Natural products are secondary metabolites produced by living organisms (such as plants, animals, or microorganisms) through natural selection during the process of evolution. They often possess novel chemical structures and diverse biological activities. Natural products have been recognized as an important source for discovering antitumor drugs. According to statistical data [2], approximately 60% of small molecule antitumor drugs launched between 1981 and 2019 are derived from or closely related to natural products, among which representative examples include paclitaxel, vinblastine, trabectedin, and eribulin.

Eribulin (1, also known as Halaven) is a novel small-molecule chemotherapeutic agent developed by Eisai Pharmaceuticals (Fig. 14.1). Clinically, it is administered in the form of mesylate salt, namely eribulin mesylate [3]. As a potent tubulin inhibitor, eribulin exerts its antitumor effect by inhibiting tubulin polymerization and microtubules' assembly, thereby inducing cell cycle arrest at the G2/M phase in cancer cells. In 2010, eribulin was approved by the U.S. Food and Drug Administration (FDA) as a single-agent chemotherapy drug for the treatment of patients with locally advanced or metastatic breast cancer who had previously received at least two chemotherapy regimens (anthracycline or taxane). Subsequently, it gained approval for marketing in multiple countries and regions, including Europe, the Americas, and Asia. In 2019, eribulin was officially approved in China by the National Medical Products Administration. Recently, the indications for eribulin have been expanded to various other cancers such as soft tissue sarcoma and liposarcoma.

Eribulin is a simplified analog of the marine natural product halichondrin B [4]. Although the structure of eribulin has been greatly simplified compared to halichondrin B, it still possesses a complex molecular framework, consisting of

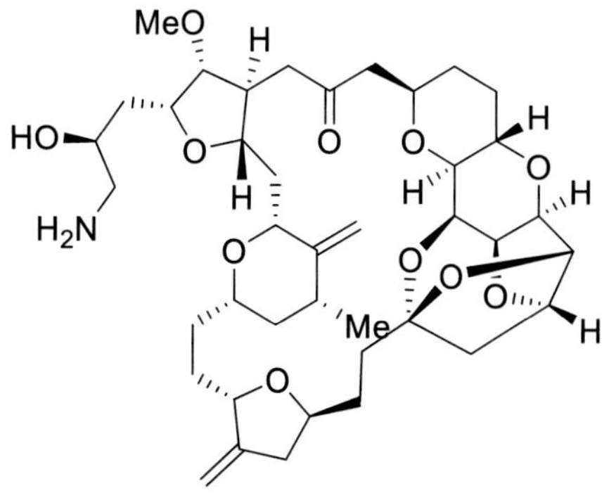

FIGURE 14.1 The structure and fundamental information of eribulin.

Drug name	Eribulin mesylate
Trade name	Halaven
Original manufacturer	Eisai
Drug type	Cancer chemotherapy drugs (Tubulin inhibitors)
Indications	Metastatic breast cancer, liposarcoma
Dosage form/ Administration route	Injection/intravenous drip
Approved countries	United States, Europe, Japan, India, China, etc.

nine-ring systems and nineteen chiral centers, which renders it an extremely complex and challenging synthetic target. It is worth noting that eribulin cannot be obtained through either extraction from natural sources or semisynthesis. In addition, biosynthesis is also not applicable to it. That means chemical synthesis is the sole method to access eribulin. Indeed, eribulin is currently the most complex nonpeptide small molecule drug obtained through chemical synthesis [5] and thus has been recognized as the "Mount Everest" of chemical synthesis in the pharmaceutical research area. Among the currently known antitumor drugs, eribulin stands out due to its unusual development process, which not only highlights the crucial role of synthetic chemists in drug discovery but also showcases the remarkable courage and ingenuity of humanity in recognizing and reforming nature. This chapter will provide a detailed account of the development process of eribulin, including its discovery, chemical synthesis, antitumor mechanism, pharmacological characteristics, and clinical applications, which enables readers to acquire a comprehensive understanding of this unique antitumor agent.

14.2 Antitumor mechanism of eribulin

For an improved comprehension of the antitumor mechanism of eribulin, the first section will provide a brief introduction to the structure and function of tubulin, the relationship between tubulin and tumors, and the commonly seen tubulin inhibitors.

14.2.1 Structure and function of microtubules

A microtubule is a long tubular organelle structure assembled by tubulin in eukaryotic cells. It is the major component of the cellular cytoskeleton and is characterized by its hollow tubular structure [6]. The basic building block of microtubule assembly is the heterodimer of tubulin, comprising α-tubulin and β-tubulin (Fig. 14.2). During microtubule assembly, α-tubulin and β-tubulin first form an αβ-dimer of approximately 8 nm in length. These dimers then longitudinally aggregate to form protofilament, which expands into layers by increasing laterally, ultimately closing into a microtubule composed of 13 protofilaments [7]. Microtubules possess polarity due to the alternating arrangement of α- and β-tubulin within their protofilaments. The end of the microtubule where β-tubulin is exposed is referred to as the plus end (+), while the end where α-tubulin is exposed is referred to as the minus end (−). This structural characteristic of microtubules confers them with dynamic properties of assembly and disassembly [8]. Under certain conditions, one end of the microtubule undergoes assembly, leading to elongation, while the other end undergoes disassembly, resulting in shortening. When the rates of assembly and disassembly are balanced, the length of the microtubule remains stable. Due to their inherent structural feature and dynamic properties, microtubules play significant roles in maintaining cell morphology, cell division, signal transduction, and material transport.

Microtubules play a crucial role in cell division. When cells transition from interphase to division phase, the cytoplasmic microtubular network of interphase cells undergoes disintegration, leading to the depolymerization of microtubules into tubulin subunits, which are subsequently reassembled and polymerized to form spindle. During the process of mitosis, the spindle apparatus exerts force on the chromosomes, facilitating their movement toward the opposite poles of the dividing cell and ultimately enabling cell proliferation. At the end of mitosis, the spindle microtubules disassemble back into tubulin, which then reassemble to form the cytoplasmic microtubular network.

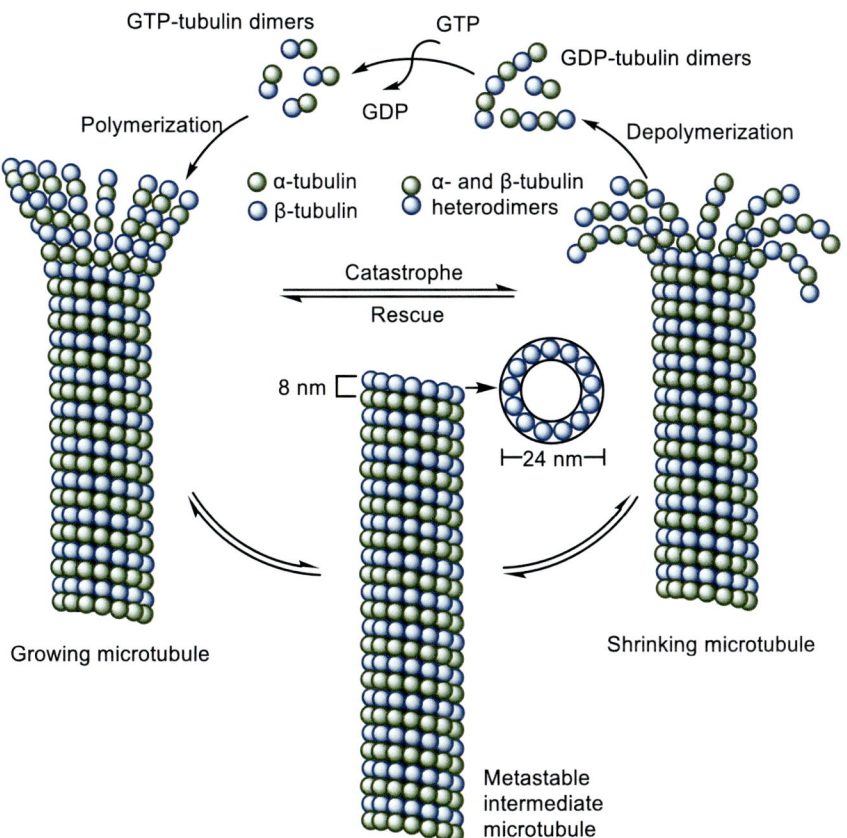

FIGURE 14.2 The constitution and structural features of microtubules.

Tumor cells are characterized by rapid proliferation, and their mitotic process occurs frequently with a notably shorter cell cycle compared to normal cells. Therefore, disrupting the microtubules in tumor cells and preventing their proper functioning during mitosis can impede cell division and proliferation, leading to growth inhibition and cell death. Consequently, tubulin, which constitutes the microtubules, has been recognized as an important target for the development of antitumor drugs. Indeed, various microtubule-targeting agents have been proven to be effective antitumor drugs.

14.2.2 Tubulin inhibitors

According to their mechanism of action, tubulin inhibitors can be divided into two types [9,10]. One is tubulin destabilizing agents, which primarily inhibit tubulin polymerization, preventing the formation of spindle microtubules. This leads to the arrest of tumor cells in the G2/M phase, inhibiting their division and proliferation. Representative drugs include colchicine, vinblastine, and maytansine. The other is tubulin stabilizing agents, which mainly inhibit tubulin depolymerization, disrupting the process of cell mitosis and triggering tumor cell death. Representative drugs include paclitaxel and ixabepilone (Fig. 14.3). Of note, most of the currently known tubulin inhibitors are derived from natural products or their derivatives. Based on the different binding sites of tubulin inhibitors, they can also be classified into several subtypes that target the colchicine site, vinca site, maytansine site, taxane site, laulimalide site, and pironetin site [11,12]. It is worth mentioning that due to their distinct binding sites, these tubulin inhibitors exhibit a certain degree of complementarity in clinical use, which makes them less likely to develop cross-resistance, thus providing more therapeutic options for antitumor treatment.

14.2.3 The mechanism of action of eribulin

Eribulin is a structurally simplified derivative of the natural product halichondrin B that has been proven as a tubulin polymerization inhibitor. In vitro experiments have shown that eribulin possesses comparable antitumor activity to halichondrin B [13]. Further mechanistic studies reveal that eribulin binds with high affinity to the plus end of microtubules

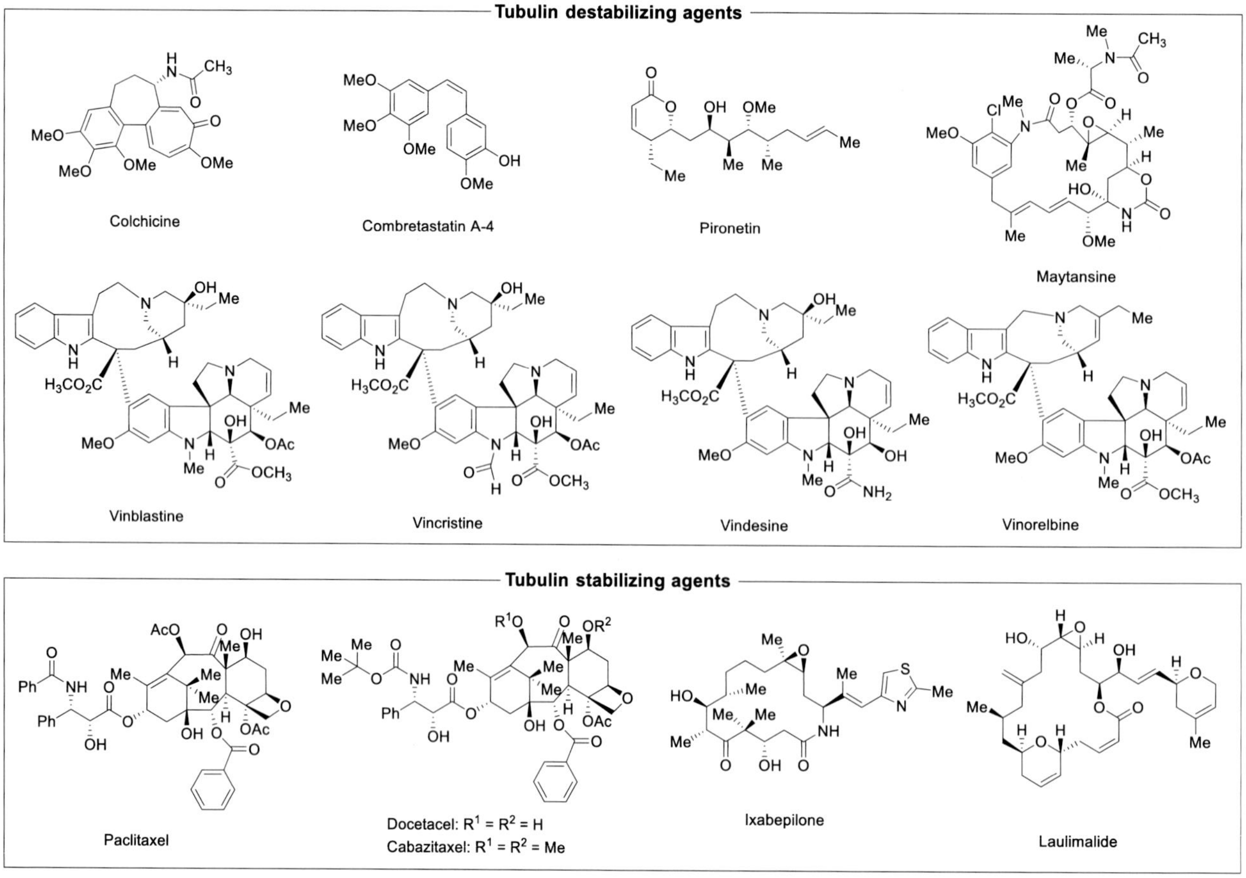

FIGURE 14.3 Common tubulin inhibitors.

[14]. This binding impedes microtubule protein polymerization, disrupting the dynamic balance between microtubule assembly and disassembly. As a result, it inhibits the formation of the mitotic spindle during cell division and ultimately induces tumor cell death (Fig. 14.4). Additionally, eribulin induces nonfunctional aggregates of tubulin without affecting the depolymerization process at the minus end of microtubules. Overall, eribulin exhibits a distinct mode of action compared to other tubulin inhibitors, thus demonstrating its uniqueness in antitumor treatment [15]. Consequently, the U.S. FDA approved eribulin mesylate for commercial use in 2010, especially for the treatment of locally advanced or metastatic breast cancer in patients who have previously received at least two chemotherapy regimens (anthracycline- or taxane-based therapies).

14.3 The development process of eribulin

14.3.1 Discovery and chemical synthesis of antitumor natural product halichondrin B

As mentioned above, eribulin is an antitumor agent derived from the marine natural product halichondrin B through structural simplification [16]. In the mid-1980s, Uemura and coworkers identified a series of structurally complex polyether macrolide compounds from the species *Halichondria okadai*, which were collectively named halichondrins (Fig. 14.5) [17,18]. It was revealed that most members of halichondrins exhibit significant inhibitory activity against melanoma cells B-16. Among them, halichondrin B (2) showed the most potent activity with an extremely low IC_{50} value of 0.093 ng/mL [19]. Furthermore, halichondrin B has also demonstrated strong inhibitory activity against various tumor cells (such as leukemia cells P-388, melanoma cells B-16, and leukemia cells L1210) in animal models, significantly improving mouse survival rates and median survival time at very low dosages. Shortly after, the National Cancer Institute (NCI) of the United States conducted a systematic evaluation of the biological activity of halichondrin B on 60 tumor cell lines. It was found that the antitumor mechanism of halichondrin B is analogous to that of known microtubule inhibitors such as vincristine and paclitaxel. However, they bear some differences in the binding sites and modes

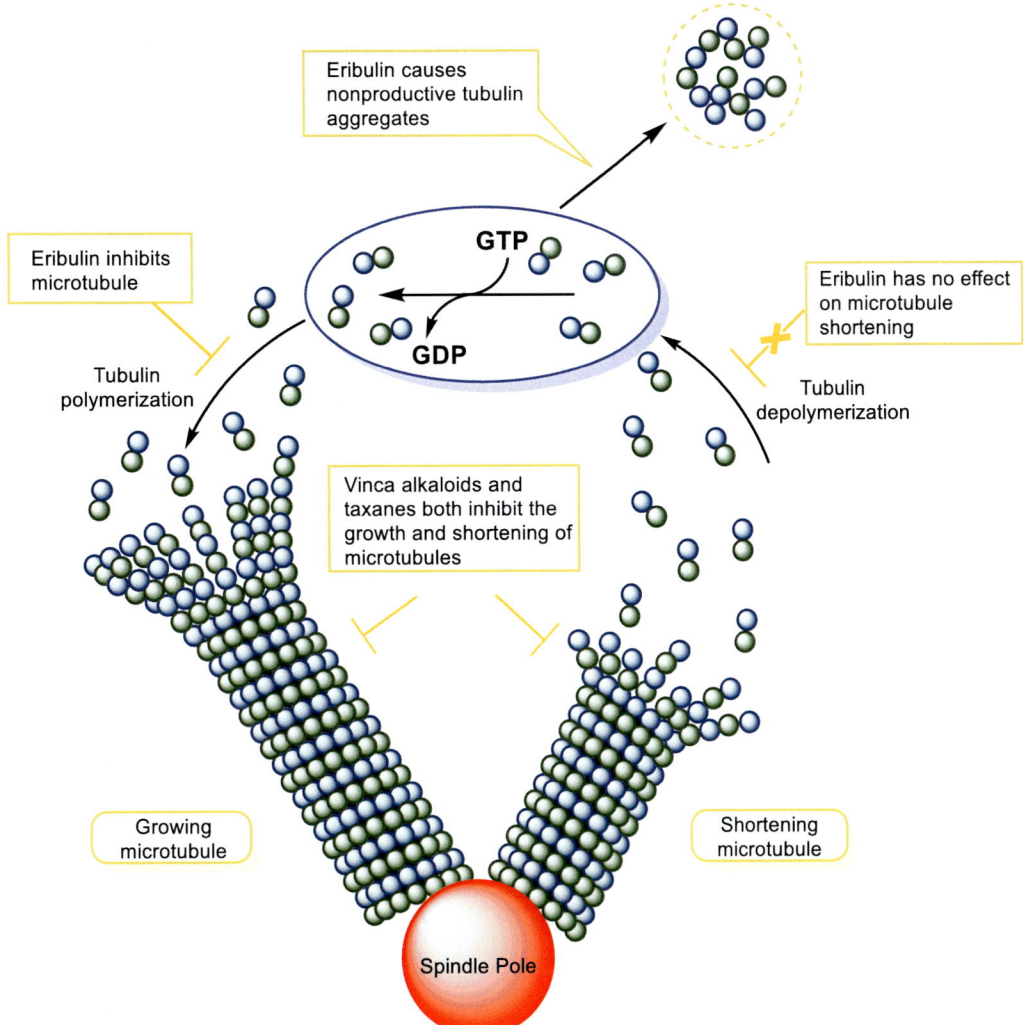

FIGURE 14.4 Antitumor mechanism of action of eribulin.

of action, indicating a low likelihood of cross-resistance among these microtubule inhibitors [20]. Since its discovery, halichondrin B has attracted widespread attention from both the academic and industrial communities due to its potent antitumor activity and unique mechanisms of action. However, the natural abundance of halichondrin B is extremely low, with only 20 milligrams of halichondrin B extracted from one ton of sponge (2×10^{-8} w/w). Given the difficulties and high costs associated with the collection of sponges, it is impossible to meet the clinical research demands for halichondrin B through conventional extraction from natural sources. Therefore, the chemical synthesis of halichondrin B became the only viable approach to address this challenge.

From a perspective of synthetic chemistry (Fig. 14.5), halichondrin B absolutely represents a daunting synthetic target. Structurally, halichondrin B can be roughly divided into two parts: the left polyether domain (blue) and the right macrocyclic domain (green), which are connected at the C_{29} and C_{30} positions. The molecule consists of 15 rings and 32 stereogenic centers, including two spirocyclic stereocenters. Apparently, the successful synthesis of halichondrin B entails not only the efficient assembly of the polycyclic framework but also the precise control of the stereochemistry of all stereogenic centers. Due to their significant biomedical potential, halichondrin B and related natural products have attracted widespread interest from the synthetic community over the past several decades. Professor Kishi and his research team from Harvard University have made remarkable contributions in this field. In 1992, they successfully achieved the first total synthesis of halichondrin B (Fig. 14.6) [21]. On the basis of this achievement, they further collaborated with Eisai Pharmaceutical Company to conduct systematic structure-activity relationship (SAR) studies on halichondrin B, which has ultimately led to the discovery of eribulin [22].

Norhalichondrin A: $R^1 = R^2 = OH$
Norhalichondrin B: $R^1 = R^2 = H$
Norhalichondrin C: $R^1 = H$, $R^2 = OH$

Halichondrin B: R = H
Halichondrin C: R = OH

Homohalichondrin A: $R^1 = R^2 = OH$
Homohalichondrin B: $R^1 = R^2 = H$
Homohalichondrin C: $R^1 = H$, $R^2 = OH$

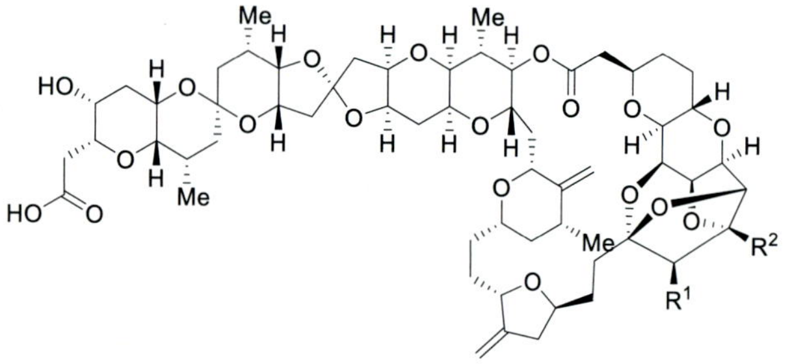

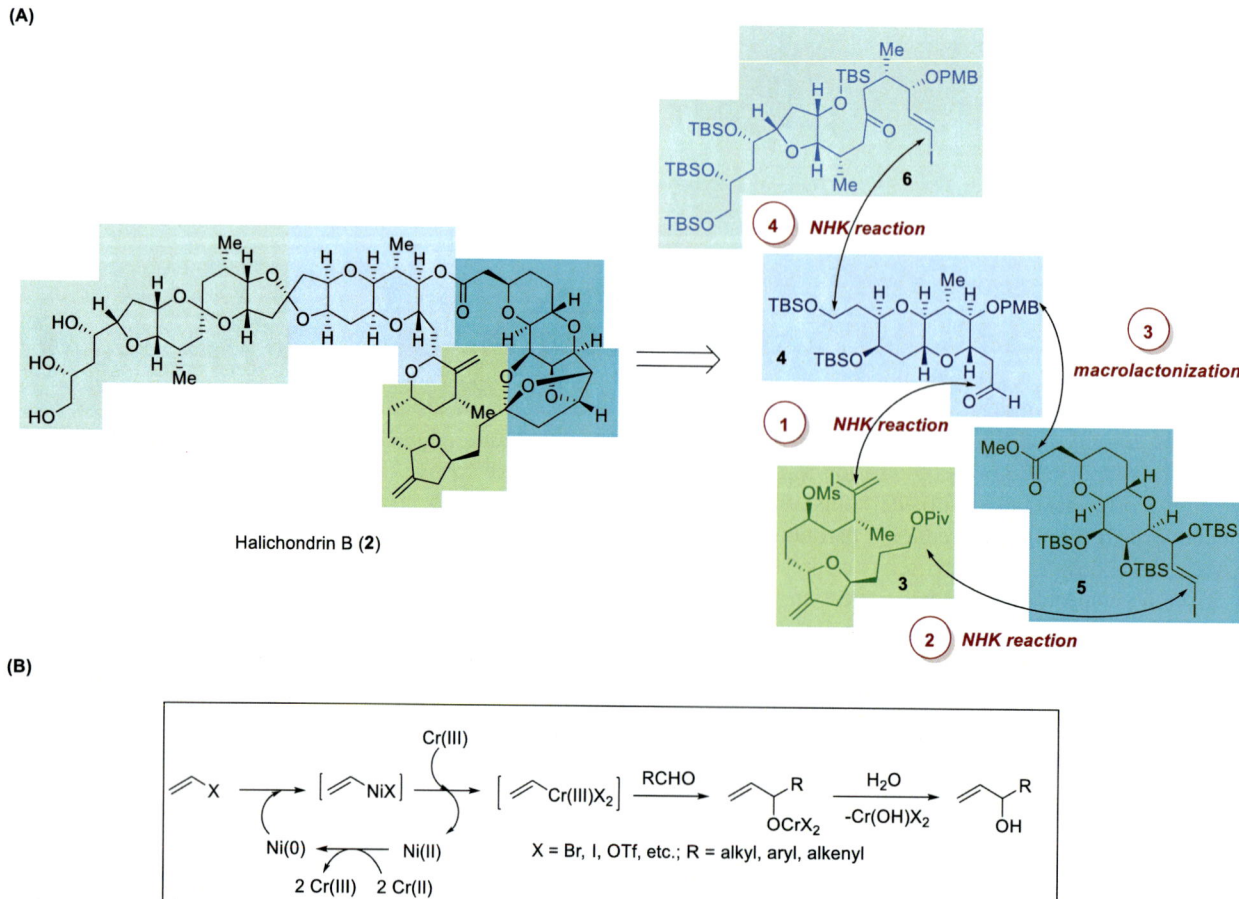

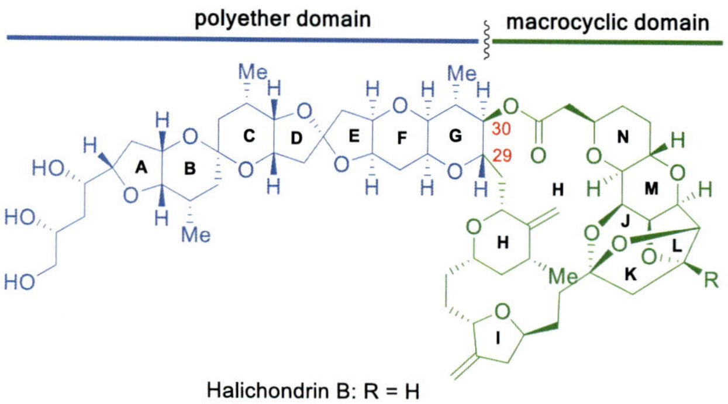

Inhibitory activity against melanoma cells B-16

compounds	IC_{50}(ng/mL)
Norhalichondrin A	5.2
Halichondrin B	0.093
Halichondrin C	0.35
Homohalichondrin A	0.26
Homohalichondrin B	0.1

FIGURE 14.5 Structure and activity of halichondrin B and its homologs.

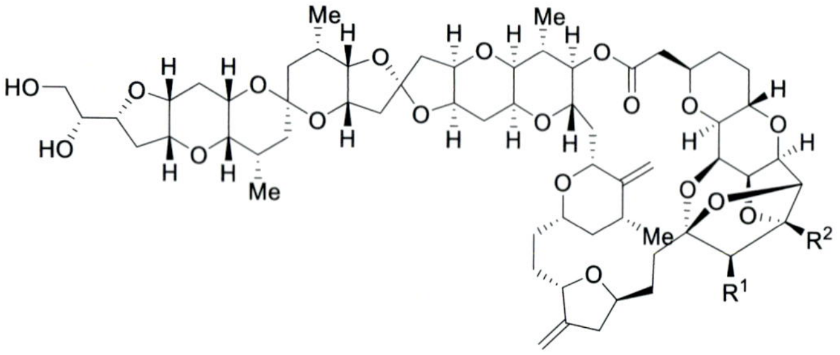

FIGURE 14.6 Kishi's synthetic strategy for halichondrin B and key reactions. (A) Retrosynthetic analysis of halichondrin B. (B) Nozaki–Hiyama–Kishi (NHK) reaction.

Kishi and coworkers developed a convergent synthetic route to access halichondrin B (Fig. 14.6A). Simply, the target molecule has been synthesized from four fundamental fragments (3−6), featuring Nozaki−Hiyama−Kishi (NHK) reaction and macrolactonization as the key elements [21]. NHK reaction was initially developed by Nozaki and Hiyama in the 1970s. The reaction features a Barbier-type addition between an alkyl halide and an aldehyde in the presence of excess chromium (II) chloride, which results in the formation of an allylic alcohol derivative [23]. Subsequently, Kishi and coworkers optimized this reaction and found that the addition of a catalytic amount of nickel salt could significantly accelerate the reaction rate and improve the efficiency. Consequently, the reaction was eventually named Nozaki−Hiyama−Kishi reaction (Fig. 14.6B) [24]. Due to the mild conditions and excellent chemoselectivity toward aldehydes, the NHK reaction has been recognized as a powerful tool for constructing allylic alcohol derivatives and found extensive applications in the synthesis of natural products and pharmaceutical molecules [25].

The pivotal steps in Kishi's total synthesis of halichondrin B are illustrated in Fig. 14.7. Initially, fragments 3 and 4 were combined together through NHK reaction. Subsequently, a base-promoted intramolecular S_N2 cyclization was employed to construct the tetrahydropyran derivative 7. Removal of the pivaloyl protecting group followed by the Dess−Martin oxidation reaction furnished aldehyde 8. Compound 8 was then coupled with alkene iodide 5 through an NHK reaction, and the resulting product underwent Dess−Martin oxidation to give compound 9. Next, deprotection of the *para*-methoxybenzyl (PMB) protecting group, hydrolysis of the methyl ester, and Yamaguchi macrolactonization reaction proceeded sequentially, leading to the formation of compound 10. Subsequently, a couple of steps were adopted to obtain the cage-like motif presented in compound 11, featuring a tandem Michael addition/hemiketalization reaction as the key step. Upon the treatment with Dess−Martin reagent, compound 11 readily converted to aldehyde 12, which then underwent NHK reaction followed by Dess−Martin oxidation to generate α,β-unsaturated ketone 13. At this stage, the deprotection of the *tert*-butyldimethylsilyl (TBS) group induced a tandem hemiketalization/Michael addition, which afforded intermediate 14. Finally, the removal of PMB group followed by acid-promoted hemiketalization resulted in halichondrin B (2). Thus, starting from commercially available materials, the Kishi group has achieved the first total synthesis of halichondrin B through a total of 92 steps (47 longest linear steps (LLS)) in an overall yield of 0.12%−0.22%.

Besides halichondrin B, the Kishi group has also successfully accomplished the total synthesis of some other congeners such as halichondrin C [26] and halichondrin A [27]. Of note, several other groups have also made notable contributions to this field. For example, in 2009, the Phillips group achieved the first total synthesis of norhalichondrin B (dechloro-halichondrin B) in 37 LLS [28]. In 2021, the Nicolaou group also completed the total synthesis of norhalichondrin B in 23 LLS [29]. In addition, a number of synthetic studies on this family of natural products have also been reported over the past decades [30−38]. However, most of them only allow for accessing some fragments en route to the targets, which indicates the great challenges associated with the total synthesis of halichondrins.

14.3.2 Study on the structure-activity relationship of halichondrin B - discovery process of eribulin

Although the Kishi group has successfully achieved the first total synthesis of Halichondrin B, both the long synthetic steps and low overall efficiency make it less applicable for obtaining ample natural samples for preclinical and clinical research. This seems to verify a long-standing bias regarding the total synthesis of complex natural products, that is, it primarily serves as a platform for synthetic chemists to showcase their exceptional synthetic skills, rather than addressing practical issues encountered in drug development. However, Kishi and coworkers did not stop at this stage. Instead, after completing the total synthesis of halichondrin B, they collaborated with Eisai Pharmaceutical Company to conduct a systematic biological evaluation of some key synthetic intermediates en route to Halichondrin B. Fortunately, they found that compound 11 displayed potent in vitro antitumor activity against human colon cancer cells (DLD-1) with an IC_{50} value of 4.6 nM (Fig. 14.8) [19]. Further studies revealed that it also functioned as a microtubule polymerization inhibitor, which rendered it a promising leading compound for further development. On the other hand, there were also notable differences between compound 11 and halichondrin B in their antitumor effects. For instance, while tumor cells treated with low concentration (10 nM) of halichondrin B could maintain a "complete mitotic arrest" for 10 hours even after drug washout in a cell culture system, compound 11 failed to give a similar result, even with a higher concentration (1 μM) [22,39]. Moreover, it is regrettable that compound 11 did not demonstrate the expected antitumor activity in animal models. This finding implies that, on one hand, it is feasible to develop structurally simplified analogs of halichondrin B that possess potent in vitro antitumor activity; On the other hand, it is imperative to conduct systematic SAR studies on halichondrin B to simplify its chemical structure while preserving in vivo antitumor activity.

Encouraged by the discovery of compound 11, the Kishi group continued their collaboration with Eisai Pharmaceutical Company to conduct a comprehensive and systematic SAR study on halichondrin B. As mentioned

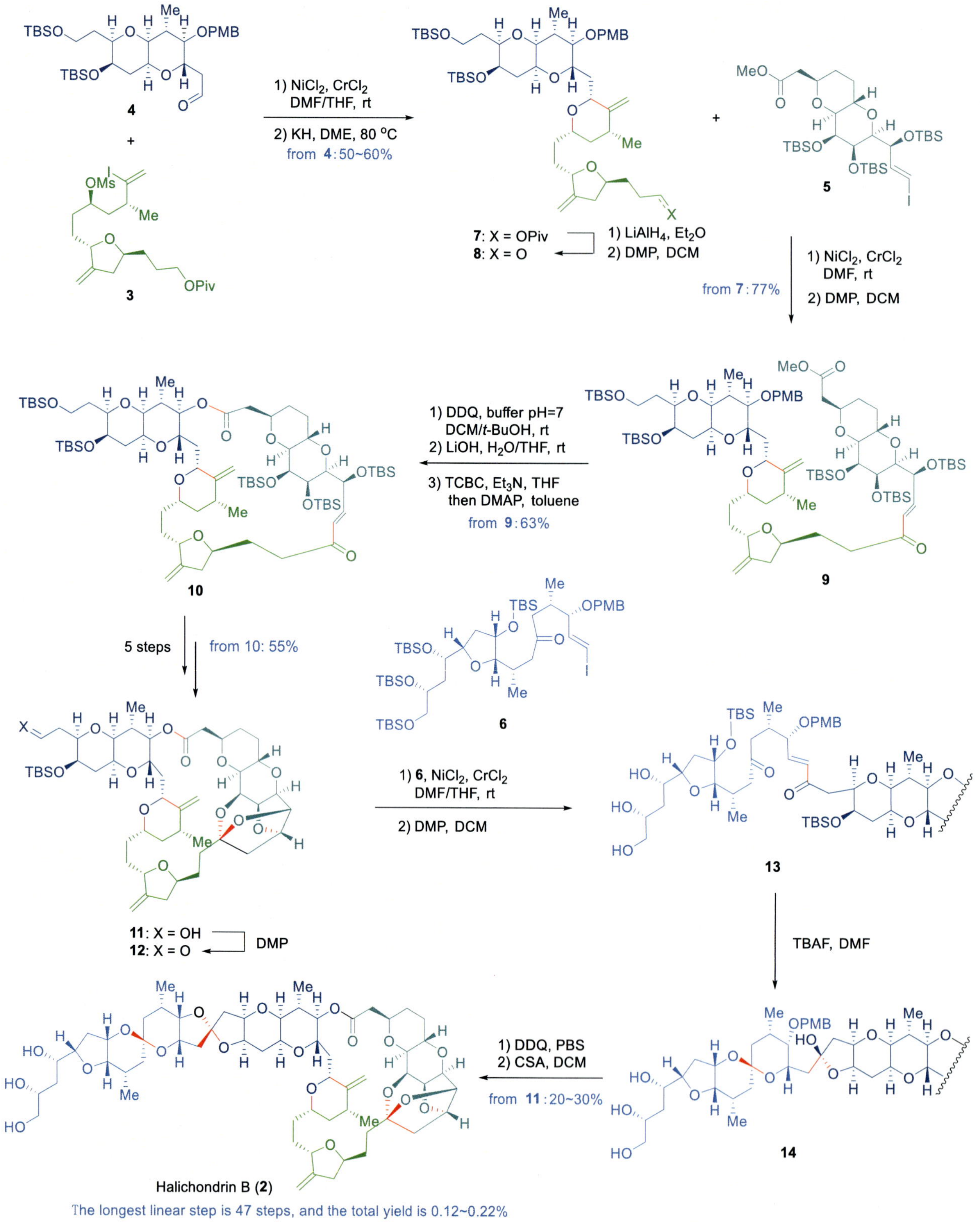

FIGURE 14.7 Total synthesis of halichondrin B.

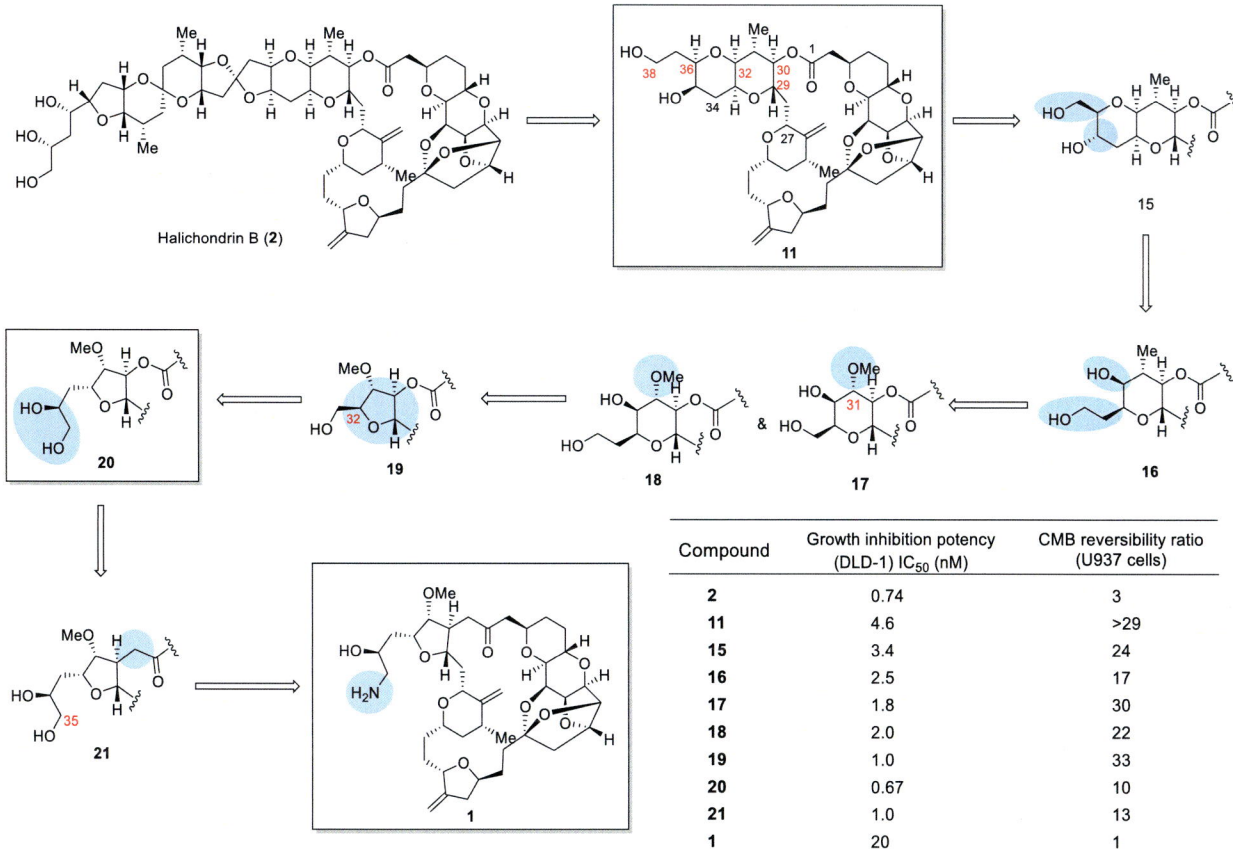

FIGURE 14.8 SAR study of halichondrin B.

above, the structure of halichondrin B can be roughly divided into two parts, the macrocyclic domain and the polyether domain, between which the former is supposed to be the key pharmacophore for its antitumor activity. This assumption is substantiated by the fact that all naturally occurring halichondrins displaying potent antitumor activity share a relatively conserved macrocyclic domain, while their polyether parts exhibit notable structural difference (as shown in Fig. 14.5). Moreover, the discovery of compound 11 also strongly supports this assumption as it bears the same macrocyclic domain as halichondrin B but a greatly simplified polyether moiety. In this context, simplification of the cyclic polyether domain is an ideal starting point for conducting the SAR study of halichondrin B. Notably, to facilitate the evaluation of in vivo antitumor activity of the synthesized analogs, researchers adopted an in vitro cell model to characterize the compounds' ability to maintain "complete mitotic block (CMB)" after washout treatment, which turned out to be well correlated to their in vivo antitumor activity [39].

Based on the above rationalization, Kishi and coworkers conducted multiple rounds of structural modifications on the $C_{30}-C_{38}$ region of compound 11 while keeping the macrocyclic domain (C_1-C_{30}) unchanged. Fortunately, this strategy was proven to be successful. While we would not discuss the details of the entire process of the SAR study, some crucial results are depicted in Fig. 14.8. Firstly, by shortening the side chain at the C_{36} position of compound 11 and altering the stereochemistry of the hydroxyl group at the C_{35} position, the researchers obtained a new analog 15, which retained both in vitro and in vivo antitumor activity. Next, they discovered that compound 16, which only keeps one tetrahydropyran ring, also displayed similar biological activity to compound 11. This result indicated that the bicyclic moiety of 11 could be further simplified to a monocyclic ring. Subsequently, a systematic study of the substituents on the tetrahydropyran ring was conducted. By replacing the methyl group at C_{31} with a methoxy group, compounds 17 and 18 were obtained, both of which preserved the in vitro antitumor activity. It should be noted that the introduction of a methoxy group onto the tetrahydropyran ring can improve the synthetic accessibility of the analog, with the suitable monosaccharide precursor used as the starting material [40].

Furthermore, by comparing the structures and biological activity of norhalichondrin A (Fig. 14.8) and halichondrin B, Kish and coworkers proposed a bold optimization strategy by replacing the tetrahydropyran ring in compounds 17 or 18 with a tetrahydrofuran ring. This structural modification aims to reduce the conformational flexibility of the macrocyclic domain and lock it into an "active conformation". Fortunately, this idea worked well in practice, as the designed analog 19 exhibited improved anti-tumor activity compared to compounds 17 and 18.

More excitingly, further modification of the side chain at C_{32} resulted in the identification of compound 20, which displayed nearly equal in vitro antitumor activity compared to the natural product halichondrin B. It appears that the extension of the side chain at C32, together with the inversion of the stereochemistry, has a positive impact on the antitumor activity. However, both compounds 17 and 20 (the most promising pyran- and furan-containing analogs) did not exhibit the expected in vivo antitumor activity in a xenograft model of human melanoma (LOX). Although this phenomenon could be attributed to several underlying reasons, the most plausible one is that the macrocyclic lactone moiety of these compounds is susceptible to hydrolysis by the action of enzymes in living organisms, leading to the loss of their antitumor activity. Guided by this hypothesis, Kish and coworkers adopted a bioisosteric approach and replaced the lactone moiety with some more stable structural units, such as amides, ethers, and ketones. Among them, ketone 21 demonstrated potent antitumor activity in various human tumor cell models (breast cancer MDA-MB435, colon cancer COLO-205, melanoma LOX, and ovarian cancer NIH: OVCAR-3 cell lines) and was thus identified as one of the promising candidates (known as ER-076349) for subsequent clinical investigation. Finally, the researchers replaced the primary alcohol at C_{35} with a primary amine, providing compound 1 as the other drug candidate (known as ER-E7389). Although compound 1 exhibited slightly lower in vitro antitumor activity compared to compound 21, it displayed better "complete mitotic arrest" maintenance, even surpassing the natural product itself. To further improve the water solubility of compound 1, the researchers chose to prepare it in the form of methanesulfonic acid salt and named it eribulin mesylate. Eribulin mesylate can easily dissolve in water at pH 3−7. It has an acceptable oral bioavailability in mice (7%), and an average distribution volume of 43−114 L/m^2. The half-life ($t_{1/2}$) is about 40 hours. Thus, after multiple rounds of structural optimization, the researcher eventually identified an ideal drug candidate applicable for further clinical studies [41].

14.3.3 Study on the process chemistry of eribulin

Having identified eribulin, the next key task was to realize its scalable synthesis to meet the demands of clinical research. The original total synthesis route developed by the Kishi group, although capable of producing halichondrin B and analogs at a milligram scale, faced considerable challenges in scaling up due to the excessively long synthetic sequences and the need for multiple-column chromatography purifications of synthetic intermediates. To address this issue, the Kishi group devoted great efforts to developing a more concise, practical, and scalable synthetic route for eribulin in collaboration with Eisai Pharmaceuticals. As a result, several generations of synthetic routes have been established, which allowed for the production of eribulin at varying scales ranging from milligrams to kilograms [42].

Based on their previous synthesis of halichondrin B, Kishi and coworkers developed a convergent synthetic strategy for eribulin, in which the target was also divided into three fragments of similar sizes, namely fragments 22, 23, and 24. Among them, fragments 22 and 24 are closely similar to those (3 and 5) used in the synthesis of halichondrin B, while fragment 23 needs to be synthesized from scratch. According to their synthetic blueprint, eribulin could be assembled from these three fragments through sequential NHK reaction, nucleophilic addition, and NHK reaction, followed by late-stage functional group transformations (Fig. 14.9). At this stage, the main objective was to successfully synthesize the three fundamental fragments 22−24 in a scalable manner. To address this challenge, Kishi and coworkers have iteratively optimized the synthetic processes for these fragments to meet the demands of industrial-scale production. The next section will provide a concise overview of the optimization process for each fragment, with an emphasis on the optimal synthetic routes.

14.3.3.1 Synthesis of fragment 22

In total, Kishi and coworkers have developed four different synthetic routes for fragment 22 and its equivalent 22′ (Fig. 14.10). The first-generation route mainly followed the approach applicable for a similar fragment in the synthesis of halichondrin B [21]. Starting from L-arabinose (25), fragment 22′ was obtained with the longest linear sequence of 22 steps and an overall yield of 7%. In 2002, the Kishi group reported a more concise synthetic approach [43], using alcohol 26 as the starting material. This route only required 13 LLS to access fragment 22′ with an overall yield of 12%. Unlike the first-generation route that relied on a chiral pool as the starting material, the second approach

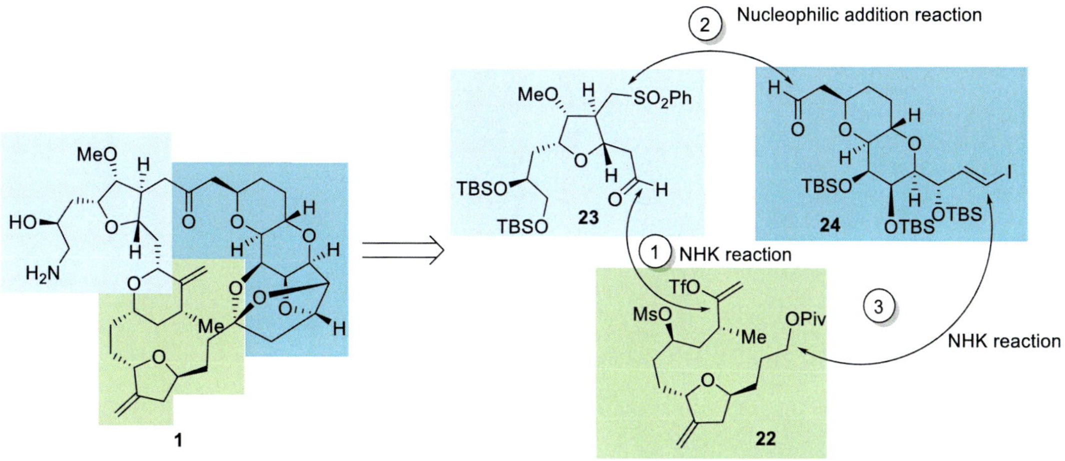

FIGURE 14.9 Overall synthetic strategy of eribulin.

employed classic asymmetric reactions to construct the chiral centers. This eliminated the need for tedious functional group adjustments, resulting in a more concise and efficient process. However, an inherent drawback associated with this approach is that some reactions only show moderate diastereoselectivity, which necessitates the use of column chromatography to separate the diastereoisomers. To address this issue, Kishi and coworkers developed the third-generation route [44], using epoxy compound 27 as the starting material, which allowed for the access of fragment 22 in the longest linear sequence of 15 steps and an overall yield of 2%−3%. Although the overall yield of this route is not very high, it offers some advantages such as reduced column chromatography and improved reproducibility, making it suitable for kilogram-scale synthesis of fragment 22. Besides, the Kishi group also accomplished the fourth-generation synthesis of fragment 22 using D-(−)-quinic acid (28) as the starting material [45]. Although this route appears to be the longest (33 LLS) among the four approaches mentioned above, all of the involved synthetic intermediates require only recrystallization for purification.

In view of its appreciable balance between efficiency and practicality, the third generation of approaches has been selected to achieve the kilogram-scale synthesis of fragment 22 (Fig. 14.10B). Starting from dihydrofuran 29, the corresponding cyclic hemiacetal is obtained through a hydration reaction under acidic conditions, which then undergoes a Barbier-type addition with the in situ-generated vinylstannane reagent, resulting in compound 30. Subsequently, the primary alcohol of 30 is selectively protected with the bulky diphenyl *tert*-butyldimethylsilyl group, and the resulting product is subjected to chiral column separation [46], yielding optically pure compound 31. Upon treatment with p-toluenesulfonyl chloride and triethylamine, compound 31 is smoothly converted to the key intermediate 32, which exhibits a high enantiomeric excess (ee) value.

In parallel, the other key fragment 40 is prepared from the epoxide 27 in a couple of steps. Firstly, compound 27 is subjected to Jacobsen hydrolytic kinetic resolution to provide the desired enantiomer 33 in >99% ee [47]. Subsequently, compound 33 undergoes a tandem ring-opening/intramolecular lactonization with diethyl malonate (34) to provide lactone 35. After decarboxylation followed by methylation, compound 36 is obtained as a single diastereoisomer. Upon the treatment with N,O-dimethylhydroxylamine hydrochloride (37) in the presence of AlMe$_3$, 36 is readily converted to Weinreb amide 38. The newly generated secondary hydroxyl group is then protected with TBS, resulting in compound 39. Oxidative cleavage of the terminal double bond of 39 yields the aldehyde 40. At this stage, the union of fragments 40 and 32 is achieved through NHK coupling, leading to the formation of compound 41 [48]. Subsequently, compound 41 readily undergoes an intramolecular cyclization in the presence of silica gel to give the furan derivative 42. Grignard addition to Weinreb amide 42 provides the corresponding methyl ketone, which then undergoes kinetic deprotonation with potassium bis(trimethylsilyl)amide (KHMDS) followed by trapping with phenyl triflimide to yield enol triflate 43. Finally, the target fragment 22 could be obtained from 43 through sequential deprotection and protection manipulations.

14.3.3.2 Synthesis of fragment 23

Kishi and coworkers also developed four synthetic routes for fragment 23 and related compounds 23′/23″ (Fig. 14.11A). The first-generation route utilizes L-arabinose (25) as the starting material [40] and allows for the synthesis of fragment 23′ in 18 LLS with an overall yield of 7%. However, this approach requires multiple-column chromatography operations to purify stereoisomers, making it less suitable for large-scale production. The second route begins with the chiral compound 44 [41], which

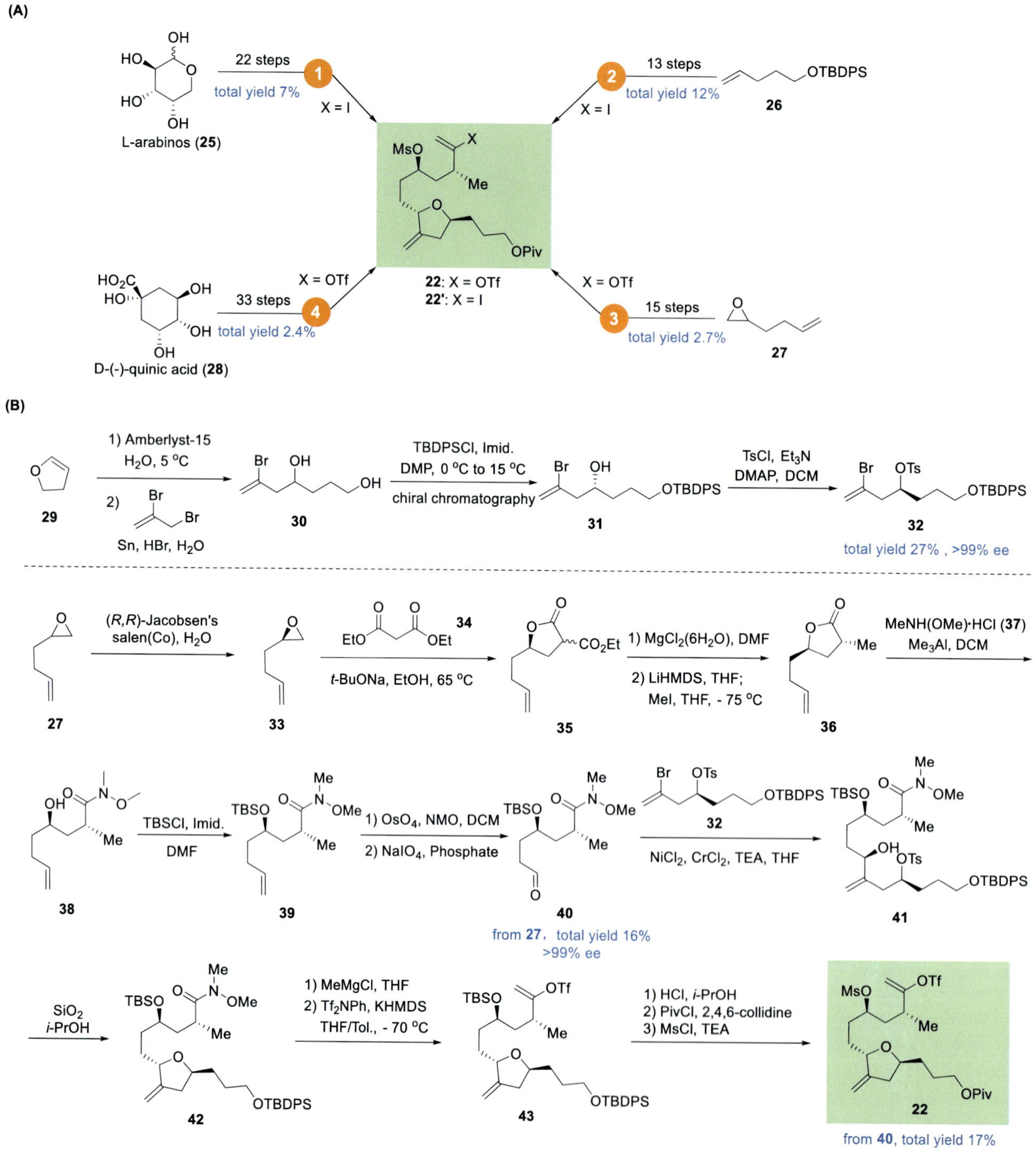

FIGURE 14.10 Synthesis of fragment 22. (A) Summary of the synthetic route of fragment 22. (B) kilogram-scale synthetic route of fragment 22.

possesses the desired stereochemistry at the C34 position. The other chiral centers in fragment 23″ are introduced through the combination of asymmetric synthesis and substrate control. This route takes 16 LLS and has an overall yield of 9%. The fine stereochemical control in this route significantly reduces the need for column chromatography. To further improve the synthetic efficiency and practicality, Kishi and coworkers subsequently developed the third-generation [49] and fourth-generation [50] synthetic routes using D-(+)-glucurono-3,6-lactone (45) as the starting material. Both of these routes leverage chiral pool strategies and asymmetric reactions to improve overall efficiency. Notably, the fourth-generation route, despite consisting of 20 LLS, completely eliminates the need for column chromatography operations. Instead, only recrystallization is used for the purification of the key intermediates, which renders it applicable for the kilogram-scale synthesis of eribulin.

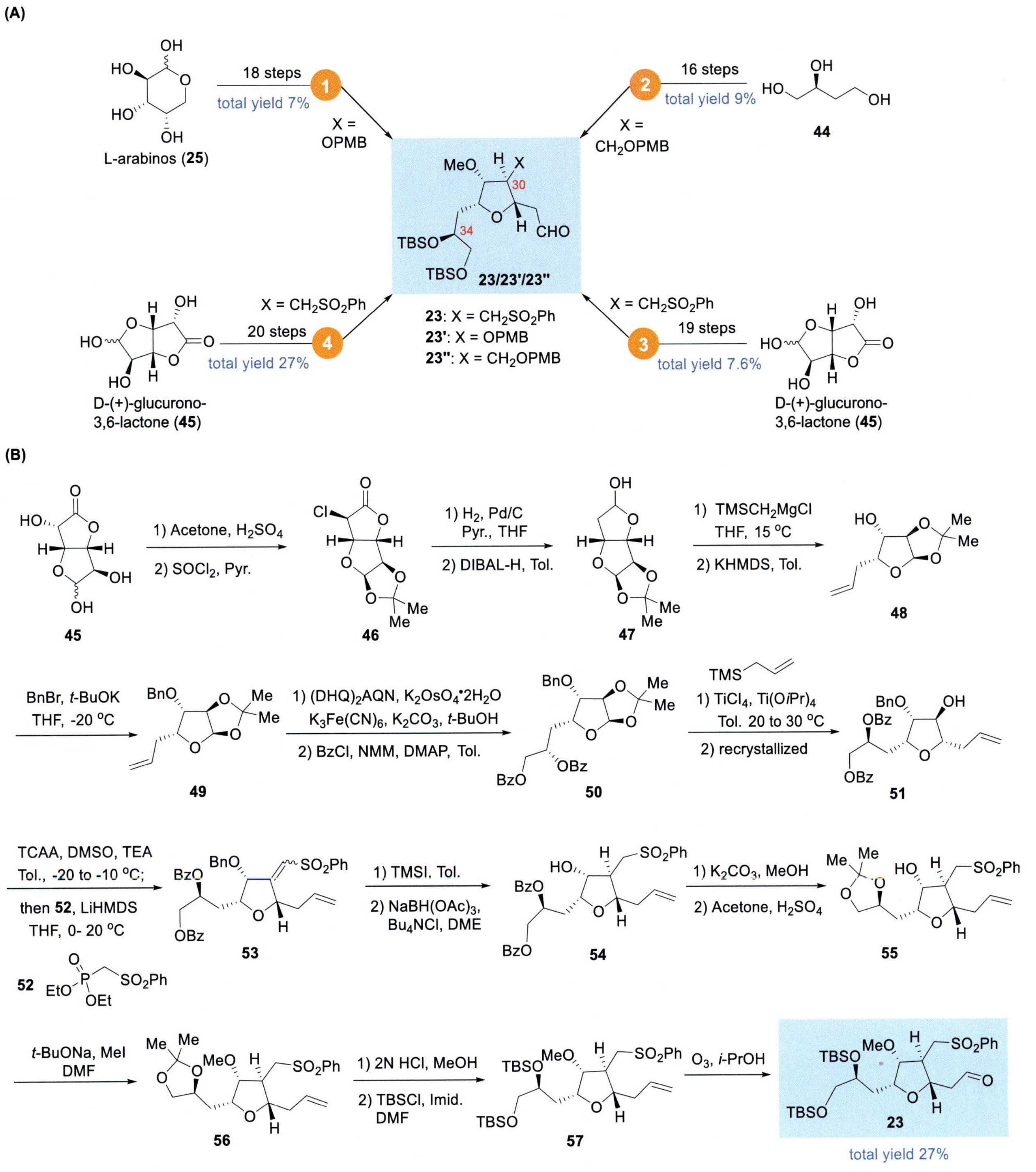

FIGURE 14.11 Synthesis of fragment 23. (A) Summary of the synthetic route of fragment 23. (B) kilogram-scale synthetic route of fragment 23.

The optimal synthetic route for fragment 23 is illustrated in Fig. 14.11B [50]. Starting from D-(+)-glucurono-3,6-lactone (45), the vicinal diol is firstly protected as the corresponding acetonide, which then undergoes chlorination to yield compound 46. Subsequently, the chloride atom is removed through catalytic hydrogenation, and the resulting product is further reduced with DIBAL-H to give hemiketal 47. Compound 47 can be converted to alkene 48 through Peterson olefination. Protecting the secondary hydroxyl group of 48 with a benzyl group results in the formation of 49, which then undergoes a Sharpless asymmetric dihydroxylation reaction followed by benzoylation to afford the compound 50. Next, Lewis acid-promoted C-glycosidation is adopted to introduce an allylic side chain onto compound 50, and the resulting product undergoes consecutive Moffat oxidation and Horner–Wadsworth–Emmons reactions, generating vinyl sulfone 53. Removal of the benzyl group of 53 followed by hydroxy-directed conjugate reduction leads to the formation of compound 54. Subsequently, a series of protecting-group manipulations are implemented to obtain the compound 57. Finally, the terminal double bond of 57 is cleaved through ozonolysis, leading to the formation of fragment 23.

14.3.3.3 Synthesis to fragment 24

For fragment 24, there are also four different routes to access it (Fig. 14.12A). The first-generation route is similar to the one used in the synthesis of halichondrin B, which takes 31 LLS and has an acceptable overall yield of 3.3% [21]. In comparison, with the commercially available L-gulonic acid γ-lactone (59) as the starting material [51], the second-generation route allows for the access of fragment 24 in 16 LLS, significantly improving the overall efficiency. Building on this achievement, the Kishi group further developed the third-generation approach, which enables the synthesis of fragment 24 in 12 LLS with an overall yield of 11%. Based on this route, fragment 24 could be obtained at a hundred-gram scale [52]. Despite the great success, the chemists from Eisai Inc. continued to optimize the synthetic process toward fragment 24, which has culminated in the establishment of the fourth-generation route [53]. With the cheap D-(−)-gulono-1,4-lactone (60) as the starting material, the fourth-generation route includes 12 LLS, with an overall yield of 2.3%. Although the overall yield of the last synthetic route is lower than others, its greater economic viability and scalability make it particularly suitable for industrial manufacturing.

The optimized synthetic route for fragment 24 is shown in Fig. 14.12B [53]. Firstly, the vicinal diol in D-(−)-gulono-1,4-lactone (60) is protected as the corresponding biscyclohexylidene lactone. Subsequently, reduction of the lactone moiety with DIBAL-H followed by Wittig reaction yields the methoxy alkene ether 64, which then undergoes tandem dihydroxylation/hemiketalization to give compound 65. Next, selective removal of one of the cyclohexylidene moieties followed by full protection of the free hydroxyl group with an acetyl group results in the formation of 66. C-Glycosidation of 66 with 3-trimethylsilyl-4-pentenoate (67) in the presence of Lewis acid leads to the formation of 68, which, upon treatment with sodium methoxide, undergoes global deacetylation, double bond migration, and oxy-Michael addition to form the diol-pyran derivative 69. Oxidative cleavage of the neighboring diol in 69 yields aldehyde 70, which then reacts with the vinyl bromide 71 through an NHK reaction to obtain allylic alcohol 72. At this stage, the remaining cyclohexylidene ring is then cleaved under acidic conditions, and the liberated hydroxyl groups are protected as their corresponding silyl ethers. Finally, vinylsilane 73 could be converted to vinyl iodide 74 through an electrophilic substitution, and the latter, upon treatment with DIBAL-H, is readily reduced to aldehyde 24.

14.3.3.4 The late-stage synthesis of eribulin

Having all requisite fragments secured in a scalable manner, the next task is to sequentially assemble these fragments together and complete the final target molecule. To achieve this goal, Kishi and coworkers have developed two generations of synthetic routes. Because these two routes share many overlapped steps, we will focus on the second one. Firstly, fragments 22 and 23 are coupled together through an asymmetric NHK reaction, and the resulting product then undergoes intramolecular Williamson ether cyclization followed by deprotection to give compound 76. Subsequently, deprotonation of sulfone 76 followed by 1,2-addition with fragment 24 yields the corresponding secondary alcohol, which then undergoes double Dess–Martin oxidation to afford compound 77 [54]. Upon the treatment with samarium diiodide, the sulfone moiety of 77 is readily removed, and the resulting product undergoes intramolecular asymmetric NHK reaction followed by Dess–Martin oxidation to yield the macrocyclic compound 78. At this stage, all TBS protecting groups of 78 are removed with the action of tetrabutylammonium fluoride (TBAF), and the liberated hydroxyl group could engage in tandem Michael addition/ketalization to provide compound 79. Lastly, the primary alcohol of 79 readily undergoes selective trifluoromethanesulfonylation followed by the substitution with ammonium hydroxide to give the corresponding primary amine derivative, which, upon the treatment with methylsulfonic acid, yields eribulin mesylate as the final product. Thus, starting from the commercially available starting material 42, the entire synthetic route to eribulin consists of 60 synthetic steps (34 LLS) and the overall yield ranges from 1% to 6.7%. Compared to the original total synthesis of halichondrin B, both the overall efficiency and practicality of the synthesis of eribulin have been improved notably. Thus, after years of collaboration between Kishi's research group and Eisai Pharmaceutical Company, they have successfully addressed the great challenge associated with the scalable synthesis of eribulin (Fig. 14.13).

In conclusion, the practical synthesis of eribulin largely follows the convergent strategy previously employed for the total synthesis of halichondrin B, with the NHK reaction serving as the key step for the assembly of several key

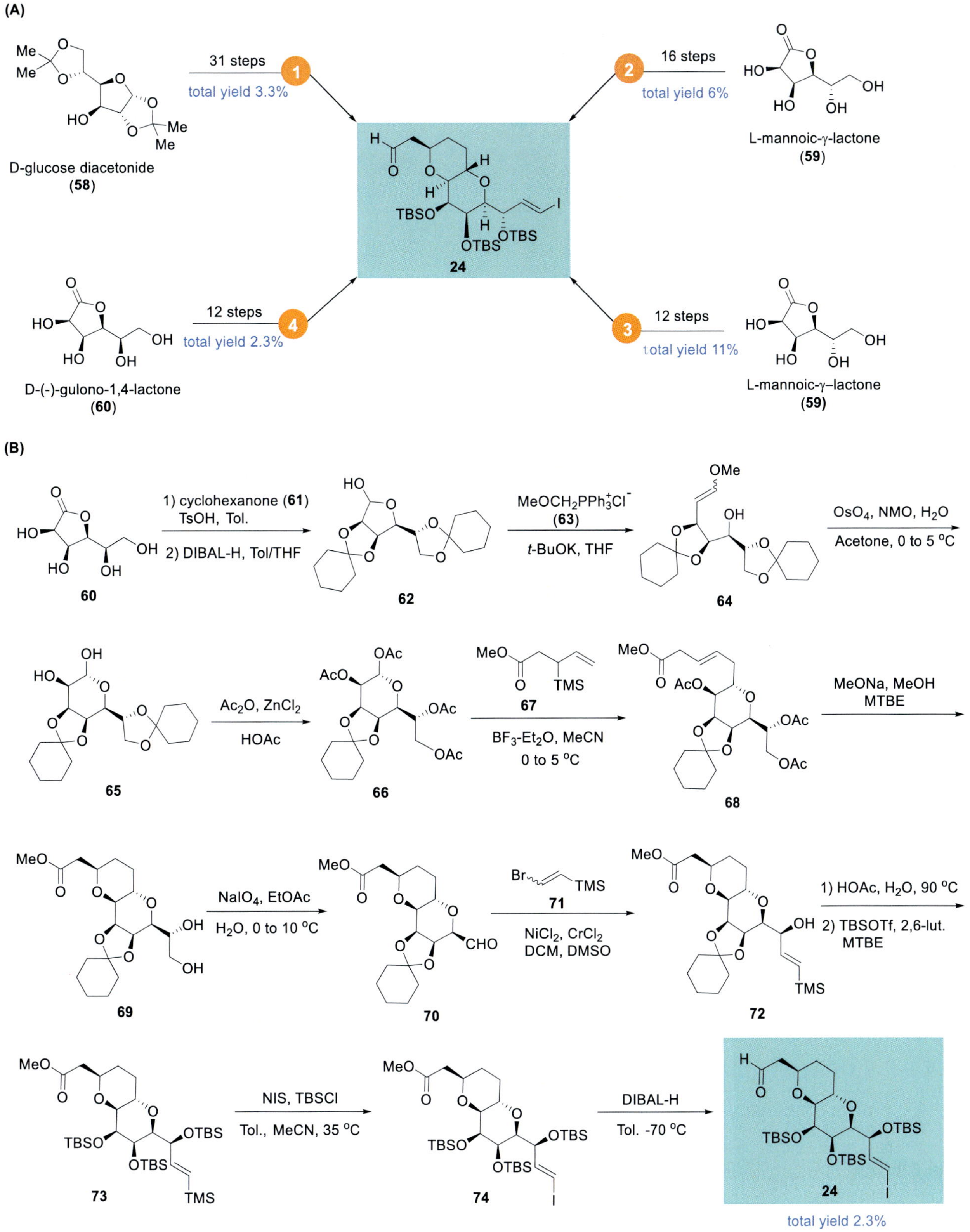

Antitumor drug eribulin **Chapter | 14** 341

FIGURE 14.12 Synthesis of fragment 24. (A) Summary of the synthetic route of fragment 24. (B) kilogram-scale synthetic route of fragment 24.

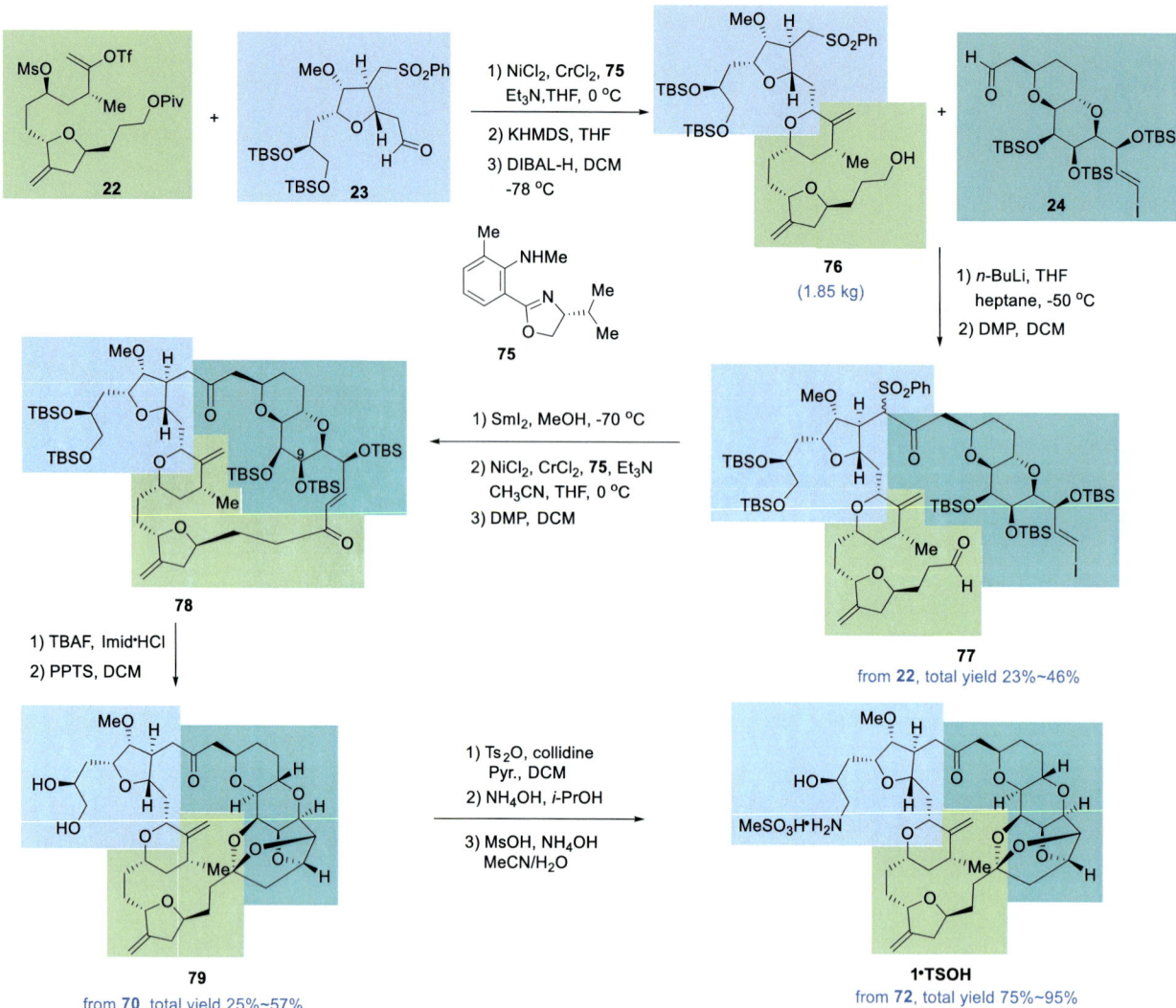

FIGURE 14.13 Study of eribulin synthetic process.

fragments. Various tactics, including chiral pools, chiral separation, and asymmetric synthesis, are employed to introduce the required stereogenic centers in a highly stereoselective manner. Both the efficiency and practicality of the synthetic routes have been significantly improved through continuous optimization, which eventually allows for the kilogram-scale synthesis of eribulin. Of note, eribulin is the most complex small-molecule drug produced by chemical synthesis to date and has been recognized as the "Mount Everest of chemical synthesis in the pharmaceutical world."

14.4 Pharmacological characteristics of eribulin

14.4.1 Pharmacodynamics of eribulin

In vitro studies have demonstrated the remarkable eribulin's inhibitory activity against the proliferation of various tumor cell lines [13,19]. For instance, the average IC_{50} values of eribulin against prostate cancer cell lines DU145 and LNCaP, colon cancer cell lines COLO 205 and DLD-1, human histiocytic lymphoma cell line U937, acute promyelocytic leukemia cell line HL-60, and LOX melanoma cell line range from 0.09 to 9.5 nM, with an average of 1.8 nM. This is 2–4 times stronger than the activity of vinblastine and paclitaxel. Eribulin exhibits significant inhibition against breast cancer cell line MDA-MB-435 at subnanomolar level (IC_{50} = 0.09 nM), which is much more potent than vinblastine (IC_{50} = 0.59 nM) and paclitaxel (IC_{50} = 2.5 nM). Inhibition experiments on nonsmall cell lung cancer cell lines A549 (wild-type p53) and Calu-1 (p53-deficient) demonstrate that eribulin exhibits non-p53-dependent anticancer activity within the range of 0.5 pM [55]. Additionally, eribulin shows no cytotoxicity against quiescent human fibroblast cells IMR-90, indicating that its inhibition of tumor cell growth at low concentrations primarily occurs during the cell division and proliferation stages, rather than through nonspecific cytotoxicity [3]. It is worth mentioning that although eribulin exhibits nearly identical activity to the natural product halichondrin B in the NCI 60-cell line screening, it demonstrates enhanced efficacy in interactions with microtubules and in vivo anticancer activity. Furthermore, it exhibits reduced toxicity in granulocyte-macrophage colony-forming units.

Eribulin has also demonstrated excellent antitumor effects in preclinical animal experiments. Results from the xenograft tumor inhibition experiments in mice (breast, lung, ovarian, colon, melanoma, pancreatic, and fibrosarcoma) indicate that eribulin can achieve tumor regression, relief, and extended lifespan at significantly lower doses than the maximum tolerated dose (MTD). Compared to paclitaxel, eribulin exhibits significant in vivo antitumor effect against breast cancer MDA-MB-435, colon cancer COLO 205, and LOX melanoma at lower doses (0.05–1.0 mg/kg) when administered through intravenous or intraperitoneal injection. In the MDA-MB-435 animal model, tumor regression was observed on the 14th day after treatment with 0.25–1.0 mg/kg of eribulin, achieving >95% tumor inhibition on the 42nd day without apparent cytotoxicity. Moreover, compared to paclitaxel, eribulin demonstrates a wider therapeutic window in vivo (fivefold vs. twofold in the LOX melanoma model, and fourfold vs. sevenfold in breast cancer MDA-MB-435 model). This characteristic ensures that increasing the dose of eribulin within the clinical safety window can improve the antitumor effect and facilitate the complete eradication of residual tumor cells [56].

14.4.2 Pharmacokinetics and toxicology of eribulin

The pharmacokinetic study in preclinical trials revealed that Eribulin exhibited a rapid distribution phase followed by a prolonged elimination phase, with an average half-life ($t_{1/2}$) of approximately 40 hours. Within the dosage range of 0.25–4.0 mg/m^2, the area under the concentration-time curve and maximum plasma concentration of the drug demonstrate a linear correlation with the dosages. The steady-state volume of distribution for this drug ranges from 43 to 114 L/m^2, and the plasma clearance rate ranges from 1.16 to 2.42 L/h/m^2, indicating a slow elimination process. Eribulin exhibits weak binding to plasma proteins, with a protein binding rate of 49%–65% within the concentration range of 100–1000 ng/mL in human plasma. The plasma protein binding rate after multiple administrations of eribulin is comparable to the level with a single dose. No accumulation was observed after weekly administration. Eribulin is primarily eliminated through biliary excretion. After administering ^{14}C-eribulin to patients, approximately 82% of the dose is eliminated in the feces and 9% is eliminated in the urine, indicating that renal clearance is not the major approach of eribulin [57].

Eribulin demonstrated nonmutagenicity in the Ames test (a test for mutagenicity of chemicals). However, positive results were observed in the mouse lymphoma mutation assay and rat bone marrow micronucleus test. No study has been conducted on the effects of eribulin on fertility in humans or animals (genetic toxicity). However, repeated-dose toxicity studies in dogs and rats showed that eribulin could impair male fertility. Furthermore, carcinogenicity studies have not been conducted for eribulin (such studies are generally not required for anticancer drugs).

14.5 Clinical research and safety evaluation of eribulin
14.5.1 Clinical research of eribulin
14.5.1.1 Phase I clinical study

Four phase I clinical trials have been conducted with patients who bear advanced solid tumors, including colorectal cancer, ovarian cancer, uterine cancer, renal cancer, liver cancer, and lung cancer and had received chemotherapy treatment. The first study by Synold et al. included a total of 40 patients, with evaluable data for 38 patients. Eribulin was administered via intravenous infusion on days 1, 8, and 15, with a chemotherapy cycle lasting 28 days [58]. The MTD was determined to be 1.4 mg/m^2. The second study by Tan et al. enrolled 21 patients, with the dose of eribulin escalating to 0.25, 0.5, 1, 2, 2.8, and 4 mg/m^2 [59]. Eribulin was administered via intravenous infusion over 1 hour every 21 days, and the MTD was determined to be 2.0 mg/m^2. The third study by Goel et al. included 32 patients with advanced solid tumors in a phase I clinical trial [60]. The starting dose of eribulin was 0.25 mg/m^2, with a maximum dose of 1.4 mg/m^2. Eribulin was administered via intravenous infusion on days 1, 8, and 15 over 1 hour, with a chemotherapy cycle lasting 28 days. The determined MTD was 1.0 mg/m^2. Minami et al. reported a phase I clinical study that enrolled 15 patients with advanced solid tumors [61]. Eribulin was administered via intravenous injection on days 1 and 8, with a chemotherapy cycle lasting 21 days. The recommended dose for phase II clinical research was ultimately determined to be 1.4 mg/m^2. The most common adverse reactions during treatment included neutropenia, fatigue, nausea, and peripheral neuropathy.

14.5.1.2 Phase II clinical study

In 2009, Vahdat et al. reported the results of a phase II clinical study [62]. This study was an open-label, single-arm clinical trial that enrolled a total of 103 patients with metastatic breast cancer who had previously received anthracycline- and taxane-based chemotherapy. The specific treatment regimen involved the administration of eribulin at a dose of 1.4 mg/m^2 via intravenous injection over 2–5 minutes, with treatment cycles occurring on days 1, 8, 15, and 28. Among the 87 evaluable patients, there were 10 cases of partial response (PR) (11.5%), 37 cases of stable disease (SD) (42.5%), and 36 cases of progressive disease (PD) (41.4%). The overall objective response rate (ORR) was 11.5% (95% CI: 5.7%–20.1%), and the clinical benefit rate (CBR) (PR + SD for more than 6 months) was 17.2% (95% CI: 10.0%–26.8%). The median duration of response (MDR), median progression-free survival (mPFS), and median overall survival (mOS) were 171, 79, and 275 days, respectively. In 2010, Cortes et al. also reported the results of a phase II clinical study [63]. This study, similar to the previous one, was an open-label, single-arm clinical trial that enrolled a total of 299 patients with locally advanced or metastatic breast cancer who had previously received anthracycline, taxane, and capecitabine chemotherapy. Out of the 299 patients, 291 received eribulin at a dose of 1.4 mg/m^2 via intravenous injection over 2–5 minutes on days 1, 8, and 21 of each treatment cycle. Among the evaluable 269 patients, 25 cases (9.3%) achieved PR, 125 cases (46.5%) had SD, and 116 cases (43.1%) showed PD. The ORR was 9.3% (95% CI: 6.1%–13.4%), and the CBR (including PR and SD lasting for more than 6 months) was 17.1%. The MDR was 4.1 months, mPFS was 2.6 months, and mOS was 10.4 months. In 2010, Iwata et al. also reported the results of a phase II clinical study [64]. This study was also an open-label, single-arm clinical trial that enrolled 80 evaluable patients with locally advanced or metastatic breast cancer. These patients received eribulin at a dose of 1.4 mg/m^2 via intravenous injection over 2–5 minutes on days 1, 8, and 21 of each treatment cycle. The results showed an overall ORR of 21.3% (95% CI: 12.9%–31.8%) and a CBR of 27.5% (95% CI: 18.1%–38.6%). The MDR was 119 days, the mPFS was 112 days, and the mOS was 331 days.

14.5.1.3 Pivotal phase III clinical study

Encouraged by the results of Phase II clinical trials, the Eisai pharmaceutical company initiated a Phase III clinical study targeting metastatic breast cancer. This is an open-label, randomized, multicenter trial that enrolled patients with locally recurrent or metastatic breast cancer ($n = 762$) [65], who had received 2–5 prior chemotherapy regimens, including anthracycline and taxane. Eligible subjects experienced disease progression within 6 months after the last chemotherapy. The eligible subjects were randomly assigned in a 2:1 ratio to receive eribulin or treatment of physician's choice (TPC). TPC included any monotherapy (cytotoxic, hormonal, and biologic) or supportive care only. The TPC group consisted of 97% chemotherapy (26% vinorelbine, 18% gemcitabine, 18% capecitabine, 16% taxane, 9% anthracycline, and 10% other chemotherapy) and 3% hormonal therapy. The study achieved its primary endpoint, demonstrating a statistically significant survival benefit for the eribulin group compared to the TPC group. The results showed a mOS of 13.1 months in the eribulin treatment group compared to 10.6 months in the control group, with a statistically significant difference ($P = 0.04$). The mPFS was 3.7 months in the eribulin group and 2.2 months in the control group, with no statistically significant difference ($P = 0.14$). The ORRs were 12% and 5% in the eribulin and control groups, respectively, showing a significant difference ($P = 0.002$). Overall, eribulin is the first single-agent chemotherapy drug that has demonstrated improved overall survival and manageable tolerability in patients with metastatic breast cancer, making it a viable treatment option for advanced cancer. Based on the results of the phase III clinical studies, eribulin was approved by the U.S. FDA in November 2010 for the treatment of metastatic breast cancer in patients who have received at least two prior chemotherapy regimens including anthracycline and taxane [4].

Currently, eribulin has emerged as a preferred therapeutic agent for advanced chemotherapy in the post--paclitaxel era. Eribulin not only significantly prolongs the overall survival of cancer patients but also exhibits a favorable efficacy and safety profile with minimal adverse effects. This provides clinicians with more diagnostic and treatment options and brings new hope to patients. In addition to metastatic breast cancer and liposarcoma, more efforts have been directed toward identifying new indications for eribulin. For instance, in 2019, Teramoto et al. conducted a clinical trial to compare the effects of eribulin and dacarbazine on smooth muscle sarcoma. The results demonstrated that eribulin treatment effectively extended overall survival [66]. With the continuous expansion of eribulin's therapeutic applications, this remarkable anticancer drug will play a more significant role in the humankind's fight against cancer.

14.5.2 Adverse effects of eribulin

Multiple phase I clinical studies have demonstrated that the most common adverse effects observed in breast cancer and liposarcoma patients receiving treatment with eribulin are neutropenia, with incidence rates increasing from 22% at low dose (1.4 mg/m^2) to 100% at high dose (4 mg/m^2). Other commonly reported adverse effects include alopecia, fatigue, peripheral neuropathy, nausea, abdominal pain, fever, and leukopenia. Peripheral neuropathy has been identified as the most frequent adverse effect leading to the discontinuation of eribulin treatment in clinical practice. Overall, eribulin demonstrates good tolerability as an antineoplastic agent [67].

14.6 Conclusion

Since the 1950s, the discovery and development of new antitumor agents has emerged as a hot subject in the drug research area. Not surprisingly, the magnificent development process of eribulin renders it a unique paradigm in the development history of contemporary drug research (Fig. 14.14). Eribulin is derived from halichondrin B, a marine natural product showing extremely attractive medicinal potential in the initial biological evaluation. However, its further development as an antitumor drug has been severely constrained due to its extremely difficult accessibility from natural resources. To address this challenge, synthetic chemists first completed the total synthesis of halichondrin B and then conducted a systematic SAR study on it, which eventually led to the discovery of eribulin with a simplified molecular architecture, improved synthetic accessibility, and enhanced drug properties. This process, which involved over 20 years of continuous perseverance and effort, successfully transformed a seemingly dead-end natural product into a great antitumor drug for the benefit of mankind. It fully demonstrates the courage and wisdom of humankind in "understanding and transforming nature." Furthermore, the development of eribulin offers a paradigm for the synergistic collaboration between academia and industry. The research team led by Professor Kishi made significant contributions to the discovery of eribulin, as well as related SAR study and synthetic chemistry. What they have demonstrated is not only their superb synthetic skill but also their venerable determination and courage to turn a seemingly impossible task into reality. Meanwhile, Eisai Pharmaceuticals also plays a pivotal role in this long adventure journey. Their unique strategic vision and unwavering support from beginning to end are indispensable for the ultimate success of eribulin.

On the other hand, the tale of eribulin once again showcases the significance of natural products as important sources for the discovery of new drugs and lead compounds. Over the past two decades, various new technologies and approaches have emerged in the field of drug research, leading to constant evolution and change in the drug development paradigm. In comparison, traditional natural product-oriented drug development has gradually fallen out of favor with pharmaceutical companies. However, nowadays major pharmaceutical companies have to face a dilemma: despite the increasing investment in drug development, the timeline for bringing new drugs to market continues to lengthen [67,68]. Although many factors may account for this phenomenon, one undeniable reason is that the efficiency and success rate of discovering drugs and leads have not been significantly improved with the application of new technologies. Fortunately, natural product-oriented drug research has been evolving continuously in recent years, owing to the rapid advancements in related research fields such as chemistry, biology, pharmaceuticals, and artificial intelligence. Some of the previously limiting factors, such as prolonged research cycles and high costs, are being addressed. This revitalizes the field with new vigor. In conclusion, as the adage goes, "all things in their being are good for something," the immense value of natural products is sufficient to encourage researchers to overcome the difficulties and challenges encountered during their research process. This is also the continuous driving force behind the advancement of natural product-oriented drug research.

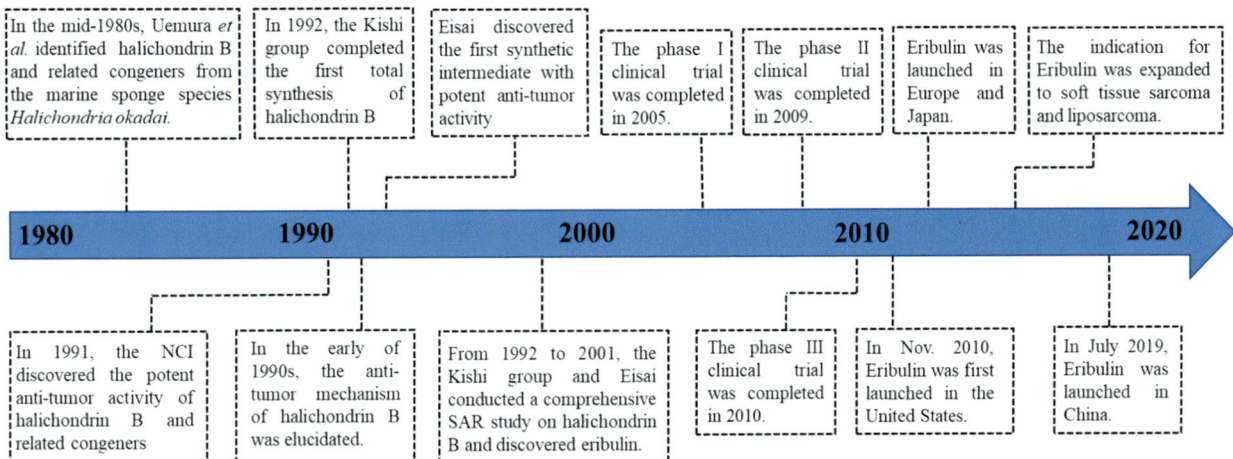

FIGURE 14.14 Summary of major events in the development history of eribulin.

References

[1] Siegel RL, Miller KD, Jemal A. Cancer statistics, 2020. CA: Cancer J Clin 2020;70(1):7−30.
[2] Newmna DJ, Cragg GM. Natural products as sources of new drugs over the nearly four decades from 01/1981 to 09/2019. J Nat Prod 2020;83(3):770−803.
[3] Huyck TK, Gradishar W, Manuguid F, et al. Eribulin mesylate. Nat Rev Drug Discov 2011;10(3):173−4.
[4] Ledford H. Complex synthesis yields breast-cancer therapy. Nature 2010;468(7324):608−9.
[5] https://www.chemistryworld.com/features/organic-odysseys-/8670.article.
[6] Jordan MA, Wilson L. Microtubules as a target for anticancer drugs. Nat Rev Cancer 2004;4(4):253−65.
[7] Zhai ZH, Wang XZ, Ding MX. Cell biology. Beijing: Higher Education Press; 2008. p. 328−9.
[8] Li JN, Jiang JD. Biological characteristics and drug research of microtubules. J Pharm Sci 2003;38(4):311−15.
[9] Kingston DGI. Tubulin-Interactive natural products as anticancer agents. J Nat Prod 2009;72(3):507−15.
[10] Shang H, Pan L, Yang S, et al. Research progress on tubulin inhibitors. J Pharm Sci 2010;45(9):1078−88.
[11] Shuai W, Wang G, Zhang YW, et al. Recent progress on tubulin inhibitors with dual targeting capabilities for cancer therapy. J Med Chem 2021;64(12):7963−90.
[12] Dumontet C, Jordan M. Microtubule-binding agents: a dynamic field of cancer therapeutics. Nat Rev Drug Discov 2010;9(10):790−803.
[13] Swami U, Chaudhary I, Ghalib MH, et al. Eribulin-a review of preclinical and clinical studies. Crit Rev Oncol Hemat 2012;81(2):163−84.
[14] Jordan MA, Kamath K, Manna T, et al. The primary antimitotic mechanism of action of the synthetic halichondrin E7389 is suppression of microtubule growth. Mol Cancer Ther 2005;4(7):1086−95.
[15] Jain S, Vahdat LT. Eribulin mesylate. Clin Cancer Res 2011;17(21):6615−22.
[16] Zongru G. Chemically synthesized complex natural remodeling drug Eribulin. J Pharm Sci 2015;50(9):1197−202.
[17] Uemura D, Takahashi K, Yamamoto T, et al. Norhalichondrin A: an anti-tumor polyether macrolide from a marine sponge. J Am Chem Soc 1985;107(16):4796−8.
[18] Hirata Y, Uemura D. Halichondrins-anti-tumor polyether macrolides from a marine sponge. Pure Appl Chem 1986;58(5):701−10.
[19] Towle MJ, Salvato KA, Budrow J, et al. In vitro and in vivo anticancer activities of synthetic macrocyclic ketone analogues of Halichondrin B. Cancer Res 2001;61(3):1013−21.
[20] Bai RL, Paull KD, Herald CL, et al. Halichondrin B and homoHalichondrin B, marine natural products binding in the vinca domain of tubulin. J Biol Chem 1991;266(24):15882−9.
[21] Aicher TD, Buszek KR, Fang FG, et al. Total synthesis of Halichondrin B and norHalichondrin B. J Am Chem Soc 1992;114(8):3162−4.
[22] Allred TK, Manoni F, Harran PG. Exploring the boundaries of "Practical": de novo syntheses of complex natural product-based drug candidates. Chem Rev 2017;117(18):11994−2051.
[23] Okude Y, Hirano S, Hiyama T, et al. Grignard-type carbonyl addition of allyl halides by means of chromous salt. A chemospecific synthesis of homoallyl alcohols. J Am Chem Soc 1977;99(9):3179−81.
[24] Jin H, Uenishi J, Christ WJ, et al. Catalytic effect of nickel(II) chloride and palladium(II) acetate on chromium(II)-mediated coupling reaction of iodo olefins with aldehydes. J Am Chem Soc 1986;108(18):5644−6.
[25] Furstner A. Carbon-carbon bond formation involving organochromium(III) reagents. Chem Rev 1999;99(4):991−1045.
[26] Yamamoto A, Ueda A, Bremond P, et al. Total synthesis of halichondrin C. J Am Chem Soc 2012;134(2):893−6.
[27] Ueda A, Yamamoto A, Kato D, et al. Total synthesis of halichondrin A, the missing member in the halichondrin class of natural products. J Am Chem Soc 2014;136(13):5171−6.
[28] Jackson KL, Henderson JA, Motoyoshi H, et al. A total synthesis of norHalichondrin B. Angew Chem Int Ed 2009;48(13):2346−50.
[29] Nicolaou KC, Pan S, Shelke Y, et al. A highly convergent total synthesis of norHalichondrin B. J Am Chem Soc 2021;143(49):20970−9.
[30] Kim S, Salomon RG. Total synthesis of halichondrins: highly stereoselective construction of a homochiral pentasubstituted H-ring pyran intermediate from α-D-glucose. Tetrahedron Lett 1989;30(46):6279−82.
[31] Cooper AJ, Salomon K. Total synthesis of halichondrins: highly stereoselective construction of a homochiral pentasubstituted H-ring pyran intermediate from α-D-glucose. Tetrahedron Lett 1990;31(27):3813−16.
[32] Burke SD, Buchanan JL, Rovin JD. Synthesis of a C(22)→C(34) halichondrin precursor via a double dioxanone-to-dihydropyran rearrangement. Tetrahedron Lett 1991;32(32):3961−4.
[33] Cooper AJ, Pan W, Salomon RG. Total synthesis of Halichondrin B from common sugars: an F-ring intermediate from D-glucose and efficient construction of the C1 to C21 segment. Tetrahedron Lett 1993;34(51):8193−6.
[34] Horita K, Hachiya S, Nagasawa M, et al. Synthetic studies of Halichondrin B, an anti-tumor polyether macrolide isolated from a marine sponge. 1. Stereoselective synthesis of the C1-C13 fragment via construction of the B and A rings by kinetically and thermodynamically controlled intramolecular michael reactions. Synlett 1994;5(1):38−40.
[35] Lambert WT, Hanson GH, Benayoud F, et al. Halichondrin B: synthesis of the C1-C22 subunit. J Org Chem 2005;70(23):9382−98.
[36] Henderson JA, Jackson KL, Phillips AJ. Highly functionalized pyranopyrans from furans: a synthesis of the C27 − C38 and C44 − C53 subunits of norHalichondrin B. Org Lett 2007;9(25):5299−302.
[37] Yadav JS, Reddy CN, Sabitha G. Synthesis of the C38−C54 spiroketal segment of Halichondrin B. Tetrahedron Lett 2012;53(20):2504−7.
[38] Belanger F, Chase CE, Endo A, et al. Stereoselective synthesis of the halaven C14−C26 fragment from D-Quinic acid: crystallization-induced diastereoselective transformation of an α-Methyl nitrile. Angew Chem Int Ed 2015;54(17):5108−11.

[39] Yu MJ, Kishi Y, Littlefield BA. Discovery of E7389, a fully synthetic macrocyclic ketone analog of Halichondrin B. In: Cragg GM, Kingston DGI, Newman DJ, editors. Anticancer agents from natural products. 2nd ed. Boca Raton, FL: CRC Press/Taylor & Francis; 2012. p. 317–45.

[40] Seletsky BM, Wang Y, Hawkins LD, et al. Structurally simplified macrolactone analogues of Halichondrin B. Bioorg Med Chem Lett 2004;14(22):5547–50.

[41] Zheng W, Seletsky BM, Palme MH, et al. Macrocyclic ketone analogues of Halichondrin B. Bioorg Med Chem Lett 2004;14(22):5551–4.

[42] Yu MJ, Zheng WJ, Seletsky BM. From micrograms to grams: scale-up synthesis of Eribulin mesylate. Nat Prod Rep 2013;30(9):1158–64.

[43] Choi HW, Nakajima K, Demeke D, et al. Asymmetric Ni(II)/Cr(II)-mediated coupling reaction: catalytic process. Org Lett 2002;4(25):4435–8.

[44] Austad BC, Benayoud F, Calkins TL, et al. Process development of Halaven®: synthesis of the C14-C35 fragment via iterative Nozaki-Hiyama-Kishi reaction-Williamson ether cyclization. Synlett 2013;24(3):327–32.

[45] Chase C., Endo A., Fang F.G., et al. Methods for the synthesis of Halichondrin B analogs and their intermediates. WO2009046308 A1, 2009.

[46] Pedeferri M, Zenoni G, Mazzotti M, et al. Experimental analysis of a chiral separation through simulated moving bed chromatography. Chem Eng Sci 1999;54(17):3735–48.

[47] Tokunaga M, Larrow JF, Kakiuchi F, et al. Asymmetric catalysis with water: efficient kinetic resolution of terminal epoxides by means of catalytic hydrolysis. Science 1997;277(5328):936–8.

[48] Stamos DP, Sheng XC, Chen SS, et al. Ni(II)/Cr(II)-mediated coupling reaction: beneficial effects of 4-tert-butylpyridine as an additive and development of new and improved workup procedures. Tetrahedron Lett 1997;38(36):6355–8.

[49] Choi H, Demeke D, Kang FA, et al. Synthetic studies on the marine natural product Halichondrins. Pure Appl Chem 2003;75(1):1–17.

[50] Yang YR, Kim DS, Kishi Y. Second generation synthesis of C27-C35 building block of E7389, a synthetic Halichondrin analogue. Org Lett 2009;11(20):4516–19.

[51] Duan JJW, Kishi Y. Synthetic studies on Halichondrins: a new practical synthesis of the C.l-C.12 segment. Tetrahedron Lett 1993;34(47):7541–4.

[52] Stamos DP, Kishi Y. Synthetic studies on Halichondrins: a practical synthesis of the C.1-C.13. Tetrahedron Lett 1996;37(48):8643–6.

[53] Chase CE, Fang FG, Lewis BM, et al. Process development of Halaven®: synthesis of the C1-C13 fragment from D-(−)-Gulono-1,4-lactone. Synlett 2013;24(3):323–6.

[54] Austad BC, Calkins TL, Fang FG, et al. Commercial manufacture of Halaven®: chemoselective transformations en route to structurally complex macrocyclic ketones. Synlett 2013;24(3):333–7.

[55] Kimura T, Synold T, Mahaffey CM, et al. E7389, a novel antimicrotubule agent with potent p53-independent induction of p27, Bcl2 phosphorylation and cytotoxicity in nonsmall cell lung cancer (NSCLC). Proc Am Soc Clin Oncol 2003;22 [abstr2804].

[56] Dabydeen DA, Burnett JC, Bai R, et al. Comparison of the activities of the truncated Halichondrin B analog NSC 707389 (E7389) with those of the parent compound and a proposed binding site on tubulin. Mol Pharmacol 2006;70(6):1866–75.

[57] Qing Y. Eribulin mesylate, a new anti-metastatic breast cancer drug. Chin J N Drugs 2012;21(1):1–5.

[58] Synold TW, Morgan RJ, Newman EM, et al. A phase I pharmacokinetic and target validation study of the novel anti-tubulin agent E7389: a California cancer consortium trial. 2005 ASCO Annual Meeting Proceedings. J Clin Oncol 2005;23(16 Suppl.):3036.

[59] Tan AR, Runbin EH, Walton DC, et al. Phase I study of Eribulin mesylate (E7389) administered once every 21 days in patients with advanced solid tumors. Clin Cancer Res 2009;15(12):4213–19.

[60] Goel S, Mita AC, Mita M, et al. A phase I study of Eribulin mesylate (E7389), a mechanistically novel inhibitor of microtubule dynamics, in patients with advanced solid tumors. Clin Cancer Res 2009;15(12):4207–12.

[61] Minami H, Mukohara T, et al. A Phase I study of Eribulin mesylate (E7389) in patients with refractory cancers. Eur J Cancer Suppl 2008;6(12):140-140.

[62] Vahdat LT, Pruitt B, Fabian CJ, et al. Phase II study of Eribulin mesylate, a Halichondrin B analog, in patients with metastatic breast cancer previously treated with an anthracycline and a taxane. J Clin Oncol 2009;27(18):2954–61.

[63] Cortes J, Vahdat L, Blum JL, et al. Phase II study of the Halichondrin B analog Eribulin mesylate in patients with locally advanced or metastatic breast cancer previously treated with an anthracycline, a taxane and capecitabine. J Clin Oncol 2010;28(25):3922–8.

[64] Iwata H, Aogi K, Masuda N. Efficacy and safety of eribulin in Japanese patients (Pts) with advanced breast cancer. 2010 ASCO Annual Meeting I. J Clin Oncol 2010;28(15, Suppl.):1081.

[65] Twelves C, Loesch D, Jl BLUM, et al. A Phase III study (EMBRACE) of Eribulin mesylate versus treatment of physician's choice in patients with locally recurrent or metastatic breast cancer previously treated with an anthracycline and a taxane. 2010 ASCO Annual Meeting II. J Clin Oncol 2010;28(18, Suppl.):CRA1004.

[66] Fujimoto E, Takehara K, Tanaka T, et al. Uterine leiomyosarcoma well-controlled with Eribulin mesylate. Int Canc Conf J 2019;8(1):33–8.

[67] Scannell J, Blanckley A, Boldon H, et al. Diagnosing the decline in pharmaceutical R&D efficiency. Nat Rev Drug Discov 2012;11(3):191–200.

[68] Abou-Gharbia M, Childers WE. Discovery of innovative therapeutics: today's realities and tomorrow's vision. 2. Pharma's challenges and their commitment to innovation. J Med Chem 2014;57(13):5525–53.

Chapter 15

Targeted protein kinase inhibitor imatinib

Lijie Peng[1] and Ke Ding[1,2]
[1]*College of Pharmacy, Jinan University, Guangzhou, P.R. China,* [2]*Shanghai Institute of Organic Chemistry, Chinese Academy of Sciences, Shanghai, P.R. China*

Chapter outline

- 15.1 Protein kinases (PKs) and protein kinase inhibitors (PKIs) as antineoplastic agents   349
  - 15.1.1 Introduction   349
  - 15.1.2 Protein kinases   350
  - 15.1.3 Composition and catalytic mechanism of protein kinase   350
  - 15.1.4 Classifications and design of PKIs   354
- 15.2 Medicinal chemistry of imatinib   362
  - 15.2.1 Bcr-Abl and CML   362
  - 15.2.2 Molecular design and structure optimization   363
  - 15.2.3 Structure-activity relationship   366
  - 15.2.4 Synthesis of imatinib   367
  - 15.2.5 Pharmacokinetics and pharmacodynamics of imatinib   369
  - 15.2.6 Drug safety and drug-drug interaction   370
  - 15.2.7 Clinical efficacy and expansion of indications   371
- 15.3 Imatinib resistance and solutions   373
  - 15.3.1 Clinical mechanisms of imatinib resistance   373
  - 15.3.2 Next-generation drugs to overcome imatinib resistance   374
- 15.4 Summary   382
- References   382

15.1 Protein kinases (PKs) and protein kinase inhibitors (PKIs) as antineoplastic agents

15.1.1 Introduction

The genesis and progression of cancer represent profoundly intricate processes, the thorough exploration of which has persisted for over a century. Presently, clinical cancer management primarily involves three therapeutic modalities: surgical intervention, radiotherapy, and pharmacotherapy. Among these modalities, the development of antineoplastic agents commenced in the latter half of the 20th century. Preceding the 1980s, the mechanistic action of anticancer agents primarily targeted DNA synthesis and cell division, giving rise to agents such as antimetabolites, alkylating agents, and microtubule destabilizers. Despite demonstrating efficacy, these traditional cytotoxic chemotherapeutic agents exhibit limited selectivity for tumor cells, resulting in significant adverse effects toward vigorously proliferating normal cells, such as bone marrow, hair follicles, and gastrointestinal cells.

Post-1990s, concomitant with the advancements in human genomics, proteomics, and oncobiology, considerable strides have been made in comprehending the oncogenic processes at the molecular level. Several specific biological targets within tumor cells or their microenvironments have been identified and validated, thereby ushering in the era of targeted antineoplastic agents. Compared to conventional chemotherapeutic agents, targeted therapies exhibit enhanced specificity, efficacy, and reduced side effects, thus propelling cancer treatment toward precision and personalized medicine.

By the end of 2020, more than 110 targeted drugs had been approved by the US Food and Drug Administration (FDA), accounting for over 60% of newly launched antineoplastic drugs, including monoclonal antibodies and small molecule inhibitors. Depending on their respective targets, targeted therapies can be classified into various categories, including PKIs, ubiquitin-proteasome inhibitors, epigenetic modifiers, tumor metabolism modulators, apoptosis inducers, and DNA damage repair agents. Among these, PKIs represent the most extensively researched category.

In 1998, the first monoclonal antibody targeting human epidermal growth factor receptor-2 (HER2), trastuzumab, was approved by the FDA for the treatment of HER2-positive breast cancer patients. Its success marked a milestone in cancer-targeted therapy and driven the development of large-molecule PKIs. Subsequently, in 2001, the approval of the small molecule inhibitor, which targets the breakpoint cluster region-abelson (Bcr-Abl) PK, imatinib, for the treatment of Bcr-Abl-positive chronic myeloid leukemia (CML), not only provided the proof of principle that cancer can be treated by targeting the underlying molecular defects but also fueled the small molecule PKI discovery.

15.1.2 Protein kinases

Kinases are a family of enzymes that catalyze the transfer of phosphate groups from adenosine triphosphate (ATP) to specific substrates (Fig. 15.1), thus causing phosphorylation and in turn regulating various cellular processes, including gene transcription, protein translation, cell differentiation, and signal transduction. Virtually, the deregulation of kinase function through environmental and genetic alterations is linked to the development of a large diversity of diseases such as cancer, immunodeficiency, metabolic, cardiovascular, and infectious diseases.

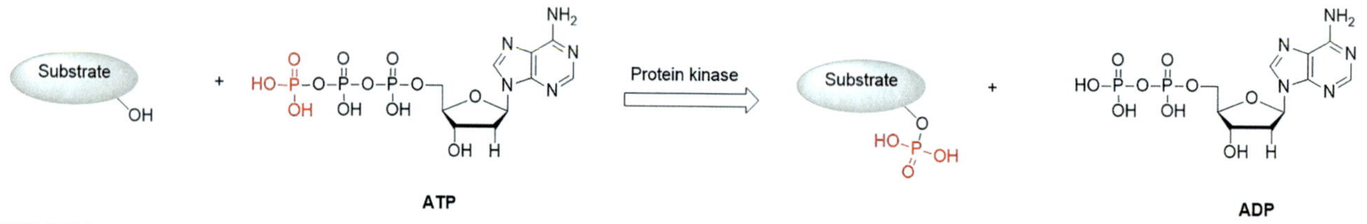

FIGURE 15.1 Function of protein kinase.

Based on their substrate specificity, kinases can be categorized into PKs, lipid kinases, carbohydrate kinases, and nucleotide kinases. The PKs family is among the largest and most investigated groups, with 518 members being encoded by about 2.5% of the human genome [1]. According to the types of residues phosphorylated of their substrates, PKs can be further divided into serine/threonine PKs (385 members), tyrosine PKs (90 members), and tyrosine kinase (TK)-like protein enzymes (43 members). Among these, the typical drug target is predominantly TKs, including receptor tyrosine kinases and nonreceptor tyrosine kinases (NRTKs).

The concept of developing PKIs originated in the late 1950s to early 1960s when partial characteristics, cascade signaling pathways, and functions of PKs were just being elucidated. The emergence of small molecule inhibitors targeting kinases began in the early 1980s [2], with the first reported inhibitor targeting the epidermal growth factor receptor (EGFR), followed by numerous small molecule inhibitors targeting different kinases. The success of PKIs was initially validated in clinical contexts with the approval of trastuzumab in 1998 and imatinib in 2001 by the US FDA. Presently, PKs have now become the second most important group of drug targets after G-protein-coupled receptors [3], and developing PKIs has been proven to be an effective strategy in targeted cancer therapy.

The marketed PKIs comprise both large-molecule and small-molecule varieties. Large molecule inhibitors, primarily monoclonal antibodies and fusion proteins such as rituximab and aflibercept, exhibit excellent specificity. However, their target mainly consists of receptor-type PKs situated on cell membranes, necessitating exclusive intravenous administration and resulting in elevated costs. In contrast, small molecule inhibitors can target nonreceptor PKs, are conveniently administered orally, and are relatively more cost-effective. Consequently, small-molecule PKIs constitute the cornerstone of targeted anticancer drugs. As of the end of 2023, more than 80 small molecule PKIs have been approved by the FDA, primarily indicated for cancer treatment.

15.1.3 Composition and catalytic mechanism of protein kinase

Since the resolution of the crystal structure of the catalytic domain of the first PK (protein kinase A, PKA) in 1991 [4], over 6000 crystal structures related to PKs have been reported. PKs have a small amino-terminal lobe and a large carboxyl-terminal lobe that contain several conserved α-helices and β-strands. The N-lobe and C-lobe form a cleft that serves as a docking site for ATP, and peptide substrates bind at the edge of the ATP-binding pocket [5] (Fig. 15.2). Although the primary sequences of PKs exhibit considerable diversity, there exists a high conservation in their three-dimensional structures, particularly within the catalytic domain responsible for ATP binding. This catalytic domain ranges from 250 to 300 amino acid residues, corresponding to about 30 kD.

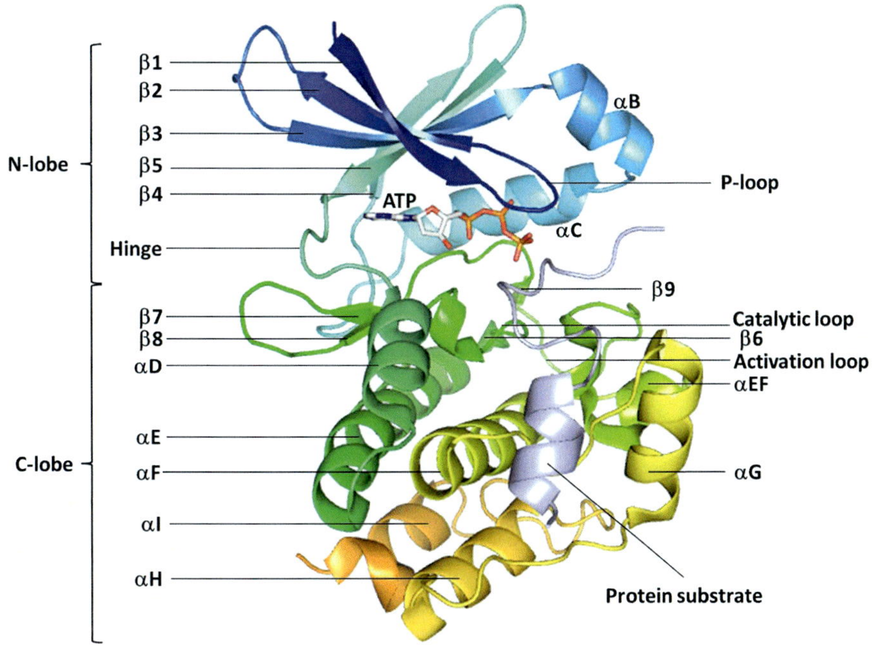

FIGURE 15.2 Catalytic domain of PKA (PDB: 4dh3).

The catalytic domain can be divided into several smaller subdomains based on their functions, and some specific residues play crucial roles in maintaining the active conformation of PKs and facilitating the binding of ATP to achieve catalytic function. Here is a detailed description:

15.1.3.1 Hinge

The hinge is a segment connecting the small and large lobes and is composed of 6–7 residues. It interacts with the adenine moiety of ATP through hydrogen bonds. Specifically, the exocyclic N6 of ATP forms a hydrogen bond with the carbonyl backbone of the first hinge residue (E121) as depicted for active PKA, and the adenine N1 of ATP forms another hydrogen bond with the backbone amide of the third hinge residue (V123) as depicted for PKA (Fig. 15.3). Most ATP-competitive kinase inhibitors also make hydrogen bonds with the backbone residues of the hinge.

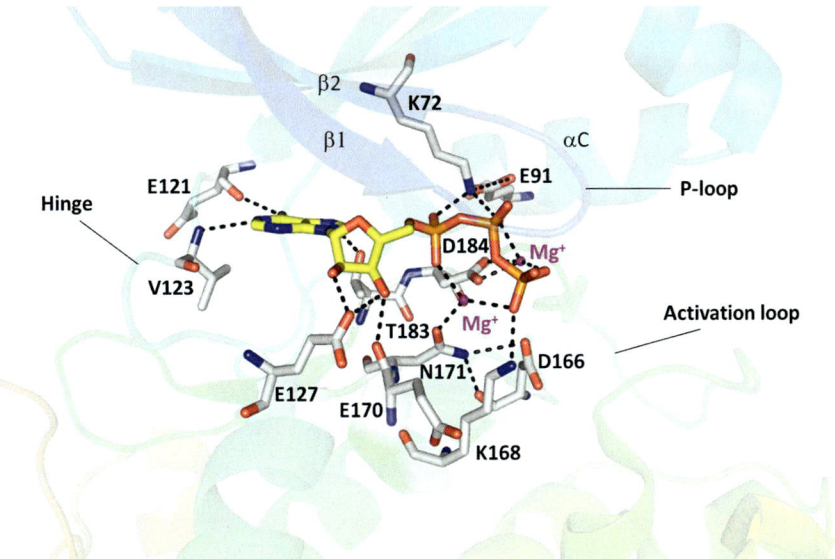

FIGURE 15.3 ATP-binding site of PKA (PDB: 4dh3).

15.1.3.2 N-lobe

Although both small N- and large C-lobes contribute to nucleotide binding, most of the interaction involves the N-lobe.

15.1.3.2.1 P-loop (phosphate-binding loop)

The P-loop, the most flexible part of the lobe, occurs between the β1- and β2-strands. It is glycine-rich and contains the conserved GxGxxG signature, which was found to stabilize the β and γ phosphate groups of ATP. Additionally, there is often a valine residue following the GxGxxG motif, which also interacts hydrophobically with the adenine base of ATP and many small molecule inhibitors.

15.1.3.2.2 Lysine (K) on β3

The lysine residue (K72 for PKA) of the β3-strand holds the α- and β-phosphates of ATP in position.

15.1.3.2.3 Glutamic acid (E) near the middle of the αC helix

Glutamic acid (E) forms a salt bridge with the lysine (K) of the β3. The presence of a salt bridge is a prerequisite for the formation of the active state of the kinase, known as the "αC-helix$_{in}$" conformation. For example, E91 forms an electrostatic bond with K72 of active PKA. The absence of this electrostatic bond leads to the "αC-helix$_{out}$" conformation, rendering the kinase in an inactive state. However, it should be noted that the αC-helix$_{in}$ conformation is necessary but not sufficient for the expression of full kinase activity, as the activated kinases are also regulated by the activation loop of the C-lobe.

15.1.3.2.4 Gatekeeper residue

The gatekeeper residue is the last residue at the end of the β5-strand immediately before the hinge. It controls the access of inhibitors to the hydrophobic pocket adjacent to the adenine binding site [6,7] and is a crucial determinant for the binding affinity and selectivity of inhibitors. Approximately 77% of PKs have a relatively large (e.g., Phe, Leu, and Met) gatekeeper residue, while the others have smaller gatekeeper residues (e.g., Val and Thr).

15.1.3.3 C-lobe

The C-lobe makes a major contribution to protein/peptide substrate binding and also participates in nucleotide binding.

15.1.3.3.1 The second residue on β7

It is located at the bottom of the adenine binding pocket and interacts hydrophobically with the adenine base of ATP and ATP-competitive inhibitors.

15.1.3.3.2 The catalytic loop

It is proximal to the β6- and β7-strands, consisting of HRDxxxxN (His-Arg-Asp-xxxx-Asn) sequence. The aspartic acid (D) residue in this loop plays a central role in catalysis (Fig. 15.4). It acts as a base, abstracting the proton from the hydroxyl group of the protein substrate, thereby facilitating the nucleophilic attack of oxygen on the γ-phosphate group of ATP. Additionally, the asparagine (N) residue in this loop chelates one magnesium ion (Mg^{2+}) [8]. Most kinase catalytic reactions require the participation of two magnesium ions.

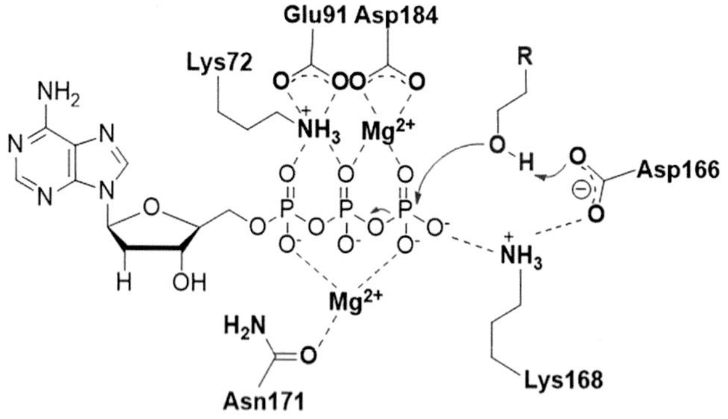

FIGURE 15.4 Catalytic mechanism of protein kinase.

15.1.3.3.3 Activation segment

The activation segment of nearly all kinases begins with the Asp-Phe-Gly (DFG) motif and ends with the APE motif, generally 35–40 residues long (Fig. 15.5). The center of the activation segment, which is its most diverse part in various PKs in terms of length and sequence, is known as the activation loop, which plays a crucial role in regulating substrate binding and the conformational activity of the PK. This loop in many PKs contains one or more

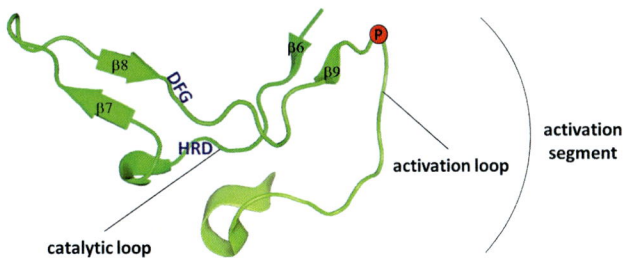

FIGURE 15.5 Structure of catalytic loop and activation segment.

phosphorylatable residues. Phosphorylation of specific residues can result in various conformational changes. The activation segment exhibits an open or extended conformation in all active enzymes, with DFG-D side chain pointing toward the ATP-binding site and coordinating the second Mg^{2+}, corresponding to the "DFG_{in}" conformation. Whereas in many dormant enzymes, the activation segment adopts a closed conformation, with DFG-D extending in the opposite direction away from the active site, corresponding to the "DFG_{out}" conformation. A small number of kinases may also exhibit an inactivated state with α-helix$_{out}$ and DFG_{in} conformation (Fig. 15.6).

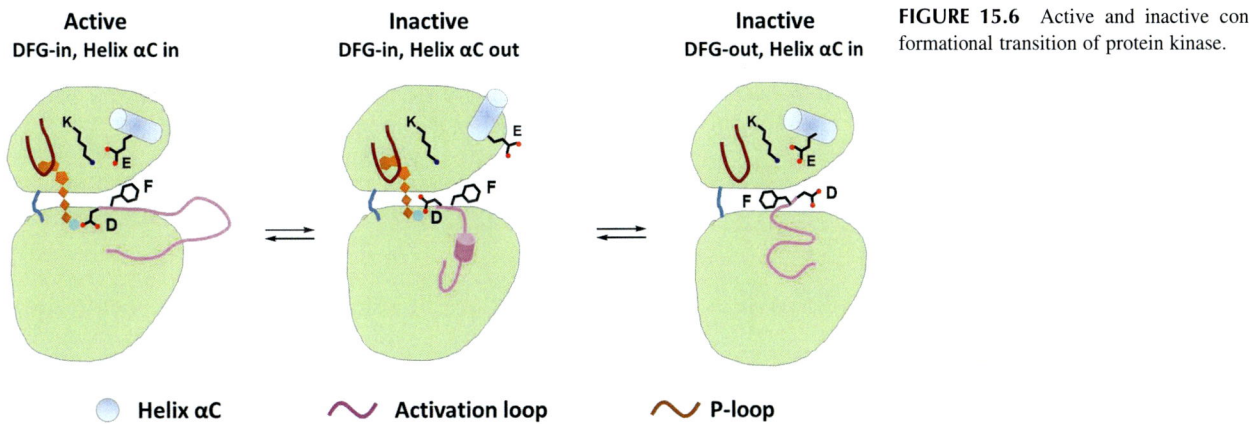

FIGURE 15.6 Active and inactive conformational transition of protein kinase.

In addition to the fingerprint residues K/E/D/D, His-Arg-Asp (HRD), and DFG motifs mentioned above, 16 functionally important hydrophobic residues make up PK skeletal assembly, classified into three categories: the catalytic spine (C-spine, 8 residues), the regulation spine (R-spine, 5 residues), and the shell (3 residues) based on their local spatial pattern alignment [9,10].

The C-spine participates in the positioning of ATP, and the R-spine determines the activate/inactivate enzyme states and interacts with protein substrates to enable catalysis. The shell residues strengthen and stabilize the regulatory spine of most PKs. These hydrophobic skeletons also contribute to the interactions of many ATP competitive inhibitors with targeted kinase. Table 15.1 lists the residues that make up the catalytic and regulatory spines and shells of human Abl.

TABLE 15.1 Key hydrophobic residues in the Abl catalytic domain.

Category	Location	Symbol	Residue
Regulation spine	β4-strand	RS4	L301
	αC-helix	RS3	M290
	Activation loop DFG-F	RS2	F382
	Catalytic loop HRD-H	RS1	H361
	αF-helix	RS0	D421
R-Shell	Two residues upstream from the gatekeeper	Sh3	I313
	Gatekeeper	Sh2	T315
	αC-β4 back loop	Sh1	V299

(Continued)

TABLE 15.1 (Continued)

Category	Location	Symbol	Residue
Catalytic spine	β3-strand Axk-A	CS8	A269
	β2-strand V	CS7	V256
	β7-strand	CS6	L370
	β7-strand	CS5	V371
	β7-strand	CS4	C369
	αD-helix	CS3	L323
	αF-helix	CS2	L428
	αF-helix	CS1	L432

An intact regulation spine is required for the formation of the active PK conformation. The superposition of the R-spine and shell residues of active and inactive Abl show that most components are nearly superimposable (0.6 Å) except for Phe382, which is displaced from that of active Abl by 9 Å and lead to a broken R-spine in the inactive conformation (Fig. 15.7).

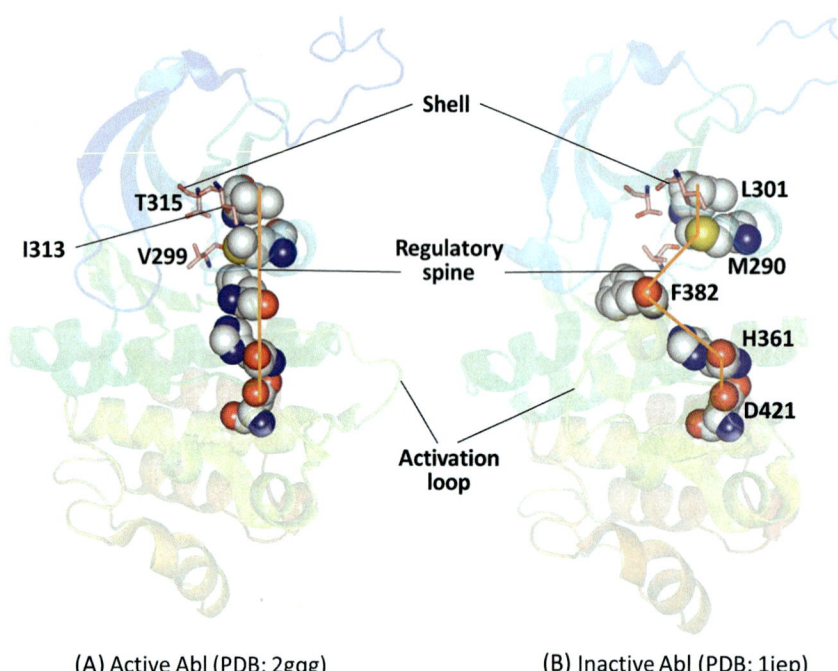

FIGURE 15.7 Shell and regulatory spine of Abl.

(A) Active Abl (PDB: 2gqg)   (B) Inactive Abl (PDB: 1iep)

15.1.4 Classifications and design of PKIs

In terms of the structural understanding of active/inactive kinase regulatory mechanisms [11,12], a variety of PKIs were developed. Based on their binding modes with targeted kinases, PKIs can be classified into three major categories: ATP-competitive inhibitors, allosteric inhibitors, and covalent kinase inhibitors.

Structural investigations have revealed the conservation of the catalytic domain, encompassing the ATP-binding site, across various PKs. Therefore, achieving target selectivity presents the primary challenge in the design of small molecule PKIs. The unique structural features of various binding pockets within targeted kinases should be strategically exploited to develop more selective inhibitors.

The binding pocket occupied by the majority of PKIs within the catalytic domain of PKs is typically subdivided into the front pocket (FP) and the back pocket (BP) (Fig. 15.8). The specific details are listed in Table 15.2.

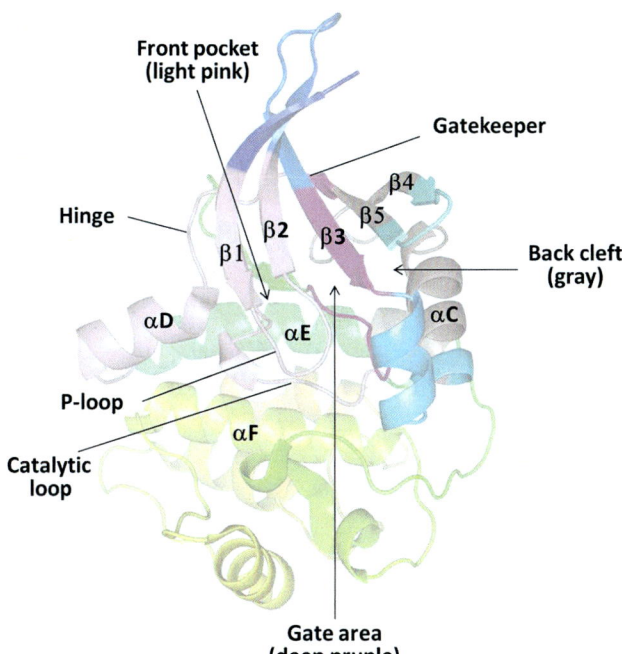

FIGURE 15.8 Drug-binding pocket of PKA (PDB: 4dh3).

TABLE 15.2 Categories and location of ligand-binding pockets within PK catalytic domain.

Front pocket	AP	Adenine pocket
	FP-I	Between the large lobe xDFG motif and the solvent-exposed hinge residues
	FP-II	Between the small lobe β3-strand near the ceiling of the cleft and the glycine-rich loop
Back pocket	Gate area	Between the β3-strand of the small lobe and the proximal section of the activation segment including the DFG of the large lobe
	Back cleft	The αC-β4 back loop, the β4- and β5-strands of the small lobe, and the αE-helix within the large lobe

Among, the gate area consists of two pockets: the smaller BP-I-A located near the top of the gatekeeper region, and the larger BP-I-B located in the middle of the gatekeeper region, controlling the entrance to the back cleft. The back cleft is further divided into several subpockets (Fig. 15.9). The size of the gatekeeper residue significantly influences the volume and accessibility of the back cleft. For instance, when the gatekeeper residue is relatively small, such as Gly/Ala/Ser/Cys/Thr/Val, the back cleft exhibits a larger volume and is easily accessible to ligands. Conversely, when the gatekeeper residue is of medium size, such as Ile/Leu/Met/Gln, the volume of the back cleft is slightly reduced, but ligands can still enter. However, if the gatekeeper residue is a large residue like Phe/Tyr, the back cleft becomes markedly constricted, posing challenges for ligand occupancy.

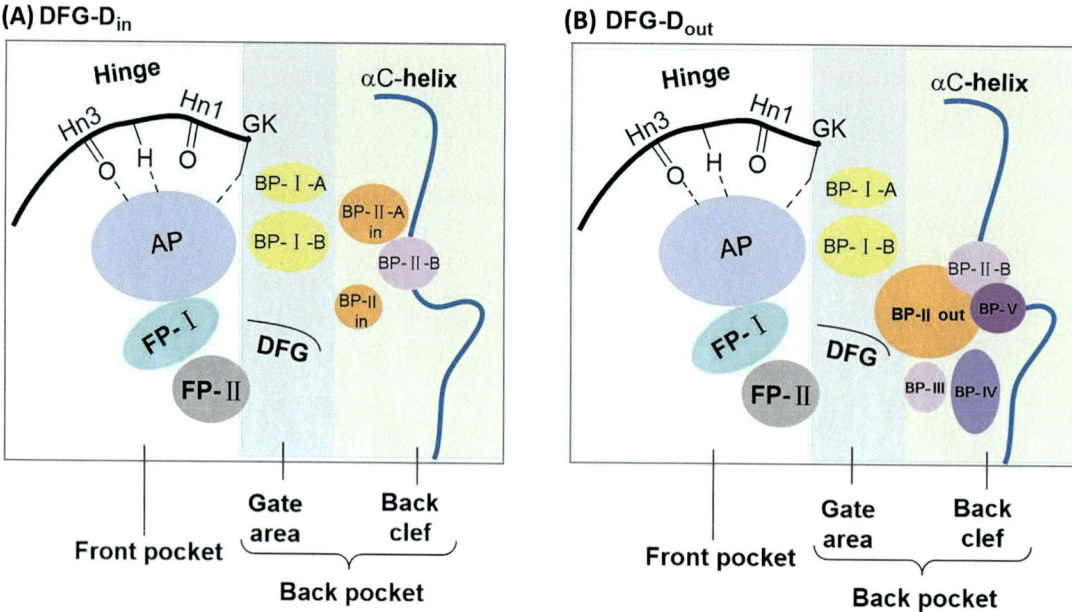

FIGURE 15.9 Ligand-binding pockets of the protein kinase catalytic domain.

During the transition of the kinase catalytic domain from the activated DFG$_{in}$ conformation to the inactivated DFG$_{out}$ conformation, corresponding alterations occur in the binding pockets for ligands. Specifically, significant changes occur in the BP. The original subpockets BP-II-in and BP-II-A-in within the BP disappear, giving rise to new subpockets BP-II-out, BP-III, BP-IV, and BP-V. Among them, BP-II-out emerges as a hydrophobic pocket exposed by the movement of the phenylalanine (F) residue in the DFG motif conformational shift. BP-III is located at the bottom of the pocket. BP-IV and BP-V partially extend into the solvent region (Fig. 15.9).

In the development of small molecule PKIs, structure-based drug design has consistently held a pivotal role. The crystal structures of PKs bound to ATP provide invaluable insights into amino acid residues and their conformational alterations, serving as essential templates for designing drugs targeting these kinases. Moreover, comparative analyses of amino acid variances and binding pockets among diverse kinases have been extensively employed to enhance the activity and selectivity of inhibitors, thus playing a crucial role in the successful development of PKI drugs.

15.1.4.1 ATP-competitive inhibitors

ATP-competitive inhibitors bind reversibly to the ATP-binding pocket of PKs and typically exhibit steady-state enzyme competitive inhibition with respect to ATP. Therefore, most ATP-competitive inhibitors contain a heterocyclic scaffold, which mimics the interactions of the adenine moiety of ATP by forming multiple hydrogen bonds with the hinge residues. The representative heterocyclic scaffolds as hinge-binding elements for FDA-approved PKI drugs are shown in Fig. 15.10. The compound libraries designed with these structural features have become vital sources of lead compounds for kinase inhibitors discovery.

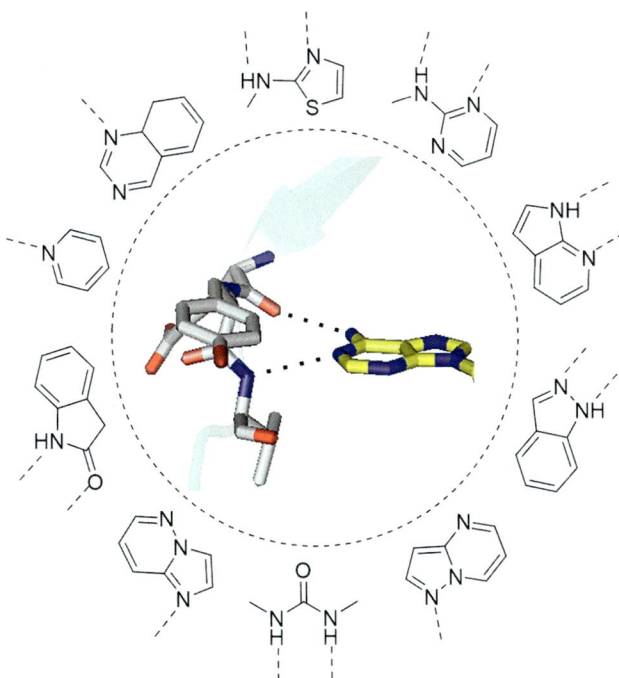

FIGURE 15.10 Typical heterocyclic scaffolds of known PKIs.

Based on the conformational state of the kinase they interact with, ATP-competitive kinase inhibitors can be further classified into three types: Type I, Type $I_{1/2}$, and Type II.

15.1.4.1.1 Type I inhibitors

Type I inhibitors bind to the active conformation (α-helix$_{in}$, DFG$_{in}$) of PKs. The general pharmacophore model for Type I PKIs is shown in Fig. 15.11, with a heterocyclic core that occupies the adenine region and forms 1–3 hydrogen bonds with the hinge region, two hydrophobic groups that occupies the FP and BP, respectively. Additionally, a hydrophilic group is generally directed toward the solvent region to modulate the pharmacokinetic properties of the compound.

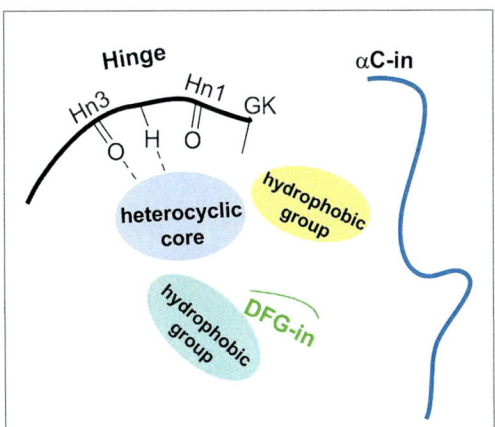

FIGURE 15.11 Binding mode of Type I inhibitors.

Type I inhibitors constitute the predominant class among FDA-approved kinase inhibitors (Fig. 15.12), including EGFR inhibitors gefitinib and erlotinib; Bcr-Abl inhibitor dasatinib; anaplastic lymphoma kinase (ALK) inhibitors brigatinib and lorlatinib; and VEGFR inhibitors pazopanib, vandetanib, and lenvatinib. The design of dasatinib will be discussed in detail below.

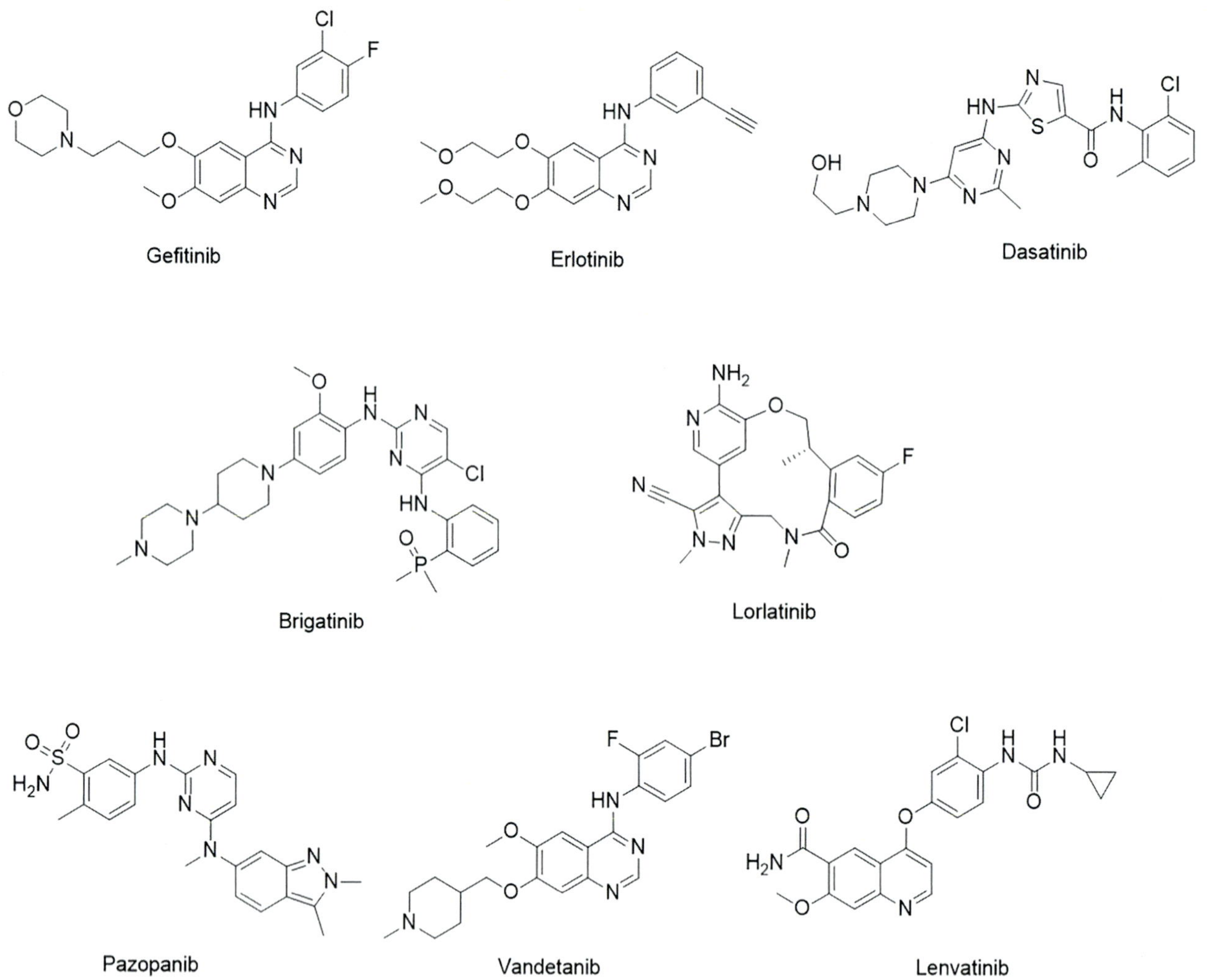

FIGURE 15.12 Representatives of Type I inhibitors.

15.1.4.1.2 Type I½ inhibitors

Type I½ inhibitors are a hybrid of the Type I and II classes and bind to the inactive conformation (α-helix$_{out}$, DFG$_{in}$) of PKs (Fig. 15.13).

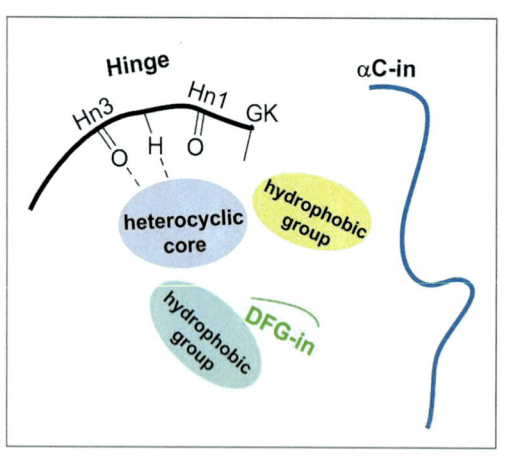

FIGURE 15.13 Binding mode of Type I½ inhibitors.

In the existing FDA-approved kinase inhibitors, there are approximately 10 drugs that belong to the Type I½ inhibitors (Fig. 15.14), including EGFR inhibitor lapatinib; ALK inhibitors crizotinib, ceritinib, and alectinib; B-Raf inhibitors vemurafenib, dabrafenib, and encorafenib; and CDK4&6 inhibitors palbociclib, abemaciclib, and ribociclib.

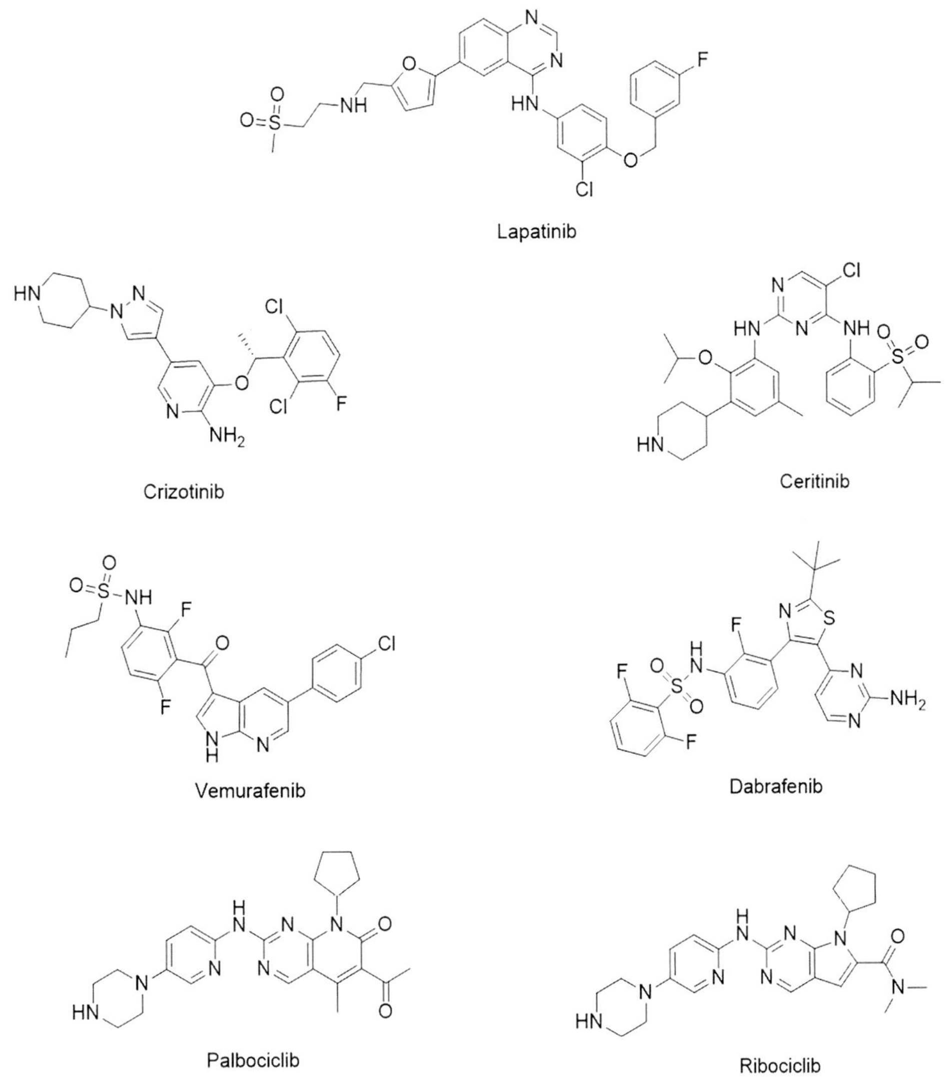

FIGURE 15.14 Representatives of Type I½ kinase inhibitors.

15.1.4.1.3 Type II inhibitors

Type II inhibitors primarily bind to an inactive (α-helix$_{in}$, DFG$_{out}$) conformation of a kinase, where the Asp (D) residue rotates outward and the Phe (F) residue rotates inward, resulting in a larger BP available for drug binding. Additionally, the backbone N—H group of the DFG-Asp and the C=O group of conserved Glu in the α-helix are available to form hydrogen bonds with the ligand that occupies hydrophobic pocket III (Fig. 15.15).

360 Medicinal Chemistry and Drug Development

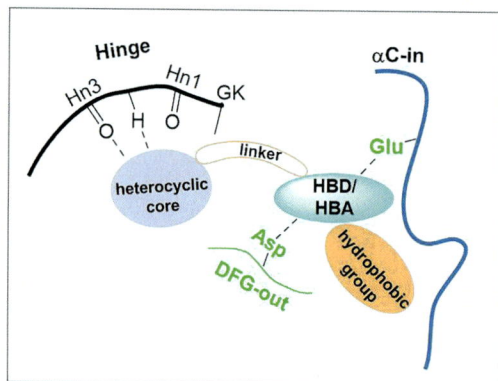

FIGURE 15.15 Binding mode of Type II inhibitors.

The representatives of Type II FDA-approved kinase inhibitors include Bcr-Abl inhibitors such as imatinib, nilotinib, and ponatinib, as well as VEGFR inhibitors such as sunitinib and sorafenib (Fig. 15.16). The design of imatinib will be discussed in detail below.

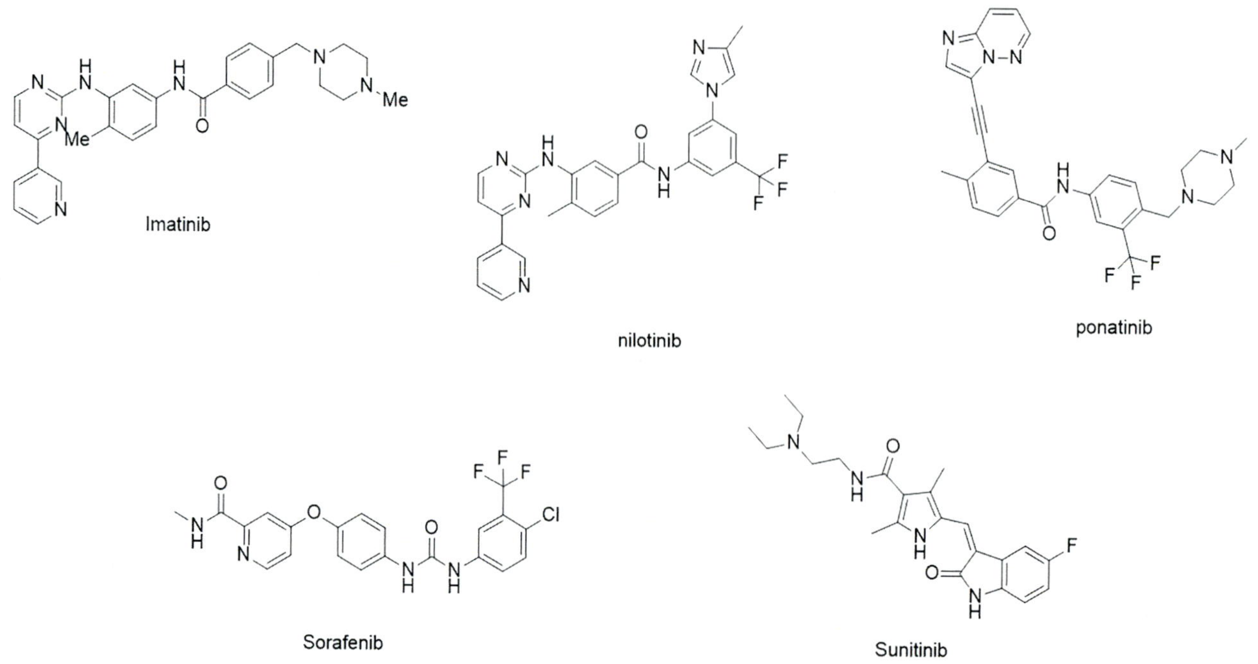

FIGURE 15.16 Representatives of Type II kinase inhibitors.

As mentioned above, both Type I and Type II inhibitors feature a foundational scaffold that binds to the hinge region. However, Type II inhibitors distinguish themselves by forming specific hydrogen bonding and hydrophobic interactions facilitated by the DFG residues within the activation loop. Therefore, the rational design of Type II inhibitors often involves a hybrid approach, wherein typical Type II fragments are incorporated into the hinge-binding scaffolds of Type I inhibitors [13]. Taking ponatinib, for example, the detailed design process will be discussed below.

15.1.4.2 Allosteric inhibitors

By definition, the allosteric inhibitors bind to allosteric pockets outside the highly conversed ATP pocket. Owing to the greater variation of this location, allosteric inhibitors have the potential to exhibit greater selectivity and the ability to overcome resistance to ATP-competitive inhibitors. However, the discovery of the allosteric inhibitors is extremely challenging, as reflected by the fact that some of the reported allosteric pockets are only identified serendipitously by crystallographic analysis. Recently, based on the structural features of the allosteric site or its endogenous substrates, rational design has been performed to introduce allosteric regulation into normally unregulated enzymes [14], leading to the discovery of allosteric modulators trametinib and asciminib. The discovery process of asciminib will be discussed in detail below.

15.1.4.3 Covalent inhibitors

Covalent inhibitors can form reversible or irreversible covalent bonds with their target enzyme, typically reacting with nucleophilic cysteine residues. Mechanically, it is likely that noncovalent interactions position the small molecule in a productive orientation within the ATP binding pocket that allows accessible nucleophilic cysteine of targeting kinases to attack the electrophilic portion of the drug to form a covalent adduct. Covalent inhibitors have the potential to increase the residence time of PKIs on the kinase targets and subsequently lead to increased selectivity, higher potency, and reduced risk of off-target effects and toxicity. Although covalent irreversible drugs are somewhat disfavored as a drug class owing to safety and toxicity concerns, since the approval of the first covalent EGFR inhibitors afatinib [15] in 2013, a collection of covalent PKIs have been FDA-approved, such as Bruton's tyrosine kinase (BTK) inhibitors acalabrutinib, ibrutinib, and zanubrutinib; EGFR inhibitors dacomitinib; and ErbB2 inhibitor neratinib, as well as osimertinib inhibiting the T790M EGFR (Fig. 15.17).

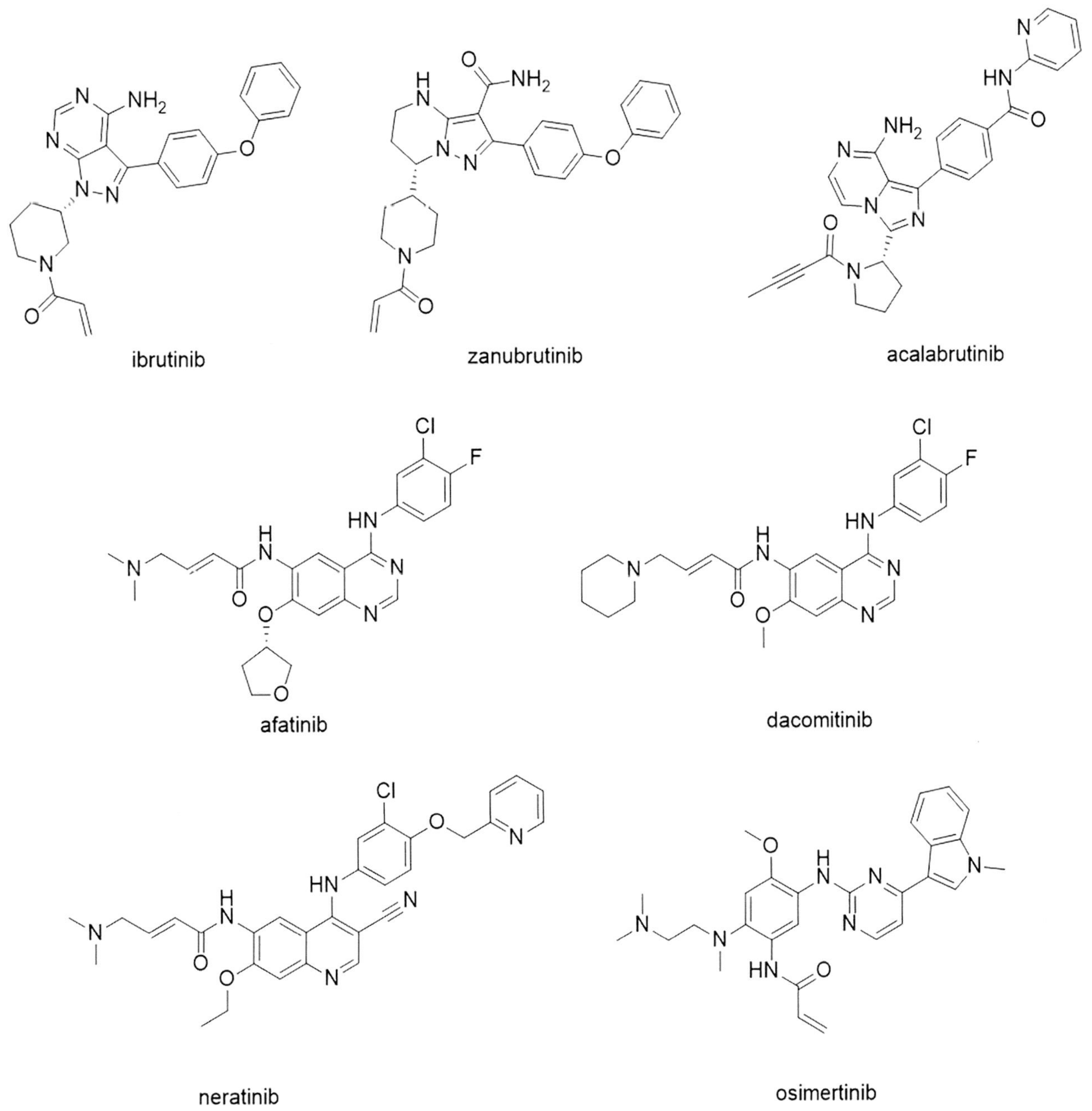

FIGURE 15.17 Representatives of the covalent inhibitors.

The design strategy for covalent kinase inhibitors involves combining the electrophilic warhead groups with a noncovalent compound with reasonable selectivity. A variety of warheads specifically targeting various nucleophilic protein residues, most commonly cysteine and lysine residues, have been developed, facilitating the systematic design of covalent PKIs (Table 15.3).

TABLE 15.3 Representative warheads targeting specific residues in kinases and their reaction mechanisms.

Warhead	Targeting residues	Kinetic property	Addition reaction
(acrylamide)	Cys	Irreversible covalent	
(cyanoacrylamide)	Cys	Reversible covalent	
(sulfonyl fluoride)	Lys, Tyr	Irreversible covalent	
(oxaziridine)	Met	Irreversible covalent	

15.2 Medicinal chemistry of imatinib

Imatinib, also known as Gleevec or Glivec, is the first small molecule PKI. It was developed by Novartis Pharmaceuticals and was approved by the FDA for the treatment of CML in 2001 [16]. The discovery of imatinib was a culmination of intensive research endeavors during the 1990s focused on the development of targeted antineoplastic agents. This progress was further propelled by the concurrent advancement of high-throughput drug screening methodologies.

15.2.1 Bcr-Abl and CML

CML is a hematological stem cell disorder characterized by excessive proliferation of cells of the myeloid lineage [17], constituting approximately 15% of adult leukemias, with a global annual incidence ranging between 1 and 2 per 100,000 individuals. The disease progresses through three distinct phases: chronic phase, accelerated phase, and acute phase [18,19]. The chronic phase typically lasts 3–5 years, with approximately half of the patients transitioning to the accelerated phase within 6–12 months, eventually culminating in the acute phase. Alternatively, the remaining patients may progress directly to the acute phase, leading to death within 3–6 months. Untreated patients exhibit a median survival period of around 3 years, whereas those newly diagnosed and treated with interferon therapy demonstrate a median survival of 5–6 years.

The hallmark of CML is the Philadelphia chromosome (Ph-chromosome), a shortened version of chromosome 22, found in approximately 95% of patients with CML. It was initially identified by Peter Nowell and David Hungerford in 1960 [20] and provided the first evidence of a specific genetic change associated with human cancer. In 1973, Janet Rowley confirmed that the Ph-chromosome originated from a reciprocal translocation between the long arms of chromosome 9 and chromosome 22 [21]. Specifically, the Abelson (Abl) proto-oncogene of chromosome 9q34 and the breakpoint cluster region (Bcr) gene of chromosome 22q11 undergo a specific translocation and recombination, ultimately giving rise to the Bcr-Abl fusion gene. Depending on the specific breakpoints of the Bcr gene, three major isoforms of Bcr-Abl can be produced, including 190, 210, and 230 kDa proteins (Fig. 15.18), which are respectively associated with different types of leukemia. Among, p210 Bcr-Abl is typically associated with CML patients, whereas p190 Bcr-Abl and p230 Bcr-Abl are commonly found in cases of acute lymphoblastic leukemia (ALL) [22] and chronic neutrophilic leukemia [23], respectively. Therefore, understanding the specific molecular characteristics of BCR-ABL variants is essential for accurate diagnosis and treatment selection in patients with BCR-ABL-positive leukemias.

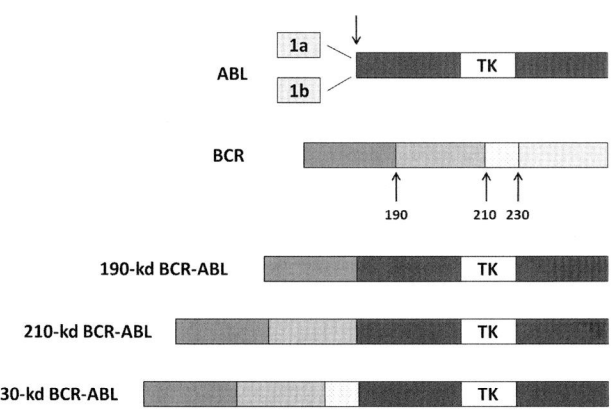

FIGURE 15.18 Structure of Bcr-Abl fusion protein.

In 1980, David Baltimore and others validated that the product of the Abl leukemia virus proto-oncogene, v-Abl, exhibits tyrosine-PK activity [24]. Subsequently, it was determined that the recombined Bcr-Abl protein also falls within the NRTK family [25]. Moreover, the Bcr-Abl fusion protein disrupts the autoinhibitory mechanism inherent in the native Abl protein structure, resulting in sustained activation of the Abl protein [26]. Subsequent experiments demonstrated that the expression of p210 Bcr-Abl in a murine model induces the onset of CML [27] and this pathogenicity is directly associated with its kinase activity [28]. Furthermore, the aberrant activation of the Bcr-Abl fusion protein leads to dysregulated signaling pathways [29] (Fig. 15.19) that ultimately promote cell proliferation, inhibit apoptosis, and contribute to the development of leukemia.

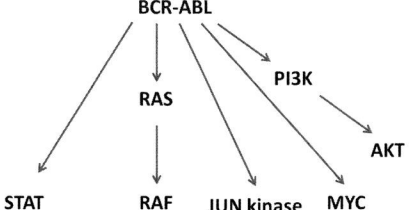

FIGURE 15.19 Main signaling pathway of Bcr-Abl kinase.

Consequently, Bcr-Abl kinase emerged as the predominant etiological factor underlying CML, prompting the exploration of selective kinase inhibitors targeting Bcr-Abl as a promising therapeutic approach for CML. However, during the mid-1980s, doubts prevailed regarding the druggability of PKs, with the development of selective inhibitors targeting specific PKs perceived as a tough challenge owing to the intracellular abundance of ATP at millimolar levels and the structural and functional homologies shared among various kinases. However, advancements in cancer biology and structural biology spurred efforts to identify kinase inhibitors, while high-throughput kinase screening and feasible model cell assays also accelerated the process of kinase inhibitor development, ultimately culminating in the discovery of imatinib targeting Bcr-Abl.

15.2.2 Molecular design and structure optimization

The discovery of imatinib involves the construction of a drug-like compound library and investigations of classical structure-activity relationships (SARs) in medicinal chemistry. The concept of "drug-likeness" serves as a valuable tool in guiding the design and optimization of small molecule drug candidates, aiding researchers to prioritize compounds with the highest likelihood for clinical success while minimizing failure risk in drug development [30]. In the 1990s, based on the analysis of orally administered small molecule drugs that had successfully progressed through clinical trials, researchers derived empirical "drug-likeness" principles. For instance, the widely employed Lipinski's Rule of Five [31] posits that a molecule's molecular weight should be less than 500 Da, it should possess no more than 5 hydrogen bond donors, no more than 10 hydrogen bond acceptors, a log$P$ value below 5, and no more than 10 rotatable bonds. Compounds adhering to these criteria are more likely to exhibit desirable pharmacokinetic properties and enhanced oral bioavailability. Subsequently, researchers incorporated the principles of "lead-like compounds" to construct molecule libraries [32]. These principles advocate for compounds with moderate affinity (affinity $>$ 0.1 μmol/L), molecular weight $<$ 350, and clog$P$ $<$ 3. Such lead-like compounds are amenable to extensive derivatization through straightforward synthetic chemistry in subsequent stages, facilitating their optimization into more drug-like candidates.

The pharmaceutical company Ciba Geigy initiated multiple kinase inhibitor projects targeting Bcr-Abl and protein kinase C (PKC). PKC, a Ser/Thr PK, is known to inhibit histamine release from human basophils. Based on a comprehensive review of literature and patents [33], a class of phenylaminopyrimidine (PAP) compounds exhibiting antiinflammatory activity was identified, although the underlying mechanism remains elusive. To probe whether these molecules mediate their antiinflammatory effects via PKC inhibition, researchers constructed a compound library based on the PAP scaffold under the guidance of the "lead-like compound" principle. This scaffold, characterized by low molecular weight, facilitates synthesis and allows for derivatization, rendering it an excellent lead framework. A systematic SAR study examined the impact of substituents on both the pyrimidine and phenyl rings on kinase activity [34]. The results validated this PAP scaffold's ability to bind to the ATP pocket of PKCα (K_i = 3.2 μmol/L for compound **1**, Fig. 15.20), thus classifying it as an ATP-competitive kinase inhibitor.

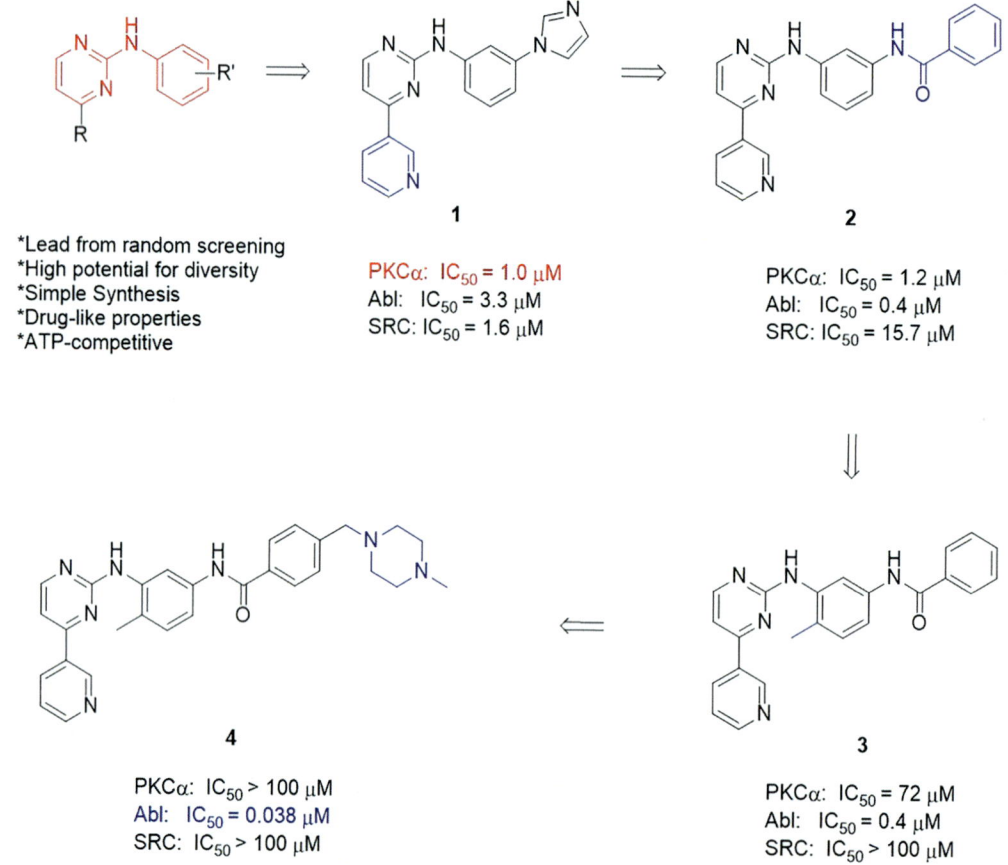

FIGURE 15.20 Optimization process for imatinib.

Of particular note is that the pyrimidine ring in the PAP scaffold is essential for activity, as the removal of any nitrogen atom from the ring results in a complete loss of activity (compounds **6**, **7**, and **5**). Additionally, the presence of a hydrogen atom on the aniline nitrogen is crucial for kinase inhibition, as its replacement with a methyl group absolutely abolishes activity (compound **8** vs compound **5**, Fig. 15.21).

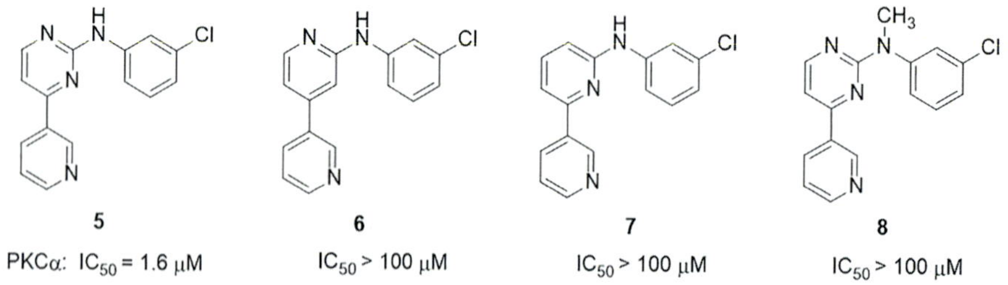

FIGURE 15.21 Structure of compound 5−8.

Based on the above SAR investigation, it is inferred that the N1 of the pyrimidine ring may serve as a hydrogen bond acceptor, while the adjacent hydrogen atom of the amine group also serves as a hydrogen bond donor. Furthermore, this interaction mode involving dual hydrogen bonds with the target enzyme requires that the hydrogen bond donor and acceptor in the molecule maintain a *cis* configuration (Fig. 15.22). However, due to steric hindrance from the adjacent hydrogen atoms on the pyridine and phenyl rings, these groups are inclined to adopt a *trans* configuration in compounds **6** and **7**, thereby failing to meet the requirements and consequently rendering both compounds completely inactive.

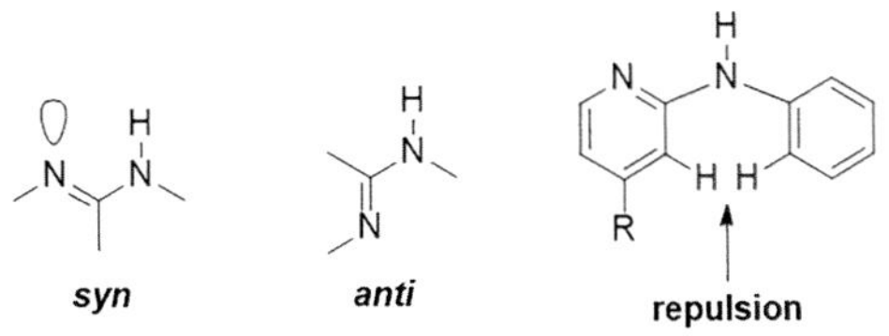

FIGURE 15.22 Conformation of the H-bonding part of PAPs.

Given high sequence homology of the ATP binding domain among PKs, subsequent investigations revealed that the lead compound **1** also exerts inhibitory effects on other kinases [35], with the following activity hierarchy: PKCα (1.0 μmol/L) > SRC (1.6 μmol/L) > Abl (3.3 μmol/L) > PKCδ (21 μmol/L) > EGFR and PKA (>100 μmol/L). Thus, as a lead compound targeting Abl kinase, further optimization should aim to enhance its selectivity for the target enzyme.

Further SAR studies on the substituents on the phenyl ring revealed that compound **2**, with a benzamide group at the 3-position, showed increased selectivity and activity against TK Abl (Abl: $IC_{50} = 0.4$ μmol/L, PKCα: $IC_{50} = 1.2$ μmol/L, SRC: $IC_{50} = 15.7$ μmol/L). Subsequently, the introduction of a flag-methyl group at the 6-position of the phenyl ring led to the corresponding compound **3**, which exhibited a significant decrease in inhibitory activity against PKCα and SRC (Abl: $IC_{50} = 0.4$ μmol/L, PKCα: $IC_{50} = 72$ μmol/L, SRC: $IC_{50} > 100$ μmol/L), thereby further enhancing its selectivity for Abl kinase. This result may be attributed to the incorporation of the flag-methyl group, which augmented the twist angle between the phenyl and pyrimidine rings, consequently altering and stabilizing the preferred conformation of this molecular class (Fig. 15.23). Such conformational restriction is crucial for the selective binding of the compound **3** to Abl kinase.

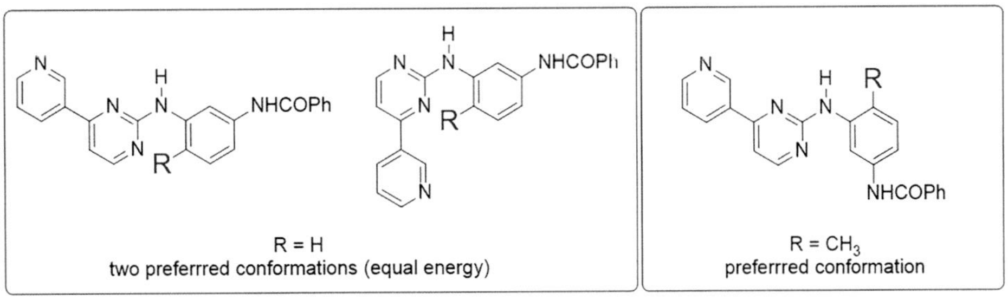

FIGURE 15.23 Increase of selectivity and analysis of the conformation.

Compound **3** exhibits low solubility in water (2 mg/L at pH 4 with log$P$ 4.2), thereby hindering its ability to manifest inhibitory effects on Abl kinase at the cellular level. To improve solubility, the polar side chain at the *para* position of the acylamino phenyl group, such as *N*-methyl piperazine, was introduced with the anticipation that it would extend into the solvent region of the kinase. Furthermore, to avoid potential toxicity associated with aromatic amine compounds, the piperazine moiety was linked to the aromatic phenyl ring via a methylene spacer. The resulting optimal compound **4**, imatinib, exhibited increased kinase activity and selectivity (Abl: $IC_{50} = 0.038$ μmol/L, PKCα: $IC_{50} > 100$ μmol/L, SRC: $IC_{50} > 100$ μmol/L), as well as improved solubility and oral bioavailability (200 mg/L at pH 4 with log$P$ 3.1). Consequently, imatinib was identified as the most promising candidate for clinical development.

Subsequently, Brian Druker's team conducted preclinical trials of imatinib for the treatment of CML [36]. At the enzymatic level, imatinib demonstrated inhibition of the phosphorylation of v-Abl, Bcr-Abl, and c-Abl substrates, with IC50 values of 0.038, 0.025, and 0.025 μmol/L, respectively. At the cellular level, it inhibited the phosphorylation of v-Abl and Bcr-Abl kinases with IC_{50} values of 0.25 μmol/L and displayed high selectivity against more than 10 other kinases tested (except platelet-derived growth factor receptor (PDGFR) at the cellular level with IC_{50} value of 0.3 μmol/L). Furthermore, experimental data show that this high selectivity can be translated into a very specific Bcr-Abl-dependent tumor-growth inhibition at the cellular and animal level. Additionally, in colony-forming assays, using ex vivo peripheral blood and bone marrow samples from CML patients, imatinib shows selective inhibition of Ph-chromosome-positive colonies (92%–98%). Subsequent extensive cell and animal studies, based on Bcr-Abl positive expression, corroborated that imatinib achieved the therapeutic effect of treating CML by inhibiting the kinase function of Bcr-Abl [16].

15.2.3 Structure-activity relationship

The crystal structure of the Bcr-Abl complex with imatinib (PDB: 1iep) demonstrates that imatinib induces and specifically binds to the inactivated conformation of the Abl kinase [37] (α-helix$_{in}$, DFG$_{out}$) (Fig. 15.24), in contrast to the typically activated conformation of the kinase upon ATP binding (similar to the ADP-bound Abl protein complex, PDB: 2g2i). The predominant distinction between these two binding states lies in imatinib's posterior extension into the pocket formed by the rotation of the DFG motif, thereby establishing multiple interactions with the target enzyme to stabilize its inactivated conformation. Simultaneously, the phosphorylated residue Tyr393 on the activation loop extends toward the active pocket of Abl, forming a hydrogen bond with Asp363 of the HRD motif in the catalytic loop, effectively mimicking the conformation of the original substrate peptide and thus occluding the binding of exogenous proteins.

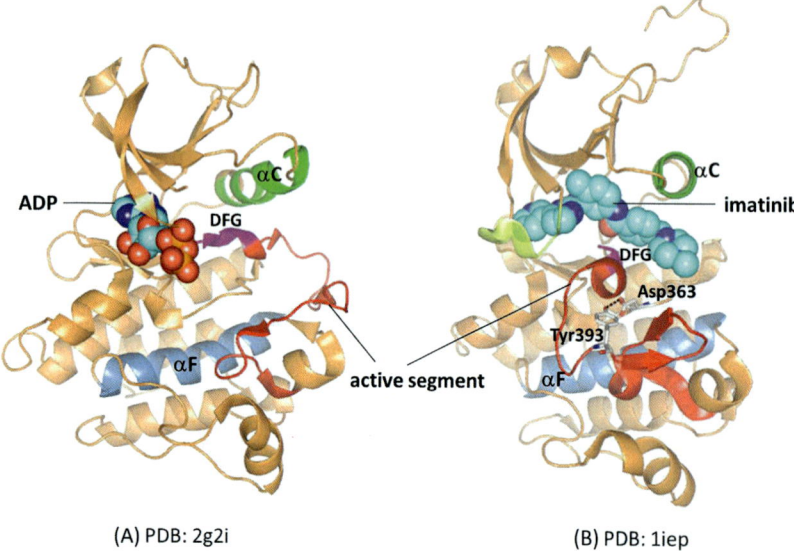

FIGURE 15.24 Active conformation (left) and inactive conformation (right) of Abl.

Specifically, imatinib occupies the AP, BP-I, BP-IIout, and BP-IV binding pockets of the kinase catalytic domain (Fig. 15.25). The nitrogen atom of the pyridine group forms crucial hydrogen bonds with Met318 in the hinge region, while the N1 of the pyrimidine group participates in a hydrogen bond network with the conserved residues Lys271, Glu286, Asp381, and two water molecules. The pyrimidine amine group also acts as a hydrogen bond donor, forming a hydrogen bond with the hydroxyl group of the crucial gatekeeper residue Thr315, thereby allowing molecule to enter

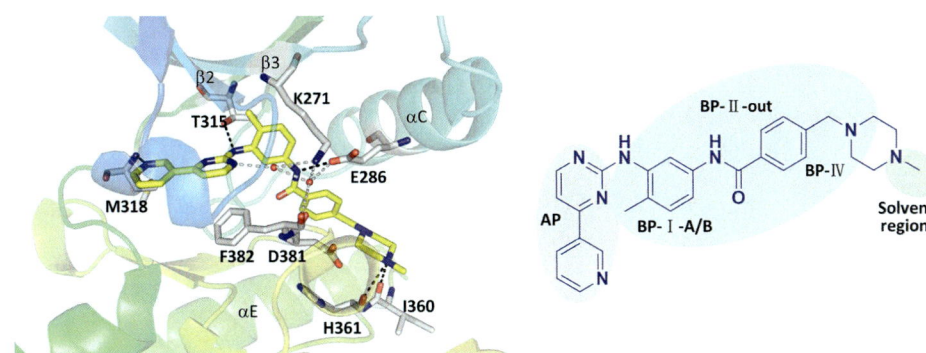

FIGURE 15.25 Cocrystal structure and binding mode of Abl with imatinib (PDB: 1iep).

the BP. The amide linker interacts with Glu286 in the αC-helix and Asp381 in the DFG motif of the activation loop. The phenyl group enters the back hydrophobic cavity (BP-IIout), displacing the DFG motif that originally occupied this position, promoting the protein to adopt the inactivated DFG$_{out}$ conformation. The methyl group at the adjacent position of the amine imposes steric hindrance, compelling the pyrimidine ring along with the pyridine ring to undergo a certain degree of torsion, thereby stabilizing the preferred conformation of the molecule, which coincides with the pharmacophoric conformation of imatinib binding to the inactivated Abl. Additionally, the nitrogen atom of the piperazine ring is protonated under physiological conditions and forms a hydrogen bond with the carbonyl groups of His316 and Ile360, further reinforcing the binding of imatinib to Abl.

In conclusion, the multiple interactions between imatinib and the Abl kinase effectively explain the structural optimization process of imatinib (Fig. 15.20). Firstly, the initial PAP core of compound **1** possesses typical "drug-like" features, containing hydrogen bond donors/acceptors, prevalent in the design of ATP-competitive kinase inhibitors. Secondly, in the transformation from compound **1** to compound **2**, the incorporation of the benzamide moiety is crucial in inducing and stabilizing the inactive conformation of the kinase and enhancing selectivity. Thirdly, in the transformation from compound **2** to compound **3**, the introduction of a 6-position methyl moiety fixes the molecule's pharmacophoric conformation, further enhancing kinase selectivity. Lastly, in the transformation from compound **3** to compound **4**, the introduction of the *N*-methylpiperazine moiety imparts good solubility embedded in the hydrophobic pocket rather than extended toward the protein's exterior, resulting in de-solvation effects. However, the augmentation of hydrogen bond interactions effectively offsets the energy loss, thus contributing to the overall stabilization of the complex.

This "imatinib-like" (α-helix$_{in}$, DFG$_{out}$) kinase conformation represents a typical action mode observed in type II ATP-competitive inhibitors. The dynamic equilibrium between kinase phosphorylation and dephosphorylation governs intracellular kinase activity. Notably, imatinib can bind and stabilize the inactive conformation of the Abl kinase only during transient dephosphorylation of its activation segment, thereby exerting its inhibitory effect [38]. In contrast to highly homologous activate conformations, the inactivated states of PKs exhibit considerable structural diversity, thereby affording imatinib relatively high selectivity for Bcr-Abl kinase. The mechanistic elucidation has significantly influenced the design of subsequent PKIs [39,40]. Moreover, the elucidation of the cocrystal structure depicting imatinib bound to Bcr-Abl kinase offers crucial insights into the mechanisms underlying imatinib resistance arising from Bcr-Abl mutations. This understanding lays a foundation for the development of novel inhibitors aimed at overcoming imatinib resistance.

15.2.4 Synthesis of imatinib

Many synthetic methodologies for the production of imatinib have been documented in the literature. The representative is the route advanced by Juerg Zimmermann [41] (Fig. 15.26).

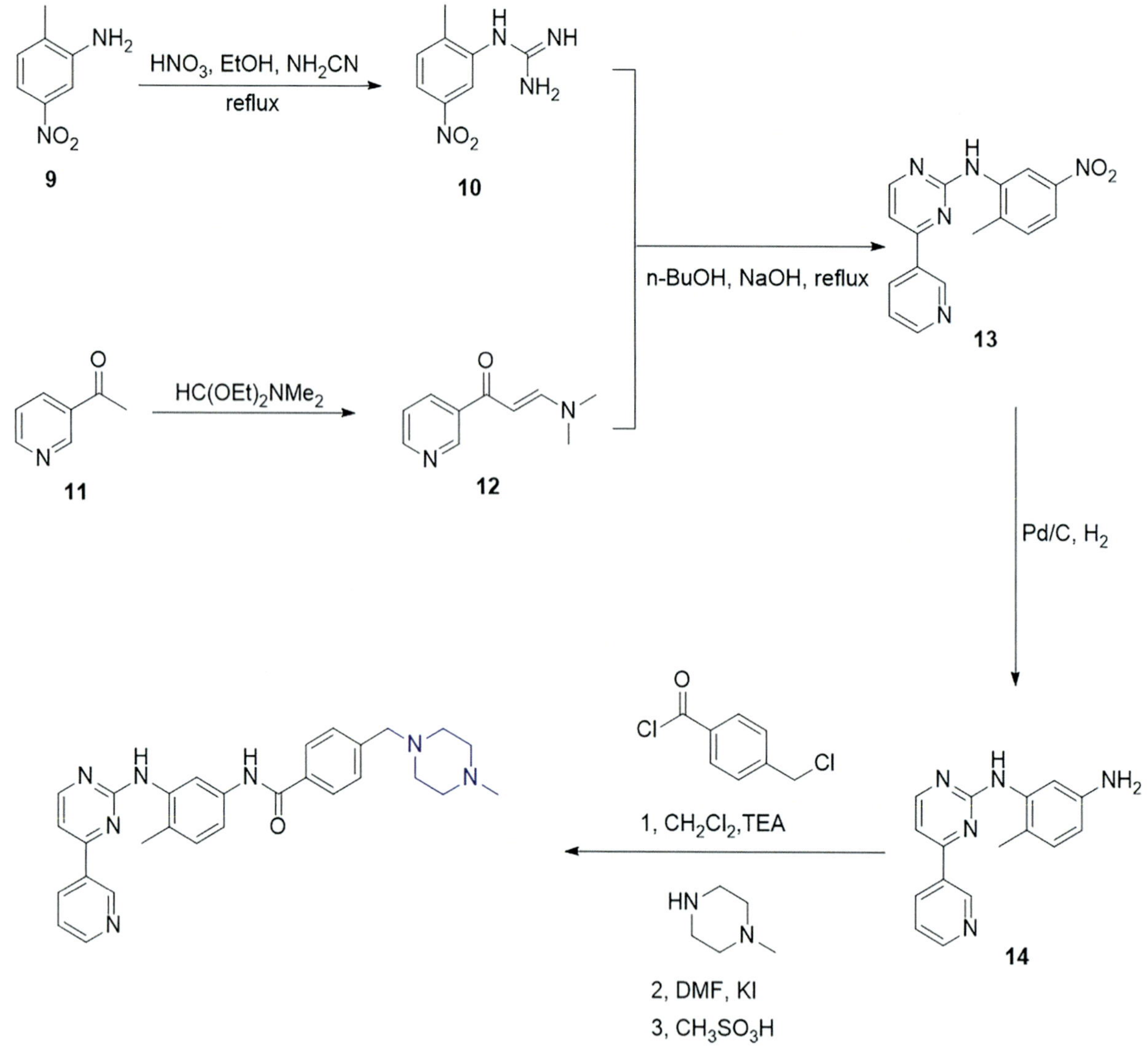

FIGURE 15.26 Synthetic scheme of imatinib.

Initially, the reaction between a phenylamine derivative **9** and cyanamide yielded guanidine **10**, while 3-acetylpyridine reacted with *N,N*-dimethylformamide-diethylacetal to generate enaminone **12**. Subsequently, the PAP core was constructed by the reaction of guanidine **10** and enaminone **12**. Catalytic hydrogenation of the nitro group in **13** resulted in the amine **14**, which was acylated with the corresponding acid chloride to give the amide, followed by nucleophilic substitution of *N*-methylpiperazine, ultimately yielding the desired imatinib. Further, salt formation with methanesulfonic acid results in the production of imatinib methanesulfonate.

During the early stages of development, imatinib was recognized to target three distinct kinases, thereby offering a wide array of potential indications for clinical trials. However, unlike many cancers characterized by multifaceted dysregulation of various genes and signaling cascades, CML stands out as a malignancy primarily driven by a singular aberrant signaling pathway. Moreover, in contrast to the intricate response evaluation necessitated by solid tumors, the therapeutic efficacy for hematologic malignancies, including CML, can be readily assessed through straightforward endpoint measurements such as blood cell counts. Consequently, CML emerged as the initial choice for clinical trials. This indication selection not only facilitated expedited development but also contributed significantly to the successful advancement of imatinib as a therapeutic agent.

15.2.5 Pharmacokinetics and pharmacodynamics of imatinib

In terms of physicochemical characteristics [42], imatinib is a quadrivalent base with acid dissociation constant (pK_a) values ranging from 1.52 to 8.07. Thus, imatinib is freely soluble in water at pH 5.5 or less, and solubility in aqueous buffer decreases as the pH increases. The drug has sparingly soluble solubility (50 μg/mL at pH 7.4 with log$P$ 1.99), and nearly insoluble at pH 8.0. Imatinib dissolves readily in polar solvents like methanol and ethanol but has diminished solubility in organic solvents of low polarity. Furthermore, imatinib demonstrates stability when exposed to artificial gastric fluid (1 hour at pH 1.2 and temperature 37°C), with no observable hydrolysis of the amide bond.

15.2.5.1 ADME

Pharmacokinetic studies of imatinib in healthy volunteers and patients with CML, gastrointestinal stromal tumor (GIST), and other cancers show that orally administered imatinib is well absorbed and has an absolute bioavailability of 98% irrespective of the oral dosage form (solution, capsule, tablet) or dosage strength (100 mg, 400 mg) [43]. Food has no relevant impact on the rate or extent of bioavailability.

In phase I clinical trials conducted in CML patients [44], 64 adult patients (47 in the chronic phase and 17 in the advanced phase or with acute leukemia) received oral imatinib with the dose gradually increased from 25 to 750 mg once daily in a stepwise manner (14 steps), eventually escalating to 800 and 1000 mg twice daily. The results obtained show that imatinib exposure (area under the drug-time curve and maximum concentration) was dose-proportional after oral administration for the dose range of 25–1000 mg. There was a 1.5- to 3-fold drug accumulation at steady-state after repeated once-daily dosing. Pharmacokinetic parameters for the 400 mg dose are shown in Table 15.4. On day 1, the imatinib time to reach C_{max} (t_{max}) was 3.1 ± 2.0 hours and C_{max} was 1907 ± 355.0 ng/mL. Terminal half-life $t_{1/2\beta}$ was 14.8 ± 5.8 hours. After continuous administration for 28 days, at steady state, a mean C_{max} of 2596 ± 787 ng/mL was obtained, with a plasma through concentration of 1215.8 ± 750.2 ng/mL, which exceeds the 50% inhibitory concentration required to inhibit proliferation of Bcr-Abl–positive leukemic cells.

TABLE 15.4 Pharmacokinetic parameters for imatinib 400 mg in CML patients on day 1 and at steady state.

Parameter	Day 1 of administration	Steady state (day 28)
C_{max} (ng/mL)	1907.5 ± 355.0	2596.0 ± 786.7
T_{max} (h)	3.1 ± 2.0	3.3 ± 1.1
AUC_{24} (μg·h/mL)	24.8 ± 7.4	40.1 ± 15.7
AUC_{∞} (μg·h/mL)	38.8 ± 15.9	81.9 ± 45.0
$t_{1/2\beta}$ (h)	14.8 ± 5.8	19.3 ± 4.4
CL/F (L/h)	12.5 ± 7.2	11.2 ± 4.0
V_z/F (L)	236.0 ± 76.5	295.0 ± 62.5
Through concentration (ng/mL)	Not calculated	1215.8 ± 750.2
Time above 1 μmol/L (h)	Not calculated	49.3 ± 17.1

AUC_{24}, area under the plasma concentration-time curve from 0 to 24 hours; AUC_{∞}, AUC from time zero to infinity; CL/F, apparent total plasma clearance of drug after oral administration; C_{max}, peak plasma concentration; $t_{1/2\beta}$, terminal elimination half-life; T_{max}, time to reach Cmax; V_z/F, apparent volume of distribution during terminal phase after oral administration.

In vitro studies indicate that, at clinically relevant concentrations, imatinib is approximately 95% bound to plasma proteins, predominantly albumin and α1-acid glycoprotein. Imatinib is widely distributed into tissues, with a distribution volume of approximately 435 L. However, the ability of imatinib to penetrate the blood-brain barrier is limited, resulting in approximately 100-fold lower concentration in the cerebrospinal fluid (CSF) compared to that in the plasma [45]. Moreover, imatinib serves as a substrate for the drug transmembrane transporter P-glycoprotein. Therefore, the expression level of this transporter influences the oral bioavailability of imatinib and is involved in imatinib resistance [46].

Metabolic studies [47] in humans indicate that the main circulating metabolite of imatinib is the *N*-desmethylated piperazine derivative, with approximately 10% of the area under the curve (AUC) for imatinib. In addition, multiple oxidative metabolites are generated, including the 4-*N*-oxide of piperazine, pyridine *N*-oxide, methyl hydroxylation, and benzylic amine oxidation (Fig. 15.27). In vitro metabolic research in human liver microsomes has confirmed that the phase I oxidation of imatinib is mainly catalyzed by hepatic CYP3A4 and CYP3A5 isoenzymes, while other CYP2D6, CYP2C9, CYP2C19, and CYP1A2 metabolic enzymes play a minor role. The phase II metabolic pathway mainly involves the glucuronidation of imatinib and its primary metabolites.

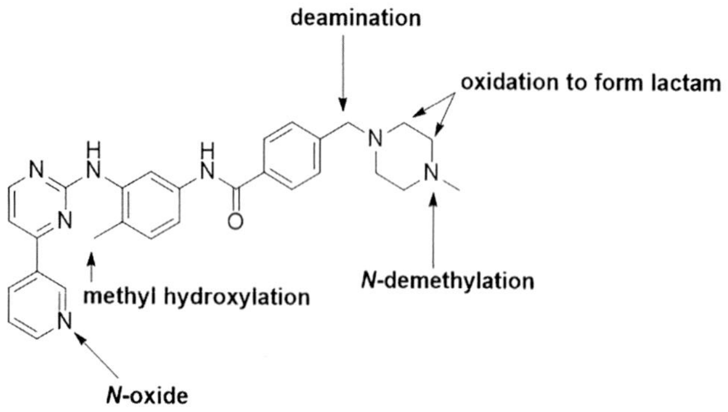

FIGURE 15.27 Metabolites of imatinib.

Imatinib is excreted mainly via the feces, mostly as metabolites. Imatinib was orally administered to healthy volunteers, approximately 80% of the dose was eliminated within 7 days, with 67% of the dose found in the feces and 13% in the urine. Unchanged imatinib accounts for 28% of the recovered dose, and the primary metabolite accounts for 13%. Furthermore, the primary metabolite has in vitro potency similar to that of the parent imatinib, but with a longer elimination half-life of approximately 40 hours.

15.2.5.2 Pharmacokinetics in special groups

The results from a phase I study for the treatment of 31 children with CML [48] showed that plasma concentrations at steady-state and mean AUC in children after once-daily administration of imatinib 260 and 340 mg/m^2 were comparable to the values reported in adults given daily doses of imatinib 400 and 600 mg, respectively. In patients with CML, no effect of sex on imatinib pharmacokinetics was found; however, the clearance of imatinib has been shown to correlate with bodyweight. In patients with varyingly impaired hepatic function [49], the imatinib exposure showed large interpatient variability. Additionally, due to cumulative dose-limiting toxicities, the clinically recommended maximum dose for patients with mild hepatic impairment is 500 mg daily. For patients with moderate and severe hepatic impairment, the occurrence of grade 3–4 adverse reactions increases when the dose of imatinib is 300 mg daily, therefore requiring a reduction in the clinically recommended dose compared to the standard dose. In patients with renal impairment [50], the imatinib exposure is increased, and there is an unexpected decline in plasma clearance. However, patients experienced no unexpected or serious toxicities with imatinib 600 or 800 mg daily. Thus, no dose adjustments are currently recommended.

15.2.6 Drug safety and drug-drug interaction

Drug safety assessment serves as an integral part of the development of new drugs and therapeutics, including the evaluation of adverse events, hematologic assessment, biochemical testing, urinalysis, and physical examination. Toxicity was graded in accordance with the Common Toxicity Criteria of the National Cancer Institute.

Phase I clinical trials showed [51] that imatinib was generally well tolerated without a maximal tolerated dose identified. The most frequent adverse effects were nausea (55%), vomiting (41%), and edema (41%), most of these were grade 1 (mild) or grade 2 (moderate). Grade 4 neutropenia and thrombocytopenia occurred in 40% and 33% of patients, respectively. There was some evidence of an increased incidence of toxic effects at the higher doses of imatinib, especially at 800–1000 mg per day.

Drug−drug interactions (DDIs) pose a major problem to patient safety. Evaluating potential DDIs is crucial to decrease adverse drug events. Some of the most common DDIs result from alterations in drug metabolism through interactions with cytochrome P450 enzymes. As previously noted, imatinib is metabolized mainly by the CYP3A4 and CYP3A5 isoenzymes. Thus, interactions may occur between imatinib and inhibitors or inducers of these enzymes, leading to changes in the plasma concentration of imatinib.

On the one hand, when imatinib is coadministered with inhibitors of these enzymes (such as cimetidine, ketoconazole, cyclosporine, and grapefruit juice), the metabolism of imatinib decreases and its plasma concentrations increase. For example, following administration of 200 mg imatinib alone or with ketoconazole 400 mg, mean C_{max} and AUC_{24} increased significantly by 26% and 40%, respectively. Also, apparent clearance decreased, with a mean reduction of 28.6%. On the other hand, the imatinib exposure decreases, when imatinib is coadministered with inducers of these enzymes (such as rifampicin, dexamethasone, phenobarbital, phenytoin, carbamazepine, and St. John's wort). For example, following administration of a single dose of imatinib alone or with multiple doses of rifampicin, the imatinib clearance increased by nearly fourfold, with decreased C_{max} (54%) and AUC_{24} (68%) [52].

In addition, human liver microsome studies have shown that imatinib competitively inhibits CYP3A4/5, CYP2C9, and CYP2D6, with inhibition constant (K_i) values of 8, 27, and 7.5 μmol/L, respectively. Imatinib is also the substrate and inhibitor of the P-glycoprotein transporter. Therefore, imatinib can also alter the pharmacokinetic properties of other coadministered drugs by inhibiting metabolic enzymes and/or cellular transporters. For example, in a study of 20 patients in CML, the administration of imatinib increased the mean C_{max} of simvastatin (lipid-lowering agent, a CYP3A4 substrate) twofold and the AUC_{∞} 3.5 fold, compared with simvastatin alone. Clearance of simvastatin was reduced by 70%, and the mean half-life was prolonged from 1.4 to 3.2 hours [53]. Therefore, the substrates of these enzymes (such as simvastatin, warfarin, and cyclosporine) should be administered with caution when together with imatinib.

In summary, imatinib has favorable pharmacokinetic properties, including a terminal elimination half-life of approximately 18 hours and a good oral bioavailability of up to 98%, which permits once-daily oral administration. When reaching a steady state with 400 mg once-daily oral administration, the mean plasma concentration of imatinib remains above the level needed for the Abl kinase inhibition in vitro, thereby leading to normalization of hematological parameters in the majority of CML patients, regardless of baseline white blood cell (WBC) count. Furthermore, the need for caution should be underlined when coadministering imatinib in consideration of potential DDIs.

15.2.7 Clinical efficacy and expansion of indications

15.2.7.1 Clinical efficacy of imatinib in the treatment of CML

Based on its antileukemic activity in preclinical models, Novartis conducted a Phase I trial of imatinib in June 1998 in patients with CML in the chronic phase in whom treatment with interferon alfa had failed or who could not tolerate this drug. The primary endpoint of the dose-escalation study was to identify the safety and tolerability of imatinib, but surprisingly, its substantial activity against CML was synchronously observed. Of the 54 patients treated with daily doses of 300 mg or more of imatinib within 4 weeks, 53 (98%) had complete hematological responses and 29 (54%) had major or minor cytogenetic responses, including 17 (31%) with major responses and 7 (13%) of these had complete cytogenetic remissions. The median time to the best cytogenetic response was approximately 5 months.

In the Phase I trial, a maximum inhibition-effect model was used to describe the relationship between pharmacodynamic (PD) (WBC reduction) and PK parameters. The results clearly demonstrated that the initial hematologic response depends on the administered dose for patients with CML. In the 400-mg group, levels of the drug that killed CML cells in vitro correlated well with clinical response and serum drug levels. Furthermore, there was substantial in vivo inhibition of the enzymatic activity of Bcr-Abl at the 400-mg dose, as demonstrated by decreased phosphorylation of CRKL, a substrate of Bcr-Abl [54]. Therefore, the recommended daily dose of at least 400 mg for future studies was required for maximal PD effect.

On the basis of the substantial activity of imatinib in patients in the chronic phase, Novartis also evaluated the effects of imatinib in patients who had CML in blast crisis and in patients with Ph-chromosome-positive ALL [55]. There was a relatively decreased overall response rate (70%) and complete remission rate (20%) due to other complex molecular abnormalities replacing the sole Bcr-Abl aberration underlying in these cases. Therefore, it is likely that imatinib will need to be combined with other therapies to achieve maximal therapeutic benefits for these patients.

In late 1999, Phase II clinical trials were conducted to characterize the efficacy and safety profiles of imatinib in a large group of patients at different phases of CML [56−58]. The comprehensive results (as shown in Table 15.5) indicated that imatinib induced distinct response rates in three phases of CML, with reduced efficacy associated with disease progression.

TABLE 15.5 Efficacy of imatinib in patients at different phases of CML.

CML patients	Daily dose	Complete hematologic response	Major cytogenetic response	Progression-free rates	Overall survival rates	Toxicity
In late-chronic phase (N = 524)	400 mg	95%	60%	89% (18-month)	95% (18-month)	Nonhematologic toxic effects were generally mild or moderate, hematologic toxicity was manageable.
In accelerated phase (N = 181)	400 mg or 600 mg	69%	24%	59% (12-month)	74% (12-month)	
In blast crisis (N = 229)	600 mg	31%	16%	–	–	

The Phase III clinical trial of imatinib was initiated in 2000 [59] to compare the efficacy of imatinib (400 mg/d) with that of the most effective therapy of interferon alfa combined with cytarabine in newly diagnosed chronic-phase CML. After a median follow-up of 19 months, imatinib was significantly superior to interferon alfa plus cytarabine in terms of hematologic and cytogenetic response rates, tolerability, and freedom from progression to accelerated-phase or blast-crisis CML (Table 15.6). Moreover, in the design of crossover to the alternative group, imatinib has been shown to be an effective rescue therapy for patients who have no response to combination therapy.

TABLE 15.6 Rates of observed hematologic and cytogenetic responses.

Response	Initial treatment		Crossover treatment	
	Imatinib (N = 553)	Interferon alfa plus cytarabine (N = 553)	From imatinib to interferon alfa plus cytarabine (N = 11)	From interferon alfa plus cytarabine to imatinib (N = 318)
Complete hematologic	95.3%	55.5%	27.3%	82.4%
Major cytogenetic	85.2%	22.1%	0	55.7%
Complete cytogenetic	73.8%	8.5%	0	39.6%
Partial cytogenetic	11.4%	13.6%	0	16.0%

The level of cytogenetic response was defined by the percentage of Philadelphia-chromosome–positive cells in metaphase: complete response, 0%; partial response, 1%–35%. A major cytogenetic response was defined as a complete or partial response.

Consequently, imatinib had only been in clinical trials for 3 years and was approved as a first-line therapy in newly diagnosed chronic-phase CML in May 2001 [60]. After more than 10 years of follow-up, the phase IV trial confirmed the long-term efficacy and safety of imatinib. The estimated overall survival rate at 10 years was 83.3% and no unacceptable cumulative or late toxic effects were observed.

15.2.7.2 Expansion of clinical indications

Subsequent studies have shown that imatinib is a multitargeted kinase inhibitor. In addition to inhibiting Bcr-Abl kinase, imatinib also targets the same array of other TKs, including PDGFR, colony-stimulating factor-1 receptor, discoidin domain receptors 1 and 2, and the proto-oncogene c-KIT, albeit with differing potencies. Given the relevance of these target enzymes to the specific diseases, imatinib has subsequently been approved for the treatment of GISTs associated with gain-of-function mutations in c-KIT [61]; Ph-chromosome-positive ALL; myeloproliferative diseases associated with PDGFR rearrangements; aggressive systemic mastocytosis with FIPIL1-PDGFRα fusion kinase and without c-KIT D816V mutation; and dermatofibrosarcoma protuberans [3].

15.3 Imatinib resistance and solutions

15.3.1 Clinical mechanisms of imatinib resistance

Cancer drug resistance remains a major challenge in medical oncology, arising from diverse mechanisms broadly classified into two categories. The first is directly related to the target kinase itself (on-target), including kinase overexpression and mutations. Among these, kinase mutations are the predominant mechanism of resistance to PKIs in targeted therapy. The second category is not inherently related to the target itself (off-target) but achieves resistance through bypass signaling. Targets implicated in bypass resistance exhibit relative diversity, whereas drug-resistant mutations associated with the target itself often follow specific patterns.

For ATP-competitive small molecule kinase inhibitors, the resistant mutations frequently occur at sites of drug interaction proximal to the ATP-binding domain. For example, mutations in key residues located deep within the ATP pocket and gatekeeper mutations in the hinge region represent the most prevalent locations associated with acquired resistance. The conserved DFG motif at the end of the activation loop and the solvent-front region are also relatively common regions for mutations. Additionally, mutations may sometimes occur infrequently at the distal end of the ATP-binding domain that does not directly bind to a kinase inhibitor.

For covalent small molecule kinase inhibitors, the mutations of residues involved in covalent bond formation are the most frequent mutations, directly leading to the disruption of the covalent interaction and consequent resistance. For example, mutations in cysteine residue predominantly induce resistance to irreversible EGFR and BTK inhibitors by disrupting the formation of covalent adducts and decreasing the binding affinity.

Despite the remarkable therapeutic efficacy of imatinib in CML treatment, approximately 3%−4% of newly diagnosed patients in the chronic phase fail to achieve a complete hematological response. Furthermore, 20%−25% of those who attain complete hematological response or complete cytogenetic remission, or both, eventually develop resistance and cease to respond to the drug. Additionally, patients in the accelerated or blastic phase exhibit even higher nonresponse rates, approximately 40%−50% and 80%, respectively [62]. This absence of response to imatinib is attributed to various Bcr-Abl-dependent and/or independent resistant mechanisms [63−65]. Among these, point mutations in the Abl-kinase domain seem to be the more frequent resistance mechanism [66,67], accounting for 60%−80% of imatinib resistance cases. Currently, over 100 point mutations have been identified clinically, with the most common point mutations in four major regions of the kinase domain shown in Fig. 15.28.

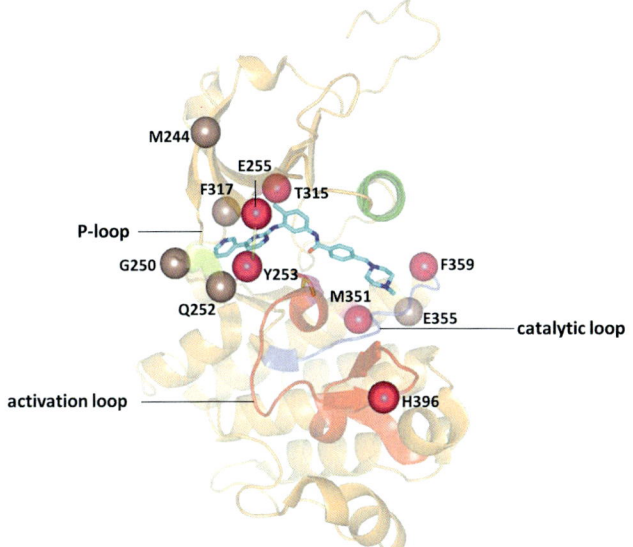

FIGURE 15.28 Representative mutation sites of Bcr-Abl kinase (red spheres: high occurrence rate; brown spheres: relatively high occurrence rate).

15.3.1.1 ATP binding pocket: T315I, F317V/L, etc

Among these mutations, the gatekeeper T315I mutation exhibits the highest prevalence in clinical patients (15%–20%). Substitution of threonine at position 315 with isoleucine results in a loss of the crucial hydrogen bond interaction between the hydroxyl group of original T315 and imatinib. Additionally, the hydrophobicity and larger sizes of the isoleucine at this position result in steric clashes, preventing imatinib from binding to the mutant Abl structures. Furthermore, the T315I mutation favors the active conformation of Abl kinase, thereby enhancing its affinity for ATP binding. Consequently, the T315I mutation severely diminishes imatinib's inhibitory efficacy on Abl kinase, resulting in a substantial decrease in affinity by up to 3000-fold.

15.3.1.2 Phosphate binding loop: E255K/V, Y253H/F, Q252H/R, G250E, etc

The binding between the phosphate binding loop and imatinib is primarily stabilized by water-mediated hydrogen bonding with residues Y253 and N322, as well as hydrophobic interactions. Mutations in this region markedly reduce the sensitivity of the P-loop to recognize imatinib. For instance, the Y253 mutation disrupts the hydrogen bond between imatinib and N322, resulting in decreased binding affinity and loss of inhibitory effect.

15.3.1.3 Catalytic domain: M351T, F359V, V379L, etc

M351 interacts with the SH2 domain of Abl kinase, stabilizing the DFG_{out} form of Abl catalytic domain. Conversely, mutations proximal to M351 prevent Abl from adopting the specific conformation required for high-affinity imatinib binding.

15.3.1.4 Activation loop: H396P/R, etc

The activation loop regulates kinase activity. Mutations in this loop stabilize active DFG_{in} conformation that is inaccessible to imatinib, consequently displaying moderate resistance to imatinib.

Similar resistance mutations, such as those occurring in the ATP binding pocket (T670I and V654A) and the activation loop (N822K, D816E/H/V, D820E/G/Y, and A829P), also have been observed in c-KIT, another target of imatinib for treating GISTs. As in Abl, the gatekeeper T670I mutation is more prevalent in clinical cases. Correspondingly, the observed PDGFR mutation T674I is equivalent to the Abl T315I mutation, leading to reduced effectiveness of imatinib.

In summary, a large number of clinical mutations have been observed in response to imatinib exposure. While some of these mutations directly affect the binding of imatinib to the target kinase, the majority decrease the occupancy of the DFG_{out} conformation of the protein, which is the preferred binding state for imatinib. The deviation of equilibrium from this state is believed to be the primary determinant of the loss in binding efficacy.

15.3.2 Next-generation drugs to overcome imatinib resistance

Based on the specific resistant mechanisms encountered in disease treatments, various strategies have been devised to overcome the clinical resistance of imatinib [68,69]. Here, we mainly introduce the development of next-generation kinase inhibitors aimed at achieving superior efficacy, particularly against the observed clinical mutations associated with resistance. Taking the Bcr-Abl kinase as a case, the development of novel drugs unfolds as follows.

1. Nilotinib [70], a derivative of benzamide, is developed based on the rational drug design of imatinib (Fig. 15.29). The initial assumption for imatinib was that the polar hydrophilic *N*-methylpiperazine moiety would extend into the solvent region outside the protein. However, the crystal structure of the complex showed that most of this group is buried inside the catalytic hydrophobic pocket, which is unfavorable for binding energy contribution. Therefore, researchers attempted to explore the topological adaptability of the posterior pocket in the DFG_{out} conformation with other moieties, while preserving the PAP pharmacophore of imatinib. Initially, the amide group was replaced by sulfonamide or urea to maintain hydrogen-bonding interactions with D381 and E286, but the resulting series of derivatives exhibited poor activity or pharmacokinetic properties, thus impeding further optimization efforts [71]. However, by interchanging the carbonyl and amino positions within the amide bond, a reversed amide was obtained, and it still maintained the two hydrogen bonding interactions of the original pattern. Additionally, the highly electronegative trifluoromethyl group at the end phenyl ring is situated perfectly within the posterior hydrophobic pocket, with one of the electronegative fluorine atoms forming an electrostatic interaction with the adjacent (3 Å) positively charged carbon atom of carbonyl of the Ala380 peptide backbone [72]. Furthermore, the introduction of the methylimidazole ring at the terminus improved the drug-like properties of the entire molecule, including improvements in water solubility and oral absorption (Fig. 15.30). Consequently, this led to the nilotinib (AMN107). Compared to

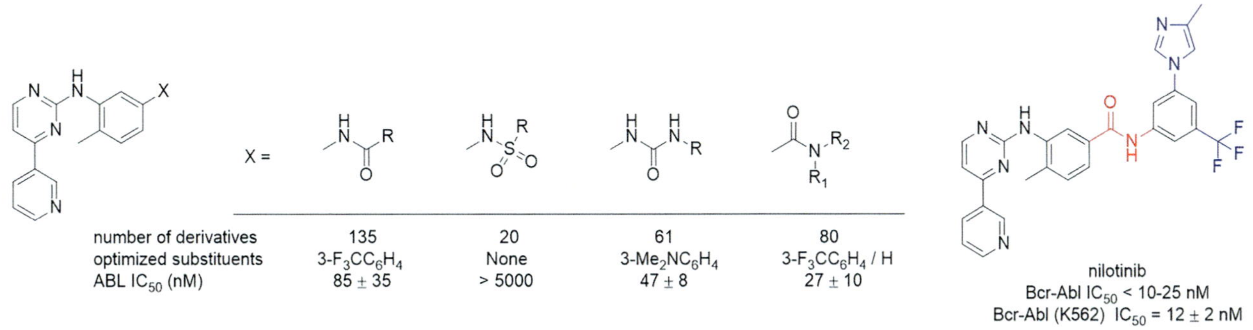

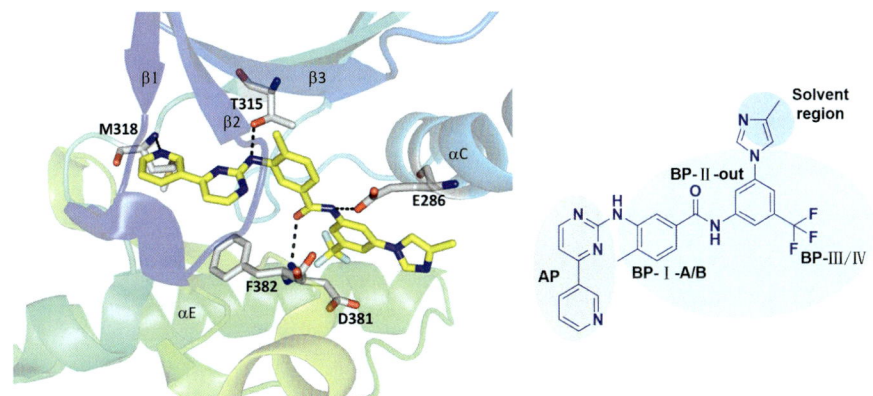

FIGURE 15.29 Optimization process for nilotinib.

FIGURE 15.30 Cocrystal structure and binding mode of Abl with nilotinib (PDB: 3cs9).

imatinib, nilotinib exhibits higher selectivity and affinity for Abl protein with a prolonged retention time of up to 200 minutes (imatinib has only 28 minutes). Therefore, nilotinib is at least 10-fold more potent than imatinib against wild-type Bcr-Abl kinase (IC_{50} 20 vs 194 nM) and has shown enhanced inhibitory activity against Bcr-Abl overexpressing K562 and Ba/F3 cells with IC_{50} values of 12 and 25 nM, respectively. Additionally, nilotinib potently inhibited the majority (32/33) of imatinib-resistant Bcr-Abl mutants (IC_{50} < 10−1000 nM). But the autophosphorylation of the T315I mutant was unaffected by nilotinib (IC_{50} > 10 μM) [73].

Compared to the binding of imatinib with Abl, the crystallographic studies of nilotinib suggest subtle differences in the mode of binding to Abl. Nilotinib lacks the two hydrogen bonds formed by the nitrogen atom of the piperazine ring and requires less change in the conformation of the protein C-terminus, thereby leading to a better topological fit to the Abl protein. In terms of physicochemical properties [74], nilotinib has higher lipophilicity (log$P$ 4.9 vs 3.1) and significantly reduced basicity (pK_1 5.6 vs 7.8), but the solubility of the hydrochloride salt is not high (0.29 mg/mL). Therefore, the recommended clinical dose of nilotinib (400 mg BID) is higher than that of imatinib. Nilotinib was approved in 2007 for the treatment of adult patients with chronic-phase and accelerated-phase CML who are resistant to or intolerant of imatinib [75,76]. Subsequent head-to-head clinical studies revealed that key response rates for nilotinib were significantly superior to those observed with imatinib [77], leading to its approval for newly diagnosed CML patients in 2010.

2. Dasatinib, also known as BMS-354825, is a 2-aminopyrimidine thiazole-5-carboxamide derivative developed by Bristol−Myers Squibb and was approved in 2006 for use in CML patients. Dasatinib originated from inhibitors targeting the Src family kinases, including Src, Lck, and Yes [78,79]. Initially, modifications of substituents at three positions on aminothiazole-5-carboxamide core resulted in compound 15 (Fig. 15.31), which exhibited moderate kinase activity (IC_{50} = 35 nM) but limited cellular activity (IC_{50} = 884 nM). Given that bulky moiety (e.g., cyclopropane) on the amide led to decreased activity, a structurally rigid 2-aminopyrimidine analog 16 was subsequently designed, which showed significantly improved kinase and cellular activity (hLck: IC_{50} = 0.096 nM, K562: IC_{50} = 1.6 nM). Subsequently, various hydrophilic groups were introduced at the tail of compound 16 with the aim of improving potency and ADME properties [80]. Finally, dasatinib displayed potent inhibitory activity against Abl/Lck kinase and K562 cell lines with IC_{50} values of less than 1 nM.

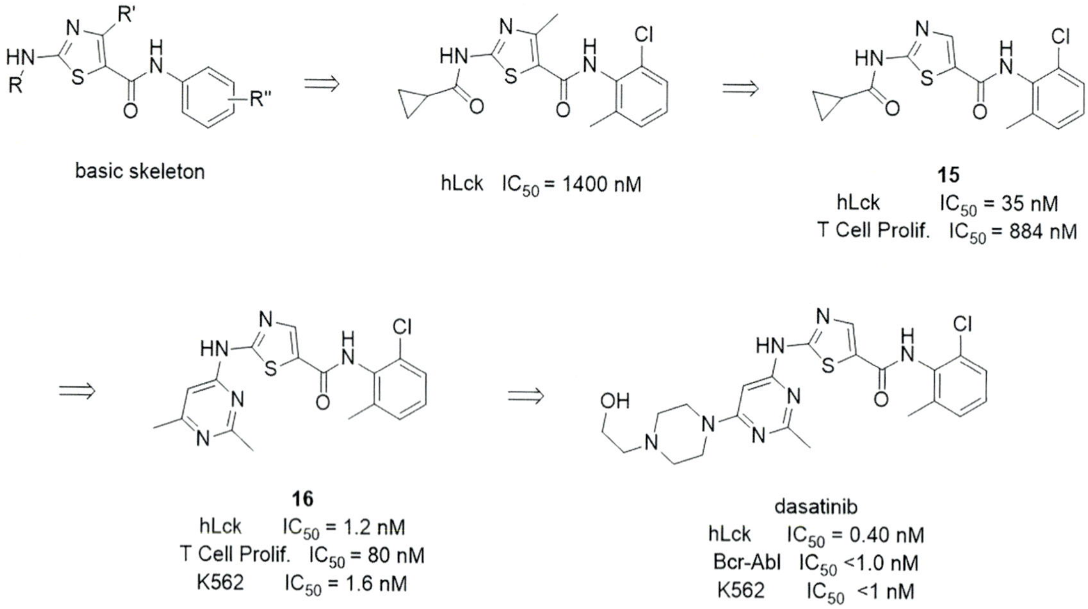

FIGURE 15.31 Optimization process for dasatinib.

Dasatinib belongs to Type I inhibitors [81] and binds to the activated conformation of Abl kinase (Fig. 15.32). The aminothiazole moiety occupies the adenosine pocket (AP) and forms two crucial hydrogen bond interactions with the Met318 of the hinge region. The 2-chloro-6-methylphenyl ring occupies the hydrophobic pocket of the gatekeeper region (FP-I-A/B), and the amide nitrogen forms a hydrogen bond with the gatekeeper Thr315. The ethoxy-substituted piperazine group is directed toward the surface-exposed region.

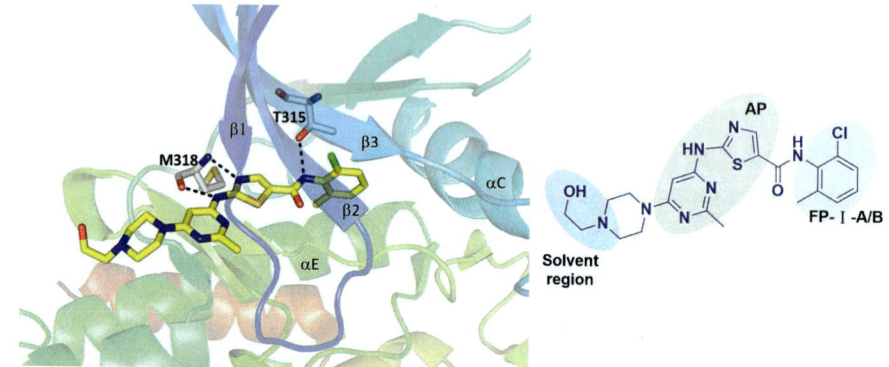

FIGURE 15.32 Cocrystal structure and binding mode of Abl with dasatinib (PDB: 2gqg).

Compared to Type II inhibitors, dasatinib imposes less stringent conformational requirements on Abl for kinase inhibition, thereby resulting in a significant increase in activity against wild-type Bcr-Abl (IC_{50} = 0.8 nmol/L), about 325- and 16-fold more potent than imatinib and nilotinib [82], respectively. Thus, the clinical dosage of dasatinib (100 mg QD) is also lower. In addition, the kinase activity of imatinib-resistant Abl isoforms (18/19) was effectively inhibited in the low nanomolar range. The sole isoform that exhibited clear resistance to dasatinib was the T315I mutant, which retained kinase activity even in the presence of μM concentrations of the compound [83]. Dasatinib has been approved for use in patients with Ph-chromosome-positive CML and ALL who are resistant to or intolerant of imatinib [84], as well as in newly diagnosed CML patients [85].

It is worth noting that the Type I mechanism of binding to the activated kinase conformation also reduces the kinase selectivity of dasatinib. It also exhibits an additional inhibitory effect on Src family kinases, c-KIT, and PDGFRβ, leading to potential side effects such as immunosuppression and increased risk of infectious disease.

3. Bosutinib, a 4-anilino-3-quinolinecarbonitrile derivative [86], was launched in 2012. Initially, the SAR study was performed with an aim to discover a potent Src kinase inhibitor [87]. The selectivity of the compound for Src kinase was markedly enhanced by the introduction of the cyano group and the optimization of the substituents on the aniline ring. Further enhancements in activity were achieved by introducing the N-methylpiperazine ring, ultimately leading to the more potent bosutinib (SKI-606) [88] (Fig. 15.33). The further screening revealed that bosutinib is also active against Bcr-Abl, with an IC_{50} value of 5 nM for the inhibition of K562 cell proliferation, making it 15-fold more potent than imatinib (IC_{50} = 88 nM), and it also effectively prolongs the survival of mice harboring wild-type Bcr-Abl [89,90]. Additionally, in vitro and in vivo studies have demonstrated that bosutinib exhibits activity against multiple imatinib-resistant Bcr-Abl mutants except those harboring the T315I gatekeeper mutation [91]. Additionally, bosutinib has shown efficacy against imatinib-resistant CML [92].

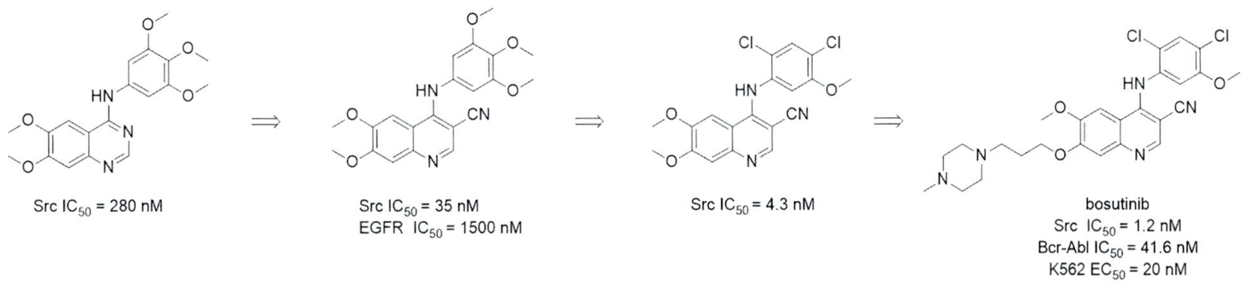

FIGURE 15.33 Optimization process for bosutinib.

The cocrystal structure [93] (Fig. 15.34) shows that bosutinib binds to the DFG_{in} conformation of Abl, where the quinoline core occupies the adenosine pocket (AP), with the N1 atom forming a key hydrogen bond with gatekeeper Met318. The 2,4-dichloro-5-methoxyaniline is oriented at approximately 65° to the plane of the quinoline core, binding to the back hydrophobic pocket (BP-I) of the gatekeeper area. The flexible N-propyl-N-methylpiperazine group is oriented toward the surface solvent region, with the methoxy oxygen participating in a hydrogen bond mediated by water with Asn322. While imatinib, nilotinib, and dasatinib all form hydrogen bonds with Thr315, the cyano group of bosutinib interacts via van der Waals forces with Thr315 and forms a hydrogen bond network with Asp381, mediated by a water molecule (PDB: 4mxo).

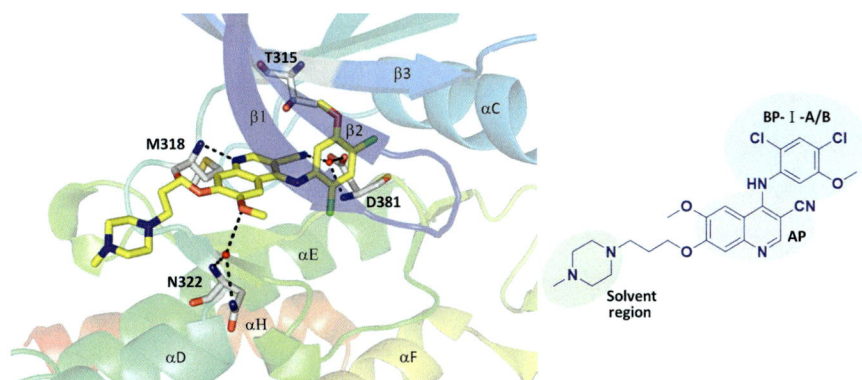

FIGURE 15.34 Cocrystal structure and binding mode of Abl with bosutinib (PDB: 4mxo).

4. Ponatinib, a member of the benzoylethynyl derivative class, was launched in 2012 for the treatment of CML patients carrying the Bcr-Abl^{T315I} mutation or those who have exhibited resistance to other Bcr-Abl inhibitors [94]. The discovery of ponatinib started from AP24149, a Type I and dual Abl/Src inhibitor [95] with a *trans*-ethylene linker on a purine scaffold [96]. (Fig. 15.35). Initially, the hybrid strategy was performed to develop DFG_{out}-targeted Abl kinase inhibitors based on AP24149 template, by coupling with typical N-arylbenzamide fragment of Type II inhibitors. Moreover, the incorporation of rigid, rod-shaped acetylene linkage further reduced the steric repulsion with the enlarged Ile315 side chain of the T315I mutant. Subsequently, modifications were made to the purine and phenyl ring

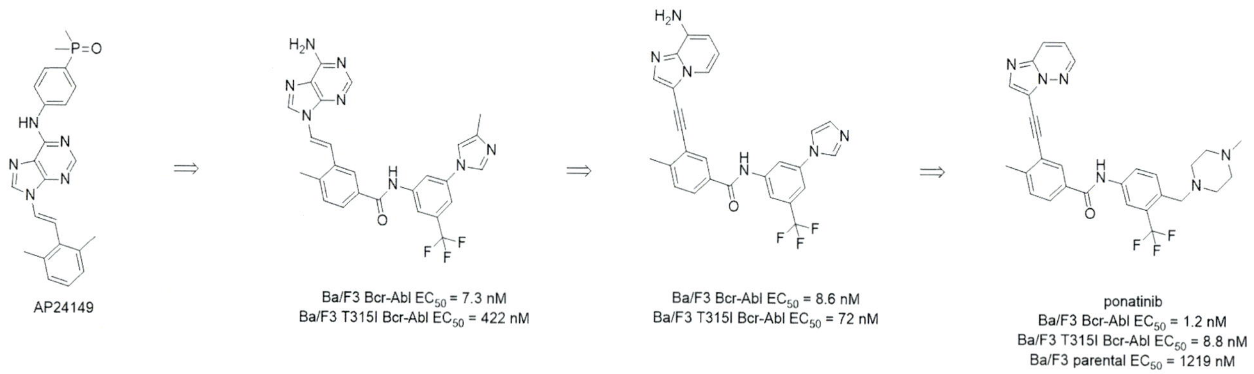

FIGURE 15.35 Optimization process for ponatinib.

substituents to optimize potency and pharmacokinetic properties and ultimately led to ponatinib (AP24534) [97]. It exhibited low nM cellular potency against cell lines expressing either native Bcr-Abl or T315I mutant Bcr-Abl. Ponatinib also significantly prolonged survival in an aggressive mouse model of CML driven by the T315I mutant. In addition, ponatinib also potently inhibited the proliferation of all clinically relevant Abl mutants in cell-based assays, characterizing it as the first pan-Bcr-Abl inhibitor. The cocrystal structure [98] (Fig. 15.36) reveals that the imidazo[1,2-b]pyridazine ring occupies the AP and interacts through hydrogen bond with the hinge region; the methylphenyl group occupies the back hydrophobic pocket (BP-II-out); the amide forms hydrogen bonds with Asp381 and Glu286; the trifluoromethyl phenyl group tightly occupies the hydrophobic pocket induced by the DFG$_{out}$ conformation (BP-III); and the N-methylpiperazine group occupies a solvent-accessible pocket (BP-IV) and forms hydrogen bonds with Ile360 and His361 (similar to imatinib). Among, the key structural elements necessary for achieving high potency against T315I mutation is the presence of rigid and less sterically demanding acetylene linker, which effectively overcomes steric hindrance and forms favorable van der Waals interactions with Ile. In contrast, when the ethynyl group is replaced with a saturated ethyl group, the cellular activity against Ba/F3 (Bcr-Abl^{T315I}) decreases by nearly 34-fold.

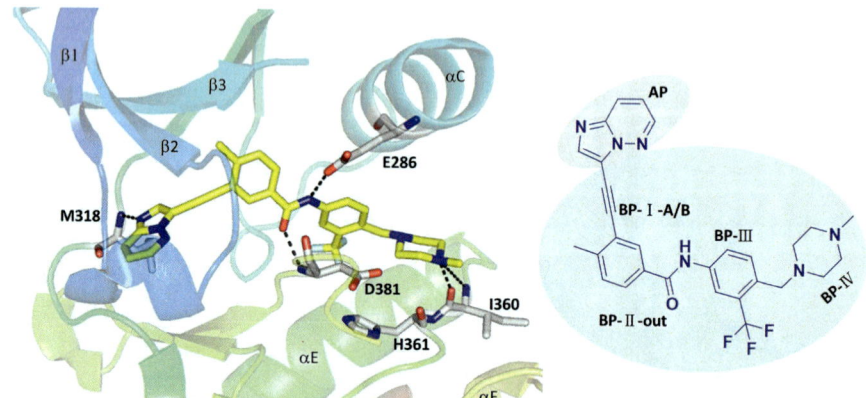

FIGURE 15.36 Cocrystal structure and binding mode of Abl with Ponatinib (PDB: 3oxz).

However, the selectivity of ponatinib is relatively modest, as it exhibits activity against other kinases such as FGFR, c-KIT, PDGFR, VEGFR, Ret, Tie2, and Flt3 families, thereby associating with the risk of hepatotoxicity and arterial thrombosis [99,100].

Based on the structure of ponatinib, the authors' team further explored 1H-pyrazolo[3,4-b]pyridine-based heterocyclic core serving as hinge binder (Fig. 15.37), which allowed to form two hydrogen bonds with the hinge region, thereby enhancing the binding affinity with the Abl protein. As a result, the representative olverembatinib (GZD824, HQP1351) was obtained [101], demonstrating broad-spectrum inhibitory activity against native Bcr-Abl and Bcr-Abl mutants, including T315I, in both in vitro and in vivo models. Olverembatinib became the first drug conditionally approved by the National Medical Products Administration for the treatment of CML patients carrying the Bcr-Abl^{T315I} mutation in November 2021. Two years later, olverembatinib received further approval for the treatment of CML patients with other PKI resistance and intolerance.

HN
N
N
H
N
N
N
O
F
F
F
GZD 824
T315I Bcr-Abl IC50 = 0.68 ± 0.11 nM
Ba/F3: Bcr-Abl EC50 = 1.0 ± 0.3 nM
Ba/F3: T315I Bcr-Abl EC50 = 7.1 ± 1.3 nM

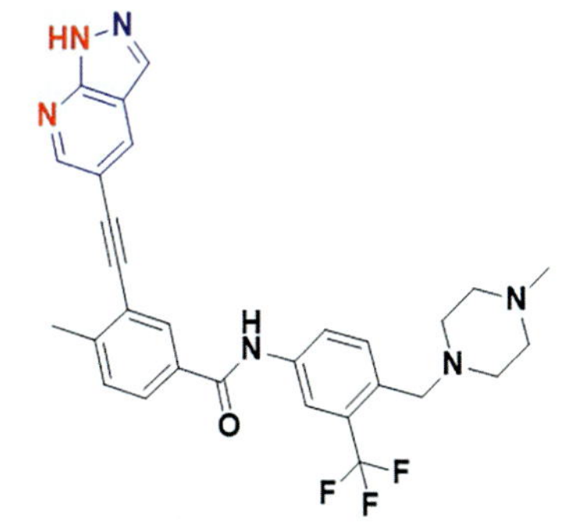

FIGURE 15.37 Chemical structure of olverembatinib.

As described above, several second and third-generation Abl-targeted inhibitors have, to some extent, overcome imatinib resistance induced by multiple Abl mutations. However, drugs with different binding modes exhibit varying sensitivity to specific point mutations in the ATP-binding domain. For example, nilotinib and ponatinib, which bind to inactive conformation of Abl, are more sensitive to mutations in the phosphate-binding loop. Conversely, dasatinib, which binds to the active conformation of Abl, is more susceptible to mutations in the hinge region. In general, while these approved targeted drugs have shown efficacy, they still pose a tremendous challenge due to the occurrence of resistance induced by additional point mutations.

5. Asciminib

   In addition to ATP competitive inhibitors, another class of drugs developed to override the Bcr-Abl T315I mutation binds to the allosteric pocket, known as the myristate pocket, which is located at the C-terminus of the Abl kinase, away from the ATP-binding site (Fig. 15.38).

ATP pocket
myristate pocket

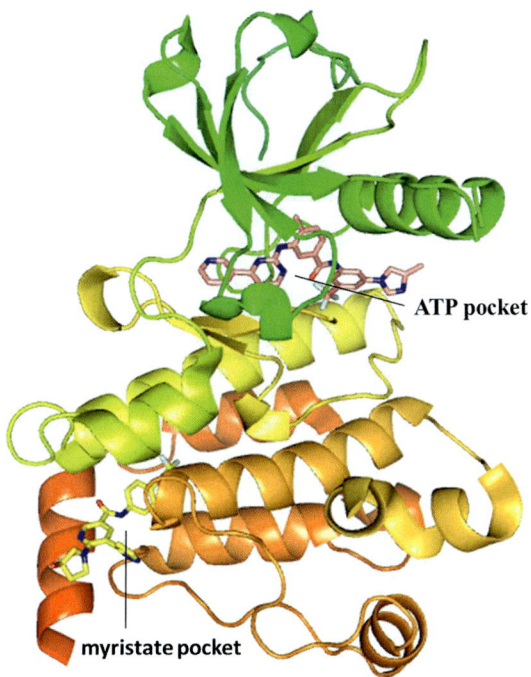

FIGURE 15.38 Cocrystal structure of Abl with asciminib and nilotinib.

Initially, through a cell-based phenotypic screening strategy, Novartis discovered a 4,6-disubstituted pyrimidine compound, GNF-2 [102] (Fig. 15.39), which exhibits specific cytotoxicity against Ba/F3 cells with high expression of Bcr-Abl (IC$_{50}$ = 0.576 μM), and displays no toxicity against nontransformed cells. It inhibits the activity of Bcr-Abl kinase (IC$_{50}$ = 0.26 μM) and also exhibits inhibitory effects on some imatinib-resistant Bcr-Abl mutant forms.

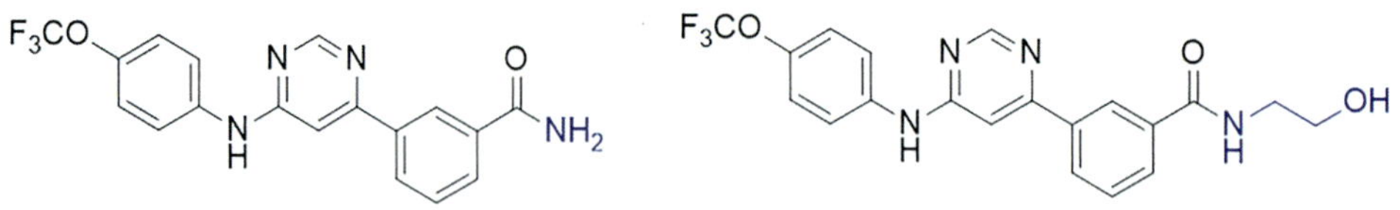

	GNF-2	GNF-5
Abl SH1	IC$_{50}$ > 10 μM	IC$_{50}$ > 10 μM
Abl SH3SH2SH1	0.009 μM	0.017 μM
Ba/F3 Bcr-Abl^{wt}	GI$_{50}$ 0.576 μM	GI$_{50}$ 0.145 μM
Ba/F3 Bcr-Abl^{T315I}	> 10 μM	> 10 μM

FIGURE 15.39 Chemical structure of GNF-2 and GNF-5.

The X-ray crystallographic study indicates that GNF-2 is an allosteric inhibitor, mimicking the substrate myristate and potently binding to the myristate pocket (Fig. 15.40) with its trifluoromethoxy group buried deeply in the hydrophobic pocket formed by Leu448, Ala452, and Leu360, while the amide group is directed toward the protein surface. The nitrogen atom on the pyrimidine ring forms a hydrogen bond with Tyr454, mediated by a water molecule, and the amine group forms a hydrogen-bond network with Ala452 and Glu481, also via a water molecule. These unique binding interactions ensure the remarkable selectivity of GNF-2 toward Bcr-Abl (PDB: 3k5v). Further optimization of GNF-2, by replacing the tail amine with a hydroxyethylamine, resulted in GNF-5 with improved cellular potency (IC$_{50}$ = 0.145 μM) and more favorable pharmacokinetic properties [103]. However, both compounds failed to show inhibitory activity against Ba/F3 cells harboring the Bcr-Abl T315I mutant (GI$_{50}$ > 10 μM).

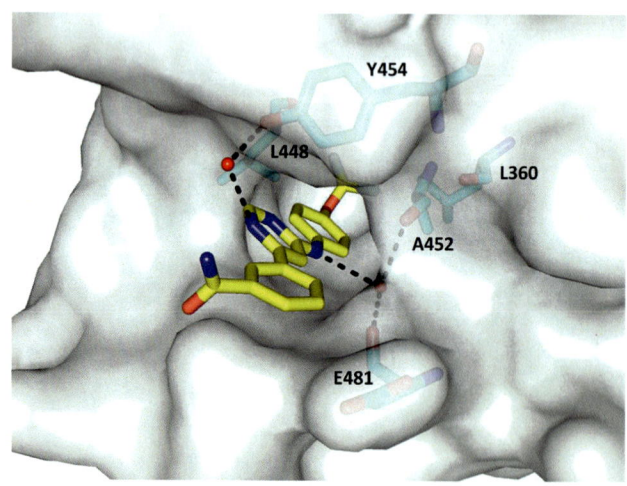

FIGURE 15.40 Cocrystal structure of GNF-2 in Myristate pocket of Abl (PDB: 3k5v).

Next, the fragment-based screening using nuclear magnetic resonance (NMR) [104] and further structure-based optimization (Fig. 15.41) led to asciminib [105] (ABL001), with a K_d value of 0.5–0.8 nM and 100-fold greater potency over that of GNF-2, which was launched to treat CML and Ph-chromosome-positive ALL in October 2021. Consistent with GNF-2, the cocrystal structures revealed that the trifluoromethoxy group of asciminib adopted almost identical binding poses. However, the open-chain amide linkage, which replaced the original pyrimidine amine structure, formed two hydrogen bond interactions mediated by water molecules (Fig. 15.42). The pyridine ring extending outside the pocket, along with its connected imidazole and 3-hydroxy pyrrole, established an extensive hydrogen bonding network

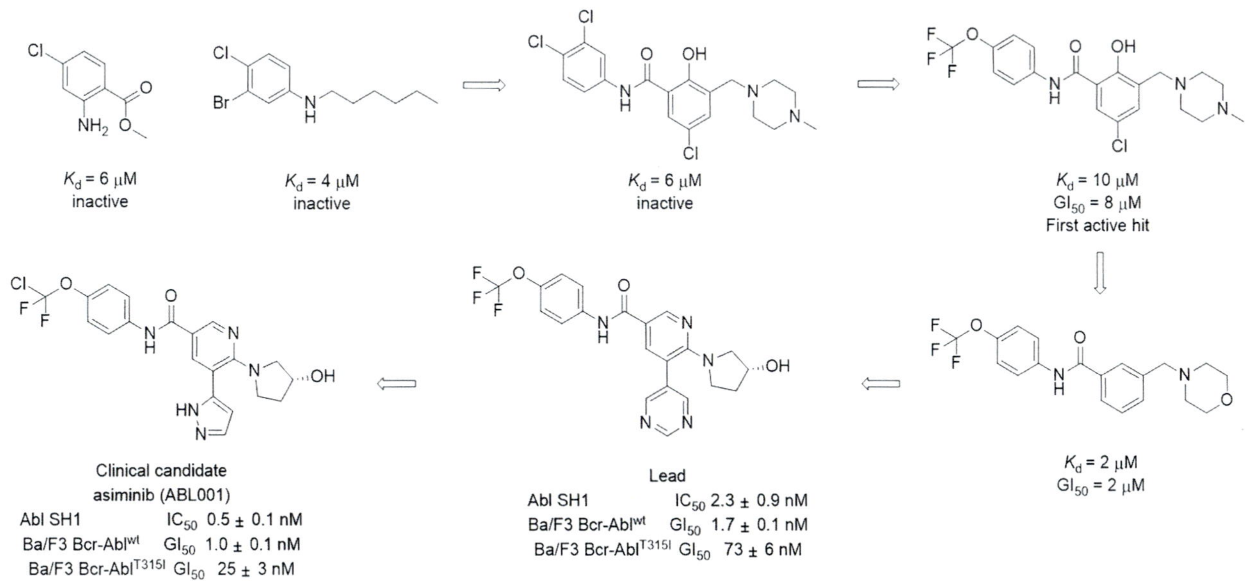

FIGURE 15.41 Optimization process for asciminib.

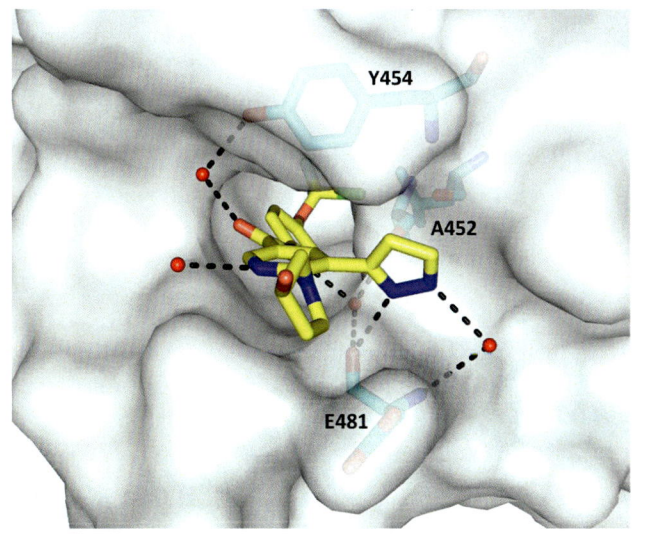

FIGURE 15.42 Cocrystal structure of asciminib in myristate pocket of Abl (PDB: 5mo4).

with surrounding polar residues, significantly enhancing the molecule's affinity. More importantly, asciminib exerts its activity via an allosteric mechanism effectively in the low nanomolar concentration range against wild-type Bcr-Abl, as well as PKI-resistant Bcr-Abl mutations, including T315I. Meanwhile, ATP-site inhibitors, such as nilotinib, have been suggested to be effective against asciminib-resistant mutations. Furthermore, combination therapy of asciminib and nilotinib can inhibit the emergence of resistance caused by the Bcr-Abl-driven mutation [106]. Currently, asciminib is mainly used to treat adult patients in the chronic phase of Ph-chromosome-positive CML who have previously received at least two TK inhibitors, and it is also used to treat patients carrying the Bcr-Abl^{T315I} mutation.

In summary, the newly developed Bcr-Abl kinase inhibitors represent significant therapeutic advancements in tackling clinical imatinib resistance. However, most of these PKIs function as multitarget inhibitors, lacking the relative selectivity within the kinase family. Furthermore, as clinical usage progresses, acquired drug resistance commonly arises due to secondary or tertiary kinase point mutations. Therefore, the development of kinase inhibitors with high potency, selectivity, and novel action mechanisms remains still an urgent need in both clinical and experimental practice.

15.4 Summary

The remarkable success of imatinib against CML, as the first marketed small molecule kinase inhibitor, could be attributed to three critical factors, including clear clinical indications, excellent drug properties, and precise patient selection. Firstly, Bcr-Abl kinase had been confirmed as a specific target for treating CML, leading to the goal of developing Abl-targeted inhibitors. Secondly, although the discovery of imatinib started from an empirical screening of compound libraries with a fortuitous element, the PAP scaffold-based compound libraries using a rational drug design strategy determined its favorable drug-likeness. Moreover, the selection of appropriate patients carrying the Bcr-Abl fusion gene (easily identified through the Philadelphia chromosome) for clinical trials ensured the maximum clinical benefit and the most promising outcomes of trials. Additionally, data monitoring of clinical endpoints, such as specific hematological and cytological responses, as well as biomarkers, is simple and feasible. Subsequently, based on comprehensive kinase activity profiling, the clinical use of imatinib was rapidly extended to other indications besides CML.

Imatinib represents a therapeutic breakthrough of molecularly targeted therapy in cancer and accelerates the development of small molecule PKIs. However, kinase selectivity and resistance remain the two major challenges.

In terms of selectivity of PKIs, firstly, most PKIs are still multitarget inhibitors and seem to be generally more effective, given that most cancers are mainly caused by dysregulation of multiple signaling pathways. In fact, poor selectivity of PKIs greatly restricts their usage for indications other than cancer. Secondly, it is worth noting that Type II inhibitors are not intrinsically more selective than Type I inhibitors, although the inactive conformation of PKs commonly shares less structural similarity than their active conformation. Compared with ATP competitive inhibitors, both allosteric inhibitors and covalent inhibitors, which bind to less-conserved allosteric pockets and form specific covalent binding with target kinases, respectively, may offer a potentially complementary strategy to improve the selectivity of PKIs.

In addition, due to the inherent genetic instability of cancer cells, new mutations will continue to emerge, leading to acquired resistance to existing drugs. In recent years, newly developed targeted protein degradation technologies have emerged as novel therapeutic paradigms [107], with representative proteolysis targeting chimeras (PROTACs) technology. Different from enzymatic inhibition of traditional PKIs, PROTACs impede the whole biological function of the target protein by binding to the target protein and inducing subsequent proteasomal degradation. Therefore, PROTACs not only have the potential to overcome the clinical resistance of PKIs caused by point mutations in the kinase but also have the advantages of improving selectivity and specificity. Moreover, PROTAC affords an additional opportunity to degrade so-called undruggable targets, such as transcription factors and scaffold proteins. So far, a variety of PROTAC-based kinase degraders have entered into clinical trials, underscoring the huge therapeutic potential of PROTAC in cancer treatment.

In conclusion, although numerous obstacles and challenges persist, the advent of PKIs in cancer therapy has led to a paradigm shift in cancer treatment approaches. However, only a small subset of the human kinome has been studied, with PKIs reported. Hence there is an urgent need to develop new chemical probes to explore the functions of the other unknown kinases and promote the kinase-based drug development.

References

[1] Manning G, Whyte DB, Martinez R, et al. The protein kinase complement of the human genome. Science 2002;298:1912–34.
[2] Cohen P. Protein kinases—the major drug targets of the twenty-first century. Nat Rev Drug Discov 2002;1:309–15.
[3] Roskoski RJ. Properties of FDA-approved small molecule protein kinase inhibitors. Pharmacol Res 2019;144:19–50.
[4] Knighton DR, Zheng JH, Ten Eyck LF, et al. Crystal structure of the catalytic subunit of cyclic adenosine monophosphate-dependent protein kinase. Science 1991;253:407–14.
[5] Hanks SK, Quinn AM, Hunter T. The protein kinase family: conserved features and deduced phylogeny of the catalytic domains. Science 1988;241:42–52.
[6] Shah K, Liu Y, Deirmengian C, et al. Engineering unnatural nucleotide specificity for Rous sarcoma virus tyrosine kinase to uniquely label its direct substrates. Proc Natl Acad Sci U S A 1997;94:3565–70.
[7] Liu Y, Shah K, Yang F, et al. A molecular gate which controls unnatural ATP analogue recognition by the tyrosine kinase v-Src. Bioorgan Med Chem 1998;6:1219–26.
[8] Herberg FW, Yonemoto W, Taylor SS. The catalytic subunit of cAMP-dependent protein kinase. Springer Berlin Heidelberg; 1993.
[9] Kornev A, Haste N, Taylor S, et al. Surface comparison of active and inactive protein kinases identifies a conserved activation mechanism. Proc Natl Acad Sci U S A 2006;103:17783–8.
[10] Kornev AP, Taylor SS, Eyck LFT. A helix scaffold for the assembly of active protein kinases. Proc Natl Acad Sci U S A 2008;105:14377–82.
[11] Johnson LN, Noble MEM, Owen DJ. Active and inactive protein kinases: structural basis for regulation. Cell 1996;85:149–58.

[12] Huse M, Kuriyan J. The conformational plasticity of protein kinases. Cell 2002;109:275–82.
[13] Lu XY, Cai Q, Ding K. Recent developments in the third generation inhibitors of Bcr-Abl for overriding T315I mutation. Curr Med Chem 2011;18:2146–57.
[14] Shaoyong, Xinheng, Duan, et al. Allosteric modulator discovery: from serendipity to structure-based design. J Med Chem 2019;62:6405–21.
[15] Barf T, Kaptein A. Irreversible protein kinase inhibitors: balancing the benefits and risks. J Med Chem 2012;55:6243–62.
[16] Capdeville R, Buchdunger E, Zimmermann J, et al. Glivec (STI571, imatinib), a rationally developed, targeted anticancer drug. Nat Rev Drug Discov 2002;1:493–502.
[17] Sawyers CL. Chronic myeloid leukemia. N Engl J Med 1999;340:1330–40.
[18] Ahuja H, Bareli M, Arlin Z, et al. The spectrum of molecular alterations in the evolution of chronic myelocytic leukemia. J Clin Invest 1991;87:2042–7.
[19] Sill H, Goldman JM, Cross NCP. Homozygous deletions of the p16 tumor-suppressor gene are associated with lymphoid transformation of chronic myeloid leukemia. Blood 1995;85:2013–16.
[20] Nowell PC, Hungerford DA. A minute chromosome in human chronic granulocytic leukemia. Science 1960;132:1497.
[21] Rowley JD. A new consistent chromosomal abnormality in chronic myelogenous leukaemia identified by quinacrine fluorescence and giemsa staining. Nature 1973;243:290–3.
[22] Faderl S, Garcia-Manero G, Thomas DA, et al. Philadelphia chromosome-positive acute lymphoblastic leukemia- current concepts and future perspectives. Rev Clin Exp Hematol 2002;6:142–60.
[23] Radaelli F, Calori R, Ripamonti C, et al. Treatment of myeloproliferative syndrome with hydroxyurea. Ann Hematol 1996;73:205.
[24] Witte ON, Dasgupta A, Baltimore D. Abelson murine leukaemia virus protein is phosphorylated in vitro to form phosphotyrosine. Nature 1980;283:826–31.
[25] Konopka JB, Watanabe SM, Witte ON. An alteration of the human c-abl protein in K562 leukemia cells unmasks associated tyrosine kinase activity. Cell 1984;37:1035–42.
[26] Nagar B, Hantschel O, Young MA, et al. Structural basis for the autoinhibition of c-Abl tyrosine kinase. Cell 2003;112:859–71.
[27] Daley G, Van Etten R, Baltimore D. Induction of chronic myelogenous leukemia in mice by the P210bcr/abl gene of the Philadelphia chromosome. Science 1990;247:824–30.
[28] Lugo T, Pendergast A, Muller A, et al. Tyrosine kinase activity and transformation potency of bcr-abl oncogene products. Science 1990;247:1079–82.
[29] Pendergast MA. The Abl family kinases: mechanisms of regulation and signaling. Adv Cancer Res 2002;85:51–100.
[30] Eddershaw PJ, Beresford AP, Bayliss MK. ADME/PK as part of a rational approach to drug discovery. Drug Discov Today 2000;5:409–14.
[31] Lipinski A, Lombardo F, Dominy BW, et al. Experimental and computational approaches to estimate solubility and permeability in drug discovery and development settings. Adv Drug Deliv Rev 2001;46:3–26.
[32] Teague SJ, Davis AM, Leeson PD, et al. The design of leadlike combinatorial libraries. Angew Chem Int Ed Engl 1999;38:3743–8.
[33] Paul R, Hallett WA, Hanifin JW, et al. Preparation of substituted N-phenyl-4-aryl-2-pyrimidinamines as mediator release inhibitors. J Med Chem 1993;36:2716–25.
[34] Zimmermann J, Caravatti G, Mett H, et al. Phenylamino-pyrimidine (PAP) derivatives: a new class of potent and selective inhibitors of protein kinase C (PKC). Arch Pharm 1996;329:371–6.
[35] Zimmermann J, Buchdunger E, Mett H, et al. Potent and selective inhibitors of the Abl-kinase: phenylamino-pyrimidine (PAP) derivatives. Bioorg Med Chem Lett 1997;7:187–92.
[36] Druker BJ, Tamura S, Buchdunger E, et al. Effects of a selective inhibitor of the Abl tyrosine kinase on the growth of Bcr – Abl positive cells. Nat Med 1996;2:561–6.
[37] Schindler T. Structural mechanism for STI-571 inhibition of abelson tyrosine kinase. Science 2000;289:1938–42.
[38] Nagar B. Crystal structures of the kinase domain of c-Abl in complex with the small molecule inhibitors PD173955 and imatinib (STI-571). Cancer Res 2002;62:4236–43.
[39] Liu Y, Gray NS. Rational design of inhibitors that bind to inactive kinase conformations. Nat Chem Biol 2006;2:358–64.
[40] Tong M, Seeliger MA. Targeting conformational plasticity of protein kinases. ACS Chem Biol 2015;10:190–200.
[41] Zimmermann J.D.R.. Pyrimidin derivatives and process for their preparation: EP, EP0564409 A1. 1993-03-15 [2000-01-19].
[42] Schran H, Peng B, Lloyd P. Clinical pharmacokinetics of imatinib. Clin Pharmacokinet 2005;44:879–94.
[43] Peng B, Dutreix C, Mehring G, et al. Absolute bioavailability of imatinib (GlivecÂ®) orally versus intravenous infusion. J Clin Pharmacol 2004;44:158–62.
[44] Peng B. Pharmacokinetics and pharmacodynamics of imatinib in a phase I trial with chronic myeloid leukemia patients. J Clin Oncol 2004;22:935–42.
[45] Petzer AL, Gunsilius E, Hayes M, et al. Low concentrations of STI571 in the cerebrospinal fluid: a case report. Br J Haematol 2015;117:623–5.
[46] Mahon F-X. MDR1 gene overexpression confers resistance to imatinib mesylate in leukemia cell line models. Blood 2003;101:2368–673.
[47] Gschwind H-P, Pfaar U, Waldmeier F, et al. Metabolism and disposition of imatinib mesylate in healthy volunteers. Drug Metabol Disposit 2005;33(10):1503–12.
[48] Champagne MA. Imatinib mesylate (STI571) for treatment of children with Philadelphia chromosome-positive leukemia: results from a Children's Oncology Group phase 1 study. Blood 2004;104:2655–60.

[49] Ramanathan RK, Egorin MJ, Takimoto CHM, et al. Phase I and harmacokinetic study of imatinib mesylate in patients with advanced malignancies and varying degrees of liver dysfunction: a study by the national cancer institute organ dysfunction working group. J Clin Oncol 2008;26:563−9.

[50] Ramanathan RK, Egorin MJ, Takimoto CHM, et al. Phase I and pharmacokinetic study of imatinib mesylate in patients with advanced malignancies and varying degrees of renal dysfunction: a study by the national cancer institute organ dysfunction working group. J Clin Oncol 2008;26:570−6.

[51] Druker BJ, Talpaz M, Resta DJ, et al. Efficacy and safety of a specific inhibitor of the BCR-ABL tyrosine kinase in chronic myeloid leukemia. N Engl J Med 2001;344:1031−7.

[52] Bolton A, Peng B, Hubert M, et al. Effect of rifampicin on the pharmacokinetics of imatinib mesylate (Gleevec, STI571) in healthy subjects. Cancer Chemother Pharmacol 2004;53:102−6.

[53] O'Brien SG, Meinhardt P, Bond E, et al. Effects of imatinib mesylate (STI571, Glivec) on the pharmacokinetics of simvastatin, a cytochrome P450 3A4 substrate, in patients with chronic myeloid leukaemia. Br J Cancer 2003;89:1855−9.

[54] Oda T, Heaney C, Hagopian JR, et al. Crkl is the major tyrosine-phosphorylated protein in neutrophils from patients with chronic myelogenous leukemia. J Biol Chem 1994;269:22925−8.

[55] Druker BJ, Sawyers CL, Kantarjian H, et al. Activity of a specific inhibitor of the BCR-ABL tyrosine kinase in the blast crisis of chronic myeloid leukemia and acute lymphoblastic leukemia with the philadelphia chromosome. N Engl J Med 2001;344:1038−42.

[56] Kantarjian H, Sawyers C, Hochhaus A, et al. Hematologic and cytogenetic responses to imatinib mesylate in chronic myelogenous leukemia. N Engl J Med 2002;346:645−52.

[57] Talpaz M, Silver RT, Druker BJ, et al. Imatinib induces durable hematologic and cytogenetic responses in patients with accelerated phase chronic myeloid leukemia: results of a phase 2 study. Blood 2002;99:1928−37.

[58] Sawyers CL, Hochhaus A, Feldman E, et al. Imatinib induces hematologic and cytogenetic responses in patients with chronic myelogenous leukemia in myeloid blast crisis: results of a phase II study. Blood 2002;99:3530−9.

[59] O'brien SG, Guilhot F, Larson RA, et al. Imatinib compared with interferon and low-dose cytarabine for newly diagnosed chronic-phase chronic myeloid leukemia. N Engl J Med 2003;348:994−1004.

[60] Hochhaus A, Larson RA, Guilhot F, et al. Long-term outcomes of imatinib treatment for chronic myeloid leukemia. N Engl J Med 2017;376:917−27.

[61] Demetri GD, Mehren MV, Blanke C, et al. Efficacy and safety of imatinib mesylate in advanced gastrointestinal stromal tumors. N Engl J Med 2002;347:472−80.

[62] Crugnola M, Castagnetti F, Breccia M, et al. Five-year follow-up of patients receiving imatinib for chronic myeloid leukemia. N Engl J Med 2006;355:2408−17.

[63] Hochhaus A, Kreil S, Corbin AS, et al. Molecular and chromosomal mechanisms of resistance to imatinib (STI571) therapy. Leukemia 2002;16(11):2190−6.

[64] Sandra WC-J, Valerie G, Gabriele F, et al. Imatinib (STI571) resistance in chronic myelogenous leukemia: molecular basis of the underlying mechanisms and potential strategies for treatment. Mini Rev Med Chem 2004;4:285−99.

[65] Gorre EM, Mohammed M, Ellwood K, et al. Clinical resistance to STI-571 cancer therapy caused by BCR-ABL gene mutation or amplification. Science 2001;293:876−80.

[66] Shah NP, Nicoll JM, Nagar B, et al. Multiple BCR-ABL kinase domain mutations confer polyclonal resistance to the tyrosine kinase inhibitor imatinib (STI571) in chronic phase and blast crisis chronic myeloid leukemia. Cancer Cell 2002;2:117−25.

[67] O'hare T, Eide CA, Deininger M. Bcr-Abl kinase domain mutations, drug resistance, and the road to a cure for chronic myeloid leukemia. Blood 2007;110:2242−9.

[68] Bikker JA, Brooijmans N, Wissner A, et al. Kinase domain mutations in cancer: implications for small molecule drug design strategies. J Med Chem 2009;40:1493−509.

[69] Ellis LM, Hicklin DJ. Resistance to targeted therapies: refining anticancer therapy in the era of molecular oncology. Clin Cancer Res 2009;15:7471−8.

[70] Weisberg E, Manley PW, Breitenstein W, et al. Characterization of AMN107, a selective inhibitor of native and mutant Bcr-Abl. Cancer cell 2005;7:129−41.

[71] Manley PW, Breitenstein W, Bruggen J, et al. Urea derivatives of STI571 as inhibitors of Bcr-Abl and PDGFR kinases. Bioorg Med Chem Lett 2004;14:5793−7.

[72] Olsen JA, Banner DW, Seiler P, et al. Fluorine interactions at the thrombin active site: protein backbone fragments H-C(alpha)-C = O comprise a favorable C-F environment and interactions of C-F with electrophiles. Chembiochem 2004;5:666−75.

[73] Weisberg E, Manley P, Mestan J, et al. AMN107 (nilotinib): a novel and selective inhibitor of BCR-ABL. Br J Cancer 2006;94:1765−9.

[74] Tanaka C, Yin O, Sethuraman V, et al. Clinical pharmacokinetics of the BCR-ABL tyrosine kinase inhibitor nilotinib. Clin Pharmacol Ther 2009;87:197−203.

[75] Kantarjian HM, Giles F, Gattermann N, et al. Nilotinib (formerly AMN107), a highly selective BCR-ABL tyrosine kinase inhibitor, is effective in patients with Philadelphia chromosome-positive chronic myelogenous leukemia in chronic phase following imatinib resistance and intolerance. Blood 2007;110:3540−6.

[76] Coutre PL, Ottmann O, Giles F, et al. Nilotinib (formerly AMN107), a highly selective BCR-ABL tyrosine kinase inhibitor, is active in patients with imatinib-resistant or -intolerant accelerated-phase chronic myelogenous leukemia. Blood 2008;111:1834−9.

[77] Hochhaus A, Rosti G, Cross N, et al. Frontline nilotinib in patients with chronic myeloid leukemia in chronic phase: results from the European ENEST1st study. Leukemia 2016;30:57−64.

[78] Wityak J, Das J, Moquin RV, et al. Discovery and initial SAR of 2-amino-5-carboxamidothiazoles as inhibitors of the Src-family kinase p56 (Lck). Bioorg Med Chem Lett 2003;13:4007–10.

[79] Chen P, Norris D, Das J, et al. Discovery of novel 2-(aminoheteroaryl)-thiazole-5-carboxamides as potent and orally active Src-family kinase p56 (Lck) inhibitors. Bioorg Med Chem Lett 2004;14:6061–6.

[80] Lombardo LJ, Lee FY, Chen P, et al. Discovery of N-(2-chloro-6-methyl- phenyl)-2-(6-(4-(2-hydroxyethyl)-piperazin-1-yl)-2-methylpyrimidin-4-ylamino) thiazole-5-carboxamide (BMS-354825), a dual Src/Abl kinase inhibitor with potent antitumor activity in preclinical assays. J Med Chem 2004;47:6658–61.

[81] Tokarski JS, Newitt JA, Chang CY, et al. The structure of Dasatinib (BMS-354825) bound to activated ABL kinase domain elucidates its inhibitory activity against imatinib-resistant ABL mutants. Cancer Res 2006;66:5790–7.

[82] O'hare T. In vitro activity of Bcr-Abl inhibitors AMN107 and BMS-354825 against clinically relevant imatinib-resistant Abl kinase domain mutants. Cancer Res 2005;65:4500–5.

[83] Shah NP, Tran C, Lee FY, et al. Overriding imatinib resistance with a novel ABL kinase inhibitor. Science 2004;305(5682):399–401.

[84] Hochhaus A, Baccarani M, Deininger M, et al. Dasatinib induces durable cytogenetic responses in patients with chronic myelogenous leukemia in chronic phase with resistance or intolerance to imatinib. Leukemia 2008;22:1200–6.

[85] Kantarjian HM, Shah NP, Cortes JE, et al. Dasatinib or imatinib in newly diagnosed chronic-phase chronic myeloid leukemia: 2-year follow-up from a randomized phase 3 trial (DASISION). Blood 2011;119:1123–9.

[86] Boschelli DH. 4-Anilino-3-quinolinecarbonitriles: an emerging class of kinase inhibitors. Curr Top Med Chem 2002;2:1051–63.

[87] Kim LC, Song L, Haura EB. Src kinases as therapeutic targets for cancer. Nat Rev Clin Oncol 2009;6:587–95.

[88] Boschelli DH, Ye F, Wang YD, et al. Optimization of 4-phenylamino-3-quinolinecarbonitriles as potent inhibitors of Src kinase activity. J Med Chem 2001;44:3965–77.

[89] Golas JM, Arndt K, Etienne C, et al. SKI-606, a 4-anilino-3-quinolinecarbonitrile dual inhibitor of Src and Abl Kinases, is a potent antiproliferative agent against chronic myelogenous leukemia cells in culture and causes regression of K562 xenografts in nude mice. Cancer Res 2003;63:375–81.

[90] Boschelli F, Arndt K, Gambacorti-Passerini C. Bosutinib: a review of preclinical studies in chronic myelogenous leukaemia. Eur J Cancer 2010;46:1781–9.

[91] Rix L, Rix U, Colinge J, et al. Global target profile of the kinase inhibitor bosutinib in primary chronic myeloid leukemia cells. Leukemia 2009;23:477–85.

[92] Doan V, Wang A, Prescott H. Bosutinib for the treatment of chronic myeloid leukemia. Am J Health Syst Pharm 2015;72:439–47.

[93] Levinson NM, Boxer SG, Ramani R. Structural and spectroscopic analysis of the kinase inhibitor bosutinib and an isomer of bosutinib binding to the Abl tyrosine kinase domain. PLoS One 2012;7:e29828.

[94] O'hare T, Shakespeare WC, Zhu X, et al. AP24534, a pan-BCR-ABL inhibitor for chronic myeloid leukemia, potently inhibits the T315I mutant and overcomes mutation-based resistance. Cancer Cell 2009;16:401–12.

[95] Wang Y, Shakespeare WC, Huang WS, et al. Novel N9-arenethenyl purines as potent dual Src/Abl tyrosine kinase inhibitors. Bioorg Med Chem Lett 2008;18:4907–12.

[96] Huang WS, Zhu X, Wang Y, et al. 9-(Arenethenyl)purines as dual Src/Abl kinase inhibitors targeting the inactive conformation: design, synthesis, and biological evaluation. J Med Chem 2009;52:4743–56.

[97] Huang WS, Metcalf CA, Sundaramoorthi R, et al. Discovery of 3-[2-(imidazo[1,2-b]pyridazin-3-yl)ethynyl]-4-methyl-N-{4-[(4-methylpiperazin-1-yl)methyl]-3-(trifluoromethyl)phenyl}benzamide (AP24534), a potent, orally active pan-inhibitor of breakpoint cluster region-abelson (BCR-ABL) kinase including the T315I gatekeeper mutant. J Med Chem 2010;53:4701–19.

[98] Zhou T, Commodore L, Huang WS, et al. Structural mechanism of the Pan-BCR-ABL inhibitor ponatinib (AP24534): lessons for overcoming kinase inhibitor resistance. Chem Biol Drug Des 2011;77:1–11.

[99] Cortes JE, Kantarjian H, Shah NP, et al. Ponatinib in refractory Philadelphia chromosome-positive leukemias. N Engl J Med 2012;367:2075–88.

[100] Cortes JE, Kim DW, Pinilla-Ibarz J, et al. A phase 2 trial of ponatinib in Philadelphia chromosome-positive leukemias. N Engl J Med 2013;369:1783–96.

[101] Ren X, Pan X, Zhang Z, et al. Identification of GZD824 as an orally bioavailable inhibitor that targets phosphorylated and nonphosphorylated breakpoint cluster region2abelson (Bcr-Abl) kinase and overcomes clinically acquired mutation-induced resistance against imatinib. J Med Chem 2013;56:879–94.

[102] Adrian FJ, Ding Q, Sim T, et al. Allosteric inhibitors of Bcr-abl-dependent cell proliferation. Nat Chem Biol 2006;2:95–102.

[103] Deng X, Okram B, Ding Q, et al. Expanding the diversity of allosteric Bcr-Abl inhibitors. J Med Chem 2010;53:6934–46.

[104] Jahnke W, Grotzfeld RM, Pelle X, et al. Binding or bending: distinction of allosteric Abl kinase agonists from antagonists by an NMR-based conformational assay. J Am Chem Soc 2010;132:7043–8.

[105] Schoepfer J, Jahnke W, Berellini G, et al. Discovery of asciminib (ABL001), an allosteric inhibitor of the tyrosine kinase activity of BCR-ABL1. J Med Chem 2018;61:8120–35.

[106] Wylie AA, Schoepfer J, Jahnke W, et al. The allosteric inhibitor ABL001 enables dual targeting of BCR-ABL1. Nature 2017;543:733–7.

[107] Bondeson DP, Mares A, Smith I, et al. Catalytic in vivo protein knockdown by small-molecule PROTACs. Nat Chem Biol 2015;11:611–17.

Chapter 16

A case study of the irreversible covalent epidermal growth factor receptor (EGFR) inhibitor—afatinib

Yongping Yu and Wenteng Chen
College of Pharmaceutical Sciences, Zhejiang University, Hangzhou, Zhejiang Province, P.R. China

Chapter outline

- **16.1 Preface**   387
- **16.2 Epidermal growth factor receptor and quinazoline-based small molecule inhibitors**   388
  - 16.2.1 Epidermal growth factor receptor   388
  - 16.2.2 Quinazoline-based small molecule epidermal growth factor receptor inhibitors   388
  - 16.2.3 Resistance mutations for epidermal growth factor receptor   390
- **16.3 Drug design based on covalent inhibition strategies**   390
  - 16.3.1 Introduction to covalent inhibition strategies   390
  - 16.3.2 Covalent strategies based on the mechanism of Michael reaction [16]   392
  - 16.3.3 Covalent strategies based on addition-elimination or oxidation mechanisms   392
  - 16.3.4 Covalent strategies based on reversible covalent mechanisms   392
- **16.4 Development of covalent irreversible EGFR inhibitor—afatinib**   393
  - 16.4.1 The application of covalent strategy in the development of small molecule EGFR inhibitors   393
  - 16.4.2 The discovery of the covalent irreversible EGFR inhibitor—afatinib   402
  - 16.4.3 The pharmacokinetics, pharmacodynamics, and adverse reactions of afatinib   406
  - 16.4.4 Summary of structure-activity relationship of covalent EGFR inhibitor   407
- **16.5 Synthesis of afatinib**   408
  - 16.5.1 Mitsunobu reaction   408
  - 16.5.2 Dimroth rearrangement   409
  - 16.5.3 The Horner-Wadsworth-Emmons reaction   409
  - 16.5.4 Laboratory medicinal chemical synthetic route-modular synthesis approach   409
  - 16.5.5 Commercial synthetic route-sequential synthesis approach   411
- **16.6 Summary and knowledge expansion**   411
  - 16.6.1 Summary of this chapter   411
  - 16.6.2 Knowledge expansion   411
- **References**   415

16.1 Preface

Afatinib, developed by Boehringer Ingelheim Pharmaceuticals, was launched in the United States in July 2013 and in China in February 2017. As the first approved irreversible tyrosine kinase (TK) inhibitor, afatinib is primarily used for the treatment of locally advanced or metastatic nonsmall cell lung cancer (NSCLC) patients with epidermal growth factor receptor (EGFR) gene-sensitive mutations and without previously receiving small molecule inhibitor treatment targeting the EGFR. Additionally, it is indicated for patients with locally advanced or metastatic squamous histology NSCLC who experienced disease progression during or after platinum-based chemotherapy.

Main component chemical name: (S, E)-N-(4-((3-chloro-4-fluorophenyl) amino)-7-((tetrahydrofuran-3-yl) oxy) quinazolin-6-yl)-4-(dimethylamino) but-2-enamide
Chemical formula: $C_{24}H_{25}ClFN_5O_3$ (free base), $C_{32}H_{33}ClFN_5O_{11}$ (maleate salt)
Molecular weight: 485.9380 (free base), 718.0884 (maleate salt)
Melting point: 100 – 102 °C
Trade name: Gilotrif

Afatinib is a 4-anilinoquinazoline that irreversibly binds to the ErbB family, such as EGFR and ErbB2. By blocking the interaction between endogenous adenosine triphosphate (ATP) molecules and these receptors, afatinib inhibits the phosphorylation of EGFR and stops the downstream signaling pathways, thereby persistently suppressing tumor cell proliferation and growth. Clinically, afatinib has brought greater survival benefits to a wide range of lung cancer patients in contrast to the first-generation reversible EGFR inhibitors.

In this chapter, we will discuss several key aspects of the development of afatinib, providing background information on the application of small molecule EGFR inhibitors in the treatment of NSCLC, particularly to the medicinal chemistry on the development of EGFR inhibitors. The contents cover the description of EGFR signaling pathway, the design of small molecule EGFR inhibitors based on covalent strategies, lead compound optimization, discovery and synthesis of afatinib, and the progress in clinic treatment of EGFR resistance mutations.

16.2 Epidermal growth factor receptor and quinazoline-based small molecule inhibitors

16.2.1 Epidermal growth factor receptor

In the 1950s, Stanley Cohen, a researcher at Vanderbilt University in the United States, serendipitously discovered an active factor that could promote the growth of epidermal cells at the time of studying the nerve growth factor. This active factor was then named epidermal growth factor. Further research revealed that the corresponding receptor for this active factor was the EGFR. EGFR is a member of the human EGFR family including HER1 (erbB1, EGFR), HER2 (erbB2, NEU), HER3 (erbB3), and HER4 (erbB4). EGFR is a large transmembrane protein with a molecular weight of approximately 170 kDa. Its precursor consists of 1210 amino acids. After translation, the mature EGFR involves 1186 amino acid residues. EGFR consists of three regions from the N-terminus to the C-terminus, including the extracellular domain (ectodomain), the transmembrane domain, and the intracellular domain [1,2] (Fig. 16.1).

In the absence of a ligand, EGFR primarily exists as a monomer. Upon ligand binding to the extracellular ligand-binding domain, EGFR undergoes oligomerization, forming either homodimers or heterodimers with other members of the receptor family. Following the dimerization, the intracellular TK domain of EGFR binds with one molecule of ATP, stimulating the catalytic activity of the intracellular TK. This resulted in autophosphorylation of multiple tyrosine residues (Tyr1016, Tyr1092, Tyr1110, Tyr1172, and Tyr1197) on EGFR, providing sites for various downstream molecules and initiating downstream signaling pathways, such as the RAS/MAPK/ERK pathway, PI3K-AKT pathway, and EGFR-STAT2 pathway that participate in cell proliferation and differentiation processes [3] (Fig. 16.2).

Lung cancer harboring EGFR gene-sensitive mutants is a key finding. EGFR mutations are present in approximately 10%–15% of NSCLC patients of Caucasian and 40% of Asian patients [4]. Among them, mutations in exons 18–21 of the EGFR gene, especially the deletion mutation of the frame amino acid in exon 19 (Del19) and the point mutation in exon 21 (L858R), account for approximately 90% of NSCLC. EGFR mutations cause abnormal activation of TK, leading to uncontrolled cellular behaviors and ultimately resulting in the developed NSCLC. Moreover, overexpression of EGFR in lung cancer is closely associated with poor prognosis. For instance, high levels of EGFR expression render patients insensitive to conventional chemotherapy drugs, i.e., cisplatin. Therefore, inhibition of the aberrant EGFR signaling pathway represents one of the effective strategies for the treatment of NSCLC in the clinic.

16.2.2 Quinazoline-based small molecule epidermal growth factor receptor inhibitors

With the rapid technical development of protein crystallography, the precise detection of target protein binding with small molecules and electronic characteristics has provided insightful structure information that is particularly useful for drug discovery. For various kinases, although their ATP binding site in the intracellular domain of EGFR is highly

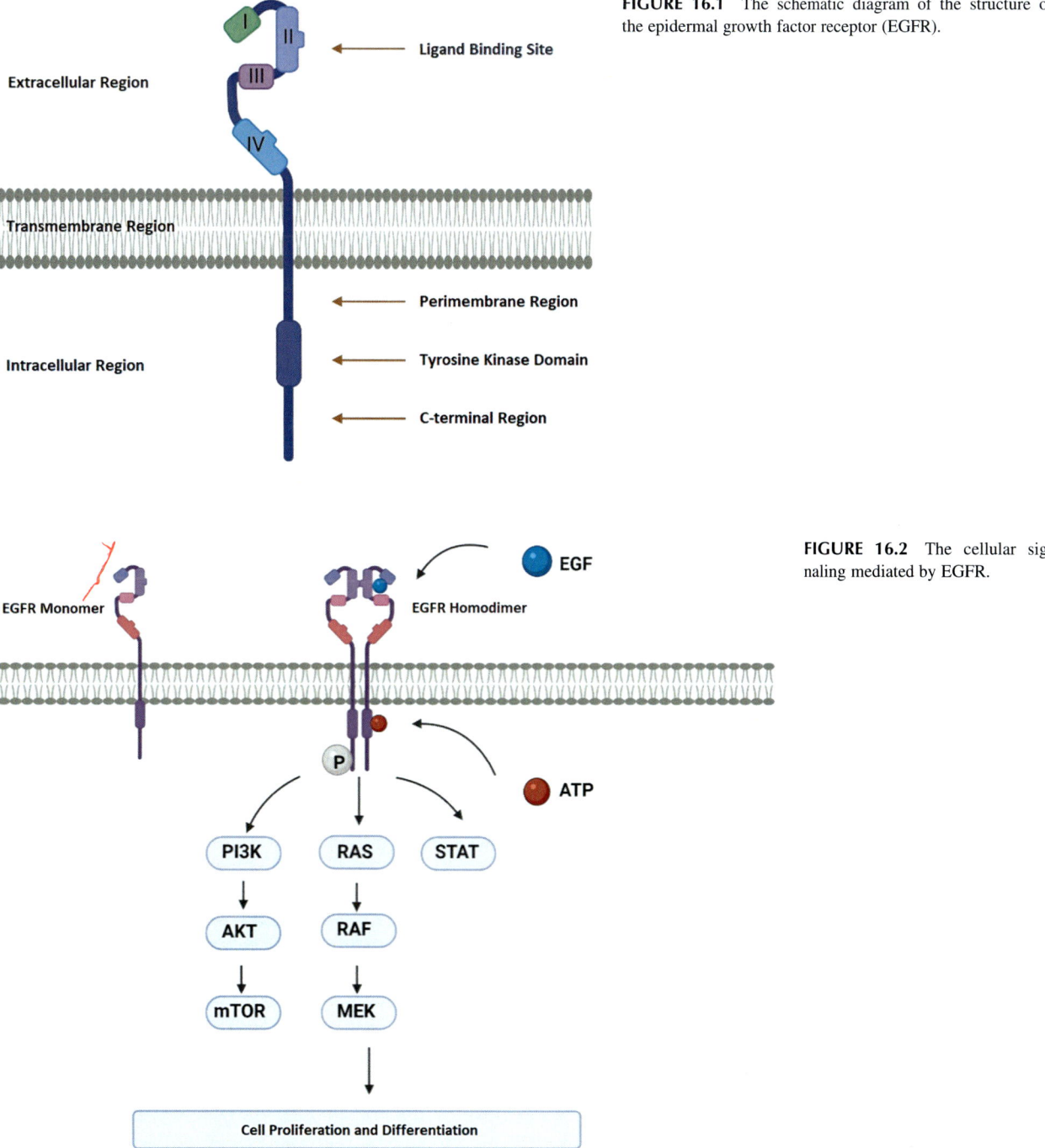

FIGURE 16.1 The schematic diagram of the structure of the epidermal growth factor receptor (EGFR).

FIGURE 16.2 The cellular signaling mediated by EGFR.

conserved, there are still minor differences in most of them when watching into the three-dimensional protein structure. This enables the scientists to successfully design EGFR-specific small molecule inhibitors, which fully compete with the endogenous ATP binding to the TK domain of EGFR, thereby specifically blocking EGFR phosphorylation and downstream signaling pathway, ultimately achieving the goal of inhibiting tumor cell proliferation and growth. Initially, designing small molecule EGFR inhibitors mainly involved heterocyclic scaffold compounds, such as quinazoline, quinoline, indole, and indazole, to mimic the purine ring of endogenous ATP, and anticipated to competitively occupy the purine ring binding site of the TK domain. Since 2003, this design strategy achieved great success [5], leading to the launch of first-generation reversible EGFR inhibitors, such as gefitinib [6,7], erlotinib [8], and icotinib [9] (Table 16.1). Their structures all belong to the 4-anilinoquinazoline.

TABLE 16.1 First-generation EGFR inhibitors for the treatment of NSCLC.

Chemical structure	Developing companies	Development status
Iressal (Gefitinib)	AstraZeneca	Listed in the United States in 2003
Tarceva (Erolitinib)	OSI Pharmaceuticals/Roche/San Francisco Gene Technology Corporation	Listed in the United States in 2004
Conmana (Icotinib)	Betta Pharmaceuticals	Listed in China in 2011

The first-generation reversible EGFR inhibitors to the ATP binding domain are manifested through weaker and reversible intermolecular forces such as hydrogen bonding, van der Waals forces, and hydrophobic interactions. The limitations of these inhibitors, such as insufficient efficacy and durability in clinical settings, quickly become apparent. Notably, the reversibility of the binding forces is correlated with drug's effect at its concentration at the binding site. When the administrated drug concentration is continuously decreased through elimination from the human body, the biological function of the target protein will be constantly restored, making it impossible for the reversible drug to maintain a sustained therapeutic efficacy that could lead to drug resistance. Albeit the response ratio of the first-generation reversible EGFR inhibitors is 60%−70% in clinical settings, advanced patients after 9−14 months of treatment have developed resistance to the drugs, and then the resistance became a great challenge for a selection of optimal therapeutic regimen of NSCLC.

16.2.3 Resistance mutations for epidermal growth factor receptor

Further studies disclosed that 50% of NSCLC patients with gefitinib resistance have the T790M mutation, which is a substitution of threonine at 790 of the EGFR exon 20 with methionine. It was initially believed that the substitution of threonine with methionine creates a steric hindrance due to the larger side chain of methionine, thus preventing the binding of small molecule inhibitors to the EGFR TK domain. On the basis, it was suggested that decreasing the steric hindrance of the first-generation of EGFR inhibitors might increase their inhibitory activities against the T790M. Further investigation revealed that the T790M mutation improved the binding affinity of endogenous ATP to EGFR. These results indicate that decreasing the steric hindrance of launched drugs is unlikely to effectively compete with ATP binding to the EGFR^{T790M}. To address the EGFR^{T790M} resistance, second-generation covalent irreversible EGFR inhibitors emerged. Since then, the development of covalent inhibitors has become a highlight and breakthrough in the design of drugs targeting EGFR [10].

16.3 Drug design based on covalent inhibition strategies

16.3.1 Introduction to covalent inhibition strategies

The design of covalent inhibitors mainly utilizes electrophilic groups, also known as "warheads" in the molecule to form a covalent bond with specific amino acid residues on the target protein, thereby irreversibly inhibiting the biological function of the target protein. Compared to reversible inhibitors, covalent inhibitors have several pharmacological advantages: (1) Covalent inhibitors exhibit higher biochemical reaction efficiency. The binding affinity between the covalent inhibitor and the target protein could be enhanced via forming covalent chemical bonds with the target protein. (2) Covalent inhibitors have prolonged efficacy. Due to the mechanism of chemical covalent binding, the pharmacokinetics of the drug is not entirely correlated with its pharmacodynamics. Even if free covalent inhibitors can be rapidly cleared by the body's metabolism and excretory organs, the drugs covalently bound to the target protein can still maintain sufficient potency. (3) Covalent inhibitors demonstrate high selectivity. The electrophilic warhead in the molecular structure can selectively react with nucleophilic side chains of specific amino acid residues on the target protein, thereby enhancing the binding affinity between the molecule and the target protein.

The binding process between covalent inhibitors and the target protein is usually divided into two steps. First, the inhibitor noncovalently binds to a specific binding pocket region of the target protein, forming a noncovalent binding complex E-I. This process brings the electrophilic group of the inhibitors close to the active covalent binding site on the target protein. Subsequently, specific electrophilic groups in the noncovalent binding complex E-I react covalently with nucleophilic amino acid residues on the target protein, such as thiol groups on the cysteine residue side chain, hydroxyl groups on the serine/threonine residue side chains, phenolic hydroxyl groups on the tyrosine residue side chain, and amino groups on the lysine residue side chain, forming stable covalent bonds and ultimately generating a covalent complex E-I (Fig. 16.3) [11]. One of the key points in the design of covalent inhibitors is the selection of electrophilic warheads (groups). Common electrophilic warheads mainly include cyanide, vinyl sulfone, thiosemicarbazone, ketones, acrylamide, quinone, alkynyl amide, propargylic acid, and sulfonyl fluoride (Fig. 16.4).

In addition, achieving the pharmacological advantages of covalent inhibitors requires the rational design of the inhibitors, ensuring that the drug molecules can precisely target the active pocket of the target protein without affecting the activity of other proteins and avoiding off-target activities [12]. Based on the medicinal chemistry practice for developing such molecules, the following points are considered crucial: (1) Selecting appropriate drug targets. Currently, commonly used methods involve the use of bioinformatic techniques to analyze the characteristics of amino acids in the active site of the target protein, determining whether there are differences between the binding sites of the target protein and those in other proteins of the same family. Rational drug design can then address these differences and avoid nonspecific covalent binding between the drug and other proteins in the same family. (2) A thorough understanding of the electrophilic activity of covalent inhibitors and the nucleophilicity of amino acid residues in the target protein. The designed covalent inhibitors should not only possess electrophilic reactive groups in a chemical sense but also have an appropriate distance between this electrophilic group and the covalent binding site on the target protein. This distance ensures moderate chemical reactivity between small molecules and the biological target, preventing rapid clearance [13–15].

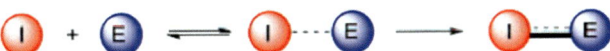

FIGURE 16.3 Mechanism of covalent inhibitors.

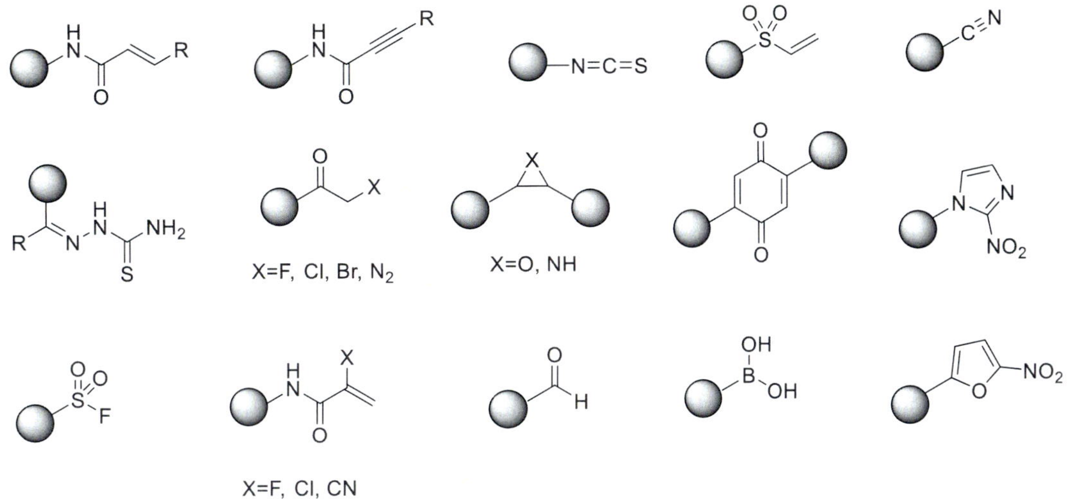

FIGURE 16.4 Chemical structure of electrophilic warhead used in covalent inhibitor design.

Common covalent inhibitors often utilize reactions such as Michael addition, addition-elimination substitution reactions, oxidation reactions, and reversible covalent reactions (such as disulfide bonds) to achieve covalent binding between compounds and the target protein.

16.3.2 Covalent strategies based on the mechanism of Michael reaction [16]

Some electrophilic warheads such as acrylamides, propargylamides, and vinyl sulfone groups readily undergo Michael reactions with the nucleophilic thiol group on the cysteine side chain. This results in the formation of stable thioether covalent bonds, irreversibly inhibiting the biochemical activity of the target protein (Fig. 16.5). Acrylamide fragments are the most commonly used electrophilic reaction warheads, often employed in the design of covalent inhibitors for TK. The β-position of α, β-unsaturated acrylamides or α, β-unsaturated propargylamides is adjacent to cysteine residues located near the active site. The appropriate distance, along with the strong nucleophilicity of the cysteine thiol group, allows for specific covalent inhibition of the target protein.

16.3.3 Covalent strategies based on addition-elimination or oxidation mechanisms

Electrophilic warheads such as sulfonyl fluoride are commonly used in the design of covalent irreversible inhibitors. Compared to the more common and highly reactive sulfonyl chloride, sulfonyl fluoride has a longer biological half-life and strikes a suitable balance between biocompatibility (mainly water stability) and protein reactivity [17]. Furthermore, compared to sulfonyl chloride, the high electronegativity of the fluorine atom enhances the resistance of sulfonyl fluoride to reduction. As shown in Fig. 16.6A, the nucleophilic group of the target protein attacks the sulfur atom of the sulfonyl fluoride, resulting in the release of fluoride ions and undergoing an addition-elimination reaction. In addition to reacting with the hydroxyl group on serine residues, sulfonyl fluoride can also modify residues such as threonine, lysine, tyrosine, cysteine, and histidine [18,19].

2-Nitrofuran-based structures are a newly discovered class of electrophilic warheads. Due to the strong electron-withdrawing effect of the nitro group, the carbon atom adjacent to it is susceptible to being attacked by the cysteine thiol group in the target protein. This leads to an addition − elimination reaction and the formation of a covalent bond, thus irreversibly inhibiting the activity of the target protein (Fig. 16.6B) [20]. Additionally, other compounds containing sulfhydryl groups can undergo oxidation reactions with cysteine, forming disulfide bonds and consequently irreversibly inhibiting the activity of the target protein (Fig. 16.6C).

16.3.4 Covalent strategies based on reversible covalent mechanisms

With the in-depth study of covalent binding mechanisms, electrophilic warheads such as cyanide and carbonyl groups can reversibly bind to the target protein. This type of reversible covalent interaction lies between irreversible and reversible covalent bonds. Reversible covalent inhibitors have the advantages of longer duration of action and lower effective concentrations compared to irreversible covalent inhibitors while reducing the toxic risks associated with off-target effects. Compared to conventional irreversible covalent inhibitors, these reversible covalent inhibitors have lower toxicity and better pharmacokinetic properties, making them a recent research hotspot. Among them, the carbonyl group is a classic electrophilic warhead in reversible covalent inhibitors. The electro-positivity of the carbonyl carbon atom makes it susceptible to nucleophilic attack, resulting in an additional reaction on the α-carbonyl group to form a stable half-ketone structure and inhibit the function of the target protein (Fig. 16.7A) [21].

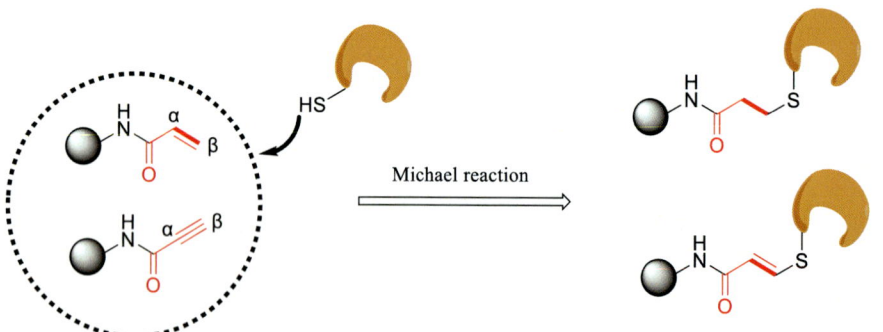

FIGURE 16.5 Covalent strategy based on Michael reaction mechanism.

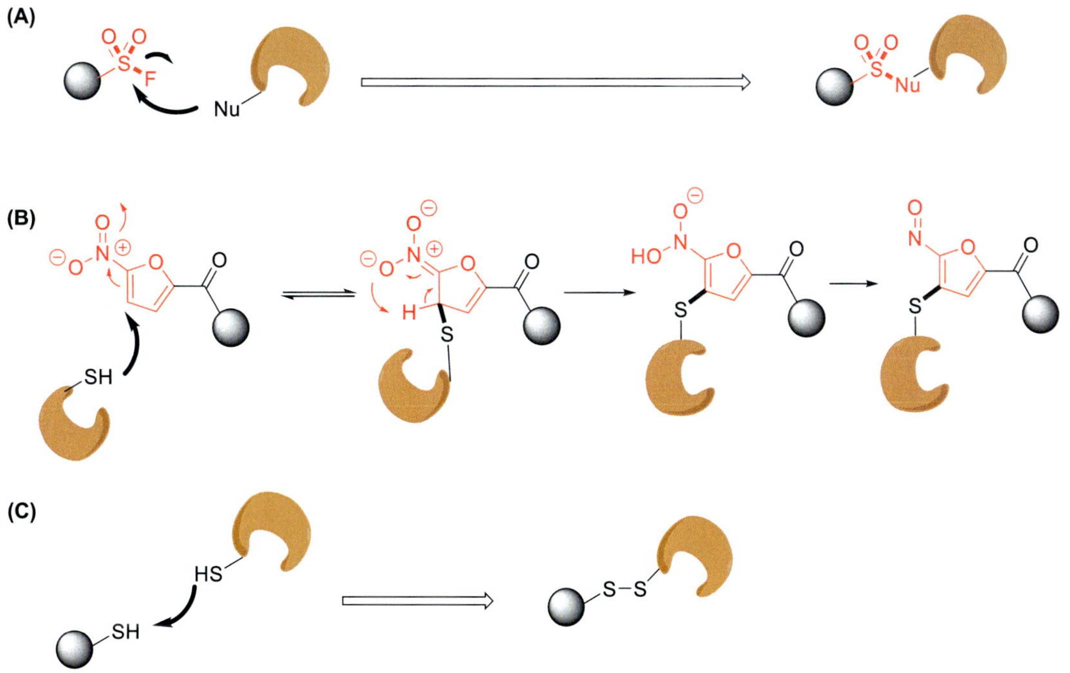

FIGURE 16.6 Covalent strategies based on addition-elimination or oxidation mechanisms. (A) Mechanism based on addition-elimination; (B) Mechanism based on substitution on 2-nitrofuran motif. (C) Mechanism based on oxidation reaction.

Boric acid and epoxides are also common electrophilic warheads in the design of reversible covalent inhibitors (Fig. 16.7B). The boron atom in boric acid has an empty p orbital that can form a coordination bond with the hydroxyl group on the amino acid side chain, covalently generating a borate ester, which exerts inhibitory effects on the target protein [22]. Epoxides are electrophilic warheads containing a three-membered oxygen ring (Fig. 16.7C). The high ring strain makes them vulnerable to nucleophilic attack. They undergo alkylation reactions with nucleophilic groups on the target protein. Additionally, the hydroxyl group on the serine side chain near the target protein can further undergo an addition reaction with the carbonyl group, forming a stable half-ketone intermediate to collectively inhibit the function of the target protein [23].

Furthermore, research has found that introducing electron-withdrawing groups, such as cyanide, at the α-position of the classic electrophilic warhead acrylamide fragment (Fig. 16.7D) can enhance both the electrophilicity of the acrylamide warhead for reacting with the cysteine thiol group and the acidity of the α-H. This allows the reverse reaction of Michael addition to occur under physiological conditions, leading to a reversible covalent process. In addition to the modification at the α-position of the acrylamide fragment affecting the reactivity of the electrophilic warhead, the steric hindrance of the β-position group can also regulate the rate of α-H elimination, thereby adjusting the rate of the reverse reaction of Michael addition. The larger the steric hindrance of the β-position group, the more difficult it is for α-H to be eliminated by the base, resulting in a lower rate of the reverse reaction of Michael addition and thus increasing the interaction time between the drug molecule and the target protein [24,25].

16.4 Development of covalent irreversible EGFR inhibitor – afatinib

16.4.1 The application of covalent strategy in the development of small molecule EGFR inhibitors [26–28]

The early design of covalent irreversible EGFR inhibitors was based on the scaffold of reversible EGFR inhibitors, such as 4-anilinoquinazoline or 4-anilino-3-cyanoquinolines. An electrophilic warhead was introduced at a suitable position of the inhibitor's structure, which could react specifically with the cysteine residue near the ATP-binding domain. This approach relied on the high specificity of cysteine residues in certain positions among different protein kinases, including EGFR, ErbB2, and ErbB4. By forming a covalent bond with the cysteine residue, the inhibitors could reduce the impact of the T790M mutation and enhance their inhibitory effect on the mutant EGFR kinase. The proposed research approach mainly stems from several assumptions. Firstly, among the protein kinases encoded by the human genome, 211 kinases have cysteine residues near their ATP-binding domain. However, the positions of these cysteine residues vary depending on the kinase type. For example, cysteine is present at position 797 in EGFR, position 805 in ErbB2, and position 803 in

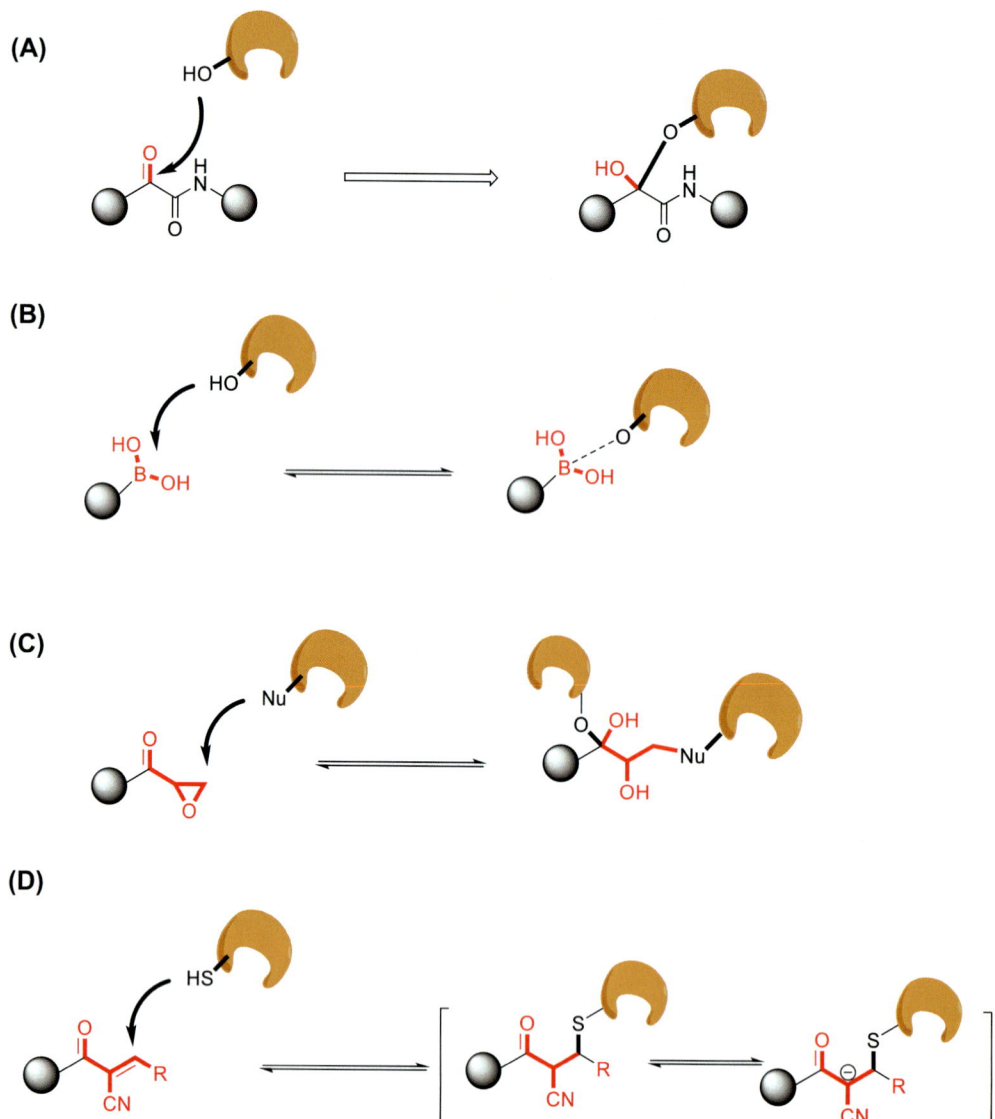

FIGURE 16.7 Covalent strategies based on reversible covalent mechanisms. (A) Covalent hydroxy-addition reaction on α-ketoamide: (B) Covalent hydroxy-addition reaction with boric acid motif; (C) Covalent reaction with epoxides: (D) Reversible thia-Michael addition to an α-cyanoacrylamide.

ErbB4. However, in other kinases, cysteine residues are almost absent at these positions. This high specificity of the site is a prerequisite for developing cysteine covalent inhibitors. Furthermore, the design of covalent inhibitors retains the basic core structure of reversible EGFR inhibitors, which allows for selectivity and reversibility of the inhibitor binding to the EGFR kinase active site. By using highly selective electrophilic warheads, nonspecific covalent binding of the drug molecule to off-target proteins can be avoided, reducing the potential for unforeseen toxic side effects. Additionally, the biosynthesis of EGFR has a longer cycle, and the use of covalent inhibitors can lower the dosage and frequency of drug administration for patients, further reducing the likelihood of off-target effects and drug−drug interactions. Based on these considerations, extensive medicinal chemistry research has been conducted on the design of EGFR kinase covalent inhibitors via introducing acrylamides, butynamides, vinylsulfonamides, α-substituted acetamides, alkynyl thiophene rings, 3-aminopropanamides, thiols, disulfides, boronic acids, or other electrophilic warheads.

16.4.1.1 Acrylamides [29−31]

Acrylamide is a common Michael acceptor that can undergo covalent binding with nucleophilic groups such as cysteine. Based on the molecular docking results of the first-generation EGFR inhibitor, David's team selected C-6 site of the quinazoline core that is close to the position 797 cysteine residue. They introduced an α, β-unsaturated acrylamide electrophilic warhead, designed and synthesized 6-acrylamide-4-anilinoquinazoline **1** (**PD 168393**, Fig. 16.8). Protein mass spectrometry studies showed that **1** could form a covalent binding product with the target protein EGFR in a 1:1 ratio, confirming the rationality of covalent inhibitor design. Although this class of molecules did not progress to clinical trials, subsequent research has built upon the experience gained from PD 168393 and continued to explore the chemical modification of the existing α,β-unsaturated acrylamide fragment for influencing the covalent inhibitory effect of compounds.

Further research on α, β-unsaturated amide electrophilic warheads has revealed that introducing a methyl group on the *N*-position of acrylamide does not affect the covalent binding of the inhibitor with the target protein. For example, **2** maintains high inhibitory activity against EGFR kinase ($IC_{50} = 0.17$ nM, Fig. 16.9). However, when the α-position of the electrophilic warhead is substituted with an alkyl group, it hinders the enhancement of the covalent inhibitory effect. Compound **3**, for instance, exhibits a significantly reduced inhibitory activity against EGFR kinase ($IC_{50} = 1.6$ nM). On the other hand, when the β-position of the electrophilic warhead is substituted with an electron-withdrawing acyl group, it allows the compound to maintain its covalent inhibitory effect. Compound **4** demonstrates good inhibitory activity against EGFR kinase ($IC_{50} = 0.61$ nM).

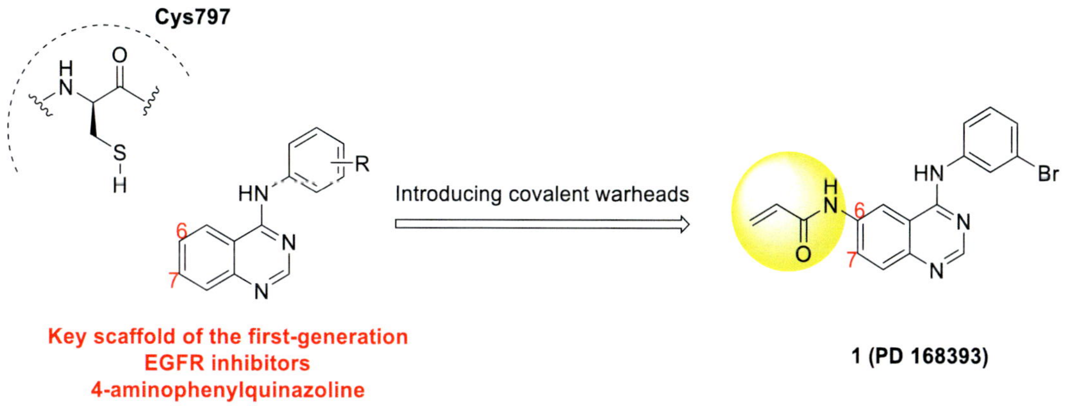

FIGURE 16.8 Design of irreversible inhibitor PD 168393 with acrylamide-based electrophilic warhead [29].

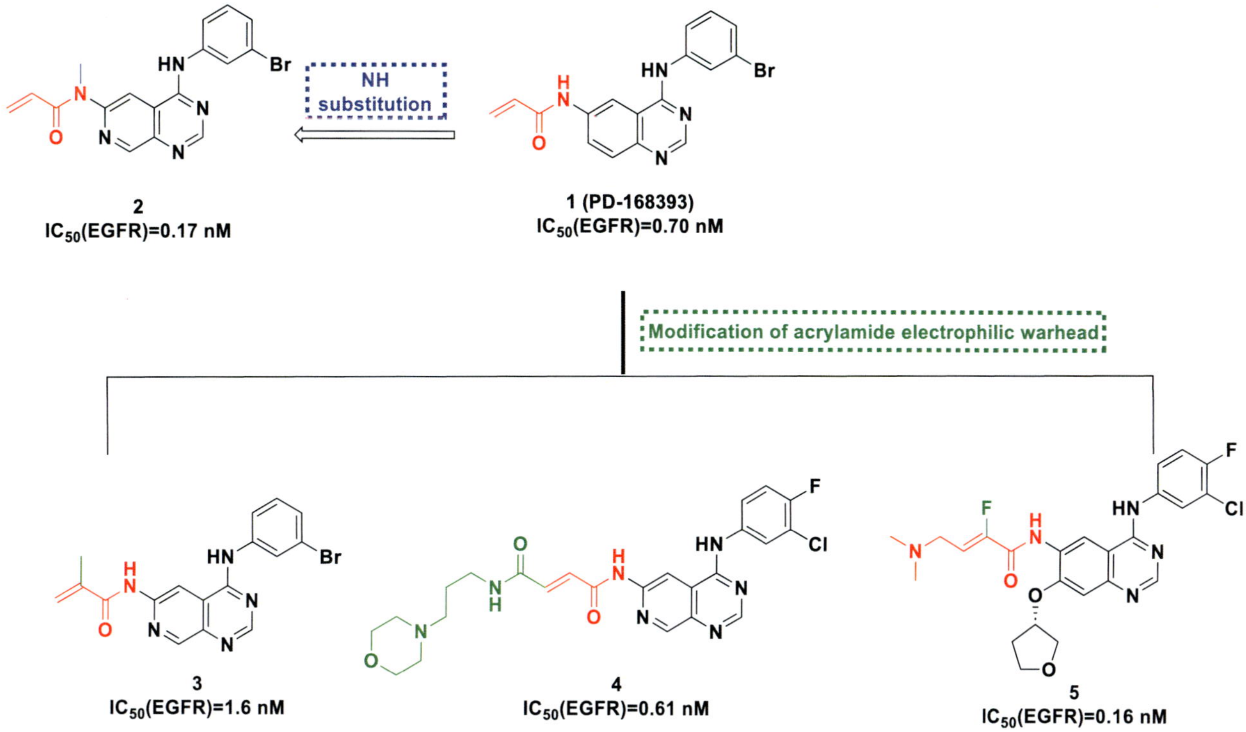

FIGURE 16.9 Structure-activity relationship of acylamide electrophilic warhead.

Unlike alkyl substitution, introducing a fluorine atom at the α-position of the acrylamide electrophilic warhead allows the inhibitor to maintain its covalent binding mode with the target protein and exhibits significant advantages in pharmacokinetics and safety. The main reasons for this are as follows: Firstly, the fluorine atom has a small atomic radius ($rF = 1.35 \times 10^{-10}$ m, $rH = 1.20 \times 10^{-10}$ m), being considered as a nonclassical electron-withdrawing group compared to hydrogen. When the fluorine atom replaces the hydrogen atom in the molecule, the overall size of the molecule remains relatively unchanged, which does not affect its binding with the target protein. For example, compound **5** maintains its inhibitory activity against EGFR kinase ($IC_{50} = 0.16$ nM, Fig. 16.9). Secondly, due to the higher bond energy of the C-F bond (483 kcal/mol) compared to the C-H bond (416 kcal/mol), fluorinated compounds exhibit increased metabolic stability against oxidation. Additionally, the fluorine atom has a high electronegativity, which increases the electrophilicity of the α, β-unsaturated amides at the β-position and promotes the Michael addition reaction with thiol group on cysteine. Finally, the introduction of fluorine atom enhances the lipophilicity and permeability of compounds, enabling its absorption and diffusion in the body. Compared to nonfluorinated substitutions, compound **5** exhibits significantly improved oral bioavailability in mice, reaching 84.7%. In a xenograft mouse model of NSCLC (NCI-H1975), compound **5** also demonstrates more potent antitumor activity, with a relative tumor volume increment rate (*T/C*) of only 19.5%. (*T/C* ratio: An evaluation index for antitumor activity, calculated as $T/C\ (\%) = T_{RTV}/C_{RTV} \times 100$, where T_{RTV} represents the relative tumor volume of the test group and C_{RTV} represents the relative tumor volume of the group with vehicle).

16.4.1.2 Butynamides [32,33]

Like acrylamides, butynamide is also a common electrophilic warhead that can undergo Michael addition reactions with nucleophilic groups such as electron-rich thiols to form covalent bonds. The research team at Wyeth Pharmaceuticals retained the 4-anilinoquinazoline core, like the acrylamide derivatives. They introduced a 2-butynamide electrophilic warhead at the C6 position of the quinazoline core and designed CL-387785 (**6**, Fig. 16.10). Computer molecular docking simulation showed that the butynamide warhead at the C6 position of the quinoline core pointed toward Cys[797], and the nearby residue Lys[728] serves as a basic center to catalyze the Michael addition reaction between butynamide and cysteine (Fig. 16.10). However, similar to the unsubstituted acrylamide, subsequent pharmacokinetic, pharmacological, and toxicological studies revealed that compound **6** had low solubility, resulting in low oral bioavailability in vivo. Some pathological changes were also observed in the kidneys of mice in the high-dose group. As a result, compound **6** did not undergo further preclinical studies.

To improve the pharmacokinetic properties of compound **6**, the research team at Wyeth Pharmaceuticals introduced some water-soluble groups, such as *N,N*-dimethylamino or *N*-methylpiperazine, at the end of the butynamide warhead, resulting in compounds **7–10**. It was found that the tertiary amine introduced at the end of the butynamide not only regulated the physicochemical properties of the compounds but also provided a basic catalytic center for the covalent binding of the butynamide fragment with the cysteine residues of the target protein (Fig. 16.11).

16.4.1.3 Vinylsulfonamides [30]

Vinylsulfonamide has been used as an alternative electrophilic warhead to α,β-acylamide warheads. The Denny research team introduced vinylsulfonamide warheads at the C6 position of both the quinazoline and 3-cyanoquinolines, resulting in compounds **11–13** (Fig. 16.12A). These compounds containing vinylsulfonamide warheads exhibit a similar mechanism of action to the acrylamide-substituted quinazolines, as they can undergo Michael addition reactions with the thiol group of cysteine residues (Fig. 16.12B).

The in vitro results confirmed that compounds **11–13** can irreversibly inhibit EGFR kinase activity. However, the vinylsulfonamide series were found to be unstable in vivo, which hindered further drug development studies.

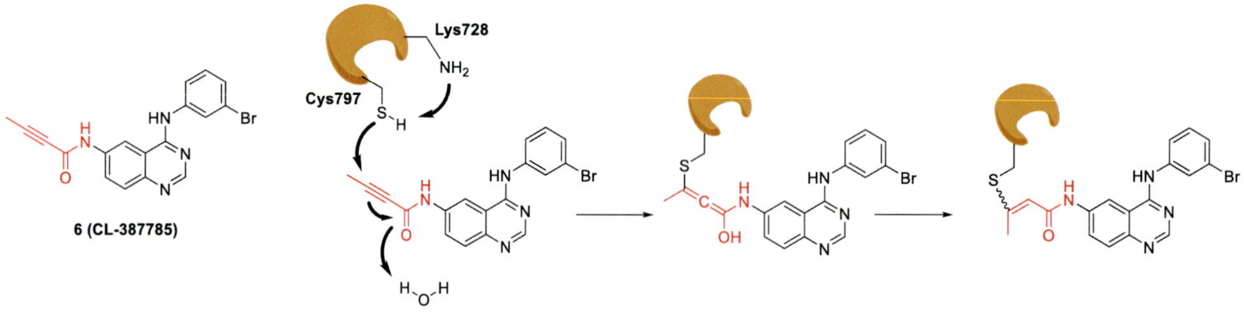

FIGURE 16.10 Covalent irreversible EGFR inhibitors containing butynamide electrophilic warheads.

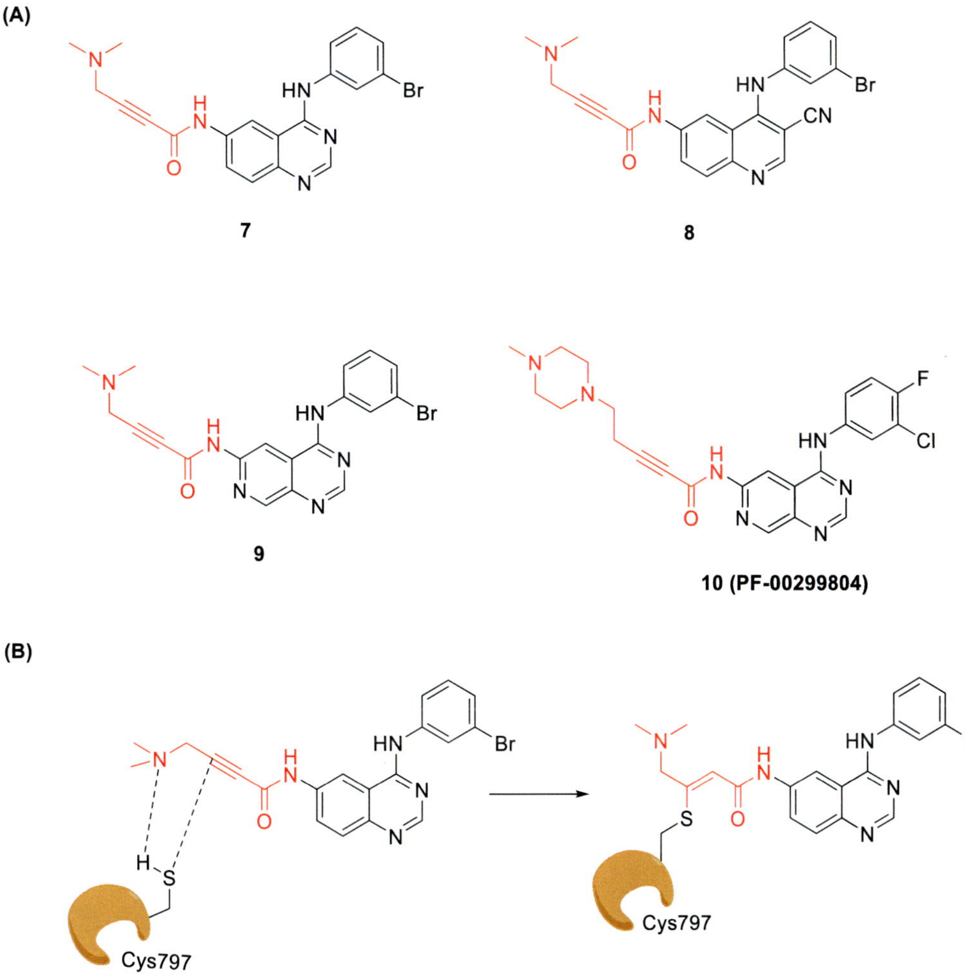

A case study of the irreversible covalent epidermal growth factor receptor (EGFR) inhibitor—afatinib Chapter | 16   397

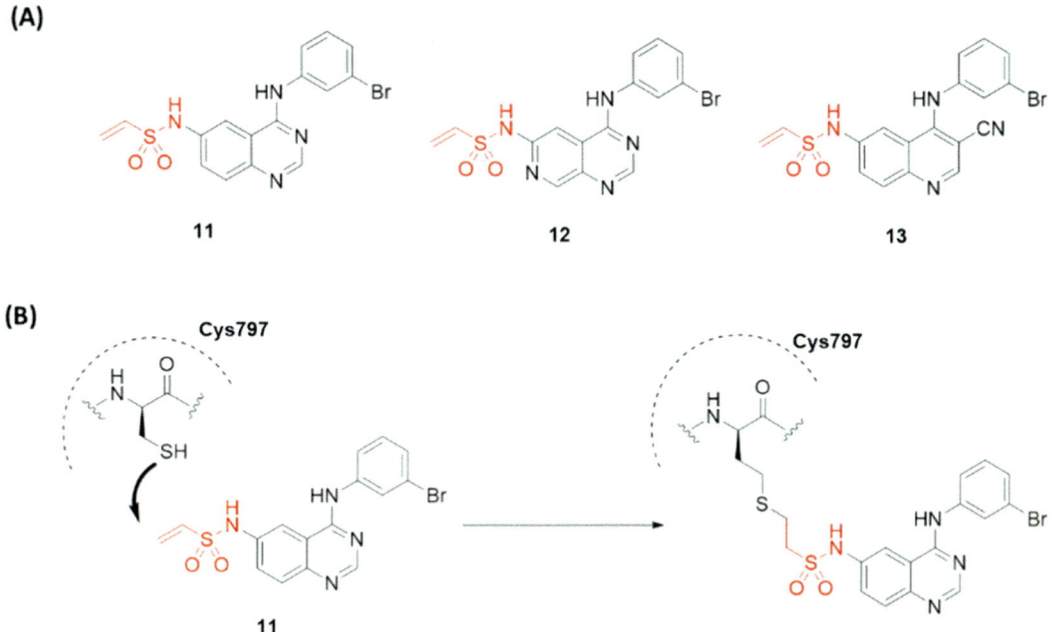

FIGURE 16.11 Structure of the covalent irreversible binding mechanism of EGFR inhibitors containing water-soluble fragments and butynamide electrophilic warheads.

FIGURE 16.12 (A) Structure of EGFR covalent irreversible inhibitors containing vinylsulfonamide warheads. (B) Mechanism of thio-Michael reaction to vinylsulfonamide warhead.

16.4.1.4 α-Substituted acetamides [34]

Based on nucleophilic substitution and in situ elimination mechanisms, the research team led by Alessio Lodola introduced some easily leaving groups, such as methoxy, chloride, phenoxy, or aryloxy, at the α-position of the C6 acetamide moiety on the quinazoline. Through substitution reactions with the thiol group of cysteine residues, these leaving groups form stable covalent bonds. (Fig. 16.13A).

Comparing the reactivity of these electrophilic warheads with glutathione, it was found that (Fig. 16.13B) α-chloroacetamide (**15**) exhibited a higher reactivity than α-methoxyacetamide (**14**) and α-aryloxyacetamides (**16−18**). α-aryloxyacetamide electrophilic warheads showed a better balance between reactivity with cysteine and inhibition activity against EGFR kinase. The covalent inhibition of EGFR kinase activity by pentafluorophenoxyacetamide electrophilic warhead (**18**) with strong electron-withdrawing substituents is irreversible, whereas the covalent inhibition of EGFR kinase activity by orthofluorophenoxyacetamide electrophilic warhead (**17**) with weak electron-withdrawing substituents is partially irreversible.

16.4.1.5 Alkynyl thiophene rings [35]

Uehling's team discovered a class of 6-ethynylthieno[3,2-d]pyrimidines **19** and **20** (Fig. 16.14A) that can effectively and irreversibly inhibit the activity of EGFR/ErbB2/ErbB4. Although these molecules do not incorporate classical electrophilic warheads, X-ray crystallography and mass spectrometry analysis confirmed that the ethynyl end can form a covalent bond with the cysteine residue in the active site of EGFR kinase. Furthermore, by employing a modification strategy similar to α,β-unsaturated amides warheads, the introduction of basic fragments such as pyrrole at the end of the ethynyl group serves as a basic center to regulate the efficiency of the covalent reaction (Fig. 16.14B), thereby enhancing the covalent inhibitory activity against EGFR kinase.

16.4.1.6 3-Aminopropanamides [36]

Unsaturated olefins or alkynes are commonly recognized as electrophilic warheads in the design of covalent inhibitors. However, the high reactivity of unsaturated bonds themselves poses risks of metabolic degradation and off-target

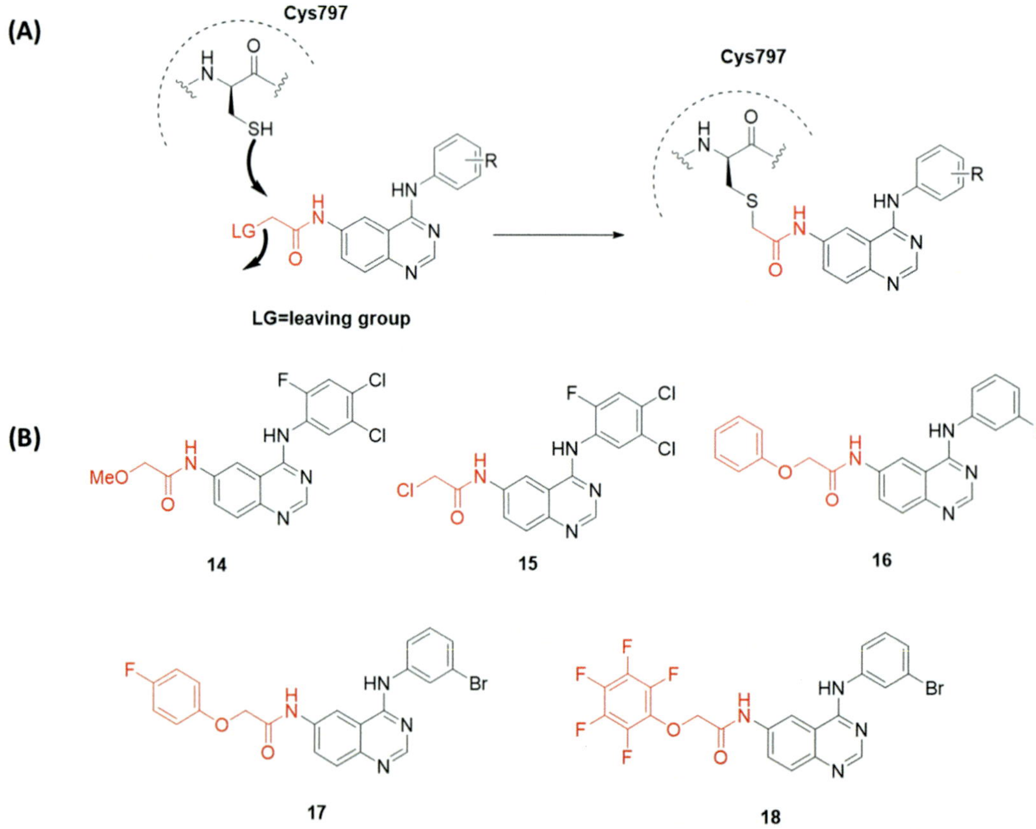

FIGURE 16.13 The covalent binding mechanism of α-substituted acetamide electrophilic warheads (A) and the chemical structures of representative inhibitors (B).

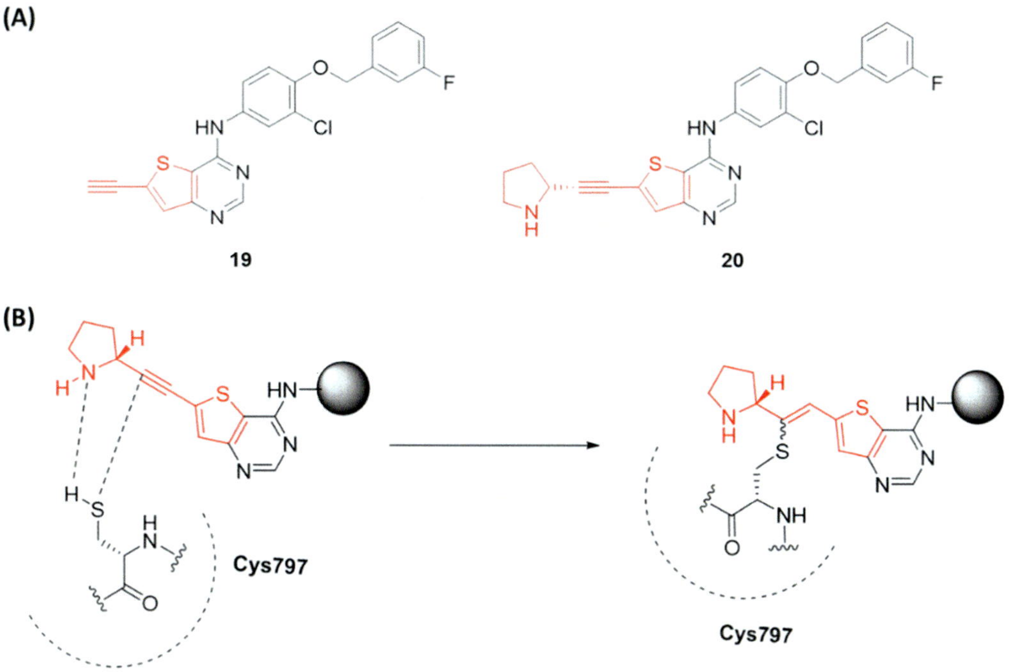

FIGURE 16.14 Covalent EGFR inhibitors with alkynyl thiophene ring warheads (A) and covalent binding mechanism (B).

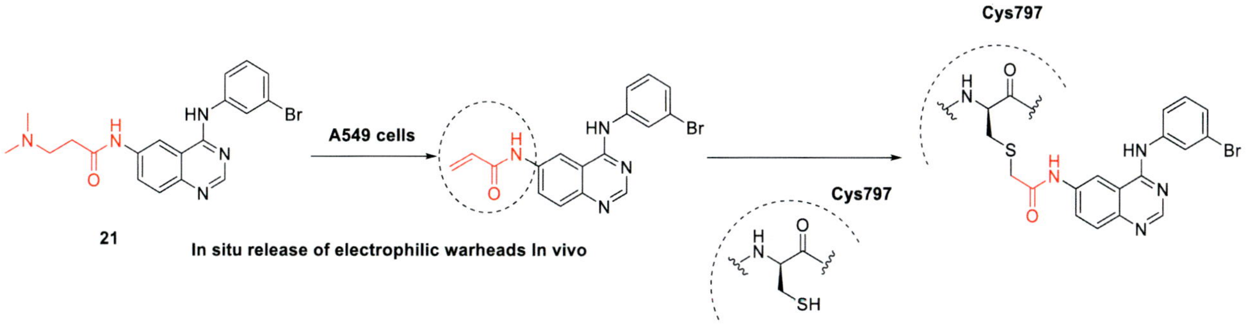

FIGURE 16.15 Schematic representation of the covalent binding between 3-aminopropionamide inhibitor **21** and the cysteine residue at the active site of EGFR kinase.

covalent binding. β-Aminoethyl ketones, also known as Mannich bases, can undergo an in situ β-elimination reaction via reverse-Michael addition under physiological conditions, generating α,β-unsaturated amides. These amides can then covalently bind to nucleophilic amino acid residues on target proteins. From a design perspective, these Mannich bases are prodrugs that by introducing "protected" electrophilic warheads can reduce the risk of covalent binding with nontarget proteins. The Marco team introduced a 3-aminopropanamide fragment at the C6 position of the quinazoline core and designed a compound **21** with covalent inhibitory activity based on the in situ generation of α, β-unsaturated amide electrophilic warheads. In the physiological environment inside cells, compound **21** can release the acrylamide structure and further covalently bind to the cysteine residue in the active site of EGFR kinase, thereby achieving proliferation inhibitory activity on NCI-H1975 cells with high expression of EGFR$^{L858R/T790M}$ (Fig. 16.15).

16.4.1.7 Thiols and disulfides [36–38]

The Singh and Parke-Davis teams designed a class of adenosine thiol analogs (**22**, Fig. 16.16) through homology modeling of the binding mode between ATP and cAMP Ser/Thr kinases, as well as the similar binding mode of the base portion of ATP molecules in various kinases.

Molecular docking studies have shown that the 2′-thiol group of adenosine can undergo an oxidation reaction with the cysteine side chain of EGFR to form a stable disulfide bond. The rate of EGFR enzyme inactivation saturates with increasing concentrations of adenosine thiol, and the inactivation of EGFR enzyme exhibits time dependence, which is a characteristic of covalent inhibition.

Furthermore, disulfur heterocycles can also serve as covalent reaction warheads. Bolognesi and Melchiorre's team designed compound **23** (Fig. 16.17) by introducing a lipoic acid fragment at the C6 position of the 4-anilinoquinazoline core. Compound **23** utilizes the dithiol heterocycle to undergo a thio-disulfide heterocycle exchange with the cysteine side chain of EGFR kinase, forming a stable covalent disulfide bond and prolonging the interaction time with the target protein. Additionally, lipoic acid, as a type of natural antioxidant, can induce apoptosis by regulating the balance between antiapoptotic and proapoptotic proteins. Therefore, strategies based on lipoic acid fragments can inhibit tumor cell proliferation through multiple mechanisms to overcome tumor resistance.

Similar covalent binding mechanisms can also be achieved with sulfur-containing electrophilic warheads such as isothiazolinones **24**, benzoisothiazolinones **25**, and thiadiazoles **26**. These compounds form stable disulfide bonds with cysteine residues of the target protein through their sulfur-containing core, resulting in covalent inhibition. Among them, quinazoline derivatives with thiadiazole electrophilic warheads have been shown to exhibit potent partial irreversible inhibition against EGFR kinase (Fig. 16.18).

16.4.1.8 Boric acids [39,40]

The boron atom consists of $2s^2 2p^1$, and it can form covalent molecules through sp^2 hybridization. Boron also has an empty orbital, and boron can act as a Lewis acid under physiological pH conditions. It can accept lone pairs of electrons from heteroatoms such as oxygen (O) and sulfur (S) to form tetrahedral coordination complexes with sp^3 hybridization.

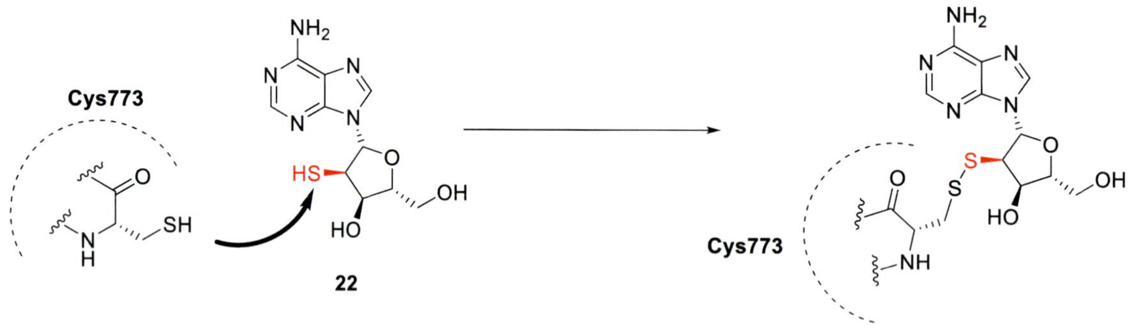

FIGURE 16.16 Covalent binding diagram of thiol inhibitor **22** with EGFR cysteine residue Cys[773].

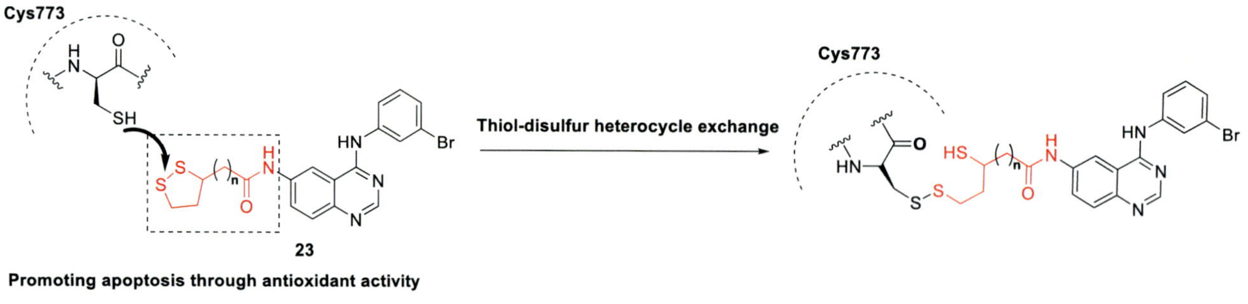

FIGURE 16.17 Schematic representation of the covalent binding between **23** containing lipoic acid and the cysteine side chain thiol of EGFR.

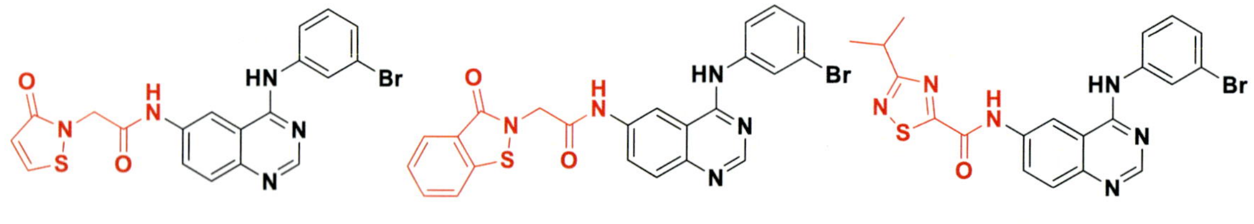

FIGURE 16.18 Other covalent EGFR inhibitors based on the mechanism of disulfide bond formation.

The coordination bonds between boron and heteroatoms in these types of complexes are often relatively strong (the bond energies of B−S and B−O bonds are approximately 24 and 18 kcal/mol, respectively), with strengths ranging between hydrogen bonds (with bond energies of 3−10 kcal/mol) and C−S covalent bonds (with a bond energy of 65 kcal/mol). Therefore, the Nakamura team introduced boronic acid electrophilic warheads at the C6 position of the 4-arylamine quinazoline core through different connecting chains and identified compound **27** (Fig. 16.2). Molecular docking simulations showed that boronic acid can form a stable B−O coordination bond with side chain carboxyl group of the conserved Asp^{800} in the EGFR kinase, exhibiting irreversible inhibitory effects (Fig. 16.19).

16.4.1.9 Others [35,41]

To further investigate the structure-activity relationship of electrophilic warheads and their covalent inhibitory effects, the Carmi team designed a series of moderately reactive electrophilic warheads (Fig. 16.20). This includes epoxy based on nucleophilic addition (**28−30**), carbamates based on carbamylation (**31**), and cyanides based on Pinner reaction (**32**). Among them, the inhibitory effect of epoxy-based electrophilic warheads (compounds **28−30**) on EGFR kinase activity is irreversible and comparable to acrylamide-based electrophilic warheads (**1**). On the other hand, carbamates (**31**) and cyanides (**32**) show partially irreversible inhibition. Similar to the acrylamide substitution, the introduction of a basic water-soluble piperidine moiety at the end of the epoxy fragment can enhance the inhibitory activity of compound 30 against gefitinib-resistant cell line NCI-H1975.

2-Nitroimidazole derivatives are a class of antitumor pharmacophores that target hypoxia in tumors. Within the hypoxic regions of tumors, 2-nitroimidazole undergoes four-electron reduction, generating a hydroxylamine intermediate, which is further reduced to nitrene. The nitrene can covalently bind to cysteine residues in the target protein, exerting

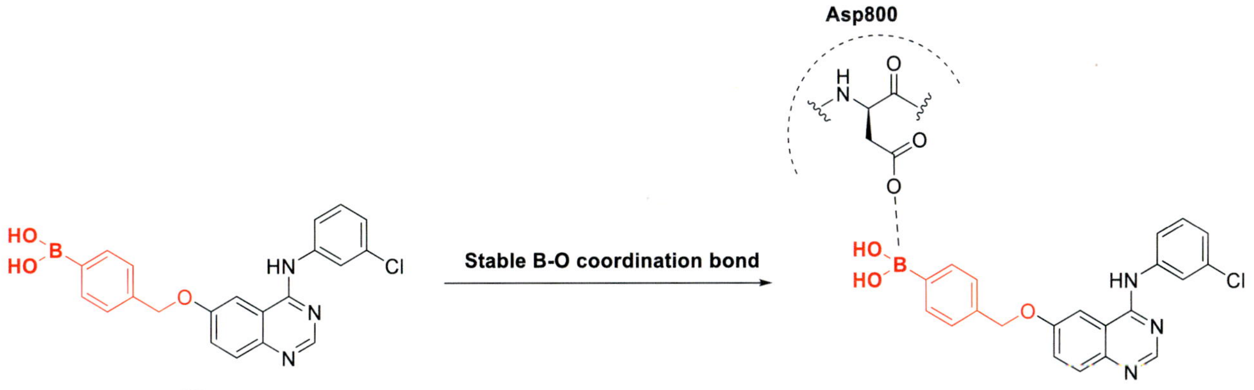

FIGURE 16.19 Binding mode of boronic acid-based electrophilic warhead with the carboxyl group of Asp^{800} side chain on EGFR.

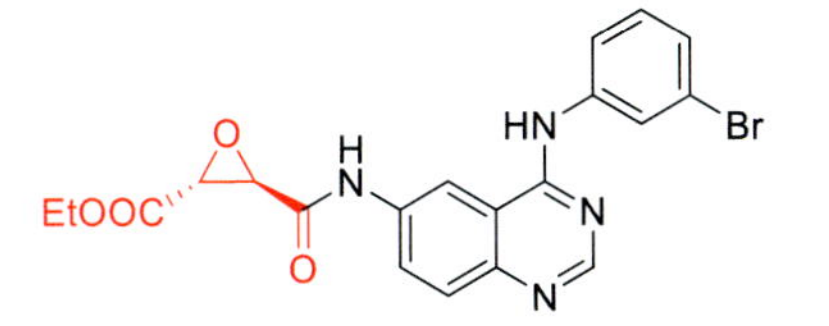

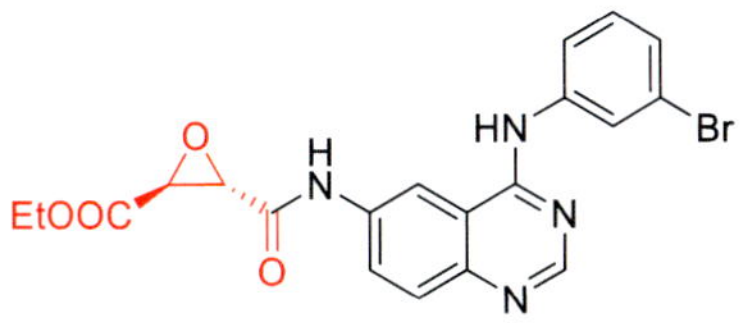

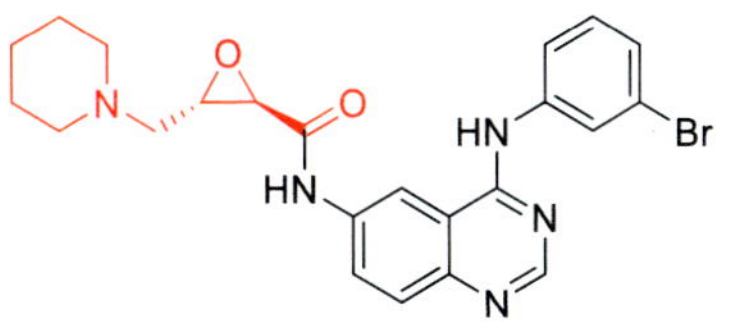

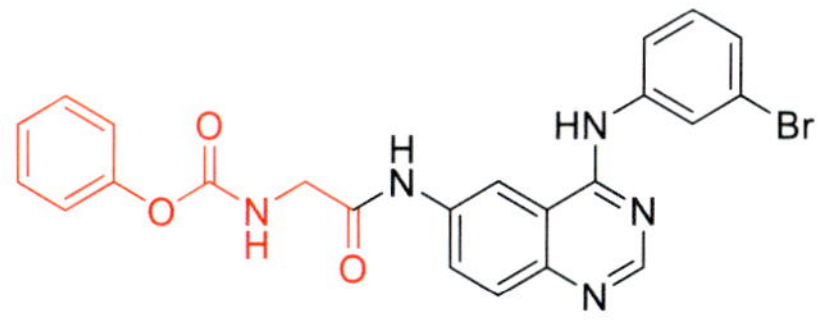

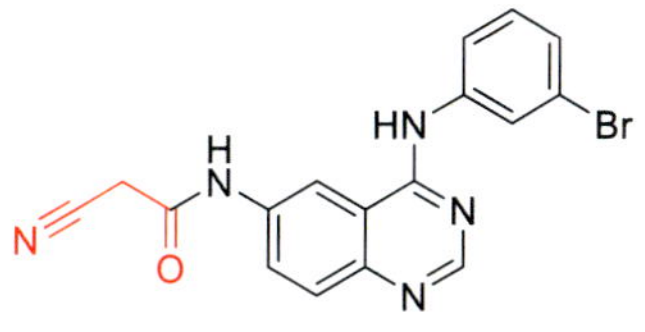

FIGURE 16.20 Other electrophilic warheads based on different mechanisms.

its anticancer effects (Fig. 16.21). Based on this reduction − activation mechanism, the 2-nitroimidazole fragment has also been developed as an electrophilic warhead for the design of EGFR covalent inhibitors. For example, by introducing a 2-nitroimidazole electrophilic warhead at the C-6 position of the quinazoline, the desired compound **33** demonstrated to undergo covalent binding with the cysteine residue of EGFR kinase through in vitro reduction activity experiments.

16.4.2 The discovery of the covalent irreversible EGFR inhibitor − afatinib

The discovery of afatinib, a covalent irreversible EGFR inhibitor with the acrylamide electrophilic warhead demonstrated significant advantages in the covalent inhibition (Fig. 16.22). In 1997, the David team retained the quinazoline core and introduced the acrylamide electrophilic warhead at the C-6 or C-7 position of the core [29]. The designed covalent irreversible inhibitors of the PD series maintained their inhibitory activity against EGFR kinase, with IC_{50} values in the nanomolar range. However, the efficiency of covalent inhibition was affected by the introduction of the electrophilic warhead at different positions of the quinazoline core. Western blotting revealed that PD 168393 with the acrylamide side chain at the C-6 position of the quinazoline core still inhibited EGFR kinase phosphorylation after 8 hours of elution. On the other hand, when the α,β-acrylamide electrophilic warhead was shifted to the C7 position of the quinazoline core, compound PD 160768 maintained the irreversible inhibitory activity but showed a slower rate of interaction with the target protein. The David team also used acetyl as a control group and found that compound PD 174265 restored EGFR kinase phosphorylation after 8 hours of elution, indicating that the acrylamide electrophilic

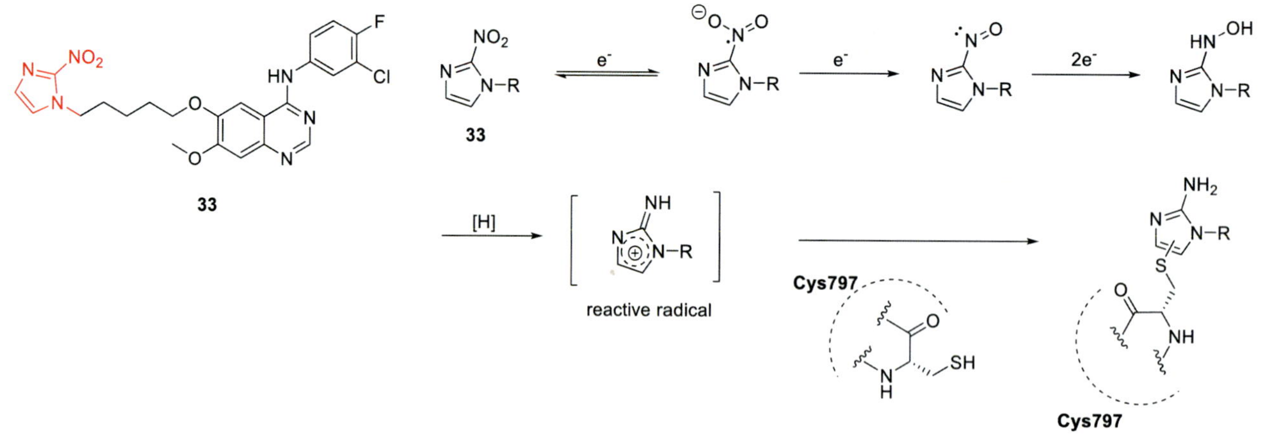

FIGURE 16.21 Covalent binding diagram of the 2-nitroimidazole electrophilic warhead based on the reduction − activation mechanism.

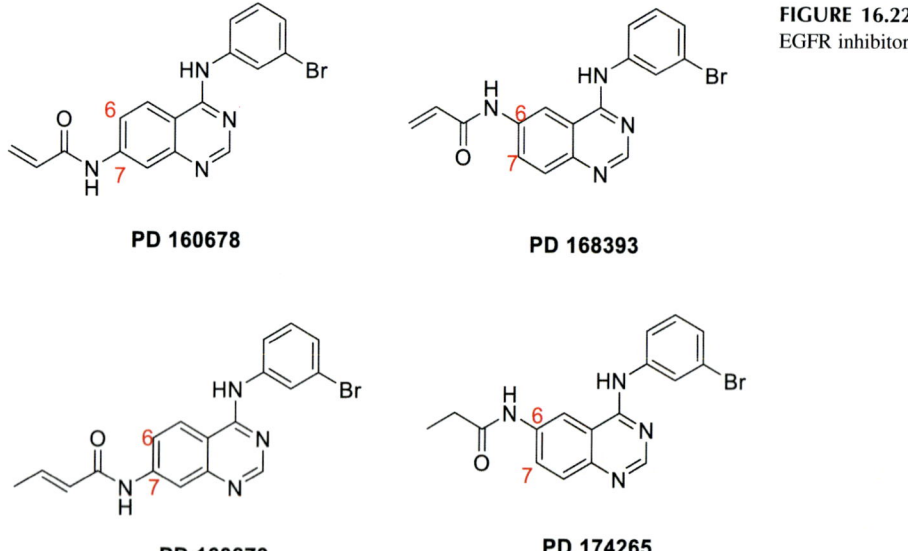

FIGURE 16.22 The PD series of covalent irreversible EGFR inhibitors developed by the Parke-Davis team.

A case study of the irreversible covalent epidermal growth factor receptor (EGFR) inhibitor—afatinib Chapter | 16 403

warhead contributed to the compound's covalent irreversible inhibition. Although PD 168393 was considered the prototype of covalent irreversible EGFR inhibitors, this class of molecules did not progress to clinical research primarily due to the low solubility and low oral bioavailability. Subsequent research work was inspired by the design concept of PD 168393 and focused on exploring the improvements in the physical and chemical properties of inhibitors around the α,β-acrylamide fragment.

To further improve the oral bioavailability of PD 168393, the research team at Wyeth Pharmaceuticals [42–44] introduced solubilizing groups at the end of the acrylamide electrophilic warhead at the C6 position of the quinazoline core. Various solubilizing groups such as *N,N*-dimethylamino, *N,N*-diethylamino, piperidine, morpholine, and *N*-methylpiperidine were designed and incorporated into a series of quinazoline derivatives **34–39** (Fig. 16.23). The results showed that directly modifying the β-position of acrylamide with water-soluble groups like *N,N*-dimethylamino (**34**) or morpholine (**35**) did not improve the inhibition activity against EGFR. However, compounds **36–39**, where the solubilizing fragments were attached to the acrylamide α- or β-position through a methylene linker, maintained inhibitory activity against EGFR kinase. Among them, the modification at the β-position of the warhead with the solubilizing fragment was the most favorable one. The *N,N*-dimethylamino modification at the end of the electrophilic warhead not only improved the solubility but also acted as a basic center of a tertiary amine, facilitating the covalent binding of the acrylamide electrophilic warhead with cysteine residues (Fig. 16.24). These structural modifications significantly enhanced the oral absorption and in vivo antitumor activity of compound **36**. In a xenograft mouse model, compound **36** showed a significant inhibition of tumor proliferation with an inhibition rate of up to 90% after continuous oral administration for 10 days, while the compound PD 168393 exhibited only 60%–70% tumor inhibition rate.

Wyeth Pharmaceuticals further investigated the introduction of the acrylamide electrophilic warhead on the 3-cyanoquinazoline core of **40**, which also possesses EGFR kinase inhibitory activity. They replaced the 3-bromoaniline at the C4 position with 3-chloro-4-fluoroaniline and introduced an ethoxy group at the C7 position, resulting in compound **41** (Fig. 16.25). Compound **41** maintained good kinase inhibitory activity and antitumor cell proliferation activity. In a xenograft mouse model, compound **41** significantly inhibited tumor proliferation with an inhibition rate of 90% after continuous oral administration for 20 days. Compound **41** was then selected for further clinical studies as the

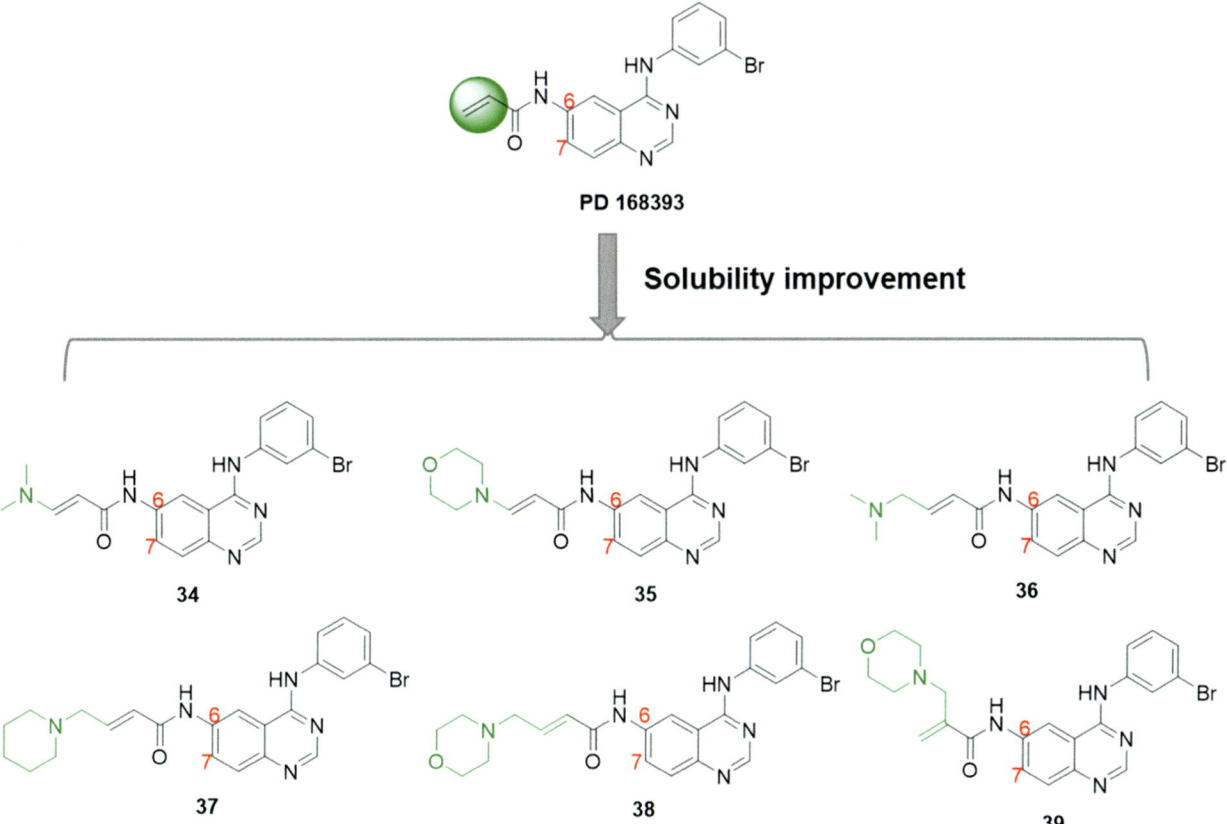

FIGURE 16.23 Water-soluble modifications based on the acrylamide electrophilic warhead by Wyeth Pharmaceuticals.

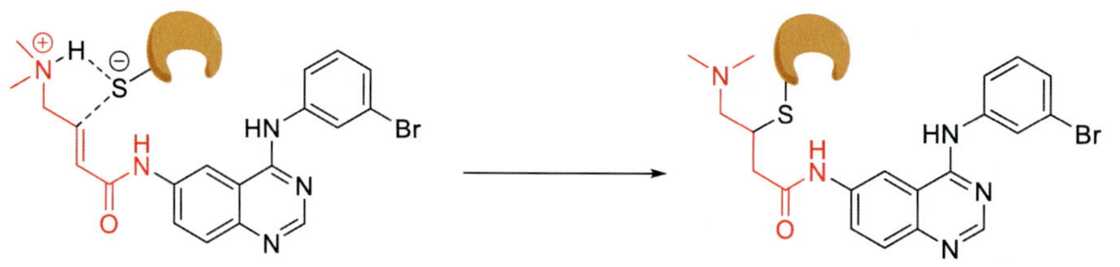

FIGURE 16.24 Modification of electrophilic warhead α,β-acrylamide with tertiary amines catalyze Michael addition reaction.

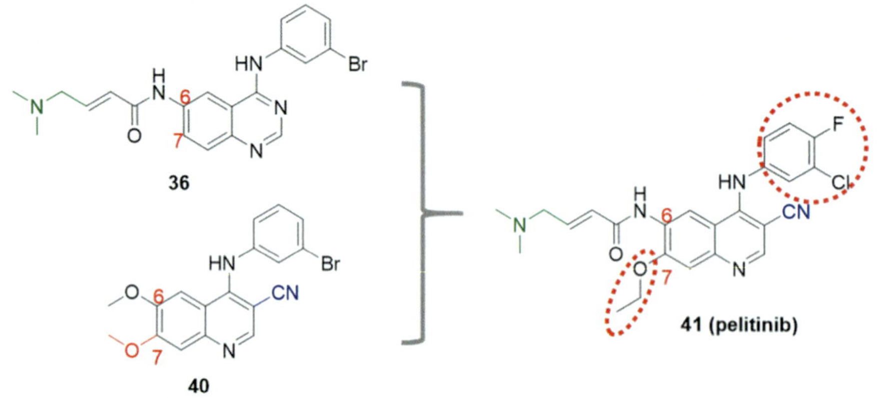

FIGURE 16.25 Design of 3-cyanoquinazoline derivative and covalent EGFR inhibitor pelitinib.

research code EKB-569 [45] (common name pelitinib). It belongs to a class of irreversible EGFR/ErbB2 inhibitors, selectively inhibiting the TK activity of EGFR and ErbB2. However, due to significant drug-related adverse reactions observed in Phase III clinical trials, the development process of pelitinib was terminated by the researchers.

At the same time, to improve the oral bioavailability of PD 168393, the research team at Parke-Davis Pharmaceutical Company attempted to introduce solubilizing groups, such as a morpholine moiety, at the C7 position of the quinazoline core. Although the solubilizing group has a bulky steric hindrance, the covalent binding between the acrylamide at the C6 position of compound **42** and the cysteine residue of EGFR was not affected, thus maintaining the covalent irreversible inhibition of EGFR kinase (Fig. 16.26). Additionally, the researchers replaced the C-4 substitution of compound **42** with 3-chloro-4-fluoroaniline, and the para position of the phenyl ring was substituted with a fluorine atom to block the metabolic site. The corresponding compound **43** exhibited slightly improved inhibitory activity against EGFR kinase (Fig. 16.26). However, when the solubilizing group at the C7 position was connected to the quinazoline core via a carbon atom, compound **44** (Fig. 16.26) maintained its inhibitory activity against EGFR kinase but almost completely lost its inhibitory activity against cell proliferation. This is possibly due to metabolic cleavage at the benzyl position of quinazoline. The research team at Parke-Davis Pharmaceutical Company then selected compound **43** for further studies. It was found that compound **43** had an effective dose as low as 5 mg/kg in a xenograft mouse model of human epidermal carcinoma (A431), with a tumor inhibition rate of up to 96% and no significant adverse reactions such as weight loss. Finally, compound **43** was confirmed as a candidate for clinical trials under the research code CI-1033 (generic name canertinib) [46]. However, in Phase II clinical trials, patients experienced adverse reactions such as thrombocytopenia, skin allergies, and severe vomiting, leading to the termination of the drug development process once again.

Drawing on the research experiences of erlotinib and canertinib, the medicinal chemists at Boehringer Ingelheim Pharmaceuticals retained the 4-arylamine substituted quinazoline structure. They introduced a 3-chloro-4-fluoroaniline group at the C-4 position of the core and an electrophilic acrylamide warhead with a terminal N,N-dimethylamine motif at the C-6 position. The C-7 position was modified with an oxygen-containing side chain. Among these modifications, the introduction of a (S)-tetrahydrofuran-3-yl oxygen group at the C-7 position resulted in compound **45** with potent EGFR inhibition (Fig. 16.27). Its inhibitory activity against EGFR$^{L858R/T790M}$ double mutant kinase is significantly 100-fold better than that of the first-generation EGFR inhibitor gefitinib. Compound **45** can significantly inhibit tumor proliferation in the NCI-H1975 xenograft mouse model of gefitinib-resistant human NSCLC. At an oral dose of 20 mg/kg, the T/C value is 12% [48] (T/C value <40% indicates effectiveness). Based on the excellent in vitro and in vivo activity mentioned above, compound **45** was quickly selected for clinical research in NSCLC. It was assigned the research code BIBW-2992 and the generic name afatinib. After extensive clinical trials, afatinib (brand name Gilotrif) became the first irreversible TK inhibitor approved globally and was launched in the United States in 2013, as well as in China in 2017. Afatinib is indicated for

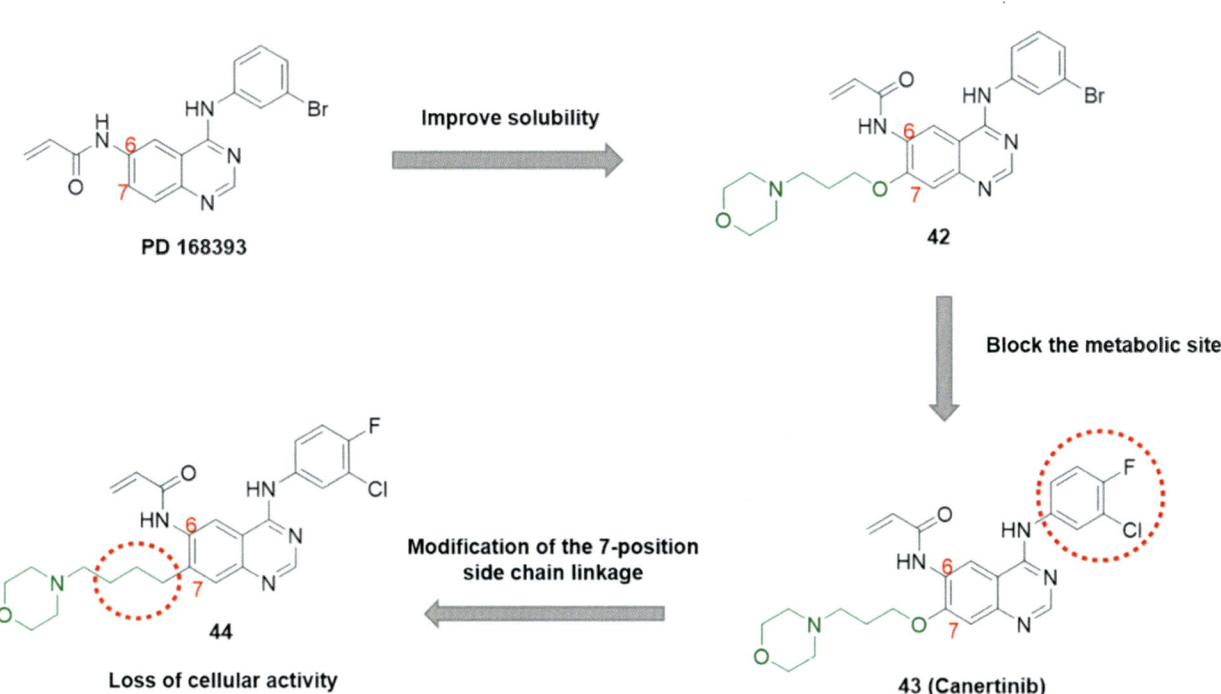

FIGURE 16.26 Design of 4-arylamine quinazolines EGFR covalent inhibitor canertinib.

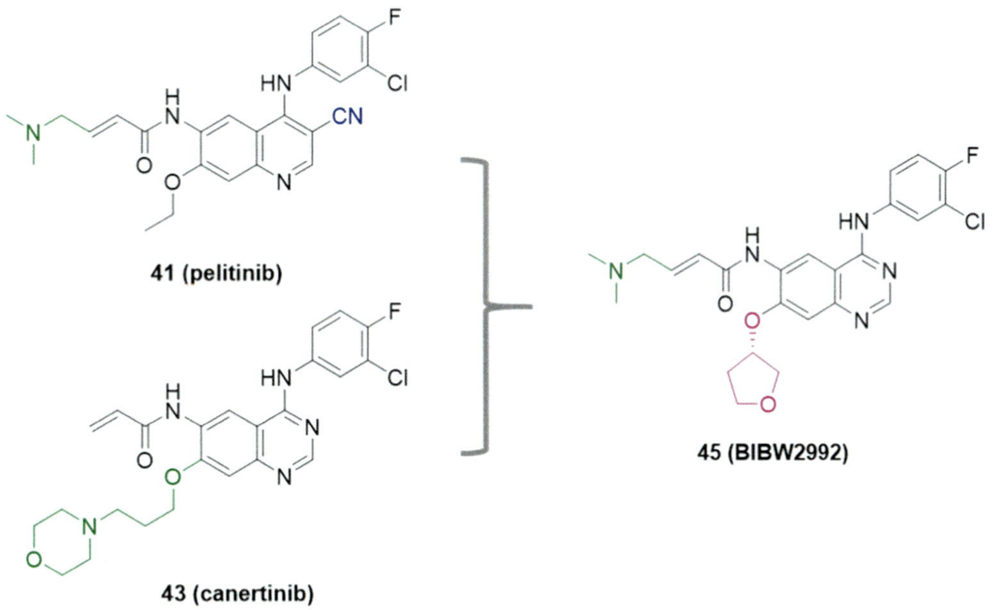

FIGURE 16.27 Design of the 4-arylamine substituted quinazoline EGFR covalent inhibitor afatinib (BIBW2992) [47].

the treatment of locally advanced or metastatic NSCLC patients with EGFR gene mutation sensitivity who have not received prior treatment with EGFR TK inhibitors, as well as for the treatment of locally advanced or metastatic squamous histology NSCLC patients who have disease progression during or after platinum-based chemotherapy.

The binding mode of afatinib (BIBW2992) with the EGFR protein complex crystal structure is shown in Fig. 16.28:

Quinazoline structure: It is an important core structure that closely mimics the purine ring of endogenous ATP molecules. It competes with ATP in the kinase domain, which is a key part of the mechanism of action of the compound. The N-1 on the quinazoline ring forms a hydrogen bond with Met^{763} of the kinase, and the N-3 forms a hydrogen bond with the hydroxyl group on the side chain of Thr^{766} through a water molecule.

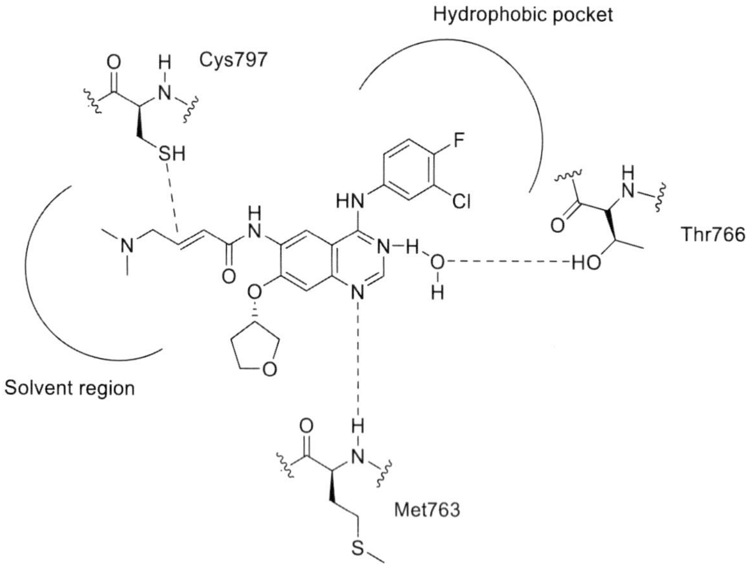

FIGURE 16.28 The schematic diagram of the binding mode of afatinib to EGFR kinase.

4-Arylamine group: The 3-chloro-4-fluoroaniline at the C-4 position of the core forms intermolecular interactions with Val^{726} and Thr^{766}, occupying the hydrophobic cavity of the protein kinase binding site.

Electrophilic acrylamide warhead at the C-6 position of the core: The acrylamide at the C-6 position plays a crucial role in the antitumor activity of afatinib. It acts as an electrophilic warhead and forms irreversible covalent bonds with the cysteine residues (Cys^{797} in EGFR and Cys^{805} in ErbB2), thereby irreversibly inhibiting the kinase activity of EGFR.

Site for improvement of physicochemical properties: At the end of the acrylamide at the C-6 position, there is an N,N-dimethylamino group connected by a methylene group. This modification improves the physicochemical properties of afatinib. Moreover, the N,N-dimethylamino group acts as a deprotonating agent for the cysteine residues, enhancing solubility and catalyzing intramolecular nucleophilic substitution reactions. The C-7 position of the quinazoline core is located at the entrance of the kinase binding pocket, pointing to the solvent region. The (S)-tetrahydrofuran-3-yl oxygen group at the C-7 position improves the solubility of afatinib.

16.4.3 The pharmacokinetics, pharmacodynamics, and adverse reactions of afatinib [49,50]

The metabolism and elimination pathways of covalent inhibitors in the body primarily involve fecal excretion rather than urinary excretion. They exhibit a high binding rate to plasma proteins and have significant tissue distribution. Moreover, most covalent inhibitors undergo oxidative metabolism catalyzed by cytochrome enzymes, which necessitates consideration of potential drug − drug interactions during clinical use.

(**Plasma protein binding rate**: It refers to the percentage of drug bound to plasma proteins after absorption into the bloodstream. It is an important pharmacokinetic parameter that influences the distribution, metabolism, and excretion of drugs, thereby affecting their potency and duration of action).

Preclinical pharmacokinetic studies have demonstrated that following oral administration of afatinib, the time to peak plasma concentration (T_{max}) in rats was 1–4 hours. The relative bioavailability in rats is 44.5%, with the drug mainly distributed in the liver, spleen, testes, and a small amount in the central nervous system and retina. Afatinib exhibits unsaturated binding to plasma proteins, with a protein binding rate of approximately 91.8%−94.9% when the drug concentration ranges from 0.05 to 0.5 μM. In rats, afatinib is primarily eliminated through fecal excretion, mainly as the prototype drug, accounting for 50% of the total excretion. Afatinib does not inhibit cytochrome P450 (CYP) isoforms (CYP1A1/2, 2A6, 2B6, 2C8, 2C9, 2C19, 2D6, 2E1, 3A4, and 4A11) and dose not the inducer of CYP isoforms (CYP1A2, 2B6, 2C8, 2C9, 2C19, and 3A4). It is a substrate of P-glycoprotein (P-gp) and exhibits moderate inhibition on the P-gp drug efflux pump.

In studies conducted on healthy volunteers and patients with advanced solid tumors, the oral administration of afatinib once daily resulted in peak plasma concentrations (C_{max}) between 2 and 5 hours. Steady-state levels were achieved after 8 days, with a half-life of 37 hours, indicating the suitability of once-daily dosing. The absorption of afatinib is reduced when taken with food. Its metabolism rate is low, primarily undergoing elimination as the prototype drug through fecal excretion, and only approximately 5% being excreted in the urine. Afatinib primarily binds to plasma proteins in a covalent manner, with a binding rate of approximately 95%. The pharmacokinetic characteristics of afatinib remain consistent across different patient populations, with no significant influence on factors such as age, race, smoking status, or liver function. However, female patients and those with lower body weight may exhibit increased pharmacokinetic parameters. The blood concentration of afatinib is influenced by renal function, with approximately a 50% increase in the area under the concentration-time curve (AUC) observed in patients with severe renal impairment. Afatinib is minimally affected by drug interactions involving biotransformation and has minimal metabolism *via* CYP enzymes. However, concurrent treatment with P-gp transporter inhibitors or inducers can affect the pharmacokinetic characteristics of afatinib. At a dose of 50 mg, afatinib does not exhibit potential proarrhythmic effects.

(**AUC**: It refers to the time as the horizontal coordinate, the blood concentration as the vertical coordinate, and the discharged curve as the blood concentration-time curve after administration. The area between the axis and the concentration-time curve is named AUC. It represents the total amount of drug in the body over time after administration, with a larger AUC indicating higher drug utilization).

The clinical trial LUX-Lung 7 conducted a head-to-head comparison between second-generation afatinib and first-generation EGFR-targeting drug gefitinib for the treatment of EGFR mutation-positive NSCLC patients who had not received prior treatment. The results demonstrated that first-line therapy with afatinib significantly reduced the risk of lung cancer progression by 26% compared to gefitinib. Furthermore, the improvement in progression-free survival (PFS) was more pronounced in the afatinib-treated group than in the gefitinib-treated group. Additionally, a significant number of patients in the afatinib-treated group experienced objective response rate (ORR). These positive findings highlight the clinical advantages of afatinib over first-generation EGFR inhibitors.

Adverse reactions associated with afatinib are more prevalent. Commonly observed side effects include diarrhea, rash, oral mucositis, paronychia, decreased appetite, epistaxis, pruritus, and xerosis. Taste alteration, dehydration, cystitis, cheilitis, fever, nasal congestion, hypokalemia, conjunctivitis, hepatic dysfunction, hand-foot syndrome, muscle spasms, and renal impairment are frequently reported. Corneal inflammation and pneumonia are rare occurrences. It is worth noting that rash is also considered a positive indicator of the efficacy of afatinib, as this adverse reaction primarily stems from the potent inhibition of wild-type EGFR kinase. Clinical trials have demonstrated that appropriately reducing the dosage can significantly decrease the incidence of adverse reactions while maintaining comparable therapeutic efficacy.

16.4.4 Summary of structure-activity relationship of covalent EGFR inhibitor

Based on the literature reports on 4-anilinoquinazolines (or 4-anilino-3-cyanoquinolines)-based irreversible EGFR TK inhibitors and the research of small molecule-protein X-ray crystal structures, the main structure-activity relationship of covalent EGFR inhibitors is summarized in Fig. 16.29.

Part A: The nitrogen atom at position 1 of the quinazoline ring forms a strong hydrogen bond with the Met[769] residue of the EGFR kinase, which is crucial for the activity of the inhibitor. When the nitrogen atom at position 1 is replaced by a carbon atom, the activity of the inhibitor is decreased by more than 3700-fold.

Part B: Substitution at position 2 of the quinazoline is detrimental to the activity of the inhibitor. Even with small substituents such as methyl group, the activity is almost lost.

Part C: The nitrogen atom at the 3-position of the quinazoline ring can form a hydrogen bond with Thr[766] through a water molecule. When X = C and Y = H, the activity is reduced by 200-fold. However, when X = C and Y = CN, which corresponds to 4-anilino-3-cyanoquinoline derivatives, the inhibitor still exhibits potent inhibitory activity. This could be because the cyano group can interact with the hydroxyl group of Thr[766] without the involvement of a water molecule.

Part D: The aniline group at the 4-position of the quinazoline occupies a hydrophobic cavity in the binding site. Modification of this aniline group plays an important role in the affinity and selectivity of the inhibitor. The aniline group with a bulkier steric can increase the affinity of the inhibitor toward ErbB2 while significantly reducing its affinity for EGFR. Therefore, the selectivity of these inhibitors can be achieved by structural modification on this site.

Part E: Introducing an electrophilic warhead at this position can form a covalent interaction with the cysteine side chain near the ATP binding site of EGFR. The formation of a covalent bond prolongs the action of the inhibitor and enhances its effectiveness.

Part F: Similar to Part E, this position is exposed to the solvent region, making it an important site for optimizing the physicochemical properties of the inhibitor and improving its pharmacokinetics and pharmacodynamics. Increasing

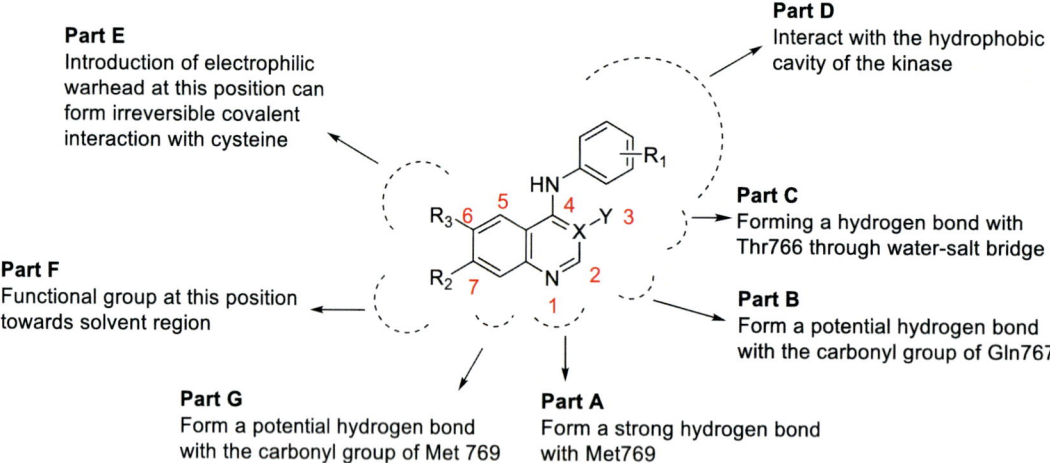

FIGURE 16.29 Structure-activity relationship of covalent EGFR inhibitors.

the hydrophilicity of the substituent at this site can significantly improve the physicochemical properties of the inhibitor, favoring its development as a drug candidate.

Part G: X-ray crystal structure studies of small molecule-protein complexes indicate a potential hydrogen bond interaction between this site and the carbonyl group of Met^{769}. Substituent modifications at this position are detrimental to the activity of the inhibitor, and larger substituents may also hinder the interaction between the enzyme and the inhibitor.

16.5 Synthesis of afatinib

The chemical structure of Afatinib can be divided into two key components. One part consists of a 4-arylamine quinazoline core (A), while the other part is the N,N-dimethylaminobut-2-enoic acid side chain (B). Afatinib can be synthesized through various methods, primarily categorized into the following two synthetic routes (Fig. 16.30): (1) Laboratorial medicinal chemical synthesis route-modular synthesis approach; first, the quinazoline core is constructed, followed by condensation with the N,N-dimethylaminobut-2-enoic acid fragment to form the amide bond, ultimately yielding Afatinib. (2) Commercial synthesis route: sequential synthesis approach; first, the N,N-dimethylaminobut-2-enoic acid fragment is connected, and then the arylamine is installed at the C-4 position of quinazoline core, yielding Afatinib.

The aforementioned synthetic methods involve the following significant organic chemical reactions:

16.5.1 Mitsunobu reaction

The substitution of primary and secondary alcohols with nucleophiles in the presence of a dialkyl azodicarboxylate and a trialkyl- or triaryl phosphine is known as the Mitsunobu reaction (Fig. 16.31). In 1967, Mitsunobu reported a new method for the condensation of acids and alcohols to form esters using triphenylphosphine (PPh$_3$) and diethyl azodicarboxylate (DEAD). When the substrate is a secondary alcohol, the configuration of the carbon atom connecting to the hydroxyl group undergoes inversion. This type of reaction is widely employed in organic synthesis and can be represented as follows:

The Mitsunobu reaction exhibits the following characteristics: (1) Both primary alcohols and secondary alcohols can undergo the Mitsunobu reaction, with the configuration of the chiral center in secondary alcohols being inverted. (2) The pK_a value of the nucleophilic reagent's proton must be lower than the pK_a value of the betaine intermediate (~13) to allow the proton transfer from the nucleophile to the intermediate. Otherwise, the proton of the nucleophilic reagent cannot be captured by the intermediate. (3) Oxygen-containing nucleophilic reagents primarily yield esters and ethers, while sulfur-containing nucleophilic reagents mainly afford thioethers. Common nitrogen-containing nucleophilic reagents include amides, hydroxylamines, heterocyclic nitrogen, and azoimides. (4) Low-polarity solvents such as tetrahydrofuran, diethyl ether, dichloromethane, and toluene are favorable for the reaction. (5) PPh$_3$ and P(n-Bu)$_3$ are the most commonly used phosphine ligands, and the frequently employed azodicarboxylate reagents are DEAD and DIAD.

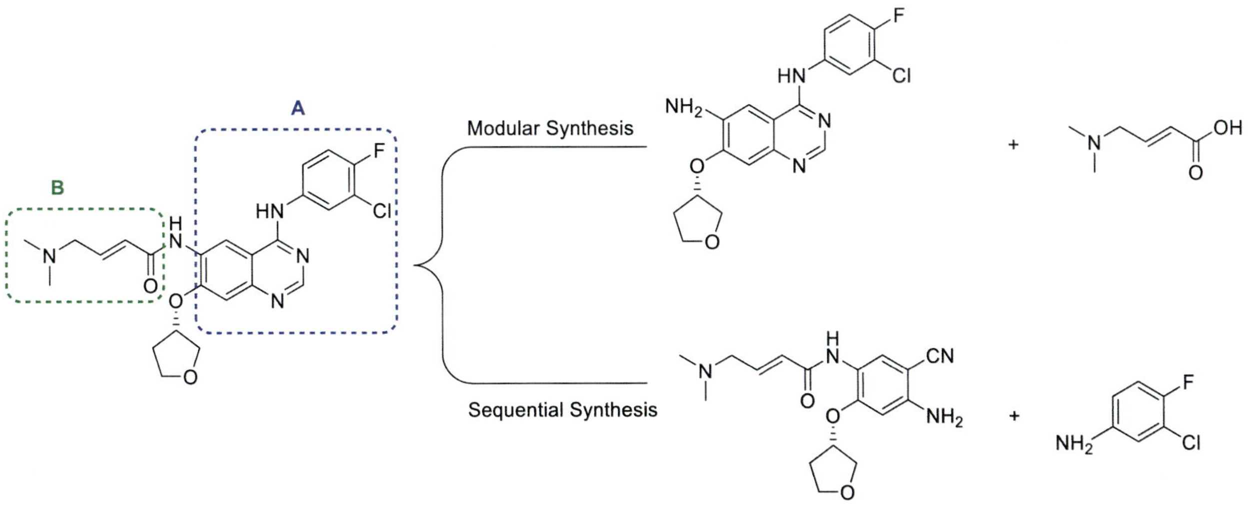

A case study of the irreversible covalent epidermal growth factor receptor (EGFR) inhibitor—afatinib **Chapter | 16** **409**

FIGURE 16.30 Retro-synthetic analysis of afatinib.

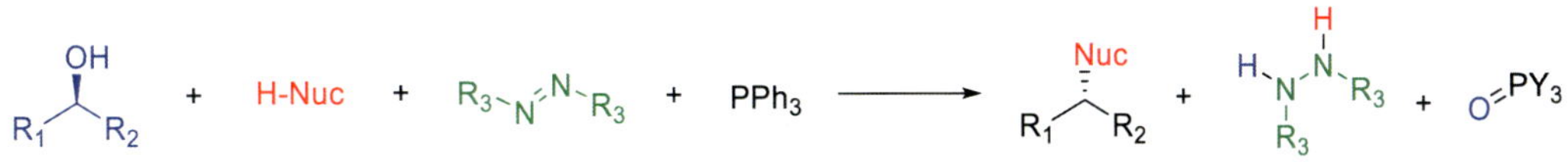

FIGURE 16.31 The general formula for the Mitsunobu reaction.

16.5.2 Dimroth rearrangement

The base-catalyzed rearrangement or translocation of exo- and endo-cyclic heteroatoms on a heterocyclic ring is generally referred to as the Dimroth rearrangement (Fig. 16.32). The Dimroth rearrangement is generally classified into two types: translocation of heteroatoms within rings of fused systems (Type I) and translocation of exo-and endocyclic heteroatoms in a heterocyclic ring (Type II). The Type II rearrangement is more observed, and this reaction can be catalyzed by acids, bases, heat, or light. Its reaction can be represented as follows:

Several factors can influence the Dimroth rearrangement reaction: (1) The number of nitrogen atoms in the heterocycle enhances the electrophilicity of the ring and facilitates the nucleophilic addition reaction in the initiating step. (2) The pH of the reaction system affects the rearrangement rate. (3) Substituents with electron-withdrawing groups are more likely to facilitate the nucleophilic catalyst's attack in the initiating step, thereby accelerating the Dimroth rearrangement. (4) The relative thermal stability of the substrate and product would also influence the reaction.

16.5.3 The Horner-Wadsworth-Emmons reaction

The Horner-Wadsworth-Emmons (HWE) reaction, also known as the Horner-Wadsworth-Emmons olefination, is a synthetic method for the preparation of alkenes. It is an improvement over the classic Wittig reaction. In this reaction, a stable phosphonate carbanion is used instead of a phosphorus ylide. The reaction of aldehydes or ketones with stabilized phosphonate carbanions leads to olefins with excellent *E*-selectivity (Fig. 16.33). The phosphonate ester participating in the reaction typically requires an electron-withdrawing group attached to the α-carbon. This facilitates the elimination of a four-membered cyclic intermediate to form the alkene. The byproduct *O,O*-dialkylphosphate is soluble in water and can be easily separated by aqueous extraction.

16.5.4 Laboratorial medicinal chemical synthetic route-modular synthesis approach

The original patents from Boehringer Ingelheim Pharmaceuticals (WO0250043 and WO03094921) describe the modular synthesis approach for the preparation of afatinib. The crucial approach involves the construction of the quinazoline core, followed by sequential functional group modifications at C-7 and C-6 positions of the quinazoline core.

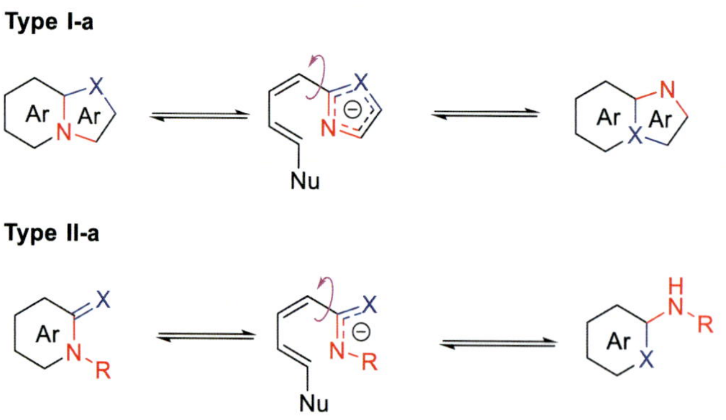

410 Medicinal Chemistry and Drug Development

FIGURE 16.32 The general formula for the Dimroth rearrangement reaction.

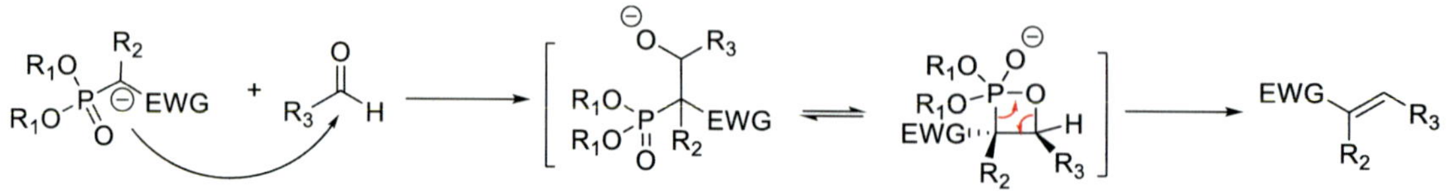

FIGURE 16.33 The reaction mechanism of the Horner-Wadsworth-Emmons (HWE) reaction.

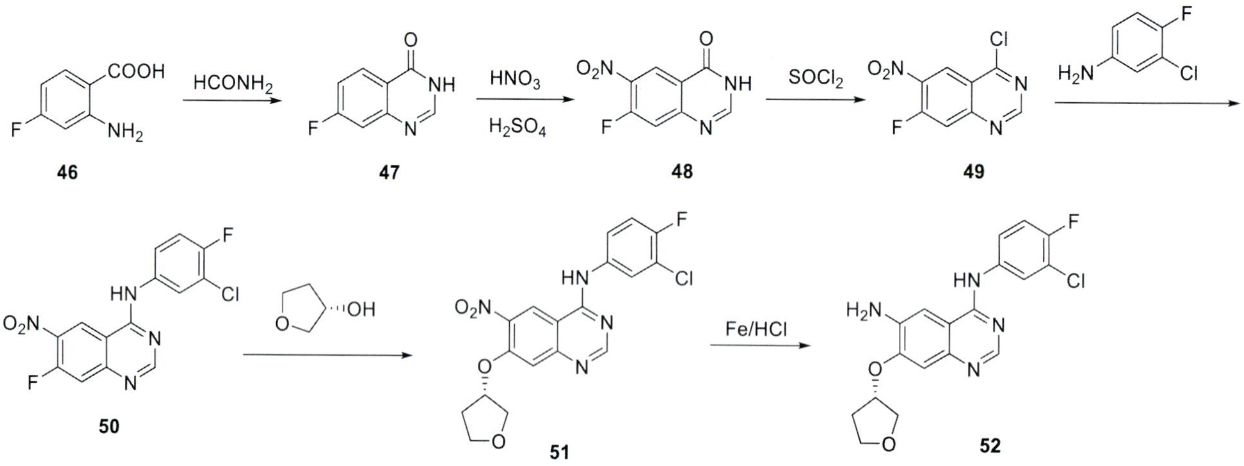

FIGURE 16.34 Synthesis of the 4-arylamine quinazoline core **52**.

The synthesis of the 4-arylamine quinazoline core **52** starts from 2-amino-4-fluorobenzoic acid **46**. The acid undergoes a cyclization reaction with formamide at high temperature to form 7-fluoroquinazolinone **47**. Nitration of 7-fluoroquinazolinone **47** occurs by treating it with fuming nitric acid and concentrated sulfuric acid, resulting in the formation of 6-nitro-7-fluoroquinazolinone **48**. Then, 6-nitro-7-fluoroquinazolinone **48** was chlorinated by sulfoxide chloride to obtain 4-chloro-6-nitro-7-fluoroquinazolinone **49**. Reaction of 4-chloro-6-nitro-7-fluoroquinazolinone **49** with 3-chloro-4-fluoroaniline yields the crucial intermediate 6-nitro-4-[(3-chloro-4-fluorophenyl) amino]-7-fluoroquinazoline **50**. Under the action of potassium *tert*-butoxide, the fluorine atom at the C-7 position of intermediate **50** is replaced by (*S*)-3-hydroxytetrahydrofuran, leading to the formation of the ether product **51**. The reduction of the nitro group at C-6 position of intermediate **51** is achieved under the condition of hydrochloric acid/iron powder, resulting in the formation of the crucial 4-arylamine quinazoline core **52** (Fig. 16.34).

The quinazoline core **52** undergoes a condensation reaction with bromocrotonyl chloride to form the intermediate **53**, which is then subjected to an amination reaction with dimethylamine to yield the target compound, afatinib. The overall yield for this route is 18% (Fig. 16.35).

The synthesis of the side chain at the C-6 position of afatinib can also be achieved through the classic HWE reaction. The condensation reaction between the key precursor **52** and 2-(diethylphosphono) acetic acid leads to the formation of the intermediate **54**. Subsequently, compound **54** undergoes an HWE reaction with (dimethylamino)-acetaldehyde diethyl acetal under alkaline conditions to yield afatinib. The overall yield of this route is 28% (Fig. 16.36).

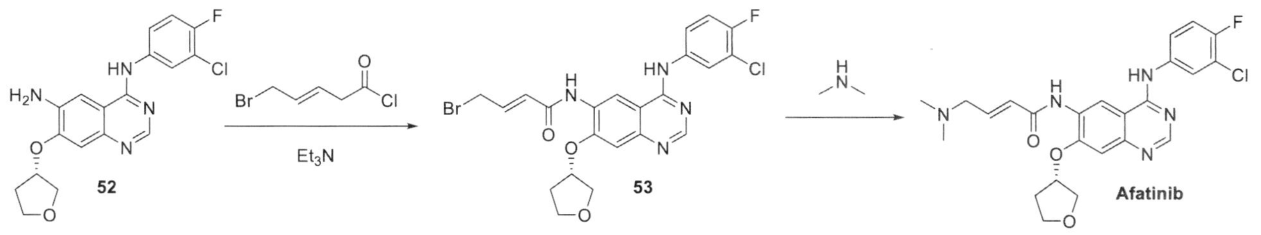

FIGURE 16.35 The synthesis of afatinib according to the original research route developed by Boehringer Ingelheim.

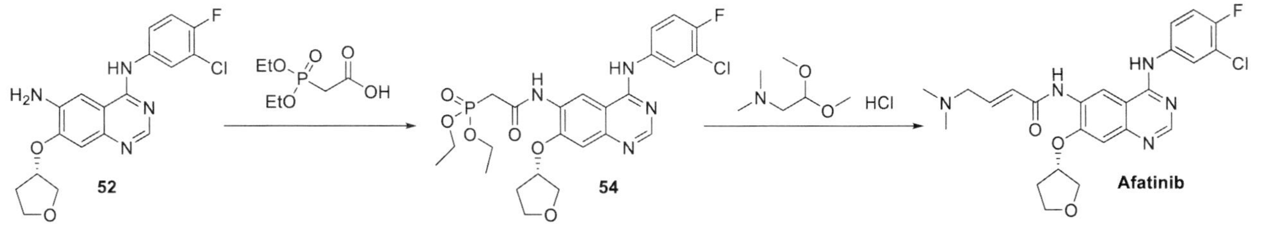

FIGURE 16.36 The synthesis of afatinib based on the Horner-Wadsworth-Emmons (HWE) reaction.

16.5.5 Commercial synthetic route-sequential synthesis approach

The above synthesis steps are typically lengthy and the route involves several quinazoline intermediates. These intermediates exhibit poor solubility in organic solvents, thereby limiting the overall synthesis yield. Through a review of synthetic literature on similar compounds, it has been found that the Dimroth rearrangement reaction is a favorable method for constructing the quinazoline ring system [51]. Researchers reported that the introduction of the quinazoline core via the Dimroth rearrangement reaction successfully addressed the issue of low solubility of quinazoline intermediates (CN103254156). Starting with the cost-effective 4-hydroxybenzonitrile **55**, a nitration reaction yields 2-nitro-4-cyanophenol **56**. Mitsunobu reaction between **56** and (R)-3-hydroxytetrahydrofuran produces the intermediate **57**. The nitro group of **57** is catalytically reduced by Pd/C to obtain 3-amino-4-[(S)-(tetrahydrofuran-3-yl) oxy]benzonitrile **58**. Intermediate **58** undergoes acylation with N,N-dimethylaminocrotonic chloride to yield the intermediate **59**. Intermediate **59** undergoes a secondary nitration and nitro group reduction to obtain intermediate **61**, which is then condensed with DMF-DMA to form 2-[(N,N-dimethylamino)methylamino]-4-[(S)-(tetrahydrofuran-3-yl)oxy]-5-[[4-(N,N-dimethylamino)-1-oxo-2-buten-1-yl]amino]benzonitrile **62**. Intermediate **62** undergoes the Dimroth rearrangement with 3-chloro-4-fluoroaniline at 120°C–130°C to generate the desired product afatinib, with an overall yield of 36%. This synthesis route is suitable for large-scale production (Fig. 16.37).

16.6 Summary and knowledge expansion

16.6.1 Summary of this chapter

With the rapid development of molecular detection techniques and the discovery of different driver genes, NSCLC has become a heterogeneous disease composed of different molecular subtypes, and the treatment of lung cancer has entered the era of targeted therapy. EGFR is an important driver of NSCLC, and the development of small molecule inhibitors targeting EGFR provides a new approach for the treatment of NSCLC. This chapter provides a theoretical guide for further molecular design by introducing the structure and function of EGFR, the design and structure-activity relationship study of quinazoline-based EGFR inhibitors, and the design principles and strategies of covalent inhibitors in the design of EGFR inhibitors. As the first approved irreversible EGFR inhibitor, afatinib has become a paradigm of successful application of covalent inhibition strategy in drug design. Afatinib was discovered during the modification of the electrophilic warhead, and the interaction mode between covalent irreversible inhibitors and enzymes is also elucidated, providing research ideas and experience for the design of covalent irreversible inhibitors targeting other targets [10].

16.6.2 Knowledge expansion

Although afatinib has overcome $EGFR^{T790M}$ mutation to some extent, it also exhibits inhibitory effects on wild-type EGFR, leading to significant dose-dependent adverse reactions such as rash and diarrhea. This greatly limits its clinical

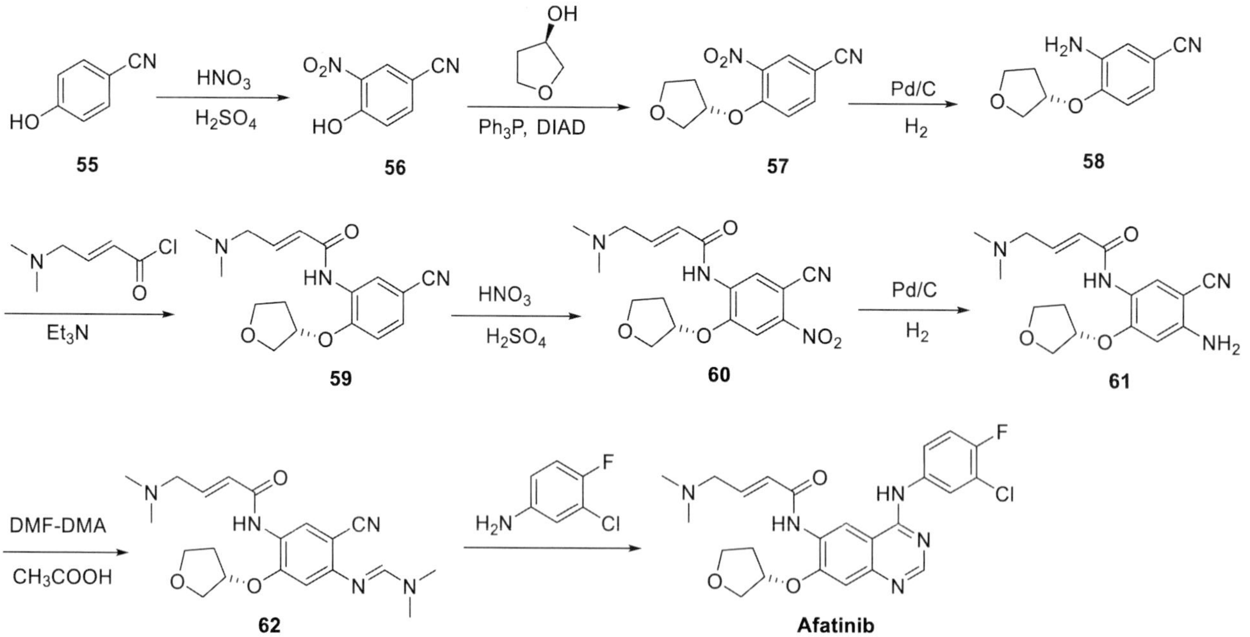

FIGURE 16.37 Larege-scale synthesis pathway of afatinib.

application and reduces patient compliance. Therefore, it is necessary to develop new inhibitors that selectively target the EGFR^{T790M} mutation without affecting the normal function of the wild-type EGFR protein.

16.6.2.1 Research progress on selective small molecule inhibitors for EGFR^{T790M} mutation

Analysis of the protein structure of EGFR^{T790M} mutation reveals that the amino acid residue located at the entrance of the binding pocket (gatekeeper) is mutated from threonine to methionine. These two amino acid residues have significant differences in hydrophobicity, with methionine having higher lipophilicity than threonine. Based on this hypothesis, researchers at the Dana-Farber Cancer Institute of Harvard University discovered a class of aminopyrimidines that selectively inhibits the mutant EGFR^{T790M} while exhibiting weak inhibition against wild-type EGFR. One representative compound is WZ-4002 [52]. Subsequently, pharmaceutical companies such as AstraZeneca, Clovis, and Novartis have conducted research on developing new generation of EGFR inhibitors based on this aminopyrimidine scaffold, and have successfully developed new drugs (Table 16.2) [53].

Osimertinib (trade name Tagrisso) developed by AstraZeneca is a selective and irreversible EGFR inhibitor targeting the EGFR^{T790M} mutation. It overcomes acquired resistance issues caused by drugs such as erlotinib, gefitinib, and afatinib. Osimertinib obtained approval for marketing in the United States and China in November 2015 and March 2017, respectively. It is used as a first-line treatment for advanced or metastatic NSCLC patients with EGFR mutation, and it is the first approved third-generation EGFR inhibitor. Studies have demonstrated that first-line treatment with osimertinib in EGFR mutation-positive advanced NSCLC patients leads to longer PFS and overall survival (OS) compared to other EGFR-TKIs. Furthermore, the efficacy and safety of osimertinib in combination with platinum-based chemotherapy (pemetrexed) were evaluated in the AURA 3 clinical trial for patients with EGFR T790M-positive advanced NSCLC and brain metastases following previous treatment with EGFR-TKIs. The results showed significant improvement in ORR for patients with brain metastases [54,55].

Rociletinib (CO1686) is a third-generation irreversible EGFR inhibitor developed by Clovis Oncology. It selectively inhibits sensitive mutations and T790M resistance mutations of EGFR. In May 2014, it was designated as the breakthrough therapy by the FDA and was intended for use as a monotherapy in the second-line treatment of NSCLC patients with the T790M mutation. However, the results of Phase III clinical trials showed an ORR of only around 30%, significantly lower than the expected 60%. Additionally, Rociletinib exhibited two severe adverse effects, including hyperglycemia and QT prolongation on electrocardiogram. In April 2016, the Oncologic Drugs Advisory Committee of the FDA voted 12:1 against the approval of Rociletinib.

Olmutinib (trade name Olita) is a third-generation EGFR irreversible inhibitor developed by Hanmi Pharmaceutical. It was launched in South Korea in May 2016 and is primarily used for the treatment of locally advanced or metastatic

TABLE 16.2 Selective EGFR inhibitors targeting EGFR^{T790M} mutation.

Chemical structure	Developing companies	Targeted receptors	Development status
Osimertinib	AstraZeneca	EGFR-sensitive mutations (19del21, L858R) and T790M mutation	FDA Approval (2015)
Rociletinib	Clovis Oncology	EGFR-sensitive mutations (19del21, L858R) and T790M mutation	Phase III, discontinued (2016)
Olmutinib	Hanmi Pharmaceuticals	EGFR sensitive mutations (19del21, L858R) and T790M mutation	Launched in South Korea (2016)
Almonertinib	Jiangsu Hansoh Pharma	EGFR-sensitive mutations (19del21, L858R) and T790M mutation	Launched in China (2020)
Avitinib	ACEA Pharma	EGFR-sensitive mutations (19del21, L858R) and T790M mutation	Phase III
Alflutinib	Shanghai Allist Pharmaceuticals Co. Ltd	EGFR-sensitive mutations (19del21, L858R) and T790M mutation	Phase III

NSCLC patients with the EGFR^{T790M} mutation who have previously received EGFR-TKIs. In the same year, serious adverse reactions were observed during the clinical trials, leading Boehringer Ingelheim to discontinue further research on Olmutinib, as well as return the global development and commercialization rights to Hanmi Pharmaceutical.

Almonertinib (trade name Almele) is the world's second and China's first third-generation irreversible EGFR inhibitor developed by Jiangsu Hansoh Pharma. It received approval from the China National Medical Products Administration in March 2020 for the treatment of advanced NSCLC patients with the T790M mutation who have previously received EGFR-TKIs. Clinical trial results demonstrated an ORR of 68.9% and a disease control rate (DCR) of 93.4% for Almonertinib. The median PFS (mPFS) reached 12.3 months, and the incidence of adverse effects associated with Almonertinib was minimal. Moreover, Almonertinib exhibited the ability to penetrate the blood-brain barrier, enabling the suppression of brain lesions with an impressive response rate of 61.5% in patients with brain metastases. The successful market launch of Almonertinib not only overcomes significant technical challenges in the development of urgently needed clinical therapeutics but also fills the gap in domestically developed third-generation EGFR-TKIs in China. It brings long-term and high-quality survival prospects for patients with advanced NSCLC [56].

(DCR refers to the proportion of patients with solid tumors whose tumors have either shrunk or remained stable for a certain period. It includes cases of complete response, partial response, and stable disease).

Since the approval of the first third-generation irreversible EGFR inhibitor osimertinib in 2013, numerous third-generation EGFR-TKIs have entered clinical trials. These include naquotinib, nzartinib, PF-06747775, TAS-121, and lazertinib, among others. However, after the approval of osimertinib, clinical trials on naquotinib, nzartinib, PF-06747775, and TAS-121 gradually terminated due to various factors.

The development of third-generation irreversible EGFR inhibitors has gradually shifted to China. Currently, besides Almonertinib, there are at least 10 drug candidates in the clinical trial stage, such as avitinib, furmonertinib, TQB3804, BPI-361175, QLH11811, HS10375, H02, and DAJH-1050766.

16.6.2.2 The emergence of $EGFR^{T790M/C797S}$ double mutations and design strategies for allosteric inhibitors

While osimertinib has improved the selectivity against the $EGFR^{T790M}$ resistance mutation through the optimization of aminopyrimidine core and addressing the adverse effects caused by targeting wild-type EGFR, prolonged drug exposure leads to the inevitable occurrence of acquired resistance mediated by the secondary $EGFR^{C797S}$ mutation. Among patients receiving osimertinib, 20%−40% will develop the Del19/T790M/C797S or L858R/T790M/C797S triple mutations. When the T790M and C797S mutations are in a *trans* configuration (on different alleles), cells only show resistance to the third-generation EGFR-TKIs but remain sensitive to the combination of first- and third-generation EGFR-TKIs. However, the sensitivity to the combination of first- and third-generation EGFR TKIs is still to be explored. Conversely, when the T790M and C797S mutations are in a *cis* configuration (within the same allele), cells exhibit resistance to all available EGFR-TKIs, whether used alone or in combination. Genetic testing of osimertinib-resistant patients has revealed that the *cis* configuration of T790M and C797S mutations is rare, while the *trans* configuration occurs more frequently and is associated with higher occurrence rates [57].

The three generations of EGFR-TKIs targeted the ATP-binding pocket of EGFR, making them ATP-competitive inhibitors. However, the issue of drug resistance caused by the mutability of the ATP pocket inevitably affects the therapeutic efficacy. The allosteric sites of target proteins provide a new approach to combat kinase resistance [58−60] (Fig. 16.38). Allosteric sites exhibit structural diversity and conformational inducibility among members of the target protein family, which can overcome the problem of poor selectivity of the ATP-competitive inhibitors. Therefore, the use of non-ATP-competitive inhibitors holds promise for reversing C797S-mediated drug resistance.

Based on the three-dimensional structure of proteins, a class of allosteric EGFR inhibitors, **EAI-045** and **JBJ-04-125-02**, which primarily target the allosteric sites of EGFR, were developed by the Dana-Farber Cancer Institute at Harvard Medical School [61,62]. These inhibitors, in combination with cetuximab, have been investigated for the treatment of NSCLC with the C797S mutation. Currently, such allosteric inhibitors are in the phase of clinical trials (Fig. 16.39).

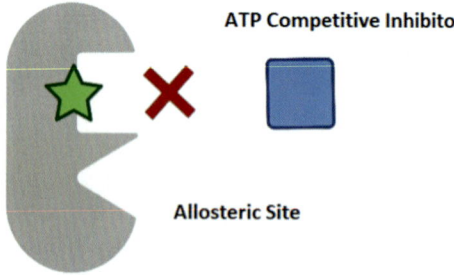
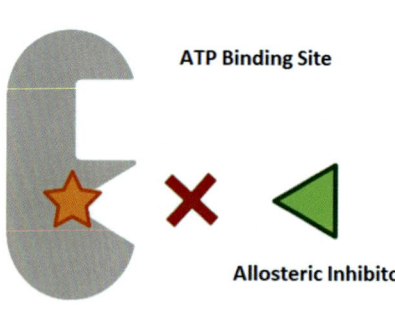

FIGURE 16.38 Schematic representation of the binding modes of ATP-competitive inhibitors and allosteric inhibitors.

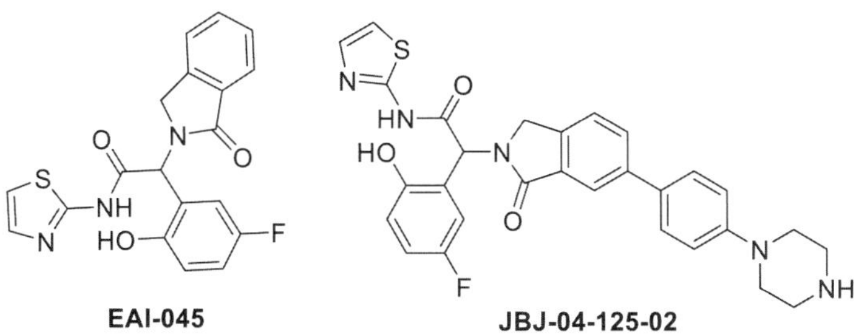

FIGURE 16.39 The structure of EGFR allosteric inhibitors **EAI-045** and **JBJ-04-125-02**.

References

[1] Ogiso H, Ishitani R, Nureki O, et al. Crystal structure of the complex of human epidermal growth factor and receptor extracellular domains. Cell 2002;110(6):775.
[2] Seshacharyulu P, Ponnusamy MP, Haridas D, et al. Targeting the EGFR signaling pathway in cancer therapy. Expert Opin Ther Targets 2012;16(1):15.
[3] Goffin JR, Zbuk K. Epidermal growth factor receptor: pathway, therapies, and pipeline. Clin Ther 2013;35(9):1282.
[4] Irmer D, Funk JO, Blaukat A. EGFR kinase domain mutations-functional impact and relevance for lung cancer therapy. Oncogene 2007;26(39):5693.
[5] Ke EE, Wu YL. EGFR as pharmacological target in EGFR-mutant non-small-cell lung cancer: where do we stand now? Trends Pharmacol Sci 2016;37(11):887.
[6] Lynch TJ, Bell DW, Sordella R, et al. Activating mutations in the epidermal growth factor receptor underlying responsiveness of non-small-lung cancer to gefitinib. N Engl J Med 2004;350(21):2129.
[7] Cohen MH, Williams GA, Sridhara R, et al. United States Food and Drug Administration Drug Approval summary: Gefitinib (ZD1839: Iressa) tablets. Clin Cancer Res 2004;10(4):1212.
[8] Zhou C, WU YL, Chen G, et al. Erolitinib versus chemotherapy as first-line treatment for patients with advanced EGFR mutation-positive non-small-cell lung cancer (OPTIMAL, CTONG-0802): a multi-center, open-label, randomized, phase 3 study. Lancet Oncol 2011;12(8):735.
[9] Shi Y, Zhang L, Liu X, et al. Icotinib versus gefitinib in previously treated advanced non-small-cell lung cancer (ICOGEN): a randomized, double-blind phase 3 non-inferiority trial. Lancet Oncol 2013;14(10):953.
[10] Kobayashi S, Boggon TJ, Dayaram T, et al. EGFR mutation and resistance of non-small-cell lung cancer to gefitinib. N Engl J Med 2005;352(8):786.
[11] Dong HR, Subiding T, Wang X, et al. Research progress of covalent inhibitors. Chin J Org Chem 2018;38(9):2296.
[12] Potashman MH, Duggan ME. Covalent modifiers: an orthogonal approach to drug design. J Med Chem 2009;52(5):1231.
[13] Barf T, Kaptein A. Irreversible protein kinase inhibitors: balancing the benefits and risks. J Med Chem 2012;55(14):6243.
[14] Gehringer M, Laufer SA. Emerging and re-emerging warheads for targeted covalent inhibitors: applications in medicinal chemistry and chemical biology. J Med Chem 2019;62(12):5673.
[15] Singh J, Petter RC, Baillie TA, et al. The resurgence of covalent drugs. Nat Rev Drug Discov 2011;10(4):307.
[16] Jackson PA, Widen JC, Harki DA, et al. Covalent modifiers: a chemical perspective on the reactivity of α, β-unsaturated carbonyls with thiols via hetero-Michael addition reactions. J Med Chem 2017;60(3):839.
[17] Narayanan A, Jones LH. Sulfonyl fluorides as privileged warheads in chemical biology. Chem Sci 2015;6(5):2650.
[18] Moss DE, Berlanga P, Hagan MM, et al. Methanesulfonyl fluoride (MSF): a double-blind, placebo-controlled study of safety and efficacy in the treatment of senile dementia of the Alzheimer type. Alzheimer Dis Assoc Discord 1999;13(1):20.
[19] Gushwa NN, Kang S, Chen J, et al. Selective targeting of distinct active site nucleophiles by irreversible Src-family kinase inhibitors. J Am Chem Soc 2012;134(50):20214.
[20] Haag SM, Gulen MF, Reymond L, et al. Targeting STING with covalent small-molecule inhibitors. Nature 2018;559(7713):269.
[21] Njoroge FG, Chen KX, Shih NY, et al. Challenges in modern drug discovery: a case study of boceprevir, an HCV protease inhibitor for the treatment of hepatitis C virus infection. Acc Chem Res 2008;41(1):50.
[22] Dorsey BD, Iqbal M, Chatterjee S, et al. Discovery of a potent, selective, and orally active proteasome inhibitor for the treatment of cancer. J Med Chem 2008;51(4):1068.
[23] Demo SD, Kirk CJ, Aujay MA, et al. Antitumor activity of PR-171, a novel irreversible inhibitor of the proteasome. Cancer Res 2007;67(13):638.
[24] Miller RM, Paavilainen VO, Krishnan S, et al. Electrophilic fragment-based design of reversible covalent kinase inhibitors. J Am Chem Soc 2013;135(14):5298.
[25] Krishnan S, Miller RM, Tian B, et al. Design of reversible, cysteine-targeted Michael acceptors guided by kinetic and computational analysis. J Am Chem Soc 2014;136(36):12624.
[26] Blair JA, Rauh D, Kung C, et al. Structure-guide development of affinity probes for tyrosine kinases using chemical genetics. Nat Chem Biol 2007;3(4):229.

[27] Leproult E, Barluenga S, Moras D, et al. Cysteine mapping in conformationally distinct kinase nucleotide binding sites: application to the design of selective covalent inhibitors. J Med Chem 2011;54(5):1347.
[28] Carmi C, Lodola A, Rivara S, et al. Epidermal growth factor receptor irreversible inhibitors: chemical exploration of the cysteine-trap portion. Mini-Rev Med Chem 2011;11(12):1019.
[29] Fry DW, Bridges AJ, Denny WA, et al. Specific, irreversible inactivation of the epidermal growth factor receptor and erbB2, by a new class of tyrosine kinase inhibitor. Proc Natl Acad Sci USA 1998;95(20):12022.
[30] Smaill JB, Showalter HDH, Zhou H, et al. Tyrosine kinase inhibitors. 18. 6-Substituted 4-anilinoquinazolines and 4-anilinopyrido[3,4-d] pyrimidines as soluble, irreversible inhibitors of the epidermal growth factor receptor. J Med Chem 2001;44(3):429.
[31] Xia G, Chen W, Zhang J, et al. A chemical tuned strategy to develop novel irreversible EGFR-TK inhibitors with improved safety and pharmacokinetic profiles. J Med Chem 2014;57(23):9889.
[32] Discafani CM, Carroll ML, Floyd MB, et al. Irreversible inhibition of epidermal growth factor receptor tyrosine kinase with in vivo activity by N-[4-(3-bromophenyl) amino]-6-quinazolinyl]-2-butyamide (CL-387,875). Biochem Pharmacol 1999;57(8):917.
[33] Wood ER, Shewchuk LM, Ellis B, et al. 6-Ethynylthieno[3,2-d]-and 6-enhynylthieno[2,3-d]pyrimidin-4-anilines as tunable covalent modifiers of ErbB kinases. Proc Natl Acad Sci USA 2008;105(8):2773.
[34] Carmi C, Cavazzoni A, Vezzosi S, et al. Novel irreversible epidermal growth factor receptor inhibitors by chemical modulation of the cysteine-trap portion. J Med Chem 2010;53(5):2038.
[35] Waterson AG, Petrov KG, Homberger KR, et al. Synthesis and evaluation of aniline headgroups for alkynyl thienopyrimidine dual EGFR-ErbB-2 kinase inhibitors. Bioorg Med Chem Lett 2009;19(5):1332.
[36] Carmi C, Galvani E, Vacondio F, et al. Irreversible inhibition of epidermal growth factor receptor activity by 3-aminopropanamides. J Med Chem 2012;55(5):2251.
[37] Singh J, Dobrusin EM, Fry DW, et al. Structure-based design of a potent, selective and irreversible inhibitor of the catalytic domain of the erbB receptor subfamily of protein tyrosine kinases. J Med Chem 1997;40(7):1130.
[38] Antonello A, Tarozzi A, Morroni F, et al. Multitarget-directed drug design strategy: a novel molecule designed to block epidermal growth factor receptor (EGFR) and to exert proapoptotic effects. J Med Chem 2006;49(23):6642.
[39] Ban HS, Usui T, Nabeyama W, et al. Discovery of boron-conjugated 4-anilinoquinazoline as a prolonged inhibitor of EGFR tyrosine kinase. Org Biomol Chem 2009;7(21):4415.
[40] Rablen PR. Large effect on borane dissociation energies resulting from coordination by Lewis bases. J Am Chem Soc 1997;119(35):8350.
[41] Cheng W, Zhu S, Ma X, et al. Design, synthesis and biological evaluation of 6-(nitroimidazole-1H-alkyloxyl)-4-anilinoquinazolines as efficient EGFR inhibitors exerting cytotoxic effects both under normoxia and hypoxia. Eur J Med Chem 2015;89:826.
[42] Palmer BD, Trumpp-kallmeyer S, Fry DW, et al. Tyrosine kinase inhibitors. 11. Soluble analogues of pyrrolo- and pyrazoloquiniazolines as epidermal growth factor receptor inhibitors: synthesis, biological evaluation, and modeling of the mode of binding. J Med Chem 1997;40(10):1519.
[43] Wissner A, Mansour TS. The development of HKI-272 and related compounds for the treatment of cancer. Arch Pharm Chem Life Sci 2008;341(8):465.
[44] Tsou HR, Mamuya N, Johnson BD, et al. 6-Substituted-4-(3-bromophenylamino)quinazolines as putative irreversible inhibitors of the epidermal growth factor receptor (EGFR) and human epidermal growth factor receptor (HER2) tyrosine kinases with enhanced antitumor activity. J Med Chem 2001;44(17):2719.
[45] Wissner A, Overbeek E, Reich MF, et al. Synthesis and structure-activity relationships of 6,7-disubstituted 4-anilinoquinoline-3-carbonitriles. The design of an orally active, irreversible inhibitor of the tyrosine kinase activity of the epidermal growth factor receptor (EGFR) and the human epidermal growth factor-2 (HER2). J Med Chem 2003;46(17):49.
[46] Smaill JB, Rewcastle GW, Loo JA, et al. Tyrosine kinase inhibitors. 17. Irreversible inhibitors of the epidermal growth factor receptor: 4-(Phenylamino) quinazoline- and 4-(phenylamino) pyrido[3,2-d] pyrimidine-6-acrylamides bearing additional solubilizing functions. J Med Chem 2000;43(7):1380.
[47] Li D, Ambrogio L, Shimamura T, et al. BIBW2922, an irreversible EGFR/HER2 inhibitor highly effective in preclinical lung cancer models. Oncogene 2008;27(34):4702.
[48] Himmelsbach F, Langkopf E, Blech S, et al. Quinazoline derivatives as inhibitors of human EGF tyrosine kinase. WO2002050043, 2002. (b) Solca F, Amelsberg A, Stehle G, et al. Quinazoline derivatives for the treatment of cancer diseases. US8404697, 2013.
[49] Katakami N, Atagis S, Goto K, et al. LUF-lung 4: a phase II trial of afatinib in patients with advanced non-small-cell lung cancer who progressed during prior treatment with erlotinib, gefitinib, or both. J Clin Oncol 2013;31(27):3335.
[50] Sequist LV, Yang JCH, Yamamoto N, et al. Phase III study of afatinib or cisplatin plus pemetrexed in patients with metastatic lung adenocarcinoma with EGFR mutations. J Clin Oncol 2013;31(27):3327.
[51] Yu S, Dirat O, Early and late-stage process development for the manufacture of dacomitinib. Comprehensive Accounts of Pharmaceutical Research and Development: From Discovery to Late-Stage Process Development Volume 1, Chapter 9, 235-252. ACS Symposium Series, Vol. 1239.
[52] Zhou W, Ercan D, Chen L, et al. Novel mutant-selective EGFR kinase inhibitors against EGFR^{T790M}. Nature 2009;462(7276):1070.
[53] Nagasaka M, Zhu VW, Lim SM, et al. Beyond osimertinib: the development of third-generation EGFR tyrosine kinase inhibitors for advanced EGFR$^+$ NSCLC. J Thorac Oncol 2021;16(5):740.

[54] Finlay MRV, Anderton M, Ashton S, et al. Discovery of a potent and selective EGFR inhibitor (AZD9291) of both sensitizing and T790M resistance mutations that spares the wild type form of the receptor. J Med Chem 2014;57(20):8249.

[55] Carlisle JW, Ramaligam SS. Role of osimertinib in the treatment of EGFR-mutation positive non-small-cell lung cancer. Future Oncol 2019;15(8):805.

[56] Yang JCH, Camidge DR, Yang CT, et al. Safety, efficacy, and pharmacokinetics of almonertinib (HS-10296) in pretreated patients with EGFR-mutated advanced NSCLC: a multicenter, open-label, phase 1 trial. J Thorac Oncol 2020;15(12):1907.

[57] Thress KS, Paweletz CP, Felip E, et al. Acquired EGFR [C797S] mutation mediates resistance to AZD9291 in non-small cell lung cancer harboring EGFR [T790M]. Nat Med 2015;21(6):560.

[58] Lu S, Li S, Zhang J. Harnessing allostery: a novel approach to drug discovery. Med Res Rev 2014;34(6):1242.

[59] Lu S, Shen Q, Zhang J. Allosteric methods and their applications: facilitating the discovery of allosteric drugs and the investigation of allosteric mechanism. Acc Chem Res 2019;52(2):492.

[60] Pisa R, Kapoor TM. Chemical strategies to overcome resistance against targeted anticancer therapeutics. Nat Chem Biol 2020;16(8):817.

[61] Jia Y, Yun CH, Park E, et al. Overcoming EGFR(T790M) and EGFR(C797S) resistance with mutant-selective allosteric inhibitors. Nature 2016;534(7605):129.

[62] To C, Jang J, Chen T, et al. Single and dual targeting of mutant EGFR with an allosteric inhibitor. Cancer Discov 2019;9(7):926.

Chapter 17

Medicinal chemistry and process development of the antibreast cancer drug tamoxifen

Hai-Bing Zhou[1,2] and Xiaoyu Ma[1,2]

[1]*Department of Hematology, Zhongnan Hospital of Wuhan University, Wuhan, P.R. China,* [2]*School of Pharmaceutical Sciences, Wuhan University, Wuhan, P.R. China*

Chapter outline

17.1 Estrogen receptors and breast cancers	**419**
17.1.1 Breast cancer	419
17.1.2 Estrogens and estrogen receptors	420
17.1.3 Estrogen receptor-positive breast cancer and drug targets	422
17.1.4 Selective estrogen receptor modulators	422
17.2 The medicinal chemistry of the selective estrogen receptor modulator tamoxifen	**423**
17.2.1 Discovery of tamoxifen — serendipity and opportunity	423
17.2.2 The mechanism of action and structure-activity relationship of tamoxifen	425
17.2.3 Structure-activity relationship of tamoxifen	427
17.2.4 In vivo metabolic characteristics of tamoxifen	432
17.2.5 Tamoxifen drug interactions	435
17.2.6 Synthesis and process of tamoxifen	435
17.3 Clinical investigations of tamoxifen	**438**
17.3.1 Clinical indications of tamoxifen	438
17.3.2 Studies on tamoxifen resistance	439
17.3.3 Adverse reactions of tamoxifen	442
17.4 Summary, knowledge expansion, and references	**442**
17.4.1 Historical significance of tamoxifen	442
17.4.2 Other drugs targeting estrogen receptor pathway for breast cancer treatment	443
References	**445**

17.1 Estrogen receptors and breast cancers

17.1.1 Breast cancer

Breast cancer is a malignancy that originates from breast tissue, with the earliest recorded cases dating back to around 1600 BCE. The ancient Egyptians documented numerous instances of breast cancer, inscribing them on stone walls and papyrus scrolls. Similar records of breast cancer have also been found in ancient Greece and Rome [1].

Whether in developed or developing countries, breast cancer remains the most common malignant tumor in women, posing a significant threat to their physical well-being [2]. According to the latest statistics, there were approximately 2.26 million new cases of breast cancer worldwide in 2020, surpassing lung cancer (2.21 million cases) for the first time and becoming the leading cancer globally. Breast cancer constitutes around 25% of all female cancer cases and ranks first in terms of mortality, accounting for 15% of all cancer deaths among women. China is a major breast cancer country, with about 420,000 new cases in 2020, causing nearly 120,000 deaths [3].

Based on the expression of hormone receptors (HR) and human epidermal growth factor receptor 2 (HER2), breast cancer is classified into different subtypes as follows:

1. Luminal A subtype: Hormone receptor positive/human epidermal growth factor receptor negative (HR^+/$HER2^-$) breast cancer.

2. Luminal B subtype: Hormone receptor positive/human epidermal growth factor receptor 2 positive ($HR^+/HER2^+$) breast cancer.
3. HER2-enriched subtype: Hormone receptor negative/human epidermal growth factor receptor 2 positive ($HR^-/HER2^+$) breast cancer.
4. Basal-like subtype: Hormone receptor negative/human epidermal growth factor receptor 2 negative ($HR^-/HER2^-$) breast cancer, also known as triple-negative breast cancer.

Among them, estrogen receptor (ER) positive patients (ER^+ breast cancer) account for approximately 70% of all breast cancer cases [4].

In the early days, there were limited regimens available for the effective treatment of breast cancer, and the disease was often regarded as incurable. Fortunately, while society progressed and there was a continuous understanding of breast cancer in depth, the range of treatment options expanded, leading to significant therapeutic outcomes. The primary treatment modalities currently include surgical intervention, radiation therapy, chemotherapy, and endocrine therapy. Since ER^+ breast cancer comprises around 70% of all breast cancer patients, endocrine therapy targeting the ER signaling pathway has become one of the mainstay approaches in clinical management [5].

Endocrine therapy, also known as hormone therapy, capitalizes on the close relationship between certain cancers and abnormal hormone levels. It involves the administration of hormones or hormone antagonists to modify the specific physiological conditions on which tumor growth depends, thereby inhibiting cancer progression. The roots of endocrine therapy for breast cancer can be traced back to 1836, when Cooper observed a correlation between tumor growth and the menstrual cycle. From 1896 to 1901, Beatson reported favorable outcomes in three advanced breast cancer cases treated with oophorectomy; Boyd performed the first combined oophorectomy and mastectomy for breast cancer. In 1905, Lett reported the results of a clinical investigation involving 99 breast cancer patients treated with oophorectomy and demonstrated the therapeutic efficacy of removing hormone-related tissues in patients. These findings establish a clear link between breast cancer and endogenous hormones. Subsequently, in 1944, Haddow discovered that high-dose synthetic estrogens yielded favorable therapeutic effects in advanced breast cancer patients, and at the same time, Nathanson reported the beneficial effects of diethylstilbestrol in advanced patients. These studies revealed the close association between estrogen and breast cancer. With further research on estrogen-related mechanisms and the development of related small molecule drugs, selective estrogen receptor modulators (SERMs), such as tamoxifen, have been extensively employed as targeted endocrine therapies for breast cancer since 1980 [6].

17.1.2 Estrogens and estrogen receptors

Estrogens are vital endocrine hormones present in the human body. Estrogens play a regulatory role in nearly all cells, tissues, and organs, particularly in the endocrine system, bone tissue [7,8], the nervous system [9,10], and the cardiovascular system [11]. Previously, it was believed that estrogens only played key roles in promoting and maintaining female reproductive and secondary sexual characteristics. However, a recent study has also revealed their significant contributions to normal physiological activities in males [12].

Endogenous estrogens primarily include estrone, estradiol (E_2), and estriol (Fig. 17.1). Estrone and estradiol are directly secreted by the ovaries in females, and estriol is a metabolite of estrone and estradiol. Among these three hormones, estradiol exhibits the most effective activity, while estrone and estriol have approximately 1/3 and 1/10 activity of estradiol, respectively [13].

Estrogens exert their biological effects through various signaling pathways, primarily mediated by ER (Fig. 17.2), which play a crucial role in their physiological regulation. This process can be divided into four steps: (1) Extracellular estrogens, such as estradiol, enter the cell nucleus and selectively bind to ER to form a complex of ER ligand receptors.

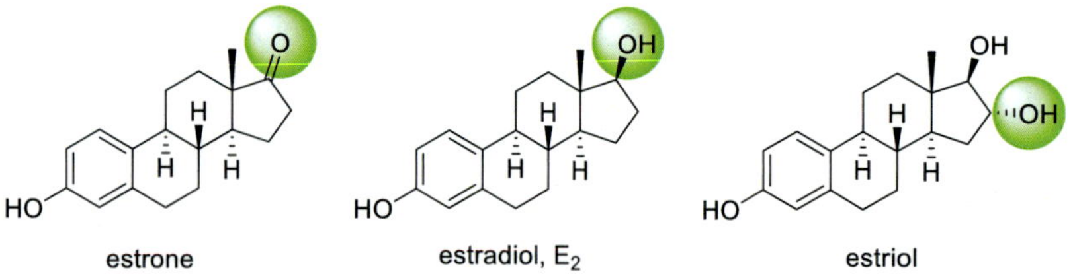

FIGURE 17.1 Endogenous estrogens estrone, estradiol, and estriol.

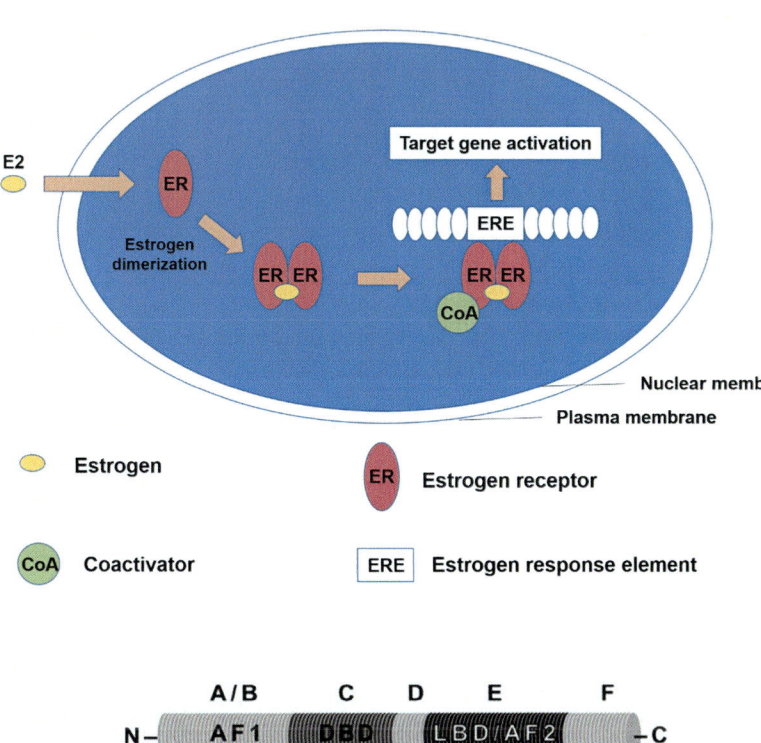

FIGURE 17.2 The mechanism and functional domains of estrogen receptors in the biological effects of estrogen.

(2) Subsequently, the conformation changes of the ER were induced, leading to the formation of homodimers or heterodimers and activation of the ER. (3) Then, activated ER binds to specific coactivator molecules, forming a complex of ligand-receptor-coactivator. (4) This complex further binds to estrogen response elements located in the promoter region, initiating the expression and transcription of target genes. In addition, ER can also interact with other transcriptional regulators, such as Sp1 or the activating protein AP-1, to modulate the transcription process of genes.

ERs are a class of nuclear receptors that are structurally classified as A-E fragments and functionally defined as four regions (Fig. 17.2) [14]. The AB region constitutes the *N*-terminal transcriptional activation domain, known as AF-1 (activation function 1), which activates the transcription of target genes by interacting with basal transcription factors, other transcription factors, and cofactors. The C region is the deoxyribonucleic acid (DNA) binding domain (DBD), responsible for binding to DNA. The D region is the hinge domain, which is associated with ER dimerization. The E region is the ligand binding domain, plays a crucial role in the specific binding of estrogens or SERMs, and is also an important site for ER dimerization. Additionally, the terminal of the E region contains another structural domain, AF-2, which is a transcriptional activation domain, as well as AF-1. AF-2 and AF-1 synergistically regulate the activation of target gene expression by binding to ligands [15].

In the 1960s, Jensen revealed the ERα subtype [16], and lately, it was believed that there was only one subtype of ER until the ERβ subtype was identified in the 1990s, leading to a broader understanding of ER and ER signaling pathways [17]. Recent research has demonstrated the significant differences in the distribution and functions of ERα and ERβ subtypes in the human body. ERα is mainly found in the uterus and breast and is also present in the central nervous system, bone, and cardiovascular system, while ERβ is widely distributed in various tissues and organs, such as the colon, pancreas, prostate, and adipose tissue [18,19]. The ERα and ERβ share highly structural similarities. For instance, their DBDs and ligand binding domains have homologies of 95% and 59%, respectively, and exhibit similar affinities for ER ligands [20]. Functionally, ERα primarily promotes cell proliferation, which is considered one of the triggers for breast cancer, leading ERα to be regarded as an important target for therapeutic intervention. Although the research on the functions of ERβ is relatively limited, it is commonly believed to exert opposite effects to ERα, with reports that ERβ can inhibit cell proliferation and may have protective effects on the nervous system [21]. Therefore, the balance of estrogen plays a crucial role in maintaining the growth and health of humanity. Recent studies revealed that serious conditions, such as osteoporosis, leukemia, myocardial infarction, and neurodegenerative diseases, are associated with abnormal regulation of estrogen secretion and expression levels of ER in the body.

17.1.3 Estrogen receptor-positive breast cancer and drug targets

The induction of breast cancer by estrogen can typically be explained through the following two aspects:

1. Estrogen, *via* signaling pathways mediated by ER, upregulates the transcription activation or transcription inhibition of certain genes associated with cancer. This is the primary cause of estrogen-induced related cancers.
2. Estrogen metabolism involves a series of redox reactions, generating a large number of oxygen-free radicals that cause lipid and genetic information oxidation damage and mutations [22–24].

The estrogen signaling pathway is one of the main causes of breast cancer. Based on the estrogen signaling pathway, three treatment targets related to breast cancer have been identified, and their drugs or small molecule modulators have been developed, as depicted in Fig. 17.3, including (1) aromatase inhibitors (AIs), which inhibit the endogenous synthesis pathway of estrogen, thereby reducing the levels of estrogen in the body and mitigating the ER overexpression-related diseases in tissues and organs; (2) drugs that act on the ER primarily, which include anti-estrogen agents known as SERMs, selective ER downregulators (SERDs), and estrogenic dimers; and (3) coactivator binding inhibitors, which suppress the binding of ligand-receptor complexes to coactivators, thereby preventing subsequent gene transcription and expression.

17.1.4 Selective estrogen receptor modulators

SERMs are structurally diverse compounds that bind to the ER and act as estrogen agonists or antagonists, depending on the target tissue and the hormone's internal environment. Ideally, SERMs should act as ER agonists in bone, liver, or the cardiovascular system and as ER antagonists in the mammary gland. They can elicit both ER agonist and antagonist effects in some tissues and organs, such as the uterus. This particular mechanism ensures, to the greatest extent possible, the safety of SERMs for other organs and tissues in the treatment of breast cancer. The selective effect of SERMs is mainly attributed to the following aspects:

1. The expression levels and distribution of ERα and ERβ are different in various tissues and organs. For instance, ERα and ERβ exhibit similar expression levels in breast cells and skeletal cells, albeit less pronounced compared to breast cells. ERα predominantly regulates the proliferative activity of uterine cells, while ERβ regulates that of prostate cells [25].
2. ERα and ERβ possess distinct physicochemical properties. ERα has a larger ligand-binding pocket; ERβ is more susceptible to inhibition by drugs, potentially due to the less stable conformation of the activated ERβ compared to ERα [26,27].
3. ERα and ERβ exert differential effects in different tissues.
4. Variations in the levels of coactivators and corepressors among different organs are significant [28].

Currently, there are four generations of SERMs being used in clinical practice: first-SERM such as tamoxifen and 4-hydroxytamoxifen (4-OHT); second-SERM including toremifene and raloxifene; third-SERM like lasofoxifene and bazedoxifene; and fourth-SERM such as acolbifene (Fig. 17.4).

The development of first-SERM, tamoxifen, has a milestone significance in targeted endocrine therapy for cancer, chemoprevention of breast cancer, and the advancement of this class of medications.

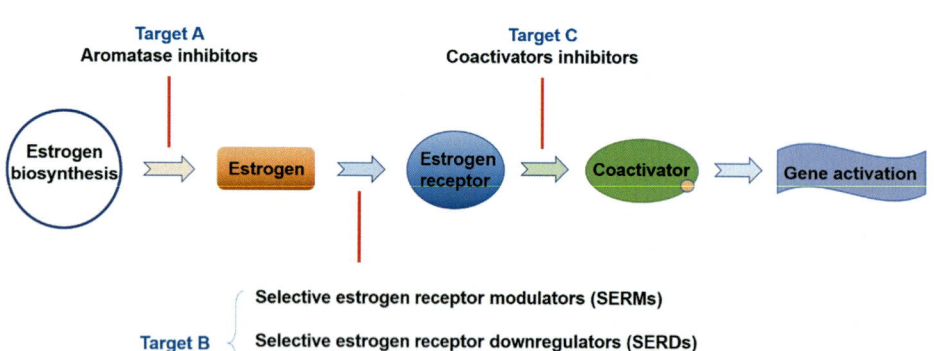

FIGURE 17.3 Targets and medications associated with the estrogen signaling pathway.

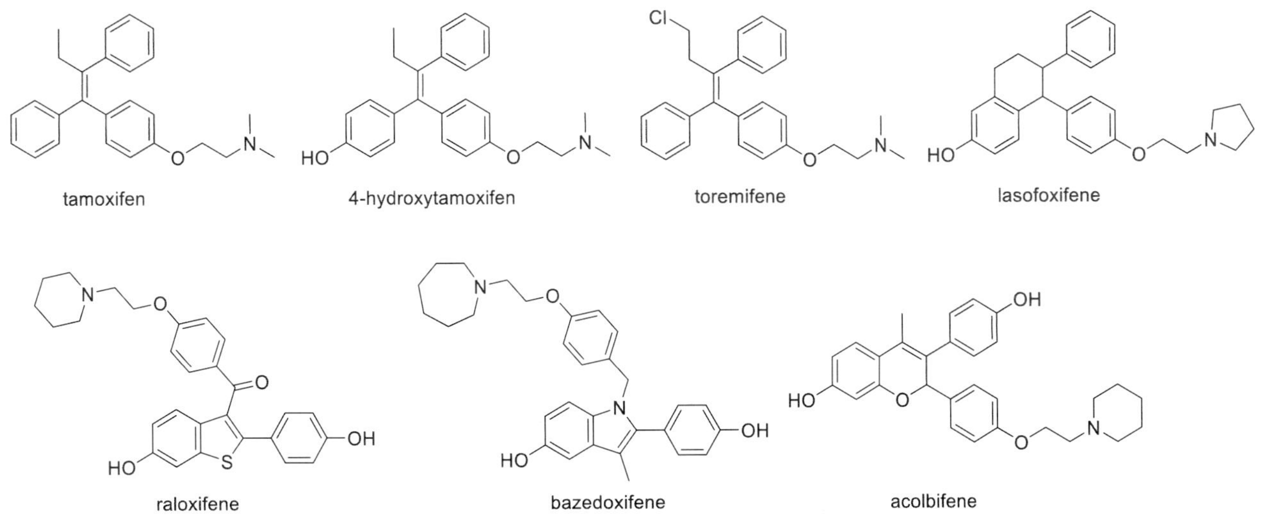

FIGURE 17.4 SERMs currently used in clinical practice.

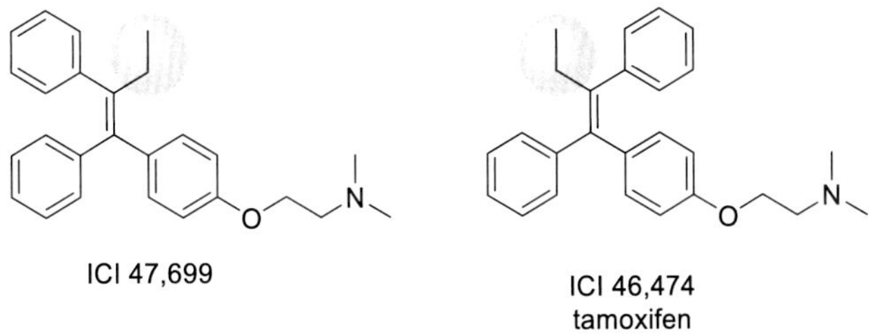

FIGURE 17.5 Tamoxifen (ICI 46,474) and isomer (ICI 47,699).

17.2 The medicinal chemistry of the selective estrogen receptor modulator tamoxifen

17.2.1 Discovery of tamoxifen — serendipity and opportunity

As a SERM, tamoxifen was approved by the United Kingdom's Medicines and Healthcare Products Regulatory Agency for the treatment of breast cancer in 1973. In the 1950s, contraceptive pills had a vast market in the United States, and scientists began to explore antiestrogenic drugs that could inhibit ovulation for human birth control plans. In 1958, Lerner discovered the first nonsteroidal antiestrogenic compound—MER25 (ethamoxy-triphetol), and observed its antifertility activity in animals. Subsequently, many pharmaceutical companies began synthesizing and screening compounds for postcoital contraception projects. In 1962, the Cheshire Royal Chemical Industry Pharmaceutical Division in the United Kingdom discovered a triphenylethylene compound in a fertility-related project led by Dr. Walpoleb and aimed to develop a new contraceptive. However, in vivo tests showed that this compound did not inhibit human ovulation but instead exhibited some ovulation-promoting effects.

In 1966, Harper et al. published a meaningful result revealing that the *cis* and *trans* isomers of the triphenylethylene structure possessed different or even opposite biological properties. This peculiar physiological phenomenon was demonstrated in animal studies. Further investigations showed that the *cis* isomer (ICI 47,699) could be considered a simple ER agonist, while the *trans* isomer (ICI 46,474, later named tamoxifen) exhibited complex ER agonistic or antagonistic activities (Fig. 17.5). In the rat, ICI 46,474 displayed weak estrogenic activity at low doses but exhibited significant antiendogenous and -exogenous estrogen effects at high doses. However, in mice, both isomers acted as ER agonists, with ICI 46,474 even demonstrating stronger agonistic effects.

Although the use of triphenylethylene as a contraceptive drug was not successful, fortunately, Dr. Walpole was also involved in the project of anticancer drug development. At the moment, scientists had already realized the potential association between estrogen and breast cancer and made an effort to synthesize the first batch of estrogen-like compounds, such as diethylstilbestrol (DES) and its diacetate. High doses of DES, dienestrol, and triphenylchlorethylene were used in clinical investigations for the treatment of breast cancer patients (Fig. 17.6). The results revealed that these estrogen-like compounds indeed exhibited a certain therapeutic effect on breast cancer. It is now known that high doses of estrogen-like compounds exert anticancer effects by producing negative feedback regulation on the release of

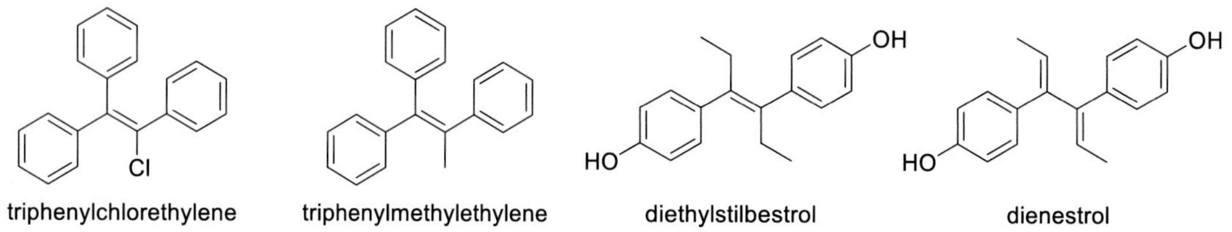

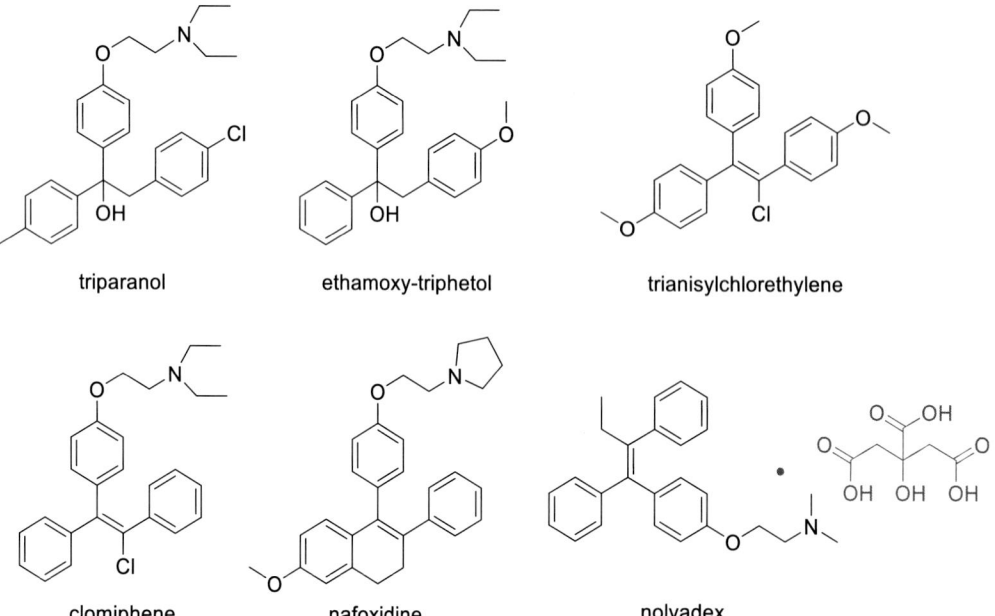

FIGURE 17.6 Nonsteroidal ICI estrogen drugs used in early clinical trials for breast cancer.

FIGURE 17.7 Early nonsteroidal antiestrogen drugs.

endogenous estrogens by the hypothalamus. This finally confirmed the correlation between estrogen and breast cancer, suggesting that the ER could be a potential therapeutic target for breast cancer. In the late 1960s, with a further understanding of the ER, it was realized that estrogen actually played a role in promoting the development of breast cancer.

As research on estrogen antagonists progressed, a number of nonsteroidal estrogen antagonists were synthesized and tested for biological activities. Ultimately, it was found that these hormone-like drugs had significant side effects. In 1950, Lerner and his colleagues reported the first nonsteroidal antiestrogen molecule, triparanol, which can clinically decrease cholesterol levels (Fig. 17.7). Triparanol had a similar molecule-skeleton to tamoxifen; however, it was found to be able to increase the circulating sterol levels and thus cause cataracts in young women, leading to its discontinuation in clinical use. Subsequently developed ER antagonists such as MER25 and clomiphene, also known as MRL41, were also discontinued due to their significant adverse effects. Under the persistence of Walpole and others, in 1974, ICI Pharmaceuticals agreed to continue research and further clinical investigations of ICI 46,474 for the treatment of breast cancer and as an ovulation inducer in the United Kingdom. Fortunately, results disclosed that ICI 46,474 was effective in the treatment of advanced breast cancer and had fewer adverse effects compared to the administration of high-dose hormone therapy. This study was a key milestone in the successful development of tamoxifen.

Another key person in the development of hormone-based antibreast cancer drugs is Dr. V.C. Jordan, who conducted pharmacological research related to triphenylethylene while in college. After obtaining his doctorate in pharmacology from the University of Leeds in 1972, he continued to explore the mechanism of action of ICI 46,474 with the support of the pharmaceutical division of ICI, actively promoting its clinical trial investigations because he confirmed the breast tumor survival that depends on the existing estrogen of tumor cells in mice. He observed that the tumor volume reduction in rats administered by ICI 46,474 specifically occurred in those ovaries surgically removed rats [29]. He believed that ICI 46 474 held promise as a pharmacological means of treating and preventing breast cancer, although this idea was still controversial at the time. Dr. Jordan further demonstrated that short-term administration of ICI 46,474 did not prevent tumor formation, but long-term administration could inhibit the development of breast tumors through a rat

TABLE 17.1 Development history of tamoxifen.	
1836	Cooper observed a correlation between tumor growth and the menstrual cycle.
1901	Boyd performed the first combined surgery of ovarian and breast removal for breast cancer, with positive postoperative results.
1905	Lett further confirmed a certain connection between breast cancer and endogenous hormones.
1944/1949	Haddow and Walpole discovered the beneficial effects of high doses of synthetic estrogens in advanced breast cancer.
1950s	Contraceptive pills had a significant market presence in the United States.
1958	Lerner identified the first nonsteroidal antiestrogen compound, MER2.
1962	The Walpole research team synthesized triphenylethylene, but it lacked contraceptive effects.
1966–1967	Harper discovered the selective action of triphenylethylene, specifically related to its *trans*-isomer ICI 46,474 and *cis*-isomer ICI 47,699.
1971	Klopper found that ICI 46,474 could even aid in fertility.
1971	Walpole and Cole initiated clinical trials of ICI 46,474 for treating breast cancer, showing promising results in late-stage breast cancer treatment.
1973	ICI designated ICI 46,474 as tamoxifen and obtained approval in the UK for breast cancer treatment.
1976	Jordan confirmed that ICI 46,474 could inhibit tumor cell growth in rats.
1977	The FDA approved tamoxifen for the treatment of late-stage diseases in postmenopausal women.
1980	Jordan discovered that long-term use of tamoxifen citrate could prevent the development of breast tumors.
1987–1992	Jordan found that ICI 46,474 had different regulatory effects on various human tissues, leading to its designation as a "selective estrogen receptor modulator."

tumor model at the University of Leeds [30]. In 1973, ICI named ICI 46,474 tamoxifen citrate (trade name Nolvadex) and received approval in the United Kingdom for the treatment of breast cancer. On December 30, 1977, the United States Food and Drug Administration (FDA) also approved tamoxifen for the treatment of advanced diseases in postmenopausal women, thus promoting its broader application in the treatment and prevention of breast cancer.

With the extensive promotion of this drug and further research, it became evident that estrogen played a critical role in the development of the cardiovascular system and bones in humans. Dr. Jordan and his colleagues began to worry about the potential adverse effects resulting from long-term estrogen deficiency caused by tamoxifen treatment. Fortunately, all subsequent research demonstrated that long-term use of tamoxifen not only did not lead to osteoporosis or heart disease, but it also appeared to reduce the incidence of osteoporosis and heart disease in rodent models [31]. Further studies revealed that each isomer of tamoxifen selectively exhibited estrogenic or antiestrogenic effects at specific sites. Therefore, these compounds were named SERMs. In his subsequent career, Dr. Jordan dedicated himself to the research of SERMs and drug resistance and further elucidated the relationship between estrogen and breast cancer [32]. Due to his outstanding contributions in the field of tamoxifen and SERM-based breast cancer treatment, he has been honored with numerous accolades and is referred to as the "Father of Tamoxifen" (Table 17.1).

17.2.2 The mechanism of action and structure-activity relationship of tamoxifen

17.2.2.1 Mechanism of tamoxifen binding to estrogen receptors

In 1946, Schueler proposed a hypothesis (Fig. 17.8) that compounds with estrogenic activity should be structurally similar to estradiol, i.e., they should have a rigid and inert skeleton with a large volume, and the distance between the two groups (phenolic or alcohol hydroxyl) capable of forming hydrogen bonds at both ends should be 14.5 Å, which would be able to mimic the binding of estradiol to the ER in vivo, and compounds that meet this distance should have estrogenic activity. For example, *trans*-diethylstilbestrol possesses this structural feature and is a class of ER agonists, while its *cis*-isomer has a corresponding distance of 7.2 Å and has no estrogenic activity.

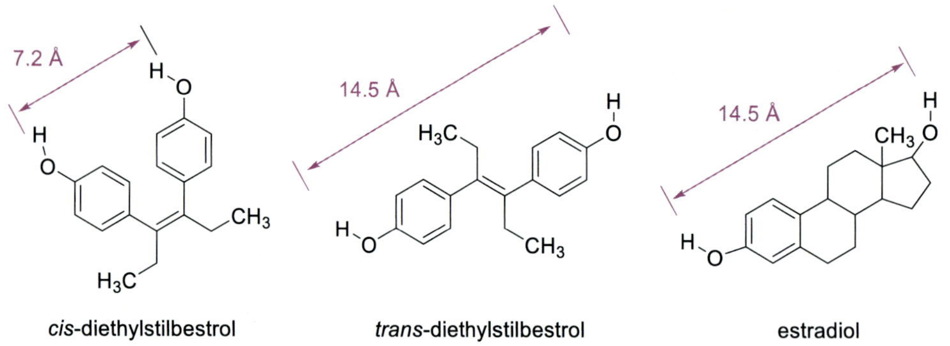

FIGURE 17.8 Comparison of the distance between estradiol hydroxyl and diethylstilbestrol hydroxyl groups.

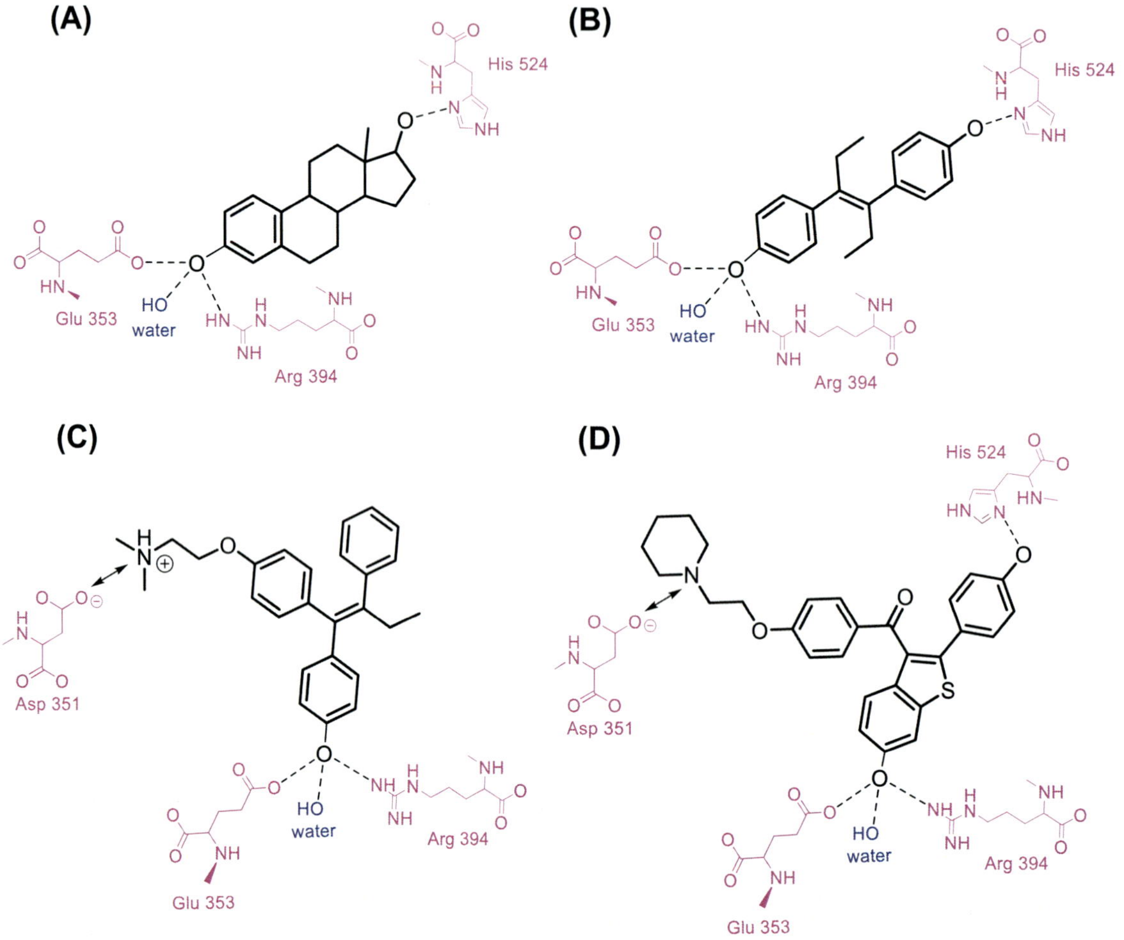

FIGURE 17.9 Comparison of the binding patterns between estradiol (A), *trans*-diethylstilbestrol (B), 4-hydroxytamoxifen (C), and raloxifene (D) with estrogen receptors.

In the complex formed by estradiol and ERα (Fig. 17.9A), the hydroxyl group at C_{17} of estradiol interacted with the His524 residue in the binding site of the ER, forming a hydrogen bond. Additionally, the hydroxy group at C_3 formed hydrogen bonds with Glu353, Arg394, and a water molecule. These tight interactions allowed estradiol to adopt a specific conformation upon binding to ERα, enabling subsequent gene regulation. Jordan's study in 1999 examined the crystal structure of *trans*-diethylstilbestrol (DES) binding to ERα (Fig. 17.9B), and DES effectively mimicked the binding mode of estradiol with ERα. In the binding mode of *trans*-DES, the two hydroxyl groups perfectly simulated the binding mode of estradiol with ERα, interacting with Glu353, Arg394, and His524 residues. This allowed *trans*-DES to exhibit estrogen-like activity. However, when comparing *trans*-DES with 4-hydroxytamoxifen (a major metabolite and active component of tamoxifen in the human body), it was observed that although the phenolic hydroxyl group in the structure of 4-hydroxytamoxifen could also effectively mimic the binding mode of estradiol with the ERα pocket, the lack of a second phenolic hydroxyl group prevented the formation of a corresponding interaction with ERα (Fig. 17.9C). Furthermore, the basic amino side chain of 4-hydroxytamoxifen extended to a different position and formed a new interaction with Asp351. Fig. 17.9D depicts the binding schematic of raloxifene, which is another SERM. Raloxifene, designed as a second-generation SERM based on the mechanism of tamoxifen and following Schueler's hypothesis, can be considered an analog of tamoxifen. Raloxifene retains the two crucial hydroxyl groups and the key basic amino side chain responsible for tamoxifen's antiestrogenic action while utilizing a benzothiophene structure to stabilize the *trans* isomer of tamoxifen, thus avoiding the issue of *cis-trans* isomerism. Similarly, in a study comparing *trans*-DES and 4-hydroxytamoxifen binding conformations to ERα (Fig. 17.9), it was found that the phenolic hydroxyl group of 4-hydroxytamoxifen exhibited similar interactions with *trans*-DES, simulating the hydrogen bonding with Glu353, Arg394, and a water molecule. However, due to the presence of the C ring and side chain in the structure, a series of amino acids in the binding pocket, such as Ala350, Asp351, and Trp383, underwent positional changes. This indicates that 4-hydroxytamoxifen induces a conformational difference in the ligand-binding pocket of ERα compared to estradiol and *trans*-DES, as observed in the secondary structure [33].

In fact, at the tertiary structure level, the mode of ER binding induced by 4-hydroxytamoxifen is also distinct from that of *trans*-diethylstilbestrol and estradiol. The ligand-binding domain (LBD) of the ER consists of twelve helices arranged in a sandwich-like structure, with a hydrophobic cavity in the middle for ligand binding and two parallel β-folds on either side. The spatial conformation of Helix12 (H12) plays a critical role in the receptor's agonistic or antagonistic activity. As shown in Fig. 17.10A, upon binding to estradiol, ERα undergoes a folding of H12, resulting in the formation of a hydrophobic pocket on the protein surface, which represents the agonist conformation. Subsequently, the receptor dimerizes and recruits coactivators or transcription factors to initiate gene regulatory processes. However, both tamoxifen and raloxifene possess a long basic side chain that can directly interact with H12. This basic side chain replaces the original position of H12, pushing it aside and preventing the formation of the hydrophobic pocket, thereby generating an antagonistic conformation. Consequently, the ligand-binding region fails to recruit transcriptional coactivators, leading to the loss of functions to initiate gene regulation (Fig. 17.10B and C) [34,35].

17.2.3 Structure-activity relationship of tamoxifen

17.2.3.1 Modifications on the nitrogen atom

The basic aminoalkyl chain on the triphenylethylene scaffold plays a pivotal role in the antiestrogenic activity of tamoxifen (Fig. 17.11). Agouridas et al. attempted to modify the basic aminoalkyl chain and synthesized a number of fluorinated derivatives of triphenylethylene in 2006 [36]. However, their activities were not satisfactory. For example, fluoride compounds **1a-c** exhibited binding affinities to the ERα approximately one order of magnitude lower than tamoxifen and almost completely lost their antagonistic activity against the ER, while nonfluorinated analogs **2a-c** showed binding potency comparable to tamoxifen. Based on the results, it was speculated that the trifluoromethyl substitution on the aminoalkyl chain in **1a-c** reduced the basicity of tamoxifen, thereby decreasing the binding ability to the ligand pocket and the inhibitory activity against ERα.

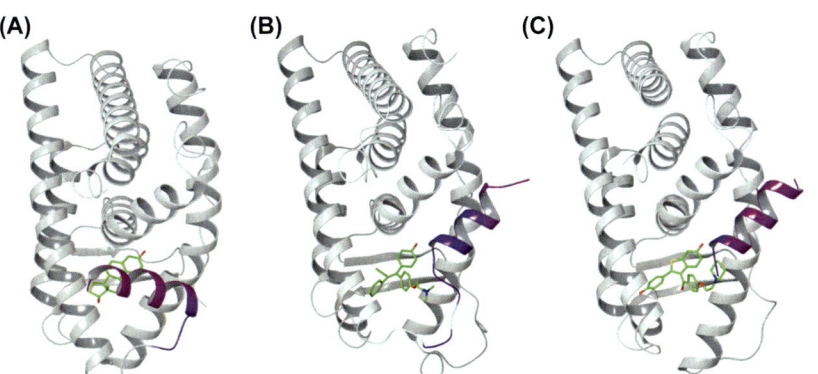

FIGURE 17.10 Complexes of ERα with estradiol (A), 4-hydroxytamoxifen (B), and raloxifene (C).

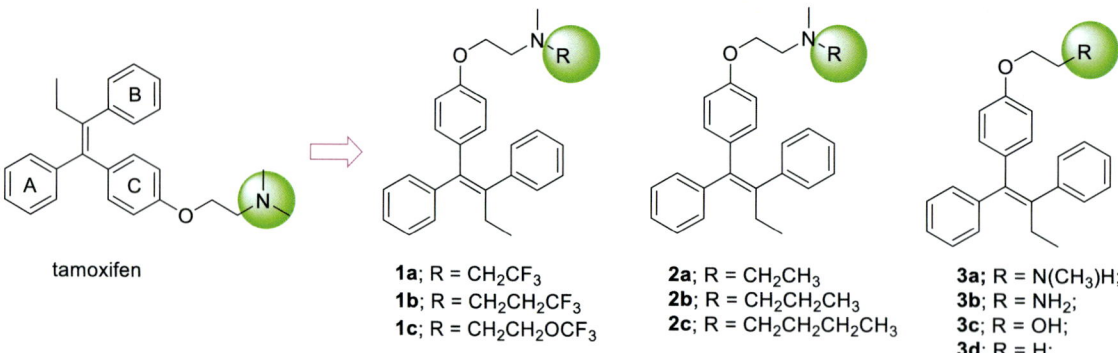

FIGURE 17.11 Derivatives of tamoxifen with structural modifications to the *N,N*-dimethyl moiety.

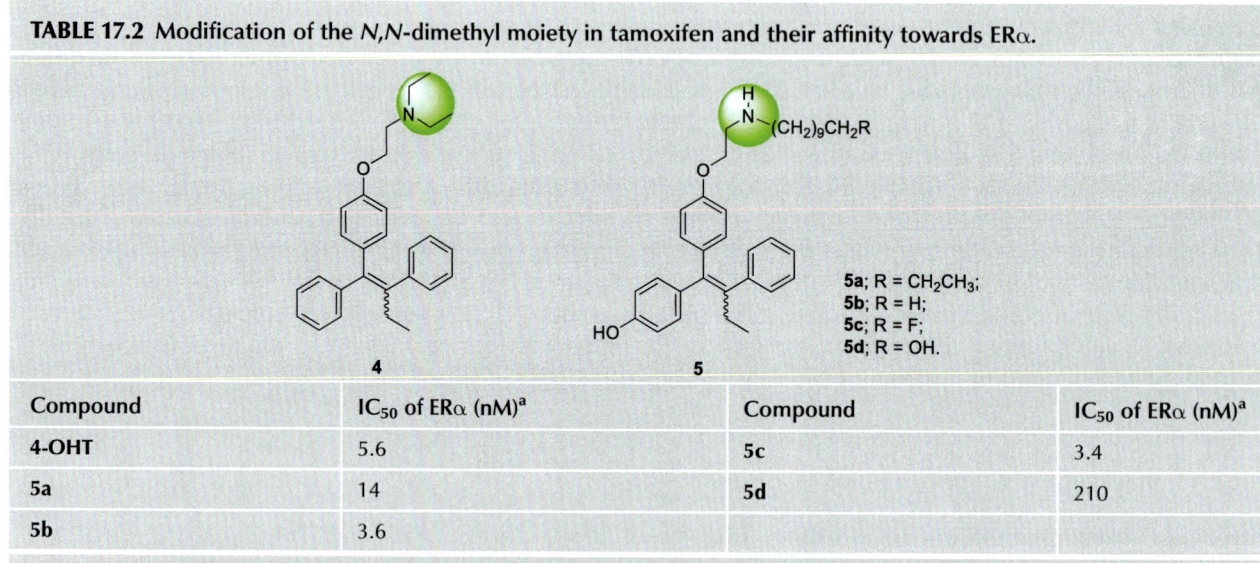

TABLE 17.2 Modification of the *N,N*-dimethyl moiety in tamoxifen and their affinity towards ERα.

Compound	IC$_{50}$ of ERα (nM)[a]	Compound	IC$_{50}$ of ERα (nM)[a]
4-OHT	5.6	5c	3.4
5a	14	5d	210
5b	3.6		

[a]Due to the diverse sources of activity data and variations in the types and values of the tested activities across different literatures and tables, it should note that the data may not be entirely consistent or standardized.

Furthermore, during the investigation of tamoxifen metabolites, it was found that removal of the methyl group from the nitrogen atom (compounds **3a-b**) or deletion of the *N,N*-dimethyl group (compounds **3c-d**) on the nitrogen atom gradually decreased the binding affinity to ERα, transforming them into weak ER antagonists [37]. These results indicated that the *N,N*-dimethyl group in the structure of tamoxifen is crucial for its antiestrogenic activity.

Compound **4**, as illustrated in Table 17.2, is a derivative of tamoxifen in which the *N*-methyl group has been replaced with an ethyl group. Affinity testing revealed that compound **4** exhibits approximately half the binding affinity to the ER compared to tamoxifen [38]. In 2004, Shoda et al. attempted to introduce a long alkyl chain on the amine group of 4-hydroxytamoxifen, aiming to induce protrusion in the ligand-binding pocket and destabilize the ER, thereby further inhibiting its interaction with coactivators. These modifications led to the synthesis of a group of SERDs with pure antagonistic activity, among which compound **5a** demonstrated the most potent activity. Compound **5b**, on the other hand, represents a further derivation of compound **5a**, exhibiting a binding affinity to ERα (IC$_{50}$ = 3.6 nM) comparable to that of 4-hydroxytamoxifen (IC$_{50}$ = 5.6 nM). Subsequently, the introduction of a fluorine atom at the end of the alkyl chain in compound **5c** resulted in an increased binding affinity to ERα (IC$_{50}$ = 3.4 nM), which enhanced the degradation activity toward ERα. Finally, the introduction of a hydrophilic hydroxyl group at the end of the alkyl chain led to compound **5d**, which exhibited decreased binding affinity to ERα (IC$_{50}$ = 210 nM) as well as diminished activity in degrading ERα protein. These findings demonstrated the critical role played by the long basic side chain of tamoxifen in its pharmacological activity [39,40].

17.2.3.1.1 Alteration of the aminoethoxy side chain

Compound **6** is a tamoxifen deoxy analog that exhibited antitumor growth activity similar to tamoxifen. Compound **7** is a metabolite found in canine bile in tamoxifen metabolism assays and exhibits a slightly weaker binding affinity for ERα than tamoxifen; however, compound **7** displays an ER agonistic activity [36]. Compound **8** is a derivative with the side chain removed and is a weaker ER agonist than compound **7** [41] (Fig. 17.12). These data, on the other hand, confirm that the aminoethoxy side chain of tamoxifen is essential for its antiestrogenic activity and that the triphenylethylene is converted into an agonist when the side chain disappears or only the phenolic hydroxyl group is retained.

17.2.3.1.2 Derivatives of tamoxifen with an A-ring substitution

Among the A-ring substituted compounds of tamoxifen, compound **9a** has about 100 times higher binding affinity for ERα than that of tamoxifen and is comparable to estradiol. Compound **9a** (4-hydroxytamoxifen), one of the major metabolites of tamoxifen, is also identified as the main active form of tamoxifen in humans. Compound **9b** (droloxifene) is a derivative of tamoxifen used in clinical practice that has been reported to have a 10- to 64-fold higher binding affinity for ERα than tamoxifen and exhibit a stronger antiestrogenic effect. Compound **9c** involves two hydroxyl groups on the A ring binding to ERα with a comparable binding affinity to that of estradiol. Compound **9d** displays a hydroxyl group that is not directly attached to the benzene ring, and its ERα binding affinity is 80 times that of tamoxifen and strongly promotes the proliferation of MCF-7 tumor cells through its ERα agonistic activity. Compound **9e** has a 20-fold higher ERα affinity and 100-fold higher antiproliferative activity than that of tamoxifen. Compound **9f** introduces a methyl substitution onto the A ring, resulting in reduced ERα affinity and antiproliferative activity. Compounds **9g-9j** are ER antagonists with binding affinity for ERα roughly 1–5 times higher than that of tamoxifen, and their anti-MCF-7 cell proliferative activity is comparable to that of tamoxifen, except for **9j**, which is significantly stronger than that of tamoxifen, like compound **9e**. Compound **9k** has an affinity for ERα comparable to that of tamoxifen but is a weak agonist [41] (Fig. 17.13).

These results demonstrate that A-ring substitution can significantly increase the binding affinity and antiproliferative activity of tamoxifen. The introduction of hydroxyl, iodine, and aldehyde groups shows the best effects, while the introduction of chlorine and fluorine has a minimal impact on activity. However, the introduction of a methyl group leads to a reversal of activity.

17.2.3.1.3 Tamoxifen derivatives with benzene ring modification

In 2003, Wenckens and colleagues replaced the phenyl group connected to the basic amino side chain in the structure of tamoxifen with an imidazole ring. Simultaneously, the B-ring was modified with substituted phenyl or heteroaromatic groups. The results disclose the obvious differences in ERα binding affinity depending on the position of the substituent in the imidazole ring. Most of the 4-substituted imidazoles exhibit good binding ability with ERα but are weaker than tamoxifen ($IC_{50} = 0.1\ \mu M$). The best one is compound **12d** ($IC_{50} = 0.2\ \mu M$). Compound **11**, which is structurally similar to tamoxifen, shows a lower binding affinity to ERα ($IC_{50} = 2.8\ \mu M$) than tamoxifen. Although

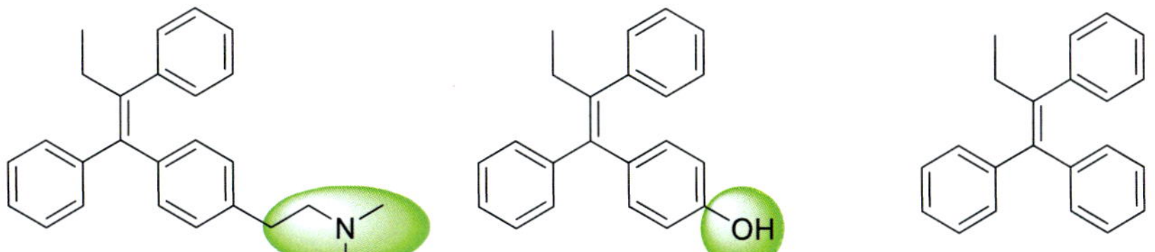

FIGURE 17.12 Derivatives of tamoxifen lacking the aminoethoxy side chain.

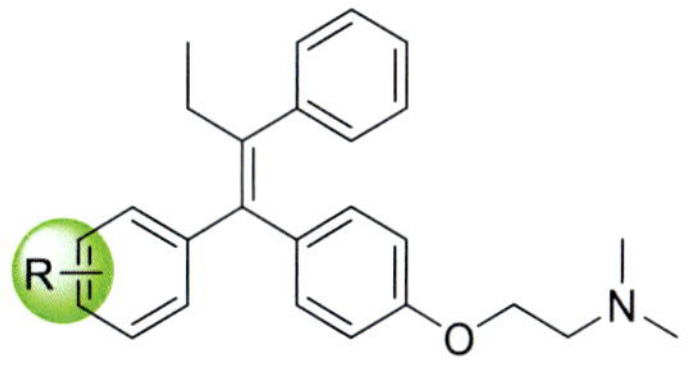

FIGURE 17.13 Tamoxifen derivatives with an A-ring substitution.

9a; R = 4-OH;
9b; R = 3-OH;
9c; R = 3,4-diOH;
9d; R = 4-CH$_2$OH;
9e; R = 4-CHO;
9f; R = 4-CH$_3$;
9g; R = 4-F;
9h; R = 4-Cl;
9i; R = 4-Br;
9j; R = 4-I;
9k; R = 4-SH.

compound **12a** exhibits better activity than compound **11**, its binding affinity (IC$_{50}$ = 1.1 μM) is still lower than that of tamoxifen. Most of these compounds display anti-MCF-7 cell growth comparable to tamoxifen, while their ERα binding affinities are lower than tamoxifen. This suggests that the 4-substituted imidazole derivatives of tamoxifen do not significantly affect its antiestrogenic activity. It is also observed that compound **13** does not exhibit anti-MCF-7 cell activity, possibly due to substantial changes in the side chain position [42] (Table 17.3).

17.2.3.1.4 Ethyl-modified tamoxifen derivatives

Compound **14a-d** and compound **15a-h** are derivatives of tamoxifen and 4-hydroxytamoxifen with ethyl modifications. Among them, **14a** exhibits binding affinity to ERα comparable to *trans*-tamoxifen but inferior inhibitory activity against ERα compared to tamoxifen [43]. Compound **14b** demonstrates antiproliferative activity against MCF-7, MDA-MB-231, M21, and HT-29 cells, which is equivalent to tamoxifen [44]. Compound **14c** exhibits 2−3 times higher binding affinity to ERα compared to tamoxifen [45]. Compound **14d**, which features an additional hydroxy group on the ethyl moiety, shows an obviously decreased binding affinity to ERα compared to tamoxifen [46].

When the ethyl group in the structure of 4-hydroxytamoxifen was replaced with chloroethyl, chloropropyl, etc., it was found that the binding affinity of compounds **15a** and **15c** for ERα was comparable to that of 4-hydroxytamoxifen and higher than that of compounds **15e** and **15g**, and the activities of other compounds showed a large decrease in comparison with that of 4-hydroxytamoxifen (Table 17.4). These results suggest that appropriate modification of the ethyl group of tamoxifen will have less overall effect on its ERα binding activity and antitumor cell proliferation activity, which is not as significant as that of other sites, but the group should not be too large [47].

17.2.3.1.5 Double-bonded immobilized tamoxifen derivatives

The structure of tamoxifen involves a double bond with two stereoisomers, *cis* and *trans*, that display opposite biological activities. This phenomenon has prompted medicinal chemists to develop antiestrogenic compounds without isomers. A large number of studies have been carried out to immobilize the double bond of tamoxifen using the cyclization approach. Some representative compounds are shown in Fig. 17.14. The results reveal that compound **16**, which cyclizes the ethyl group of tamoxifen on the same side of the double bond as the A ring, displays comparable ERα binding activity to that of tamoxifen and slightly better antiproliferative activity than tamoxifen in MCF-7 cells. Compounds **17a-b** are structurally similar to compound **16** and have antiproliferative activity close to, but slightly

TABLE 17.3 Structure and binding affinity of pyrazole derivatives of tamoxifen for ERα.

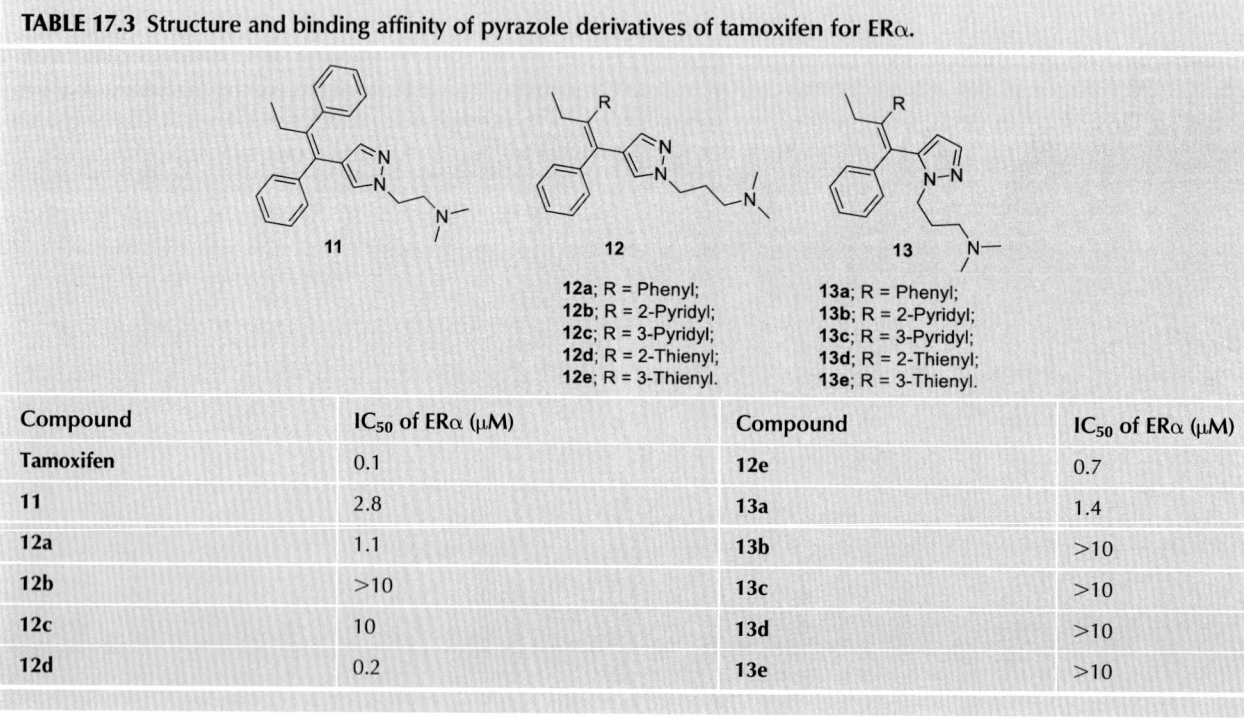

Compound	IC$_{50}$ of ERα (μM)	Compound	IC$_{50}$ of ERα (μM)
Tamoxifen	0.1	12e	0.7
11	2.8	13a	1.4
12a	1.1	13b	>10
12b	>10	13c	>10
12c	10	13d	>10
12d	0.2	13e	>10

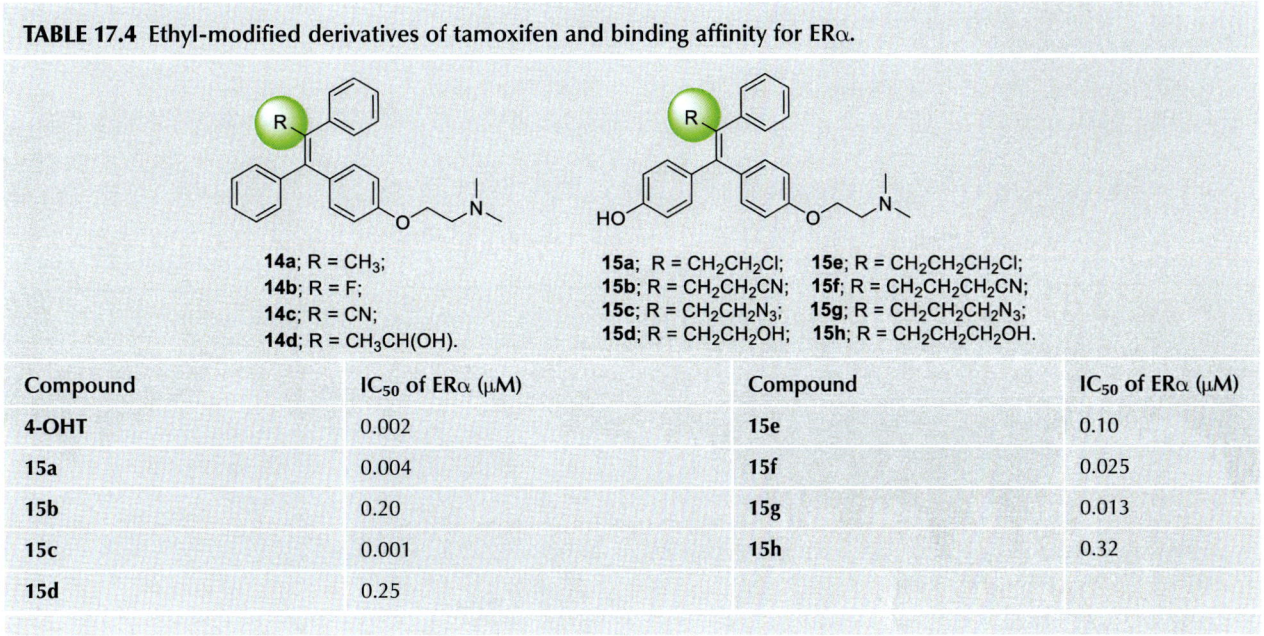

TABLE 17.4 Ethyl-modified derivatives of tamoxifen and binding affinity for ERα.

14a; R = CH₃;
14b; R = F;
14c; R = CN;
14d; R = CH₃CH(OH).

15a; R = CH₂CH₂Cl; 15e; R = CH₂CH₂CH₂Cl;
15b; R = CH₂CH₂CN; 15f; R = CH₂CH₂CH₂CN;
15c; R = CH₂CH₂N₃; 15g; R = CH₂CH₂CH₂N₃;
15d; R = CH₂CH₂OH; 15h; R = CH₂CH₂CH₂OH.

Compound	IC₅₀ of ERα (μM)	Compound	IC₅₀ of ERα (μM)
4-OHT	0.002	15e	0.10
15a	0.004	15f	0.025
15b	0.20	15g	0.013
15c	0.001	15h	0.32
15d	0.25		

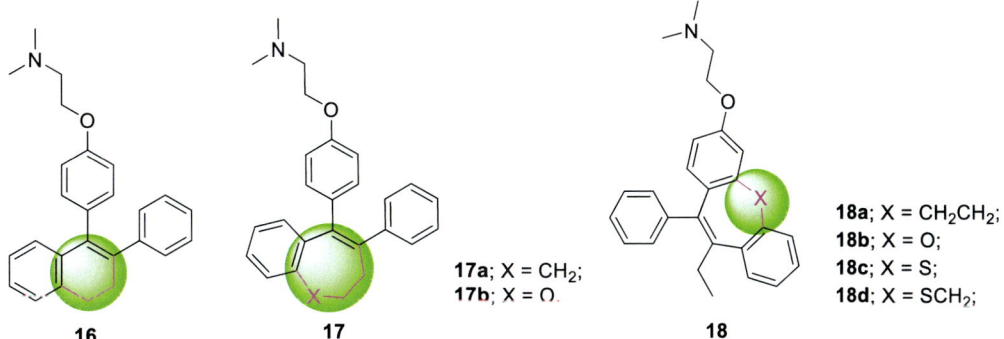

17a; X = CH₂;
17b; X = O.

18a; X = CH₂CH₂;
18b; X = O;
18c; X = S;
18d; X = SCH₂;

FIGURE 17.14 Tamoxifen derivatives with a fixed double bond.

weaker than, that of tamoxifen [48,49]. Compound **18** is cyclized on the other side of the double bond and has an obviously lower binding affinity for ERα. The binding affinity of compounds **18d** and **18b** are only 1/5 and 1/300 of that of tamoxifen, respectively, and the affinity of compounds **18a** and **18c** is about 1/50 − 1/20 of that of tamoxifen, suggesting that immobilizing the A-ring and ethyl group could avoid the creation of the *cis*-isomer and is probably more suitable for immobilizing the benzene ring than for immobilizing the structure of tamoxifen with a benzene ring on the other side of the double bond [50].

17.2.3.1.6 Double bond-reduced tamoxifen derivatives

Compounds **19** and **20** are products of tamoxifen following the reduction of the double bond (Fig. 17.15). Compound **19** is the metabolite A of tamoxifen with a 1/30 ERα binding affinity [51,52]. There are chiral isomers after the reduction of compound **20**, and all chiral isomers have a lower binding affinity than tamoxifen. These results indicate the importance of the double bond in tamoxifen, and saturation of it decreases the binding affinity of the molecule to the ER [53] (Fig. 17.15).

The structure-activity relationship of tamoxifen is summarized in Fig. 17.16. Of course, in addition to these patterns on the figure, the *trans*-isomer of tamoxifen is another key to the antiestrogenic effects of tamoxifen.

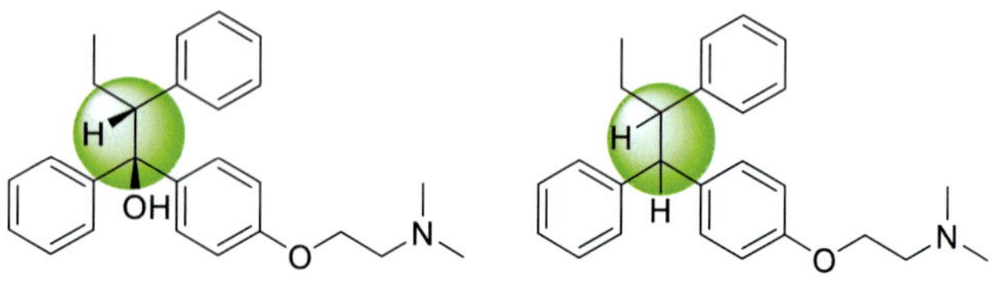

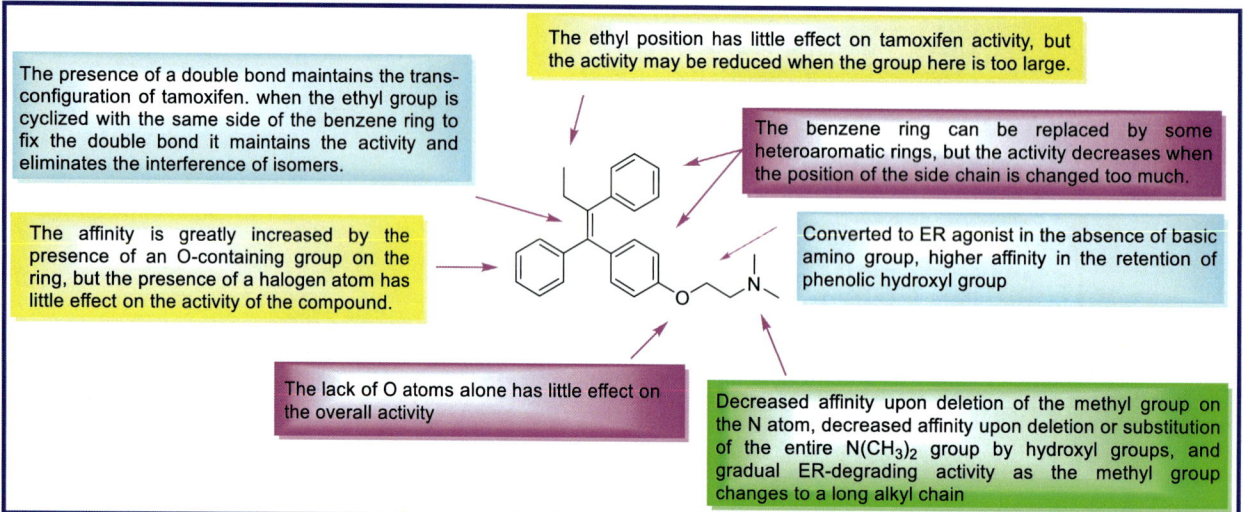

FIGURE 17.15 Tamoxifen derivatives with a reduced double bond.

FIGURE 17.16 Structure-activity relationship of tamoxifen.

17.2.4 In vivo metabolic characteristics of tamoxifen

Tamoxifen can be effectively absorbed after oral administration and is extensively metabolized in the body. Studies in rats and dogs revealed that, after oral administration, approximately 53% of tamoxifen passes through the bile as a conjugate out of the liver and into the intestine, followed by reabsorption of up to 69% of the tamoxifen conjugate through the hepatic-intestinal recirculation. Due to the hepatic-intestinal circulation and its high binding affinity to serum proteins, tamoxifen has a half-life of up to 7 days. The metabolites of tamoxifen in the body are shown in Table 17.5.

Table 17.6 shows the major pharmacokinetic parameters of three common SERM analogs. Tamoxifen citrate is rapidly absorbed after oral administration and has a high bioavailability, approaching 100%. Its maximum concentrations are reached in the blood in 6–7 hours. A second peak in the blood occurred on day 4 or later, probably caused by hepatic-intestinal circulation and high binding to serum proteins, which allows a half-life of up to 7 days. The structure of toremifene is similar to that of tamoxifen, and the pharmacokinetic indices are also similar to those of tamoxifen. Significantly different from toremifene and tamoxifen, raloxifene has a different metabolic pathway with much lower oral bioavailability and half-life, and the highest concentration is reached in the blood after 0.5 hour of oral administration.

In humans, tamoxifen is metabolized by hepatic cytochrome P450 enzymes to the active metabolites 4-hydroxytamoxifen and N-desmethyl-4-hydroxytamoxifen (4-hydroxy-N-desmethyltamoxifen/endoxifen, EDF) to exert its pharmacological effects (Fig. 17.17). These two metabolites have 30–100 times higher receptor binding capacity than tamoxifen and can effectively inhibit ER^+ breast cancer cells in humans [37,54,55].

The detailed metabolic process of tamoxifen is depicted in Fig. 17.18, involving several Phase I and Phase II metabolic enzymes involving CYP2D6, CYP3A4, and CYP3A5. Tamoxifen undergoes two main metabolic pathways in the liver, including: (1) approximately 40% of tamoxifen is metabolized via demethylation by CYP3A4 and CYP3A5 to form N-desmethyltamoxifen (N-DES-TAM). A portion of N-desmethyltamoxifen is further demethylated by CYP3A4 and CYP3A5 to generate N,N-didesmethyltamoxifen. Another portion of tamoxifen is hydroxylated by CYP2D6 to produce the more potent metabolite, N-desmethyl-4-hydroxytamoxifen. Due to structural changes caused by demethylation, N-desmethyl-4-hydroxytamoxifen exhibits a weaker affinity for ER. However, its antiestrogenic activity is 30 times

TABLE 17.5 Metabolites of tamoxifen in the body.

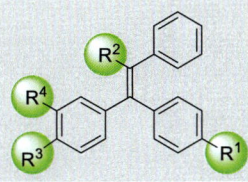

Compound	R₁	R₂	R₃	R₄
Tamoxifen	-O(CH₂)₂N(CH₃)₂	-C₂H₅	-H	-H
Metabolite A (ICI 46 929)	-O(CH₂)₂N(CH₃)₂	-C₂H₅	-H	-H
Metabolite B (ICI 79 280)	-O(CH₂)₂N(CH₃)₂	-C₂H₅	-OH	-H
Metabolite C	-O(CH₂)₂N(CH₃)₂	-C₂H₅	-OH	-OCH₃
Metabolite D (ICI 77 307)	-O(CH₂)₂N(CH₃)₂	-C₂H₅	-OH	-OH
Metabolite E (ICI 141 389)	-OH	-C₂H₅	-H	-H
Metabolite X (ICI 55 548)	-O(CH₂)₂NHCH₃	-C₂H₅	-H	-H
Metabolite Y (ICI 142 269)	-O(CH₂)₂OH	-C₂H₅	-H	-H
Metabolite Z (ICI 142 268)	-O(CH₂)₂NH₂	-C₂H₅	-H	-H
Metabolite N-oxide	-O(CH₂)₂N(CH₃)₂ (N→O)	-C₂H₅	-H	-H

TABLE 17.6 In vivo pharmacokinetics of tamoxifen with two SERMs drugs.

Characterization	Tamoxifen citrate	Toremifene	Raloxifene
Bioavailability	~100%	~100%	2%
CYP450 metabolizing enzyme	CYP2D6, CYP3A4/3A5	CYP3A	/[a]
Binding rate of plasma protein	97%	99.5%	98% – 99%
Half-life	5–7 day	5–6 day	27.7 h
T_{max}	6–7 h	2–4 h	0.5 h
Fecal excretion rate	92%	Main pathway	Main pathway
Urine excretion rate	4%	10%	<6%

[a]Raloxifene may not undergo metabolism via the CYP450 enzyme pathway.

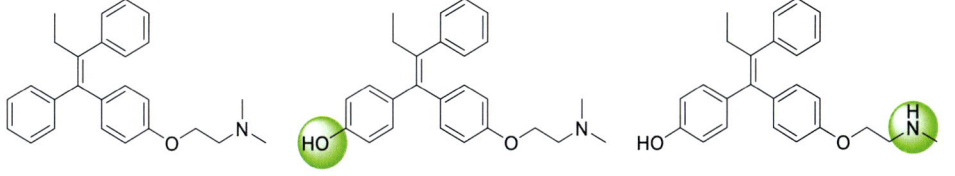

FIGURE 17.17 Tamoxifen and major active metabolites in vivo.

tamoxifen   4-Hydroxytamoxifen   endoxifen

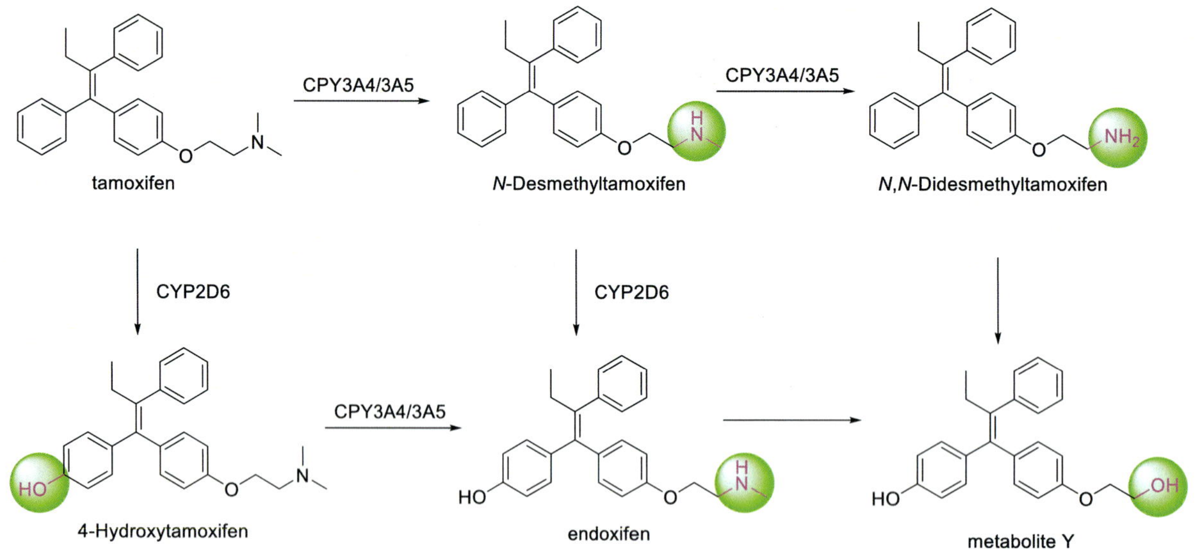

FIGURE 17.18 The main metabolic pathway of tamoxifen in the body.

higher than that of tamoxifen. (2) The alternative metabolic pathway involves the hydroxylation of tamoxifen by CYP2D6, leading to the formation of the more potent antiestrogenic metabolite, 4-hydroxytamoxifen (4-OH-TAM). 4-Hydroxytamoxifen can also be demethylated by CYP3A4 to generate N-desmethyl-4-hydroxytamoxifen. Similar to tamoxifen, both 4-hydroxytamoxifen and N-desmethyl-4-hydroxytamoxifen exist in *cis* and *trans* (or E/Z) configurations. Clinical investigations showed that the *trans* isomer is the primary metabolite responsible for the antiestrogenic effects of tamoxifen.

17.2.4.1 4-Hydroxytamoxifen (metabolite B)

Assays confirmed that 4-hydroxytamoxifen has a high binding capacity for ERα, which is about 100 times higher than that of the parent compound tamoxifen and is comparable to estradiol [56]. In addition, 4-hydroxytamoxifen possesses a stronger inhibitory effect on breast cancer cells, which is 50–100 times more potent than that of tamoxifen [57], but 4-hydroxytamoxifen has a shorter half-life in vivo compared with that of tamoxifen, and it is easily metabolized, which may affect its efficacy in vivo [30].

17.2.4.2 N-Desmethyltamoxifen

Initially, 4-hydroxytamoxifen was thought to be the major metabolite in patients; however, Adam et al. demonstrated that N-desmethyltamoxifen is also a major metabolite [58] and has a plasma half-life of approximately 14 days, which is twice that of tamoxifen [59]. It has been shown that the relative ERα binding affinity, antifertility activity, and antiestrogenic properties of N-desmethyl tamoxifen are comparable to, or slightly weaker than, the potency of tamoxifen, and its pharmacological effects are similar to those of tamoxifen [37].

17.2.4.3 N-Desmethyl-4-hydroxytamoxifen

N-Desmethyl-4-hydroxytamoxifen, a hydroxylated tamoxifen metabolite, is a potent antiestrogenic agent. Data indicate that, as an ER antagonist, N-desmethyl-4-hydroxytamoxifen has approximately 100 times the affinity and 30 times the inhibitory activity of the tamoxifen prodrug. Tamoxifen has some potency in inducing ER degradation when used, and it is the N-desmethyl-4-hydroxytamoxifen that induces ERα degradation at the transcriptional level that accounts for the potency. In humans, N-desmethyl tamoxifen is the major metabolite of tamoxifen, followed by N-desmethyl-4-hydroxytamoxifen and 4-hydroxytamoxifen tamoxifen, and the latter two are the main forms of tamoxifen that exert antiestrogenic effects and anticancer activity in humans [54,55].

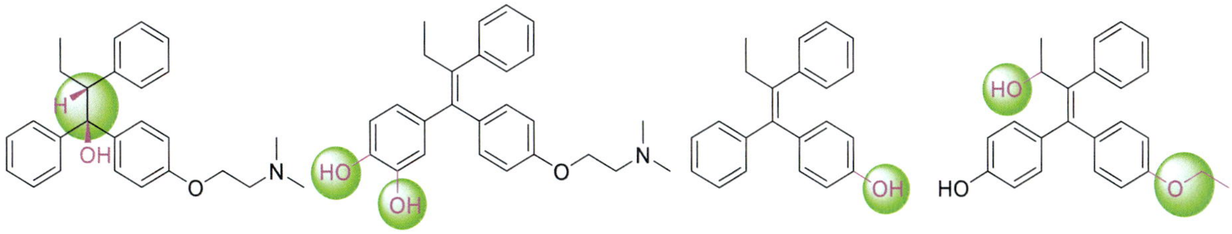

metabolite A   metabolite D   metabolite E   metabolite F

FIGURE 17.19 Some minor metabolites of tamoxifen in the body.

17.2.4.4 N,N-didesmethyl tamoxifen and metabolite Y

After *N*-desmethyl tamoxifen was identified as the major metabolite circulating in human serum, the metabolite was subsequently found to be further demethylated to *N,N*-desmethyl tamoxifen, and then finally deaminated and converted to metabolite Y. Metabolite Y is present in the serum of either normal or high-dose tamoxifen-treated patients, and both are weak antiestrogens that are capable of exerting an inhibitory effect on the ER in tumors [37,47,64].

In addition, tamoxifen also produces several other metabolites with varying levels of activity (Fig. 17.19). However, these compounds are generally present in low concentrations or are only detected in animals, with limited pharmacological research conducted in patients.

17.2.5 Tamoxifen drug interactions

CYP2D6 is the major enzyme in the metabolism of tamoxifen to produce *N*-desmethyl-4-hydroxytamoxifen; therefore, tamoxifen should be administered with caution when combined with drugs involving CYP2D6 activity. The drugs that affect the absorption and metabolism of tamoxifen, as well as its binding affinity to ER, can affect the therapeutic efficacy of tamoxifen. The defined specifics of tamoxifen-drug interactions include: (1) antidepressants: paroxetine may lead to a decrease in tamoxifen efficacy by inhibiting CYP2D6 activity; (2) phenobarbital: phenobarbital analogs may reduce the bioavailability of tamoxifen and increase the metabolic inactivation of tamoxifen by inducing enzyme/transporter inducers, thereby decreasing its steady-state blood concentration; (3) antacids, cimetidine, famotidine, ranitidine, etc., can change intragastric pH and cause tamoxifen enteric-coated tablets to decompose prematurely, which has an irritating effect on the stomach. Therefore, combined with the above drugs, there should be a 1−2 hours interval; (4) vitamin K: Combining with antivitamin K drugs has increased the effect of anticoagulant drugs, increasing the risk of bleeding; (5) cyclophosphamide, fluorouracil, methotrexate, and tamoxifen all have the side effect of increasing the risk of thrombosis, and the combination will exacerbate the risks; (6) tamoxifen may competitively inhibit the metabolism of cyclosporine, thereby increasing its blood levels; and (7) tamoxifen may decrease letrozole blood levels by inducing cytochrome P450 enzymes.

17.2.6 Synthesis and process of tamoxifen

As an aforementioned demonstration, the tamoxifen involved a double bond and thereby resulted in *cis* and *trans* isomers that exhibit different physicochemical properties, potencies, and, at some point, opposite activity. Therefore, the chemical process of synthesis should be well developed, and there are currently two main methods reported based on whether or not the two isomers need to be separated, i.e., (1) synthesizing a mixture of the two isomers; and (2) synthesizing tamoxifen in a single *trans* isomer. The representative synthetic methods are discussed in this chapter.

17.2.6.1 Synthesis of a mixture of two isomers of tamoxifen

The most important part of tamoxifen synthesis is the synthesis of the triphenylethylene skeleton. Depending on the method used to synthesize the triphenylethylene backbone, the reported syntheses of mixtures of tamoxifen isomers can be classified into three categories, ranging from simple to complex: (1) synthesis of the triphenylethylene skeleton by McMurry coupling reaction; (2) synthesis of triphenylethylene skeletons by nucleophilic addition and elimination reactions; and (3) synthesis of tamoxifen by nucleophilic substitution.

17.2.6.1.1 Synthesis of tamoxifen by McMurry coupling reaction

A McMurry coupling reaction is an organic reaction in which two molecules of a ketone or aldehyde are coupled to an olefin in the presence of titanium chloride (e.g., titanium tetrachloride) and a reducing agent (e.g., zinc powder). In this method, benzophenone-containing substituents on the benzene ring and phenylacetone are used as substrates for the direct synthesis of tamoxifen using the McMurry coupling reaction, or the tamoxifen analogs were first synthesized, and then the substituents on the benzene ring were converted to N,N-dimethylethoxy side chains to obtain tamoxifen [60,61] (Fig. 17.20). The synthesis of tamoxifen *via* the McMurry coupling reaction is convenient, whereas the McMurry coupling reaction is the main limiting factor of yield in this method, with a value of about 55% reported in the literature.

17.2.6.1.2 Synthesis of tamoxifen by nucleophilic addition

The key step in this method is the nucleophilic addition of carbonyl groups to produce hydroxyl compounds during the synthesis of the triphenylethylene skeleton, followed by the elimination of the hydroxyl groups to produce tamoxifen. In this route, phenylacetyl chloride and anisole are generally used as raw materials for the acylation, alkylation, and demethylation reactions, and basic side chains are introduced to generate 1-ethyl diphenylethanone containing substituent groups on the benzene ring, and then nucleophilic substitution is used to generate the intermediate 1-(4-(2-(dimethylamino)ethoxy)phenyl)-1,2-diphenylbutan-1-ol. This intermediate subsequently undergoes an elimination reaction in an acidic environment to form tamoxifen [62] (Fig. 17.21).

In addition, tamoxifen can also be produced by nucleophilic addition and elimination reactions of benzophenone analogs with propylbenzene in the presence of alkalies.

17.2.6.1.3 Synthesis of tamoxifen by nucleophilic substitution

In this route, phenol was used as a raw material to produce tamoxifen through substitution, alkylation, and finally an elimination reaction (Fig. 17.22). This method has shorter steps but involves more complex reactions [63].

17.2.6.2 Synthesis of single trans tamoxifen

A single *trans* isomer is more difficult to synthesize than a mixture of isomers. Based on the separation of *cis* and *trans* isomers, the synthesis of tamoxifen can be divided into three categories: resolution to obtain single *trans* tamoxifen, isomerization to obtain *trans* tamoxifen, and selecting chiral raw materials to obtain *trans* tamoxifen directly through asymmetric synthesis.

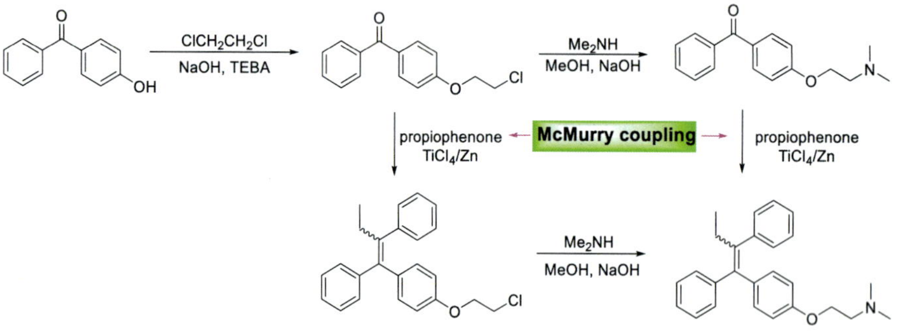

FIGURE 17.20 Synthesis of tamoxifen by McMurry coupling reaction.

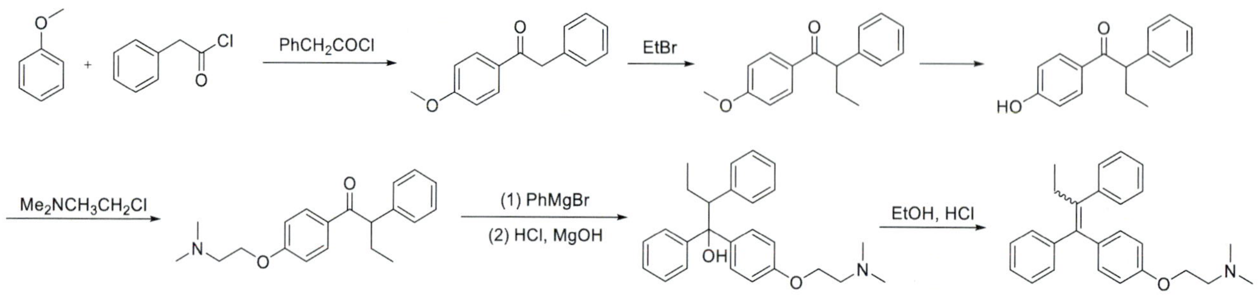

FIGURE 17.21 Synthesis of tamoxifen by nucleophilic addition.

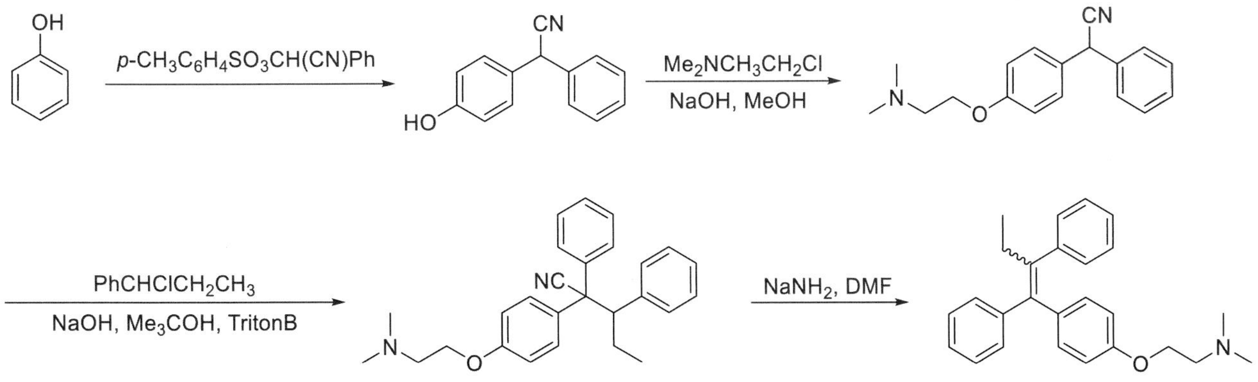

FIGURE 17.22 Synthesis of tamoxifen by nucleophilic substitution reaction.

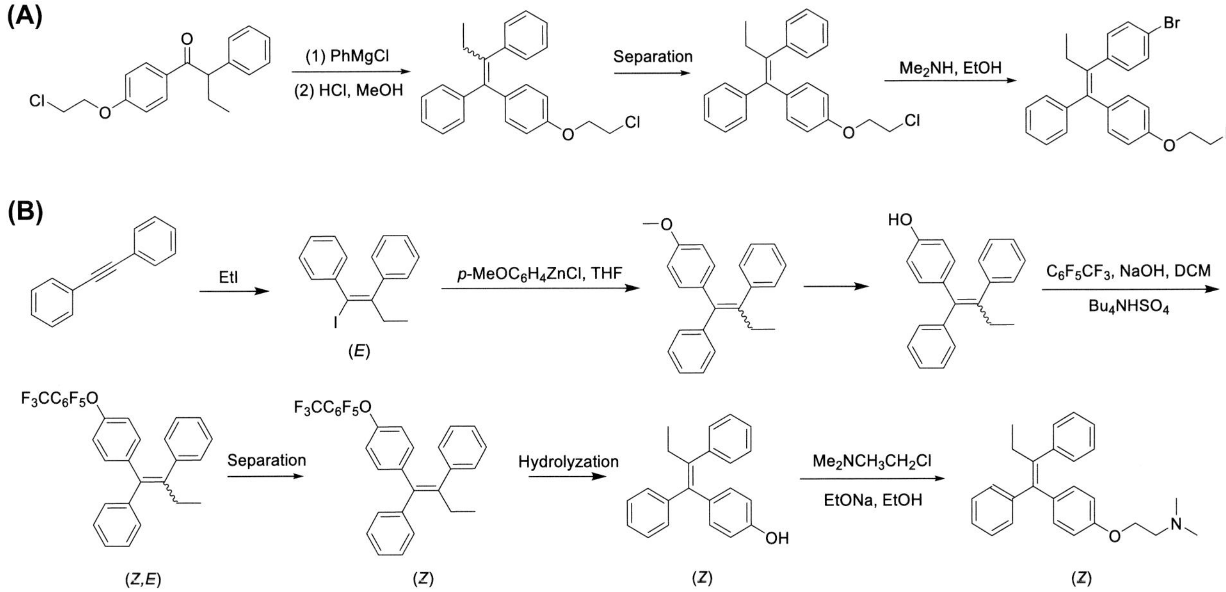

FIGURE 17.23 The synthesis of *trans*-tamoxifen through separation.

17.2.6.2.1 Resolution to obtain *trans*-tamoxifen

Resolution refers to the process of separating the two isomers to obtain a single isomer by appropriate methods based on the differences in physical and chemical properties, and the methods usually used include induced crystallization of crystal species, biochemical methods, or reacting with a resolution agent to split the product and then decomposing it into the original compound. The separation method is one of the most reported methods for the synthesis of tamoxifen, in which a single *trans* isomer is obtained by separation the intermediate in the synthesis of tamoxifen, and the *trans* tamoxifen is subsequently synthesized from the intermediate in the single configuration [64] (Fig. 17.23).

17.2.6.2.2 Isomerization to obtain *trans*-tamoxifen

Two isomers may be transformed into each other in a particular environment, which is called isomerization. Al-Hassan reported that the *cis* isomer can be converted to the *trans* isomer under acidic conditions during the synthesis of tamoxifen, and in this way, the reaction can be controlled to obtain almost pure *trans*-tamoxifen [65] (Fig. 17.24).

17.2.6.2.3 Asymmetric synthesis to obtain *trans*-tamoxifen

The asymmetric synthesis of tamoxifen is based on the catalytic addition of trimethyl(phenylethynyl)silane to give an *E*-type intermediate, and then directly synthesized *trans*-tamoxifen *via* a multistep substitution (Fig. 17.25). In this

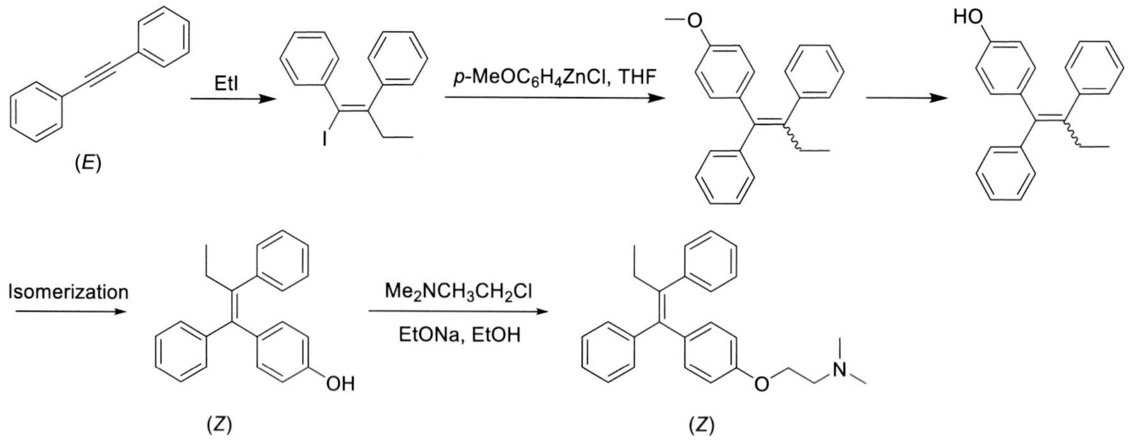

FIGURE 17.24 The synthesis of *trans*-tamoxifen through isomerization.

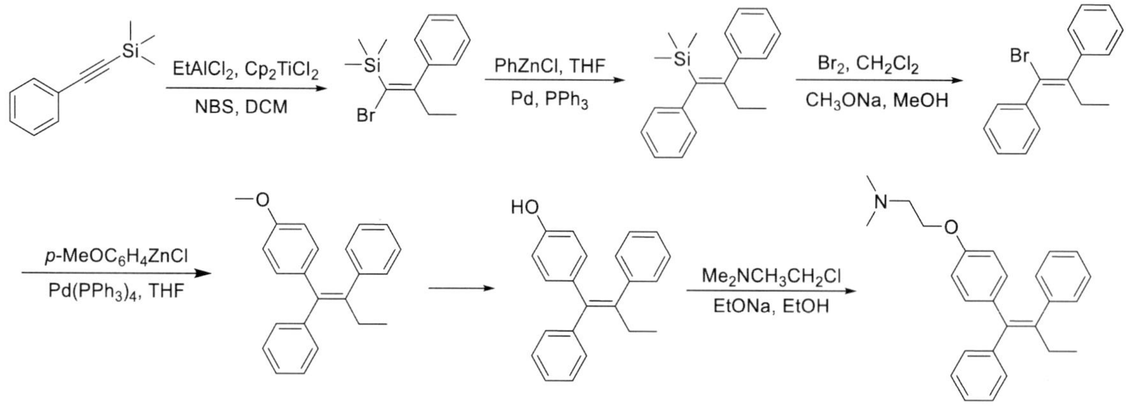

FIGURE 17.25 Asymmetric synthesis of *trans*-tamoxifen.

process, the first-step product is obtained without considering the effect of isomers, but the reagents used are expensive and not suitable for mass production [66].

17.3 Clinical investigations of tamoxifen
17.3.1 Clinical indications of tamoxifen

The effective rate of tamoxifen in the treatment of breast cancer patients is approximately 30%, while ER-positive patients are more effective and negative patients are tolerated. No matter how pre- and postmenopausal patients can be treated, the effect of postmenopausal medication is better than that of premenopausal and younger patients. In the 1970s, almost all of the initial clinical investigations of tamoxifen were designed for the treatment of metastatic breast cancer. The results showed that the treatment efficacy of tamoxifen was the same as that of high-dose estrogen therapy, but with significantly fewer adverse effects [67,68]. In recent times, tamoxifen has been used to treat patients with all stages of breast cancer as the gold standard of antihormone treatment for breast cancer between 1980 and 2000. Clinical statistics showed that breast cancer mortality rates remained essentially unchanged from 1975 to 1990 but declined by nearly 20% between 1990 and 2000, and two-thirds of this decline should be attributed to the use of tamoxifen.

When tamoxifen was used as an adjuvant treatment for premenopausal women with ER$^+$ breast cancer patients, the efficacy was positively correlated with the duration of tamoxifen treatment. The major benefit of taking tamoxifen was a reduction in mortality in the second decade after breast cancer diagnosis. One year of tamoxifen as adjuvant therapy did little or nothing for recurrence or survival, whereas 5 years of tamoxifen medication resulted in a nearly 40% reduction in mortality for patients with late-stage breast cancer [67,69], and 10 years of tamoxifen medication resulted in a

50% reduction in mortality in the second decade after diagnosis. Taking tamoxifen for 10 years was associated with a 25% and 29% reduction of recurrence and mortality, respectively, compared with taking tamoxifen for 5 years.

Clinically, tamoxifen is mainly used for the treatment and prevention of breast cancer as well as local breast ductal carcinoma. In addition, tamoxifen, as a modulator targeting ER, can also be used for the clinical treatment of infertility, ovarian cancer, polycystic ovary syndrome (PCOS), and other gynecological diseases.

Ovarian cancer is the most common cause of cancer death in women, with high mortality and morbidity due to early clinical absence of symptoms, late diagnosis, and treatment resistance. Like many breast cancers, some ovarian cancer cells also have ER and require estrogen to grow and metastasize. Researchers tested tamoxifen hormone therapy in women with advanced ovarian cancer and showed that tamoxifen was able to block the physiological actions of estrogen and was able to respond to a small percentage of recurrent ovarian cancers that did not respond to chemotherapy.

In addition, PCOS is a common endocrine disorder in women of childbearing age, characterized by anovulation or sporadic ovulation, clinical or biochemical hyperandrogenism, and polycystic ovaries. The main treatment methods are to adjust the endocrine disorder and induce ovulation. Since tamoxifen has some ovulation-promoting effects, studies have treated patients with PCOS with tamoxifen. The results showed the efficacy of tamoxifen alone was not significantly different from that of clomiphene citrate, but in patients with clomiphene citrate-resistant PCOS, combo tamoxifen significantly improved the treatment efficacy of clomiphene citrate alone.

In addition to the diseases closely related to ER, studies have also shown that tamoxifen has a certain therapeutic effect on colorectal cancer, colon cancer, bladder cancer, pancreatic cancer, lung cancer, etc. Tamoxifen has also been studied for the potential treatment of traumatic periodontitis, postmenopausal osteoporosis, inhibition of paralyzed fibroblast DNA and collagen synthesis, and antiearly pregnancy or other diseases.

17.3.2 Studies on tamoxifen resistance

Despite the proven therapeutic efficacy of tamoxifen in breast cancer patients, the majority of patients with advanced breast cancer eventually become resistant to endocrine therapy, and there remains a persistent risk of recurrence in breast cancer patients who have been treated with endocrine therapy. Specifically, approximately 50% of patients with locally advanced or metastatic ER^+ breast cancer are refractory to endocrine therapy (de novo resistance) [70]. Along with the long-term treatment of endocrine therapies such as tamoxifen, about 25% of patients with early-stage ER^+ breast cancer develop acquired resistance after 10 years, and almost all patients with metastatic ER^+ breast cancer develop secondary resistance to endocrine therapies after long-term treatment, even if they are initially sensitive to endocrine drug therapy. Thus, the emergence of resistance has become a challenge for hormone therapy. Although the mechanism by which tumors develop resistance to tamoxifen is still not completely understood, researchers have proposed several theories. For instance, tamoxifen treatment resistance is possible because of its pharmacological properties, mutations in the LBD of the ER, increased aromatase activity, activation of growth factor receptors, activation of signaling pathways related to cell survival and the cell growth cycle, cellular stress, and aberrant expression of ER coactivators that may all contribute to the development of primary or acquired resistance to tamoxifen in breast cancer [71,72].

17.3.2.1 Conversion of tamoxifen metabolites to estrogen receptor agonists

Tamoxifen is locally metabolized to a variety of metabolites, of which metabolite E (Fig. 17.22) is a weak ER agonist with the loss of the basic side chain. It has been found that the *trans* isomer of tamoxifen in metabolism can undergo a conformational shift to its *cis* isomer of a weak ER agonist in vivo [73]. Therefore, it is suggested that this conformational change during metabolism into an estrogen agonist is an important reason for the development of tamoxifen resistance [74].

17.3.2.2 Loss of estrogen receptors

One more possible mechanism for the development of tamoxifen resistance is the loss of ER in patients. Estrogen is one of the triggers of ER^+ breast cancer as well as one of the reasons for promoting the progression of the disease, whereas 15%–20% of patients with metastatic breast cancer are primarily diagnosed as ER-positive, but eventually with the growth of the tumor, they may gradually lose ER, which will lead to the development of cellular resistance to tamoxifen. The growth of such ER-deficient tumor cells will no longer be dependent on estrogen in the body, but will instead be upregulated by gene amplification or overexpression of human epidermal growth factor receptor 2 or other receptor proteins, which in turn sustains the tumor growth through the rest of the pro-growth pathways [75,76].

For such resistance due to growth factor receptor overexpression, it is possible to restore the sensitivity of tumor cells to endocrine therapy by inhibiting the growth factor receptor pathway. However, ER continues to be expressed and active in the majority of patients resistant to endocrine therapy, which is associated with abnormalities in *ESR1*, the relevant genome encoding the ERα protein in humans, as detailed below.

17.3.2.3 Alterations in the ESR1 genome and structural mutations in the estrogen receptor

ESR1 is a related gene encoding the ERα protein in humans. Several abnormalities of the *ESR1*-related genome, such as gene amplification, genomic mutations, and missense point mutations, are present in breast cancer, and recent studies have identified these genomic alterations as a key reason for the development of endocrine drug resistance [77]. Reports on metastatic ER^+ breast cancer have shown that *ESR1* mutations have a total mutation frequency of 12% in patients on long-term endocrine therapy [78] and are mainly focused on aggregated missense mutations capable of affecting the ligand-binding structural domain of the ER. Most of these mutations lead to structural or conformational changes in the LBD of the ER and subsequent ligand-independent constitutive activation, with subsequent resistance to endocrine therapy.

ESR1 gene alterations are categorized as amplifications, missense mutations, and gene rearrangements. Compared to amplification and rearrangement of the *ESR1* genome, the clinical cause of endocrine resistance is more likely to be related to missense mutations in the *ESR1* genome. A missense mutation occurs when a codon coding for one amino acid becomes a codon coding for another amino acid after a base substitution, thus changing the amino acid type and sequence of the polypeptide chain. Moreover, the vast majority of mutations are missense mutations that occur within the ER-LBD, allowing for nondependent constitutive activation of the ligand of the receptor in question. This resistance accounts for 35%–40% of the overall acquired resistance. In 1991, William et al. found that there are two types of mutants: dominant-positive receptors (transcriptionally active in the absence of estrogen) or dominant-negative receptors, in clinical breast cancer tissues with structural domains and physiological functions different from those of the wild-type ER [79]. Dominant-negative receptors are transcriptionally inactive and are not able to be activated by stimulation of estrogens or estrogenic drugs. On the contrary, dominant-positive receptors have reduced dependence on estrogen or other ligands and would have the potential to stimulate breast tumor growth in the absence of estrogen. They can then bind to coactivators in the absence of estrogen to maintain transcriptional activation and promote breast tumor cell growth, making it difficult for endocrine therapy to be effective in the treatment of the latter ER^+ breast cancer patients.

Later, several research groups identified mutant LBDs that activate ERα through circular transfer through high-throughput DNA sequencing. These mutations were found in 25%–30% of breast cancer cases, and they allowed the ERα to remain active. As a result, cancer cells with these mutations no longer require estradiol for growth, which makes them resistant to AIs. The mutations likewise make it more difficult to treat with standard antiestrogens that inhibit cancer cells, such as the SERM tamoxifen. Despite the loss of antiproliferative or ER antagonistic effects of tamoxifen, they appear to continue to maintain their ER binding affinity and continue to modulate the growth of drug-resistant ER^+ breast cancer cells. After that, with the discovery of further research, it was found that mutations in *ESR1* are commonly located in the region of the gene encoding the ligand-binding structural domain, and several of the common mutations include Y537S, D538G, Y537N, Y537C, and L536R. The mutations at positions 537 and 538 generate particularly pronounced resistance [80]. The main mutant sites in the three mutation domains of the ligand-binding sites, pharmacological phenotypes, and possible mechanisms of ERα mutations are shown in Fig. 17.26 and Table 17.7.

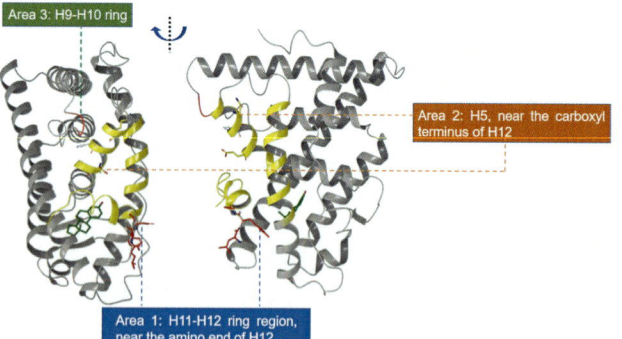

FIGURE 17.26 Mutation sites in the ligand-binding domain of ERα (regions 1–3).

TABLE 17.7 Major activating mutation sites of the mutation domains, their pharmacological phenotypes and possible mechanisms of action.

Region of mutation	Mutant site	Pharmacological characteristics	Possible mechanisms
H11-H12 ring region, near the amino end of H12	Y537S, Y537N, Y537C, Y537D	Strong intrinsic activity and antiestrogen receptor antagonist activity and resistance Y537S > Y537N-Y537C	Strong hydrogen bonding on D351 stabilizes the AF2 conformation and allows better folding of the ring region
	D538G	Moderately strong intrinsic activity; antiestrogen receptor antagonist activity easily reversible	Flexibility to connect to H12 allows for better folding of the ring area
	L536R, L536H, L536P, L536Q	Moderately strong intrinsic activity; antiestrogen receptor antagonist activity not readily reversible	Replacement of leucine with hydrophilic residues eliminates loss of hydrophobicity due to water exposure
H5, near the carboxyl terminus of H12	E380Q	Weak strength intrinsic activity; antiestrogen receptor antagonist activity easily reversible	Elimination of Coulomb repulsion with two acidic residues in H12
H9-H10 ring	S463P	Moderately strong intrinsic activity; antiestrogen receptor antagonist activity easily reversible	Potential stabilization of dimer interfaces and/or flexible recycling and possible realization of further intra-domain interactions

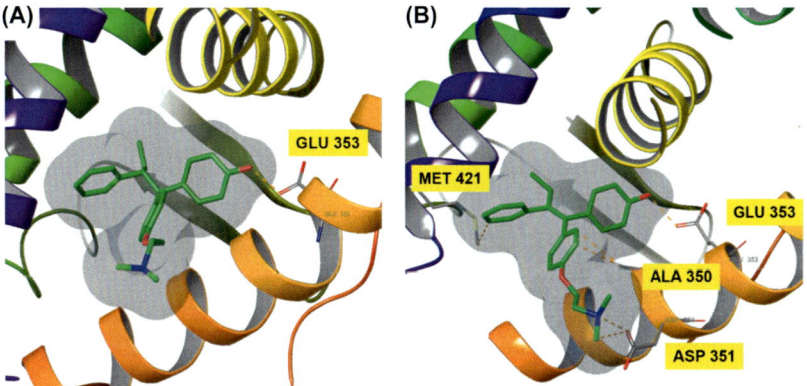

FIGURE 17.27 (A) Conformation of 4-hydroxytamoxifen bound to the ERα mutant Tyr537Ser; (B) Conformation of 4-hydroxytamoxifen bound to the ERα mutant Asp538Gly.

The mechanism by which ERα mutations confer resistance involves alterations in hydrogen bonding between the helices of ER, elongation of the hinge region between Helix 11 and Helix 12, decreased hydrophobicity, and changes in electrostatic repulsion, among others (Table 17.7). In the wild-type binding region of the receptor, the amino acid residues at positions 537 and 538 are Tyr and Asp, respectively. However, in the mutated binding region of the receptor, position 537 becomes Ser, and position 538 is replaced by Gly. These mutations increase the flexibility of the ER, thereby reducing its binding affinity for tamoxifen. Further crystallographic biology studies indicated that the Tyr537Ser mutation induces the increased flexibility of the receptor protein and forms a new hydrogen bond between Ser537 and Asp351 within the ER, which reduces the binding affinity of tamoxifen for the ER and forms an agonist rather than an antagonist conformation within the receptor, leading to the development of resistance [81] (Fig. 17.27).

17.3.2.4 Resistance due to activation of the estrogen membrane receptor pathway

ERα36, a variant of ERα, is a membrane receptor that exerts effects on the nongenomic estrogen signaling pathway. Compared with ERα, ERα36 lacks two transcriptional activation regions, AF-1 and AF-2, but retains the DNA-binding structural domain and part of the dimerization and estrogen-binding structural domains of ERα. ERα36 functionally mediates an estrogen signaling pathway that is completely different from that of ERα. It is usually anchored to the cell membrane by coupling with some membrane proteins, which has a stronger stimulatory effect on the growth of breast cancer cells and is associated with the development of a variety of tumors, including breast cancer, endometrial cancer, colorectal cancer, liver cancer, and gastric cancer. In breast cancer patients, about 40% of ERα$^+$ breast cancers also express ERα36, and ERα36 was also expressed in ER$^-$ breast cancer patients. The results reveal, when acting on ERα36-expressing cells, tamoxifen not only failed to inhibit the growth of MCF-7 cells transfected with the ERα36 gene but also stimulated the proliferation of MCF-7 cells and improved the ability of cells to migrate and invade in vitro, whereas knockdown of the ERα36 gene restored the sensitivity of MCF-7 cells to tamoxifen. Studies have reported that the resistance to tamoxifen in patients with ERα36 overexpression may be related to ERα36-associated signaling pathways such as MAPK/ERK, PI3K/AKT, and EGFR, and that tamoxifen combined with a kinase inhibitor may be an effective therapeutic regimen for this group of breast cancer patients [76].

17.3.2.5 Resistance due to activation of pathways other than estrogen receptors

In addition to the various factors directly related to the ER pathway aforementioned above, some cellular and biological response-related factors affected by endocrine therapy, such as increased expression of coactivators, alterations in the growth factor pathway and the cellular kinase or stress response kinase pathway, increased levels of phosphorylation, and increased activity of ER and coregulators, have all been associated with acquired endocrine resistance. The kinase pathway, as well as the amplification and/or overexpression of cell cycle regulators or anti-apoptotic factors, can provide alternative signaling pathways or routes for tumor cell proliferation in the presence of ER pathway inhibition [76]. Preclinical investigations have shown that up-regulation of positive cell cycle regulators, especially those controlling G1 phase progression, and down-regulation of negative cell cycle regulators can inhibit the antitumor cell proliferative effects of endocrine therapies, leading to tamoxifen resistance. Finally, various components of the tumor microenvironment and several other relevant factors have likewise been identified as being associated with acquired endocrine resistance.

17.3.3 Adverse reactions of tamoxifen

In addition to the challenges of drug resistance, another issue plaguing the clinical treatment efficacy of tamoxifen is adverse reactions. Clinical studies have shown that tamoxifen can cause adverse effects, including hot flashes and vasodilatory symptoms, osteoporosis, depression, venous thromboembolism, and endometrial cancer [82]. Endometrial cancer is the most serious and is directly related to the various side effects of tamoxifen. In the mid-1980s, tamoxifen was found to promote the growth of endometrial cancer in the laboratory, and it was predicted to increase a woman's risk of developing endometrial cancer [83]. After long-term follow-up clinical observation and examination, it has indeed been confirmed to be true that tamoxifen statistically increased the odds of endometrial cancer in postmenopausal women by three to five times [84]. This may again be related to the fact that tamoxifen, as a SERM analog, has a mild agonistic effect on ER in endometrial cells.

Tamoxifen has also been shown to have some genotoxicity, causing chromosomal aberrations and increased micronucleus formation [85], as well as tumors in the rat liver, but fortunately, these safety concerns have not been detailed in the long-term treatment of tamoxifen in clinical settings [86].

17.4 Summary, knowledge expansion, and references

17.4.1 Historical significance of tamoxifen

As a failed contraceptive, tamoxifen was successfully turned into a drug for the prevention and treatment of breast cancer, becoming a first-in-class drug for the treatment of breast cancer patients. Tamoxifen alone and combo regime therapy have saved the lives of hundreds of thousands of women around the world. To date, tamoxifen has become the gold standard as targeted therapy for all stages of breast cancer, including male breast cancer, and is also an effective therapeutic agent for a wide range of other ER-associated tumors or other diseases [69].

Extensive research on tamoxifen and related nonsteroidal antiestrogens, such as raloxifene, has opened up the clinical application of SERMs. With this deepening understanding, researchers are constantly realizing their pharmacological effects, making the application of endocrine therapy more and more widespread. To date, SERMs have shown good therapeutic efficacies or therapeutic prospects for a wide range of ER-related diseases in humans, particularly in women.

For example, raloxifene, a second-generation SERM, was also a failed antibreast cancer drug, but in subsequent applications, it was turned to target ER in human bone and cardiovascular tissue and became the first SERM to be successfully used in the treatment of postmenopausal osteoporosis in women and indirectly in the prevention of breast cancer [87].

In conclusion, the development of tamoxifen perfected targeted endocrine cancer therapy and subsequently facilitated the development of selective ER down-regulators and AIs, as well as the successful chemoprevention of breast cancer. Since then, tamoxifen has become an essential backbone for the design and synthesis of SERMs, and the study of its specific pharmacological effects and metabolites has become an important part of the development of this class of drugs. Intensive research on the SERMs has brought new hope for drug discovery for diseases previously thought to be incurable.

17.4.2 Other drugs targeting estrogen receptor pathway for breast cancer treatment

In addition to SERMs, there are two other types of drugs targeting ER: SERDs and AIs.

SERDs and SERMs have some similarities in molecular structure, which consists of a hydrophobic nucleus and a long side chain (Fig. 17.28). However, in terms of physiological function, SERDs are a class of complete antagonists that have strong inhibitory activity on ER in all tissues, and they are a new class of compounds with strong antagonistic properties. The mechanism of action of SERDs is similar to that of SERMs in that they also inhibit ER binding to coactivators and subsequent transcriptional activation by blocking estrogen binding to the ER, but they are more potent inhibitors of estradiol activity, can completely inhibit estradiol activity, and can inhibit breast cancer cells that have acquired resistance to tamoxifen.

Fulvestrant and elacestrant, as SERDs, are the only FDA-approved selective ER downregulators for the treatment of breast cancer. Unlike tamoxifen, fulvestrant and elacestrant antagonize all ERs due to their long side chains [88,89]. However, the oral bioavailability of fulvestrant is very low, requiring intramuscular administration, and its clinical use is limited.

Aromatase is also known as cytochrome P450 monooxygenase. Aromatase catalyzes the conversion of androstenedione or testosterone to estradiol and estrone in vivo, mainly by removing the carbon at the 19-position [90]. This step is the final and critical step in the synthesis of endogenous estrogens in the body. AIs, as inhibitors of aromatase, can interrupt the pathway of estrogen synthesis in the body, producing a reduction in endogenous estrogen levels. They are currently the first-line therapeutic agents for estrogen-dependent diseases such as breast cancer. There are two main classes of AIs in clinical use [91] (Fig. 17.29):

1. Steroidal inhibitors, which inhibit aromatase activity as an irreversible process; the main drugs are exemestane and formestane.
2. Nonsteroidal inhibitors: Most of these drugs contain triazoles in their structure, which inhibit the synthesis of endogenous estrogen by using heteroatoms to bind with iron atoms in hemoglobin. The major drugs are anastrozole and letrozole.

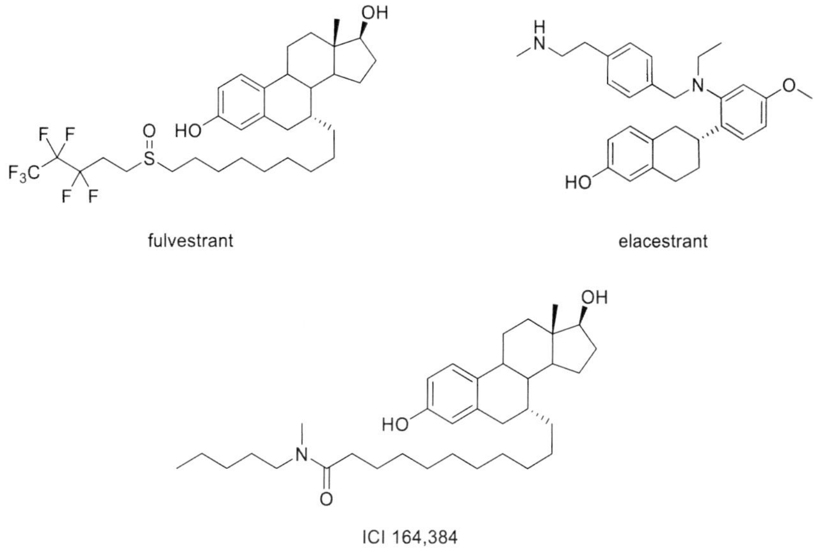

FIGURE 17.28 Selective estrogen receptor downregulators.

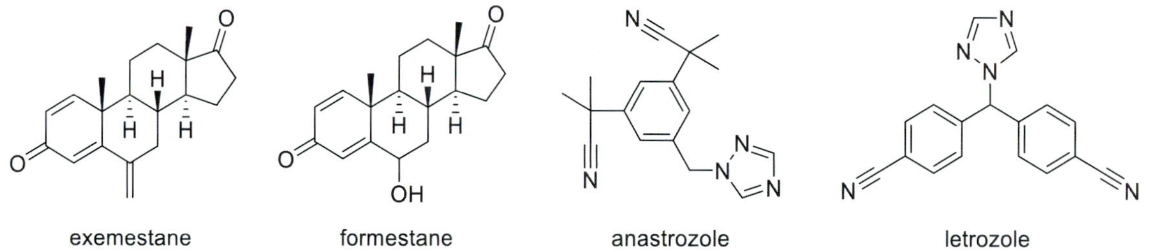

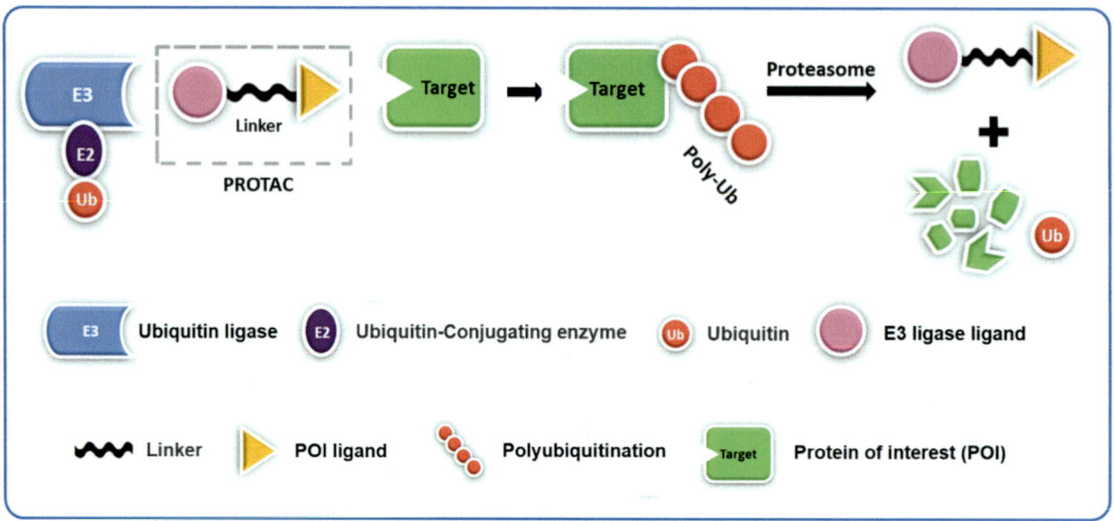

FIGURE 17.29 Some commonly used aromatase inhibitors.

FIGURE 17.30 Schematic of the principle of protein degradation by PROTACs.

In addition, protein hydrolysis targeting chimeras (PROTACs) has become one of the hot directions of drug research in recent years [92]. Protein degradation is an important process of protein renewal in cells that is closely related to cell proliferation, differentiation, functional expression, and apoptosis. Most proteins will be degraded through the ubiquitin-proteasome system, a process that achieves ubiquitination labeling of proteins through a triple enzyme cascade (E1-E2-E3), and the ubiquitin-labeled proteins are subsequently broken down by proteolytic enzymes into smaller peptides, amino acids, and reusable ubiquitin.

PROTAC technology is a powerful mode of protein degradation discovered in the study of chemical biology and drug processes. PROTACs are bifunctional molecules consisting of a ligand for a target protein of interest and a ligand for an E3 ubiquitin ligase, connected by a chain (linker) of variable length and structure. PROTACs induce a ternary complex with the target protein, E3 ligase, and ubiquitination labeling of the target protein, which is subsequently degraded through the ubiquitination pathway [93]. PROTACs essentially degrade the target protein rather than inhibiting its activity. Unlike conventional inhibitors, PROTACs do not require a strong binding ability of the target protein ligand, which, to some extent, may circumvent the problem of drug resistance that accompanies conventional inhibitors. In addition, the inhibition and degradation functions of PROTACs are more selective, and they can differentiate between some homologous proteins in the human body. Moreover, PROTACs make it possible to degrade so-called "undruggable' target proteins" (Fig. 17.30).

There is a large number of research on PROTACs for cancer treatment, but due to their molecular weight and solubility, they are still in the early stages. In 2019, Arvinas developed the world's first PROTAC drug, ARV-110, which selectively targets the androgen receptor and is intended to be used for the treatment of desmoplasia-resistant prostate cancer and received fast-track approval from the FDA. Preliminary activity data have been obtained from a Phase II clinical study of ARV-110, which demonstrated excellent safety, tolerability, and oral bioavailability. In the same year, Arvinas reported the development of a second PROTAC drug, ARV-471, which was also approved to enter clinical trial studies. This molecule targets the degradation of the ER and is intended to be used for the treatment of locally advanced or metastatic ER$^+$/HER2$^-$ breast cancer, and it is expected to be the first drug in the class of PROTACs to be approved for the treatment of breast cancer.

References

[1] Bland K.I., Iii E.M. C., Klimberg V.S. Chapter 1 - history of the therapy of breast cancer. Breast (Fifth Ed), 2018:1-19.

[2] Kamangar F, Dores GM, Anderson WF. Patterns of cancer incidence, mortality, and prevalence across five continents: defining priorities to reduce cancer disparities in different geographic regions of the world. J Clin Oncol Off J Am Soc Clin Oncol 2006;24:2137—50.

[3] Hyuna S, Jacques F, Rebecca LS, et al. Global cancer statistics 2020:Globocan estimates of incidence and mortality worldwide for 36 cancers in 185 countries. CA Cancer J Clin 2021;73:209—49.

[4] Sorlie T, Perou CM, Tibshirani R, et al. Gene expression patterns of breast carcinomas distinguish tumor subclasses with clinical implications. Proc Natl Acad Sci U S A 2001;98:10869—74.

[5] Katzenellenbogen JA, Mayne CG, Katzenellenbogen BS, et al. Structural underpinnings of oestrogen receptor mutations in endocrine therapy resistance. Nat Rev Cancer 2018;18:377—88.

[6] Cheung KL. Endocrine therapy for breast cancer: an overview. Breast 2007;16:327—43.

[7] Syed F, Khosla S. Mechanisms of sex steroid effects on bone. Biochem Biophys Res Commun 2005;328:688—96.

[8] Gennari L, Becherini L, Falchetti A, et al. Genetics of osteoporosis: role of steroid hormone receptor gene polymorphisms. J Steroid Biochem Mol Biol 2002;81:1—24.

[9] Behl C. Oestrogen as a neuroprotective hormone. Nat Rev Neurosci 2002;3:433—42.

[10] Rasmuson S, Nasman B, Carlstrom K, et al. Increased levels of adrenocortical and gonadal hormones in mild to moderate alzheimer's disease. Dement Geriatric Cognit Disord 2002;13:74—9.

[11] Hanke H, Hanke S, Bruck B, et al. Inhibition of the protective effect of estrogen by progesterone in experimental atherosclerosis. Atherosclerosis 1996;121:129—38.

[12] Heldring N, Pike A, Andersson S, et al. Estrogen receptors: how do they signal and what are their targets. Physiol Rev 2007;87:905—31.

[13] Kuiper GG, Carlsson B, Grandien K, et al. Comparison of the ligand binding specificity and transcript tissue distribution of estrogen receptors alpha and beta. Endocrinology 1997;138:863—70.

[14] Shao W, Brown M. Advances in estrogen receptor biology: prospects for improvements in targeted breast cancer therapy. Breast Cancer Res BCR 2004;6:39—52.

[15] Webb P, Nguyen P, Valentine C, et al. The estrogen receptor enhances AP-1 activity by two distinct mechanisms with different requirements for receptor transactivation functions. Mol Endocrinol 1999;13:1672—85.

[16] Jensen EV, Jacobsonk HI. Basic guides to the mechanism of estrogen action. Recent Progr Hormone Res 1962;18:387—414.

[17] Mosselman S, Polman J, Dijkema R. ER beta: identification and characterization of a novel human estrogen receptor. FEBS Lett 1996;392:49—53.

[18] Minutolo F, Macchia M, Katzenellenbogen BS, et al. Estrogen receptor beta ligands: recent advances and biomedical applications. Med Res Rev 2011;31:364—442.

[19] Zoubina EV, Smith PG. Expression of estrogen receptors alpha and beta by sympathetic ganglion neurons projecting to the proximal urethra of female rats. J Urol 2003;169:382—5.

[20] Ponglikitmongkol M, Green S, Chambon P. Genomic organization of the human oestrogen receptor gene. EMBO J 1988;7:3385—8.

[21] Huang B, Warner M, Gustafsson JA. Estrogen receptors in breast carcinogenesis and endocrine therapy. Mol Cell Endocrinol 2015;418(Pt 3):240—4.

[22] Cavalieri EL, Kumar S, Todorovic R, et al. Imbalance of estrogen homeostasis in kidney and liver of hamsters treated with estradiol: implications for estrogen-induced initiation of renal tumors. Chem Res Toxicol 2001;14:1041—50.

[23] Chakravarti D, Mailander PC, Li KM, et al. Evidence that a burst of DNA depurination in SENCAR mouse skin induces error-prone repair and forms mutations in the H-ras gene. Oncogene 2001;20:7945—53.

[24] Devanesan P, Todorovic R, Zhao J, et al. Catechol estrogen conjugates and DNA adducts in the kidney of male Syrian golden hamsters treated with 4-hydroxyestradiol: potential biomarkers for estrogen-initiated cancer. Carcinogenesis 2001;22:489—97.

[25] Pike AC, Brzozowski AM, Hubbard RE, et al. Structure of the ligand-binding domain of oestrogen receptor beta in the presence of a partial agonist and a full antagonist. EMBO J 1999;18:4608—18.

[26] Paige LA, Christensen DJ, Gron H, et al. Estrogen receptor (ER) modulators each induce distinct conformational changes in ER alpha and ER beta. Proc Natl Acad Sci U S A 1999;96:3999—4004.

[27] Hall JM, Mcdonnell DP. The estrogen receptor beta-isoform (ERbeta) of the human estrogen receptor modulates ERalpha transcriptional activity and is a key regulator of the cellular response to estrogens and antiestrogens. Endocrinology 1999;140:5566—78.

[28] Shang Y, Brown M. Molecular determinants for the tissue specificity of serms. Science 2002;295:2465—8.

[29] Jordan VC. Effect of tamoxifen (ICI 46 474) on initiation and growth of DMBA-induced rat mammary carcinomata. Eur J Cancer 1976;12:419—24.

[30] Jordan VC, Allen KE. Evaluation of the antitumour activity of the non-steroidal antioestrogen monohydroxytamoxifen in the DMBA-induced rat mammary carcinoma model. Eur J Cancer 1980;16:239—51.

[31] Jordan VC, Phelps E, Lindgren JU. Effects of anti-estrogens on bone in castrated and intact female rats. Breast Cancer Res Treat 1987;10:31—5.

[32] Ariazi EA, Cunliffe HE, Lewis-Wambi JS, et al. Estrogen induces apoptosis in estrogen deprivation-resistant breast cancer through stress responses as identified by global gene expression across time. Proc Natl Acad Sci U S A 2011;108:18879—86.

[33] Shiau AK, Barstad D, Loria PM, et al. The structural basis of estrogen receptor/coactivator recognition and the antagonism of this interaction by tamoxifen. Cell 1998;95:927–37.

[34] Brzozowski AM, Pike AC, Dauter Z, et al. Molecular basis of agonism and antagonism in the oestrogen receptor. Nature 1997;389:753–8.

[35] Heldring N, Nilsson M, Buehrer B, et al. Identification of tamoxifen-induced coregulator interaction surfaces within the ligand-binding domain of estrogen receptors. Mol Cell Biol 2004;24:3445–59.

[36] Agouridas V, Laios I, Cleeren A, et al. Loss of antagonistic activity of tamoxifen by replacement of one N-methyl of its side chain by fluorinated residues. Bioorg Med Chem 2006;14:7531–8.

[37] Jordan VC. Metabolites of tamoxifen in animals and man: identification, pharmacology, and significance. Breast Cancer Res Treat 1982;2:123–38.

[38] Watts CK, Murphy LC, Sutherland RL. Microsomal binding sites for nonsteroidal anti-estrogens in MCF 7 human mammary carcinoma cells. Demonstration of high affinity and narrow specificity for basic ether derivatives of triphenylethylene. J Biol Chem 1984;259:4223–9.

[39] Shoda T, Okuhira K, Kato M, et al. Design and synthesis of tamoxifen derivatives as a selective estrogen receptor down-regulator. Bioorg Med Chem Lett 2014;24:87–9.

[40] Shoda T, Kato M, Harada R, et al. Synthesis and evaluation of tamoxifen derivatives with a long alkyl side chain as selective estrogen receptor down-regulators. Bioorg Med Chem 2015;23:3091–6.

[41] Legros N, Leclercq G, Mccague R. Effect of estrogenic and antiestrogenic triphenylethylene derivatives on progesterone and estrogen receptors levels of MCF-7 cells. Biochem Pharmacol 1991;42:1837–41.

[42] Wenckens M, Jakobsen P, Vedso P, et al. N-alkoxypyrazoles as biomimetics for the alkoxyphenyl group in tamoxifen. Bioorg Med Chem 2003;11:1883–99.

[43] Mccague R, Rowlands MG, Grimshaw R, et al. Evidence that tamoxifen binds to calmodulin in a conformation different to that when binding to estrogen receptors, through structure-activity study on ring-fused analogues. Biochem Pharmacol 1994;48:1355–61.

[44] Malo-Forest B, Landelle G, Roy JA, et al. Synthesis and growth inhibition activity of fluorinated derivatives of tamoxifen. Bioorg Med Chem Lett 2013;23:1712–15.

[45] Carpenter C, Sorenson RJ, Jin Y, et al. Design and synthesis of triarylacrylonitrile analogues of tamoxifen with improved binding selectivity to protein kinase C. Bioorg Med Chem 2016;24:5495–504.

[46] Foster AB, Jarman M, Leung OT, et al. Hydroxy derivatives of tamoxifen. J Med Chem 1985;28:1491–7.

[47] Chao EY, Collins JL, Gaillard S, et al. Structure-guided synthesis of tamoxifen analogs with improved selectivity for the orphan ERRgamma. Bioorg Med Chem Lett 2006;16:821–4.

[48] Mccague R, Kuroda R, Leclercq G, et al. Synthesis and estrogen receptor binding of 6,7-dihydro-8-phenyl-9-[4-[2-(dimethylamino)ethoxy] phenyl]-5h-benzocycloheptene, a nonisomerizable analogue of tamoxifen. X-ray crystallographic studies. J Med Chem 1986;29:2053–9.

[49] Lloyd DG, Hughes RB, Zisterer DM, et al. Benzoxepin-derived estrogen receptor modulators: a novel molecular scaffold for the estrogen receptor. J Med Chem 2004;47:5612–15.

[50] Acton D, Hill G, Tait BS. Tricyclic triarylethylene antiestrogens: dibenz[b,f]oxepins, dibenzo[b,f]thiepins, dibenzo[a,e]cyclooctenes, and dibenzo[b,f]thiocins. J Med Chem 1983;26:1131–7.

[51] Gulino A, Pasqualini JR. Binding and biological responses of antiestrogens in the fetal and newborn uteri of guinea-pig. J Steroid Biochem 1981;15:361–7.

[52] Gulino A, Pasqualini JR. Heterogeneity of binding sites for tamoxifen and tamoxifen derivatives in estrogen target and nontarget fetal organs of guinea pig. Cancer Res 1982;42:1913–21.

[53] Mccague R, Leclercq G. Synthesis, conformational considerations, and estrogen receptor binding of diastereoisomers and enantiomers of 1-[4-[2-(dimethylamino)ethoxy]phenyl]-1,2-diphenylbutane (dihydrotamoxifen). J Med Chem 1987;30:1761–7.

[54] Maximov PY, Mcdaniel RE, Jordan VC. Tamoxifen: pioneering medicine in breast cancer. Basel: Springer; 2013.

[55] Shagufta, Ahmad I. Tamoxifen a pioneering drug: an update on the therapeutic potential of tamoxifen derivatives. Eur J Med Chem 2018;143:515–31.

[56] Jordan VC, Collins MM, Rowsby L, et al. A monohydroxylated metabolite of tamoxifen with potent antioestrogenic activity. J Endocrinol 1977;75:305–16.

[57] Coezy E, Borgna JL, Rochefort H. Tamoxifen and metabolites in MCF7 cells: correlation between binding to estrogen receptor and inhibition of cell growth. Cancer Res 1982;42:317–23.

[58] Adam HK, Douglas EJ, Kemp JV. The metabolism of tamoxifen in human. Biochem Pharmacol 1979;28:145–7.

[59] Patterson JS, Settatree RS, Adam HK, et al. Serum concentrations of tamoxifen and major metabolite during long-term nolvadex therapy, correlated with clinical response. Eur J Cancer 1980;(Suppl 1):89–92.

[60] Bristol M.C. Process for the preparation of tamoxifen:EP0126470. 1984-11-28[2022-2-12]. https://worldwide.espacenet.com/patent/search?q=pn%3DEP0126470A1.

[61] Nat R.D. Preparation of tamoxifen:Ep0168175. 1986-01-15[2022-2-12]. https://worldwide.espacenet.com/patent/search?q=pn%3DEP0168175A1.

[62] Schickaneder H.L. 1,1,2-triphenyl-but-1-enederivatives' process for their and their use as pharmaceutical agents:Ep0054168. 1982-06-23[2022-2-12]. https://www.freepatentsonline.com/EP0054168.pdf.

[63] Brittain D.R. Verfahren zur Herstellung von 1,1,2triphenyl-alk-1-enen:DE2252879. 1973-05-03[2022-2-12]. https://worldwide.espacenet.com/patent/search?q=pn%3DDE2252879A1.

[64] Double J. Tamoxifen and analogues thereof:Wo1997026234. 1997-07-24[2022-2-12]. https://www.freepatentsonline.com/WO1997026234.pdf.
[65] Al-Hassan MI. Synthesis of *cis*- and *trans*-tamoxifen. Synth Commun 1987;17:1247−51.
[66] Miller RB, Al-Hassonm MI. Stereospecific synthesis of (z)-tamoxifen via carbometalation of alkynylsilanes. J Org Chem 1985;50:2121−3.
[67] Cole MP, Jones CT, Todd ID. A new anti-oestrogenic agent in late breast cancer. An early clinical appraisal of ICI46474. Br J Cancer 1971;25:270−5.
[68] Ingle JN, Ahmann DL, Green SJ, et al. Randomized clinical trial of diethylstilbestrol versus tamoxifen in postmenopausal women with advanced breast cancer. N Engl J Med 1981;304:16−21.
[69] Jordan VC. Tamoxifen: catalyst for the change to targeted therapy. Eur J Cancer 2008;44:30−8.
[70] Clarke R, Tyson JJ, Dixon JM. Endocrine resistance in breast cancer—an overview and update. Mol Cell Endocrinol 2015;418(Pt 3):220−34.
[71] Early Breast Cancer Trialist' Collaborative Group (EBCTCG). Effects of chemotherapy and hormonal therapy for early breast cancer on recurrence and 15-year survival: an overview of the randomised trials. Lancet 2005;365:1687−717.
[72] Xiao T, Li W, Wang X, et al. Estrogen-regulated feedback loop limits the efficacy of estrogen receptor-targeted breast cancer therapy. Proc Natl Acad Sci U S A 2018;115:7869−78.
[73] Bilimoria MM, Assikis VJ, Muenzner HD, et al. An analysis of tamoxifen-stimulated human carcinomas for mutations in the AF-2 region of the estrogen receptor. J Steroid Biochem Mol Biol 1996;58:479−88.
[74] Osborne CK, Coronado E, Allred DC, et al. Acquired tamoxifen resistance: correlation with reduced breast tumor levels of tamoxifen and isomerization of *trans*-4-hydroxytamoxifen. J Natl Cancer Inst 1991;83:1477−82.
[75] Arpino G, Green SJ, Allred DC, et al. HER-2 amplification, HER-1 expression, and tamoxifen response in estrogen receptor-positive metastatic breast cancer: a southwest oncology group study. Clin Cancer Res Off J Am Assoc Cancer Res 2004;10:5670−6.
[76] Osborne CK, Schiff R. Mechanisms of endocrine resistance in breast cancer. Annu Rev Med 2011;62:233−47.
[77] Jeselsohn R, Buchwalter G, De Angelis C, et al. *ESR1* mutations-a mechanism for acquired endocrine resistance in breast cancer. Nat Rev Clin Oncol 2015;12:573−83.
[78] Jeselsohn R, Yelensky R, Buchwalter G, et al. Emergence of constitutively active estrogen receptor-alpha mutations in pretreated advanced estrogen receptor-positive breast cancer. Clin cancer Res Off J Am Assoc Cancer Res 2014;20:1757−67.
[79] Mcguire WL, Chamness GC, Fuqua SA. Estrogen receptor variants in clinical breast cancer. Mol Endocrinol 1991;5:1571−7.
[80] Merenbakh-Lamin K, Ben-Baruch N, Yeheskel A, et al. D538G mutation in estrogen receptor-alpha: a novel mechanism for acquired endocrine resistance in breast cancer. Cancer Res 2013;73:6856−64.
[81] Robinson DR, Wu YM, Vats P, et al. Activating *ESR1* mutations in hormone-resistant metastatic breast cancer. Nat Genet 2013;45:1446−51.
[82] Calster BV, Ginderachter JV, Vlasselaer J, et al. Uterine and quality of life changes in postmenopausal women with an asymptomatic tamoxifen-thickened endometrium randomized to continuation of tamoxifen or switching to anastrozole. Menopause 2011;18:224−9.
[83] Horwitz RI, Feinstein AR. Estrogens and endometrial cancer. Responses to arguments and current status of an epidemiologic controversy. Am J Med 1986;81:503−7.
[84] Davies C, Godwin J, Gray R, et al. Relevance of breast cancer hormone receptors and other factors to the efficacy of adjuvant tamoxifen: patient-level meta-analysis of randomised trials. Lancet 2011;378:771−84.
[85] Yilmaz S, Gonenc IM, Yilmaz E. Genotoxicity of the some selective estrogen receptor modulators: a review. Cytotechnology 2014;66:533−41.
[86] Jordan VC. Tamoxifen: a most unlikely pioneering medicine. Nat Rev Drug Discovery 2003;2:205−13.
[87] Hochner-Celnikier D. Pharmacokinetics of raloxifene and its clinical application. Eur J Obs Gynecol Reprod Biol 1999;85:23−9.
[88] Howell SJ, Johnston SR, Howell A. The use of selective estrogen receptor modulators and selective estrogen receptor down-regulators in breast cancer. Best Pract Res Clin Endocrinol Metab 2004;18:47−66.
[89] Defriend DJ, Howell A, Nicholson RI, et al. Investigation of a new pure antiestrogen (ICI 182780) in women with primary breast cancer. Cancer Res 1994;54:408−14.
[90] Brueggemeier RW. Aromatase inhibitors—mechanisms of steroidal inhibitors. Breast Cancer Res Treat 1994;30:31−42.
[91] Lonning PE. Pharmacological profiles of exemestane and formestane, steroidal aromatase inhibitors used for treatment of postmenopausal breast cancer. Breast Cancer Res Treat 1998;49(Suppl 1):S45−52.
[92] Burslem GM, Crews CM. Proteolysis-targeting chimeras as therapeutics and tools for biological discovery. Cell 2020;181:102−14.
[93] Pettersson M, Crews CM. Proteolysis targeting chimeras (PROTACs) - past, present and future. Drug Discov Today Technol 2019;31:15−27.

Chapter 18

Triazole antifungal drug—fluconazole

Jie Tu and Chunquan Sheng

Naval Medical University, Shanghai, P.R. China

Chapter outline

18.1 Overview of fungal infections	449	
18.1.1 Human pathogenic fungi	449	
18.1.2 Fungal cell structure and pathogenic mechanisms	450	
18.1.3 Current status and challenges of fungal infections	451	
18.2 Overview of antifungal drugs	452	
18.2.1 Antifungal antibiotics	452	
18.2.2 Azole antifungal drugs	453	
18.2.3 Allylamine antifungal drug	454	
18.2.4 Echinocandin antifungal drugs	454	
18.3 The developmental history of fluconazole	455	
18.3.1 The discovery of lead compounds: from imidazoles to triazoles	455	
18.3.2 Optimizing lead compounds: elucidating the pharmacophore of "triazole-difluorophenyl-tertiary alcohol"	457	
18.3.3 Mechanism of action of azole antifungal agents	457	
18.3.4 Protein binding mode and structure-activity relationships of fluconazole	458	
18.3.5 Research on the synthesis process of fluconazole	459	
18.3.6 Clinical application of fluconazole	460	
18.3.7 Drug resistance of fluconazole	460	
18.4 Structure optimization of fluconazole: development of new generation triazole antifungal drugs	461	
18.4.1 Development of voriconazole	461	
18.4.2 Development of isavuconazole	462	
18.4.3 The future development of triazole drugs: from triazoles to tetrazoles?	463	
References	463	

18.1 Overview of fungal infections

Fungal infection, a common disease, was highly prevalent in populations living in lower standards and damp environments during periods of relatively limited medical care. In recent years, improvements in medical care, including the extensive utilization of antineoplastic chemotherapy agents, broad-spectrum antibiotics, and immunosuppressive agents, as well as the frequent practice of organ transplantation, catheterization techniques, and other invasive surgical procedures, coupled with the occurrence of severe infectious diseases such as AIDS and pulmonary tuberculosis, have substantially compromised the normal immune function of the human body. Consequently, the incidence of fungal infections in clinical settings has been steadily on the rise.

18.1.1 Human pathogenic fungi

Fungi, a type of eukaryotic organism, are widely distributed in the natural world. It is estimated that there are approximately 6 million species in existence, with over 100,000 species formally classified. Each year, around 1500 new fungal species are discovered [1]. The majority of fungi are beneficial to humans, while only a small fraction can induce diseases in humans, animals, and plants. Currently, more than 500 fungal species are known to be pathogenic to humans (Fig. 18.1). With the widespread use of immunosuppressive agents, broad-spectrum antibiotics, and corticosteroids, along with the extensive adoption of therapeutic and diagnostic methods such as organ transplantation, radiotherapy, and catheterization, some previously nonpathogenic fungal strains have gradually evolved into opportunistic pathogens. Consequently, the incidence of fungal infections continues to rise in clinical settings.

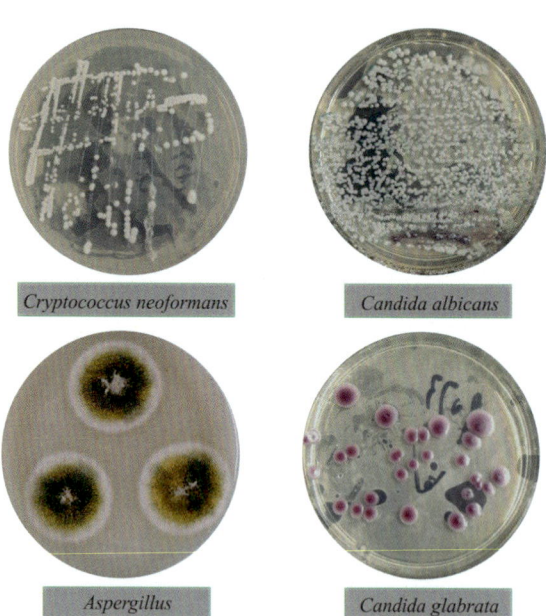

FIGURE 18.1 Morphological characteristics of common pathogenic fungi.

Human pathogenic fungi are typically categorized into three classes: anthropophilic fungi, geophilic fungi, and zoophilic fungi. Anthropophilic fungi have a higher incidence of infection and include species such as *Candida*, *Malassezia*, and *Epidermophyton*. Geophilic fungi, also known as environmental fungi, typically reside away from humans, parasitizing plants and decaying organic matter. They sporadically invade the human body, causing harm to human hosts, as exemplified by *Zygomycetes*, dimorphic fungi, and dematiaceous fungi. Zoophilic fungi, on the other hand, are referred to as indoor fungi, and individuals with compromised immune systems are more susceptible to infections by this category of fungi, including *Aspergillus* and *Penicillium*, which can occasionally trigger allergic reactions.

Diseases in humans, animals, and plants caused by fungal infections are termed mycoses. Depending on the site of fungal invasion in the human body, mycoses can be categorized into four classes: superficial mycoses, cutaneous mycoses, subcutaneous mycoses, and deep-seated mycoses. Superficial mycoses and cutaneous mycoses are collectively referred to as superficial mycoses, involving fungal infections of the skin, mucous membranes, hair, and nails, typically caused by *Epidermophyton* and superficial *Candida* species. These infections primarily affect the outermost layers of the skin, manifesting as conditions such as tinea pedis and onychomycosis, often with mild symptoms and readily diagnosable and treatable. Subcutaneous mycoses pertain to fungal infections that invade the dermis, subcutaneous tissues, and bones. These infections are usually the result of traumatic inoculation with soil or plant-associated pathogens. The lesions are typically confined to the site of inoculation or may spread to adjacent tissues, with a general absence of systemic involvement. Deep-seated mycoses, also known as invasive fungal diseases, encompass fungal infections that invade the bloodstream and disseminate throughout the body's organs and tissues, leading to systemic infections. They are characterized by high incidence and mortality rates, posing a significant challenge and area of focus in global public health research. Major fungal pathogens responsible for deep-seated infections include *Candida*, *Cryptococcus*, and *Aspergillus*, among others.

18.1.2 Fungal cell structure and pathogenic mechanisms

18.1.2.1 Fundamental structure of fungi

Fungal cells are characterized by the presence of a nucleus and nuclear pores, with linear chromosomes and nucleoli within the nucleus (Fig. 18.2). The cytoplasm contains various organelles, including mitochondria, ribosomes, rough endoplasmic reticulum, and vacuoles, although Golgi apparatus is less common. Additionally, the cytoplasm contains microfilaments composed of actin, forming the cellular cytoskeleton, as well as microtubules composed of tubulin. Unlike human cell membranes, which are rich in cholesterol, fungal cell membranes primarily consist of ergosterol, with extramembranous structures called plasmalemmasome. Differing from animal cells, fungi possess a rigid cell wall primarily composed of chitin and glucan. Fungal thalli typically exhibit a profuse branching mycelial structure, with growth occurring predominantly at the tips of hyphae. The primary targets of antifungal agents are the cell membrane and cell wall, as well as nucleic acid synthesis and function.

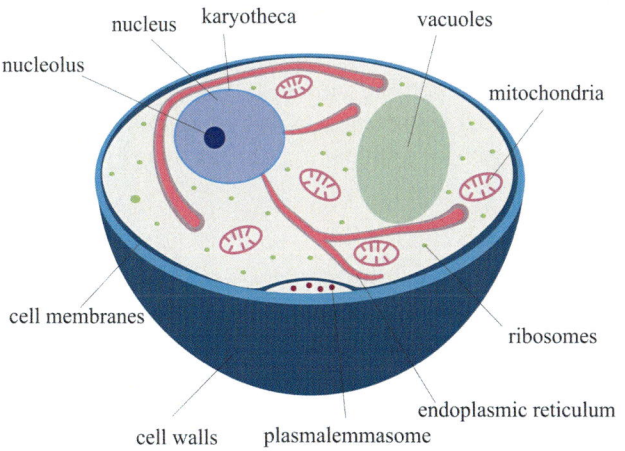

FIGURE 18.2 Basic structure of fungal cell.

18.1.2.2 Pathogenic mechanisms of fungi

Similar to other pathogenic microorganisms, fungal infections in humans result from a pathological process involving the interaction between the pathogen and the host. Fungi, leveraging their inherent genetic traits, initiate host infections through various mechanisms, including fungal adhesion to host surfaces, the release of metabolic byproducts, and the secretion of various extracellular enzymes. These actions lead to host infections and responses, ultimately resulting in a wide range of clinical pathological manifestations.

The pathogenic mechanisms underlying superficial mycoses are relatively straightforward. When fungi invade the human skin, hair, and nails, they parasitize or saprophytically colonize the keratinized tissues of the epidermis, hair, and nail plates. The fungal thalli themselves, along with their released proteolytic enzymes and other virulence factors, induce varying degrees of host inflammatory responses. This results in pathological manifestations such as erythema, scaling, itching, and swelling, encompassing conditions like tinea capitis, tinea corporis, onychomycosis, and trichomycosis. The pathogenic mechanisms of deep-seated mycoses are comparatively complex, involving multiple aspects, including fungal virulence factors, phenotypic switching, host innate and adaptive immunity, and fungal drug resistance.

18.1.3 Current status and challenges of fungal infections

Superficial fungal infections are common and widespread, with a global prevalence ranging from 20% to 25%, affecting nearly 1.7 billion individuals. In recent years, the incidence of invasive fungal infections has been steadily rising, posing a significant threat to human health, with approximately 1.5 million deaths annually. *Candida albicans* is the predominant pathogenic fungus, with a mortality rate as high as 40%, ranking fourth in nosocomial bloodstream infections. *Cryptococcus neoformans* exhibits a strong predilection for the central nervous system, frequently leading to cryptococcal meningitis, particularly prevalent among human immunodeficiency virus (HIV)-infected individuals and responsible for nearly 600,000 deaths each year. *Aspergillus* species, especially in immunocompromised patients, can readily cause invasive pulmonary aspergillosis, with a mortality rate ranging from 35% to 95%.

Fungal infections are challenging to control and prone to recurrence. The existing antifungal drug arsenal is limited in variety, associated with significant toxicity, and plagued by resistance issues. Currently, there are only four classes of antifungal drugs approved for the treatment of invasive fungal infections: polyenes (e.g., amphotericin B (AmB)), azoles (e.g., fluconazole and voriconazole), echinocandins (e.g., caspofungin and micafungin), and nucleoside analogs (e.g., 5-fluorocytosine) [2]. While these antifungal agents are widely used in clinical practice, they have several shortcomings that hinder their ability to meet clinical treatment needs. For example, AmB exhibits broad-spectrum antifungal activity but is associated with significant nephrotoxicity, limiting its use in critically ill patients. Azole antifungal drugs, while effective, carry the risk of hepatorenal toxicity, recurrence, and resistance. Echinocandins have a narrow antifungal spectrum and cannot be administered orally. Nucleoside analogs are generally ineffective when used as monotherapy and are primarily employed as part of combination therapy.

18.2 Overview of antifungal drugs

The development of antifungal drugs has spanned over half a century and has gone through four distinct phases: antifungal antibiotics, azole antifungal drugs, echinocandin antifungal drugs, and polyene antifungal drugs (Fig. 18.3) [3,4]. Given that fungi and mammalian cells are both eukaryotes, there is a need for strong selectivity to ensure safety and efficacy [5]. With the gradual maturation of target-based drug design technologies, the field of antifungal drugs has transitioned from antibiotic-based antifungals to synthetic antifungal agents.

18.2.1 Antifungal antibiotics

In the early 1950s, humanity began extracting polyene antibiotics from actinomycetes, which featured a lipophilic macrocyclic lactone ring containing 4−7 conjugated double bonds and an amino sugar moiety within their molecular structures.

In 1951, scientists isolated nystatin (Fig. 18.4) from cultures of *Streptomyces noursei*. Nystatin, a conjugated tetraene compound, became the first polyene antifungal drug employed in clinical practice. Topical nystatin applications effectively combat various fungal infections, and various topical formulations have been developed. Interestingly, due to its high toxicity, nystatin cannot be used for systemic treatment. However, because it is poorly absorbed in the gastrointestinal tract when taken orally, physicians have used it to treat local infections in the oral and gastrointestinal

FIGURE 18.3 Historical development of antifungal drugs.

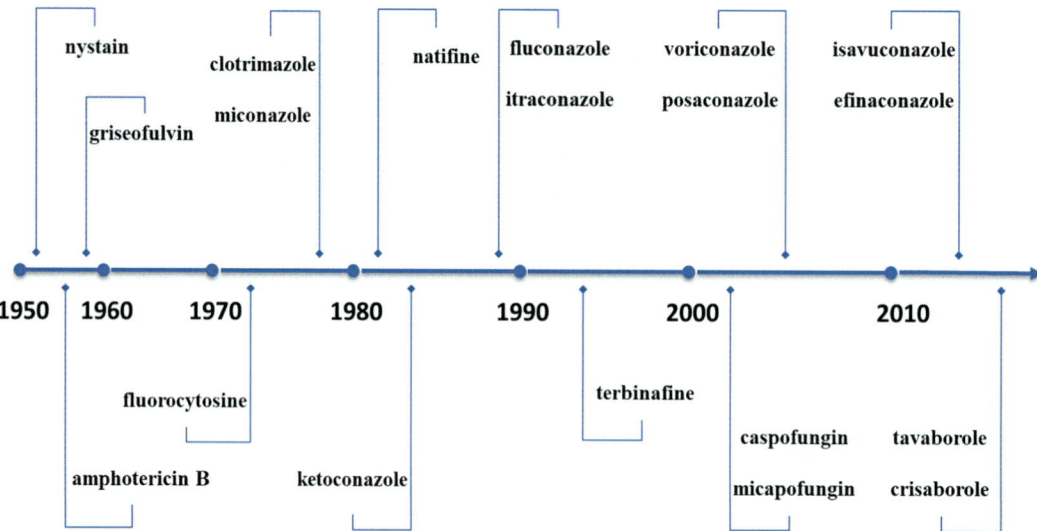

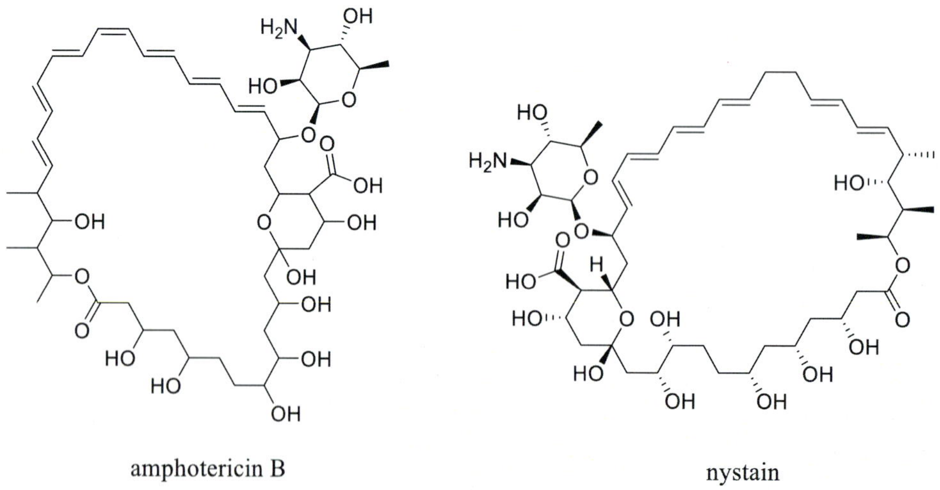

FIGURE 18.4 The chemical structures of amphotericin B and nystatin.

regions. In recent years, researchers have developed liposomal formulations of nystatin, which reduce renal toxicity while preserving its antifungal activity. The discovery of nystatin served as a starting point for the search for other polyene drugs suitable for systemic therapy.

AmB (Fig. 18.4), a heptene compound, was discovered in 1956 and rapidly approved for clinical use in 1958. Its mechanism of action involves binding to ergosterol on the fungal cell membrane, disrupting membrane permeability, leading to leakage of cellular contents, and impeding normal fungal cell metabolism, thereby inhibiting fungal growth. AmB possesses broad-spectrum antifungal activity and potent fungicidal capabilities. It remains the first-line drug for treating severe invasive fungal infections and is still considered the "gold standard" for invasive fungal infection therapy, no other antifungal drug has fully replaced its efficacy. However, its specificity for ergosterol in the fungal cell membrane is relatively low. It can also bind to cholesterol on the cell membranes of human renal tubular epithelial cells and red blood cells, contributing to its significant toxicity and limiting its clinical use. In recent years, through formulation optimization, liposomal AmB has been developed to alter drug distribution and increase plasma concentrations, thereby maintaining its fungicidal activity to some extent while reducing adverse reactions.

18.2.2 Azole antifungal drugs

Azole antifungal drugs are currently the first-line treatment for fungal infections in clinical settings. They are generally superior to antifungal antibiotics and have been developed in various formulations, including topical, oral, and intravenous administrations. Azole antifungal drugs primarily exert their effects by inhibiting the cytochrome P450-dependent enzyme, lanosterol 14α-demethylase (CYP51). This inhibition disrupts the biosynthesis of ergosterol, a crucial component of the fungal cell membrane. Simultaneously, the accumulation of methylated lanosterol inside the cell leads to alterations in various membrane-related cellular functions, ultimately resulting in the inhibition or killing of fungal cells [6]. The development of azole drugs began in the 1970s, with clotrimazole and miconazole being the earliest agents to attract significant attention due to their novel structures. These drugs share a common imidazole moiety in their chemical structure, earning them the designation of "imidazole antifungal drugs" (Fig. 18.5). Early imidazole antifungal drugs exhibited broad-spectrum antifungal activity but were associated with significant toxicity when used for invasive fungal infections, limiting their use to topical applications. In the early 1980s, scientists embarked on extensive structural modifications of these drugs to improve metabolic stability and reduce lipophilicity. This research resulted in the development of the first oral imidazole antifungal drug, ketoconazole. Compared to early imidazole antifungal drugs, ketoconazole achieved a significantly higher oral bioavailability of 75% and maintained elevated blood drug concentrations. What sets ketoconazole apart from other imidazole antifungal drugs is its versatility: it can be used for the treatment of both superficial and invasive fungal infections, administered orally or topically. This versatility significantly improves patient compliance. However, ketoconazole still exhibits adverse effects, including liver toxicity and inhibition of hormone synthesis, limiting its clinical use to some extent.

In the 1990s, research focus shifted from imidazole to triazole compounds (Fig. 18.6). Representative drugs such as fluconazole and itraconazole demonstrated high affinity for fungal cytochrome P450 enzymes, significantly reducing adverse reactions and ushering in a new era for the treatment of invasive fungal infections in humans. In 1990, fluconazole, developed by Pfizer in the United States, received Food and Drug Administration (FDA) approval for marketing. It boasts a broad antifungal spectrum, with efficacy observed in both oral and intravenous administration, and exhibits superior in vivo antifungal activity compared to ketoconazole. Itraconazole, another triazole antifungal drug introduced around the same time, offers excellent oral absorption and high lipid solubility, leading to elevated concentrations in various organs. As new pathogenic fungi and resistant strains emerged, a new generation of triazole antifungal drugs such as voriconazole, posaconazole, and isavuconazole have been developed and introduced to clinical practice [7].

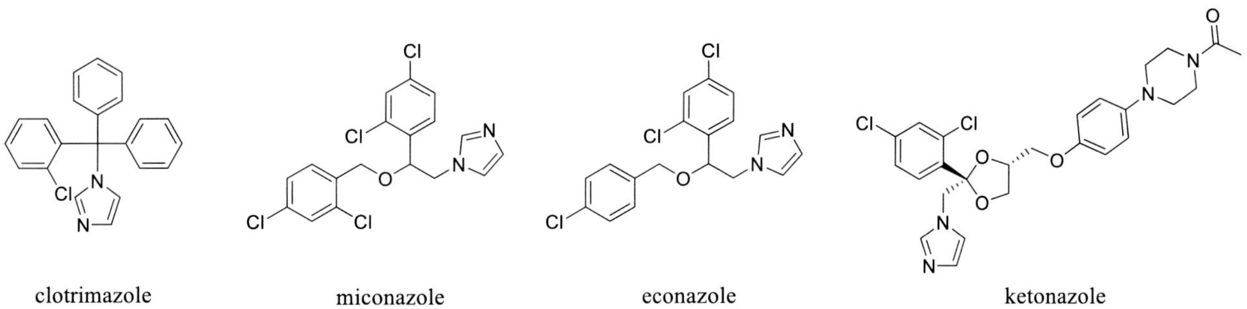

FIGURE 18.5 The chemical structures of imidazole antifungal drugs.

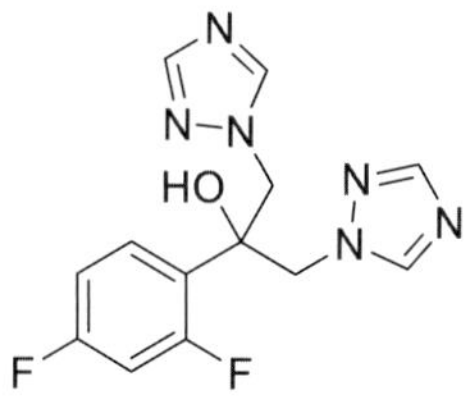

fluconazole

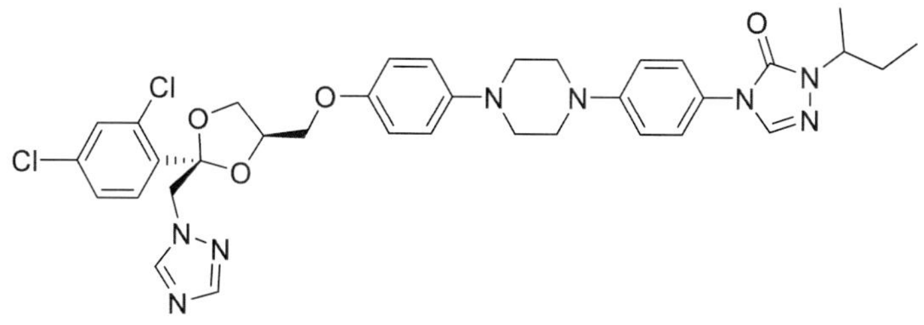

itraconazole

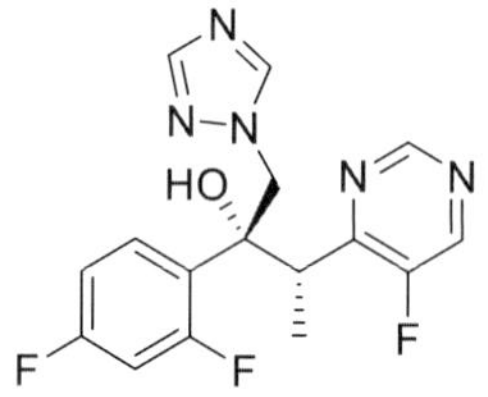

voriconazole

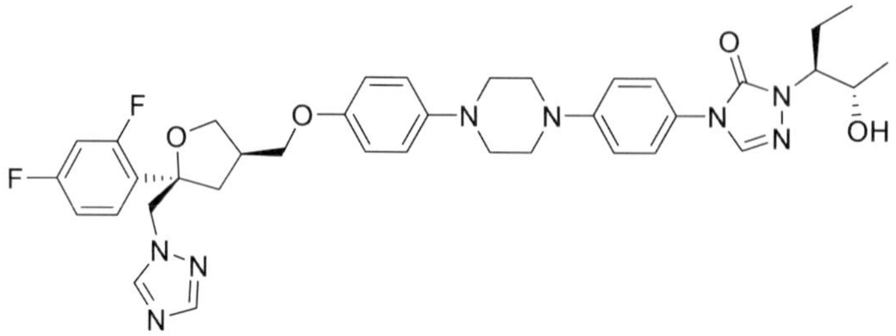

posaconazole

FIGURE 18.6 The chemical structures of triazole antifungal drugs.

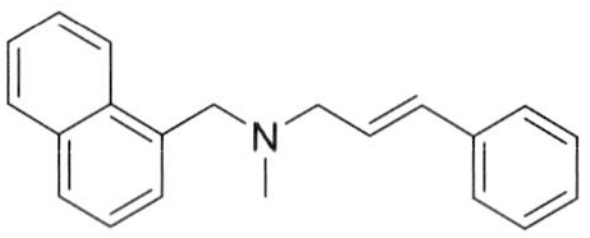

natifine

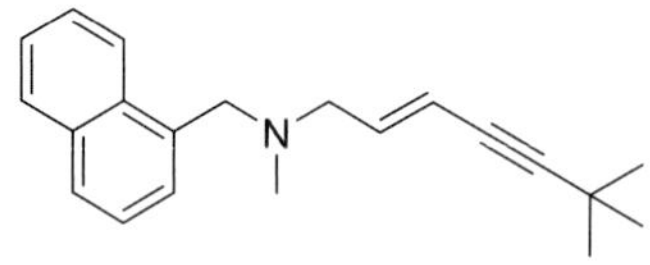

terbinafine

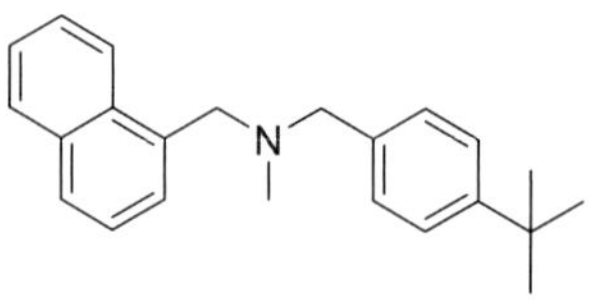

butenafine

FIGURE 18.7 The chemical structures of allylamine antifungal drugs.

18.2.3 Allylamine antifungal drug

The allylamine drugs act by inhibiting fungal squalene epoxidase, disrupting the early steps of fungal sterol biosynthesis. This disruption leads to a deficiency of ergosterol and the accumulation of squalene within fungal cells, ultimately causing fungal cell death. In 1981, researchers serendipitously discovered that the allylamine compound naftifine (Fig. 18.7) exhibited broad-spectrum antifungal activity, particularly with fungicidal effects against dermatophytes. It proved to be more effective than imidazole antifungal drugs when topically applied for the treatment of dermatophyte infections. Through extensive structural modifications and studies of antifungal activity, scientists identified terbinafine, which has an even broader spectrum of antifungal activity and can be administered topically or orally. Further modifications of terbinafine led to the development of butenafine, which has higher antifungal activity. Although butenafine lacks carbon–carbon double bonds and no longer falls within the allylamine class structurally, its mechanism of action remains similar to that of other allylamine drugs. Therefore, in clinical practice, butenafine is still classified as an allylamine antifungal drug.

18.2.4 Echinocandin antifungal drugs

Since the beginning of the 21st century, the focus of antifungal drug development has shifted toward compounds that are more selective, ensuring both safety and efficacy [8–11]. Among these, the advent of echinocandin drugs truly exemplifies the ideal state of antifungal drugs, which only target fungal-specific structures or metabolic processes without adversely affecting the host (Fig. 18.8) [8]. These drugs exhibit a low occurrence of cross-resistance, good tolerance, minimal toxicity, and few adverse effects. They also have limited drug–drug interactions. Echinocandins demonstrate excellent fungicidal activity against several common clinical *Candida* species and remain effective against

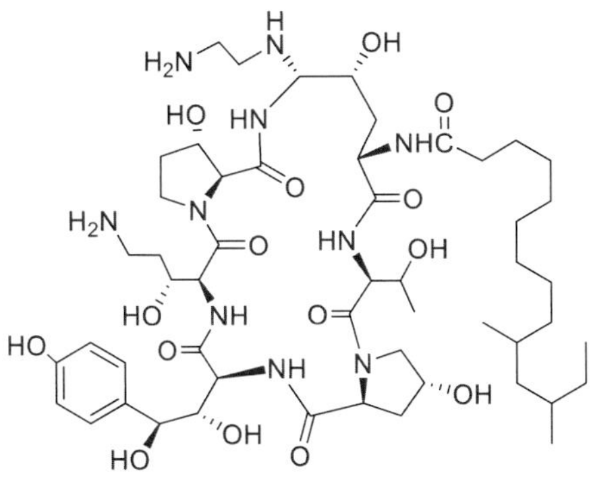

caspofungin

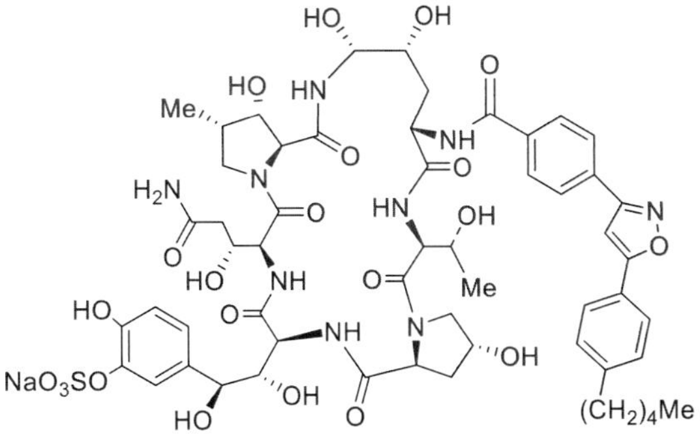

micapofungin

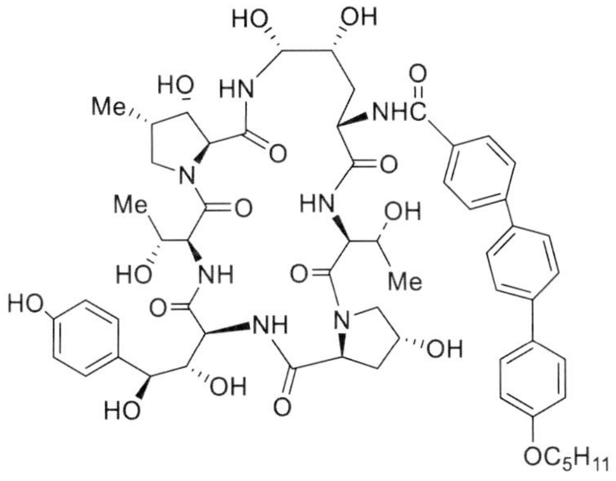

anidulafungin

FIGURE 18.8 The chemical structures of echinocandin antifungal drugs.

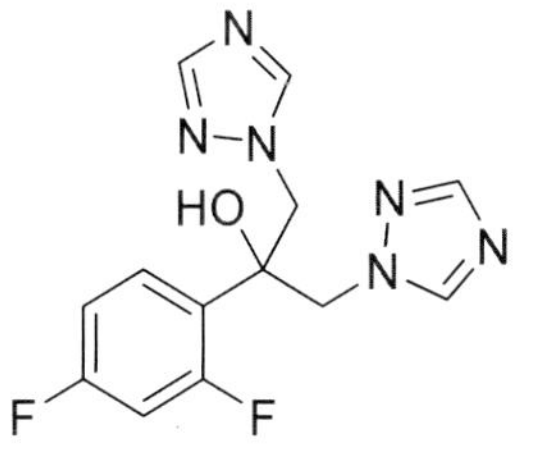

FIGURE 18.9 α-(2,4-difluorophenyl)-α-(1H-1,2,4-triazol-1-ylmethyl)-1H-1,2,4-triazole-1-ethanol.

azoles-resistant fungi. Since 2001, representative drugs such as caspofungin, micafungin, and anidulafungin have been introduced. Their drawback is that they are only available in injectable formulations and are relatively expensive, which has hindered their widespread adoption in the short term.

18.3 The developmental history of fluconazole

(Fig. 18.9)

18.3.1 The discovery of lead compounds: from imidazoles to triazoles

As early as 1944, British chemist Wooley had discovered that the compound phenylimidazole exhibited antifungal activity. However, it was not until the 1960s that this discovery began to garner the attention of other scientists. In 1967, Bayer and Janssen Pharmaceuticals independently developed pioneering antifungal prototypes: clotrimazole and miconazole. Despite the structural differences between these two compounds, they both featured the imidazole ring as a crucial moiety in their drug structures. In 1978, Janssen Pharmaceuticals developed ketoconazole, which could be taken orally. The imidazole ring and dioxolane structure were essential pharmacophores, inspiring further investigations to retain the imidazole ring and explore chemical modifications for potentially improved antifungal drugs.

In the 1970s, Pfizer initiated a research project for antifungal drugs with the aim of finding an effective treatment for invasive fungal infections. In 1974, using miconazole as a lead compound, Pfizer scientists synthesized numerous derivatives, leading to the discovery of tioconazole (Fig. 18.10). However, its drug properties were similar to miconazole, and it did not exhibit significant advantages. Both miconazole and tioconazole had more than 50% of the drug metabolized upon oral entry into the liver, with only a small fraction of free drug circulating in the body to exert its antifungal effects. In 1978, following Janssen Pharmaceuticals' announcement of the invention of ketoconazole, Pfizer immediately started a series of research efforts using ketoconazole as a lead compound. At that time, most antifungal drugs were lipophilic, making them prone to binding with fatty acids and proteins. Additionally, these antifungal drugs were rapidly metabolized, leading to low bioavailability. This limited most antifungal drugs of the time to topical applications, rendering them unsuitable for oral administration. To find a more effective antifungal drug that could be both orally and intravenously administered, Pfizer's Richardson research team replaced the dioxolane structure of ketoconazole with a polar hydroxyl group, reducing the molecule's lipophilicity. While this improved the antifungal efficacy, it still did not provide a significant advantage over ketoconazole. This was due to the researchers' limited understanding of the imidazole ring structure at the time. In 1980, Richardson proposed the idea of altering the imidazole ring to improve compound stability. Dozens of different substituents were designed to replace the imidazole ring. When the triazole ring was introduced, they finally discovered a compound that was more effective than ketoconazole. The improved activity was attributed to the triazole ring slowing down the compound's metabolism, allowing more free drugs to stay in the body and exert its antifungal effects. Inspired by this, they also introduced a triazole ring on the other side of the ketoconazole molecule to further enhance metabolic stability in the body, resulting in a compound containing two triazole rings, known by the codename UK-47265 (Fig. 18.10). This compound was particularly effective in treating severe *Candida* infections in mice.

Unfortunately, UK-47265 exhibited strong hepatotoxicity. Researchers had to further modify this structure and synthesize and screen a large number of derivatives. In 1981, the introduction of two fluorine atoms to replace two chlorine atoms on the benzene ring led to the discovery of a compound codenamed UK-49858 (Fig. 18.10). This compound, later officially named fluconazole, demonstrated antifungal activity 5–20 times higher than ketoconazole. In addition to its superior antifungal efficacy, fluconazole had a more stable metabolism, distributed evenly in tissues and the gastrointestinal tract, and had lower binding affinity to fatty acids and plasma proteins compared to other antifungal drugs. This compound did not undergo breakdown in the liver, leading to significantly slowed metabolism. After oral administration, fluconazole exhibited a particularly long duration of action, with a half-life of 29 hours, allowing for once-daily dosing in clinical practice. Approximately 90% of fluconazole was excreted unchanged in the urine and feces.

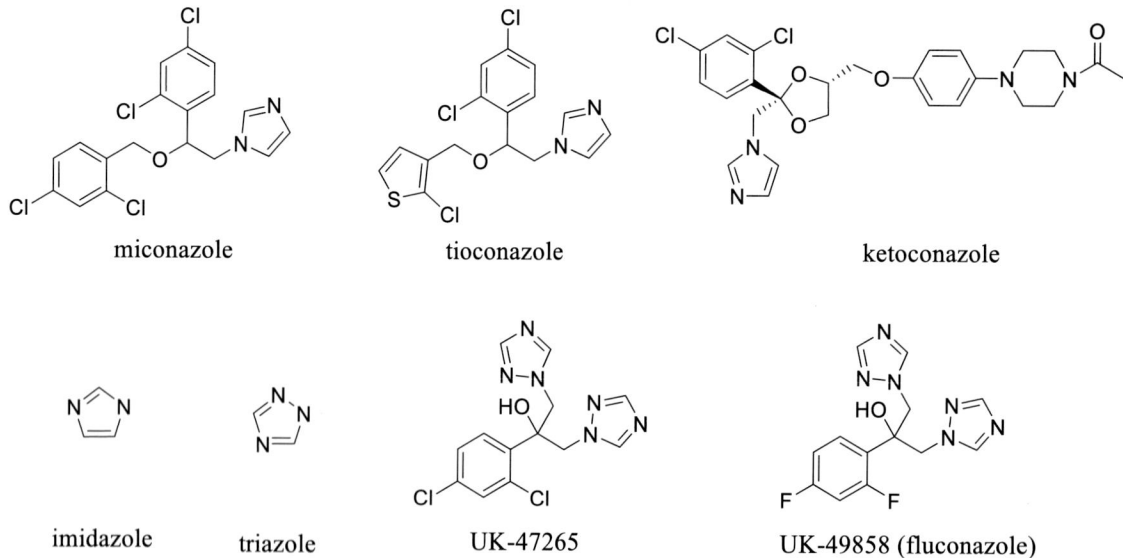

FIGURE 18.10 The discovery of lead structures in the triazole antifungal drugs.

Fluconazole had good water solubility, making it suitable for intravenous administration. Due to its small molecular weight, it could easily enter the cerebrospinal fluid, making it effective for treating fungal infections in the brain.

Following its introduction, fluconazole quickly gained widespread use and became the preferred first-line therapy. Pfizer's research team was awarded the "Queen's Award for Technological Achievement" by Queen Elizabeth II in 1991 for their contribution to the development of fluconazole.

18.3.2 Optimizing lead compounds: elucidating the pharmacophore of "triazole-difluorophenyl-tertiary alcohol"

In the molecular structures of miconazole, tioconazole, and ketoconazole all encompass the imidazole moiety. This elucidates the pivotal role of the imidazole moiety in the early stages of antifungal drug development. However, the trajectory of drug development is seldom immutable. In pursuit of formulating orally administered antifungal agents for invasive fungal infections, scientists had to challenge the prevailing consensus. Through an exhaustive examination of structure-activity relationships (SARs) involving thousands of compounds, it was discerned that replacing the imidazole moiety with a triazole ring not only enhanced the antifungal efficacy but also significantly decelerated hepatic metabolism, thereby conspicuously augmenting oral bioavailability. To mitigate the issue of excessive lipophilicity associated with imidazole drugs, substituting the dioxolane ring in ketoconazole with a hydroxyl group was instrumental in markedly enhancing the aqueous solubility of the drug molecule. Addressing safety concerns, it was only after synthesizing and screening a plethora of derivatives that the substitution of a chlorine atom on the benzene ring with a fluorine atom was discovered to drastically reduce hepatotoxicity. This culminated in the successful development of fluconazole (Fig. 18.11).

The history of the discovery of fluconazole underscores the profound impact and arduous journey of classical medicinal chemistry SAR studies in the drug development process. Over the course of nearly two decades, researchers initiated their efforts with benzimidazole as a lead compound and, through relentless structural optimizations, eventually arrived at the elucidation of the pharmacophore consisting of the "Triazole-Difluorophenyl-Tertiary Alcohol" (Fig. 18.11).

18.3.3 Mechanism of action of azole antifungal agents

Sterols constitute vital components of both fungal and mammalian cell membranes, playing a pivotal role in the function of enzymes and ion transport proteins on the membrane [12–14]. The key distinction between fungi and mammals lies in the type of sterol present in their cell membranes. Mammalian cell membranes predominantly contain cholesterol, whereas fungi are characterized by the presence of ergosterol [15].

Azole drugs exert their antifungal effects by targeting lanosterol 14α-demethylase (CYP51), a critical enzyme involved in the biosynthesis of fungal ergosterol (Fig. 18.12). The nitrogen atom of azole drugs can directly coordinate with the iron ion on the heme moiety of the fungal CYP51 enzyme, while the remaining portion interacts with amino

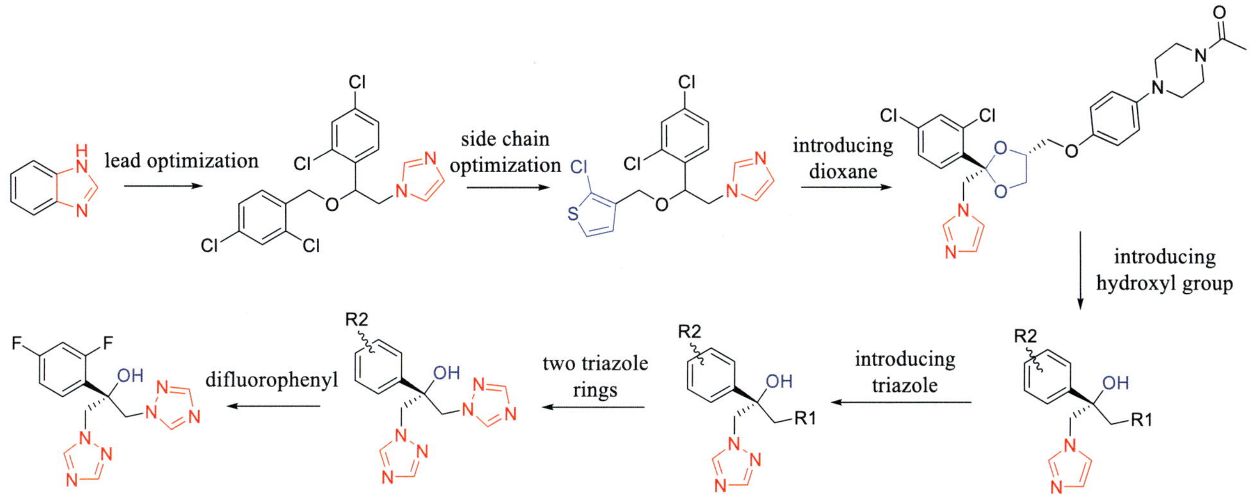

FIGURE 18.11 The developmental history of fluconazole.

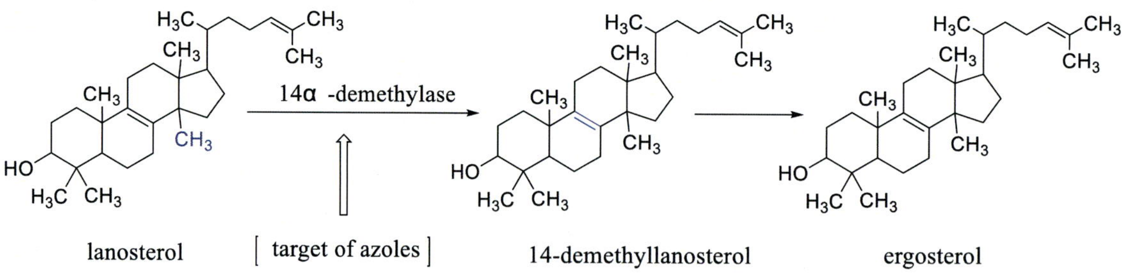

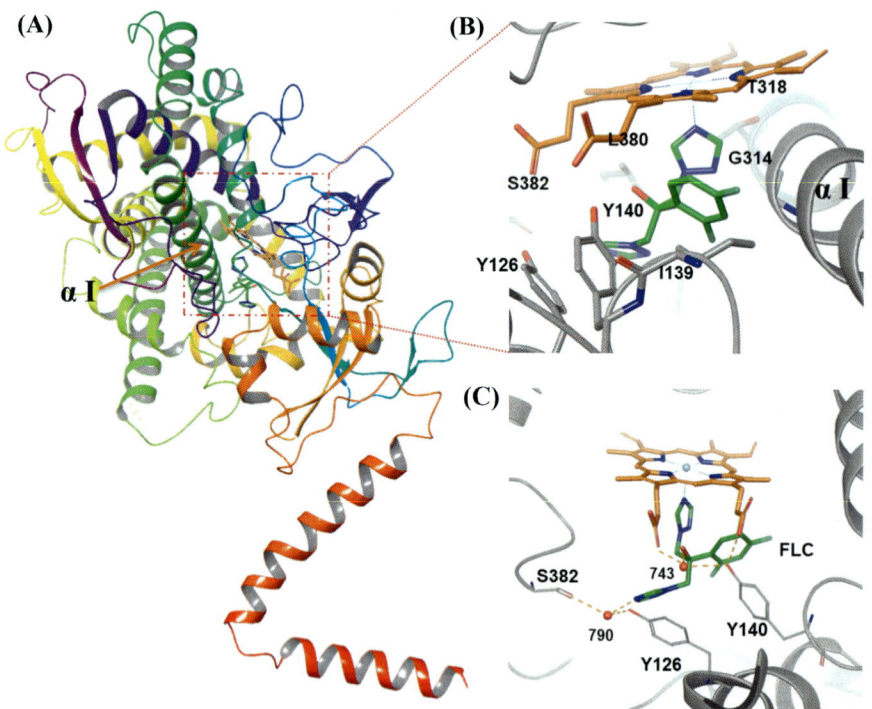

FIGURE 18.12 Biosynthesis pathway of ergosterol in the fungal cell membrane.

FIGURE 18.13 The binding mode of fluconazole with fungal CYP51 protein.

acid residues at the active site. This interaction ultimately inhibits the demethylation of lanosterol at the 14α-methyl position, allowing sterols that accumulate in the fungal cell membrane to retain their methyl groups. These sterols, lacking the precise shape and physical properties of normal ergosterol, disrupt membrane permeability, leading to content leakage and dysfunctional membrane protein activity. Consequently, this disruption culminates in fungal cell death.

18.3.4 Protein binding mode and structure-activity relationships of fluconazole

The crystal structure of fungal CYP51 protein was originally obtained through purification from *Saccharomyces cerevisiae*. In recent years, extensive research has delved into the three-dimensional structures of various pathogenic fungal CYP51 proteins, their active sites, and their binding interactions with azole drugs. As a ligand, fluconazole primarily binds to the active site of the CYP51 protein through hydrophobic interactions and hydrogen bonding (Fig. 18.13).

A substantial portion of the fluconazole molecule resides in the solvent-exposed region of the CYP51 protein's active site, resulting in robust hydrophobic interactions. Within a 4 Å radius, interactions involve 12 amino acid residues, including Tyr126, Ile139, Tyr140, Gly314, Thr318, Leu380, and Ser382. The triazole ring within the molecule is essential, as its 4-N atom coordinates with the iron ion on the heme moiety (Fe-N distance: 2−3 Å), competitively inhibiting CYP51 enzyme activity. The coordinating triazole ring is in proximity to Gly314, aiding in overall molecule binding to α-helix I (Fig. 18.13B). Substituting the triazole ring with an imidazole ring results in diminished coordination, leading to reduced antifungal activity. When other groups replace the triazole, coordination cannot occur, resulting in a loss of antifungal activity. During the binding process, water molecules can mediate hydrogen bonding interactions (Fig. 18.13C). The first water molecule, 743, facilitates a hydrogen bond network between fluconazole's hydroxyl group, Tyr140, and the heme moiety's propionate. Substituting the alcohol hydroxyl with other oxygen-containing rings, such as dioxolane or tetrahydrofuran, maintains hydrogen bonding interactions and antifungal activity (e.g., ketoconazole and itraconazole). The second water molecule, 790, mediates a hydrogen bond network between Ser382 carbonyl oxygen, Tyr126 hydroxyl, and the 4-N atom of another triazole ring. Substituting the triazole ring with groups containing nitrogen or oxygen atoms, such as ether or pyrimidine, likewise maintains hydrogen bonding interactions and antifungal activity. Furthermore, due to the group's orientation toward the heme moiety in the opposite direction, it can be replaced with a longer side chain. The difluorophenyl moiety in the molecular structure possesses a significant volume and electronegativity, primarily facilitating hydrophobic interactions. Consequently, electronegative substituents on the phenyl ring are advantageous for antifungal activity.

18.3.5 Research on the synthesis process of fluconazole

The early synthetic route for fluconazole begins with 1,2-difluorobenzene as the starting material. It proceeds sequentially through Friedel–Crafts acylation with chloroacetyl chloride and triazole substitution with 1H-1,2,4-triazole. Subsequently, it reacts with trimethyl sulfonyl chloride or trimethyl sulfonyl iodide to form an epoxide intermediate. Finally, fluconazole is obtained through the opening of the epoxide intermediate with triazole (Fig. 18.14). This method is widely used but relies on the costly and low-yield trimethyl sulfonyl chloride or trimethyl sulfonyl iodide, making it challenging to reduce the production cost of fluconazole.

Another commonly employed production process for fluconazole is depicted in Fig. 18.15. Starting with 1,3-dibromopropane (I), the carbonyl group is initially protected in the presence of toluene/ethylene glycol and catalyzed by

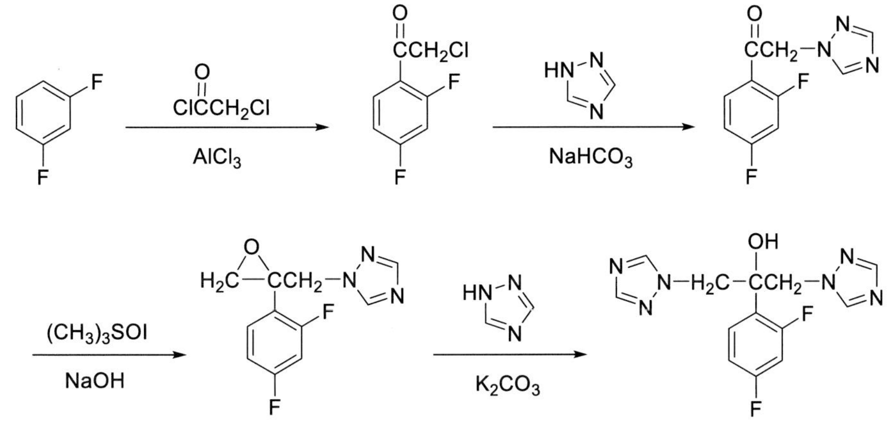

FIGURE 18.14 The synthesis pathway of fluconazole.

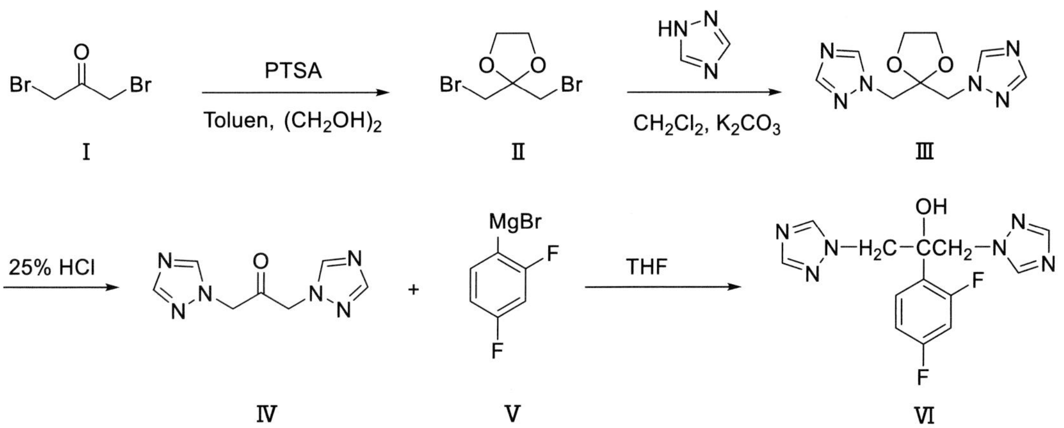

FIGURE 18.15 Synthesis process of fluconazole.

p-toluenesulfonic acid to yield 2,2-dibromo-methyl-1,3-dioxane (II). Subsequently, in a dichloromethane/K_2CO_3 system, intermediate II undergoes a reaction with 1H-1,2,4-triazole to form 1,1'-(2,2-dimethyl-1H-1,2,4-triazole-1,3-diyl) dipropane (III). Under acidic conditions, deprotection leads to 1,3-di(1H-1,2,4-triazol-1-yl)propanone (IV). Finally, the reaction with the 3,5-difluorobromobenzene-forming reagent (V) yields the end product fluconazole (VI). This synthesis route avoids the use of expensive trimethyl sulfonyl chloride or trimethyl sulfonyl iodide, exhibits good selectivity in each reaction step, and utilizes readily available and inexpensive starting materials, effectively reducing production costs. Additionally, the reaction conditions are mild, each step involves standard reaction procedures, and the final product is obtained in just four reaction steps without the need for complex or specialized equipment.

18.3.6 Clinical application of fluconazole

Fluconazole is a widely used broad-spectrum antifungal agent with therapeutic efficacy against fungal infections in both humans and animals. It is available in various forms on the market, including tablets, capsules, powder for injection, and intravenous solutions. The pharmacokinetic characteristics of intravenous administration and oral intake of fluconazole are similar. Furthermore, oral fluconazole is well-absorbed, unaffected by food, and exhibits a bioavailability exceeding 90%. Under fasting conditions, peak plasma concentrations are reached within 0.5–1.5 hours after oral administration, with blood drug levels increasing with higher oral doses. Fluconazole has a plasma protein binding rate of approximately 15%. After absorption in the body, the drug is rapidly and widely distributed, with concentrations in most body fluids and tissues exceeding 50% of concurrent blood drug levels. The highest concentration is found in the kidneys, with concentrations in saliva and sputum similar to plasma levels. In cerebrospinal fluid, concentrations are approximately 80% of concurrent plasma levels. Fluconazole can penetrate inflamed eye tissue and dialysis fluid, and it accumulates at high concentrations in the stratum corneum, dermis, and sweat secretions, sometimes surpassing plasma concentrations. Metabolism of fluconazole in the human body is minimal, primarily occurring through hepatic pathways. Over 90% of the drug is excreted via the kidneys, with approximately 80% as the unchanged parent drug and 10% as metabolites. The plasma elimination half-life of fluconazole is approximately 30 hours.

In clinical practice, fluconazole is used to treat invasive candidiasis, esophageal candidiasis, superficial fungal infections, and prophylactic treatment in patients undergoing chemotherapy and immunosuppressive therapy. Users of fluconazole should undergo regular monitoring of liver and kidney function. Furthermore, it is advisable to avoid unnecessary prophylactic use to prevent the development of drug resistance, and cross-allergic reactions may occur with other triazole antifungal drugs.

Common adverse reactions associated with fluconazole include nausea, vomiting, abdominal pain, or diarrhea. Toxic side effects are relatively mild, with occasional occurrences of skin rash, and rare instances of toxic epidermal necrolysis. Elevated liver enzymes may occur, and in some cases, liver toxicity symptoms may be observed. Dizziness, headache, and rare occurrences of hypokalemia, leukopenia, thrombocytopenia, and renal dysfunction have also been reported.

18.3.7 Drug resistance of fluconazole

In recent years, there has been an overall increase in fungal infections, and with the widespread use of antifungal drugs, some strains of *Candida* and *Aspergillus* have started to exhibit resistance to azole drugs, including fluconazole [16]. In some regions, resistance is becoming more prevalent, posing new challenges to clinical treatment. Fluconazole itself only has fungistatic activity and cannot kill pathogenic fungi, a characteristic that can contribute to the development of resistance. Fungal resistance to fluconazole primarily involves three major mechanisms: target gene mutations or overexpression, increased expression of efflux pumps, and stress adaptation.

In *Candida* species, the gene encoding CYP51 is erg11, which exhibits significant genetic polymorphism with over 100 potential mutation sites. However, only a subset of these mutations is associated with resistance to fluconazole, such as K143R and S405F. Research has shown that the biosynthesis of fungal ergosterol is regulated by numerous transcriptional activators and inhibitors, which can alter the sensitivity of *Candida* or *Aspergillus* to azole drugs by affecting the expression levels of the target protein. For example, mutations in the upc2p transcription factor gene, such as A643V, can lead to overexpression of the erg11 gene in *C. albicans*, resulting in resistance to azole drugs.

Increased expression of efflux pumps is another common mechanism of resistance to azole drugs. When efflux pump genes are overexpressed, they actively remove drug molecules from fungal cells, conferring resistance to this class of drugs. Efflux pump genes associated with resistance mainly belong to two major superfamilies: the ATP-binding cassette (ABC) superfamily and the major facilitator superfamily (MFS). In *C. albicans*, the CDR1 and CDR2 genes in the ABC superfamily and the MDR1 gene in the MFS superfamily play crucial roles in resistance to fluconazole. The transcriptional activator PDR1 can also induce resistance to azole drugs in *Candida* species by regulating the expression of the CDR1 protein.

In recent years, several proteins related to cell membrane stress responses, such as heat shock protein 90 and Sgt1, have been found to be associated with fungal resistance. Additionally, proteins related to oxidative stress and cell wall integrity stress responses, such as Yap1 and Mkk2, can reduce the sensitivity of pathogenic fungi to azole antifungal drugs such as fluconazole.

18.4 Structure optimization of fluconazole: development of new generation triazole antifungal drugs

The binding mode of fluconazole to the target enzyme CYP51 reveals that its C_3 triazole ring is situated within the substrate access channel of the active site. This elongated channel can accommodate the short side chain of fluconazole and also accommodate the long side chain of itraconazole. The development of next-generation triazole drugs based on fluconazole primarily focuses on structural optimization of the C_3 side chain [17−21].

18.4.1 Development of voriconazole

Voriconazole, developed by Pfizer, was first approved for sale in the United States in August 2002. It is a product of further structural modification of fluconazole (Fig. 18.16). In 1996, the research group led by Dickinson discovered that adding a methyl group to the propyl skeleton of fluconazole significantly enhanced its affinity for CYP51 and improved its inhibitory activity against *Aspergillus*. The minimum inhibitory concentration (MIC) value for voriconazole was found to be 12.5 μg/mL, whereas for fluconazole, it was greater than 50 μg/mL. Building upon this discovery, further structural modifications were made to the C_3 side chain. When the triazole ring was replaced with a substituted pyrimidine group, the in vitro antifungal activity increased to 0.39−3.1 μg/mL, although the in vivo activity of such compounds remained relatively poor. However, a significant improvement in antifungal efficacy was achieved when substituted pyrimidine groups were introduced. Among them, the MIC value for the 2R,3S-enantiomer with a 5-F atom reached 0.09 μg/mL. Additionally, the introduction of a fluorine atom enhanced its in vivo metabolic stability, ensuring its high antifungal activity within the body.

Voriconazole can be administered intravenously or orally and is primarily used to treat severe invasive fungal infections, caused by fluconazole-resistant *Aspergillus*, *Candida*, *Fusarium*, and *Scedosporium* species. It is rapidly and completely absorbed when taken orally, reaching peak blood concentrations within 1−2 hours of administration. Voriconazole has an oral bioavailability of approximately 96%, and its absorption is not affected by changes in gastric pH. The drug is widely distributed throughout the body, including the central nervous system, with distribution observed in the cerebrospinal fluid. Its elimination half-life in the body is approximately 6 hours, with most of it undergoing hepatic metabolism and only a small portion being excreted by the kidneys. The primary metabolite is *N*-oxide,

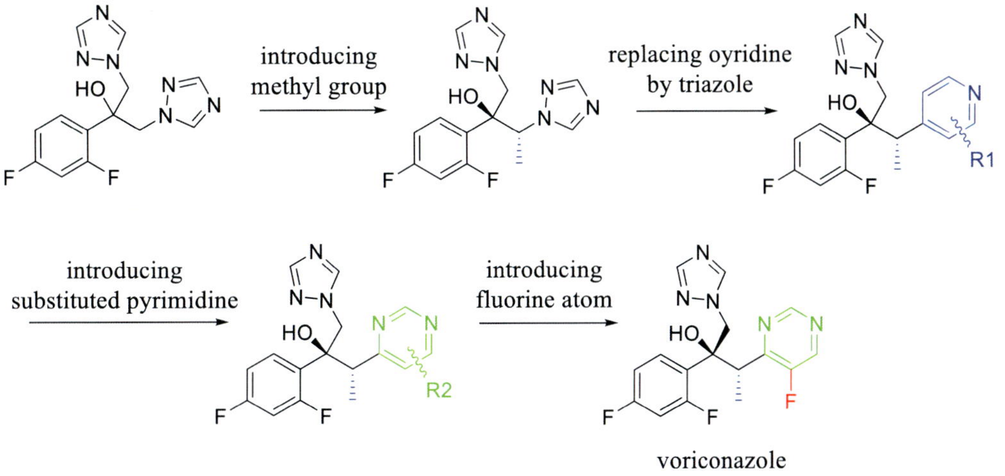

FIGURE 18.16 The development of voriconazole.

which has weak antifungal inhibitory activity and does not significantly affect the pharmacological action of voriconazole. Common adverse reactions during clinical use include visual disturbances, fever, nausea, vomiting, diarrhea, and elevated liver enzymes. Rare side effects may include allergic reactions, hyperkalemia, muscle weakness, and taste disturbances.

18.4.2 Development of isavuconazole

Isavuconazole is a novel triazole broad-spectrum antifungal medication used to treat invasive aspergillosis and invasive mucormycosis [22]. In 2001, at the 21st Symposium on Medicinal Chemistry organized by the Pharmaceutical Society of Japan, the Ohwada research group first revealed the molecular structure of isavuconazole's precursor, ravuconazole (Fig. 18.17). Ravuconazole is a new compound obtained by modifying the structure of the C_3 side chain of voriconazole while retaining the methyl group on the propyl skeleton and introducing a thiazole side chain. These modifications enhanced the molecule's affinity for fungal CYP51 proteins, broadened its antifungal spectrum, and allowed it to inhibit fungi resistant to other azole drugs. Despite its broad-spectrum antifungal activity, ravuconazole had poor oral absorption due to its high lipophilicity.

Isavuconazonium sulfate is the prodrug form of isavuconazole, developed by Astellas Pharma in Japan. It received FDA approval in 2015 and was granted orphan drug status. It is marketed under the brand name Cresemba and is available in both oral and intravenous formulations. As a prodrug, isavuconazonium sulfate not only increases the water solubility of the drug but also eliminates the renal toxicity associated with other triazole drugs (such as voriconazole) when administered intravenously due to the use of cyclodextrins to solubilize the drug. After entering the body, isavuconazonium sulfate is rapidly converted by plasma esterases into its active metabolite, ravuconazole, which has a relatively long half-life. The half-life for intravenous administration is 76–104 hours, while for oral administration, it is 56–77 hours, allowing for once-daily dosing.

Isavuconazole exhibits good antifungal activity against various fungal species, including *Aspergillus*, *Mucorales*, *Candida*, *C. neoformans*, and *Zygomycetes* species. Its activity against *Aspergillus* species (MIC range: 0.06–16 μg/mL) is comparable to that of voriconazole but superior to that of echinocandin drugs. Because it does not contain cyclodextrins associated with renal toxicity, isavuconazonium sulfate does not require dose adjustment in patients with renal impairment. It is generally well-tolerated, with common adverse reactions including nausea, vomiting, headache, abnormal liver function tests, hypokalemia, dyspnea, and edema. Rare side effects may include hepatosplenic issues, severe hypersensitivity reactions, and skin reactions.

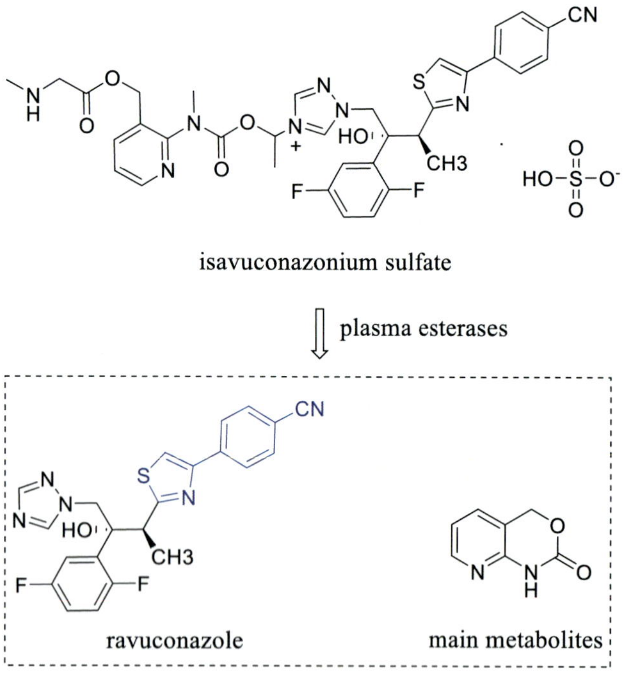

FIGURE 18.17 The in vivo metabolites of isavuconazole.

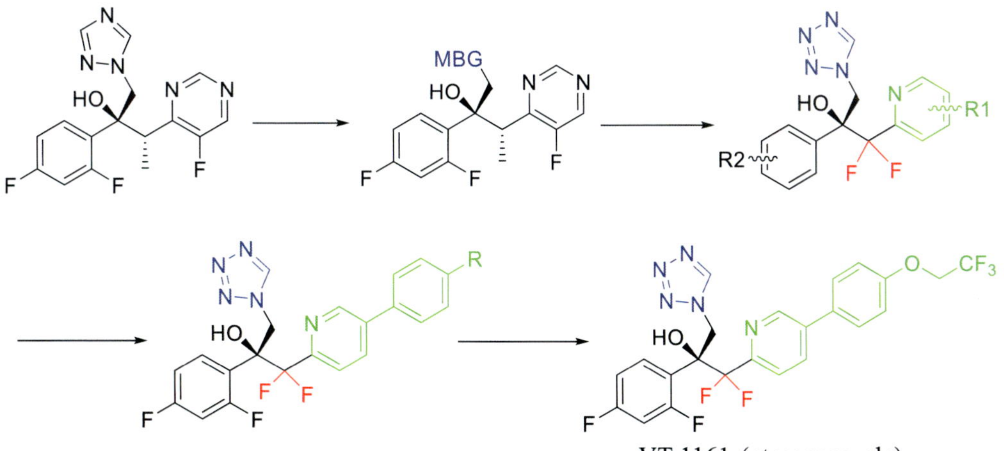

FIGURE 18.18 Development of tetrazolium antifungal drug VT-1161.

18.4.3 The future development of triazole drugs: from triazoles to tetrazoles?

Triazole drugs are primarily metabolized by the hepatic CYP450 enzyme system, particularly CYP3A4 and CYP3A5 enzymes, which can lead to hepatotoxicity. Due to the high similarity between fungal cells and human cells, the development of selective antifungal drugs poses significant challenges [23]. Recent research has revealed that replacing the triazole moiety that coordinates with iron ions in azole drugs with a tetrazole moiety can reduce the drug's affinity for CYP3A4 and enhance its selectivity for the fungal target enzyme CYP51. A representative molecule, VT-1161, has entered clinical trials. This molecule, developed by Mycovia Pharma, is a novel tetrazole antifungal clinical candidate that can be administered orally for the treatment of recurrent vulvovaginal candidiasis and onychomycosis.

In 2014, the research team led by William explored metal-binding group (MBG) on C_1 based on voriconazole. They substituted it with various imidazole, triazole, and tetrazole groups. It was discovered that when 1-tetrazole was attached to C_1, it reduced its affinity for CYP3A4 with an IC_{50} value of 32 μM (IC_{50} of voriconazole: 13 μM). However, this substitution resulted in a roughly 20-fold decrease in in vitro inhibitory activity against *C. albicans*. Consequently, optimization of the C_3 side chain was undertaken, involving the introduction of two fluorine atoms into the propyl scaffold and the replacement of the pyrimidine ring with a pyridine ring (Fig. 18.18). This modification maintained a relatively low CYP3A4 affinity (IC_{50} range: 53–74 μM) while enhancing antifungal activity. Further refinement of the C_3 side chain led to the selection of VT-1161, which exhibited a 60-fold improvement in in vitro antifungal activity compared to voriconazole. Its IC_{50} value against CYP3A4 was 65 μM, indicating a remarkable selectivity of 65,000-fold.

As a novel fungal CYP51 inhibitor, VT-1161 displayed potent inhibitory effects against various fungi. Clinical trial results demonstrated its superior efficacy in treating vulvovaginal candidiasis compared to fluconazole, with a lower recurrence rate. Due to its excellent selectivity for fungal CYP enzymes, VT-1161 is considered to have higher selectivity, fewer side effects, and greater antimicrobial potency. The emergence of VT-1161 represents another significant breakthrough in the history of antifungal drug development, continuing the evolution from "imidazole-triazole" to tetrazole. It is believed that in the near future, azole antifungal drugs will follow the path of "triazole-tetrazole."

References

[1] Reiss E, Shadomy HJ, Lyon GM. Fundamental medical mycology. Wiley-Blackwell; 2011. p. 4–30.
[2] Fu YD, Min XW, Tian SW, et al. Progress on research of antifungal drugs. Nat Product Res Dev 2006;18(2):355–61.
[3] Perfect JR. The antifungal pipeline: a reality check. Nat Rev Drug Discovery 2017;16:603–16.
[4] Liu N, Tu J, Huang Y, et al. Target- and prodrug-based design for fungal diseases and cancer-associated fungal infections. Adv Drug Deliv Rev 2023;197:114819–45.
[5] Denning DW, Bromley MJ. How to bolster the antifungal pipeline. Science 2015;347:1414–16.
[6] Sheng C, Zhang W, Ji H, et al. Structure-based optimization of azole antifungal agents by CoMFA, CoMSIA, and molecular docking. J Med Chem 2006;49:2512–25.
[7] Kofla G, Ruhnke M. Voriconazole: review of a broad spectrum triazole antifungal agent. Expert Opin Pharmacother 2005;6:1215–29.
[8] Denning DW. Echinocandin antifungal drugs. Lancet 2003;6736:14472–8.

[9] Liu N, Wang C, Su H, et al. Strategies in the discovery of novel antifungal scaffolds. Fut Med Chem 2016;8:1435−54.
[10] Livermore J, Hope W. Evaluation of the pharmacokinetics and clinical utility of isavuconazole for treatment of invasive fungal infections. Expert Opin Drug Metab Toxicol 2012;8:759−65.
[11] Brown GD, Denning DW, Gow N, et al. Hidden killers: human fungal infections. Sci Transl Med 2012;4 165-13.
[12] Brown GD, Denning DW, Levitz SM. Tackling human fungal infections. Science 2012;336:647.
[13] Liu TB, Perlin DS, Xue C. Molecular mechanisms of cryptococcal meningitis. Virulence 2012;3:173−81.
[14] Odds FC, Cheesman SL, Abbott AB. Antifungal effects of fluconazole (UK 49858), a new triazole antifungal, in vitro. J Antimicrobial Chemother 1986;4:4−9.
[15] Strushkevich N, Usanov SA, Park HW. Structural basis of human CYP51 inhibition by antifungal azoles. J Mol Biol 2010;397:1067−78.
[16] Soni N, Wagstaff A. Fungal infection. Curr Anaesth Crit Care 2005;16:231−41.
[17] Roger P, Dickinson, Bell AS, et al. Novel antifungal 2-aryl-1-(1 H -1,2,4-triazol-1-yl)butan-2-ol derivatives with high activity against Aspergillus fumigatus. Bioorg Med Chem Lett 1996;6:2031−6.
[18] Ohwada J, Tsukazaki M, Hayase T. Design, synthesis and antifungal activity of a novel water soluble prodrug of antifungal triazole. Bioorg Med Chem Lett 2003;13:191−6.
[19] Jesus G, Emilio B. Isavuconazole: a new and promising antifungal triazole for the treatment of invasive fungal infections. Fut Microbiol 2008;3:603−15.
[20] Hoekstra WJ, Garvey EP, Moore WR. Design and optimization of highly-selective fungal CYP51 inhibitors. Bioorg Med Chem Lett 2014;24:3455−8.
[21] Alia A, Sagatova. Structural insights into binding of the antifungal drug fluconazole to *Saccharomyces cerevisiae* lanosterol 14α-demethylase. Antimicrobial Agents Chemother 2015;59:4982−9.
[22] Ohwada J, Murasaki C, Yamazaki T. Synthesis of novel water soluble benzylazolium prodrugs of lipophilic azole antifungals. Bioorg Med Chem Lett 2002;12:2775−80.
[23] Lee Y, Puumala E, Robbins N, et al. Antifungal drug resistance: molecular mechanisms in *Candida albicans* and beyond. Chem Rev 2021;121:3390−411.

Chapter 19

Discovery of the antibacterial drug Linezolid and its synthetic technology research

Hong Liu and Xuewu Liang
State Key Laboratory of Drug Research, Shanghai Institute of Materia Medica, Chinese Academy of Sciences, Shanghai, P.R. China

Chapter outline

19.1 Development of antibacterial agents	465
19.2 Discovery of the antibacterial drug Linezolid	467
19.3 Bioactivity and pharmacokinetics of antibacterial drug Linezolid	472
19.3.1 Antibacterial activity of Linezolid in vitro	472
19.3.2 Antibacterial activity of Linezolid in vivo	474
19.3.3 Pharmacokinetic properties of Linezolid	475
19.3.4 The clinical efficacy of Linezolid	476
19.4 The antibacterial mechanisms of Linezolid	477
19.5 Study on structure-activity relationship of oxazolidinone antibiotics	479
19.6 Research on the synthesis process of Linezolid	484
19.7 Conclusion	486
References	486
Further reading	487

19.1 Development of antibacterial agents

As pathogens for numerous diseases, bacteria are capable of transmitting illnesses between individuals by various means, such as direct contact, through the digestive tract, via the respiratory system, or by insect bites. They exhibit strong infectivity and pose significant social harm. During the turmoil-ridden 19th century, surgical procedures were highly susceptible to bacterial infections, resulting in mortality rates as alarming as those seen in warfare. Humans lack effective strategies to combat bacterial infections. Consequently, the quest for appropriate antibacterial agents became a paramount challenge at that time. In 1867, J. Lister, the "father of antisepsis," pioneered the application of phenol in surgical procedures to prevent the occurrence of infections, which substantially reduced bacterial infection rates and saved countless lives. However, phenolic antibacterial agents could only eradicate bacteria on the surface of tissues but not within the wounds. Hence, the discovery of systemic antibacterial drugs became a new challenge. In 1910, P. Ehrlich discovered a potent antibacterial drug named Ehrlich 606 (arsphenamine), capable of killing treponema pallidum, marking the dawn of the modern era of antibacterial agents. In 1932, J. Clark from Farben co., Germany synthesized a vivid orange–red dye known as prontosil (2′,4′-diaminoazobenzene-4-sulfonamide), which is considered to be one of the first 50 drugs that changed human history. The antibacterial activity of prontosil stems from its metabolic product, sulfonamide, which subsequently led to the development of sulfonamide-derivative antibacterial drugs. Unfortunately, bacteria quickly developed resistance to sulfonamide drugs.

Undeniably, the discovery of penicillin stands as one of the most remarkable milestones in the history of human medicine, ushering in a new era of disease treatment through antibiotics. Following his vacation from July 28th to August 10th, 1928, Sir Alexander Fleming, a British bacteriologist, made an astounding observation upon examining a culture dish he had left behind before his break. He noticed that the Staphylococcus bacteria previously grown in the culture dish had been "lysed" (forming an inhibition zone) by penicillium colonies that had somehow drifted in. This keen observation led him to realize that a substance secreted by the mold had the ability to inhibit the growth of Staphylococcus, prompting him to publish his findings. It was not until 1938 that Ernst Chain, a German chemist, took notice of Fleming's publication and began collaborating with him to study and isolate the penicillin secretion capable of inhibiting Staphylococcus. Then, in 1943, Howard Florey, a British pathologist at the University of Oxford, collaborated with Chain, and after years of research, they assisted pharmaceutical companies in achieving large-scale production of penicillin, facilitating its widespread use during and after World War II. As a result of this monumental discovery, in 1945, Fleming, Florey, and Chain jointly received the Nobel Prize in Physiology or Medicine for their "discovery of penicillin and its therapeutic value." The successful development of penicillin greatly enhanced humans' ability to combat bacterial infections, providing humans with a weapon against bacteria and catalyzing the emergence of the antibiotic family. Since then, humans embarked on a journey of exploring and screening for antibiotics in microbial organisms found in nature. For instance, in 1943, Waksman and Schatz isolated streptomycin from *Streptomyces griseus*; In 1948, Pollock isolated cephalosporin from the fungal strain *Cephalosporium acremonium*; In 1949, scientists at Pfizer isolated tetracycline from soil samples; In the mid-1950s, scientists at Eli Lilly isolated vancomycin; and in 1970, chemists at Eli Lilly isolated erythromycin from Philippine soil samples, and so forth.

Simultaneously, the emergence of chemically synthesized antibacterial agents, such as aminosalicylic acid, isoniazid, and quinolones, was witnessed (Fig. 19.1) [1]. However, since the discovery of penicillin in 1928, with the continuous increase in the variety and quantity of antibiotics, the abuse of antibiotic drugs has notably escalated due to various artificial and external factors, resulting in a significant rise in drug resistance among both Gram-positive and Gram-negative bacteria. The acquisition of exogenous resistance genes in bacteria has also accelerated the development of resistant strains, drawing increasing societal attention to the issue of multidrug-resistant bacteria. Notably, Gram-positive bacteria such as methicillin-resistant *Staphylococcus aureus* (MRSA), methicillin-resistant *Staphylococcus epidermidis* (MRSE), multidrug-resistant tuberculosis (MDR-TB), vancomycin-resistant Enterococcus (VRE), and penicillin-resistant *Streptococcus pneumoniae* (PRSP) are particularly prevalent, posing significant challenges in clinical treatment. The vicious cycle of "resistance—drug development—resistance" and the ineffectiveness of existing antibacterial drugs in alleviating infections caused by new resistant strains highlight the critical importance of developing novel antibacterial agents with new structures, unique mechanisms of action, and novel targets. Furthermore, before the discovery of the oxazolidinone drug Linezolid, there was a 35-year gap in the introduction of new innovative antibacterial drugs. During this period, the emergence of multidrug-resistant strains rapidly became a severe therapeutic concern in both community and hospitals, necessitating the urgent need for new antibiotics to combat these bacterial infections. Linezolid emerged at this critical juncture.

Linezolid (trade name: Zyvox, Fig. 19.2) was the first clinically used oxazolidinone-class antibacterial agent. It was approved in 2000 for the treatment of infections caused by Gram-positive (G +) cocci, including suspected or confirmed hospital-acquired pneumonia (HAP) and community-acquired pneumonia (CAP), as well as complicated skin or soft tissue

FIGURE 19.1 The development of antibacterial agents [1].

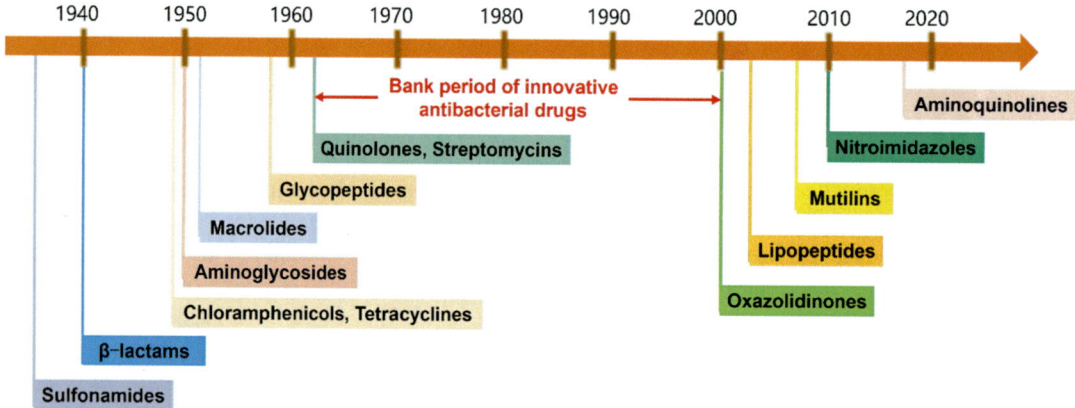

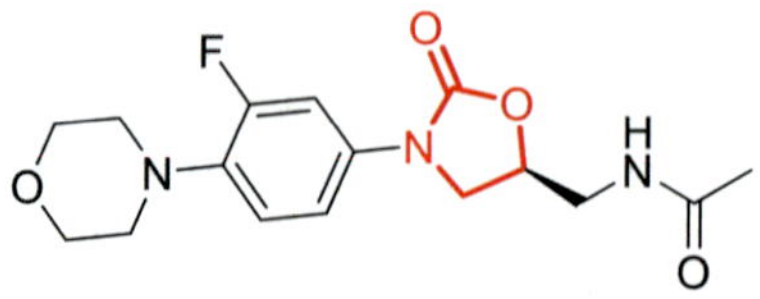

FIGURE 19.2 The chemical structure of Linezolid and its oxazolidinone scaffold.

infections (SSTI) and VRE infections. The discovery of Linezolid holds significant importance in the history of antibiotic development. It was the first drug approved for the treatment of hospital and CAP caused by drug-resistant *S. pneumoniae*. Additionally, it was the first oral medication used to treat skin infections caused by MRSA. Furthermore, it was representative of novel structural antibiotics after a gap of 35 years.

Linezolid is an inhibitor of protein synthesis, which holds similar mechanisms of action to chloramphenicol, macrolides, and lincomycin. These drugs all target the 50 S subunit of bacterial ribosomes, resulting in the termination of bacterial protein synthesis. Linezolid does not affect the activity of peptidyl transferase. Instead, it selectively binds to the 50 S subunit of the ribosome and acts specifically during the initiation of protein translation. It disrupts the formation of the 70 S initiation complex, thereby inhibiting bacterial protein synthesis. The unique mechanism of action of Linezolid makes it less prone to cross-resistance with other protein synthesis inhibitors in Gram-positive bacteria, regardless of whether the resistance is inherent or acquired. Furthermore, it does not induce bacterial resistance.

This chapter primarily focuses on the development story of Linezolid, elaborating on its discovery process, biological activity and pharmacokinetic properties, antibacterial mechanism of action, and structure-activity relationship studies. Lastly, we will provide a brief overview of the synthetic technology research on Linezolid.

19.2 Discovery of the antibacterial drug Linezolid

Linezolid was developed from chemical modifications of oxazolidinone derivatives reported by scientists from DuPont company in the United States (Fig. 19.3). In 1987, DuPont company presented a novel antibacterial scaffold "oxazolidinone" and synthesized a series of racemic 5-halomethyl-3-phenyl-2-oxazolidinone derivatives, such as compound **1**, which was reported to be effective in treating various plant diseases. Subsequent chemical modifications of compound **1** led to the discovery of compound **2** (S1623), which exhibited certain antibacterial activity against both Gram-positive and Gram-negative bacteria *in vitro* and *in vivo*. Further structural modifications on the 5-hydroxymethyl and sulfonamide functional groups of compound **2** ultimately yielded two lead compounds **3** (DuP 105) and **4** (DuP 721), with potent antibacterial activity [2–4]. Among them, compound **4** (DuP 721) showed MIC_{90} values of 4.0 μg/mL against both methicillin-resistant and penicillin-resistant *S. aureus*, which was slightly weaker antibacterial activity compared to vancomycin (MIC_{90} values were both 1.0 μg/mL).

The oxazolidinone derivatives developed by DuPont Pharmaceuticals are highly attractive antibiotics due to their broad spectrum of activity against resistant Gram-positive bacteria, without cross-resistance to existing antibiotics. Resistance strains to oxazolidinones are rare to find in laboratories. Furthermore, oxazolidinones can be fully synthesized artificially and exhibit substantial activity against Gram-positive resistant bacteria, suggesting a unique antibacterial mechanism. In animal models, oxazolidinones demonstrate high efficacy in combating infections. Preliminary pharmacokinetic assessments indicate significant plasma exposure, with drug concentrations in the plasma far exceeding the MIC_{90} values of the infecting pathogens. Moreover, these compounds possess favorable oral bioavailability, allowing for administration via both oral and intravenous routes. Before the discovery of Linezolid, most antibiotics used to

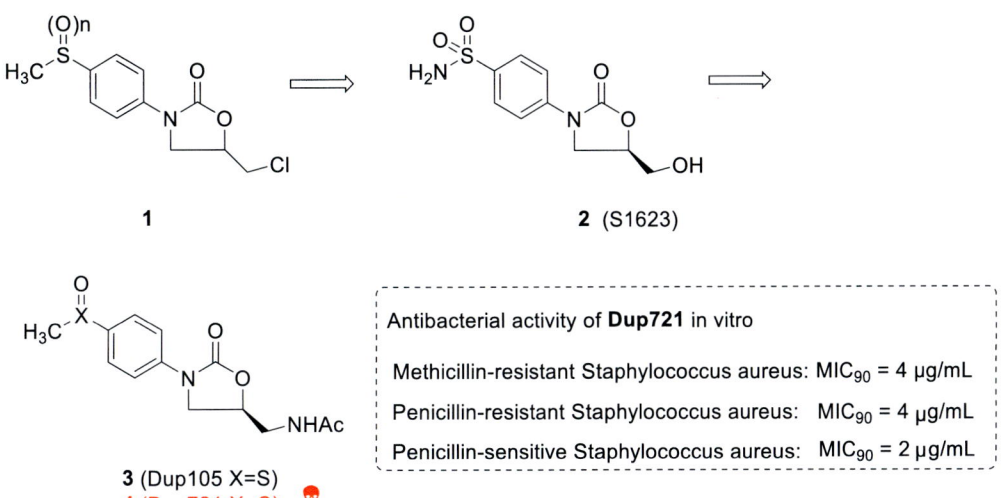

FIGURE 19.3 Origin of oxazolidinone derivatives.

treat serious gram-positive infections were only administered intravenously. Therefore, oxazolidinone derivatives offer a notable advantage in terms of pharmacokinetic properties.

Subsequently, scientists from DuPont Pharmaceuticals conducted preliminary structure-activity relationship studies on Dup 721 (Fig. 19.4) and unveiled several key rules: (1) The chirality at the C_5 position of the oxazolidinone ring must be of the *S* configuration, as compounds with the *R* configuration exhibited a significant reduction in bioactivity. (2) Substitution on the C_5 position with a 5-acetamidomethyl moiety demonstrated favorable bioactivity. (3) The presence of an N-aromatic ring served as an essential pharmacophore. These crucial structure-activity relationships (SAR) facilitated subsequent structural optimization and ultimately led to the discovery of Linezolid. Unfortunately, in 1989, DuPont Pharmaceuticals discontinued their oxazolidinone research program due to concerns about the potential toxicity of these compounds.

Upjohn company further conducted chemical modifications on the lead compound Dup 721, primarily focusing on fused-ring design around the phenyl ring to explore the effect of compounds on antibacterial activity (Fig. 19.5). As a result, they obtained several lead compounds, including **5** (PNU-82965), **6** (PNU-85055), and **7** (PNU-85112) [5–7]. It should be noted that these early analogs were prepared as racemic mixtures, which were typically half as potent as pure enantiomers because only the 5-(*S*)-enantiomer exhibited antimicrobial activity. Compound **5** (PNU-82965) played a crucial role in Upjohn's oxazolidinone project. Due to the earlier report by DuPont on the toxicity issues of Dup 721, the scientists at Upjohn company internally compared the safety of the racemic Dup 721 and PNU-82965. Three male and three female Sprague-Dawley rats were orally administered with a dose of 100 mg/kg of the racemic Dup 721 and

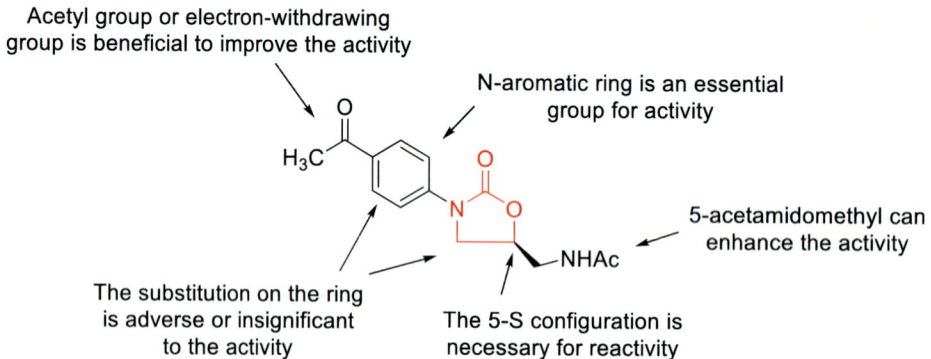

FIGURE 19.4 The preliminary SAR summary of oxazolidinone derivatives developed by DuPont. *SAR*, Structure-activity relationships.

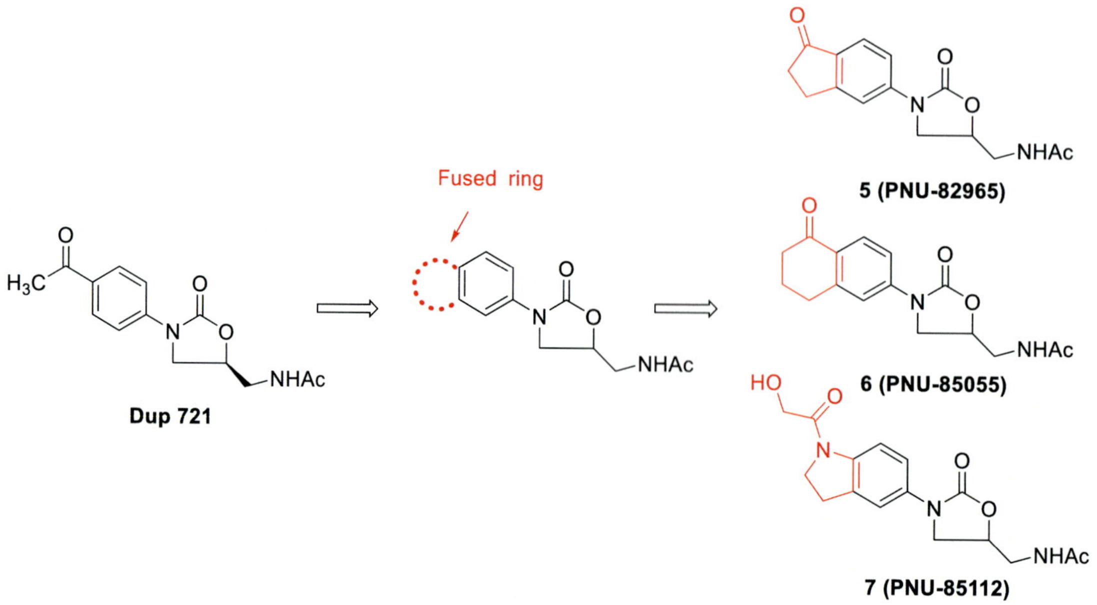

FIGURE 19.5 Structural modifications of Dup 721 by Upjohn company.

PNU-82965 twice a day for 30 consecutive days. The study results revealed poor safety of the racemic Dup 721, with one rat fatality and two rats in a moribund state. Additionally, some rats also exhibited severe progressive weight loss and bone marrow atrophy toxicity. In contrast, the rats treated with PNU-82965 only showed minimal adverse reactions, with no drug-related clinical toxic symptoms, no serum or urine side effects, or histopathological manifestations. Therefore, the scientists speculated that the fused-derivatives may provide favorable safety properties for the oxazolidinone pharmacophore. The subsequently designed compound PNU-85112 also demonstrated excellent safety, further validating the aforementioned speculation. *In vitro* antibacterial activity tests on PNU-85112 and PNU-82965 indicated a range of MIC_{90} values of 4–16 μg/mL against Staphylococcus and Enterococcus, showing a slight decrease in bioactivity compared to Dup 721. Further studies revealed that although PNU-85112 and PNU-82965 demonstrated efficacy against lethal bacterial infections in mice, they were not considered candidates for clinical trial research by pharmaceutical scientists. This is because their minimum inhibitory concentration (MIC) values and ED_{50} values were much higher than those of Dup 721 and marketed antibiotics, making it difficult to predict their clinical therapeutic effects. However, these two lead compounds indeed achieved the mid-term goal of medicinal chemists, proving that novel oxazolidinone candidates with antibacterial activity and high safety can be theoretically obtained. At this point, medicinal chemists also set high standards and selected vancomycin as the benchmark molecule (considered the last resort in clinical treatment) to develop candidates with bioactivity equivalent to or superior to vancomycin and high safety.

Afterward, scientists at Upjohn company opted to investigate the *S*-configured oxazolidinone derivatives and developed an asymmetric synthesis method for their production. As depicted in Fig. 19.6, the aniline formate ester derivatives can directly react with commercially available (*R*)-glyceryl butyrate ester under the conditions of *n*-butyllithium, yielding (*R*)-3-phenyl-5-hydroxymethyl oxazolidinone intermediate **8**. This step is known as the Manninen reaction. The hydroxymethyl oxazolidinone intermediate **8** can be easily converted to diverse (*S*)-configured oxazolidinone derivatives.

Until the end of 1992, research on oxazolidinone derivatives focused on three lead compounds: indole derivative **9** (PNU-97456), piperazine derivative **10** (PNU-97665), and cyclotriene derivative **11** (PNU-97786), as shown in Fig. 19.7

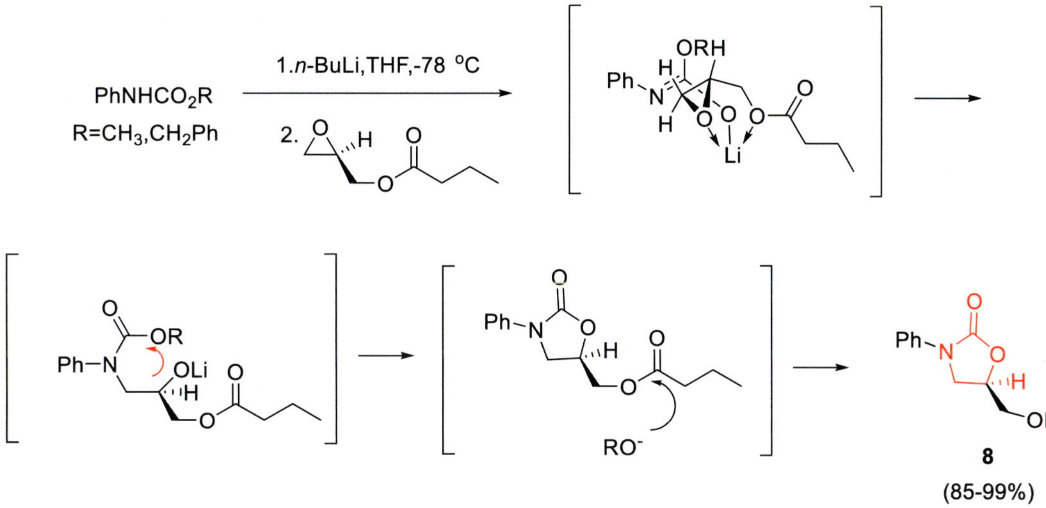

FIGURE 19.6 The construction of *S*-configured oxazolidinone derivatives by Manninen reaction.

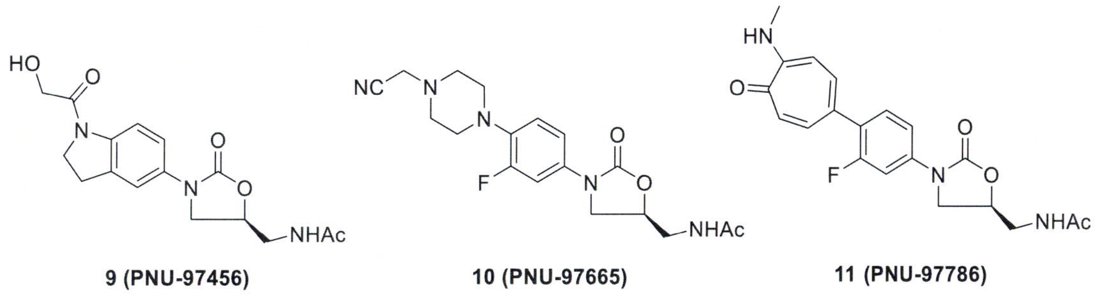

FIGURE 19.7 Representative oxazolidinone derivatives **9–11**.

[8–10]. Studies have demonstrated that indole derivatives generally exhibited good safety profiles but lower antibacterial activity. Cyclotriene derivatives showed strong antibacterial activity but poor water solubility and pharmacokinetic characteristics. Notably, piperazine derivatives demonstrated excellent antibacterial activity both *in vitro* and *in vivo* while maintaining acceptable safety profiles, water solubility, and favorable pharmacokinetic properties. Additionally, piperazine analogs are easier to obtain by chemical synthesis. These characteristics have made piperazine derivatives a hot topic in medicinal chemistry research.

Different kinds of alkyl, acyl, and sulfonyl substituents can be introduced to the remote nitrogen (N) atom of the piperazine fragment by various organic reactions, such as nucleophilic substitution, reductive amination, and amide condensation. The introduction of a hydroxyacetamide group to the remote nitrogen (N) atom of the piperazine fragment gives compound **12** (PNU-100592), which exhibited optimal drug-like characteristics. Scientists have also observed that fluorination on the phenyl ring enhances the antibacterial activity both *in vitro* and *in vivo*. However, the positively charged nature of the piperazine ring often leads to some cytotoxicity and poor absorption properties. Medicinal chemists further replaced the piperazine ring using its bioisosteric groups, resulting in the design of thiomorpholino derivative **13** (PNU-100480) and morpholino derivative **14** (PNU-100766) [11,12]. The morpholino derivative PNU-100766 is the subsequently approved antibacterial drug Linezolid (Fig. 19.8).

Two clinical candidate drugs eperezolid (compound **12**) and Linezolid (compound **14**) were initially selected by Upjohn company in their oxazolidinone project. Both compounds exhibited equal antibacterial MIC values against gram-positive pathogens to vancomycin. Moreover, Linezolid and eperezolid administered orally demonstrated comparable ED_{50} values for bacterial infection in mice to subcutaneous vancomycin administration (currently administered intravenously). Therefore, the *in vitro* and *in vivo* antibacterial activities of Linezolid and eperezolid met the criteria expected for potential drug candidates by medicinal chemists. Additionally, they were effective against penicillin- and cephalosporin-resistant *S. pneumoniae*, as well as VRE faecium. Given that all preclinical trial results for Linezolid and eperezolid indicated similar biological activity and pharmacokinetic properties, the drug development team concurrently progressed them to Phase I clinical trials in humans. Based on the pharmacokinetic parameters inferred from clinical trial data, Linezolid should be administered twice daily, while eperezolid requires thrice-daily dosing. Clearly, Linezolid was ultimately selected as the candidate drug to

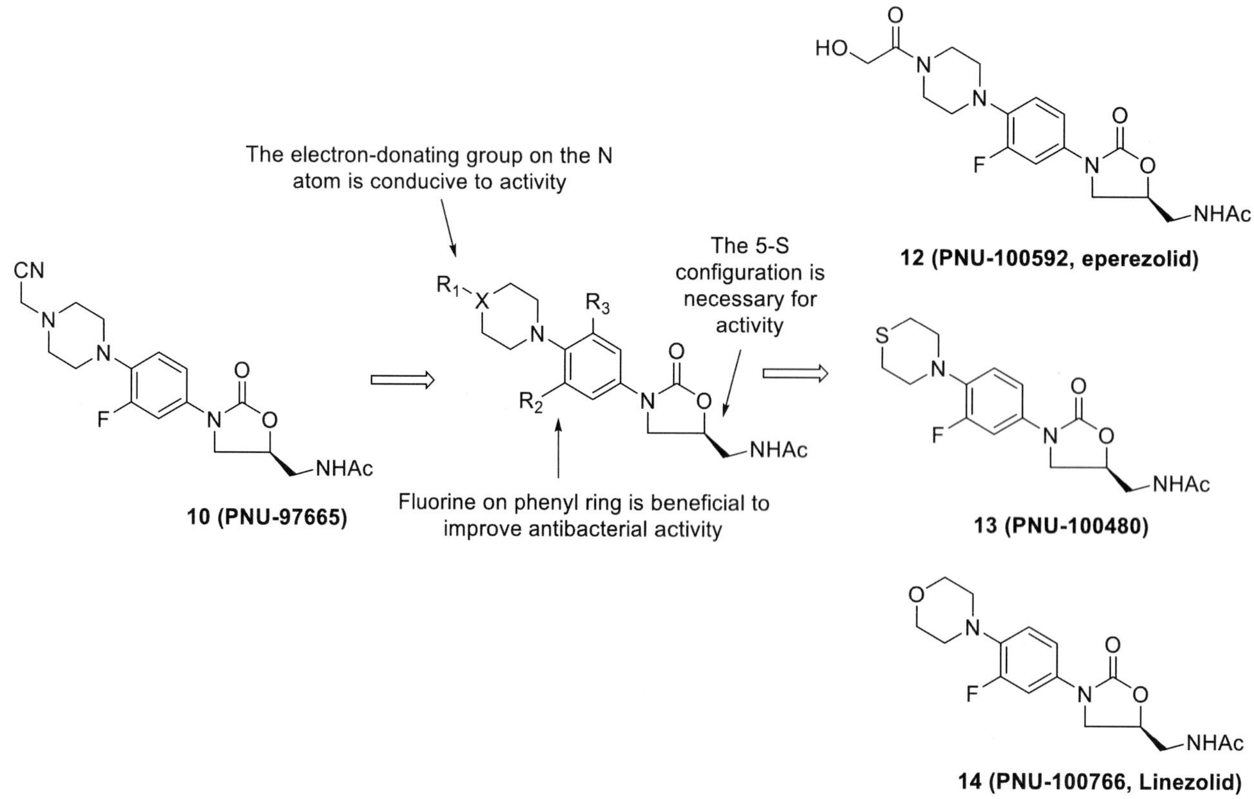

FIGURE 19.8 The discovery of the antibacterial drug Linezolid.

proceed with subsequent Phase II/III clinical trials. In 2000, it was approved for marketing in the United States under the trade name Zyvox, becoming the first oxazolidinone antibacterial drug in human history.

Fig. 19.9 briefly presents an enumeration of the pivotal lead compounds involved in the discovery process of the antibacterial drug Linezolid. In essence, DuPont Pharmaceuticals initially identified a lead compound, Dup 721, possessing potent antibacterial activity. However, Dup 721 exhibited significant *in vivo* toxicity, leading DuPont Pharmaceuticals to abandon the associated research project. On the other hand, Upjohn employed classical drug design principles to structurally modify Dup 721, aiming to discover novel candidates with potent antibacterial activity and low *in vivo* toxicity. This iterative design process ultimately yielded the desired drug, Linezolid.

It is worth mentioning that through subsequent structural modifications, two novel oxazolidinone drugs have also been approved and marketed. These two drugs are tedizolid and contezolid (MRX-I, Fig. 19.10). Tedizolid is a derivative of Linezolid and belongs to the new class of oxazolidinone antibacterial drugs. As a second-generation oxazolidinone antibiotic, tedizolid exhibits a similar mechanism of action to that of the first-generation oxazolidinone antibiotic, Linezolid. In June 2014, the U.S. Food and Drug Administration (FDA) approved tedizolid phosphate for the treatment of acute bacterial skin and skin structure infections (ABSSSI) caused by Gram-positive bacteria, including MRSA. Tedizolid is also effective against Gram-positive bacteria, including *S. aureus*, *Streptococcus pyogenes*, *Streptococcus agalactiae*, *Streptococcus anginosus*, and *Enterococcus faecalis*, and exhibits strong antibacterial activity against certain strains resistant to vancomycin and Linezolid. Tedizolid has the advantages of potent antibacterial activity, high oral

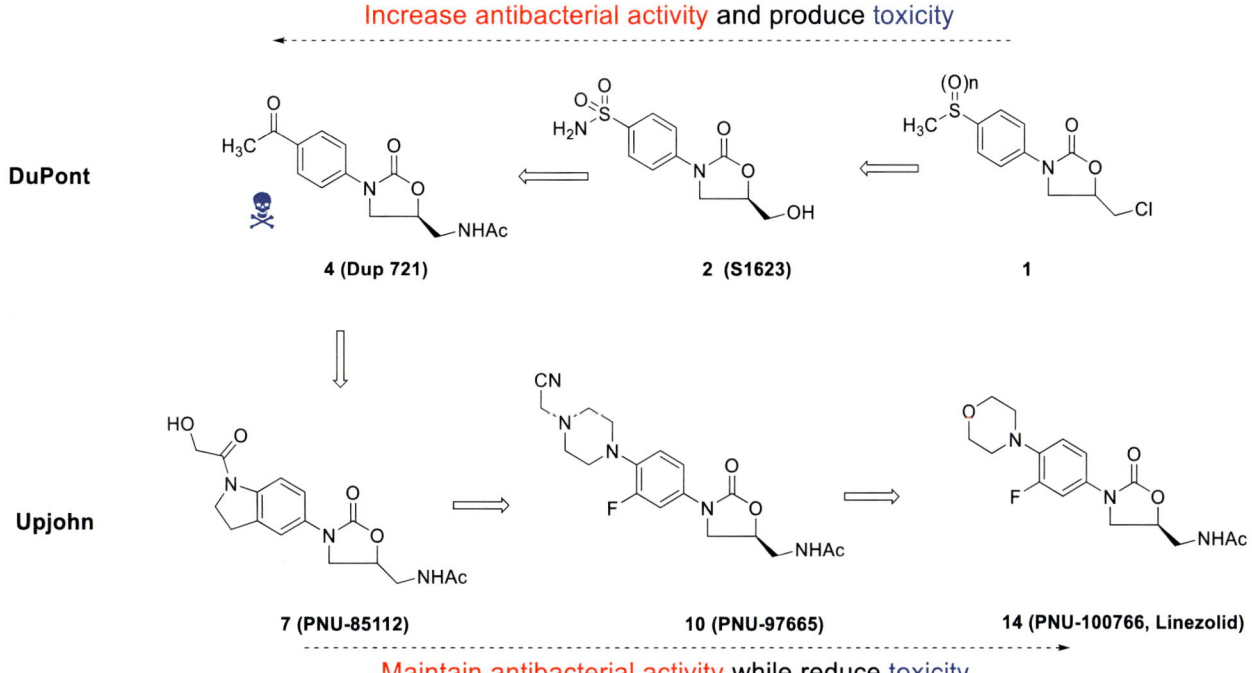

FIGURE 19.9 Drug discovery flowchart for Linezolid.

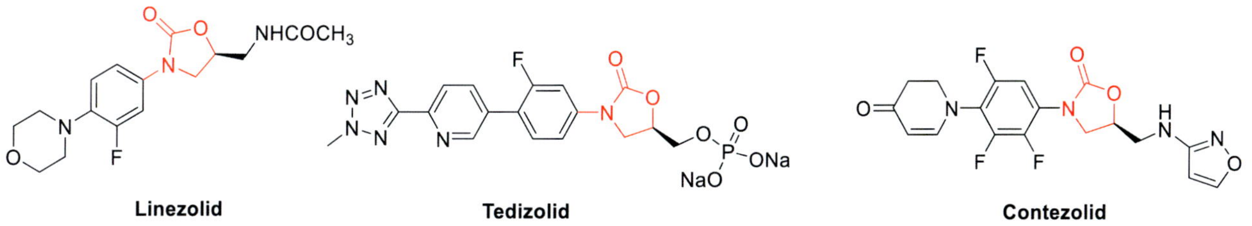

FIGURE 19.10 The approved oxazolidinone antibacterial drugs Linezolid, Tedizolid, and Contezolid.

bioavailability, long half-life, and no need for dosage adjustment based on renal or hepatic function, making it an ideal antibacterial drug.

Contezolid (MRX-I), a novel oxazolidinone antibacterial drug, is used to treat infections caused by drug-resistant bacteria such as MRSA and VRE. The structural design of contezolid aims to reduce the risk of hematological adverse reactions and monoamine oxidase inhibition associated with oxazolidinone drugs. On June 2, 2021, the National Medical Products Administration of China announced on its official website that a first-class innovative drug, contezolid tablets (trade name: Youxitai), applied by Shanghai MicuRx Pharmaceutical has been approved through the priority approval process. It is indicated for the treatment of complicated skin and soft tissue infections caused by contezolid-susceptible *S. aureus* strains (including methicillin-sensitive and resistant strains) as well as *S. pyogenes* or *S. agalactiae*.

19.3 Bioactivity and pharmacokinetics of antibacterial drug Linezolid

19.3.1 Antibacterial activity of Linezolid in vitro

The in vitro antibacterial activity and antibacterial spectrum of Linezolid are shown in Table 19.1 [13,14]. Linezolid exhibits potent antibacterial activity against both methicillin-sensitive and MRSA, which is comparable to that of vancomycin. Other studies have also confirmed that Linezolid demonstrates similar antibacterial activity against methicillin-sensitive and MRSA and *S. epidermidis in vitro*. Linezolid shows potent antibacterial activity against all tested strains of Staphylococcus, with MIC_{90} values of 2–4 μg/mL and a narrow range of MIC_{50} values, ranging from 0.5 to 4 μg/mL. Unlike the wide MIC range observed with most antibiotics, the relatively narrow MIC range of Linezolid against various strains of Staphylococcus is rare, indicating minimal differences in antibacterial activity against susceptible and resistant *Staphylococcus strains*. In comparison to other antibacterial agents, Linezolid does not exhibit cross-resistance with Staphylococcus and demonstrates even antibacterial activity against all bacteria. Obviously, Linezolid has a novel antibacterial mechanism of action.

The antibacterial assays against penicillin-sensitive and PRSP demonstrated that Linezolid exhibits approximately fourfold greater anti-*S. pneumoniae* activity than *S. aureus*. Linezolid exhibits potent antibacterial activity against both penicillin-resistant and penicillin-sensitive *S. pneumoniae*, with MIC_{90} values of 0.5 and 1.0 μg/mL, respectively. Additionally, Linezolid displays potent antibacterial activity against other Streptococcus species, such as *S. pyogenes*, with a MIC_{90} value of 1 μg/mL. The robust antibacterial activity against *S. pyogenes* of Linezolid expands its potential application in postpartum women infections.

The antibacterial activity of Linezolid against *E. faecalis* and Enterococcus faecium is particularly significant, as the treatment options for these microorganisms are limited, attracting considerable attention in the medical field. Linezolid demonstrates strong inhibition against all enterococci, including strains resistant to vancomycin. Other researchers have performed antibacterial assays against geographically diverse and multidrug-resistant enterococci, and they have observed the potent antibacterial activity of Linezolid against all tested enterococci. Linezolid has been regarded as an antibiotic suitable for the treatment of enterococcal infections.

Linezolid also demonstrates mild antibacterial activity against gram-negative pathogens, but its activity is relatively weaker than that against Gram-positive bacteria. For instance, the MIC_{90} values for Linezolid against Gram-negative bacteria 8 μg/mL for *Haemophilus influenzae* and *Legionella pneumophila*, and 4 μg/mL for *Klebsiella pneumoniae*. Furthermore, Linezolid exhibits strong antibacterial activity against mononucleosis-causing Listeria monocytogenes and corynebacterium. Interestingly, Linezolid also shows mild antibacterial activity against anaerobic bacteria, including the commonly found *Bacteroides fragilis* in intraabdominal abscesses, with a MIC_{90} value of 8 μg/mL. In a fascinating study, Linezolid has been demonstrated to show certain *in vitro* antibacterial activity against both aerobic bacteria (typically belonging to the Pasteurella genus) and anaerobic bacteria, which can cause infections after bites in animals and humans.

The *in vitro* antibacterial assays of Linezolid indicated that Linezolid has a predominantly gram-positive antibacterial spectrum. However, it also exhibits certain antibacterial activity against Gram-negative bacteria, although the antibacterial activity of Linezolid is relatively weaker than that of Gram-positive bacteria. In addition, Linezolid demonstrates strong antibacterial activity against Gram-positive anaerobic bacteria but moderate antibacterial activity against Gram-negative anaerobic bacteria.

TABLE 19.1 The in vitro antibacterial activity and antibacterial spectrum of Linezolid.

Organism[a]	Sensitivity	Agent	MIC_{90} (μg/mL)[b]
S. aureus	Methicillin-sensitive	Linezolid	4.0
		Vancomycin[c]	1.0
	Methicillin-resistant	Linezolid	4.0
		Vancomycin	2.0
S. epidermidis	Methicillin-sensitive	Linezolid	2.0
		Vancomycin	2.0
	Methicillin-resistant	Linezolid	2.0
		Vancomycin	2.0
S. pneumoniae	Penicillin-sensitive	Linezolid	1.0
		Vancomycin	≤ 0.25
	Penicillin-resistant	Linezolid	0.5
		Vancomycin	≤ 0.25
S. pyogenes		Linezolid	1.0
		Vancomycin	2.0
E. faecium	Vancomycin-susceptible	Linezolid	4.0[d]
		Vancomycin	0.5[d]
	Vancomycin-resistant	Linezolid	4.0
		Vancomycin	> 16
E. faecalis		Linezolid	4.0
		Vancomycin	2.0
H. influenzae		Linezolid	8.0
		Vancomycin	0.5
M. catarrhalis		Linezolid	4.0
		Vancomycin	1.0
Corynebacterium spp.		Linezolid	0.5
		Vancomycin	1.0
L. monocytogenes		Linezolid	2.0
		Vancomycin	1.0
B. fragilis[e]		Linezolid	8.0
		Vancomycin[c]	4.0
Peptostreptococcus spp.[e]		Linezolid	1.0
		Vancomycin	1.0

[a]From [13,14].
[b]The drug concentration at which 90% of tested bacterial strains are killed or not permitted to grow, μg/mL.
[c]Control drug.
[d]MIC_{50}.
[e]Anaerobic species.

TABLE 19.2 Representative ED_{50} values of linezolid in bacteremia and soft tissue infections in mice.

Organism	Drug	MIC (μg/mL)	ED_{50} (mg/kg)[a]
S. aureus UC6685[c]	Linezolid	2.0	3.8 (2.2–5.6)
	Vancomycin[b]	2.0	2.6 (1.4–5.0)
S. aureus UC15083[c]	Linezolid	4.0	7.0 (3.9–11.1)
	Vancomycin	1.0	3.2 (1.8–4.5)
S. aureus UC15084[c]	Linezolid	4.0	2.9 (1.8–4.4)
	Vancomycin	1.0	4.4 (2.5–6.3)
S. aureus UC12084[d]	Linezolid	1.0	4.7 (3.1–7.8)
	Vancomycin	2.0	1.8 (1.1–3.0)
S. aureus UC152	Linezolid	2.0	5.0 (3.6–17.4)
	Clindamycin	0.6	8.6 (6.3–12.0)
S. aureus UC15087[e]	Linezolid	0.5	3.8 (2.3–5.5)
	Penicillin G	8.0	> 20.0
E. faecalis UC12379	Linezolid	4.0	10.0 (6.2–19.5)
	Vancomycin	1.0	0.5 (0.3–0.8)
E. coli UC9451[c,f]	Linezolid	32.0	80.0 (ND)
	Vancomycin	0.03	0.4 (ND)
S. aureus UC9271[c,f]	Linezolid	4.0	39.0
	Vancomycin	1.0	4.7
E. faecalis UC15060[c,f]	Linezolid	4.0	11.0
	Vancomycin	2.0	16.3
B. fragilis UC12199[f]	Linezolid	4.0	46.3
	Clindamycin	1.0	200.0

[a]Dose required to cure 50% of bacteremia or eradicate 50% of the bacteria in soft tissue infections, mg/kg. Linezolid and ciprofloxacin were dosed orally. Vancomycin and Clindamycin were dosed subcutaneously. Parenthesis in table is 95% Confidence Limits.
[b]Control drug.
[c]Multidrug resistant.
[d]Methicillin-resistant.
[e]Penicillin and cephalosporin-resistant.
[f]Subcutaneous soft tissue infections.

19.3.2 Antibacterial activity of Linezolid in vivo

The antibacterial study results of Linezolid in mice are presented in Table 19.2 [13,15]. In the evaluation of a group of drug-resistant S. aureus infections, Linezolid achieved a 50% cure rate at concentrations of 2.9–7.0 mg/kg (ED_{50}). In each case, the efficacy of oral Linezolid and subcutaneous vancomycin reached the 95% confidence limit. In the antistreptococcus assays, Linezolid exhibited an ED_{50} value below 5 mg/kg against pyogenic streptococcus, as well as penicillin-resistant and cephalosporin-resistant S. pneumoniae. In a mouse model of enterococcal bacteremia, Linezolid showed an ED_{50} of 10 mg/kg, while vancomycin demonstrated stronger in vivo antibacterial activity in this model. The in vivo antibacterial activity against mouse bacteremia infections showed that Linezolid was effective against significant Gram-positive pathogens, and its in vivo antibacterial activity is not compromised by abnormal absorption, elimination, or metabolism. A comparison of Linezolid with vancomycin antibacterial activity suggests that it may be effective in treating bacterial infections in humans at clinically appropriate doses. The results of Linezolid against Gram-negative Escherichia coli infections confirmed it was not sensitive to the gram-negative spectrum in vivo and excluded the possibility that Linezolid metabolites possessed gram-negative antibacterial activity. The remaining groups in this table represent the models of soft tissue infection where the infection is localized subcutaneously and the antibiotic dosing regimen exceeds 6 days. Due to the different dosing regimens and infection sites, it is not possible to quantitatively compare the ED_{50} values between bacteremia and soft tissue infection. Linezolid showed an ED_{50} value of 39 mg/kg against *S. aureus* soft tissue infection, indicating a potential therapeutic effect in this model. In the antibacterial evaluation on Enterobacteriaceae soft tissue infection, Linezolid demonstrated comparable efficacy to vancomycin, and they are both highly effective antibiotics. Although Linezolid exhibited a moderate MIC value against *Bacillus fragilis*, it effectively cured soft tissue infections caused by *B. fragilis*, surpassing the effectiveness of the highly active antibiotic, clindamycin.

Other researchers have also observed the therapeutic efficacy of Linezolid in animal models of infection. In a rat model of *streptococcus pneumoniae*, Linezolid administered at a dose of 50 mg/kg twice daily demonstrated comparable antibacterial therapeutic effects to ceftriaxone at a dose of 100 mg/kg once daily. In a study on the efficacy of Linezolid in a squirrel model of otitis media, oral Linezolid at a dose of 25 mg/kg twice daily successfully eradicated otitis media caused by multidrug-resistant *S. pneumoniae* (MDRSP). However, Linezolid showed relatively poor effectiveness in an abdominal abscess rat model of enterococcal infection, with only a partial reduction in bacterial count observed with a dosage of 25 mg/kg. Furthermore, in a rabbit model of *S. aureus* endocarditis, Linezolid and vancomycin were directly compared for their antibacterial activity. The results indicated that Linezolid exhibited a similarly negative therapeutic effect on endocarditis as vancomycin.

19.3.3 Pharmacokinetic properties of Linezolid

The adequate oral absorption of antibacterial agents is generally crucial for providing sufficient plasma drug concentrations to eradicate diseases. To effectively exert their therapeutic effect, drugs should not undergo extensive metabolism in the animal's gastrointestinal tract and systemic circulation, as these factors would decrease the amount of parent drug available within the plasma. Additionally, antibacterial drugs should have a reasonable duration of stay in the blood and tissues to achieve therapeutic effects. Therefore, the elimination rate of drugs should not be excessively high, as it would significantly reduce the levels of parent drugs in the blood and tissues. Furthermore, antibacterial agents need to be widely distributed throughout the animal's tissues, as most infections in human bacterial diseases occur in various tissues, not just the bloodstream.

The antibacterial activity data of Linezolid on soft tissue infections provide two valuable pieces of information. Firstly, the therapeutic effects of oral Linezolid are very impressive. In a bacteremia model, the oral administration of Linezolid demonstrates equivalent antibacterial efficacy to the subcutaneous administration of vancomycin. Furthermore, when Linezolid is administered orally, it exhibits significant tissue penetration and achieves sufficient levels of drug exposure to treat recalcitrant soft tissue infections.

Linezolid is a highly promising clinical candidate for the treatment of severe gram-positive infections. It is crucial to determine the pharmacokinetic parameters of drugs in animals to predict their therapeutic efficacy. This pharmacokinetic information will have a significant impact on the design of future clinical protocols. Based on experimental data estimates, Linezolid's plasma drug concentration exceeds the MIC of the microorganism within 24 hours. The data also predicts that a twice-daily dosing regimen of 600 mg may be an effective approach in humans, which was further supported by subsequent pharmacokinetic assessments. Subjects were given 400 and 600 mg of Linezolid orally, with blood samples taken at intervals after administration to test Linezolid's plasma drug concentration levels. The 600 mg dose of Linezolid achieved the mean plasma drug concentration of 19 μg/mL, which remained at 6 μg/mL even after 12 hours. After 12 hours of dosing, the plasma drug concentration of Linezolid following a second 600 mg dose exceeded the MIC_{90} of all pathogens. This means that a twice-daily dosing regimen maintains Linezolid's plasma drug concentrations above the MIC_{90} in humans, providing maximum assurance of antibiotic effectiveness against highly challenging gram-positive pathogens throughout the dosing period [16].

Further pharmacokinetic studies have revealed that Linezolid exhibits a high bioavailability of 103%. This means that when administered at a dose of 375 mg via oral and intravenous routes, the oral administration yields a slightly larger area under the curve than the intravenous administration. This exceptional oral bioavailability is rarely observed with antibiotics, enabling a transition from intravenous to oral treatment without dosage adjustment. Consequently, doctors may consider starting treatment with the oral route, as the oral plasma drug concentration levels are comparable to those achieved through intravenous therapy [17].

In the human body, Linezolid demonstrates linear pharmacokinetic characteristics, with plasma drug concentration and the area under the curve increasing proportionally with the dose. Linezolid can be administered orally with or without food, as the presence of food does not affect the area under the curve, time to reach maximum plasma drug concentration, or the drug's bioavailability. Even with high-fat meals, the time to reach maximum plasma drug concentration is only slightly delayed, while the area under the curve remains unchanged. Linezolid exhibits a plasma protein binding rate of 31%, which is not influenced by drug concentration. Importantly, Linezolid is not metabolized by cytochrome P450 enzymes nor does it inhibit key cytochrome P450 isoforms. Linezolid is metabolized through nonenzymatic oxidation, resulting in two inactive metabolites. Linezolid is eliminated through both renal and nonrenal routes, with 80%−85% of the parent drug excreted in urine and 7%−12% excreted in the gastrointestinal tract. The pharmacokinetic parameters of Linezolid are not affected by age or gender. In summary, Linezolid exhibits favorable pharmacokinetic properties, making it suitable for clinical use [18,19].

19.3.4 The clinical efficacy of Linezolid

Linezolid, with its potent antibacterial activity, broad-spectrum coverage, and remarkable pharmacokinetic and pharmacodynamic properties, is a highly promising broad-spectrum antibiotic that has rapidly advanced into clinical research. Clinical studies primarily evaluate the efficacy of Linezolid against MRSA and VRE faecium in the treatment of pneumonia or skin infections.

In a randomized, double-blind, and multicenter trial, the efficacy of Linezolid and vancomycin in the treatment of pneumonia was directly compared. Both drugs were used in combination with Aztreonam to evaluate their efficacy against pneumonia caused by *S. pneumoniae* and *S. aureus* in hospitalized patients. The results showed that the clinical cure rate was 66.4% in the Linezolid group and 68.1% in the vancomycin group. The microbial clearance rate for Linezolid was 67.9%, compared to 71.8% for vancomycin. This indicates that Linezolid is equally effective as vancomycin in treating nosocomial pneumonia caused by Gram-positive bacteria.

In a comparative assessment of the clinical efficacy of oral Linezolid and cefuroxime axetil in the treatment of CAP, Linezolid demonstrated a cure rate of 89.6%, while cefuroxime axetil exhibited a cure rate of 90.8%. The microbial clearance rate for Linezolid was 87.8%, compared to 89.4% for cefuroxime axetil. Furthermore, a large-scale open study comparing the clinical efficacy of Linezolid and cephalosporin antibiotics revealed that the clinical cure rate for the Linezolid group was 90.8%, whereas the cure rate for the ceftriaxone/cefpodoxime group was 87.1%. These findings suggest that Linezolid is as effective as cephalosporin antibiotics in the treatment of CAP.

Skin and skin structure infections (SSSI) are characteristic of streptococcal and staphylococcal infections, which are often difficult to treat. Comparing the efficacy of oral Linezolid following intravenous Linezolid and oral dicloxacillin following intravenous oxacillin in the treatment of SSSI caused by Gram-positive bacteria, the clinical cure rates were 88.6% and 85.8%, respectively. The microbial clearance rates were 88.1% and 86.1%, respectively. In a study comparing oral Linezolid and oral Clarithromycin for uncomplicated SSSI, the clinical cure rate of Linezolid and clarithromycin was 91.1% and 92.7%, respectively. These studies confirm the suitability of Linezolid as an antibiotic for the treatment of local tissue infections.

In a clinical trial evaluating the efficacy of Linezolid in 108 cases of MRSA infections, including 64 cases of SSSI, Linezolid was administered intravenously at a dose of 600 mg twice daily, and its efficacy was compared to that of intravenous vancomycin at a dose of 1 g. In these severe infections, Linezolid demonstrated a clinical cure rate of 79%, while vancomycin exhibited a clinical cure rate of 73%. Additionally, an efficacy assessment of Linezolid against VRE showed a microbial clearance rate of 85.7%. However, this study lacked a suitable control group. Another case series evaluated Linezolid in 17 patients infected with VRE, MRSE, and MRSA. At the end of the treatment, 10 out of 17 patients survived, and the deceased individuals succumbed to complications rather than infections, indicating the highly effective therapeutic potential of Linezolid against MRSA and VRE infections.

In addition to efficacy, the clinical trials also assessed the Linezolid-associated adverse events in a large number of patients. In Phase III clinical trials, Linezolid demonstrated excellent tolerability, with transient, mild to moderate adverse events. The most commonly reported Linezolid-associated adverse events were nausea (8.3%), headache (6.5%), and diarrhea (6.2%). Other infrequent adverse reactions included vomiting, insomnia, constipation, rash, dizziness, and fever. It is worth noting that these side effects are common with antibiotic therapy, and in fact, the frequency of these events occurring in the Linezolid treatment group was very similar to that observed in other antibiotic groups within the same trial. Among patients receiving Linezolid treatment for up to 28 days, a temporary decrease in platelet count was observed in some individuals. However, within a few days after discontinuation of Linezolid treatment, the platelet count rebounded to normal levels, indicating the favorable safety profile of Linezolid as an antibiotic for the treatment of gram-positive infections.

In summary, both preclinical and clinical data demonstrate that Linezolid is a safe and effective novel antibiotic for the treatment of infections caused by Gram-positive (G +) bacteria.

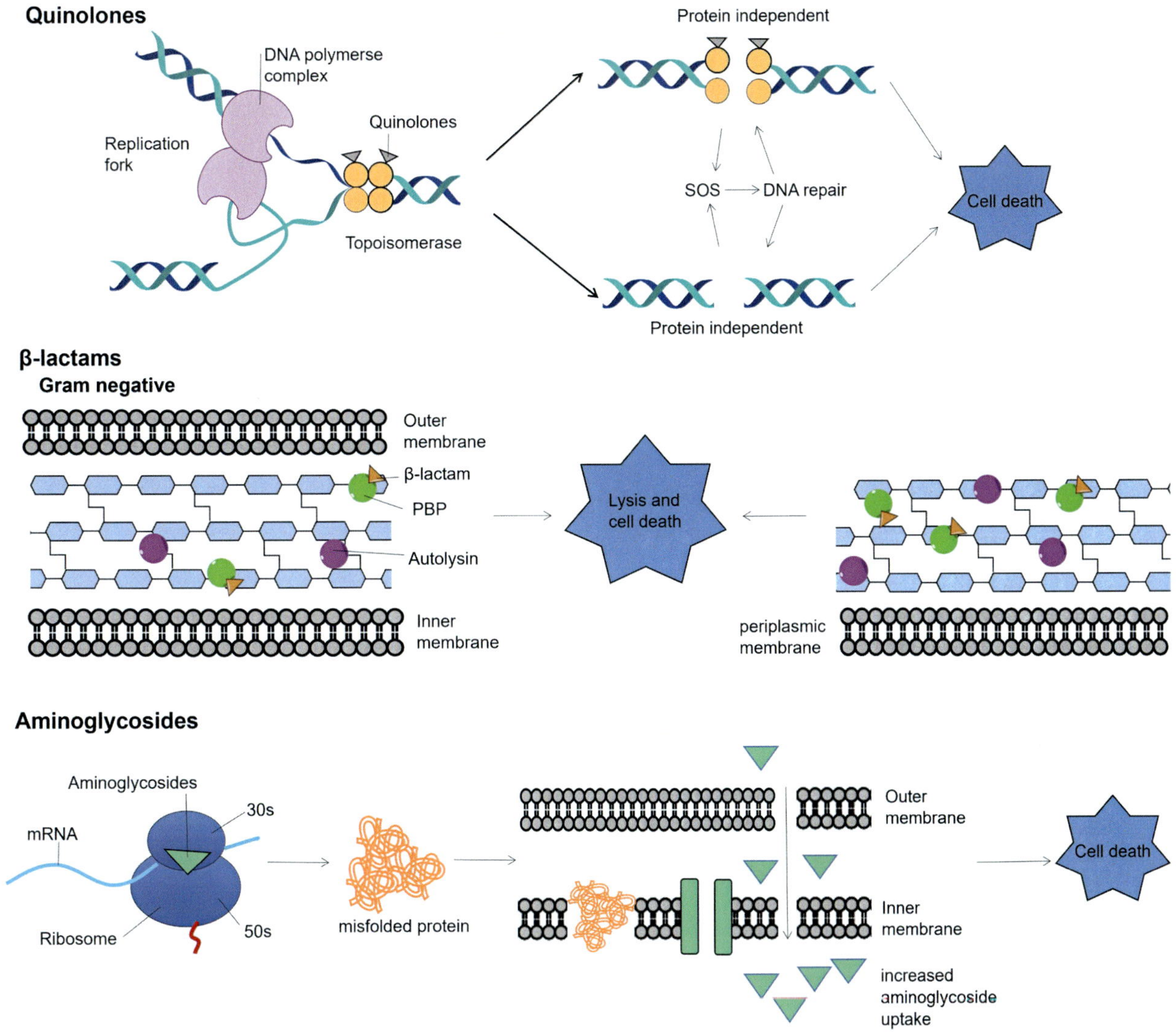

FIGURE 19.11 Antimicrobial mechanisms of common antibiotics.

19.4 The antibacterial mechanisms of Linezolid

In general, the main mechanisms of antimicrobials typically involve inhibiting bacterial growth by blocking the synthesis of ribonucleic acid (RNA), deoxyribonucleic acid (DNA), cell wall, or proteins within bacterial cells (Fig. 19.11) [20]. For example, quinolones are a novel class of synthetic antibacterial drugs featuring a 1,4-dihydro-4-oxoquinoline-3-carboxylic acid structure. Quinolone antibiotics exert their effects by binding to topoisomerase II or topoisomerase IV, thereby inhibiting DNA gyrase and causing irreversible damage to bacterial DNA, leading to double-stranded DNA breaks and bacterial cell death. Peptidoglycan is a major component of the bacterial cell wall and consists of a network structure of polysaccharides composed of alternating linear glycan chains of N-acetylglucosamine (NAG) and N-acetylmuramic acid, which undergo transpeptidation catalyzed by transpeptidases to form cross-linked structures, thus synthesizing the bacterial cell wall. Penicillin antibiotics, for instance, bind to penicillin-binding proteins on mature peptidoglycan chains, thereby inhibiting the activity of transpeptidases and preventing bacterial cell wall synthesis. This disruption in cell wall synthesis impairs cell integrity and the intracellular ability to withstand high osmotic pressure, leading to cell lysis and ultimately cell death. Aminoglycoside drugs primarily bind to the 30 S subunit of the ribosome, resulting in erroneous amino acid incorporation during peptide synthesis. These protein translation errors lead to misfolded proteins, thereby interfering with proper protein synthesis.

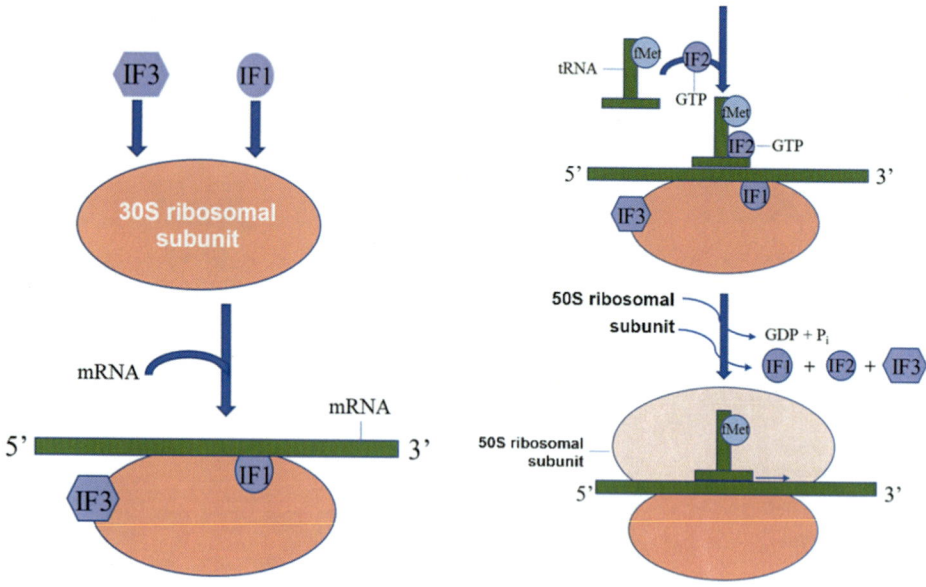

FIGURE 19.12 The process of 70 S ribosome formation [21].

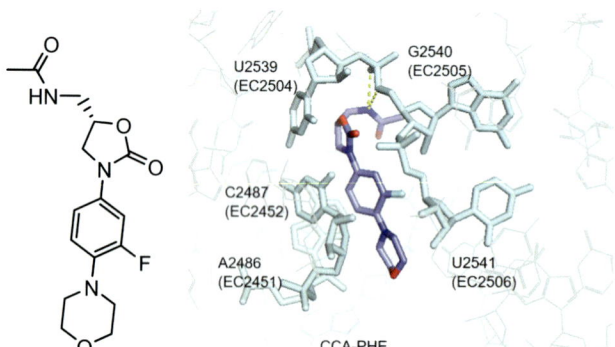

FIGURE 19.13 Crystal complex of Linezolid with the 50 S ribosomal subunit (PDB: 3CPW).

Research indicates that Linezolid is also a bacterial protein synthesis inhibitor, similar to chloramphenicol, macrolides, and lincomycin. They all act on the bacterial 50 S ribosomal subunit, leading to the termination of protein synthesis. Bacterial protein synthesis occurs in three stages: initiation, elongation, and termination. During the initiation stage, the ribosomal small subunit 30 S forms a complex with messenger RNA (mRNA), which serves as the initiation codon for the fMet-tRNA^{fmet}. The N-formylmethionine transfer RNA (fMet-tRNA)^{fmet} initiation complex then binds to the ribosomal 50 S subunit, resulting in the formation of the 70 S ribosome and completing the initiation stage of protein synthesis (Fig. 19.12). In the next stage, the fMet-tRNA complex enters the A site of the 70 S initiation complex, and with the help of peptidyl transferase, a transpeptidation reaction occurs. Formyl methionyl or peptidyl group is transferred from the P site to the amino group of the aminoacyl-tRNA in the A site, forming a peptide bond and extending the peptide chain by one amino acid. Once the peptide bond is formed, the ribosome moves one codon ahead along the mRNA. Each cycle of peptide chain elongation requires three elongation factors and two molecules of guanosine triphosphate (GTP). Guided by the mRNA codon, this process of extending the peptide chain by one amino acid is called ribosomal cycling. It continues in a repetitive manner, elongating the peptide chain until the termination codon stop codon UAA (UAA) enters the A site of the ribosome. Under the influence of GTP, the termination factor recognizes the termination codon, leading to the binding of the release factor and activation of the peptidyl transferase. This results in the hydrolysis of the ester bond between the tRNA in the P site and the peptide chain, releasing the nascent peptide chain. The 70 S ribosome dissociates into the 30 S and 50 S subunits, preparing for the next round of peptide chain synthesis.

Although the precise mechanism of action is not yet fully elucidated, studies have indicated that oxazolidinone-class drugs can bind to the 50 S ribosomal subunit, with no affinity for the 30 S subunit and no inhibition of fMet-tRNA formation, elongation, or termination steps. It is now believed that oxazolidinone-class drugs can inhibit the formation of aminoacyl-tRNA initiation complexes, thereby impeding 70 S ribosome assembly.

In 2008, Erin M. Duffy et al. reported the crystal complex of Linezolid with the ribosomal 50 S subunit, revealing its mode of action with the target protein [22]. Studies have suggested that Linezolid interacts with the active site pocket within the ribosomal peptidyl transferase center through hydrogen bonds and hydrophobic interactions (Fig. 19.13). The oxazolidinone ring stacks with the base part of U2539, resulting in favorable van der Waals interactions. The oxazolidinone ring and the C-5 acetyl amide side chain exhibit good shape complementarity with the ribosomal A-site surface near the exit tunnel. Additionally, an important hydrogen bond is formed between the NH group of the amide and the phosphate group of G2540. Structure-activity relationship studies have also indicated the crucial role of the carbonyl oxygen atom in the oxazolidinone ring as a hydrogen bond acceptor. The fluorophenyl moiety of Linezolid resides in a crevice formed by residues A2486 and C2487, known as the A-site crevice, which is a wedge-shaped pocket. In bacterial protein synthesis, this active pocket interacts with the amino acid side chain of fMet-tRNA. The drug occupies this pocket, thereby preventing the formation of the 70 S ribosome and inhibiting bacterial protein production. The fluorophenyl fragment of Linezolid engages in a typical aromatic–aromatic stacking interaction with C2487 (distance of 3.5 Å from plane to plane and 4.3 Å from center to center) and simultaneously forms a T-shaped interaction with A2486. The morpholine ring of Linezolid, on the other hand, does not exhibit significant interactions with the ribosome. From a drug design perspective, this region can be further structurally modified to fine-tune the pharmacological properties of the molecule without significantly impacting its biological activity.

19.5 Study on structure-activity relationship of oxazolidinone antibiotics

With the continuous advancement in the research of oxazolidinone derivatives, a profound elucidation of the structure-activity relationship of Linezolid has been achieved. To facilitate comprehension and memorization, the structure of Linezolid is regarded as the fundamental framework, wherein the oxazolidinone ring is designated as the A-ring, the phenyl ring as the B-ring, the morpholine ring as the C ring, and the acetyl amine methyl group as the C-5 side chain (Fig. 19.14). We systematically summarized the SAR of oxazolidinone derivatives around the fundamental framework of linezolid.

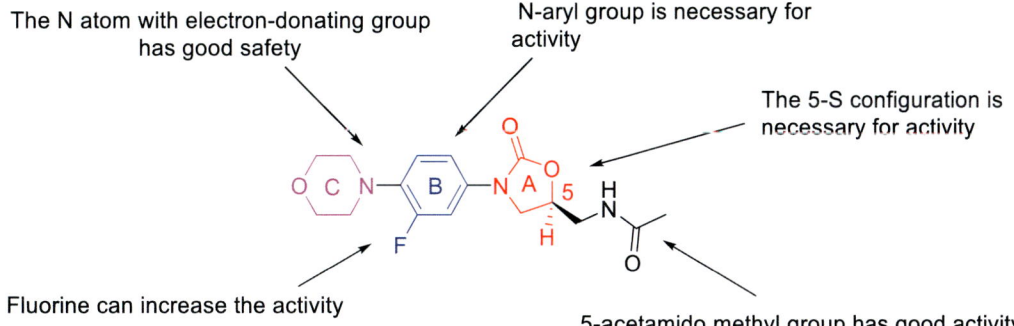

FIGURE 19.14 Research on the structure-activity relationships of oxazolidinone derivatives [23].

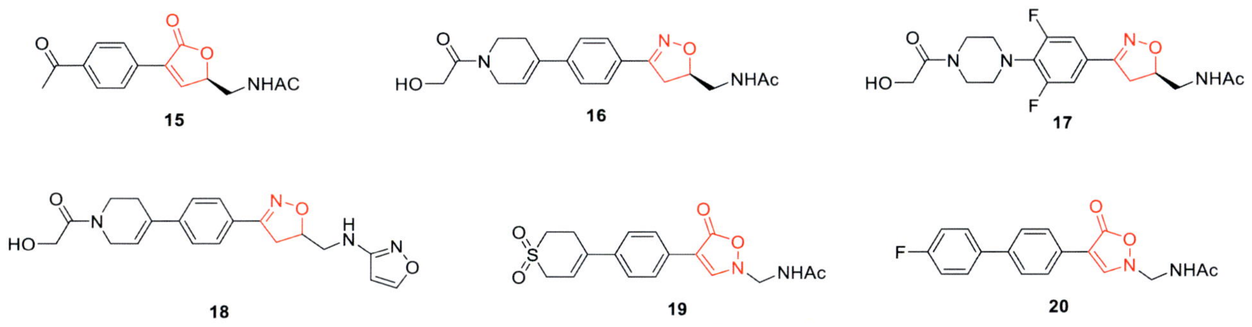

FIGURE 19.15 Oxazolidinone SAR analysis—modification on A-ring. *SAR*, Structure-activity relationships.

The A-ring serves as the core pharmacophore framework, as evidenced by the nomenclature of this class of drugs as oxazolidinone derivatives. Therefore, the structural modification of the A-ring, such as skeletal transitions, holds the utmost significance. Not only does it have the potential to significantly enhance the antibacterial activity of oxazolidinone derivatives, but it also presents the most promising opportunity for groundbreaking original research in this field. Representative achievements in the early stage of A-ring modification include the discovery of the butenolide ring in the mid-1990s, the isoxazoline ring reported by Pharmacia and Bayer in the late 1990s, and the isoxazolidinone ring reported by Bristol-Myers Squibb (BMS) in 2006.

In 1994, Roussel Uclaf, a French company, was the first to report the potent antibacterial activity of butenolide derivatives (Fig. 19.15). They synthesized the corresponding butenolide compound **15**, based on the lead compound DuP-721. Its antibacterial activity was comparable to that of DuP-721, with a MIC of 2–4 μg/mL against *S. aureus* and *S. epidermidis*. However, compound **15** exhibited slightly weaker activity against *S. pneumoniae* and *Enterococcus*. It is worth noting that the chirality at the C_5 position of the butenolide ring is crucial; only the *R* configuration is active, while the *S* configuration is inactive [24].

Pharmacia's Barbachyn reported a series of isoxazolidine ring derivatives, such as compounds **16** and **17**, with MIC of 2 and 1 μg/mL, respectively, against *S. aureus*. Both compounds displayed MIC values of 0.5 μg/mL against *S. epidermidis* and *S. pneumoniae* while exhibiting comparable *in vivo* activity to Linezolid. Research has revealed the significance of chirality at the C_5 position, where only the *R* configuration is active and the *S* configuration is inactive. The presence of the O atom in the isoxazolidine ring is essential for activity, and the introduction of fluorine atoms on the B-phenyl ring can enhance the activity. AstraZeneca also reported a series of isoxazolidine derivatives. Among them, the racemic compound **18** displayed a MIC of 4 μg/mL against MRSA and a MIC of 8 μg/mL against quinolone-resistant Enterococcus [25].

BMS researchers have reported a series of isoxazolidinone derivatives, such as compound **19**, with MIC of 0.5 μg/mL against *S. aureus* and 4 μg/mL against *H. influenzae*. In 2005, they further reported another series of isoxazolidinone derivatives, which exhibited good *in vitro* antibacterial activity. Some of these compounds demonstrated strong *in vivo* activity, for instance, compound **20** displayed MIC values of 0.03 μg/mL against *S. aureus* and 2 μg/mL against *H. influenzae*. Its *in vivo* antibacterial activity, with an $ED_{50} < 5$ mg/kg/day, surpassed that of Linezolid [26].

Early B-rings of oxazolidinone derivatives were predominantly benzene rings. Extensive research has shown that by introducing fluorine atoms into the benzene ring, the activity can be enhanced, and the pharmacokinetic properties can be improved. Using the principle of bioisosterism, the benzene ring in oxazolidinone is also commonly replaced by other aromatic heterocycles such as pyrrole, thiophene, and pyridine (Fig. 19.16). However, when the B-ring is a pyrrole, the corresponding compound **21** loses its antibacterial activity. Bayer has reported a series of compounds with B-ring consisting of thiophene and pyridine, such as compounds **22** and **23**, with MIC ranging from 0.25 to 1 μg/mL against Gram-positive bacteria [27]. Literature has also documented a series of compounds with B-rings consisting of pyridine and C-rings consisting of piperazine, which exhibit favorable activity. Compounds **24–26** possess comparable activity, with MIC values ranging from 0.5 to 8 μg/mL against *S. aureus*, stronger activity against *S. pneumoniae*, with MIC values of 0.25–1 μg/mL, and slightly weaker activity against Enterococcus, with MIC values of 2–8 μg/mL. Ring fusion strategies are frequently employed in drug modification approaches. Early literature has also reported several fused five- or six-membered tricyclic compounds by connecting the A-ring and B-ring through a C-C bond [28]. Compound **27**, among them, exhibits notable antibacterial activity, with good activity against *S. aureus* and *S. pneumoniae*, with MIC values of 2 and 0.5 μg/mL, respectively, and a MIC value of 2 μg/mL against Enterococcus. However, this compound exhibited toxicity at high doses, leading to the termination of further research.

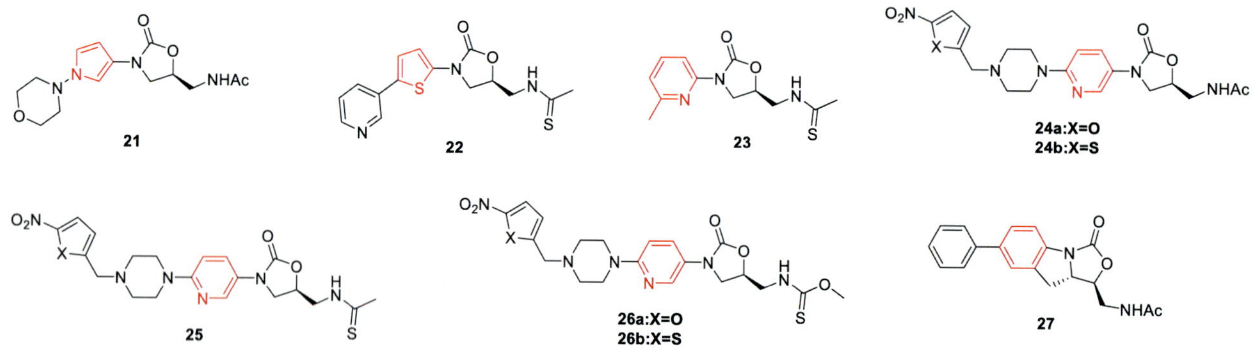

FIGURE 19.16 Oxazolidinone SAR analysis—modification on B ring. *SAR*, Structure-activity relationships.

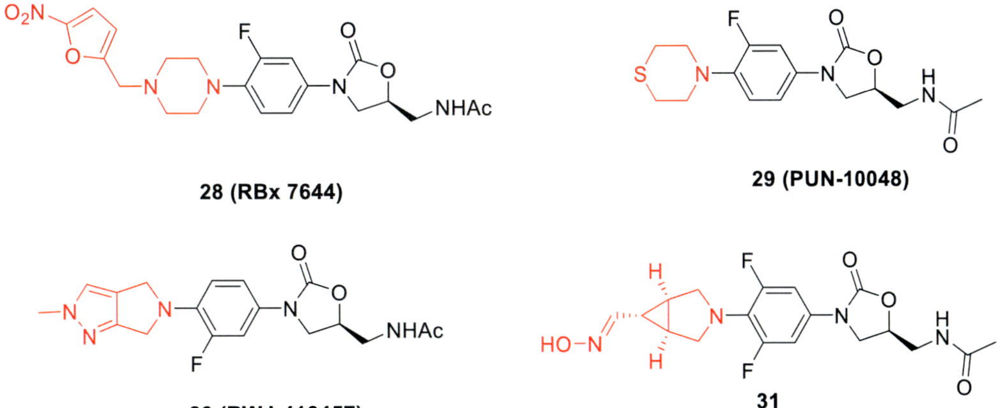

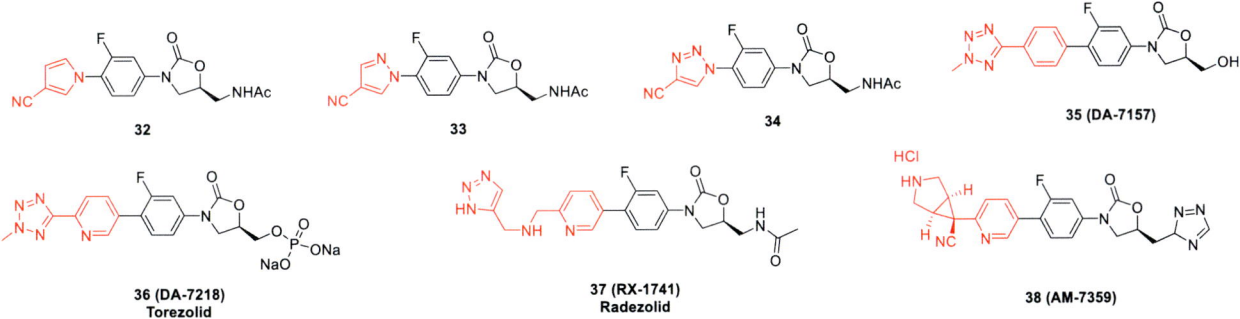

FIGURE 19.17 Oxazolidinone SAR analysis—a nonaromatic heterocycle (C ring). *SAR*, Structure-activity relationships.

FIGURE 19.18 Oxazolidinone SAR analysis—aromatic heterocycle (C ring). *SAR*, Structure-activity relationships.

The modification of the C ring is the focus of oxazolidinone research, mainly including nonaromatic heterocyclic C ring, aromatic heterocyclic C ring, and mixed C ring.

The piperazine ring is a crucial nonaromatic heterocyclic C ring, and the introduction of the piperazine ring increases the activity of oxazolidinone derivatives, improves their pharmacokinetic properties, and reduces adverse reactions. Hydroxypipexone (eperezolid) is a drug with a piperazine ring, and its activity is comparable to Linezolid. In addition, compound **28** (RBx 7644) reported by Ranbaxy has entered clinical studies, with good *in vitro* and *in vivo* antibacterial activity and favorable pharmacokinetic properties (Fig. 19.17). Replacing the morpholine ring in Linezolid with a thiomorpholine ring yields compound **29** (PNU-10048), which has a MIC value of 0.03−0.5 μg/mL for *Mycobacterium tuberculosis*. At present, PNU-10048 is in clinical trials as an antituberculosis drug. There have been many studies on the replacement of morpholine rings in Linezolid with substituted tetrahydropyrrole, and in general, the introduction of tetrahydropyrrole rings can improve the antibacterial activity of such compounds, especially against Gram-negative bacteria. The most notable of these was the discovery of compound **30** (RWJ-416457) [29]. This compound has also entered clinical trials, and its MIC values for *S. aureus*, coagulase-negative staphylococcus, *E. faecalis*, and *Enterococcus faecalis* are 1, 0.5, 0.5, and 1 μg/mL, respectively. In large-scale *in vitro* activity screening tests, RWJ-416457 is at least 2−4 times more active than Linezolid in all strains (including Gram-negative bacteria such as *Haemophilus influenzae*). In a mouse model of *S. aureus* infection, the active ED_{50} value of RWJ-416457 was 3.4 mg/kg/day, compared with 6.4 mg/kg/day for the control drug Linezolid. Merck reported compound **31** [30], which has a MIC value of 0.06−0.5 μg/mL for MRSA and 0.5 μg/mL for vancomycin-resistant and quinolone-resistant enterococci, both of which are better than Linezolid. However, this compound is less effective than Linezolid against Gram-negative bacteria such as *Moraxella catarrhalis*.

Researchers at Pharmacia have reported a series of oxazolidinone derivatives in which the C ring is substituted (or unsubstituted) pyrrole, pyrazole, triazole, and tetrazolium (Fig. 19.18) [31]. Among these compounds, the antibacterial activity of unsubstituted aromatic heterocycles is better, and when there is a smaller electron withdrawing group (such as cyanogen) substituted on the aromatic heterocycles, its activity is greatly improved. For instance, compounds **32**−**34** showed strong antibacterial activity against *S. aureus* (MICs value of < 0.5−1 μg/mL) and *H. influenzae* and

M. catarrhalis (both MIC values of 2−4 μg/mL). Furthermore, these compounds showed strong efficacy in mouse models of *S. aureus* and *S. pneumoniae* infections. Compound **36** (torezolid) reported by Dong-A in South Korea was approved by the FDA in June 2014 for the treatment of ABSSSI in adults caused by Gram-positive bacteria, including MRSA. Compared with linezolid, torezolid showed 4−8 times higher activity against a variety of common clinical bacteria, and its *in vitro* antibacterial activity against linezolid-resistant strains was increased by 4−16 times [32]. Oral and injected torezolid *in vivo* rapidly releases the original drug **35** (DA-7157), which has very good metabolic properties (half-life about 3.5 hours, bioavailability 92.8%), but also reduces myelosuppressive toxicity. Rib-X in the United States has also developed a series of substituted aromatic heterocyclic compounds, of which compound **37** (radezolid) has a half-life of 5.9 hours in rats. Rib-X announced two sets of phase II clinical data, and the clinical cure rate of radezolid in 160 patients with mild to moderate CAP reached 78%−92%, and no hematological adverse reactions were observed. In Phase II clinical trial of patients with SSSI, using Linezolid as a control, radezolid achieved a clinical cure rate of more than 90% and was safe and effective. Compound **38** (AM-7359), codeveloped by Kyorin (Japan) and Merck (United States), exhibited the most potent antibacterial activity among oxazolidinone compounds known so far. The MIC values of compound **38** against MRSA, PRSP, and VRE are 0.0625, 0.0625, and 0.25 μg/mL, respectively, which showed 16 times higher antibacterial activity than that of Linezolid. The antibacterial activity of compound **38** against Linezolid-resistant *S. aureus* in mice was 8 times that of Linezolid (ED_{99}: AM-7359 10.2 mg/kg, Linezolid 85 mg/kg).

The diversity of mixed C-ring structures adds complexity to the research process. An exemplary small molecule is compound **39** (PNU-94756), disclosed in the early patents of Pharmacia (Fig. 19.19) [6]. This compound exhibited comparable *in vitro* antibacterial activity to Linezolid, with MIC values ranging from 1 to 8 μg/mL against common Gram-positive bacteria, including MRSA, MRSE, *S. pneumoniae*, and *E. faecalis*. Furthermore, other literature reports describe compounds characterized by the connection of the B-ring and C-ring through heteroatoms (O and S), double bonds, triple bonds, or various other shorter structural units. However, the antibacterial activity of these compounds is weaker than that of Linezolid.

The study of C_5-substituents is of paramount importance in enhancing the activity, reducing toxicity, and improving the pharmacokinetic properties of oxazolidinone derivatives. Early research by DuPont demonstrated that the acetyl amide methyl group at the C_5 position is an essential and active moiety and that derivatives in the *S* configuration are effective but not those in the *R* configuration. However, as research progressed, oxazolidinone derivatives containing numerous C_5-substituents were discovered with excellent activity, which were broadly categorized into two classes: noncyclic and cyclic structures. Noncyclic structures of C_5-substituents mainly include substituted acyl amine groups, substituted thioacyl amine groups, ureas, and thioureas, while cyclic structures of C_5-substituents primarily encompass five- or six-member heterocycles containing N (or O) atoms.

Ulanowica and Brickner from Pharmacia company were the first to report on the substituted acyl amine at the C5-substituents. Compound **40** derived from eperezolid replaces two hydrogen atoms with chlorines on the C5-substituents. Its antibacterial activity against *S. aureus* and *Enterococcus species* is approximately 2−4 times that of eperezolid, but its *in vivo* efficacy is slightly weaker. Conversion of the acyl amine group to a thioacyl amine group on the C_5-substituent often improves the *in vitro* antibacterial activity of oxazolidinone derivatives. However, these compounds tend to have poor *in vivo* efficacy, pharmacokinetic properties, or higher toxicity. Thioacyl substituted compound **41b**, reported by Bayer, demonstrates enhanced antibacterial activity against *S. aureus*, *H. influenzae*, and *K. pneumoniae* compared to its acetyl derivative **41a**. Nevertheless, compound **41b** has greater toxicity than **41a**. Acyl amine substituted compound **42** (PF-00422602) reported by researchers at Pharmacia & Upjohn Inc (Pfizer Inc) exhibits a MIC value of 2 μg/mL against *S. aureus*. While maintaining potent antibacterial activity, compound **42** decreases the inhibition of monoamine oxiidase-A (MAO-A) by 10-fold and reduces bone marrow toxicity by at least twofold compared to Linezolid. Additionally, it possesses favorable pharmacokinetic properties [33].

Gravestock et al. reported a series of compounds with five-membered and six-membered heterocyclic side chains on C_5-substitutions (Fig. 19.20). Among the six-membered heterocyclic rings, compounds containing unsubstituted pyridine and pyrazine rings exhibit the strongest activity, but weaker than the corresponding C_5 acyl amine

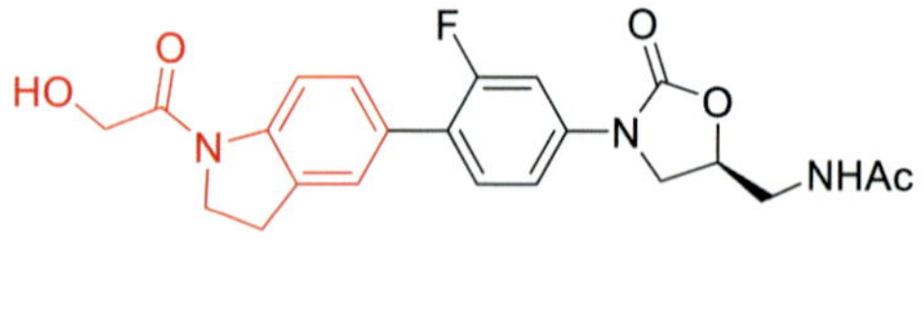

FIGURE 19.19 Oxazolidinone SAR analysis—promiscuous C ring. *SAR*, Structure-activity relationships.

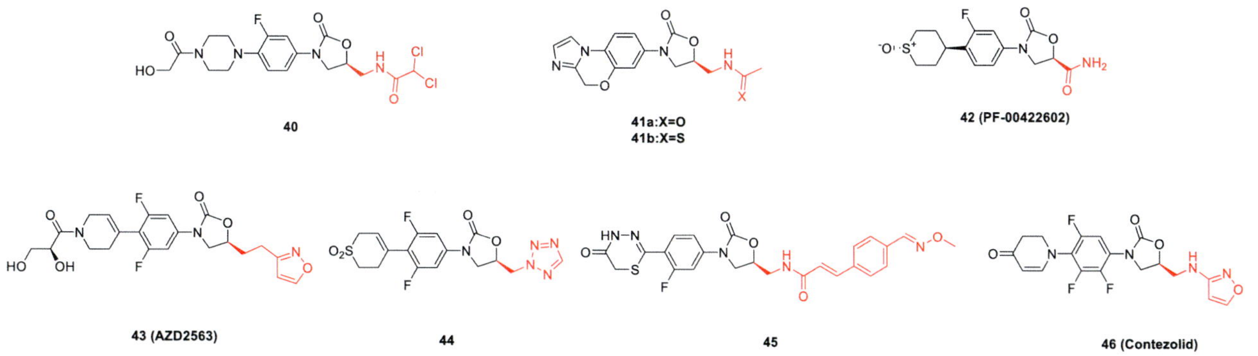

FIGURE 19.20 Oxazolidinone SAR analysis—modification of the C_5 side chain. *SAR*, Structure-activity relationships.

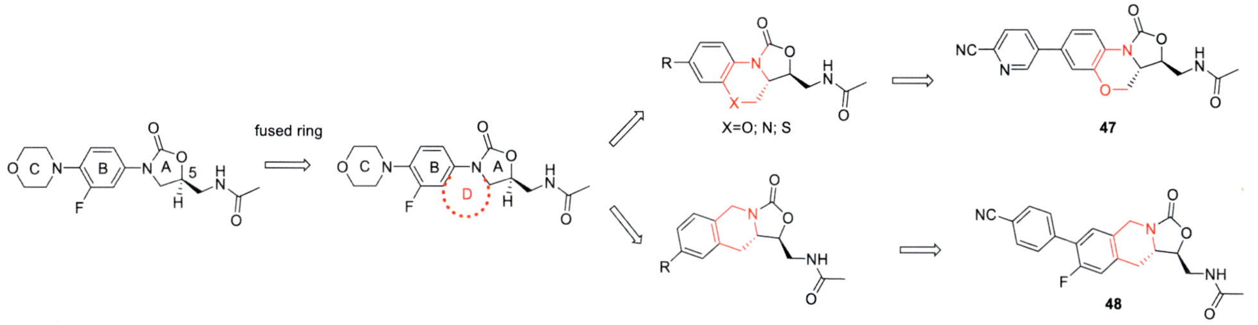

FIGURE 19.21 Oxazolidinone SAR analysis—the fusion of A- and B- ring. *SAR*, Structure-activity relationships.

compounds. In the case of the five-membered rings, a compound containing isoxazole ring demonstrates potent activity. Further structure-activity relationship studies led to the discovery of compound **43** (AZD-2563). AZD-2563 underwent clinical trials in the UK, demonstrating comparable or slightly superior *in vitro* antibacterial activity to Linezolid. In addition, it exhibited stronger antibacterial efficacy *in vivo* than Linezolid and required only once-daily dosing. Gravestock et al. reported a series of compounds containing tetrazolium moieties on C_5-substituent. For example, compound **44** showed MIC values of 0.125−0.25 μg/mL against *S. aureus*, 0.06−0.13 μg/mL against coagulase-negative staphylococci, and 0.25 μg/mL against *S. pneumoniae* and *Enterococcus species*. Additionally, it exhibited strong antibacterial activity against Gram-negative bacteria, with MIC values 2 μg/mL for both *H. influenzae* and *K. pneumoniae*. Vircuron reported some nonclassical cyclic C_5-substituted compounds. Compound **45** demonstrated MIC values of 0.06−0.125 μg/mL against *S. pneumoniae* and 0.06 μg/mL against VRE but was ineffective against Gram-negative bacteria such as *H. influenzae*. Contezolid (**46**) is an oxazolidinone drug designed by MicuRx company. Like Linezolid, it is used to treat complex skin and soft tissue infections caused by methicillin-sensitive and resistant *S. aureus*, pyogenic streptococci, or coagulase-negative staphylococci sensitive to and tolerant of cotrimoxazole. The drug was launched in China in 2021, and its C_5-substituent is also a cyclic side chain, specifically isoxazole. Contezolid is as effective as Linezolid but avoids bone marrow suppression-related toxicity. *In vitro*, it showed strong antibacterial activity against broad-spectrum Gram-positive bacteria (such as *S. aureus*, *Enterococcus species*, and streptococci), with MIC values ranging from 0.06 to 2.85 μg/mL. Structure-activity relationship studies indicate that the introduction of dihydropyridone fragment to the oxazolidinone scaffold not only enhances antibacterial effects but also significantly reduces MAO inhibition activity, suggesting that contezolid may have better safety profiles.

Additionally, there are other transformation strategies that have been extensively studied. One such strategy involves the fusion of the oxazolidinone A-ring and the benzene ring of the B-ring in various ways to construct novel tetracyclic antibiotics. Representative works in this field include the lead compound **47** reported by Yang et al. and compound **48** reported by Huang et al. (Fig. 19.21). These two compounds demonstrate distinct fusion patterns. Compound **47** exhibits a MIC of 0.25−0.5 μg/mL against MRSA, which is 8−16 times more active against Linezolid-resistant strains compared to Linezolid. In an MRSA systemic infection model, the ED_{50} value of this compound is <5.0 mg/kg, which was almost three times more potent than Linezolid. Moreover, this compound possesses favorable pharmacokinetic properties. Compound **48** demonstrates good antibacterial activity against various drug-resistant bacteria, including drug-resistant strains of tuberculosis, MRSA, MRSE, vancomycin-intermediate *S. aureus*, VRE, and some Linezolid-resistant strains, with MIC values ranging from 0.25 to 1 μg/mL. Furthermore, this compound exhibits favorable pharmacokinetic properties and stability in hepatic microsomes.

The study of SAR of oxazolidinone derivatives is instrumental in revealing the intrinsic connection between molecular structure and biological activity. The aforementioned analysis of SAR holds representativeness. To date, the discussion of SAR for oxazolidinone drugs continues to evolve and be supplemented. With continuous exploration and refinement by subsequent scientists, it is expected that more novel oxazolidinone candidates with potent antibacterial activity will be discovered.

19.6 Research on the synthesis process of Linezolid

In the synthesis process of Linezolid, the construction of the pentacyclic oxazolidinone ring and its chirality poses a highly challenging task. The efficient and rapid synthesis of this pharmacophore fragment is a crucial step in the overall synthetic route. Medicinal chemists have employed a chiral (*R*)-2-hydroxymethyl oxirane derivative as a starting material, which enables the efficient construction of the five-membered oxazolidinone fragment in a single step. This approach cleverly avoids the need for complex chiral resolution and purification steps.

The specific synthetic method is depicted in Fig. 19.22 [12,34]. Initially, the starting materials 3,4-difluoronitrobenzene (compound **49**) and morpholine (compound **50**) undergo an aromatic nucleophilic substitution reaction under weak base DIPEA conditions, giving the nitrobenzene intermediate **51** in high yield. Subsequently, the nitro group of **51** is quantitatively reduced to the corresponding aniline intermediate **52** using palladium-carbon catalysts. Intermediate **52** then undergoes an amide condensation reaction with benzyl chloroformate (CbzCl) to generate the key intermediate **53**. Here, benzyl chloroformate serves dual chemical functions: protecting and activating the amino group, as well as providing a partial structural fragment of the oxazolidinone. The reaction of intermediate **53** with (*R*)-2-hydroxymethyl oxirane derivative **54**, under strong base n-BuLi conditions and at low temperature (−78°C), results in the production of the single stereoisomeric oxazolidinone intermediate **55**. The hydroxyl group of intermediate **55** reacts with methylsulfonyl chloride to generate the methylsulfonate **56**. Subsequently, sodium azide nucleophilically attacks the sulfonate group, forming the azide intermediate **57**. Azide intermediate **57** then undergoes hydrogenation using a palladium-carbon catalyst, yielding intermediate **58**. Finally, in the presence of acetic anhydride, the amino group of intermediate **58** undergoes acetylation to afford the desired product, Linezolid. This synthesis process encompasses a total of 8 reaction steps, with an overall yield of 47%. However, it should be noted that the construction of the pentacyclic oxazolidinone ring and its chirality involves highly dangerous and harsh reaction conditions, such as ultra-low temperatures and the use of explosive reagents like sodium azide. These conditions are not conducive to the large-scale production of Linezolid in industrial settings.

The process preparation of drug production pursues simple operation, low pollution (green), low price, etc. In the subsequent many optimized process routes, it is also divided into two strategies: linear synthesis method and convergence synthesis method, both of which focus on the two key points: synthesis of oxazolidinone and the introduction of

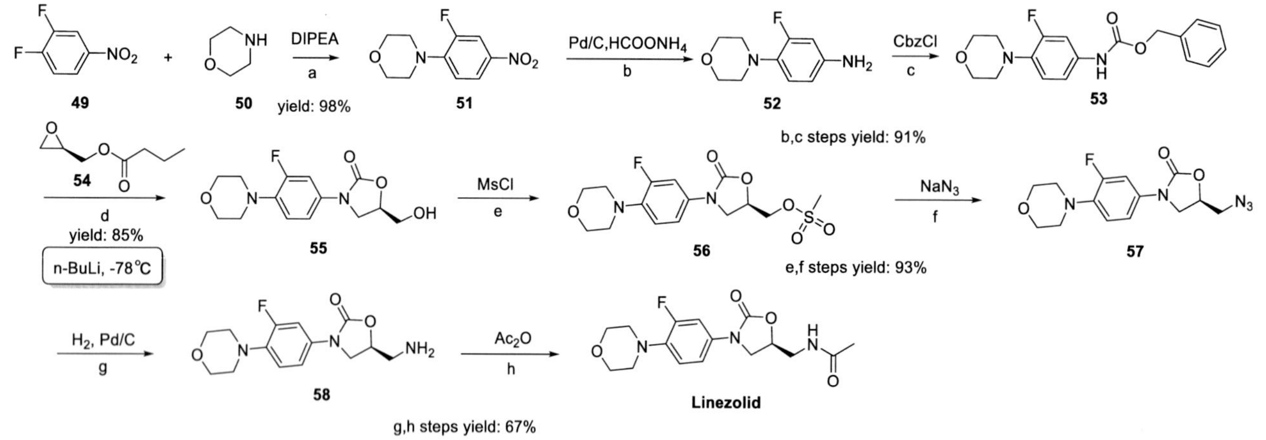

FIGURE 19.22 Original synthetic route of Linezolid.

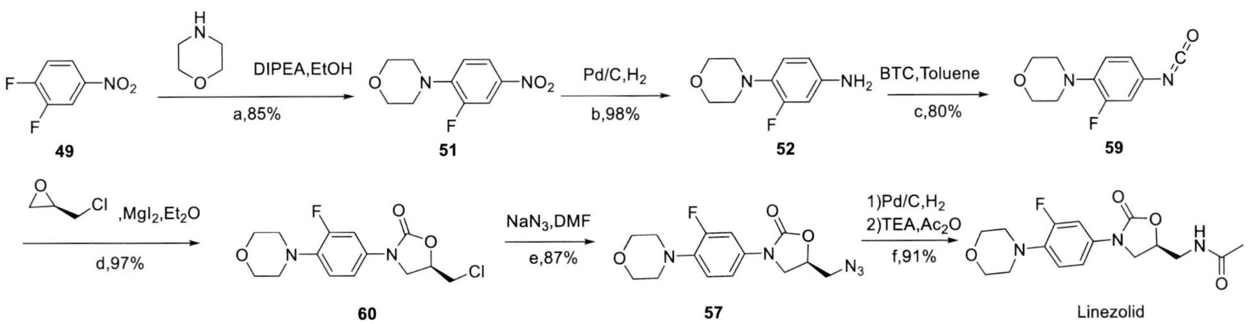

FIGURE 19.23 Optimization of the synthesis process of Linezolid (1).

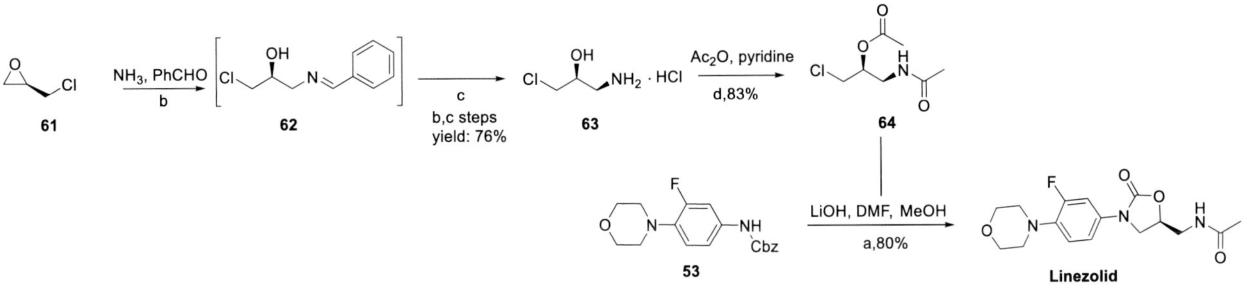

FIGURE 19.24 Optimization of the synthesis process of Linezolid (2).

the amino group (the former uses ultra-low temperature conditions, and the latter uses explosive sodium azide in the original route). In general, the synthesis of oxazolidinone is mainly accomplished through three main cyclization pathways, namely benzoxyformamide cyclization with ethylene oxide under strong base, employing carbonylation reagents, or utilizing isocyanate intermediates. Chiral center, on the other hand, is mainly accomplished by introducing chiral precursor raw materials or asymmetric catalytic synthesis. The introduction of the amino group is mostly accomplished by sodium azide reduction or through phthalimide reactions, polymerization synthesis, and other nonsodium azide processes.

Zhang X. et al. constructed the chiral center of Linezolid by using (R)-epichlorohydrin and 3-fluorophenyl isocyanate at relatively mild reaction condition. This approach provided good stereoselectivity avoided the use of methylsulfonyl chloride, and reduced the number of synthesis steps (Fig. 19.23). However, the fly in the ointment is that sodium azide is still used in the synthetic process to introduce amino groups [35].

Perrault et al. devised an alternative method to avoid the use of sodium azide. This process utilizes 3,4-difluoronitrobenzene and morpholine as starting materials, similar to the original route. Through substitution and reduction reactions, intermediate **53** is obtained. Furthermore, this method involves the use of chiral (R)-chloropropyl epoxide **61**, benzaldehyde, and ammonia water to form an imine intermediate **62**, which undergoes hydrolysis in dilute hydrochloric acid to yield a salt **63**. Intermediate **63** then undergoes a reaction with acetic anhydride to generate 2S-N-(acetyloxy-3-chloropropyl)acetamide **64**. Finally, **53** and **64** undergo cyclization reactions in the presence of lithium hydroxide, methanol, and N,N-Dimethylformamide (DMF) to yield Linezolid (Fig. 19.24) [36]. In this route, intermediate **53** reacts directly with the chiral fragment **64** in a single step to yield Linezolid, resulting in a shorter synthesis route. Moreover, the synthetic process avoids the use of sodium azide and n-butyllithium, which have significant safety concerns, making it more suitable for industrial-scale production.

Linezolid, as the first novel oxazolidinone antibacterial drug, has significant market value both domestically and internationally due to its unique antibacterial mechanism and low susceptibility to cross-resistance. Currently, pharmaceutical manufacturers worldwide are still committed to developing proprietary synthesis routes, aiming to greatly facilitate and scale up production, minimize pollution, and enable rapid market access. Furthermore, a well-established synthesis route will provide valuable assistance and new insights for the synthesis and process optimization of other oxazolidinone antibacterial drugs.

19.7 Conclusion

With the continuous growth of the variety and quantity of antibiotics, under the influence of various human factors and external factors, the widespread abuse of antibiotics has led to severe acquired drug resistance in both Gram-positive and Gram-negative bacteria. As a result, multidrug-resistant bacteria, also known as "superbugs," have emerged, including MRSA, multidrug-resistant *S. pneumoniae* (MDRSP), VRE, MDR-TB, multidrug-resistant *Acinetobacter baumannii* (MRAB), and the newly discovered *E. coli* and *K. pneumoniae* carrying the NDM-1 gene. Because most antibiotics are ineffective against them, superbugs have caused extreme harm to human health.

The new oxazolidinone drug, Linezolid, has a good effect on certain multidrug-resistant bacteria, especially for suspected or confirmed HAP, CAP, complicated SSTI, and vancomycin-resistant enterococcal (VRE) infection caused by MRSA. Linezolid has a unique antibacterial mechanism that can avoid cross-resistance with other antibiotic drugs, and it is not easy to induce bacteria to acquire drug resistance. Therefore, Linezolid has important clinical application value in the treatment of infectious diseases.

Linezolid, the first oxazolidinone-class drug, represents a pioneering and innovative drug targeting an unknown mechanism. Consequently, the research and discovery process for this novel drug encountered numerous setbacks. Initially, DuPont derived a lead compound, Dup 721, with potent antibacterial activity through iterative modifications of active compounds. Unfortunately, Dup 721 exhibited significant toxicity, leading DuPont to discontinue its research efforts. Fortunately, Upjohn persevered to conduct comprehensive investigations on the oxazolidinone structure of Dup 721. Employing classical drug design principles, Upjohn continuously modified and optimized its structure and ultimately discovered Linezolid, a drug with excellent antibacterial efficacy and safety. The discovery of Linezolid revolutionized the treatment of infections, shifting from inconvenient intravenous administration to the more convenient and patient-friendly oral route.

In the investigation of the mechanism of action of Linezolid, this drug has exhibited a distinctive antibacterial mechanism. It was not until the discovery of the crystal complex between Linezolid and the 50 S subunit of the ribosome that the interactions between Linezolid and its target were truly elucidated. This breakthrough further validated that Linezolid inhibits the formation of aminoacyl-tRNA initiation complexes, thereby blocking bacterial protein synthesis to exert its antibacterial effect.

With the deepening exploration of the SAR in the oxazolidinone derivatives, further insights into the intrinsic connections between structures and biological activities have emerged. This has led to the continuous development of novel oxazolidinone antibacterial drugs, including the newly marketed drugs tedizolid and contezolid. These emerging oxazolidinone antibiotics exhibit superior safety profiles and antibacterial efficacy compared to Linezolid, offering improved therapeutic options for bacterial infectious diseases.

The synthesis of Linezolid has been developed using various methods. An ingenious approach involves the use of a chiral (R)-2-hydroxymethyl oxirane derivative as a starting material, enabling the efficient one-step construction of the five-membered oxazolidinone ring and its chirality. This approach cleverly avoids the need for complex chiral resolution and purification steps. Furthermore, to address the harsh synthesis conditions and the use of highly toxic reagents in the original synthetic route, subsequent developments have focused on more industrially viable synthetic processes.

References

[1] Li J. Studies of small-molecule intervention on *Staphylococcus aureus* ClpP function and new antibacterial agents. Shanghai Institutes of Materia Medica, Chinese Academy of Sciences, Doctoral dissertation, 2019.

[2] Slee A, Wuonola M, Mcripley R, et al. Oxazolidinones, a new class of synthetic antibacterial agents: in vitro and in vivo activities of DuP 105 and DuP 721. Antimicrob Agents Chemother 1987;31(11):1791–7.

[3] Gregory W. Preparation of (aminomethyl)phenyloxazolidinones as antibacterial agents. US4705799, 1987.

[4] Gregory W, Brittelli D, Wang C, et al. Antibacterials. Synthesis and structure-activity studies of 3-aryl-2-oxooxazolidines. 1. The B group. J Med Chem 1989;32(8):1673–81.

[5] Park C, Brittelli D, Wang C, et al. Antibacterials. Synthesis and structure-activity studies of 3-aryl-2-oxooxazolidines. 4. Multiply-substituted aryl derivatives. J Med Chem 1992;35(6):1156–65.

[6] Brickner S. Preparation of 5β-amidomethyloxazolidin-2-ones as antibacterial agents. European Patent Organization. EP359418, 1990.

[7] Vara Prasad J, Boyer F, Chupak L, et al. Synthesis and structure-activity studies of novel benzocycloheptanone oxazolidinone antibacterial agents. Bioorg Med Chem Lett 2006;16(20):5392–7.

[8] Hutchinson D, Barbachyn M, Brickner S, et al. (Piperazinylphenyl)oxazolidinone antimicrobials. US5547950, 1996.

[9] Barcachyn M, Toops D, Ulanowicz D, et al. Synthesis and antibacterial activity of new tropone-substituted phenyloxazolidinone antibacterial agents. 1. Identification of leads and importance of the tropone substitution pattern. Bioorg Med Chem Lett 1996;6(9):1003–8.

[10] Barbachyn M, Toops D, Grega K, et al. Synthesis and antibacterial activity of new tropone-substituted phenyloxazolidinone antibacterial agents. 2. Modification of the phenyl ring - the potentiating effect of fluorine substitution on in vivo activity. Bioorg Med Chem Lett 1996;6(9):1009−14.
[11] Brickner S, Hutchinson D, Barbachyn M, et al. Synthesis and antibacterial activity of U-100592 and U-100766, two oxazolidinone antibacterial agents for the potential treatment of multidrug-resistant gram-positive bacterial infections. J Med Chem 1996;39(3):673−9.
[12] Barbachyn M, Hutchinson D, Brickner S, et al. Identification of a novel oxazolidinone (U-100480) with potent antimycobacterial activity. J Med Chem 1996;39(3):680−5.
[13] Ford C, Zurenko G, Barbachyn M. The discovery of linezolid, the first oxazolidinone antibacterial agent. Curr Drug Targets - Infect Disord 2001;1(2):181−99.
[14] Zurenko G, Yagi B, Schaadt R, et al. In vitro activities of U-100592 and U-100766, novel oxazolidinone antibacterial agents. Antimicrob Agents Chemother 1996;40(4):839−45.
[15] Edlund C, Oh H, Nord CE. In vitro activity of linezolid and eperezolid against anaerobic bacteria. Clin Microbiol Infect 1999;5(1):51−3.
[16] Turner M, Forrest A, Hyatt J, et al. Abstracts of papers, Proceedings of the 38th Interscience Conference on Antimicrobial Agents and Chemotherapy, San Diego CA, 1998. American Society for Microbiology, Washington, DC.
[17] Pawsey S, Daley-Yates P, Wajszczuk C, et al. Abstracts of papers, Proceedings of the First European Congress of Chemotherapy, 1996, Glasgow, Scotland.
[18] Welshman I, Stalker D, Wajszczuk C. Abstracts, Antiinfective Drugs Chemotherapy, 1998, 16.
[19] Wienkers L, Wynalda M, Feenstra K, et al. Abstracts of papers, Proceedings of the 39th Interscience Conference on Antimicrobial Agents and Chemotherapy, San Francisco, California, 1999. American Society for Microbiology, Washington, DC.
[20] Kohanski M, Dwyer D, Collins J. How antibiotics kill bacteria: from targets to networks. Nat Rev Microbiol 2010;8(6):423−35.
[21] Bozdogan B, Appelbaum P. Oxazolidinones: activity, mode of action, and mechanism of resistance. Int J Antimicrob Agents 2004;23(2):113−19.
[22] Ippolito J, Kanyo Z, Wang D, et al. Crystal structure of the oxazolidinone antibiotic linezolid bound to the 50S ribosomal subunit. J Med Chem 2008;51(12):3353−6.
[23] Xin Q. Design, synthesis and structure-activity relationship studies of oxazolidinone antibacterial agents. Shanghai Institutes of Materia Medica, Chinese Academy of Sciences, Doctoral dissertation, 2011.
[24] Denis A, Villette T. 5-Aryl-α, β-butenolide, a new class of antibacterial derived from the N-aryl oxazolidinone DUP 721. Bioorg Med Chem Lett 1994;4:1925−30.
[25] Barbachyn M, Cleek G, Dolak L, et al. Idetification of phenylisoxazolidin- ones as novel and viable antibacterial agents active against gram-positive pathogens. J Med Chem 2003;46(2):284−302.
[26] Snyder L, Zheng Z. Preparation of novel isoxazolinone antibacterial agents. WO2000010566, 2000.
[27] Riedl B, Haebich D, Stolle A, et al. Preparation of 3-aryl-5-aminomethyl-2-oxazolidinones as bactericides. DE19604223, 1997.
[28] Gleave D, Brickner S, Manninen P, et al. Synthesis and antibacterial activity of [6,5,5] and [6,6,5] tricyclic fused oxazolidinones. Bioorg Med Chem Lett 1998;8(10):1231−6.
[29] Paget S, Weidner-Wells M, Werblood H. Preparation of isoquinolinylphenyloxazolidinone antibacterials. WO2002064574, 2002.
[30] Fukuda Y, Hammond M. Preparation of bicyclo[3.1.0]hexane containing oxazolidinone derivatives for pharmaceutical use as antibiotics. WO2003027083, 2003.
[31] Genin M, Allwine D, Anderson D, et al. Substituent effects on the antibacterial activity of nitrogen-carbon-linked (Azolylphenyl) oxazolidinones with expanded activity against the fastidious gram-negative organisms *Haemophilus influenzae* and *Moraxella catarrhalis*. J Med Chem 2000;43(5):953−70.
[32] Jo Y, Im W, Rhee J, et al. Synthesis and antibacterial activity of oxazolidinones containing pyridine substituted with heteroaromatic ring. Bioorg Med Chem 2004;12(22):5909−15.
[33] Ulanowicz D, Brickner S, Ford C, et al. 37th Intescience Conference on Antimicrobial Agents and Chemotherapy (ICAAC), Toronto, 1997, F21.
[34] Barbachyn M, Brickner S, Hutchinson D. Preparation of substituted oxazine- and thiazineoxazolidinone antibiotics. 1995, WO9507271.
[35] Zhang X, Zhao C, Gu Y. A facile solvent-free synthesis of chiral oxazolidinone derivatives catalyzed by MgI_2 etherate: an approach to enantiopure synthesis of linezolid. J Heterocycl Chem 2009;49:1143−6.
[36] Perrault WR, Pearlman BA, Godrej DB, et al. The synthesis of N-aryl-5(S)-aminomethyl-2-oxazolidinone antibacterials and derivatives in one step from aryl carbamates. Org Process Res Dev 2003;7:533−46.

Further reading

Fischbach M, Walsh C. Antibiotics for emerging pathogens. Science 2009;325(5944):1089−93.

Chapter 20

Carbapenem antibiotic meropenem

Li Zhuorong and Cui Along
Institute of Medicinal Biotechnology, Peking Union Medical College, Beijing, P.R. China

Chapter outline

20.1 Introduction	489
20.1.1 Overview of bacterial infections	489
20.1.2 Commonly used antibacterial medications	491
20.2 Bacterial resistance and special use level antibacterial drugs	493
20.2.1 Bacterial resistance	493
20.2.2 Special use level antibacterial drugs	495
20.3 Case of meropenem	495
20.3.1 Discovery of carbapenem antibiotics	497
20.3.2 Structural optimization of carbapenem antibiotics	497
20.3.3 Discovery and structural features of meropenem	499
20.3.4 Mechanism of action of meropenem	500
20.3.5 Pharmacodynamics and pharmacokinetics of meropenem	500
20.3.6 Process synthesis of meropenem	500
20.4 The progress on other carbapenem antibiotics	502
20.4.1 Recently marketed carbapenem antibiotics	502
20.4.2 Chemical structure features and structure-activity relationship of carbapenem antibiotics	505
20.4.3 Mechanisms of carbapenem antibiotic resistance	506
20.4.4 Research features of carbapenem antibiotics	506
References	507

20.1 Introduction

20.1.1 Overview of bacterial infections

Bacterial infection refers to the process in which bacteria invade the host organism, including animals and humans, grow and reproduce, and release toxic substances that cause variable degrees of pathological reactions in the body. Therefore, bacterial infections are more likely to occur when the immune defense ability of humans or animals is weakened.

Bacteria belong to a category of prokaryotic microorganisms characterized by their small size and simple structure. Most bacteria reproduce through binary fission. In nature, bacteria are widespread. Although most bacteria are harmless and even beneficial, as they can coexist harmoniously with humans and animals, there are a considerable number of bacteria that can infect humans or animals and thus cause diseases. Common foodborne pathogenic bacteria include pathogenic *Escherichia coli*, *Salmonella*, *Shigella*, *Listeria*, *Vibrio parahaemolyticus*, *Hemolytic streptococcus*, and *Staphylococcus aureus*. Ingesting contaminated food can also lead to infection. Conditional pathogens are part of the normal bacterial flora in humans. When the gathering place changes, the immune defense ability is lowered, or under a dysbacteriosis, these conditional pathogens could be pathogenic. Currently, approximately 100 pathogenic bacteria have been identified in humans [1,2]. Fig. 20.1 shows the images of some mostly realized pathogenic bacteria, such as *S. aureus*, which is the most prevalent pathogenic bacterium on human skin and also exists in the nose and throat; *Streptococcus*, which subsists in the mouth, nose, throat, and intestinal tract; *E. coli*, which inhabits the intestinal tract; and *Pseudomonas aeruginosa*, which resides in the intestinal tract and on the skin. In addition, there is *Proteusbacillus vulgaris*, which survives in the intestinal tract and anterior urethra. Therefore, human or animal health depends largely on the survival struggle between beneficial bacteria and harmful bacteria. Beneficial bacteria gaining the upper hand allow the body's immune system to maintain its normal order.

In recent years, scientists and researchers have used the Gram staining method to identify and classify bacterial strains as either Gram-positive or Gram-negative categories. This method, established by Danish physician, Hans Christian Gram in 1884,

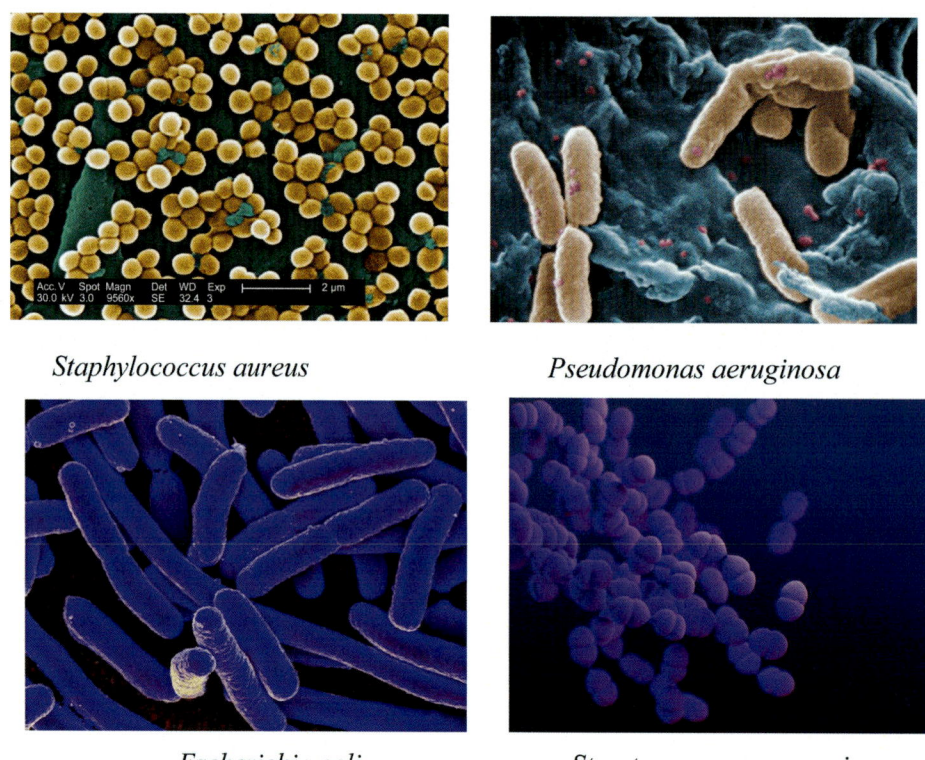

FIGURE 20.1 Common pathogenic bacteria. *Reproduced from the US CDC website, images of* Staphylococcus aureus *and* Pseudomonas aeruginosa *sourced from Janice Haney Carr, image of* Escherichia coli *sourced from the National Institute of Allergy and Infectious Diseases, image of* Streptococcus pneumoniae *sourced from Meredith Newlove.*

is a bacteriological laboratory technique. The assays consists of a cascade of steps, including staining with crystal violet and iodine, decolorizing with ethanol or acetone, and restaining with red dyes, i.e., safranin. Bacteria that retain a purple color after staining and decolorization are defined as Gram-positive strains, while the bacteria that becomes colorless after ethanol decolorization and then turn red with a red dye stain are classified as Gram-negative strains. When unstained bacteria occur, they are difficult to distinguish under a microscope because their refractive index is close to that of the background. Stained bacteria, on the other hand, have a distinct contrast with the background, allowing for clear observation of their morphology, arrangement, and certain structural features, making them suitable for classification and identification. Pathogens, such as *S. aureus, Staphylococcus epidermidis, H. streptococcus, Viridans streptococci, Enterococcus, Corynebacterium diphtheriae,* and *Bacillus anthracis* are Gram-positive bacteria. On the other hand, *E. coli, Pseudomonas species* (for example, *P. aeruginosa*), *Moraxella species* (for example, *Moraxella catarrhalis*), *Neisseria species* (for example, *Neisseria gonorrhoeae* and *Neisseria meningitidis*), *Acinetobacter species* (for example, *Acinetobacter baumannii*), *Klebsiella species* (mainly *Klebsiella pneumoniae*), *Salmonella species, Shigella species, Flavobacterium species, Proteus species, Legionella species, Yersinia species, Haemophilus influenzae, Enterobacter aerogenes, Vibrio cholerae,* and *Enterobacter cloacae* belong to Gram-negative bacteria, which account for more than 70% of clinical isolates, while Gram-positive bacteria account for less than 30%. Therefore, bacterial infections in clinical settings are mainly caused by Gram-negative bacteria [3].

Of note, bacterial invasion and successful infection depend on the individual's defense against bacterial virulence, including immune dysfunction, the number of bacteria, and other factors. For instance, intact skin and mucous membranes serve as natural barriers against bacterial invasion. When they are compromised, bacteria can easily enter the blood. The likelihood of bacterial invasion is elevated when the skin's inflamed areas or abscesses are squeezed. For example, in cases of severe burns, the wounds become the open gateways for bacteria, as skin necrosis and plasma exudation provide a favorable environment for bacterial proliferation, making bacterial infections highly probable. Damage to the urinary tract, biliary tract, gastrointestinal tract, and respiratory mucosa, coupled with the accumulation of contents and increased pressure, can facilitate bacterial entry into the bloodstream. The presence of urinary catheters, indwelling vascular catheters, and intubation during assisted respiration also make bacterial invasion more likely. In individuals with healthy immune defense, the bacteria in the human bloodstream can be rapidly cleared by defense cells, such as monocytes and neutrophils. In contrast, individuals under chronic disease conditions, i.e., liver cirrhosis, diabetes, hematological disorders, and connective tissue diseases, may experience sepsis due to metabolic disturbances and compromised humoral and cellular immune functions. The use of immunosuppressive medications and radiation therapy also contributes to the high incidence of sepsis. The usage of broad-spectrum antimicrobial drugs can suppress or eradicate bacteria that are susceptible to the drugs, but it can also facilitate the proliferation of drug-resistant bacteria, leading to sepsis.

20.1.2 Commonly used antibacterial medications

Antibacterial medications refer to drugs that have bactericidal or bacteriostatic activity *in vivo*, including various naturally occurring antibiotics as well as chemically synthesized or semisynthetic antibacterial drugs. Throughout the long history of the human-bacteria battle and continuous efforts, human beings have invented various medications to usher into a new era of human-bacteria combat, and some of these drugs have even changed the fate of mankind.

When it comes to antibiotics, one will immediately recall Alexander Fleming (August 6th, 1881 − March 11th, 1955) and penicillin, which changed the history of drug development. In 1928, Fleming, as a microbiologist, serendipitously observed that there was a zone surrounding the colonies of *Staphylococcus* in his culture dish. He thought that was caused by the substance of colonies produced by the mold. He then named the substance penicillin, although he did not know the details (Fig. 20.2). However, the clinical usage of penicillin and the start of the era of antibiotic chemotherapy are inseparable from the rediscovery of penicillin by two other scientists. Due to the urgent need to control infections on the battlefields of World War II, Howard Florey (September 24th, 1898 − February 21st, 1968) and Ernst Chain (June 19th, 1906 − August 12th, 1979) began to reexamine Fleming's discovery in 1939. They successfully isolated and purified penicillin in 1940, and through pharmacological and clinical trials, its remarkable efficacy and indications were finally confirmed, opening a new era of chemotherapy with antibiotics with an ability to industrially manufacture penicillin on a large scale in 1942 [1,2].

In fact, the time gap between Fleming's observation and Florey and Chain's successful isolation of penicillin is nearly a decade, during which research on antibiotics was neglected. Prontosil (Fig. 20.2) is the first sulfonamide drug that was discovered in 1932. Prontosil was disclosed as an effective antibacterial drug *in vivo* but not *in vitro* on dying assays against various bacteria. Scientists believed that prontosil is a prodrug that triggered a frenzy of research on the antibacterial azo dyes. It was initially believed that the azo group (−N=N−) in the prontosil's molecule was the pharmacophore that is responsible for the bacteriostatic effect. However, it was later found that only azo dyes containing sulfonamide fragments had antibacterial activity. Considering that the chemical azo group is easily cleaved to finally produce sulfonamide compounds, it was then speculated that sulfonamide was the true pharmacophore earning its antibacterial efficacy *in vivo*. Indeed, subsequent research disclosed that synthetic sulfonamides presented potent antibacterial activity *in vitro*, and para-amino benzenesulfonamide was finally isolated from the urine of patients who were administered with prontosil. Considering the universality of acylation reactions in the metabolic processes *in vivo*, it was determined that prontosil is a prodrug that is normally without antibacterial activity *in vitro*. The prodrug is only effective after being converted into active sulfanilamide in humans. Following this definition of the prodrug, several different sulfonamides were successfully discovered and developed in the following decades that effectively controlled bacterial infections of humans, such as pneumonia and meningitis infections, which had high mortality rates. Therefore, the chemically therapeutic treatment of patients with sulfonamide drugs heralded the first era in human history. In recent years, people have realized that sulfonamides are effective against a wide type of bacteria and are inexpensive and readily accessible, and therefore, some of them, such as sulfathiazole and sulfadiazine, are still widely used clinically today. Structurally, all sulfonamide drugs are close to that of para-aminobenzoic acid (PABA) and thus can compete with PABA for binding to dihydrofolate synthetase, affecting the synthesis of dihydrofolate and inhibiting the growth and reproduction of bacteria [1,2].

After recognizing the value of penicillin, scientists worldwide initiated a resurgence in the screening of antibiotics. Many new antibiotics were discovered and rapidly moved into clinical investigation and medications. This resulted in a large-scale antibiotic pharmaceutical industry in human history, fundamentally changed the treatment of infectious

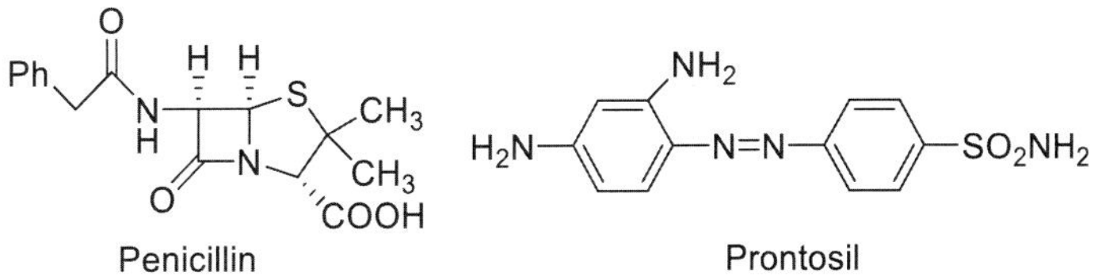

FIGURE 20.2 Chemical structures of penicillin and prontosil.

diseases, and promoted the development of chemotherapy. By the early 1950s, four major types of antibiotics, namely β-lactams, aminoglycosides, macrolides, and tetracyclines, were successfully established, marking the vigorous development of antibiotic research in the emerging field of international medical science at that time.

Currently, the widely used antibacterial drugs in clinics are the β-lactam antibiotics that are based on a β-lactam pharmacophore in their molecular structure, including penicillin, cephalosporins, recently developed cephamycin, carbapenems, and monocyclic β-lactam. Their mechanisms of action are similar as they all inhibit the synthesis of peptidoglycan by binding to penicillin-binding proteins (PBPs) in the cell wall, which causes defects in the bacterial cell wall, cell swelling, lysis, and death, taking advantage of potent bactericidal activity, low toxicity, broad-spectrum antimicrobial activity, and tolerated clinical efficacy.

Macrolide antibiotics are the ones with a macrolactone ring structure, which are effective against both Gram-positive and Gram-negative bacteria, as well as against *Mycoplasma*, *Chlamydia*, *Legionella*, *Spirochetes*, and *Rickettsia*. Currently, successful macrolide antibiotics are typically divided into three classes: the erythromycins involving 14-membered macrolides, the midecamycins, and the spiramycins taking 16-membered macrolides. Azithromycin, a derivative of erythromycin, is the first 15-member nitrogen-containing macrolide antibiotic to be marketed. The nearly launched ketolide antibiotic, telithromycin (Fig. 20.3), is a 14-membered macrolide. Of note, the broad category of macrolide antibiotics also includes 24-membered or 31-membered macrolide antibiotics, i.e., tacrolimus and sirolimus; polyene macrolide antibiotics, i.e., amphotericin B and pentamycin; and novel 18-membered macrolide antibiotics, i.e., fidaxomicin.

Aminoglycoside antibiotics have also been widely medicated in the clinic, including streptomycin, neomycin, gentamicin, kanamycin, and a derivative called amikacin. Their chemical structure consists of an aminoglycoside linked to an aminocyclitol by an oxygen bridge, resulting in superior water solubility and necessitating intravenous administration. Aminoglycoside antibiotics are primarily used for the treatment of systemic infections caused by susceptible aerobic Gram-negative bacilli. They are also used to treat severe infections caused by aerobic Gram-negative bacilli, such as meningitis, and infections in the respiratory tract, urinary tract, skin and soft tissue, gastrointestinal tract, burn, trauma, bone, and joint. Aminoglycoside antibiotics are excreted primarily in the intact form by the kidneys and accumulate significantly in the renal cortex, leading to nephrotoxicity. They also pose a damaging effect on the eighth pair of cranial nerves, causing irreversible deafness. These adverse reactions limit their clinical usage. Due to the problem of drug resistance in *Mycobacterium tuberculosis*, streptomycin has recently been prescribed to treat patients with multidrug-resistant tuberculosis. Aminoglycoside antibiotics mainly inhibit bacterial protein synthesis by acting on the A-site of the 16S ribosomal RNA (rRNA) decoding region in the 30S ribosomal subunit. Although most antibiotics that inhibit microbial protein synthesis are bacteriostatic, aminoglycoside antibiotics can exhibit bactericidal activity.

Tetracycline antibiotics are a class of broad-spectrum antibiotics produced by actinomycetes, including chlortetracycline, oxytetracycline, and tetracycline, as well as semi-synthetic derivatives such as methacycline, doxycycline, and minocycline. All of which are based on a tetracyclic scaffold. Tetracyclines are broad-spectrum bacteriostatic agents, exhibiting inhibitory effects against not only common Gram-positive and Gram-negative bacteria but also rickettsiae, chlamydiae, mycoplasmas, and spirochetes, with bactericidal activity at higher concentrations. Tigecycline (Fig. 20.3) represents a novel broad-spectrum antibiotic launched in 2005 as the first glycylcycline drug, displaying optimal activity against drug-resistant bacteria, such as methicillin-resistant *S. aureus* (MRSA). Tigecycline possesses a broad antibacterial spectrum, a long half-life, a low effective dosage, and is less prone to resistance. Tetracycline antibiotics specifically bind to the A site of the 30S subunit of the bacterial ribosome, inhibiting peptide chain elongation and affecting bacterial protein synthesis. These drugs structurally contain numerous hydroxyls, enol hydroxyl, and carbonyl

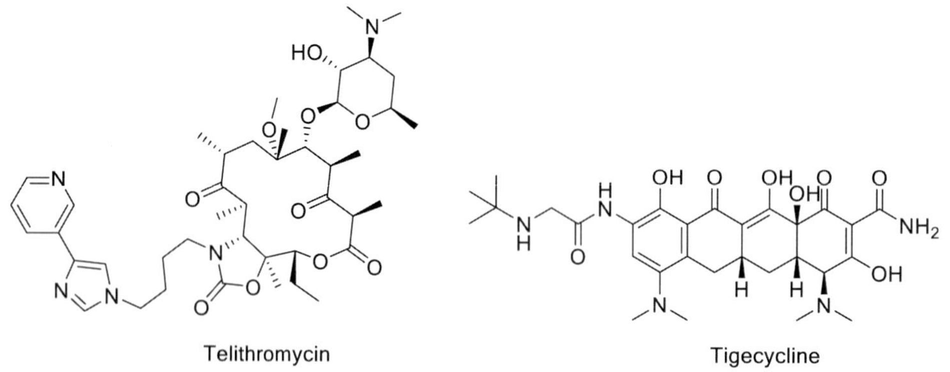

FIGURE 20.3 The chemical structures of telithromycin and tigecycline.

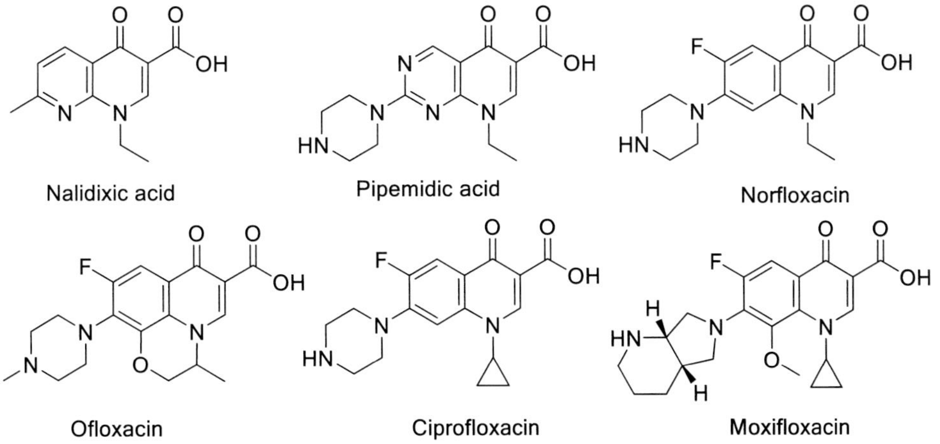

FIGURE 20.4 Chemical structures of selected quinolone antibiotics.

groups, forming complexes with calcium ions in the body, resulting in yellow deposits in bones and teeth. Administration to children can cause tooth discoloration, and in pregnant women, it may lead to discolored teeth in their offspring, as well as potential bone growth inhibition and various other adverse effects.

The above-discussed four major antibiotics are either microbial fermentation secondary metabolites or structurally modified derivatives, while sulfonamide drugs come from chemically synthesized compounds. Recently, chemically synthesized antimicrobial drugs are also including quinolones, oxazolidinones, and nitroimidazoles, as well as imidazole antifungal drugs and synthetic antitubercular drugs such as isoniazid, ethambutol, and others. Quinolones represent the most important class of artificial antibiotics, originating from the modification of chloroquine around the 1960s. Representative varieties include nalidixic acid, pipemidic acid, norfloxacin, ofloxacin, ciprofloxacin, and moxifloxacin (Fig. 20.4). The antibacterial spectrum initially targeted Gram-negative bacteria, such as *E. coli*, *Shigella*, *Klebsiella*, and a few *Proteus* strains, and is now gradually expanding to broad-spectrum activity against Gram-negative bacteria, with increased activity against Gram-positive bacteria, such as *S. aureus*, and anaerobic bacteria like *Bacteroides fragilis*. Furthermore, they have enhanced efficacy against typical pathogens such as *Mycoplasma pneumoniae*, *Chlamydophila pneumoniae*, *Legionella*, as well as *Mycobacterium tuberculosis*. Clinically, moxifloxacin is also employed as a second-line drug for tuberculosis treatment. Quinolone antibiotics selectively target bacterial DNA by acting on bacterial DNA gyrase, causing irreversible damage to bacterial DNA and halting bacterial cell division.

Additionally, owing to their low intrinsic resistance rate and effectiveness against multidrug-resistant bacteria, peptide-based antibiotics (Fig. 20.5) are increasingly gaining attention in the clinical management of infections caused by multidrug-resistant bacteria. Among them, glycopeptide antibiotics, such as vancomycin, primarily target Gram-positive resistant bacteria, while lipopeptide antibiotics, such as polymyxin, are effective against Gram-negative resistant bacteria.

20.2 Bacterial resistance and special use level antibacterial drugs

20.2.1 Bacterial resistance

Bacterial resistance is typically classified as innate or acquired resistance. The former is determined by chromosomal genes, whereby variations in bacterial cell structure and chemical composition result in innate insensitivity to certain antibiotics, such as *P. aeruginosa* displaying innate insensitivity to most antibiotics. The latter occurs due to genetic mutations in susceptible bacteria under drug pressure or the acquisition of exogenous resistance genes. For instance, *S. aureus* acquires resistance to β-lactam antibiotics after obtaining the *mecA* gene [4].

In nature, a particular strain of pathogenic bacteria (or individual bacteria) may also possess innate resistance. Prolonged antibiotic usage leads to the continuous eradication of sensitive bacterial strains, allowing resistant strains to proliferate extensively. This proliferation can ultimately lead to an increase in the resistance rate of bacteria to a particular antibiotic, potentially substituting the sensitive bacterial strain. Therefore, the misuse of antibiotics could accelerate the formation of bacterial resistance. The phenomenon of bacterial resistance always exists and is inevitable. In 2009, scientists discovered New Delhi metallo-beta-lactamase-1 (NDM-1), which even exhibits resistance to carbapenems, raising broad concerns about the issue of bacterial resistance. Currently, bacterial resistance has evolved into a serious global public health issue, with the situation in China being particularly severe.

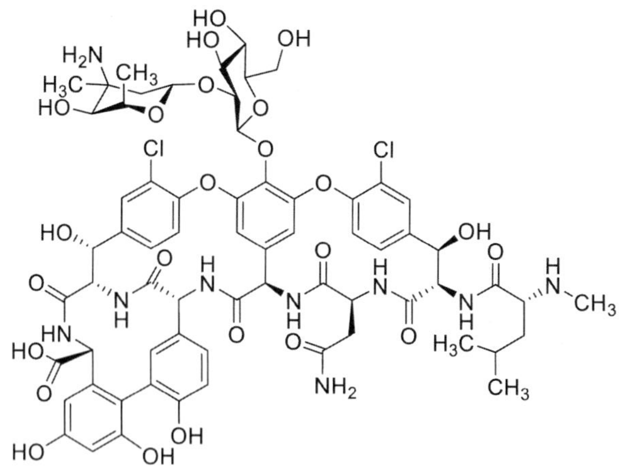

FIGURE 20.5 Chemical structures of vancomycin and polymyxin B1.

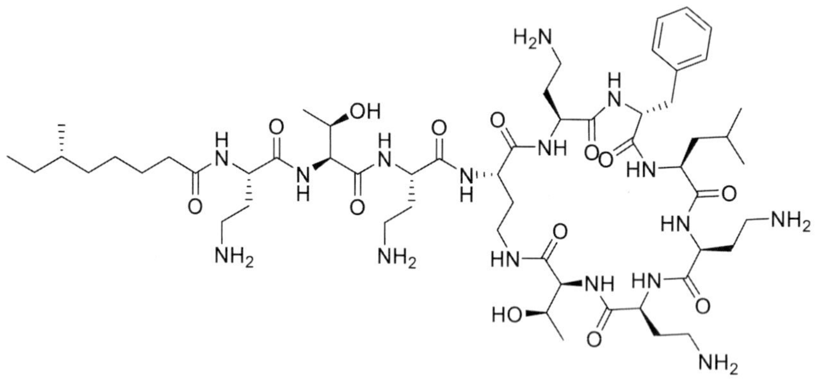

The development of bacterial resistance involves several primary mechanisms. (1) Production of inactivating enzymes: resistant strains produce inactivating enzymes that act on antimicrobial drugs, rendering them inactive. For example, strains that produce β-lactamases are resistant to β-lactam antibiotics, such as penicillin and cephalosporins, as these enzymes specifically open the β-lactam ring of these drugs, resulting in loss of antimicrobial activity. Similarly, bacteria modify the structures of aminoglycoside antibiotics through the action of phosphotransferases, acetyltransferases, and adenylyl transferases, leading to a loss of antimicrobial activity. Due to the structural similarity of aminoglycoside antibiotics, cross-resistance is commonly observed. (2) Mutation of drug targets: Mutation of drug target sites results in the drug's inability to bind or weakened affinity, leading to resistance. For instance, penicillin acts on the penicillin-binding proteins (PBPs) located on bacterial cell membranes, which have enzymatic activity and participate in cell wall synthesis, serving as the target protein for β-lactam antibiotics. Bacteria can alter the structure of these PBPs, reducing the affinity of β-lactam antibiotics to them and leading to resistance. Quinolones target bacterial DNA gyrase, and genetic mutations in bacteria can cause structural changes in the enzyme, preventing the entry of quinolones into the binding site and resulting in cross-resistance among all quinolone drugs. The target of erythromycin is the L4 or L12 protein of the 50S subunit. Mutations in the erythromycin resistance (*ery*) gene on the chromosome can lead to changes in the conformation of L4 or L12 proteins, resulting in resistance to erythromycin. The binding site of streptomycin resides on the S12 protein of the 30S subunit, and if the configuration of the S12 protein changes, preventing streptomycin from binding, it will also lead to resistance. (3) Alteration of cell wall permeability and active efflux mechanisms: For example, the outer membrane of the Gram-negative bacterial cell wall acts as a barrier, and bacteria can modify cell wall permeability, making it difficult for drugs to exert bacteriostatic effects, thereby leading to nonspecific low-level resistance.

Antimicrobial resistance exhibited by pathogens such as *S. aureus*, *Enterobacteriaceae*, *P. aeruginosa*, and *Mycobacterium tuberculosis* is a substantial challenge in the treatment of bacterial infections. In 2008, "ESKAPE" is pathogens were clinically recognized as the foremost pathogens of concern, consisting of *Enterococcus faecium*, *S. aureus*, *K. pneumoniae*, *A. baumannii*, *P. aeruginosa*, and *Enterobacter species*. The resistance displayed by these six categories of bacteria is extremely severe, and the acronym "ESKAPE" is derived from the initial letters of their Latin names [5]. In 2017, the World Health Organization (WHO) published the highest priority list of 12 pathogens that urgently require the development of new antibiotics. This group (critical) includes carbapenem-resistant *A. baumannii*, carbapenem-resistant *P. aeruginosa*, and carbapenem-resistant or extended-spectrum β-lactamase (ESBL)-producing *Enterobacteriaceae*. The second priority group (high) includes vancomycin-resistant *E. faecium*, methicillin-resistant or vancomycin-intermediate and resistant *S. aureus*, clarithromycin-resistant *Helicobacter pylori*, fluoroquinolone-resistant *Campylobacter species*, fluoroquinolone-resistant *Salmonellae*, cephalosporin-resistant or fluoroquinolone-resistant *N. gonorrhoeae*. The third priority group (medium) includes penicillin-non-susceptible *Streptococcus pneumoniae*, ampicillin-resistant *H. influenzae*, and fluoroquinolone-resistant *Shigella species*. The purpose of WHO's listing of these "priority pathogens" is to guide and encourage researchers in developing new antibiotics for these drug-resistant bacteria. Resistance to β-lactam antibiotics poses one of the most challenging problems in the treatment of clinical bacterial infections. Among these, the ESBL-producing Gram-negative bacteria is a leading cause of infections and contributes to their resistance to third-generation cephalosporins. Since their discovery in the early 1980s, they have spread worldwide and have become a significant public health concern.

20.2.2 Special use level antibacterial drugs

The overuse of antibacterial agents has significantly exacerbated the situation of bacterial resistance. The antimicrobial resistance surveillance system annual report of 2019 in China released the clinically common resistant bacteria, including methicillin-resistant *S. aureus*, methicillin-resistant *coagulase-negative staphylococci*, penicillin-resistant *S. pneumoniae*, erythromycin-resistant *S. pneumoniae*, vancomycin-resistant *E. faecium* and vancomycin-resistant *Enterococcus faecalis*, cefotaxime- or ceftriaxone-resistant *E. coli*, carbapenem-resistant *E. coli*, quinolone-resistant *E. coli*, cefotaxime- or ceftriaxone-resistant *K. pneumoniae*, carbapenem-resistant *K. pneumoniae*, carbapenem-resistant *P. aeruginosa*, and carbapenem-resistant *A. baumannii*. In 2019, the detection rate of carbapenem-resistant *A. baumannii* even reached 56%; the detection rate of carbapenem-resistant *K. pneumoniae* was 10.9%; the detection rate of third-generation cephalosporin-resistant *K. pneumoniae* was 31.9%; the detection rate of third-generation cephalosporin-resistant *E. coli* showed a slight downward trend, gradually decreasing from 59.7% in 2014 to 51.9% in 2019; the detection rate of quinolone-resistant *E. coli* showed a gradual and slow declining trend, decreasing from 54.3% in 2014 to 50.6% in 2019; the detection rate of methicillin-resistant *S. aureus* was 30.2%; the detection rates of penicillin-resistant *S. pneumoniae*, vancomycin-resistant *E. faecium*, and carbapenem-resistant *E. coli* were 1.6%, 1.1%, and 1.7%, respectively, maintaining at relatively low level in recent years; the detection rate of carbapenem-resistant *P. aeruginosa* in 2019 was 19.1%, showing a gradual downward trend over the past three years. Currently, most used antibiotics have exhibited varying degrees of resistance. Although the detection rates of some resistant strains have declined because of strict management of antimicrobial drug usage, the resistance rates of certain Gram-negative bacteria to high-grade antibiotics, such as carbapenems, still exceed 50%, potentially leading to a situation where no effective drugs are available. The inappropriately prescribed antimicrobial drugs will further aggravate bacterial resistance.

In China, it has implemented a hierarchical management system for antimicrobial drugs in clinical medication. This system consists of three levels, with the highest level defined as the special use level. The "Beijing Antibiotic Clinical Application Hierarchical Management Catalog (2021 Edition)" lists the main special-use level antibacterial drugs, including broad-spectrum tetracyclines such as tigecycline, the third-generation cephalosporins such as ceftazidime/avibactam, carbapenems such as biapenem, meropenem, imipenem/cilastatin; antibiotics for Gram-positive bacteria such as glycopeptides like vancomycin, norvancomycin, and teicoplanin, cyclic lipopeptides like daptomycin, and oxazolidinones like linezolid; antibiotics for Gram-negative bacteria such as polymyxin B, colistin, and colistin methane sulfonate; antifungal drugs such as amphotericin B, voriconazole, itraconazole, caspofungin, and micafungin. Special-use antibacterial drugs often serve as the "last line of defense" against resistant bacteria and play an important role in the treatment of critically ill patients in hospitals [6].

20.3 Case of meropenem

Penicillin and cephalosporins, the early discovered β-lactam antibiotics, have become the most widely used antibacterial drugs in clinical medication due to their remarkable efficacy in humans, high therapeutic window and tolerance, and a diverse range of treatments. Unfortunately, with their extensive clinical use and even abuse, the emergence of drug-resistant clinical pathogens has become an increasing challenge that needs to be urgently addressed. Studies have shown that the resistance to penicillin and cephalosporins mainly includes decreased outer membrane permeability, mutants in the target site of PBPs, active efflux mechanisms, and high-level expression of β-lactamases.

Carbapenems are a new type of β-lactam antibiotic that emerged in the 1970s. Compared to penicillin and cephalosporins, carbapenems exhibit stronger and broader-spectrum antibacterial activity and are tolerated by most β-lactamases. They are often considered the ultimate treatment option for multidrug-resistant Gram-negative bacterial infections. The antibacterial spectrum of carbapenems covers Gram-positive, Gram-negative, and anaerobic bacteria, as well as exhibiting potent antibacterial activity against multidrug-resistant bacteria or those producing β-lactamases. The minimum inhibitory concentration (MIC) and minimum bactericidal concentration (MBC) of carbapenems are close. However, carbapenems are ineffective against MRSA, *E. faecium*, and *Stenotrophomonas maltophilia*. Carbapenems act on penicillin-binding proteins (PBPs) to block the synthesis of bacterial cell wall peptidoglycan, leading to defects in the cell wall, bacterial cell swelling, changes in cell osmotic pressure, and cell lysis, ultimately killing bacteria. Mammalian cells do not have a cell wall structure and are not affected by such drugs; therefore, they are selectively bactericidal with minimal host cytotoxicity.

Carbapenems combine the five-membered ring of penicillin and the conjugated double-bond moiety of cephalosporin. Compared with penicillin (Fig. 20.6), the unsaturated double bonds between the C_2- and C_3-positions of carbapenems not only improved the ring tension but also greatly enhanced their antibacterial activity. Replacement of the sulfur atom in the penicillin thiazole with a carbon atom further reduces the bond angle from 120° to 108°, resulting in

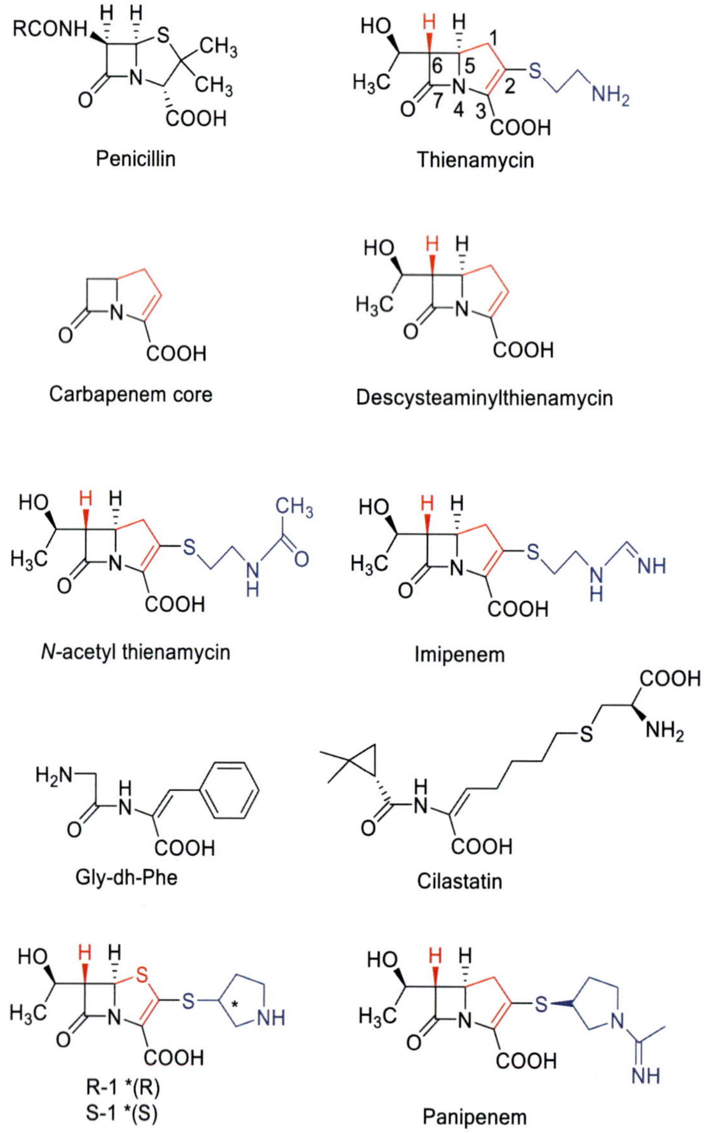

FIGURE 20.6 Chemical structures of penicillin and carbapenem antibiotics.

increased ring tension and enhanced antibacterial activity. In particular, the *trans*-configuration of β-H at the C_6-position and α-H at the C_5-position provides better binding poses for PBPs and thus improves drug stability against β-lactamases. Additionally, the *trans* α-hydroxyethyl side chain at the C_6-position extends underneath the β-lactam ring, increasing steric hindrance and further enhancing resistance to enzyme-mediated hydrolysis. Studies have revealed that it is the unique configuration of this group that endows these compounds with broad-spectrum antibacterial activity, very potent antibacterial efficacy, and the ability to resist most β-lactamases [7–9].

20.3.1 Discovery of carbapenem antibiotics

In the mid-1970s, researchers at Merck screened the isolates from soil microorganisms for the identification of inhibitors acting on peptidoglycan synthesis of both Gram-positive and Gram-negative bacteria. The first naturally occurring carbapenem compound, thienamycin, was discovered from the fermentation broth of *Streptomyces cattleya*, a soil microorganism (Fig. 20.6). In addition to thienamycin, the fermentation broth also yielded penicillin N, cephamycin C, and *N*-acetyl thienamycin. Studies indicated that the antibacterial activity of the fermentation broth against *S. aureus* was predominantly attributed to thienamycin, with *N*-acetylthienamycin demonstrating one-eighth of the antibacterial activity of thienamycin. Thienamycin demonstrated broad-spectrum antibacterial activity against methicillin-sensitive or resistant *S. aureus* and other Gram-positive bacteria, *P. aeruginosa* and other Gram-negative bacteria, as well as anaerobic bacteria like *B. fragilis*. Meanwhile, it also exhibited superior stability against most β-lactamases [10]. Since its initial report at the 16th Interscience Conference on Antimicrobial Agents and Chemotherapy (ICAAC) in 1976, carbapenem antibiotics quickly gained attention worldwide, and subsequent modifications yielded a series of carbapenem antibiotics. Thienamycin binds to PBPs, thereby inhibiting bacterial cell wall peptidoglycan synthesis and disrupting the bacterial cell wall to elicit bactericidal effects. Thienamycin exhibits high affinity to PBP1, PBP2, PBP4, PBP5, and PBP6, but has low binding affinity to PBP3. Subsequent studies revealed that the thienamycin was unstable in a higher concentration of aqueous solutions or under a solid state. For example, it was behavior as an accelerated deactivation in 10 mg/mL of water, in particular sensitive to the alkaline solutions (pH above 8.0). The nucleophilic reagents, such as hydroxylamine, cysteine, and even its own aminoethylthio side chain at the C_2-position, can take place nucleophilic substitution, which resulted in its lack of chance to be investigated and used in the clinic.

20.3.2 Structural optimization of carbapenem antibiotics

To overcome the chemical instability and challenge in the purification of thienamycin, researchers attempted to identify new derivatives with potent antibacterial activity and improved chemical stability through structural modifications. Scientists at Merck developed a method to efficiently synthesize the carbapenem core structure (Fig. 20.6) and found that it remained effective against penicillin-sensitive *S. aureus* and *E. coli*, while demonstrating diminished efficacy against penicillinase-producing strains, however, still indicating the instability against β-lactamase. Furthermore, the removal of the aminoethylthio side chain at the C_2-position, which was responsible for the instability of thienamycin, led to the synthesis of descysteaminylthienamycins (Fig. 20.6). These new derivatives exhibited antimicrobial activity comparable to that of thienamycin against penicillin-sensitive or resistant strains of *S. aureus*, *E. coli*, and *E. cloacae* in vitro. However, their activity against *P. aeruginosa* was only one-third that of thienamycin, indicating the significance of the aminoethylthio side chain for antimicrobial activity against *P. aeruginosa*, despite causing decomposition of thienamycin in solutions. Medical chemists considered derivatizing the free amino group to address this contradiction. Additionally, naturally occurring *N*-acetylthienamycin displayed reduced antibacterial activity against *P. aeruginosa*. Therefore, preserving the antibacterial activity against *P. aeruginosa* during the structural modification of the aminoethylthio side chain was crucial in designing new derivatives. Researchers believed that replacing the aminoethylthio side chain with a stronger basicity at C_2-position would generate more cationic forms at physiological pH, thus facilitating the passage of the compound through the negatively charged cell membranes of Gram-negative bacteria and could enhance the activity. Furthermore, the researchers hoped to obtain a derivative that could be easily recrystallized to facilitate purification that is necessary for the industrial production of the compound. In the 19th ICAAC in 1979, Merck's scientists reported the synthesis of an *N*-formimidoyl derivative, imipenem (MK0787, Fig. 20.6), which could be recrystallized from ethanol-water solution to obtain imipenem monohydrate. Imipenem exhibited 5–10 times higher stability in a high-concentration solution compared to thienamycin, and the decomposition rate of imipenem was less than 1% per hour in a solution of 10 mg/mL. Imipenem not only retained the antimicrobial spectrum of thienamycin but also enhanced the antimicrobial activity against *P. aeruginosa*. Due to its improved stability and activity against *P. aeruginosa*, imipenem was moved into clinical investigation [11].

Clinical trial investigation of chimpanzees and humans reveals that imipenem exhibited acceptable stability in plasma with a half-life of approximately 1 hour when dosed alone. However, only 10% urinary recovery was observed in chimpanzees, suggesting a possible metabolism pathway in the kidney, which was later confirmed to be due to the hydrolytic inactivation of imipenem by renal dehydropeptidase-I (DHP-I). The structural similarity between imipenem and the substrate of DHP-I, dehydropeptides (such as Gly-dh-Phe, Fig. 20.6), allows DHP-I to hydrolyze the β-lactam ring of imipenem, leading to low recovery of the intact drug in the urine and making it unsuitable for the treatment of urinary tract infections. Imipenem was predominantly subjected to glomerular filtration and renal tubular excretion, but it was susceptible to hydrolytic inactivation by DHP-I in the brush border of proximal renal tubular epithelial cells, resulting in only a small amount of the intact drug being recovered in urine (approximately 80% hydrolyzed), as well as the generation of nephrotoxic degradation products. Therefore, researchers have to initiate a project to find DHP-I inhibitors. The first candidate was MK0789, but it generated an injection of local irritation in animals at high concentrations. Subsequently, a new dehydropeptidase inhibitor, MK0791, was developed to replace MK0789. MK0791, also known as cilastatin, was the compound later used in combination with imipenem. Cilastatin is a potent and selective DHP-I inhibitor, and the pharmacokinetic profiles of imipenem/cilastatin combo therapy are similar to those of imipenem alone. Cilastatin itself had no antimicrobial activity but blocked the entry of imipenem into renal tubular epithelial tissue, reducing the excretion and inhibiting hydrolytic degradation of imipenem by DHP-I, thereby increasing the urinary recovery to 70%−80%. These results made the combination suitable for the treatment of urinary tract infections. In 1985, imipenem, developed by Merck, was first approved in Japan, and it received FDA approval in the United States in 1987. Imipenem exhibited high affinity for PBP1a, PBP1b, PBP2, PBP4, PBP5, and PBP6 of *E. coli*, as well as PBP1a, PBP1b, PBP2, PBP4, and PBP5 of *P. aeruginosa*, and exerted its bactericidal effect by inhibiting bacterial cell wall synthesis. The bactericidal action was primarily attributed to its binding to PBP2 and PBP1b. The intravenous imipenem/cilastatin is a broad-spectrum antibiotic. The *in vitro* studies confirmed its broad-spectrum antimicrobial activities, including Gram-negative bacteria, Gram-positive bacteria, including penicillinase-producing and non-penicillinase-producing *S. aureus*, most *Streptococcus species*, and anaerobic bacteria, while maintaining stability in the presence of most β-lactamases. It is also effective against *Nocardia species*, *Rhodococcus species*, and various species of *Listeria*; however, it shows no efficacy against MRSA and *S. maltophilia*. Among Gram-negative bacteria, many members of the *Enterobacteriaceae* family, such as *Citrobacter* and various species of *Enterobacter, E. coli, Klebsiella, Proteus, Salmonella, Serratia, Shigella*, and *Yersinia*, are sensitive to the intravenous use of imipenem/cilastatin. The activity of imipenem/cilastatin against *P. aeruginosa* is similar to that of ceftazidime. It is also active against *Acinetobacter, Campylobacter jejuni, H. influenzae*, and various *Neisseria species*. Additionally, it is effective against anaerobic bacteria, including various *Bacteroides*, whereas it shows only moderate sensitivity against *Clostridium difficile*. The post-antibiotic effect (PAE) of imipenem varies depending on the bacteria, ranging from 2.6 to 3.5 hours for *S. aureus* and approximately 1.6 hours for *P. aeruginosa*.

Imipenem carries a higher risk of inducing seizures and thus cannot be used to treat central nervous system infections. The possible neurotoxicity mechanism induced by imipenem is speculated that imipenem may disturb the binding of gamma-aminobutyric acid (GABA) to its receptors, thereby interfering with the inhibitory function of GABA that eventually results in an imbalance of excitatory and inhibitory neuronal synaptic transmission and consequently increasing the risk of seizures.

When synthesizing of carbapenem derivatives, the Japanese researchers disclosed that the C_2-position of the carbapenem contained a pyrrolidine thiol side chain (R-1, S-1, Fig. 20.6) that exhibited similar antimicrobial activity *in vitro* to that of thienamycin, prompting researchers to incorporate the pyrrolidine thiol side chain into carbapenem derivatives. In 1983, researchers reported the synthesis and *in vitro* antimicrobial activity of RS-533, a carbapenem compound with a substituted pyrrolidine thiol side chain (panipenem, Fig. 20.6). The results illustrated that panipenem exhibited superior antimicrobial activity against the most tested strains, and its activity against *P. aeruginosa* was comparable to that of thienamycin [12]. Panipenem increased its stability against DHP-I-mediated hydrolysis. However, when used alone, it tends to accumulate in the renal cortex and exhibits significant and transient nephrotoxicity. With the combination of an organic ion transfer inhibitor called betamipron, the nephrotoxicity induced by panipenem could be effectively attenuated, which was finally approved in 1994 and developed by Sankyo in Japan. Panipenem and betamipron were formulated in a 1:1 ratio by weight to create a combo formulation. Panipenem exhibits high affinity for PBP1a, PBP1b, PBP2, PBP4, PBP5, and PBP6 of *E. coli*, PBP1a, PBP1b, PBP2, PBP3, PBP4, and PBP5 of *P. aeruginosa*, and PBP1, PBP2, PBP3, and PBP4 of *S. aureus*, and it exerts bactericidal effectiveness by inhibiting bacterial cell wall synthesis. Its antibacterial spectrum is close to that of imipenem, showing potent antibacterial effects against both Gram-positive and Gram-negative bacteria, aerobic bacteria, and anaerobic bacteria. It exhibits improved activity against *S. aureus* and similar activity against *Enterococcus, Peptostreptococcus, Citrobacter, Klebsiella, E. coli, Serratia,*

Proteus, *H. influenzae*, and *B. fragilis* compared to imipenem. It has lower activity against *P. aeruginosa* compared to imipenem, and the incidence of inducing seizures is also lower than that of imipenem. Panipenem displays a PAE against both Gram-positive and Gram-negative bacteria, with growth inhibition times of 2.1, 1.7, and 1.7 hours for *S. aureus*, *E. coli*, and *P. aeruginosa*, respectively, after incubation with 4 times the MIC of panipenem for 2 hours.

20.3.3 Discovery and structural features of meropenem

Due to the broad market prospects of carbapenem antibiotics and the instability of imipenem to DHP-I in renal tubular epithelial cell brush border, researchers have intensified their efforts to develop DHP-I-resistant carbapenem antibiotics. In 1984, researchers from Merck reported the successful introduction of a β-methyl group at the C_1-position in the carbapenem scaffold (Fig. 20.7). The study showed that the addition of a β-methyl group at the C_1-position increased the antibacterial activity and the improved stability against DHP-I. At the 27th ICAAC in 1987, researchers from Sumitomo in Japan reported a novel 1β-carbapenem antibiotic, meropenem (SM-7338) (Fig. 20.7). Meropenem, a new generation of carbapenem antibiotic, was jointly developed by Sumitomo and ICI (UK) and was approved for marketing in Italy in 1994. Compared to imipenem, the introduction of a β-methyl group at the C_1-position increases the stability against DHP-I, while the presence of a dimethylcarbamoylpyrrolidinethio side chain at the C_2-position enhances the activity against Gram-negative bacteria. Meropenem has a broad spectrum of activity against Gram-positive bacteria such as *S. pneumoniae* (excluding penicillin-resistant strains) and *V. streptococci*, as well as Gram-negative bacteria including *E. coli*, *H. influenzae* (both β-lactamase positive and negative strains), *K. pneumoniae*, *P. aeruginosa*, and *N. meningitidis*. It is also effective against anaerobic bacteria such as *B. fragilis*, *Bacteroides thetaiotaomicron*, and *Peptostreptococcus*. Meropenem's activity against Gram-positive bacteria is slightly weaker than that of imipenem, but it is superior to imipenem in terms of its activity against Gram-negative bacteria. Meropenem possesses 2–8 times stronger antibacterial activity against certain Enterobacteriaceae compared to imipenem, but it is ineffective against *Xanthomonas*, *S. maltophilia*, and some *Burkholderia cepacia*. It demonstrates potent antibacterial activity against most anaerobic bacteria, which is comparable to or slightly stronger than imipenem. Meropenem does not exhibit significant accumulation in humans and thus has lower toxicity. It demonstrates a PAE against both Gram-positive and Gram-negative bacteria, lasting approximately 3 hours against *S. aureus* and *S. epidermidis*, 1.2 hours against *E. coli*, and 2.5 hours against *P. aeruginosa*.

Makoto et al. [13] conducted a structure-activity relationship investigation on meropenem (Fig. 20.7) and found that among derivatives without methyl substitution at the C_1-position, four stereoisomers generated by the two chiral centers at the 3′- and 5′-positions of the pyrrolidine ring showed strong antibacterial activity against both negative and positive bacteria, except for *P. aeruginosa*. The *cis* isomer exhibited superior activity against *P. aeruginosa* compared to the *trans* isomer, and when both the chiral centers at the 3′- and 5′-position of the pyrrolidine ring were in the *S* configuration and a dimethylaminocarbonyl group was introduced at the 5′-position, the yielded derivative showed the best activity against *P. aeruginosa*. The presence of an aminocarbonyl or dimethylaminocarbonyl group at the 5′-position did not significantly affect the stability against DHP-I. The introduction of a methyl group at the 1α-position did not improve the stability against DHP-I and even decreased the antibacterial activity, while the introduction of a methyl group at the

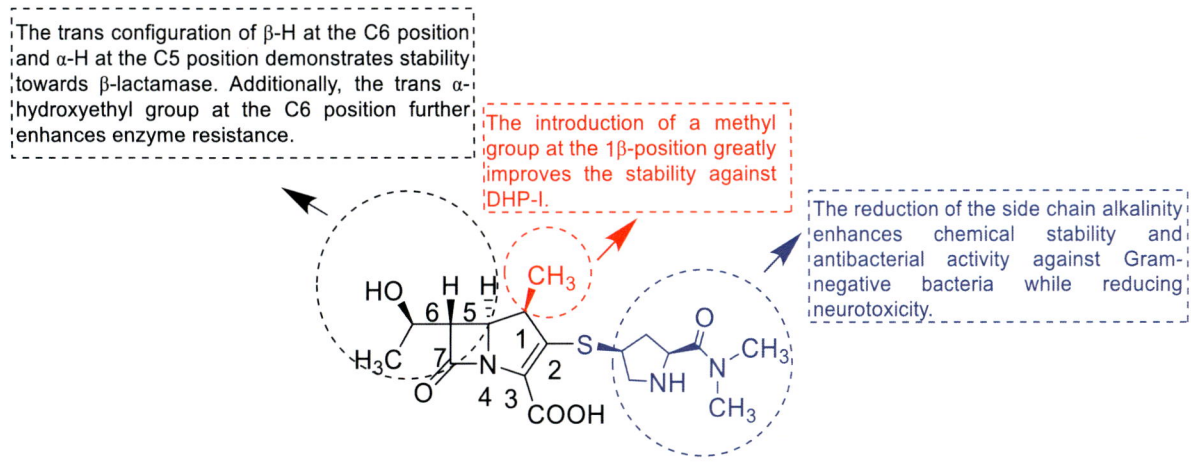

FIGURE 20.7 Structure-activity relationship of meropenem.

1β-position not only enhanced the stability against DHP-I but also increased the activity against Gram-negative bacteria, especially against *P. aeruginosa*. The introduction of a methyl group at the 1β-position in meropenem greatly improves the stability against DHP-I and reduces nephrotoxicity, obviating the need for co-administration with a DHP-I inhibitor. Meropenem easily crosses the blood-brain barrier and effectively treats central nervous system infections, with a lower incidence of seizures compared to imipenem.

The summary of the structure-activity relationship of Meropenem:

1. **Stability to β-lactamases.** The compound with a *trans* configuration between the β-H at the C_6-position and the α-H at the C_5-position in the carbapenem core demonstrates stability to β-lactamases. Additionally, the presence of a *trans*-α-hydroxyethyl side chain at the C_6-position increases the steric hindrance, further enhancing its resistance to the β-lactamase.
2. **Enhancement of antibacterial activity and drug stability.** The amino group at the C_2-position of thienamycin leads to chemical instability. Therefore, the subsequent development of clinically used compounds such as imipenem, panipenem, and meropenem involved substitutions on the amino group, reducing the alkalinity of their side chains and consequently improving their chemical stability, thus reducing central nervous system toxicity. Meanwhile, the presence of a dimethylcarbamoylpyrrolidinethio side chain at the C_2-position of meropenem enhances its antibacterial activity against *P. aeruginosa* and other Gram-negative bacteria.
3. **Resistance to DHP-I.** Meropenem is the first carbapenem antibiotic that can be used as a monotherapy. Compared to imipenem, meropenem possesses a β-methyl group at the C_1-position, which provides stability against DHP-I and improves its antimicrobial activity against Gram-negative bacteria. However, the presence of α-methyl substitution at the C_1-position does not yield the same benefits.

20.3.4 Mechanism of action of meropenem

Meropenem is a bactericidal agent that targets bacteria during their growth phase. Like the other β-lactam antibiotics, it primarily exerts its bactericidal effects by binding to PBPs located on the inner membrane of the bacterial cell walls, influencing cell wall synthesis. In Gram-negative bacteria, meropenem preferentially binds to PBP2, PBP3, and PBP4, and it shows strong binding affinity to PBP1a and PBP1b as well. It can penetrate *Enterobacteriaceae* and *P. aeruginosa*, primarily through tight binding to PBP2 and PBP3. Research suggests that the high binding affinity of meropenem to PBP3 is attributed to the C_2-position dimethylcarbamoylpyrrolidinethio side chain.

20.3.5 Pharmacodynamics and pharmacokinetics of meropenem

Meropenem is a time-dependent antimicrobial drug that requires a sustained period at a certain drug concentration to exert its bactericidal effects. This is typically represented by the percentage of time that the drug concentration remains above the MIC during the dosing interval ($\%T > MIC$). Increasing the drug concentration above 4−5 times the MIC does not necessarily increase its bactericidal effectiveness, but prolonging the exposure time with an effective drug concentration ($\%T > MIC$) significantly improves its antimicrobial efficacy in humans.

Meropenem exhibits linear pharmacokinetic characteristics, and the plasma pharmacokinetic profile is nearly identical between continuous and single-dose administration, indicating no accumulation in blood. The plasma protein binding of meropenem is very low, with a value of approximately 2%. Following administration, the drug is widely distributed in various tissues and body fluids, including cerebrospinal fluid, reaching effective concentrations. The half-life of the drug is 1.00−1.40 hours, with a plasma clearance rate of 16.70 L/h and a renal clearance rate of 11.70 L/h. Meropenem is primarily eliminated through glomerular filtration in the kidneys, with 54%−79% excreted in urine as the intact drug and 19%−27% eliminated as inactive metabolites in feces [14].

20.3.6 Process synthesis of meropenem

The current synthetic route includes the synthesis of the key side chain (Figs. 20.8 and 20.9), the synthesis of the bicyclic pharmacophore (Fig. 20.10), and the synthesis of the final product, meropenem (Fig. 20.11) [15−22]. Fig. 20.8 represents the first reported process for the synthesis of the meropenem side chain, with an overall yield of up to 71.6%. However, the reaction conditions of this route are harsh, and the operation is challenging. In addition, the reagents involved are expensive, and the cost is prohibitively high, making it unsuitable for industrial manufacturing. Matsumura et al. first synthesized the PNZ-protected thiolactone, which can be easily deprotected to obtain the key side chain of meropenem (Fig. 20.9). The meropenem side chain obtained from this route can be directly used in the

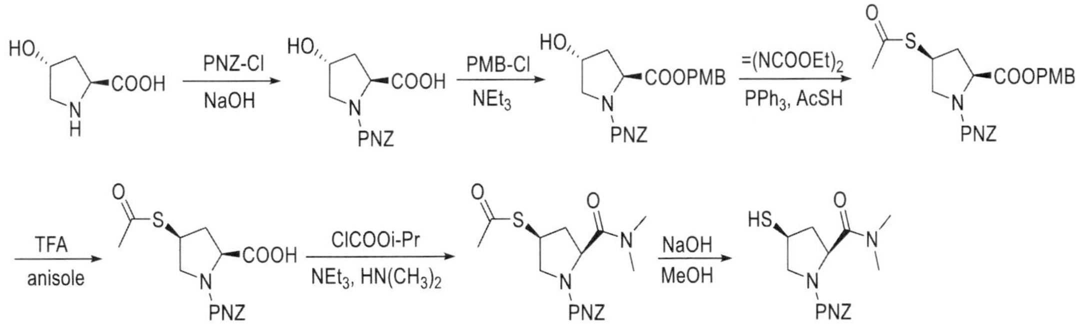

FIGURE 20.8 The first synthetic route of the side chain of meropenem.

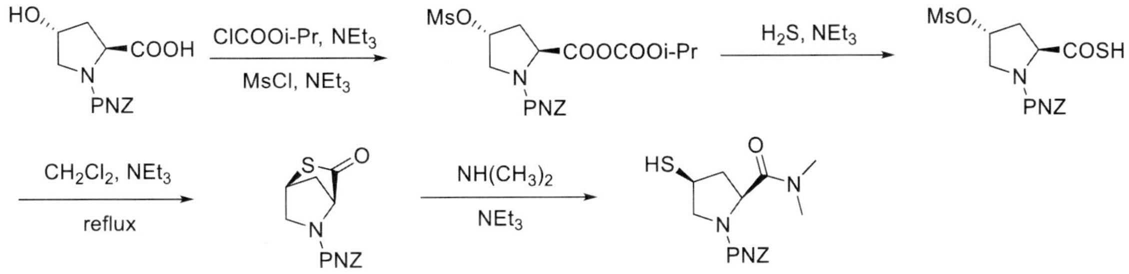

FIGURE 20.9 The synthetic route of the side chain of meropenem using thiolactone as the intermediate.

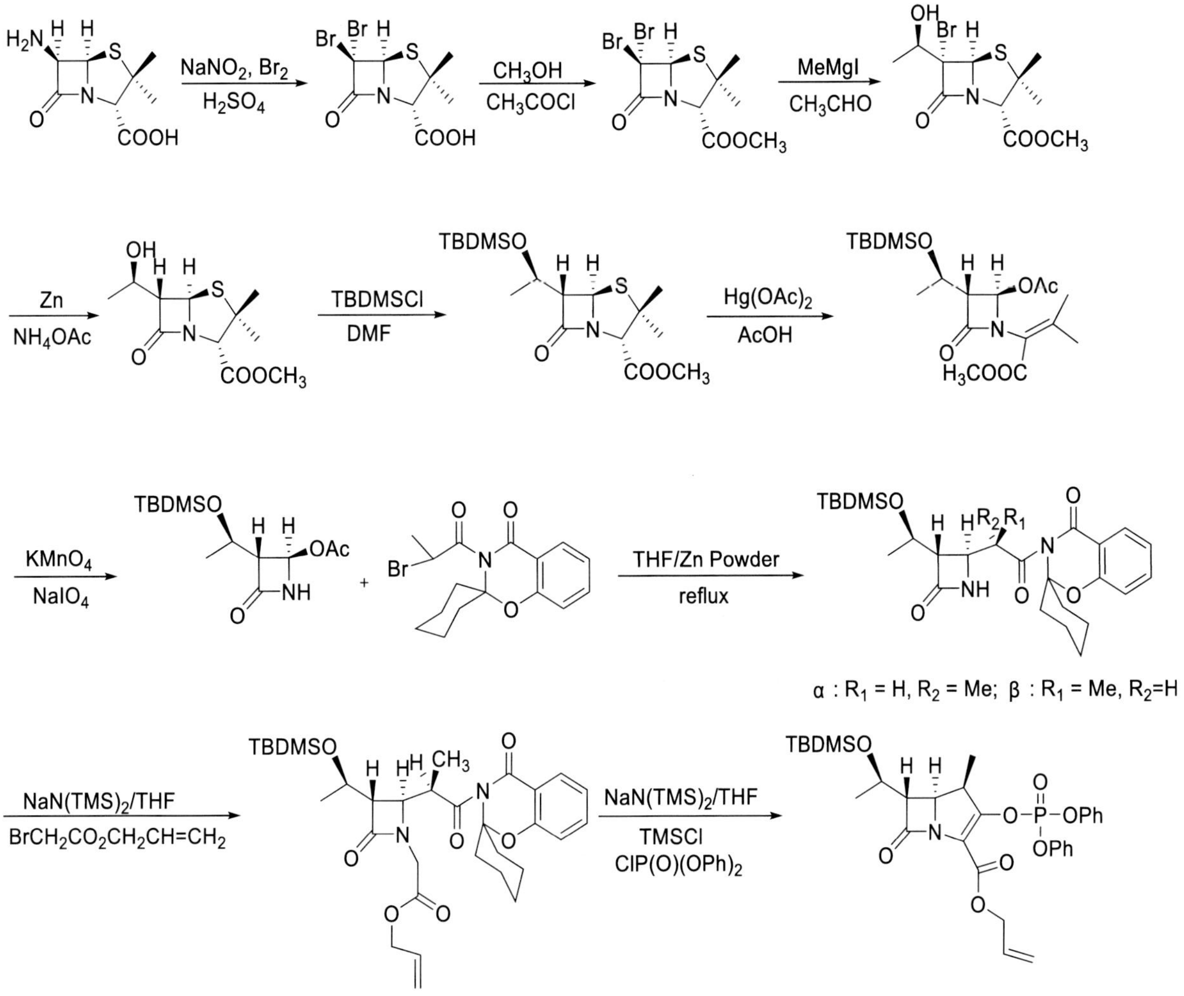

α : R_1 = H, R_2 = Me; β : R_1 = Me, R_2=H

FIGURE 20.10 The synthetic rote of the bicyclic core.

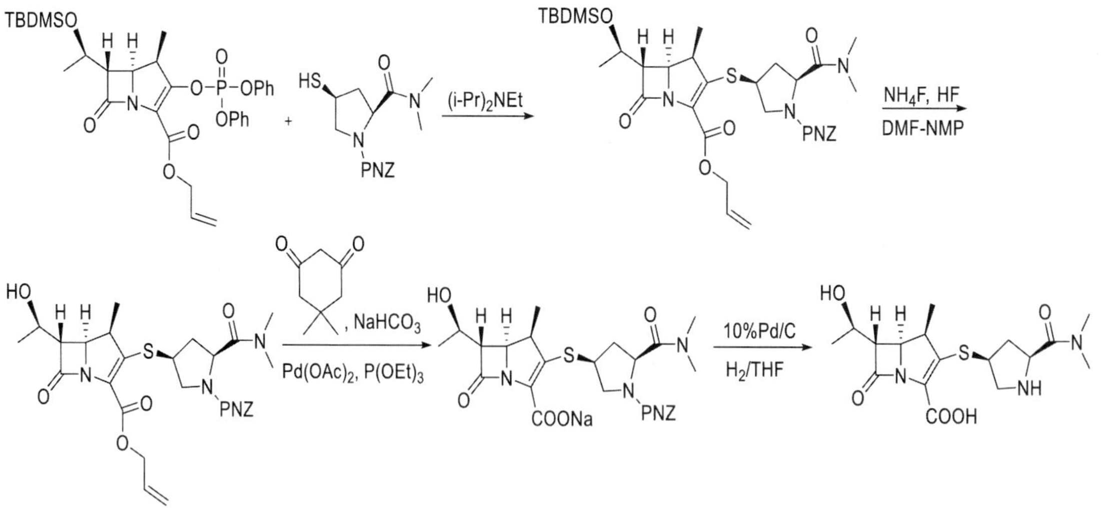

FIGURE 20.11 The synthetic route of meropenem.

subsequent reactions without purification, making the operation simpler. Besides, the reagents of this method are easily accessible, and thus, this route is suitable for industrial manufacturing. The synthesis of the bicyclic core consists of three key steps, namely the synthesis of the monocyclic β-lactam intermediate, the introduction of the 1β-methyl side chain, and the construction of the bicyclic core. The monocyclic β-lactam intermediate is synthesized in seven steps using 6-amino-penicillanic acid (6-APA) as the starting material. This method possesses several advantages, such as inexpensive and readily available starting material (6-APA), relatively simple operation, and good stereo-selectivity. The introduction of the 1β-methyl side chain is achieved by the Reformatsky reaction with good stereoselectivity and high yield. These features make this route suitable for industrial manufacturing. The bicyclic core is generated through the Dieckman reaction. Finally, the key side chain and bicyclic core react with each other to produce the desired product, meropenem. In this route, the protection groups are removed by hydrogenation over Pd/C with a high yield, making it environmentally friendly.

The synthesis of the key side chain [15]:
The synthesis of the bicyclic core [15−21]:
The synthesis of meropenem [15,22]:

Meropenem exhibits moderate adverse reactions, with good tolerance and widespread clinical application. The most frequently reported adverse effects include diarrhea (2.3%), rash (1.4%), nausea and dizziness (1.4%), injection site inflammation (1.1%), and other drug-related adverse reactions (incidence <1%). Among recipients of meropenem, 1.5%−4.3% experienced drug-related elevations in liver enzymes and platelets.

According to the 2019 CHINET surveillance of bacterial resistance across China, the resistance rates of *P. aeruginosa* to meropenem are 23.5%, *Acinetobacter species* to meropenem are 75.1%, and *K. pneumoniae* to meropenem are 26.8%. The issue of resistance to meropenem poses significant challenges to clinical antimicrobial therapy once again [3].

20.4 The progress on other carbapenem antibiotics

20.4.1 Recently marketed carbapenem antibiotics

The key feature of the new generation of carbapenem antibiotics is the introduction of a β-methyl group at the C_1-position. This structural modification greatly improves the stability of the new carbapenem antibiotics against DHP-I, thus enabling their monotherapy. Following the approval of meropenem, ertapenem (Fig. 20.12), biapenem, doripenem, and tebipenem pivoxil were also successfully launched in the US and Japan, which were developed by Merck, Wyeth, Shionogi, and Meiji Seika, respectively. All these drugs have received favorable clinical contexts. In addition, the approved carbapenem antibiotics are derivatives of meropenem with a C_2-position sulfur-containing side chain, which results in a broader antimicrobial spectrum, increased antimicrobial activity, or improved pharmacokinetic properties. These characteristics made them the first-line antibacterial agents for clinical use.

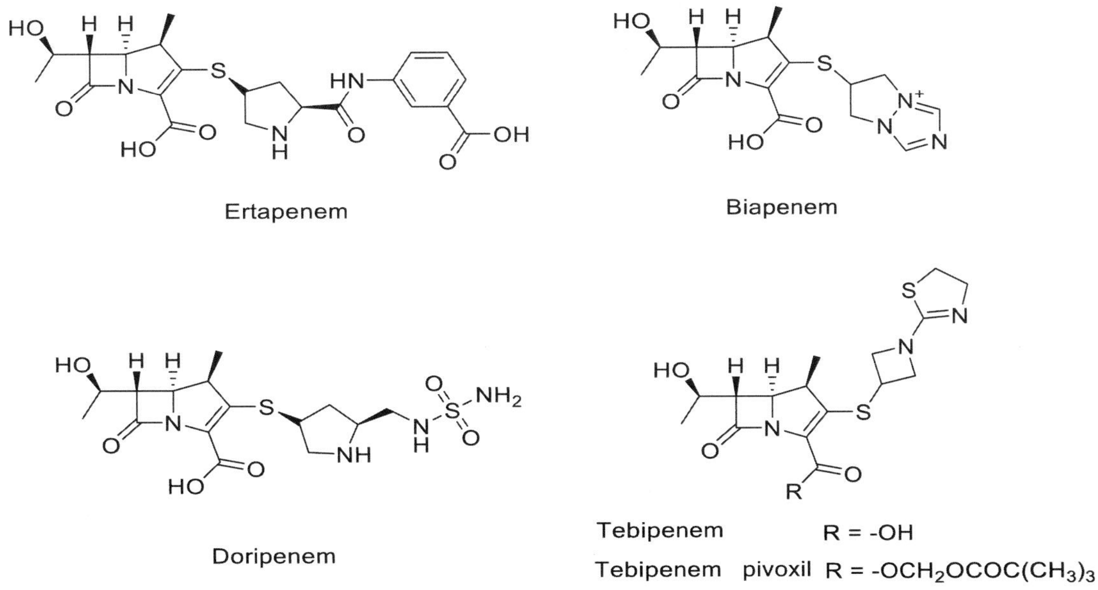

FIGURE 20.12 The chemical structures of recently marketed carbapenem antibiotics.

20.4.1.1 Ertapenem

In 1996, scientists reported a novel carbapenem antimicrobial agent named ertapenem (MK-0826; L749 345) at the 36th ICAAC. Animal studies indicated that it had a high plasma protein binding rate, a long duration of action *in vivo*, and a high concentration of the intact drug in urine, enabling it to achieve sufficient concentrations to treat bacterial infections in the urinary tract, including *P. aeruginosa*. Ertapenem is a new carbapenem antibiotic developed by Merck that was first approved by the FDA in the US in 2001. Ertapenem is a 1β-methyl carbapenem antibiotic that is stable against DHP-I and can be used as a monotherapy. The proton at the 5′-position of the pyrrole ring of ertapenem is substituted with a 3-carboxyphenylaminocarbonyl group, leading to high affinity for PBP2 and PBP3. The introduction of a benzoic acid group in the C$_2$-side chain increases lipophilicity. At the physiological pH, the benzoic acid ionizes into a carboxylate anion, resulting in a high protein binding rate and prolonged half-life of ertapenem. However, the introduction of the benzoic acid moiety leads to a decrease in antibacterial activity against *P. aeruginosa* and *Acinetobacter species* [23]. Ertapenem has a half-life of approximately 4.5 hours in primates, with 30%–40% of the intact drug excreted in the urine, allowing for a once-daily dosing regimen based on its pharmacokinetic profiles. Ertapenem exhibits high affinity for PBP1a, PBP1b, PBP2, PBP3, PBP4, and PBP5 of *E. coli*, especially PBP2 and PBP3. Ertapenem exerts bactericidal activity against Gram-negative bacteria by inhibiting bacterial cell wall synthesis. It is effective against aerobic Gram-positive bacteria such as methicillin-susceptible *S. aureus*, *Streptococcus agalactiae*, penicillin-susceptible *S. pneumoniae*, and *Pyogenic streptococci*; aerobic Gram-negative bacteria including *E. coli*, *H. influenzae* (limited to β-lactamase-negative strains), *K. pneumoniae*, *M. catarrhalis*, and *Proteus mirabilis*, and anaerobic bacteria such as *B. fragilis*, *Bacteroides distasonis*, *Bacteroides ovatus*, *B. thetaiotaomicron*, *Bacteroides uniformis*, *Clostridium*, *Eubacterium lentum*, *Peptostreptococcus*, *Porphyromonas asaccharolytica*, and *Prevotella Shan and Collins*. However, it is not effective against methicillin-resistant *S. aureus*, enterococci, *P. aeruginosa*, and *Acinetobacter species*. The PAE of ertapenem is approximately 3 hours for *S. aureus*, 1.5 hours for *E. coli*, and 2.4 hours for *S. pneumoniae*.

20.4.1.2 Biapenem

The novel carbapenem antibiotic, biapenem (LJC10627), was reported in the 29th ICAAC in 1989. It features a triazolium cationic side chain at the C$_2$-position, displaying higher activity against *Enterobacteriaceae*, *P. aeruginosa*, and *B. fragilis* but lower activity against aerobic Gram-positive bacteria as compared to imipenem. Biapenem exhibits a slightly lower affinity for PBP1b compared to imipenem, and the influence of ethylenediaminetetraacetic acid (EDTA) on the MIC value of biapenem against *P. aeruginosa* is less than imipenem, suggesting strong cellular permeability of this compound. Pharmacokinetic experiments revealed that 74% of the intact drug is excreted in urine. When used alone, biapenem provides better protection against *E. coli* and *P. aeruginosa* infections in mice compared to imipenem/cilastatin. Similarly, like ertapenem, biapenem is a 1β-methyl carbapenem antibiotic that remains stable against DHP-I and thus can be used alone [24]. Biapenem, a new carbapenem antibiotic developed jointly by Lederle in Japan and Wyeth in the US, was approved for marketing in Japan in 2002. Its most notable feature is the triazolium cationic side chain at the C_2-position, which is critical for outer membrane permeability, and thus it exhibits stronger inhibition of *P. aeruginosa* and anaerobic bacteria compared to imipenem, as well as stronger inhibition of multidrug-resistant *P. aeruginosa* compared to meropenem. Additionally, it is more effective against *Acinetobacter species* and anaerobic bacteria than ceftazidime. The mechanism of action of biapenem involves the inhibition of bacterial cell wall synthesis. It exhibits a high affinity for PBP1 and PBP4 in *S. aureus*, PBP1a, PBP1b, PBP2, PBP4, PBP5, and PBP6 in *E. coli* and *P. aeruginosa*. Besides, it also displays strong cellular permeability and minimal cross-resistance issues with other β-lactam antibiotics. Biapenem is effective against *Staphylococcus species*, *Streptococcus species*, *S. pneumoniae*, *Enterococcus species* (excluding *E. faecium*), *Moraxella*, *E. coli*, *Citrobacter species*, *Klebsiella species*, *Enterobacter species*, *Serratia species*, *Proteus species*, *H. influenzae*, *P. aeruginosa*, *Actinomyces species*, *Peptostreptococcus*, *Bacteroides species*, *Prevotella species*, and *fusobacterium*. Biapenem possesses a PAE against *P. aeruginosa*, with a growth inhibition time of 1.6 hours after incubation at 4 times the MIC for 2 hours. Moreover, biapenem exhibits low nephrotoxicity and virtually no central nervous system toxicity, making it a safer and more effective carbapenem antibiotic.

20.4.1.3 Doripenem

In 1996, Japanese researchers reported the synthesis and activity of a series of novel 1β-methyl carbapenem derivatives. It was found that the presence of an aminomethyl group at the 5′-position of the pyrrolidine ring resulted in better activity. Subsequent chemical modifications resulted in the discovery of doripenem (S-4661) with optimal antibacterial activity, which possesses a sulfamoylaminomethyl group at the 5′-position of the pyrroline ring. Doripenem showed good antibacterial activity against both Gram-positive bacteria and Gram-negative bacteria, including *P. aeruginosa*. Doripenem, like ertapenem and biapenem, is a 1β-methyl carbapenem compound and does not need to be dosed in combination with renal dehydropeptidase inhibitors [25]. Developed by Shionogi, doripenem was first approved for marketing in Japan in 2005. Doripenem exhibits different affinity for various PBPs of different bacteria, particularly exhibits high affinity for PBP1 in *S. aureus*, PBP2 and PBP3 in *P. aeruginosa*, and PBP2 in *E. coli*. Doripenem has a broad spectrum of antibacterial activity and possesses strong activity against both aerobic and anaerobic bacteria. Its activity against Gram-positive bacteria is stronger than meropenem and biapenem and comparable to imipenem; its activity against Gram-negative bacteria is stronger than imipenem and biapenem but slightly lower than meropenem. It shows sensitivity against various bacteria, including *E. coli*, *K. pneumoniae*, *P. aeruginosa*, *Bacteroides stercoris*, *B. fragilis*, *B. thetaiotaomicron*, *B. uniformis*, *Bacteroides vulgatus*, *Streptococcus intermedius*, *Streptococcus constellatus*, *Peptostreptococcus micros*, *P. mirabilis*, and *A. baumannii*.

20.4.1.4 Tebipenem pivoxil

The various carbapenem antibiotics mentioned earlier are not suitable for oral administration. Therefore, researchers aimed to develop an orally available carbapenem drug with broad-spectrum antibacterial activity, high stability against β-lactamases and DHP-I, antibiotic PAE, and high oral bioavailability. In the 38th ICAAC in 1998, Japanese scientists first reported the orally available carbapenem antibiotic L-084 (tebipenem pivoxil). The C_2-side chain of tebipenem pivoxil is a 1-(1,3-thiazolin-2-yl) azetidin-3-ylthio group, and its oral bioavailability is improved by forming an ester-type prodrug at the C_3-position. Tebipenem pivoxil lacks antibacterial activity *in vitro*, but its active metabolite, tebipenem (LJC 11 036), exhibits antibacterial activity equivalent to that of the imipenem against methicillin-sensitive *S. aureus*, with improved activity against MRSA and *S. epidermidis*. It shows high antimicrobial activity against penicillin-sensitive or resistant *S. pneumoniae* and *Streptococcus pyogenes*. It's *in vitro* antimicrobial activity against *E. coli*, *K. pneumoniae*, *Branhamella catarrhalis*, *H. influenzae*, *Enterobacter*, and *P. mirabilis* is superior to imipenem, while its activity against *Serratia marcescens* and *P. aeruginosa* is lower than imipenem. Tebipenem has strong affinity for PBP1a, PBP1b, PBP2a/2x, PBP2b, and PBP3 of *S. pneumoniae* and high affinity for PBP1b, PBP2, PBP3a, and PBP3b of *H. influenzae*. Similar to other carbapenems, tebipenem pivoxil also contains a 1β-methyl group and does not require co-administration with a renal dehydropeptidase inhibitor. Tebipenem pivoxil is a newly developed oral carbapenem antibiotic by Meiji Seika and was approved in Japan in 2009. It is the first orally bioavailable carbapenem antibiotic, where the carboxyl group at the C_3-position of tebipenem is masked as an ester (prodrug), which can be readily hydrolyzed to tebipenem after oral administration. Tebipenem (Fig. 20.12) has a broad spectrum of antimicrobial activity and shows stronger antibacterial activity against most clinically isolated strains (except for *E. faecium* and *P. aeruginosa*) compared to penicillin and cephalosporins. Compared with other injectable carbapenem antibiotics, tebipenem also exhibits similar or greater antibacterial effects.

Tebipenem pivoxil is the first drug used to treat infections caused by drug-resistant strains of *S. pneumoniae*, including persistent otitis media and bacterial pneumonia. Its inhibitory activity against *S. pneumoniae*, *E. coli*, *K. pneumoniae*, *H. influenzae*, and *Legionella pneumophila* makes it suitable for the treatment of pediatric otolaryngological and upper respiratory infections, showing superiority over reference drugs such as imipenem, cefdinir, amoxicillin, and levofloxacin. It particularly displays strong antibacterial effects against the main causative agents of pediatric infections in recent years, including penicillin-resistant *S. pneumoniae*, erythromycin-resistant *S. pneumoniae*, and *H. influenza* [26,27].

20.4.2 Chemical structure features and structure-activity relationship of carbapenem antibiotics

20.4.2.1 Stability against β-lactamases

The cis-configuration at the C_5- and C_6-positions of penicillin, as well as at the C_6-and C_7-positions of cephalosporins, makes them susceptible to hydrolysis by β-lactamases. In contrast, the thiazolidine ring in carbapenems features a carbon atom instead of a sulfur atom and an unsaturated double bond between the C_2-and C_3-positions. Particularly, the trans-configuration between the β-H at the C_6-position and the α-H at the C_5-position results in a better binding conformation for penicillin-binding proteins, thus enhancing the stability of the drug against β-lactamases. Additionally, the trans-α-hydroxyethyl side chain at the C_6-position creates steric hindrance, further augmenting its stability against β-lactamases. Currently, all the available carbapenem drugs exhibit this trans-configuration.

20.4.2.2 Antibacterial activity and stability

The presence of a free amino group at the C_2-position of thienamycin leads to chemical instability. Structural modifications at the C_2-position, such as the introduction of heterocyclic substituents like pyrrolidine, can enhance the stability of carbapenem antibiotics. Various substitutions at the C_2-position include sulfur substitution (e.g., imipenem, panipenem, meropenem, ertapenem, biapenem, doripenem, etc.), carbon substitution (e.g., ME1036, also known as CP5609, Fig. 20.13 [28]), and a tricyclic compound (e.g., sanfetrinem, Fig. 20.13 [7]). Among the sulfur substitutions, the most common approach is the introduction of a substituted pyrrolidine sulfur side chain. Introducing one or more amino or guanidino groups at the 5'-position of the pyrrolidine side chain at the C_2-position significantly enhances the antibacterial activity against MRSA and multidrug-resistant *P. aeruginosa*. For example, tomopenem (CS-023, Fig. 20.13) has a guanidino group at the pyrrolidine substituent at the C_2-position, resulting in potent antibacterial activity against MRSA and *P. aeruginosa*, but its clinical trials were terminated after Phase II [7]. In addition, altering the substituents on the pyrrolidine ring is a common strategy to enhance the affinity of carbapenems for bacterial PBPs and improve chemical stability. In recent years, it has been discovered that introducing a thiazole ring at the C_2-position exhibits better anti-MRSA activity compared to the pyrrolidine substituent, such as SM-17466, SM-197436 (Fig. 20.13), and SM-232721, which may be attributed to the weaker basicity of the thiazole ring and the improved lipophilicity conferred by the

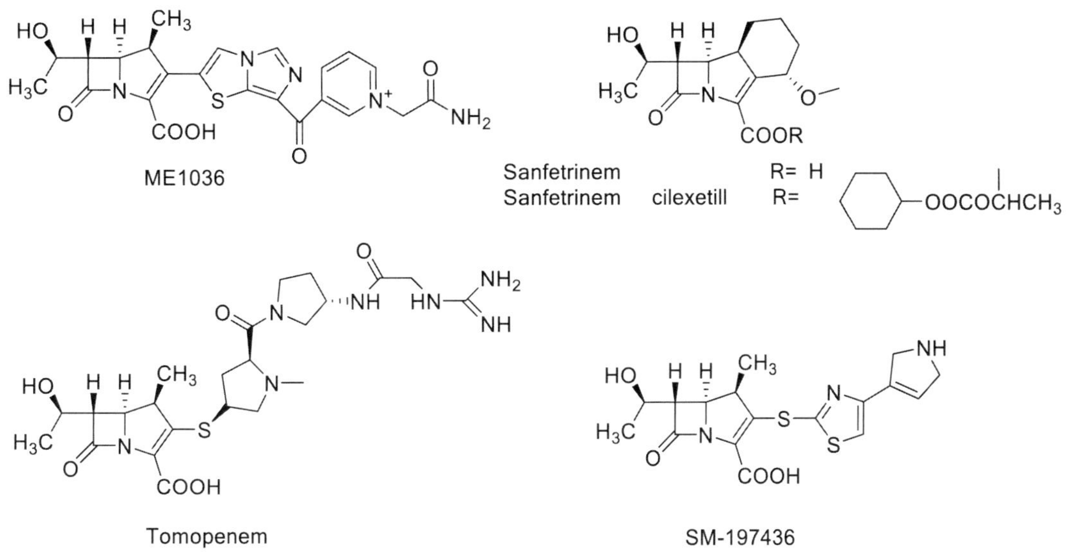

FIGURE 20.13 The chemical structures of the carbapenem antibiotics under clinical trial and clinical trial termination.

sulfur atom on the thiazole ring [29]. Furthermore, the introduction of a bicyclic moiety at the C_2-position can enhance stability against β-lactamases. The introduction of a dithiolaminomethyl ester or a 7-(1-carbamoylmethylpyridinium-3-yl) carbonyl imidazo[5,1-*b*]thiazole-2-yl group at the C_2-position significantly enhances the activity against MRSA, such as ME1036 [28]. The alkalinity of the substitution at the C_2-position also affects the inherent stability of carbapenem antibiotics. Stronger basicity leads to poorer chemical stability, while weaker basicity improves chemical stability. Therefore, lowering the basicity of the C_2-substitution group can enhance the chemical stability of the compound. Reducing the alkalinity of the C_2-substitution can enhance the molecular stability of the compound. In comparison to the amino at the C_2-position of thienamycin, the C_2-position of imipenem, meropenem, and panipenem consists of amino substitution derivatives with dissociation constants (pKa) of 9.9, 7.4, and 10.9, respectively. The reduced alkalinity of the C_2-side chain significantly improves stability [7,8,30–32].

20.4.2.3 Stability against DHP-I

Compared to imipenem, the new generation of carbapenem antibiotics, such as meropenem, ertapenem, biapenem, and doripenem display, significantly enhanced stability in the presence of DHP-I by introducing a β-methyl group at the C_1-position. They also show partially increased activity against Gram-negative bacteria. Imipenem lacks a β-methyl group at the C_1-position, making it susceptible to hydrolysis by DHP-I, resulting in the breakdown of the β-lactam ring and subsequent loss of efficacy. Therefore, the addition of cilastatin as a DHP-I inhibitor is necessary to prevent its metabolism in the kidneys, enhance efficacy, and reduce nephrotoxicity. In contrast to imipenem, panipenem, despite its enhanced stability in the presence of DHP-I, tends to accumulate in the renal cortex, exerting significant nephrotoxic effects when used alone. Therefore, its co-administration with betamipron is required to facilitate renal excretion.

20.4.2.4 Relationship between structure and toxicity

Nephrotoxicity and neurotoxicity (mainly inducing spasms and epilepsy) are the most common adverse reactions of carbapenem antibiotics. Currently, it is believed that such adverse effects are mainly associated with the side chains at the C_2- and C_3-positions, particularly the alkalinity of the amino group in the C_2 side chain, the distance between the carboxyl group and the amino group, and the spatial environment around the amino group. The substitutions on the amino group determine the alkalinity of the compound, and the stronger alkalinity of the amino group, the higher the possibility for the occurrence of nephrotoxicity and neurotoxicity. Additionally, the neurotoxicity of carbapenem drugs is also related to their specific binding and inhibitory effect on the neurotransmitter GABA. Imipenem has a high affinity for GABA, which is also the reason for its higher incidence of adverse reactions in the nervous system than other carbapenem drugs [7,8,30–32].

20.4.3 Mechanisms of carbapenem antibiotic resistance

Carbapenems demonstrate high stability against various β-lactamases and possess excellent antimicrobial effects against most cephalosporin-resistant bacteria, with the presence of a PAE. However, with the increasing clinical use, the incidence of bacterial resistance to carbapenem antibiotics is gradually increasing. The mechanisms of resistance to carbapenem antibiotics in *Enterobacteriaceae* mainly include the production of carbapenemases; the loss or reduction in the number of outer membrane proteins (OMPs), leading to decreased affinity; changes in drug target sites, primarily alterations in PBPs; and the induction of overexpression of efflux pumps. For *P. aeruginosa*, the main mechanisms of resistance to carbapenems include the production of carbapenemases, the loss of membrane porins (e.g., OprD2 mutations or deletions), and the overexpression of efflux pumps. Regarding *A. baumannii*, the major mechanisms of resistance to carbapenems are the production of carbapenemases, the reduction of OMPs, the overexpression of efflux pumps, and alterations in PBPs.

20.4.4 Research features of carbapenem antibiotics

Currently, the marketed carbapenem antibiotics have largely displayed superb stability against DHP-I-mediated hydrolysis, thus reducing the occurrence of nephrotoxicity. However, there are still several issues that need to be addressed: (1) some carbapenem antibiotics exhibit central nervous system toxicity. For example, imipenem is prone to inducing seizures with an incidence rate of up to 5%, and there have been occasional reports of seizures caused by meropenem as well. (2) Current carbapenem antibiotics are still ineffective against MRSA. (3) The carbapenemases produced by some Gram-negative bacteria, such as metallo-β-lactamases, lead to hydrolytic inactivation of carbapenem antibiotics. (4) The short half-life and rapid elimination of carbapenem antibiotics, except for ertapenem, necessitate multiple daily dosing, i.e., twice daily or more.

The strategic directions for future development of carbapenem antibiotics mainly include the following aspects [7,8,30−32].

20.4.4.1 Enhancement of activity against MRSA

MRSA produces a unique PBP2a, which has a low affinity to β-lactam antibiotics, resulting in weak or no binding with β-lactam antibiotics. Among the investigational carbapenem antibiotics, tomopenem has shown significant *in vitro* activity against MRSA, mainly due to its high affinity for MRSA PBP2a. Unfortunately, results from the subsequent clinical trial were not ideal [7].

20.4.4.2 Development of novel β-lactamase inhibitors for combinational use with carbapenem drugs

Vabomere, which was approved by the FDA in 2017, is a 1:1 combination of vaborbactam and meropenem. Vaborbactam is a β-lactamase inhibitor with no intrinsic antibacterial activity. It acts by preventing the degradation of meropenem by certain serine β-lactamases (such as *K. pneumoniae* carbapenemase, KPC). Obviously, vaborbactam does not diminish the activity of meropenem. In 2019, recarbrio (imipenem/cilastatin/relebactam) was approved by the FDA, with relebactam being a novel β-lactamase inhibitor belonging to the diazabicyclooctane class. Relebactam exhibits a broad-spectrum activity against class A and class C β-lactamases. Relebactam can protect imipenem from certain serine β-lactamases-mediated degradation, and when used in combination with imipenem, imipenem-resistant Gram-negative bacteria become more sensitive to imipenem.

20.4.4.3 Development of oral drugs

By esterifying the carboxylic group of carbapenem antibiotics, prodrugs are obtained, which can be transformed into active parent drugs by esterases in humans to exert antibacterial activity. Tebipenem pivoxil is the first clinically approved oral carbapenem antibiotic, which was launched in Japan in 2009. Sanfetrinem cilexetil is a prodrug of sanfetrinem that can be administered orally, but its development was terminated after Phase II clinical trials in 2009 [7].

20.4.4.4 Prolonging the half-life of drugs and reducing the frequency of administration through structural optimization

Among the carbapenem antibiotics currently on the market, ertapenem has the longest half-life, allowing for once-daily dosing.

In recent years, many world-renowned pharmaceutical companies have been accelerating the pace of carbapenem antibiotic development, yielding several promising candidates such as tomopenem and razupenem. However, tomopenem was discontinued after Phase II clinical trials [7], and the development of razupenem also ceased after Phase II trials due to adverse reactions [8]. Domestic research and development of new carbapenem antibiotics in China is also speeding up, and several candidates, such as benapenem and apapenem, are in the pipeline. However, there are no new antibiotics currently on the market.

References

[1] Liu JM. Sulfanilanmide and penicillin the past and present of antibacterial agents. Scientist 2014;09:21−4.
[2] Dodds DR. Antibiotic resistance: a current epilogue. Biochem Pharmacol 2017;134:139−46.
[3] Hu FP, Guo Y, Zhu DM, et al. CHINET surveillance of bacterial resistance across tertiary hospitals in 2019. Chin J Infect Chemother 2020;20 (03):233−43.
[4] Ma XL, Lu HW, Zhnag Y. Understanding the natural and acquired drug resistance of bacteria. Chin J Lab Med 2012;35(8):762−3.
[5] Rice LB. Federal funding for the study of antimicrobial resistance in nosocomial pathogens: no ESKAPE. J Infect Dis 2008;197(8):1079−81.
[6] Bao JY, Ning H, Song CS. Analysis of the special class antibacterial agents. Chin J Drug Evaluation 2018;35(05):371−5.
[7] Papp-Wallace KM, Endimiani A, Taracila MA, et al. Carbapenems: past, present, and future. Antimicrob Agents Chemother 2011;55 (11):4943−60.
[8] El-Gamal MI, Brahim I, Hisham N, et al. Recent updates of carbapenem antibiotics. Eur J Med Chem 2017;131:185−95.

[9] Liu T, Zang YS, Xiu QY. Advances in carbapenems. Chin J N Drugs Clin Rem 2013;32(12):927−31.
[10] Kahan JS, Kahan FM, Goegelman R, et al. Thienamycin, a new beta-lactam antibiotic. I. Discovery, taxonomy, isolation and physical properties. J Antibiot 1979;32(1):1−12.
[11] Leanza WJ, Wildonger KJ, Miller TW, et al. N-Acetimidoyl- and N-formimidoylthienamycin derivatives: antipseudomonal beta-lactam antibiotics. J Med Chem 1979;22(12):1435−6.
[12] Miyadera T, Sugimura Y, Hashimoto T, et al. Synthesis and in vitro activity of a new carbapenem, RS-533. J Antibiot 1983;36(8):1034−9.
[13] Sunagawa M, Matsumura H, Inoue T, et al. A novel carbapenem antibiotic, SM-7338 structure-activity relationships. J Antibiot 1990;43(5):519−32.
[14] Lian WW, Chen WQ, Yan Y, et al. Progress of pharmacokinetics/pharmacodynamics research and therapeutic drug monitoring of meropenem. Evaluation Anal Drug-Use Hospitals China 2021;21(01):121−4 128.
[15] Liu HX, Meng QW. Progress in synthesis of 1β-methyl carbapenem antibiotic meropenem. Chin J Antibiot 2009;34(05):257−62.
[16] Dininno F, Beattie TR, Christensen BG. Aldol condensations of regiospecific penicillanate and cephalosporanate enolates. Hydroxyethylation at C-6 and C-7. J Org Chem 1977;42(18):2960−5.
[17] Martel A, Daris JP, Bachand C, et al. Anhydropenicillin: a key intermediate for the stereocontrolled introduction of the 6-R-hydroxyethyl side chain of the penem and carbapenem antibiotics. Can J Chem 1987;65(9):2179−81.
[18] Tajima Y, Yoshida A, Takeda N, et al. Reaction of acetoxyazetidinones with trimethylsilylacetyl thioesters: preparation of azetidinone-thioester precursors to carbapenems. Tetrahedron Lett 1985;26(5):673−6.
[19] Fujimoto K, Iwano Y, Hirai K. From penicillin to penem and carbapenem. VI[1]): synthesis of dethiathienamycin. Tetrahedron Lett 1985;26(1):89−92.
[20] Kondo K, Seki M, Kuroda T, et al. 2-substituted 2,3-dihydro-4H-1,3-benzoxazin-4-ones: a novel auxiliary for stereoselective synthesis of 1-β-methylcarbapenems. J Org Chem 1995;60(5):1096−7.
[21] Kondo K, Seki M, Kuroda T, et al. 2-Substituted 2,3-Dihydro-4H-1,3-benzoxazin-4-ones: novel Auxiliaries for Stereoselective Synthesis of 1-beta-Methylcarbapenems(1). J Org Chem 1997;62(9):2877−84.
[22] Sunagawa M, Matsumura H, Inoue T, et al. Synthesis and biological properties of 1 beta-methylcarbapenems with N-methylpyrrolidinylthio group at C-2 position. J Antibiot 1992;45(6):971−6.
[23] Sundelof JG, Hajdu R, Gill CJ, et al. Pharmacokinetics of L-749,345, a long-acting carbapenem antibiotic, in primates. Antimicrob Agents Chemother 1997;41(8):1743−8.
[24] Ubukata K, Hikida M, Yoshida M, et al. In vitro activity of LJC10,627, a new carbapenem antibiotic with high stability to dehydropeptidase I. Antimicrob Agents Chemother 1990;34(6):994−1000.
[25] Iso Y, Irie T, Iwaki T, et al. Synthesis and modification of a novel 1 beta-methyl carbapenem antibiotic, S-4661. J Antibiot 1996;49(5):478−84.
[26] Hikida M, Itahashi K, Igarashi A, et al. In vitro antibacterial activity of LJC 11,036, an active metabolite of L-084, a new oral carbapenem antibiotic with potent antipneumococcal activity. Antimicrob Agents Chemother 1999;43(8):2010−16.
[27] Jain A, Utley L, Parr TR, et al. Tebipenem, the first oral carbapenem antibiotic. Expert Rev Anti Infect Ther 2018;16(7):513−22.
[28] Kurazono M, Ida T, Yamada K, et al. In vitro activities of ME1036 (CP5609), a novel parenteral carbapenem, against methicillin-resistant staphylococci. Antimicrob Agents Chemother 2004;48(8):2831−7.
[29] Ueda Y, Sunagawa M. In vitro and in vivo activities of novel 2-(thiazol-2-ylthio)-1beta-methylcarbapenems with potent activities against multi-resistant gram-positive bacteria. Antimicrob Agents Chemother 2003;47(8):2471−80.
[30] Xu H, Xu YL, Ma HM. Res Prog carbapenems antibiotics. Journal of Shenyang Pharmaceutical University 2007;24(06):385−8.
[31] ZHANEL GG, WIEBE R, DILAY L, et al. Comparative review of the carbapenems. Drugs 2007;67(7):1027−52.
[32] Liu YN. Essent Clin application carbapenems. Bjing: People's Medical Publishing House; 2019. p. 8−16.

Chapter 21

Antiparasitic drug praziquantel

Fuli Zhang and Zhezhou Yang
Shanghai Institute of Pharmaceutical Industry Co., Ltd., Shanghai, P.R. China

Chapter outline

21.1 Parasitic diseases	**509**
21.1.1 Parasitic diseases	509
21.1.2 Antiparasitic drugs	510
21.2 Antiparasitic drug praziquantel	**510**
21.2.1 A brief history of antischistosomal drugs	510
21.2.2 The insecticidal mechanism of action of praziquantel	513
21.2.3 Dosage and treatment duration of praziquantel	513
21.2.4 Resistance to praziquantel	514
21.3 Medicinal chemistry of praziquantel	**514**
21.3.1 Structure-activity relationship of praziquantel	514
21.3.2 Levopraziquantel	515
21.3.3 Pharmacokinetics of praziquantel and deuterated praziquantel	517
21.4 Green process for praziquantel and its levoisomer	**518**
21.4.1 Green chemistry	518
21.4.2 Synthesis of praziquantel	519
21.4.3 Synthesis of levorotatory praziquantel	522
21.5 Green chemistry future	**526**
References	527

21.1 Parasitic diseases

21.1.1 Parasitic diseases

Due to the diversity of parasitic diseases, especially their widespread distribution in developing countries in tropical and subtropical regions, they pose serious threats to human health and are one of the global concerns of public health and hygiene. Among the seven tropical diseases prioritized for prevention and control by the World Health Organization's Special Program for Research and Training in Tropical Diseases (WHO/TDR), except for leprosy and tuberculosis, the rest, such as malaria, schistosomiasis, filariasis, leishmaniasis, and trypanosomiasis, are all parasitic diseases [1]. Parasitic diseases have not only burdened a wide range of global populations but have also been transmitted in diverse forms, which have been impeding economic development in developing countries and bringing a worldwide challenge concerning social public health.

There are over 200 parasitic diseases that are prevalent globally; for instance, common species include malaria, trypanosomiasis, leishmaniasis, amebiasis, trichomoniasis, toxoplasmosis, cysticercosis, schistosomiasis, clonorchiasis, paragonimiasis, fasciolopsiasis, intestinal nematodiasis, and taeniasis. Upon transmission and infection approaches, parasitic diseases are defined as the following four types: [1]

1. Waterborne parasitic diseases
   Infection through skin contact with water contaminated with parasites, such as schistosomiasis; or due to poor sanitary conditions, poor hygiene habits, and other reasons, raw water contaminated by parasitic pathogens and infected, such as cryptosporidiosis.
2. Foodborne parasitic diseases
   The patients are infected by eating an uncooked diet or semiraw food containing parasitic pathogens; for instance, infection with clonorchiasis due to eating raw fish food; infection with pneumostomiasis due to taking raw snail and crab food; contracting trichinosis and taeniasis by eating raw animal meat; and infection with gingerchiasis and hepatic fascioliasis by eating raw aquatic plants.

3. Contacting parasitic diseases

The infected patients are directly contacted with parasitic contaminated goods and/or public facilities, such as pinworm disease, which is easy to occur in kindergartens, welfare homes, and construction sheds; trichomoniasis of the vagina can be transmitted through bathing utensils, toilets, etc.

4. Insect-borne parasitic diseases

Pathogen vectors, such as mosquitoes, flies, and cockroaches, contaminate food or utensils during foraging through contact, backvomiting, or excretion of pathogens in feces.

Schistosomiasis is typically divided into three types: Schistosomiasis japonicum, Schistosomiasis mansoni, and Schistosomiasis egypti. Schistosomiasis cercariae reproduces in suitable snails many times and eventually develops intothousands of cercariae and are released into the surrounding water. Due to production or living contact with infected water, cercaria can drill into the skin and infect people [2]. Schistosomiasis mainly resides in the liver of the host and thus causes serious organ pathological changes, such as hepatosplenomegaly, liver fibrosis, portal hypertension, hematuria, and ascites. Schistosomiasis is endemic in 76 countries and regions in Asia, Africa, and Latin America and is most severe in sub-Saharan Africa, where more than 90% of the world's infected people live. The Philippines has the highest infection rate in Asia. Through the implementation of prevention and control measures, the disease has been effectively controlled in Brazil, Venezuela, the Middle East, North Africa, and China.

Clonorchis sinensis, commonly known as hepatic fluoriasis, is a foodborne parasitic disease caused by Clonorchis sinensis parasitism in human hepatobiliary canals, mainly through raw freshwater fish and shrimp infection. The cysticercus of Clonorchis sinensis in fish fillets takes 6 seconds to be killed in water at 70°C, 15 seconds to be killed in water at 60°C and can survive for 2 hours in 3.36% acetic acid solution and 15 hours in soy sauce containing 19.3% NaCl. Therefore, raw freshwater fish and shrimp are quite dangerous to eat. Clonorchiasis can lead to biliary cirrhosis, cholangitis, cholecystitis, obstructive jaundice, bile duct stones, and pancreatitis. The disease is mainly distributed in Guangdong, Guangxi Zhuang Autonomous Region, and the "three Eastern provinces" in China, and the number of infected people has reached 12 million [3].

21.1.2 Antiparasitic drugs

Due to the wide variety of parasitic diseases, the corresponding treatment drugs are also varied [4]. For instance, artemisinin is used to treat malaria; amphotericin B is used to treat leishmaniasis; metronidazole and tinidazole are the first choices to treat amebiasis and trichomoniasis; pyrimethamine is the preferred drug for the treatment of toxoplasmosis; there is no other drug choice except nidazolide for treating cryptosporidiosis; praziquantel is the preferred drug for the treatment of cestode infections; and The classic drugs used to treat intestinal nematode diseases, such as ascariasis, ancylostomiasis, trichuriasis, and enterobiasis mainly include mebendazole, albendazole, levamisole, pyrimethamine, and ivermectin (Fig. 21.1). In the WHO's chemoprevention program for parasitic diseases, seven broad-spectrum antiparasitic drugs are recommended, namely albendazole, diethylcarbamazine, ivermectin, levamisole, mebendazole, praziquantel, and pyrimethamine (Table 21.1) [2]. These drugs are not only convenient and effective but also safe, with fewer observed adverse effects. In highly endemic areas, the safety record of these drugs ensures that it is unnecessary for patients to undergo individual diagnosis and is suitable for large-scale distribution and treatment.

21.2 Antiparasitic drug praziquantel

21.2.1 A brief history of antischistosomal drugs

In 1918, Christopherson pioneered the chemical treatment of schistosomiasis by using potassium antimonyl tartrate to treat schistosomiasis haematobia [5]. While this drug showed some efficacy in treating the disease, such as patients indications that they generally improved after treatment, with symptoms disappearing and appetite increasing, it suffered from severe adverse effects. Almost every patient receiving potassium antimonyl tartrate treatment experienced electrocardiogram changes, which could cause severe cardiac toxicity and arrhythmias. In 1961, Lei Xinghan from the Shanghai Institute of Pharmaceutical Industry developed furapromide, an oral nonantimony antischistosomal drug [6].

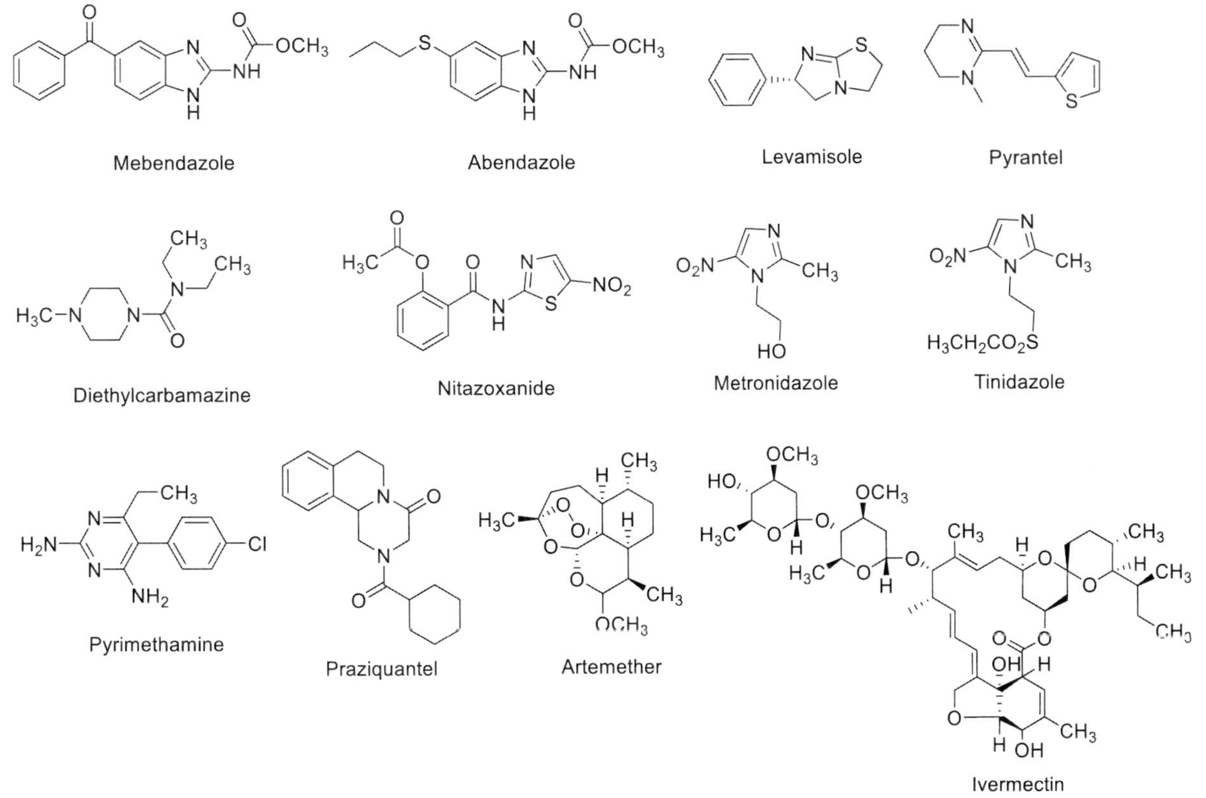

FIGURE 21.1 The chemical structure of some antiparasitic drugs.

Furapromide is active in killing both larval and adult schistosomes. The fecal examination negative rate of furapromide after 6 months of treatment for acute schistosomiasis was between 12.5% and 52.0%. During the 1960s and 1970s, furapromide was applied to many schistosomiasis patients, especially acute patients, with the noted adverse effects being gastrointestinal reactions, paroxysmal muscle spasms, and neuropsychiatric disorders. In 1963, Chinese researchers further found hexachloro-*p*-xylene exhibiting antischistosomal activity in patients, with the fecal examination negative rate reaching 50% ~ 70% after 6 months of treatment. However, it still had numerous adverse effects, and its long-term therapeutic efficacy was poor. In 1975, China approved nitrofurazone, which demonstrated good therapeutic results for *Schistosomiasis japonica*. The negative conversion rate of fecal examination after 3, 6, and 12 months of treatment was 92.4%, 87.6%, and 85.3%, respectively [7]. Unfortunately, nitrofurazone manifested clear side effects, in particular neurotoxicity and hepatotoxicity, with a relatively high incidence of jaundice, and was gradually phased out of the clinic list of drugs.

In the 1970s, the German Merck KGaA and Bayer pharmaceutical companies jointly developed the antiparasitic drug praziquantel. As a pioneer, Merck KGaA attempted to develop pyrazinoisoquinolines as sedatives; however, researchers at Bayer alternatively found that they exhibited an antiparasitic effect and further synthesized and screened over 400 compounds for evaluation of their antiparasitic activity. Fortunately, among them, praziquantel demonstrated excellent antiparasitic activity for the first time [8]. The WHO and Bayer then signed an agreement on collaboration to conduct clinical trials in Zambia, Japan, the Philippines, Brazil, and other locations, yielding encouraging outcomes. Praziquantel has significant killing effects on parasites, including schistosomes, clonorchiasis sinensis, paragonimus westermani, fasciolopsis buski, and various cestodes. With regular doses, the cure rate of praziquantel can reach 90%, which is obviously superior to other available antischistosomiasis drugs. Moreover, the oral administration action effect is fast, and the course of treatment is short; therefore, the patient is well tolerated with no observations of severe short- and long-term adverse effects. In 1980, praziquantel was first launched in Germany and quickly became the preferred drug for treating parasitic diseases such as schistosomiasis, clonorchiasis, pulmonary parasitosis, and fascioliasis. The advent of praziquantel has completely eliminated the shortcomings of

TABLE 21.1 WHO-recommended antiparasitic medicines for use in preventive chemotherapy.[a]

Parasitic diseases	Albendazole	Mebendazole	Diethylcarbamazine	Ivermectin	Praziquantel	Levamisole	Pyrimethamine
Ascariasis	√	√		(√)		√	√
Hookworm	√	√				√	√
Lymphatic filariasis	√		√				
Onchocerciasis				√			
Schistosomiasis					√		
Trichuriasis	√	√		(√)		(√)	(√)
Clonorchiasis					√		
Opisthorchiasis					√		
Paragonimiasis					√		
Strongyloidiasis	√	(√)		√			
Taeniasis					√		
Zoonotic ancylostomiasis	√	(√)		(√)		(√)	(√)
Ectoparasitic infections				√			
Enterobiasis	√	√		(√)		(√)	√
Intestinal trematodiases					√		
Toxocariasis			√	(√)			

[a] In this table, √ indicates medicines recommended by WHO for treatment of the relevant disease, and (√) indicates medicines that are not recommended for treatment but that have a (suboptimal) effect against the disease.

many antiparasitic drugs in the past, such as their high toxicity, low efficacy, and long course of treatment, which is very conducive to the development of group chemotherapy and has opened a new era of chemotherapy for parasitic diseases.

Praziquantel

Chemical Name: 2-(cyclohexylcarbonyl)-1,2,3,6,7,11b-hexahydro-4H-pyrazino[2,1-a] isoquinolin-4-one
CAS: 55268-74-1
Molecular Formula: $C_{19}H_{24}N_2O_2$
Molecular Weight: 312.41
Trade Name: Biltricide (Bayer), Cysticide (Merck KGaA), and Cesol (Merck KGaA).
Market Launch Date: Launched in Germany in 1980
Original Research Company: Merck KGaA and Bayer
Dosage Form: Tablet
Specification: 600 mg (Bayer), 500 mg (Merck KGaA), 150 mg (Merck KGaA), and 200 mg (China).
Indications: A broad-spectrum antiparasitic drug suitable for the treatment of various schistosomiasis, clonorchiasis, pulmonary parasitosis, fascioliasis, cestode infection, and cysticercosis.

21.2.2 The insecticidal mechanism of action of praziquantel

The insecticidal mechanism of action of praziquantel involves two pathways: the direct action of the drug on the worm and the immune effect on the host [9]. Praziquantel can disrupt the Ca^{2+} balance in the parasite, quickly causing the parasite body activity excitement, muscle contracture, and cortex damage, resulting in its sucker not being attached to the blood vessel wall of the host, migrating to the liver with the blood flow, affecting the nutrient absorption, excretion, and defense functions, and finally resulting in the metabolic disorders of sugar, nucleic acid, and adenosine triphosphate (ATP), ultimately leading to the death of the parasite. At the same time, the damage and peeling of the cortex also destroyed the immune mechanism of the parasite, exposed the surface epitopes, and caused the recognition and response of the host immune system, resulting in a large number of neutrophils, eosinophils, macrophages, etc., gathered around the parasite and then exerted additional specific attacks on the parasite. Since parasites are more difficult to kill than viruses and bacteria, these two action mechanisms of praziquantel insecticide are indispensable. In addition, the studies revealed that praziquantel had different effects on different stages of Schistosoma development and showed a pattern of interval change, as shown in Fig. 21.2. For example, praziquantel was effective in killing adult parasites but not in killing eggs. It can kill the miracidia quickly, but it cannot kill the sporocysts in the snail. It can kill cercariae, but it is not effective for schistosomula.

21.2.3 Dosage and treatment duration of praziquantel

Praziquantel tablets are a broad-spectrum antiparasitic medication used for the treatment of various parasitic infections, including schistosomiasis, clonorchiasis, pulmonary parasitosis, fascioliasis, cestode infection, and cysticercosis. The treatment of most parasitic diseases with praziquantel requires a short course of therapy; however, the doses are relatively high. The dosage of praziquantel tablets varies depending on the condition being treated and the age of the patient. Of note, it should be taken orally with a meal.

For adults:

1. For the treatment of schistosomiasis: 600 mg once daily for 2 days.
2. For the treatment of clonorchiasis: 1500 mg in a single dose.

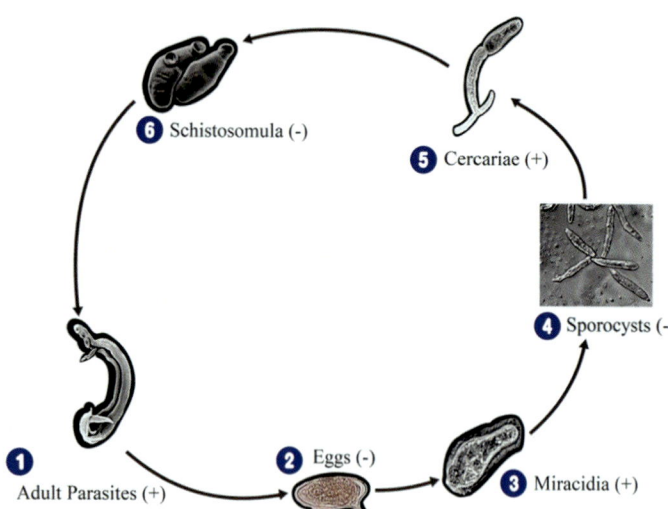

FIGURE 21.2 The effect of praziquantel on different stages of schistosoma development.

3. For the treatment of pulmonary parasitosis: 1500 mg in a single dose.
4. For the treatment of fascioliasis: 1500 mg in a single dose, followed by 750 mg daily for 10 days.
5. For the treatment of cestode infection and cysticercosis: Dosage varies depending on the parasite species and severity of the infection.

For children:
The dosage should be adjusted based on the child's weight and age. Please consult your healthcare provider for specific dosing instructions.

21.2.4 Resistance to praziquantel

Drug resistance refers to the emergence of heritable drug insensitivity in populations that were originally sensitive to the drug. The development of drug resistance is an adaptive response of parasite populations to the selective pressure of drugs. This response is physiological and heritable, involving changes in genetic genes. If an antiparasitic drug is overused, used in insufficient dosages, or due to other possible factors, it often leads to the development of drug resistance, which makes the drug ineffective in controlling parasitic infections. Fallon first induced a praziquantel-resistant strain of *Schistosoma mansoni* in mice infected with the parasite by continuously passing it through generations and treating it with subtherapeutic doses of praziquantel in the laboratory [10]. This led to the recognition that drug pressure can cause drug resistance to praziquantel in *S. mansoni*. Epidemiological studies have also found that in some endemic areas of *S. mansoni* in Africa, such as Senegal and Egypt, some patients with schistosomiasis who have been repeatedly treated with praziquantel still have difficulty being cured, which is likely due to drug resistance. However, in endemic areas of *S. japonica* in China, repeated use of praziquantel to treat schistosomiasis has not resulted in significant changes in treatment effectiveness, and no resistance to praziquantel has been found in *S. japonica* [11].

21.3 Medicinal chemistry of praziquantel

21.3.1 Structure-activity relationship of praziquantel

Using methods involving mice infected with tapeworms and *S. mansoni*, as well as in vitro cultivation of schistosomes, praziquantel was screened over 400 derivatives of 1,2,3,6,7,11b-hexahydro-4H-pyrazino[2,1-a]isoquinolin-4-one because of their antischistosomal and anthelmintic activities. These pyrazino[2,1-a]isoquinoline small molecular compounds encompassed substitutions at all positions and were extensively modified, including structural isomerism, changes in ring size, or the replacement of one or two rings with equivalent open chains. Evaluation data disclosed that none of these compounds exhibited antiparasitic effects, indicating that the pyrazino[2,1-a]isoquinoline scaffold is crucial for anthelmintic activity, also known as the pharmacophore.

In consequence, researchers from worldwide countries continued to modify the chemical structure of praziquantel; however, it was still unsatisfactory, meaning that no further breakthroughs were achieved. This suggests that the pharmacophore structure of praziquantel is unique and highly specific for anticipated antiparasite activity. The structure-activity relationship is roughly summarized as follows: [12]

1. The pyrazino[2,1-a]isoquinoline ring is the unique scaffold for insecticidal activity, and modifying the ring size or opening the ring will result in the loss of insecticidal activity.
2. The carbonyl at the C_4-position is essential. The compounds replaced by other groups have no insecticidal activity, and only thiourea replacement retains the insecticidal effect.
3. The N_2-acyl group, or thioacyl group, is necessary for insecticidal activity.
4. The introduction of methyl at C_3-position or C_6-position showed insecticidal activity; however, the activity was significantly decreased when methyl was simultaneously at both C_3-position and C_6-position.
5. When R is an aromatic ring, the unsubstituted benzene ring is the most effective, followed by thiophene and pyridine rings. If the benzene ring introduces chlorine, nitro, hydroxyl, methylamino, dimethylamino, and other substituents, the insecticidal effect will be reduced. When R is an open-chain aliphatic chain, the insecticidal activity is very low. When R was a cycloalkyl substituent, the activity increased significantly from a three-membered ring to a six-membered ring, but further increasing the ring size will reduce activity. The activity could not be further increased by introducing substituents into the six-membered ring, and the activity remained unchanged if heteroatoms O or S replaced the methylene in the six-membered ring.
6. There is an asymmetric center at the C_{11b}-position, and studies have shown that the L-isomer is an effective component of insecticides.

21.3.2 Levopraziquantel

21.3.2.1 A brief description of chiral drugs

If a compound cannot be coincident with its mirror image, the compound is called a chiral compound, and the compound and its mirror image are called enantiomers. Chirality is one of the basic properties of nature, and many basic structural units of organisms have chirality, such as proteins, polysaccharides, and nucleic acids. These biological macromolecules often have important physiological functions in the body.

Chiral drugs and their enantiomers are often absorbed, activated, or metabolized in different pathways or at different rates in vivo and often lead to different effects when they interact with the receptor. Thus, pairs of enantiomers may have significantly different biological activities, which can be roughly divided into the following cases [13,14].

1. The biological activity of a drug is produced entirely or primarily by one of these enantiomers. For example, the analgesic effect of (S)-naproxen in vitro tests was 35 times stronger than that of its (R)-isomer, and the activity of (S)-propranolol was 98 times higher than that of the corresponding (R)-isomer.
2. The two enantiomers have completely opposite biological activities. For example, the right isomer of the analgesic drug picenadol is an agonist of the opioid receptor, while the left isomer is an antagonist of the opioid receptor.
3. An enantiomer has serious toxic side effects. The most famous example is thalidomide, a drug developed by the German pharmaceutical company Grnenthal in the 1960s. The drug has been very effective in eliminating pregnancy reactions in pregnant women, but unfortunately, women who have taken it have given birth to deformed babies. Later, it was found that its (R)-isomer did have the effect of alleviating pregnancy reactions, but the (S)-isomer deformed the fetus.
4. The biological activity of the two enantiomers is different, but the combination of drugs is advantageous. For example, the antihypertensive drug (R)-Nebivolol is a β-receptor blocker, while (S)-nebivolol can reduce the resistance of peripheral blood vessels and has a protective effect on the heart. The (R)-isomer of the antihypertensive drug Indacrinone has a diuretic effect but has the side effect of increasing uric acid in the blood, while the (S)-isomer has the effect of promoting uric acid excretion and can effectively reduce the side effect of the (R)-isomer.

5. The two enantiomers have exactly the same biological activity. For example, both enantiomers of propafenone have the same antiarrhythmic effect. Administration with racemes inhibits (R)-isomer competitive inhibition of (S)-isomer elimination in vivo, resulting in a significant improvement in the bioavailability and blood concentration of the two enantiomers compared with administration with only enantiomers.

The use of optically pure drugs can reduce the dosage and metabolic burden, reduce the side effects caused by their enantiomers, and set the dose range more widely. Therefore, in 1992, the US Food and Drug Administration (FDA) mandated that before a racemic new drug is introduced to the market, it must ensure that its two enantiomers are evaluated separately for activity and toxicity. In 2006, China's National Medical Products Administration (NMPA) also issued corresponding policies and regulations.

The clinical use of chiral drugs has been increasing recently, and the market share is expanding year by year. At present, more than 1000 of the more than 1800 drugs commonly used in clinical practice are chiral drugs, accounting for 62%. Chiral drugs have the advantages of high curative effect, little side effect, and small dosage, and have become one of the main directions of new drug research in the world.

21.3.2.2 Levopraziquantel

The chiral center of the antiparasitic drug praziquantel is in the C_{11b}-position of the maternal isoquinoline ring, which has two (R)- and (S)-isomers, and its racemes are used in the clinic. However, a large number of studies have shown that (R)-praziquantel is an effective component of insecticides, while (S)-praziquantel is almost ineffective and has certain toxic side effects (Fig. 21.3).

The Chemistry Department of Chongqing Medical University evaluated the efficacy of levorotatory and dextrorotatory praziquantel in treating artificially infected mice with schistosomiasis by gavage [15]. They found that levopraziquantel at doses of 250 and 417 mg/kg achieved parasite reductions of 50.0% and 71.9%, respectively, while dextrorotatory praziquantel at the same doses only achieved 5.9% and 4.3%, respectively, demonstrating that only levopraziquantel is active while dextropraziquantel is inactive. The safety evaluation of mice and rabbits indicated that dextropraziquantel was significantly more toxic than levopraziquantel as well [16,17].

Xiao Shuhua *et al.* studied the damage caused by levorotatory and dextrorotatory praziquantels to the tegument of schistosomes using scanning electron microscopy [18]. It was found that levopraziquantel caused significant and widespread damage to the tegument, including severe swelling, fusion, erosion, and desquamation, accompanied by adhesion of host cells and obvious swelling and deformation of the discoid sensory organs. In contrast, dextropraziquantel only caused minimal damage to the tegument of schistosomes, even at higher treatment doses. These results are consistent with the observations of in vivo investigations conducted by Chongqing Medical University.

In 1985, Professor Liu Yuehan and his colleagues from the Schistosomiasis Research Laboratory of Chongqing Medical University conducted a comparative trial in Lushan County, Sichuan Province, a heavily endemic area for schistosomiasis, to evaluate the efficacy of a single-dose therapy using levorotatory and racemic praziquantel, respectively, in the treatment of schistosomiasis [19]. A total of 367 patients were included. After 3 and 6 months of treatment, the negative rates of fecal examination were 85.2% and 87.7% in the levopraziquantel group, and 72.1% and 73.6% in the racemic praziquantel group, respectively. This was the first clinical investigation concluding that levopraziquantel was more efficient than racemic praziquantel in patients, with a tolerated levopraziquantel dose as well, and no severe adverse effects were observed.

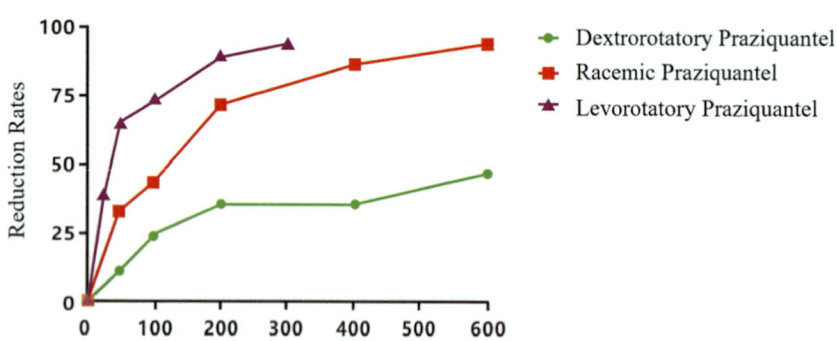

FIGURE 21.3 The parasite reduction rates of levorotatory praziquantel, dextrorotatory praziquantel, and the racemate.

Wu Minghe *et al.* further employed a randomized double-blind trial to investigate 20 mg/kg levopraziquantel and 40 mg/kg racemic praziquantel, involving 278 patients with *S. japonica* [20]. After 4 and 6 months of treatment, the negative rates of fecal examination were 94.85% and 96.27% in the levopraziquantel group, and 97.06% and 94.03% in the racemic praziquantel group, respectively. The efficacy of the two groups was relatively close.

Similar results were observed in the comparison of levorotatory and dextrorotatory praziquantel in the treatment of clonorchiasis. Wang Xiaogen *et al.* from Chongqing Medical University conducted clinical treatment by administration of 12.5 mg/kg levopraziquantel and racemic praziquantel in 70 patients with clonorchiasis [21]. The fecal examination results after 3 and 6 months of treatment showed that the negative rates were 92.9% and 92.6% in the levopraziquantel group, and 58.6% and 53.6% in the racemic praziquantel group, respectively. Once again, it demonstrated that the administration of dextropraziquantel is ineffective in patients.

21.3.3 Pharmacokinetics of praziquantel and deuterated praziquantel

Isotopes are atoms with very similar physical and chemical properties that differ in mass only because of the number of neutrons in their nuclei. Hydrogen has three isotopes: hydrogen (1H), deuterium (2H or D), and tritium (3H or T). Deuterium is one of the most widely used isotopes, and unlike tritium, it is a stable isotope of hydrogen that exists in nature and is nonradioactive. Deuterium occurs in nature at about 0.015%, and a large amount is currently isolated from water in the form of deuterium. Deuterium and hydrogen exhibit almost exactly the same physical properties; in general, the parent compound has almost the same physical and chemical properties as its deuterated derivatives, including solubility, melting point, and drug target binding affinity. When the hydrogen in a compound is replaced by deuterium, the rate of chemical reactions that activate the breaking of the C-D covalent bond can be slowed down by about 85% due to the higher energy required to break the C-D covalent bond than the C-H bond.

Deuterated drugs are drugs obtained by replacing one or more C-H bonds in specific metabolic sites with C-D bonds. Due to the deuteration of carbon, the C-D bond energy becomes lower and the strength becomes stronger, which will have certain effects on the absorption, distribution, metabolism, and excretion of drugs [22–25], and sometimes these effects may bring clinical benefits. Typically, these effects are summarized as follows: (1) Deuteration can reduce the rate of drug elimination in humans, which results in prolonging the half-life of the drug in patients, which is conducive to maintaining the effective concentration of the drug for a longer period and reducing the dosage of the drug used, and may also reduce the side effects of the drug; (2) Deuteration may also cause the drug to be oxidatively metabolized at a lower rate in the liver, allowing more prototype drugs to enter the bloodstream. In many cases, this metabolic slowing effect does not change the total clearance of the drug in the body but also helps to reduce the dose of the drug used and reduce the metabolic burden in the body. In addition, there are some drugs that cause intestinal irritation related to the dose of the drug but not to the concentration of the drug in the blood, so the results of deuteration of these drugs may also be beneficial to increase the patient's tolerance to the drug. (3) Deuterated drugs may also cause changes in drug metabolites. The metabolic mode of most drugs is relatively complex, and the cytochrome enzyme in the liver sometimes produces high-activity metabolites during phase I oxidative metabolism, and then secondary phase II metabolic reactions occur, resulting in adverse effects. The isotope effects caused by the deuteration of drugs have the potential to reduce the production of toxic metabolites or increase the production of useful active metabolites, potentially improving the therapeutic range of drugs. The phenomenon that deuterium can affect the metabolism of hydrogen in a specific metabolic site of a drug molecule has long been recognized by scientists, but it has not been used in the development of new drugs until the past decade. At present, deuterated drugs are becoming a hot field of new drug research and development, and more than ten deuterated drugs have moved into clinical trials.

Praziquantel is a hydrophobic molecule that is characterized by fast absorption, metabolism, and excretion. After oral administration, more than 80% of the drug can be quickly absorbed from the intestine. The peak time of blood drugs is about 1 hour. The drug is mainly oxidized in the liver and metabolized into monohydroxyl and polyhydroxyl metabolites (Fig. 21.4) [26], and its efficacy will be significantly decreased or disappear. The concentration of praziquantel in portal vein blood can be more than 10 times higher than that in peripheral venous blood, resulting in low oral bioavailability. Praziquantel was mainly distributed in the liver, followed by the kidney, lung, pancreas, adrenal gland, pituitary gland, salivary gland, etc., rarely passing the placenta, and there was no accumulation after repeated administration. Since the metabolism of praziquantel mainly occurs in the liver, an impaired liver can affect the metabolic process of praziquantel, resulting in increased blood concentration and a prolonged half-life. Praziquantel is primarily excreted by the kidneys as a metabolite, with 72% excreted within 24 hours and 80% excreted within 4 days.

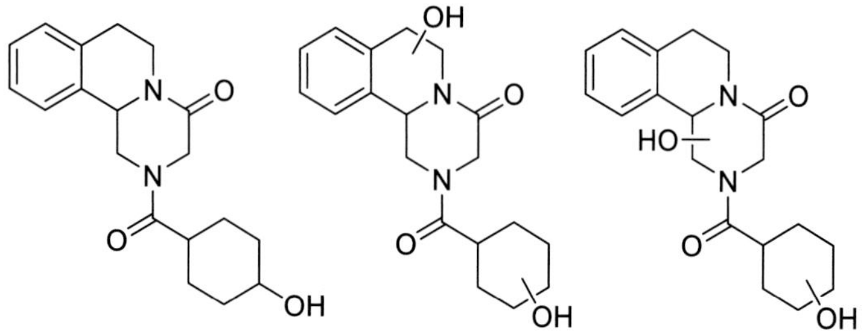

FIGURE 21.4 The main metabolites of praziquantel.

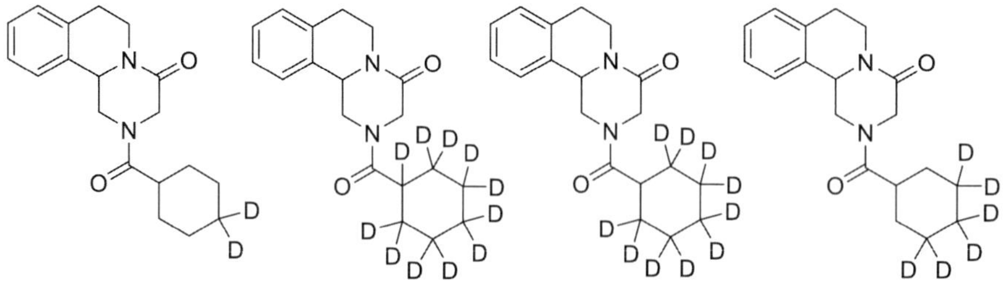

FIGURE 21.5 Deuterated forms of praziquantel.

Concert Pharmaceuticals has developed deuterated versions of praziquantel by replacing the hydrogen atoms on its cyclohexyl group with deuterium (Fig. 21.5). Certain deuterated forms of praziquantel are currently under preclinical investigation [25].

21.4 Green process for praziquantel and its levoisomer

21.4.1 Green chemistry

While chemistry creates wealth for human beings, it also brings harm to human beings. The pollution caused by the traditional chemical industry in the environment has been very serious. At present, the harmful waste produced every year in the world is as high as 300–400 million tons, which seriously threatens the survival of mankind. Whether the chemical industry can produce chemicals that are not harmful to the environment or even develop processes that do not produce waste has become an important direction of human efforts. Green Chemistry, proposed by the American Chemical Society in 1991, has become a central slogan of the U.S. Environmental Protection Agency and has received an immediate and positive response from around the world.

Green chemistry is primarily evaluated based on the safety of raw materials, energy efficiency in the process, atom economy, and environmental friendliness of products. Atom economy and the "5R" principles are the core content of green chemistry [26]. Atom economy refers to fully utilizing each atom in the reactants, thus enabling both efficient resource utilization and pollution prevention. The higher the atom utilization rate, the more each atom in the raw material can be maximized to be incorporated into the target product, resulting in less waste generated and less pollution caused to the environment. During experiments, the five "R" principles of green chemistry experiments should be followed, namely:

Reduction: reducing the use of raw materials and minimizing the generation and discharge of experimental waste.
Reuse: recycling and reusing materials.
Recycling: recovering and reusing resources to achieve "resource conservation, less pollution, and cost reduction."
Regeneration: turning waste into treasure and reusing resources. It is an effective way to reduce pollution.
Rejection: refusing to use toxic and harmful substances. For those toxic, harmful, and polluting raw materials that cannot be replaced, recycled, reused, or recovered, refusing to use them is the most fundamental way to eliminate pollution.

In 1996, the United States established the Presidential Green Chemistry Challenge Award to recognize outstanding achievements in the field of green chemistry by companies and scientists. In 1998, Paul Anastas and John C. Warner published the book "Green Chemistry: Theory and Practice" and proposed twelve principles of green chemistry: [27]

1. Prevention
    It is better to prevent waste than to treat or clean up waste after it has been created.

2. Atom Economy

   Synthetic methods should be designed to maximize the incorporation of all materials used in the process into the final product.

3. Less Hazardous Chemical Syntheses

   Wherever practicable, synthetic methods should be designed to use and generate substances that possess little or no toxicity to human health and the environment.

4. Designing Safer Chemicals

   Chemical products should be designed to effect their desired function while minimizing their toxicity.

5. Safer Solvents and Auxiliaries

   The use of auxiliary substances (e.g., solvents and separation agents) should be made unnecessary wherever possible and innocuous when used.

6. Design for Energy Efficiency

   The energy requirements of chemical processes should be recognized for their environmental and economic impacts and should be minimized. If possible, synthetic methods should be conducted at ambient temperature and pressure.

7. Use of Renewable Feedstocks

   A raw material or feedstock should be renewable rather than depleting whenever technically and economically practicable.

8. Reduce Derivatives

   Unnecessary derivatization (use of blocking groups, protection/deprotection, and temporary modification of physical/chemical processes) should be minimized or avoided if possible because such steps require additional reagents and can generate waste.

9. Catalysis

   Catalytic reagents (as selective as possible) are superior to stoichiometric reagents.

10. Design for Degradation

    Chemical products should be designed so that, at the end of their function, they break down into innocuous degradation products and do not persist in the environment.

11. Real-time analysis for Pollution Prevention

    Analytical methodologies need to be further developed to allow for real-time, in-process monitoring and control before the formation of hazardous substances.

12. Inherently Safer Chemistry for Accident Prevention

    Substances and the form of a substance used in a chemical process should be chosen to minimize the potential for chemical accidents, including releases, explosions, and fires.

Green chemistry differs from pollution control chemistry. The research object of pollution control chemistry is the chemical technology and principles for treating already polluted environments to restore them to their prepolluted state. The ideal goal of green chemistry is to eliminate pollution at its source, making the entire synthesis and production process environmentally friendly, eliminating the use of toxic and harmful substances, generating no waste, and no longer treating waste. This is a fundamental approach to eliminating pollution, marking a shift from passive to active pollution prevention efforts. Therefore, it has deeper significance compared to traditional end-of-pipe treatment.

21.4.2 Synthesis of praziquantel

As the most effective antischistosomal drug, praziquantel has attracted a large number of researchers to develop various preparation methods since its launch to achieve a more green, efficient, and environmentally friendly purpose. The parent structure of praziquantel is a fused ring system composed of a tetrahydroisoquinoline ring and a piperazine ring. The key point of synthesis lies in the construction of the two rings. Therefore, according to the order of ring formation, the synthesis strategies are mainly divided into the following three types (Fig. 21.6):

1. Construct the tetrahydroisoquinoline ring, i.e., synthesize the key intermediate 2-aminomethyl tetrahydroisoquinoline derivative.
2. First, construct the piperazine ring, and then construct the tetrahydroisoquinoline ring.
3. First, prepare the acetal intermediate, and then construct the tetrahydroisoquinoline ring and piperazine ring in one step *via* the intramolecular Pictet-Spengler reaction.

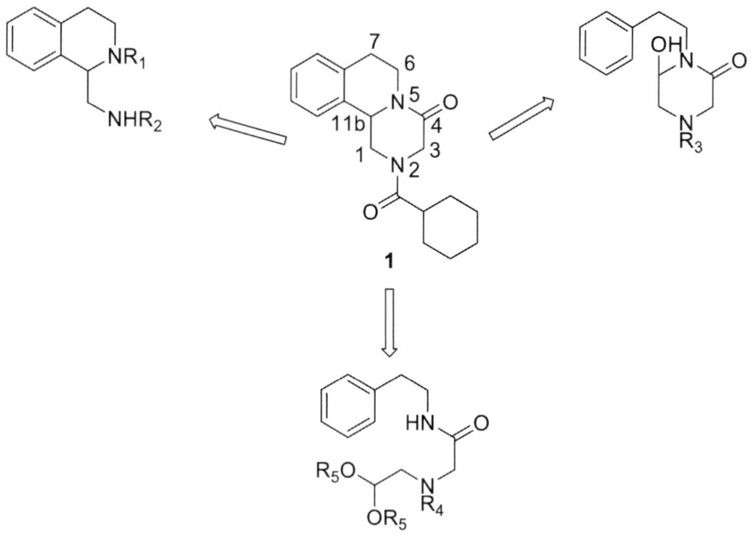

FIGURE 21.6 Preparing praziquantel through different intermediates.

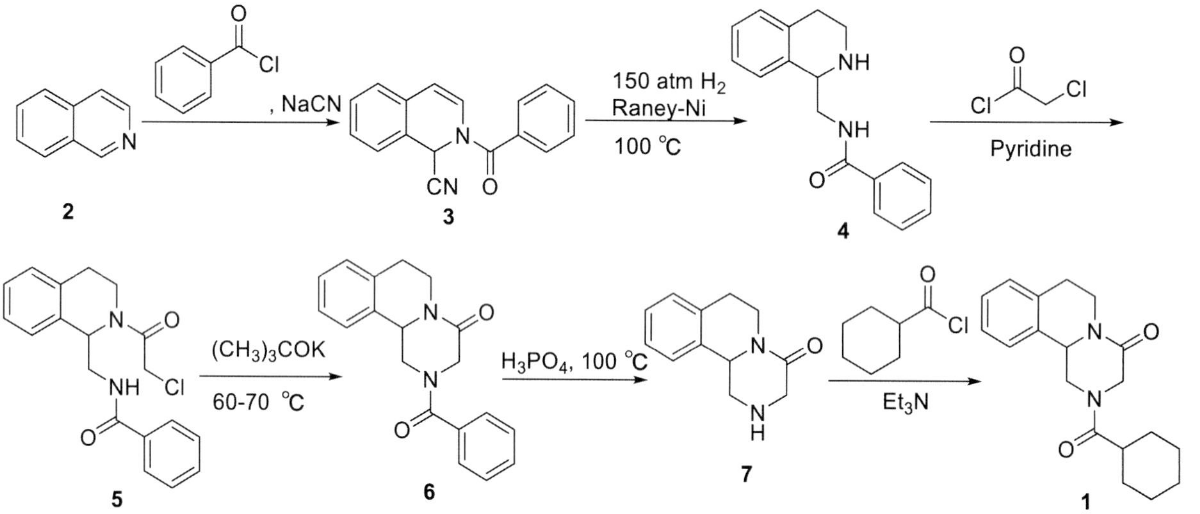

FIGURE 21.7 The synthesis process of praziquantel by German Merck KGaA company.

In the early 1970s, the German Merck KGaA and Bayer companies first disclosed the synthetic method of praziquantel, which used isoquinoline as a raw material to prepare intermediate compound **3** through the Reissert reaction [28–40]. Compound **3** was then subjected to high-pressure catalytic hydrogenation and intramolecular rearrangement to obtain compound **4**. Compound **4** was further condensed with chloroacetyl chloride, followed by cyclization and hydrolysis of the benzoyl group catalyzed by concentrated phosphoric acid to obtain compound **7**. Finally, compound **7** was condensed with cyclohexanecarbonyl chloride to obtain praziquantel (Fig. 21.7).

This process was once widely used as an industrial production method worldwide. However, it requires the use of high-pressure hydrogenation and highly toxic sodium cyanide, which brings inconvenience to the operation. At the same time, it generates a large amount of nitrogen- and phosphorus-containing waste liquid, causing serious environmental pollution. The source of the raw material isoquinoline is limited and mainly obtained through extraction and distillation from high-temperature coal tar [41]. With increasing environmental governance costs in recent years, many production companies are facing significant environmental pressure and the risk of shutting down production lines. Therefore, to build an efficient, clean, low-carbon, and circular green manufacturing system and achieve sustainable development in ecological industry and society, it has become urgent for production companies to develop a green and efficient new process for the synthesis of praziquantel.

There are many synthesis methods for praziquantel, which can be summarized as having the following disadvantages: complex synthesis reaction steps, low yield, harsh reaction conditions, expensive raw materials and reagents, or severe pollution caused by waste. Among them, Yuste reported the use of inexpensive N-benzyliminodiacetic acid compound **8** and β-phenylethylamine compound **9** as raw materials and obtained compound **10** through a melt reaction at 200°C. Compound **10** was then reduced by NaBH$_4$/CuCl$_2$, cyclized by concentrated HCl, and debenzylated by hydrogenation to obtain compound **7**. Finally, compound **7** was condensed with cyclohexanecarbonyl chloride to produce praziquantel, with a total yield of 16%. This synthesis route has inexpensive and easily available raw materials and short reaction steps, but the yield is relatively low (Fig. 21.8) [42,43].

Zhang Fuli and his team comprehensively optimized Yuste's process and made significant progress, successfully achieving industrial production (Fig. 21.9) [44].

1. Commercially available benzylamine was reacted with sodium chloroacetate with sodium hydroxide as the base to give compound **8** in high conversion. After the completion of the reaction, an aqueous solution of HCl was added to the mixture to adjust the pH at 1.3–1.8, and **8** as an amphoteric molecule could be crystallized from the reaction solution in 81% yield, which made the workup procedure simple [45].
2. A practical and efficient synthesis of compound **10** was developed from compound **8** *via* the formation of anhydride with Ac$_2$O and acylation with β-phenethylamine, followed by intramolecular cyclization with an overall yield of 93%.
3. In the preparation of compound **11**, NaBH$_4$/CuCl$_2$ was replaced by KBH$_4$/MgCl$_2$ and the quantity of the reducing agent was reduced from 5.0 equiv to 0.5 equiv. The yield of **11** was increased from 86% reported in the literature to 97%.
4. In the preparation of compound 7, HCl was replaced by *conc.* H$_2$SO$_4$. The sulfate salt of compound **12** could be separated from water by filtration, which removed the aqueous solution of H$_2$SO$_4$ and avoided the formation of the ring-opening impurity in the next step. Then the catalytic hydrogenation was performed under 1 atmosphere of hydrogen in water to afford compound **7** in quantitative yield, which made the process safe and environmentally friendly. Pd/C could also be reused ten or more times through consecutive cycles without loss of activity.
5. In the synthesis of compound **1**, NaHCO$_3$ aqueous solution was used instead of Et$_3$N to reduce the discharge of nitrogen-containing waste liquid.
6. To simplify postprocessing and reduce unnecessary product loss, a practical and efficient telescoped process for praziquantel was developed, eliminating some isolation and purification operations. The four-step telescoped process was successfully run in the pilot plant to give compound **11** an 85% overall yield from compound **8**. Similarly, compound **1** was isolated in 80% overall yield from compound **11** for the three-step sequence. This not only improved production efficiency but also ensured product quality, facilitating scale-up production.
7. The telescoped synthesis of praziquantel provided an overall yield of 68% from compound **8** with 99.7% purity after crystallization, and all the impurity levels were less than 0.1%, significantly higher than the 16% reported in the lit-

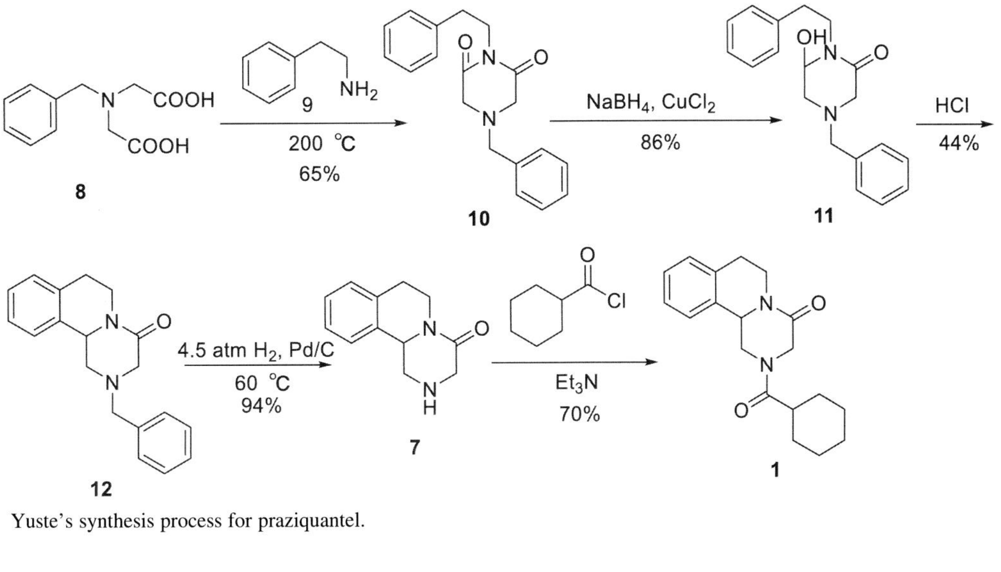

FIGURE 21.8 Yuste's synthesis process for praziquantel.

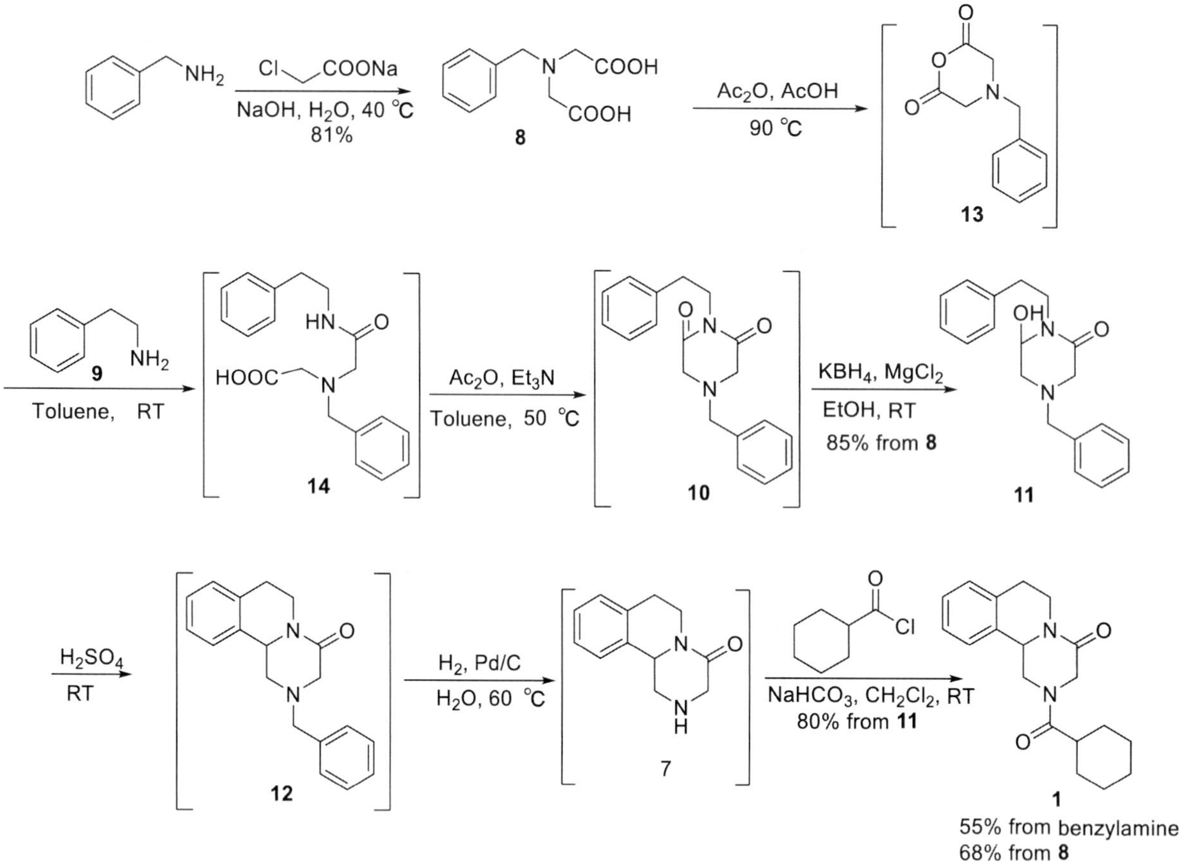

FIGURE 21.9 Zhang Fuli et al.'s synthesis process for praziquantel.

erature. Compared to the process of German Merck KGaA, the raw material cost for preparing 1 kg of praziquantel using this process was reduced by half.

8. Compared to the process of German Merck KGaA, the synthesis process for praziquantel was relatively green and environmentally friendly. It avoided the use of highly polluting H_3PO_4, significantly reducing waste generation. The reaction conditions were mild, eliminating the need for toxic reagents such as NaCN and high-temperature and high-pressure operations, thus eliminating potential safety hazards. The operation was simple, reducing equipment and energy consumption accordingly. Additionally, the raw materials were inexpensive and easily accessible.

21.4.3 Synthesis of levorotatory praziquantel

The chirality center of praziquantel is located at the C_{11b}-position of the tetrahydroisoquinoline ring, with two isomers of levorotatory (R configuration) and dextrorotatory (S configuration). At present, its racemate is mainly used in clinics. Studies have shown that (R)-praziquantel is the main active ingredient for insecticides, while (S)-praziquantel has some toxic side effects. The clinical dose of racemic praziquantel is large, such as in the treatment of schistosomiasis and clonorchiasis, which require 9 tablets and 21 tablets per day, respectively. The side effects caused by high doses are also difficult to ignore, such as headaches, nausea, abdominal pain, diarrhea, rash, gastrointestinal bleeding, and liver function damage. Racemic praziquantel has a nauseating taste. Meyer et al. sampled and investigated the bitter taste values of racemic praziquantel and (R)-praziquantel [46]. The results showed that there was a significant difference in bitter taste values between the two, indicating that these nauseating tastes were mainly caused by the inactive (S)-isomer.

In 2007, the WHO drafted the "Drug Development and Evaluation for Helminths and Other Neglected Tropical Diseases: Business Plan 2008–2013," which included a plan to develop a large-scale synthetic method for (R)-praziquantel. Due to the low cost of the raw materials for racemic praziquantel, the target population is mainly concentrated in poor regions of Asia, Africa, and Latin America. Therefore, the cost of (R)-praziquantel raw materials cannot be too high compared to the racemate. As a result, the synthesis of (R)-praziquantel in a green, efficient, and low-cost manner has become a significant challenge [47]. Although researchers from various countries have actively explored in recent years, the reported methods for synthesizing (R)-praziquantel still have significantly higher raw material costs than the racemate, such as noble metal asymmetric catalysis, chiral auxiliary induction, the chiral pool method, and enzymatic catalysis. Therefore, there has been no progress in marketing praziquantel in a single configuration. It is reported that German Merck KGaA has already conducted Phase III clinical trials for (R)-praziquantel [48].

Traditional chiral resolution is a method of chemically separating the two enantiomers in a racemate to obtain optically active products, which is also an important route for the preparation of optically pure enantiomers. Compared with asymmetric synthesis methods, chemical resolution is simple, widely applicable, and highly practical, and it is currently one of the most widespread and practical methods for the industrial production of chiral drugs.

Since praziquanamine **7** is a commonly used intermediate for the industrial production of racemic praziquantel, it is inexpensive and easily available. There have been multiple reports on the resolution of compound **7** in the literature [49–55]. Among them, Todd *et al.* developed a method with (−)-dibenzoyl-L-tartaric acid as the resolution agent for the separation of rac-**7** [49]. The (R)-**7** could be obtained in 38% yield with a 99% ee value (Fig. 21.10).

Although classical chiral resolution is an important method for the preparation of optically pure enantiomers in industry, its theoretical maximum yield is limited to 50%, and the undesired enantiomer (S)-**7** is usually discarded as waste. The German Merck KGaA company reported a method for racemization and recovery of (S)-**7** [56]. This method involves the use of tetrahydrofuran (THF) as a solvent and the action of t-BuOK to racemize (S)-**7**. However, under these conditions, only a small portion of (S)-**7** undergoes racemization, and with the prolongation of reaction time, there is a significant increase in undetermined impurities, resulting in a significant decrease in the chemical purity of (S)-**7**.

Seubert reported a method for racemization of the unwanted enantiomer (S)-**6**, which involves mixing (S)-**6** with sulfur powder, heating and melting under N_2 at 180°C to dehydrogenate, and then purifying by column chromatography to obtain compound **15** [57]. Compound **15** was then catalytically hydrogenated to obtain the racemate compound **6**. The reaction conditions were harsh, and the yield was very low (Fig. 21.11).

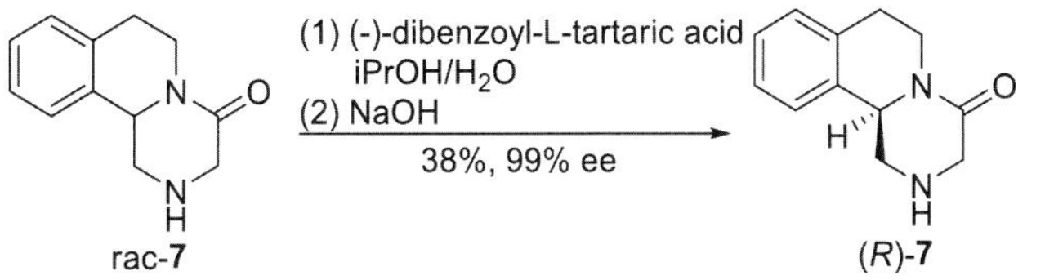

FIGURE 21.10 Resolution of praziquanamine.

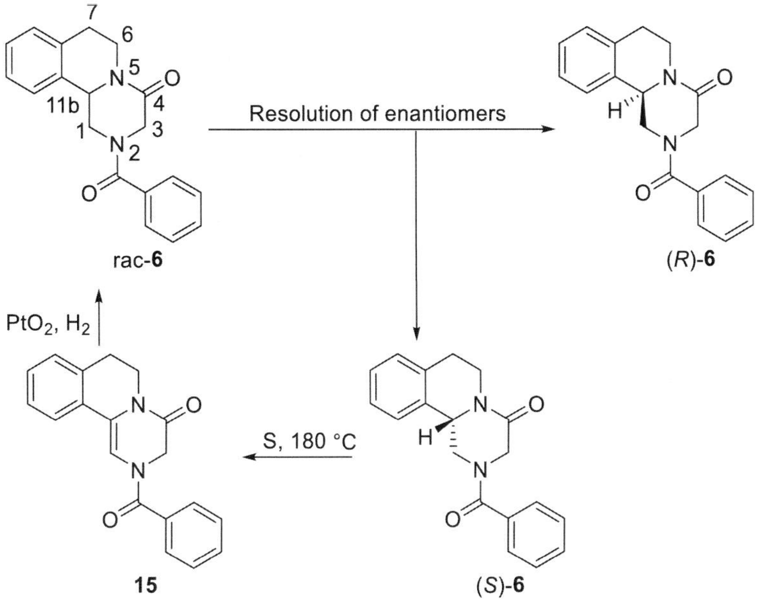

FIGURE 21.11 Racemization of (S)-**6** by dehydrogenation and hydrogenation.

Although the racemization methods mentioned above were cumbersome and inefficient, they indicated that the H at the C_{11b} position has some reactivity. Therefore, we hypothesized that dehydrogenation at the C_{11b} and C_1 positions of (S)-7 would form a C=C bond, followed by catalytic hydrogenation to reduce the double bond, achieving the purpose of racemization. Initially, the researchers attempted to react (S)-7 with conventional dehydrogenation reagents such as 2,3-dicyano-5,6-dichlorobenzoquinone (DDQ) but did not detect the formation of the target dehydrogenated product. When (S)-7 was oxidized with NaClO aqueous solution, (S)-16 was mainly formed, along with a very small amount of byproduct, which was identified as a conjugated compound 17. Subsequently, it was found that rac-7 could be obtained through hydrogenation of compound 17 (Fig. 21.12) [58]. Therefore, to convert (S)-7 into compound 17 with higher conversion, the researchers turned to other possible dehydrogenation methods.

Catalytic dehydrogenation is the reverse process of catalytic hydrogenation, and commonly used catalysts for catalytic hydrogenation, such as Pt, Pd, and Ru, can also be used as catalysts for catalytic dehydrogenation. Unlike DDQ, which accepts hydrogen to form the corresponding hydroquinone, this type of catalytic dehydrogenation method is environmentally friendly and clean, theoretically producing no waste residue, and the catalyst can be reused. However, it was usually carried out at high temperatures and used high-boiling solvents such as p-methylisopropylbenzene, nitrobenzene, and decahydronaphthalene [59–61].

The researchers first treated the (S)-7 to dehydrogenation with a catalytic amount of Pd/C at 180°C under an N_2 atmosphere. After 5 hours, the reaction mixtures were detected by high performance liquid chromatography (HPLC) using an achiral C18 column, which indicated that 70.66% of compound 17 was observed with 18.25% of "undehydrogenated" praziquanamine without conversion (Table 21.2, entry 1). When the reaction time was increased to 10 hours, the praziquanamine almost disappeared, but the content of impurities increased up to 23.82% (entry 2). In addition, an incomplete reaction was also observed by using solvents such as xylene and toluene under refluxing conditions (entries 3 and 4). Surprisingly, chiral HPLC examination of the above reaction mixtures indicated that the undehydrogenated praziquanamine had been converted to a near racemic mixture, which meant the dehydrogenation of (S)-7 to the desired compound 17 was accompanied by the racemization of (S)-7. A possible reaction mechanism for the palladium-

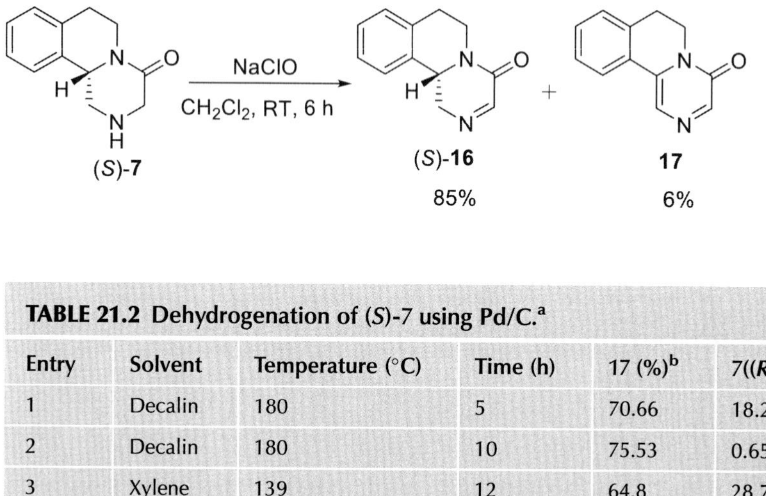

FIGURE 21.12 Dehydrogenation of (S)-7 with NaClO.

TABLE 21.2 Dehydrogenation of (S)-7 using Pd/C.[a]

Entry	Solvent	Temperature (°C)	Time (h)	17 (%)[b]	7((R)-7/(S)-7) (%)[c]	16 (%)[b]	Byproducts (%)[b]
1	Decalin	180	5	70.66	18.25 (48.0/52.0)	ND[d]	11.09
2	Decalin	180	10	75.53	0.65 (51.50/48.50)	ND	23.82
3	Xylene	139	12	64.8	28.7(49.74/50.26)	0.14	6.36
4	Toluene	110	24	55.49	40.89(49.80/50.20)	0.30	3.32
5[e]	Toluene	110	48	5.14	52.66 (0.46/99.54)	11.23[f]	30.97
6	Toluene	95	48	4.59	80.06 (0.47/99.53)	11.89[f]	3.46
7[g]	Toluene	130	48	ND	95.50(48.36/51.64)	ND	4.50

[a]Reaction conditions: 0.1 g/mL (S)-7 in solvents with 10% Pd/C (10% wt) under N_2 atmosphere.
[b]Measured by HPLC on a Waters XBridge C18 column.
[c]Measured by HPLC on a Chiralpak IC-3 column.
[d]ND = not detected.
[e]Addition of 4 equiv of styrene.
[f]The stereochemical structure of 16 was identified as an S configuration.
[g]The reaction was performed under 24 atmospheres of H_2.

catalyzed dehydrogenation of (S)-**7** concomitant with racemization is shown in Fig. 21.13. The dehydrogenation of amine (S)-**7** as a hydrogen donor could give the corresponding compound **17**, which can also act as a hydrogen acceptor and be reduced to amine enantiomer. The reaction might proceed *via* hydrogen transfer between praziquanamine and compound **17**.

To test this hypothesis, an additional experiment was carried out by adding styrene as a competing hydrogen acceptor to the reaction mixture, and in the presence of styrene, the racemization was completely inhibited (entry 5); meanwhile, the reductive product ethylbenzene was also detected by HPLC. The experimental results indicated that the competitive hydrogen acceptor styrene blocked the transfer of hydrogen between praziquanamine and compound **17** (Fig. 21.14).

On the other hand, when the reaction temperature in the dehydrogenation was dropped to 95°C, a major product with a molecular weight of 200 was obtained and identified as (S)-**16** by optical rotation, ^{1}H- and ^{13}C-NMR spectra. Moreover, no racemization of (S)-**7** or (S)-**16** was observed (entry 6). The results seemed to suggest that the catalytic dehydrogenation of (S)-**7** proceeded *via* (S)-**16**. Then, if the reaction was conducted at a higher temperature, (S)-**16** would be transformed into the more stable product compound **17**, in which the benzene ring, carbonyl group, and double bonds formed a much larger conjugated system (Fig. 21.15). Only hydrogenation of compound **17** rather than (S)-**16** could lead to the conversion of (S)-**7** to the racemic compound **7**.

Obviously, the dehydrogenation reaction endpoint was determined by the degree of racemization of (S)-**7** rather than achieving complete conversion to compound **17**. Consequently, although the racemization rate in toluene was slower compared to that with the use of xylene and decalin, target products **17** and rac-**7** were obtained with excellent conversion at relatively low reaction temperatures (entry 4). In the subsequent step, N_2 gas was replaced with H_2 to reduce **17** into rac-**1**, which was performed under 5 atmospheres of hydrogen at 50°C−60°C for 4 hours to afford a racemic mixture of (R)-**7**/(S)-**7** (49.8%/50.2%) as a deep yellow solid in quantitative yield with 92% purity.

Based on the mechanism for the racemization of (S)-**7**, a superior and one-pot racemization method was also found that treatment (S)-**7** with Pd/C under 24 atmospheres of H_2 at 130°C for 48 hours straightly accomplished a near racemic mixture in quantitative yield with 95% chemical purity (entry 7).

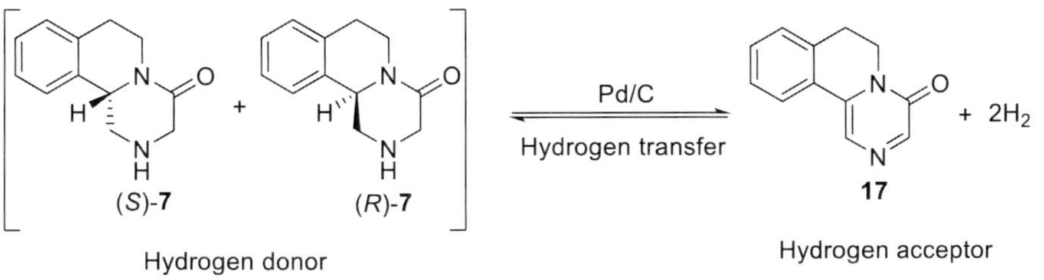

FIGURE 21.13 A possible mechanism for the palladium-catalyzed dehydrogenation of (S)-**7** along with racemization.

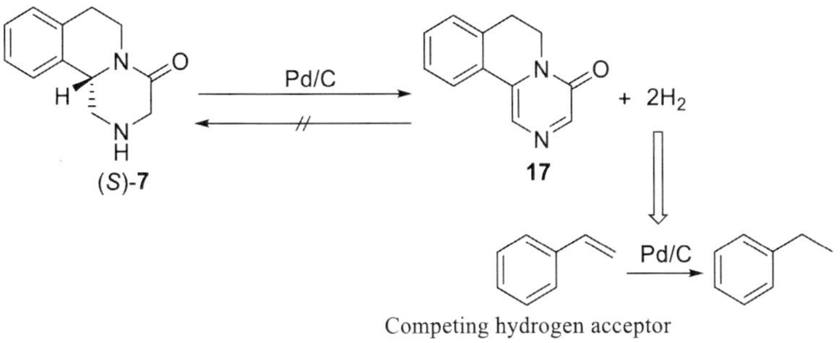

FIGURE 21.14 No racemization of (S)-**7** in the presence of styrene.

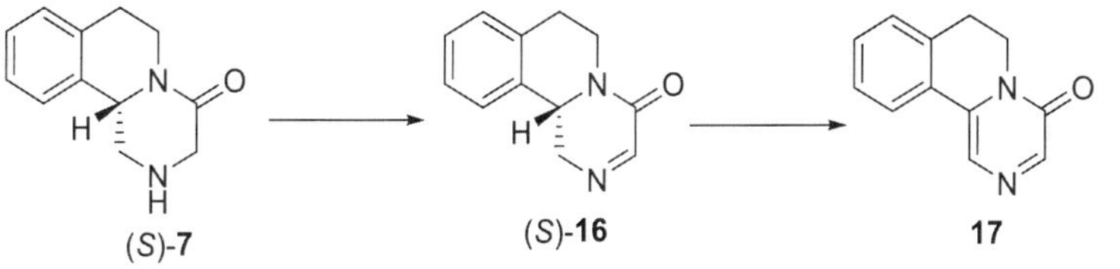

FIGURE 21.15 The two-stage dehydrogenation of (S)-**7**.

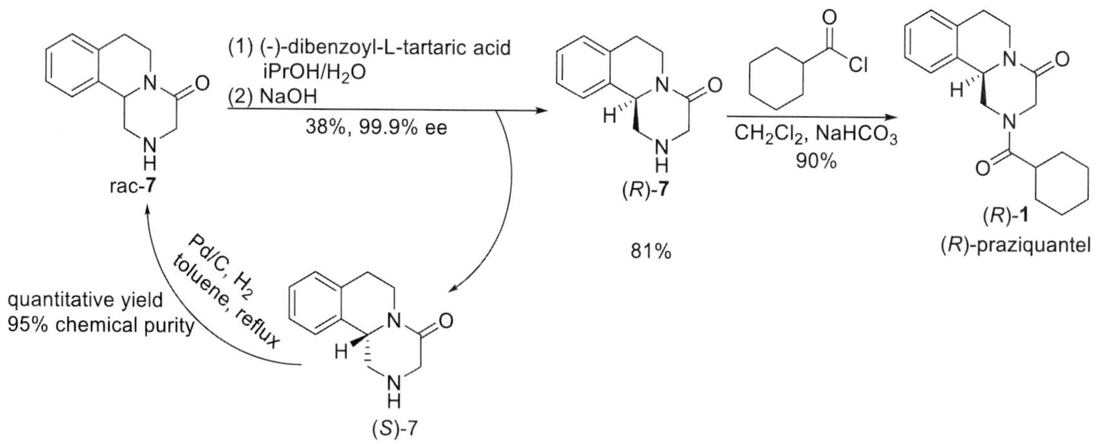

FIGURE 21.16 Synthesis of (*R*)-praziquantel.

In summary, a one-pot palladium-catalyzed procedure for racemization of (*S*)-**7** has been developed in which (*S*)-**7** was directly treated with Pd/C under H$_2$, atmosphere to obtain a racemic mixture in quantitative yield with 95% chemical purity [62–64]. In this efficient way, (*S*)-**7** was racemized, and the racemic mixture obtained was recycled into the resolution process so that the yield of (*R*)-**7** could be increased from 38% to 81%. As the (*R*)-**7**, which is the key intermediate in the synthesis of the anthelmintic drug (*R*)-praziquantel, is prepared by classical resolution of the racemate, such a concise and efficient procedure can be applied on a large scale to racemize and recycle the undesired enantiomer and is of great importance for (*R*)-praziquantel manufacture without an increase in cost compared with rac-praziquantel. In the final step, (*R*)-**7** was reacted with cyclohexanecarbonyl chloride to give (*R*)-praziquantel in 90% yield and 99.9% ee (Fig. 21.16).

21.5 Green chemistry future

Although researchers have made a lot of process optimizations for the synthesis of praziquantel from the perspective of green chemistry, there is no end to process improvement. For example, when intermediate compound **11** undergoes an acid-catalyzed cyclization reaction, it requires the use of excessively concentrated H$_2$SO$_4$, which leads to the generation of a large amount of inorganic salt waste residue in the posttreatment, which brings a certain burden to the treatment of waste gas, waste water, and waste residue in production enterprises. We could find an acid, such as solid acid, which can be used in catalytic amounts to realize quantitative conversion of the reaction, and the solid acid catalyst is also easy to recover and can be recycled many times to effectively reduce or even avoid environmental pollution.

The development of chemical science has brought a steady stream of energy and various chemical products to human society and is a powerful tool to promote human progress. The traditional chemical industry often follows a linear development model, from fossil energy to end products. People only care about how the product comes and how it is used, but no one cares about how the product disappears. However, the development of chemistry in the future must jump out of the existing model and adopt a circular thinking model, fully considering the recycling and degradation of future products from the beginning of product design.

In January 2020, Professor Julie B. Zimmerman, deputy director of the Green Chemistry and Green Engineering Center at Yale University, Paul T. Anastas, the father of green chemistry, and Walter Leitner, former editor-in-chief of Green Chemistry, published their jointly written review "Designing for a Green Chemistry Future" in Science [65]. The authors proposed twelve changes that must be made in the field of chemistry in the future, which can also be regarded as the new version of the twelve principles of green chemistry (Fig. 21.17). Essentially, the concept of waste must disappear from our design framework so that we can think from the perspective of material and energy flow. The harm caused by chemical products and production processes to the biosphere and ecosystem should be regarded as an important design defect, and the definition of performance should be extended to both functionality and sustainability. Undoubtedly, this is the goal that all chemical workers should strive for in the future.

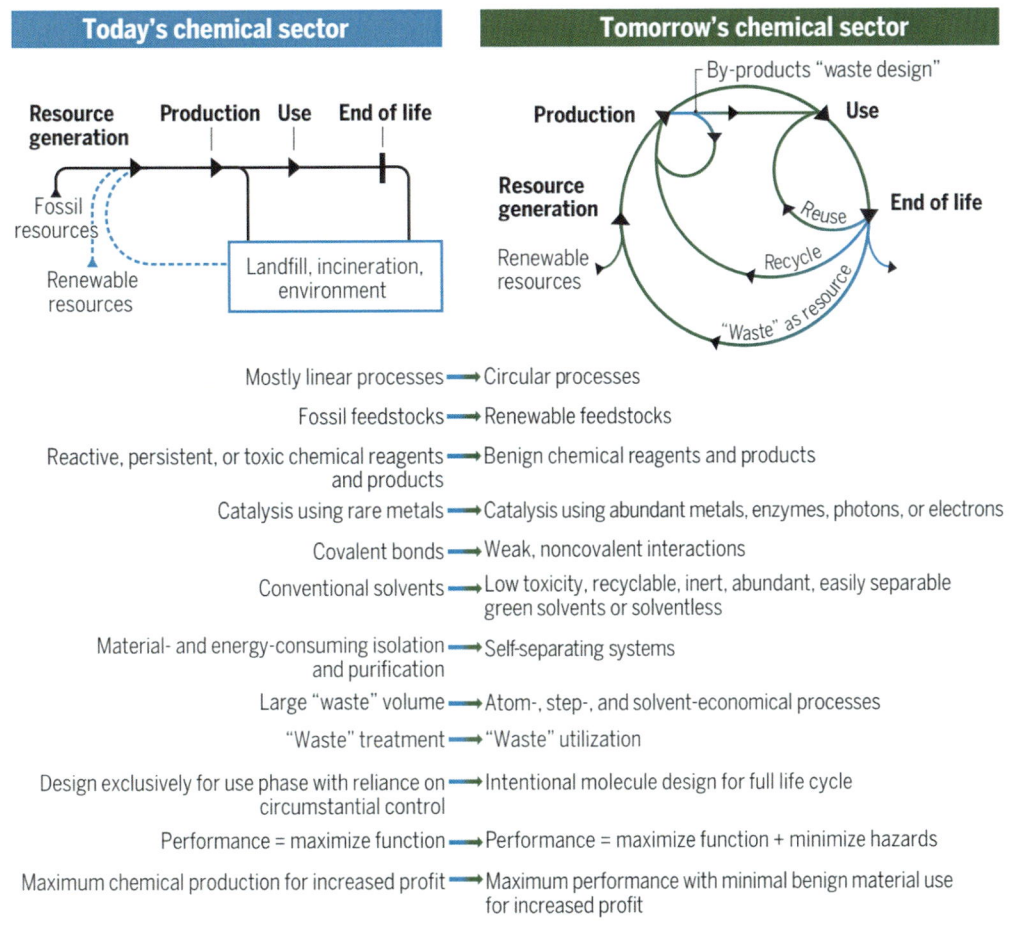

FIGURE 21.17 Characteristics of today's and tomorrow's chemical sectors [65].

References

[1] Zhou XN. Risks and prevention and control of parasitic diseases transmission in large-scale international urban activities. Shanghai: Shanghai Scientific and Technical Publishers; 2010.
[2] World Health Organization. First WHO report on neglected tropical diseases: working to overcome the global impact of neglected tropical diseases. Switzerland: WHO Press; 2010.
[3] Zhou XN. Food-borne parasitic diseases. Beijing: People's Medical Publishing House; 2009.
[4] Zhou WC. Advanced topics in medicinal chemistry. Beijing: Chemical Industry Press; 2006.
[5] Sabah AA, et al. *Schistosoma mansoni*: chemotherapy of infections of different ages. Exp Parasitol 1986;61(3):294–303.
[6] Lei XH, et al. Novel oral therapeutics effective against *Schistosomiasis japonica*. Acta Pharm Sin 1962;1962(7):429–31.
[7] Yu HZ, et al. Scanning electron microscope observation of the damage to the tegument of schistosoma japonicum caused by nitrothiourea. Chin J Parasitol Parasitic Dis 1987;5(1):68–9.
[8] Huang YX, Xiao SH. Research and application of the anthelmintic drug praziquantel. Beijing: People's Medical Publishing House; 2008.
[9] Huang YX. Arcanum of mechanism of praziquantel against schistosomes. Chin J Schistosom Control 2010;22(2):101–4.
[10] Fallon PG, et al. Diminished susceptibility to praziquantel in a senegal isolate of *Schistosoma mansoni*. Am J Trop Med Hyg 1995;74(53):61–2.
[11] Liang YS, et al. 'Studies on resistance of schistosoma to praziquantel X. Field investigation on susceptibility of schistosoma japonicum to praziquantel in china. Chin J Schistosom Control 2005;17(5):328–32.
[12] Peter A, et al. Praziquantel. Med Res Rev 1983;3(2):147–200.
[13] Lin GQ, et al. Chiral synthesis: asymmetric reactions and their applications. Beijing: Science Press; 2013.
[14] You QD, Zhou WC. Industrial technology for the preparation of chemical pharmaceuticals. Beijing: Chemical Industry Press; 2007.
[15] Li YZ, et al. Antischistosomal activity of praziquantel enantiomers and three derivatives of praziquantel. J Chongqing Med Univ 1988;1988(2).
[16] Qian YS, Quan YZ. Effects of praziquantel and its enantiomers on the physiological properties of isolated rat atrial muscle. Acta Pharm Sin 1988;23(11):812–16.

[17] Qian YS, Quan YZ. Comparison of the arrhythmogenic effects of praziquantel and its optical isomers on rabbits. Sichuan J Physiol Sci 1987;1987(1).

[18] Xiao SH, Shen BG. Scanning electron microscope observation on tegumental alteration of schistosoma japonicum induced by levo and dextro praziquantel. Chin J Parasitol Parasitic Dis 1995;18(1):46−50.

[19] Liu YH, et al. Clinical comparative observation of levo-praziquantel and praziquantel in the treatment of schistosomiasis. Sichuan J Physiol Sci 1986;1986(2).

[20] Wu MH, et al. Observation on the therapeutic effect of single-dose treatment with levo-praziquantel and praziquantel in 278 cases of *Schistosomiasis japonica*. Fudan Univ J Med Sci 1990;1990(6):469−72.

[21] Wang XG, et al. Experimental and clinical observations of the therapeutic effect of levo-praziquantel in the treatment of clonorchiosis. J Chongqing Med Univ 1989;1989(4):296−8.

[22] Blake MI, Crespi HL, Katz JJ. Studies with deuterated drugs. J Pharma Sci 1975;64(3):367−88.

[23] Foster AB. Deuterium isotope effects in studies of drug metabolism and xenobiotics: implication for drug design. Adv Drug Res 1985;1985(14):1−40.

[24] Bühring KU, et al. Metabolism of praziquantel in man. Eur J Drug Metab Pharmacokinet 1978;3(3):179−90.

[25] Julie F.L., Scott L.H., Roger D.T., *Methods of use comprising deuterated pyrazino[2,1-a]isoquinolines*, US9206179, 2014.

[26] Trost BM. Atom economy-a challenge for organic synthesis: homogeneous catalysis leads the way. Angew Chem Int Ed 1995;34(3):259−81.

[27] Anastas PT, Warner JC. Green chemistry: theory and practice. New York: Oxford University Press; 1998.

[28] Seubert J, Pohlke R, Loehich F. Synthesis and properties of praziquantel, a novel broad spectrum anthelmintic with excellent activity against schistosomes and cestodes. Experientia 1977;33(8):1036−7.

[29] Rolf P., *Pyrazino-isochinolin-derivat und verfahrenzu seiner herstellung*, DE1795728, 1964.

[30] Jan T., Georg S., *1,2,3,6,7,11b-Hexahydro-4H-pyrazino[2,1-a]isoquinolines*, US3393195, 1964.

[31] Rolf P. et al., *Anthelmintic*, US3993759, 1973.

[32] Rolf P. et al., *Pyrazinoisoquinolines as anthelmintic agents*, US3993760, 1973.

[33] Jürgen S., Herbert T., Peter A., 2-Acyl-4-oxo-pyrazinoisoquinoline derivatives and process for the preparation thereof, US4001411, 1973.

[34] Jürgen S., Herbert T., Peter A., 2-Acyl-4-oxo-pyrazinoisoquinoline derivatives and process for the preparation thereof, US4196291, 1973.

[35] Jürgen S., *2-Benzoyl-4-oxo-2,3,6,7-tetrahydro-4H-pyrazino[2,1-a]isochinolin*, DE2418111, 1974.

[36] Jürgen S. et al., *Ring substituted pyrazinoisoquinoline derivatives and their preparation*, US4051243, 1974.

[37] Jürgen S., *Verfahrenzurherstellung von 2-acyl-4-oxo-pyrazinoisochinolin-derivaten*, DE2457971, 1974.

[38] Jürgen S., *Process for the preparing (1-acylaminomethyl)-1,2,3,4-tetrahydroiso- quinolones*, US4362875, 1975.

[39] Rolf P., *Process for the preparation of 4-oxo-hexahydropyrazinoisoquinolines derivatives*, US4049659, 1975.

[40] Weinstock J, Boekelheide V. 1-Methylisoquinoline. Org Synth 1958;38:58.

[41] Chen MW, Gan LZ. Organic heterocyclic compounds. Beijing: Higher Education Press; 1990.

[42] Yuste F, et al. A short synthesis of praziquantel. J Heterocycl Chem 1986;1986(23):189−90.

[43] Brewer MD, et al. Synthesis and anthelmintic activity of a series of pyrazino[2,1-a][2]benzazepine derivatives. J Med Chem 1989;32(9):2058−62.

[44] Zhang F.L. et al., *Method for preparing 4-benzyl-1-phenethyl piperazine-2,6-diketone*, CN104230743, 2013.

[45] Fan NT. Encyclopedia of organic synthesis. Beijing: Beijing Institute of Technology Press; 1992.

[46] Meyer T. Taste, a new incentive to switch to (R)-praziquantel in schistosomiasis treatment. PLoSNegl Trop Dis 2009;3(1):e357.

[47] Woelfle M, Olliaro P, Todd MH. Open science is a research accelerator. Nat Chem 2011;2011(3):745−8.

[48] ClinicalTrials.gov home page 2021, National Library of Medicine: National Center for Biotechnology Information, Available from: https://clinicaltrials.gov/study/NCT03845140?term = Praziquantel.&page = 1&rank = 4.

[49] Todd MH, et al. Resolution of praziquantel. PLoSNegl Trop Dis 2011;5(9):e1260.

[50] Sun D.Q., *Preparation method of pyrazino amine salt and corresponding pyrazino amine with optical activity*, CN103755701, 2013.

[51] Alberto CC, et al. A straightforward and efficient synthesis of praziquantel enantiomers and their 4'-hydroxy derivatives. Tetrahedron: Asymmetry 2014;25(2):133−40.

[52] Lalit KS, et al. Design and synthesis of molecular probes for the determination of the target of the anthelmintic drug praziquantel. Bioorg Med Chem Lett 2014;24(11):2469−72.

[53] Zheng Y, et al. Development of chiral praziquantel analogues as potential drug candidates with activity to juvenile schistosoma japonicum. Bioorg Med Chem Lett 2014;24(17):4223−6.

[54] Hu C, et al. Development and validation of process for resolution of praziquantel amine for preparation of chiral praziquantel. Asian J Chem 2014;26(23):8158−62.

[55] Liu J.F., Harbeson S.L., Tung R.D., *Methods of use comprising deuterated pyrazino[2,1-a]isoquinolines*, US9206179, 2015.

[56] David M. et al., *Method for the production of praziquantel and precursors thereof*, WO2016078765, 2014.

[57] Katarzyna KK. Spectral and chemical properties of pyrazino[2,1-*a*]isoquinolin-4-one derivatives. Arch Pharm 1989;322(11):795−9.

[58] Zhao Q, et al. Tetrasubstitutedpyrazinones derived from the reaction of praziquantel with *N*-bromosuccinimide. Tetrahedron Lett 2014;55(32):4463−5.

[59] Baeckvall JE, Plobeck NA. New synthesis of the 6*H*-pyrido[4,3-*b*]carbazoles ellipticine and olivacine*via* cycloaddition of 2-phenylsulfonyl 1,3-dienes to indoles. J Org Chem 1990;55(15):4528−31.

[60] Pelcman B, Gribble GW. Total synthesis of the marine sponge pigment fascaplysin. Tetrahedron Lett 1990;31(17):2381–4.
[61] Ronald GH, et al. A new general synthesis of polycyclic aromatic compounds based on enamine chemistry. J Org Chem 1991;56(3):1210–17.
[62] Yang ZZ, et al. One-pot palladium-catalyzed racemization of (S)-praziquanamine: a key intermediate for the anthelmintic agent (R)-praziquantel. Heterocycles 2017;94(1):122–30.
[63] Zhang F.L., Yang Z.Z., *Recovery preparation method of racepiquamine*, CN107814797, 2016.
[64] Zhang F.L., Yang Z.Z., *Racemic praziquanamine recovery and preparation method*, CN107151244, 2016.
[65] Julie BZ, et al. Designing for a green chemistry future. Science 2020;367(6476):397–400.

Chapter 22

A case study on the proton pump inhibitor omeprazole

Maosheng Cheng, Jian Wang and Rui Wen
School of Pharmaceutical Engineering, Shenyang Pharmaceutical University, Shenyang, P.R. China

Chapter outline

22.1 Peptic ulcer — 531	22.3.2 The synthesis process of omeprazole — 546
22.1.1 Pathogenesis of peptic ulcer — 531	22.3.3 Structure-activity relationship of proton pump inhibitors — 549
22.1.2 Classification and clinical applications of antiulcer medications — 535	**22.4 Clinical applications of omeprazole** — 550
22.2 Why is omeprazole — 538	22.4.1 The clinical indications and safety of omeprazole — 550
22.2.1 Physiological functions and structural characteristics of proton pumps — 538	22.4.2 Omeprazole and esomeprazole — 551
22.2.2 The development process of omeprazole — 539	**22.5 Summary and knowledge expansion** — 553
22.2.3 The mechanism of action of omeprazole — 545	22.5.1 Chapter summary — 553
22.3 Medicinal chemistry of omeprazole — 546	22.5.2 Expansion of knowledge: the patent portfolio of omeprazole — 553
22.3.1 The structural characteristics of omeprazole — 546	**References** — 554

22.1 Peptic ulcer

22.1.1 Pathogenesis of peptic ulcer

Peptic ulcer (PU) is an inflammatory defect that occurs in the mucous membrane of the gastrointestinal tract, penetrating through the mucosal muscle layer and even deeper layers. It is directly associated with the digestive action of gastric acid and pepsin, hence referred to as PU. The affected sites encompass various areas such as the stomach, duodenum, gastroesophageal junction, gastrojejunostomy, or nearby areas containing gastric mucosa such as Meckel's diverticulum. Gastric ulcer (GU) and duodenal ulcer (DU) stand out as the most prevalent types [1]. Clinical symptoms predominantly manifest as epigastric pain, dyspepsia, gastrointestinal bleeding, and perforation.

In 1910, Schwartz proposed the classic theory of "no acid, no ulcer," attributing the occurrence of PUs to excessive gastric acid secretion. According to this theory, it was believed that the excessive release of gastric acid and the consequent increased activity of gastric proteases were pivotal factors in ulcer formation. Subsequently, over the following decades, mitigating the damage caused by gastric secretions has been a primary focus of research in the treatment of PUs. Against this historical backdrop, various therapeutic approaches have been developed, including acid-neutralizing agents based on the principles of acid-base neutralization, H_2 receptor antagonists that inhibit gastric acid secretion, anticholinergic agents, gastrin receptor antagonists, proton pump inhibitors (PPIs), and gastric mucosal protective agents. While these drugs can provide short-term relief for PU symptoms, they are also associated with a notable recurrence rate of ulcers.

In 1982, pathologist Warren achieved a groundbreaking milestone by successfully isolating *Helicobacter pylori* (Hp) from the stomachs of patients suffering from gastritis and GUs [2]. This pivotal discovery, accomplished in collaboration with internist Marshall, conclusively proved Hp as the etiological agent responsible for gastritis and PUs. In 1994, the National Institutes of Health convened a consensus conference in the United States, marking the first instance where the eradication of Hp was incorporated into the treatment protocol for PUs. The introduction of eradication therapy targeting Hp has significantly reduced the recurrence rate of PUs. In recognition of their exceptional contributions to the discovery of Hp and its role in the mechanisms underlying PUs, Warren and Marshall were awarded the Nobel Prize in Physiology or Medicine in 2005.

The currently widely accepted perspective posits that the occurrence and progression of PUs are multifactorial processes influenced by multiple factors, arising from an imbalance between the invasive factors affecting the gastrointestinal mucosa and the reparative factors of the mucosal barrier defense. Invasive factors include gastric acid, gastric proteases, Hp, medications, and various other contributors.

22.1.1.1 Gastric acid and gastric proteases

Gastric acid and gastric proteases are primary components of gastric fluid, playing a crucial role in food digestion and the eradication of pathogenic microorganisms within the gastric cavity. Gastric acid, chemically known as hydrochloric acid (HCl), is secreted by the parietal cells located in the gastric body and fundus. Under normal physiological conditions, the daily secretion ranges from 1 to 2 L, a process regulated by endocrine, paracrine, and neural mechanisms. During the secretion phase, the pH within the stomach drops to approximately 0.9–1.5. Sensory stimuli such as those from smell, taste, and sight from food, neural impulses are generated. These impulses first reach the reflex center and then are transmitted through the vagus nerve to the digestive organs, stimulating the secretion of digestive juices. In this process, gastrin, acetylcholine, and histamine bind to specific receptors on the basolateral membrane of parietal cells, directly participating in the regulation of gastric acid (Fig. 22.1). Gastrin is secreted into the bloodstream by G cells located in the gastric antrum. It primarily binds to receptors on enterochromaffin-like (ECL) cells within the intestine, thereby stimulating histamine release. In smaller quantities, it also attaches to cholecystokinin 2 receptors found on parietal cells, resulting in intracellular calcium release and subsequent secretion of gastric acid through a pathway mediated by calcium-dependent protein kinase. Histamine can activate histamine H_2 receptors on parietal cells, stimulating adenylate cyclase and increasing intracellular cAMP levels. This activates downstream signaling pathways involving protein kinase A, ultimately enhancing gastric acid secretion by parietal cells. Acetylcholine, secreted by the nerve endings of the gastric antrum and fundic glands, can bind specifically to M3 receptors on parietal cells, elevating intracellular calcium concentration. This directly promotes gastric acid secretion via a Ca^{2+}/calcium-dependent protein kinase pathway. Additionally, acetylcholine promotes the release of gastrin from G cells in the gastric antrum, which, in turn, downregulates the production of somatostatin by D cells in the gastric fundus. Somatostatin is an endogenous acid-inhibitory substance that indirectly enhances gastric acidity [3,4].

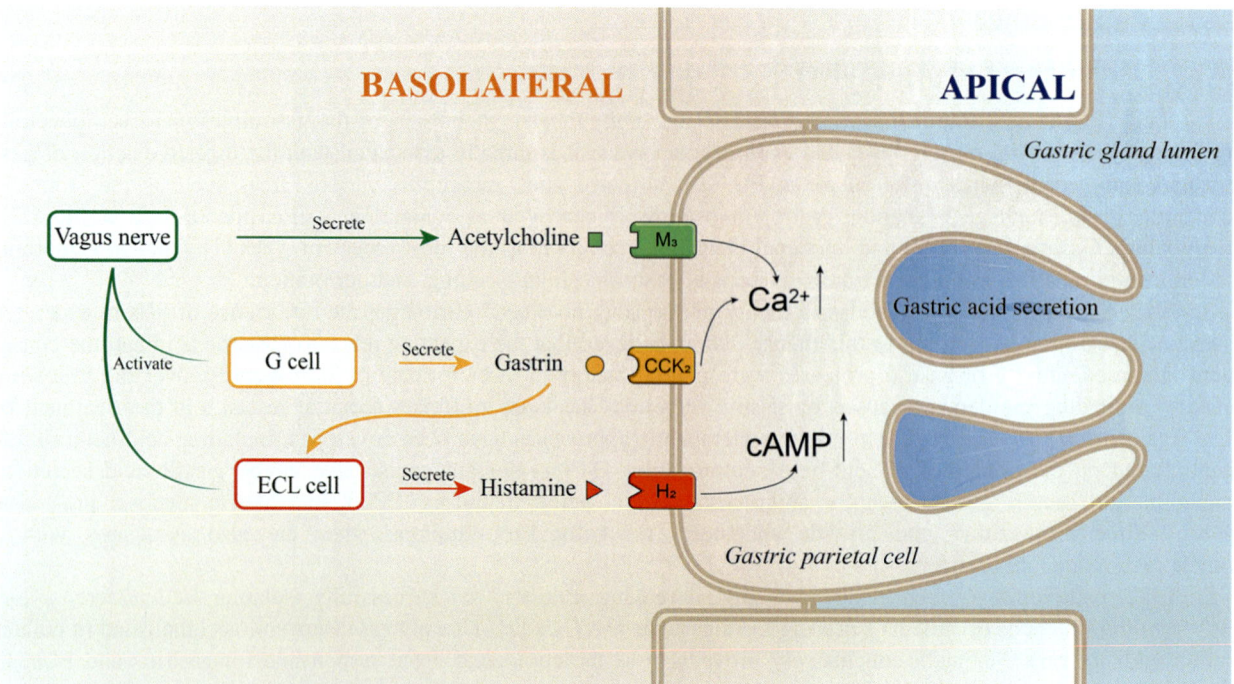

FIGURE 22.1 Regulation mechanisms of gastric acid secretion.

Gastric pepsinogen is released by the chief cells of the gastric fundus as an inactive precursor. It undergoes activation in the acidic environment of the gastric cavity, thus exerting its proteolytic function [5]. Its activity is dependent on the pH of the gastric juice, with activation being facilitated at a pH of 2−3, while activity is lost at pH values greater than 4.

Under normal physiological conditions, the surface of the gastric mucosal epithelial cells is covered by a layer of mucous-bicarbonate barrier, which has a thickness of approximately 0.5 mm. This barrier, composed mainly of glycoproteins and bicarbonate, ensures that gastric acid and pepsin can function normally without causing damage to the gastric mucosa. However, when gastric acid is excessively secreted, an excessive amount of H^+ can diffuse back and breach the mucous-bicarbonate barrier, directly stimulating the gastric mucosal epithelial cells. This exposure to gastric acid, pepsin, pathogenic microorganisms, and other invasive factors can lead to ulcer formation. DUs are characterized by high gastric acid secretion and are associated with hypergastrinemia in patients [6], as well as abnormal proliferation of parietal cells [7].

22.1.1.2 Helicobacter pylori

Hp is a microaerophilic Gram-negative bacterium that primarily colonizes the gastric mucosa and adheres to the surface of the mucosal epithelium [8]. Its global infection rate is approximately 50%, with most infected individuals showing no obvious symptoms. However, 5%−10% of infected individuals may progress to develop ulcers. The detection rates of Hp in patients with GUs and DUs are 90% and 80%, respectively [9].

The pathogenic mechanisms of Hp include colonization of the bacteria and toxin-related damage, abnormal gastric acid secretion, and the host's immune response.

22.1.1.2.1 The colonization and toxin-mediated damage caused by *Helicobacter pylori*

The survival of Hp in the stomach is facilitated by its unique physiological structures (Fig. 22.2): urease, helical structure, flagella, and adhesins.

Urease: Urease is capable of breaking down urea into alkaline ammonia and carbon dioxide, which are released into the acidic environment surrounding the bacteria to resist gastric acid erosion.

Helical structure: The helical structure of Hp allows for more efficient traversal through the mucus layer.

Flagella: Flagella serve as the motility apparatus for Hp, and an increase in the number of flagella significantly enhances its motility.

Adhesins: Adhesins enable Hp to attach to the surface of gastric epithelial cells by recognizing receptors in the mucus layer and on the epithelial cell surface, thereby overcoming the peristaltic emptying action of the stomach.

When these structures mentioned above are functional, they can also cause damage to the host organism. The ammonia released by urease disrupts the colloidal structure of the mucus layer, reducing its viscosity and elastic modulus, transforming it into a viscous solution, and thereby weakening the defensive barrier of the epithelial cells. High concentrations of ammonium salts can also directly harm the epithelial cells. Adherence to the epithelial cells facilitates the transfer of bacterial toxins into the cells, and it also allows the lipopolysaccharides on the cell wall to be recognized by Toll-like receptors (TLRs) within the cells, activating downstream transcription factor NF-κB and promoting the expression of inflammatory factors [10,11].

The cellular toxins associated with Hp include vacuolating cytotoxin A (VacA) and cytotoxin-associated protein A (CagA). (1) VacA is a secreted protein with a molecular weight of 87 kDa, composed of an N-terminal p33 domain and a C-terminal p55 domain. VacA has the ability to induce vacuolation in epithelial cells, and its mechanism of action is associated with the formation of membrane ion channels, where VacA assembles as oligomers and inserts into the lipid bilayer of the cells. (2) CagA has a molecular weight ranging from 120 to 140 kDa and is encoded within the CagA pathogenicity island (CagPAI). Following secretion into gastric epithelial cells via the type IV secretion system (T4SS), CagA can induce the secretion of inflammatory factors and cellular depolarization, promote cell apoptosis, and even initiate carcinogenesis [12].

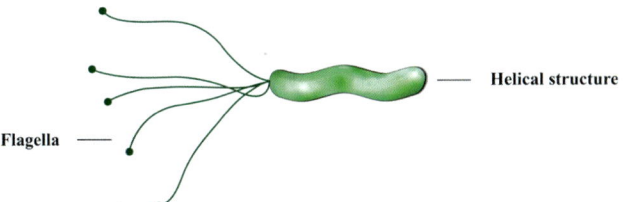

FIGURE 22.2 The morphological structure of *Helicobacter pylori*.

22.1.1.2.2 Abnormal gastric acid secretion

The impact of Hp infection on gastric acid secretion exhibits varying clinical symptoms depending on the duration and location of the infection. In chronic *H. pylori* infection, DUs are primarily associated with increased gastric acid secretion, while GUs are predominantly associated with decreased gastric acid secretion. In acute infection, both conditions manifest as reduced gastric acid levels.

Excessive gastric acid secretion in DUs is associated with the negative feedback mechanism and downregulation of neural pathways involved in gastric acid secretion blockage by Hp. Under normal physiological conditions, when the gastric gland pH is low, it stimulates the D cells of the gastric glands to secrete somatostatin, which inhibits the neighboring G cells from synthesizing gastrin through paracrine secretion. However, when the gastric epithelial cells are colonized by Hp, the urease enzyme of the bacteria hydrolyzes urea, releasing a large amount of alkaline ammonia, which raises the cell surface pH above the normal physiological range. This hampers the effective release of somatostatin and inappropriately stimulates the release of gastrin [13–15]. The latter not only promotes gastric acid secretion but also induces differentiation of ECL cells and parietal cells, further exacerbating acidification. Additionally, the inhibitory effect of Hp on the neural reflex in the basal side of the gastric antrum that downregulates gastric acid secretion is another significant factor contributing to its promotion of gastric acid secretion [16].

In GUs, Hp primarily inhibits gastric acid secretion. The mechanisms include direct interaction with parietal cells, indirect inhibition of H^+, K^+-ATPase alpha subunit transcription and translocation by secretions, activation of calcitonin gene-related peptide sensory neurons that upregulate somatostatin expression, induction of proinflammatory factor IL-1β production and inhibition of gastric acid secretion through IL-1β activated protein kinases C and its downstream signaling pathways, as well as direct neutralization of gastric acid by NH_3 generated from urease decomposition [17].

The difference in gastric acid secretion is also related to the preinfection gastric acid secretion status of patients with Hp infection. When patients before infection exhibit high gastric acid secretion, *H. pylori* colonizes the gastric antrum, stimulating gastrin secretion and further promoting gastric acid production, leading to DUs. On the other hand, when there is low gastric acid secretion, *H. pylori* colonizes the gastric body and fundus mucosa, inhibiting gastric acid production and causing stomach ulcers [18].

22.1.1.2.3 Immune response

Pathogen-associated molecular patterns present in Hp can interact with pattern recognition receptors on host cells, thereby inducing a nonspecific immune response. For example, the cell wall components lipopolysaccharide and peptidoglycan of *H. pylori* can be recognized by Toll-like receptors (TLRs) such as TLR4 and TLR2, activating downstream transcription factor NF-κB and promoting the expression of inflammatory cytokines. Additionally, VacA and neutrophil-activating protein in *H. pylori* can activate macrophages, further enhancing the inflammatory response. This nonspecific immune response at the site of gastric infection not only promotes inflammation but also directs the recruitment of neutrophils and monocytes to the infected area.

In addition, Hp can also be recognized by the immune T-cells and B-cells in the human body. The B-cell response, in particular, leads to the production of antibodies, while the T-cell response activates neutrophils and monocytes to secrete inflammatory cytokines such as IL-1β, TNF-α, IL-8, and IL-6, thereby further promoting the inflammatory response. Furthermore, activated macrophages can release nitric oxide molecules with proinflammatory effects [19,20].

22.1.1.3 Nonsteroidal antiinflammatory drugs

Long-term intake of nonsteroidal antiinflammatory drugs (NSAIDs) can induce ulcer formation. For individuals with preexisting ulcers, the use of NSAIDs can hinder the healing process or increase the recurrence rate, potentially leading to complications such as bleeding or perforation. Among patients on long-term NSAID therapy, approximately 50% show gastric and duodenal mucosal erosion or bleeding upon endoscopic examination, and 5%–30% develop PUs. Epidemiological studies have demonstrated that the risk of developing PUs in individuals who chronically use NSAIDs is 4.31 times higher compared to the control group [21].

The mechanisms underlying the development of ulcers induced by NSAIDs include.

22.1.1.3.1 Inhibit the synthesis of prostaglandins by cyclooxygenase (COX) enzymes

Prostaglandins play a vital role in promoting mucus and HCO_3^- secretion, vasodilation, and increasing mucosal blood flow, making them essential components of gastric mucosal defense. Inhibiting cyclooxygenase not only directly impairs the defensive capacity of the gastric mucosa but also indirectly enhances the involvement of 5-lipoxygenase in the metabolism of arachidonic acid. This, in turn, stimulates the release of inflammatory mediators such as TNF-α, NF-κB, and ICAM-1, thereby inducing inflammation [22].

22.1.1.3.2 Weakening the defensive capabilities of epithelial cells
NSAIDs, characterized by their amphiphilic structure, possess both hydrophilic head groups and hydrophobic tail regions. They can interact with the phospholipid bilayers of the mucus layer and epithelial cells, disrupting the hydrophobic structure of the mucus layer and cell membranes, thereby weakening the defensive capabilities of epithelial cells. This exacerbates the damaging effects caused by gastric acid and invading pathogens [23].

22.1.1.3.3 Inhibit mitochondrial oxidative phosphorylation process
Based on the "ion trapping" theory, acidic NSAIDs exist as free forms in gastric acid and possess excellent lipid solubility, allowing easy passive diffusion into the epithelial cells of the stomach and duodenum. Within the neutral environment inside the cells, they dissociate and their lipid solubility diminishes, resulting in significant intracellular accumulation. The accumulated NSAIDs within the cells can interfere with mitochondrial oxidative phosphorylation by binding to mitochondrial respiratory chain complex I, disrupting electron transfer, impeding ATP production, and causing cellular energy depletion, ultimately inducing cell apoptosis [24].

22.1.1.4 Idiopathic peptic ulcer
Idiopathic PU refers to a type of PU that occurs without a history of NSAID use or Hp infections, accounting for approximately 4%–30% of all PUs [25–30]. The pathogenesis of idiopathic PUs is complex and may be associated with the concurrent occurrence of other diseases such as gastric cancer and Zollinger-Ellison syndrome (ZES). It is also influenced by factors such as smoking, alcohol consumption, anxiety, and genetic susceptibility [31].

22.1.2 Classification and clinical applications of antiulcer medications
According to their functions, the therapeutic drugs for PUs can be categorized into several types, such as acid-neutralizing drugs that directly neutralize gastric acid, acid-suppressing drugs that inhibit gastric acid secretion, gastric mucosal protectants that enhance the defense capability of the gastric mucosa, and anti-Hp drugs. In this chapter, the focus will be on PPIs, which belong to the category of acid-suppressing drugs (Table 22.1).

1. H^+, K^+-ATPase, also known as the proton pump, is a crucial protein located on the cell membrane that facilitates the exchange of H^+ and K^+ ions between the intracellular and extracellular environments. It serves as the final step in gastric acid secretion. PPIs irreversibly bind to cysteine residues on the α subunit of H^+, K^+-ATPase through disulfide bonds, thereby inhibiting the activity of H^+, K^+-ATPase and blocking the process of gastric acid secretion. The acid-secreting function of parietal cells gradually recovers only when new proton pumps are generated or when disulfide bonds are reduced by endogenous substances. Currently, there are 8 marketed PPIs worldwide. Based on their developmental history, pharmacokinetic properties, and mode of action, they can be classified as first-generation and second-generation PPIs. The first-generation PPIs include omeprazole, lansoprazole, and pantoprazole, while rabeprazole, esomeprazole, levosulpiride, ilaprazole, and dexlansoprazole belong to the second-generation PPIs. The latter group comprises either optical isomers of the former group or demonstrates significant improvements in pharmacokinetic properties and drug-drug interactions compared to the former.

Omeprazole, developed by Astra AB (one of the predecessors of AstraZeneca), was the pioneering PPI introduced to clinical practice. It was first launched in Sweden in 1988 and made available in the United States the following year. With annual sales reaching 24.625 billion Swiss francs in 1996, it became the top-selling medication worldwide that year.

Lansoprazole, developed by Takeda Pharmaceutical Company in Japan, was first launched in 1991. It is worth mentioning that Takeda, prior to AstraZeneca, identified a promising compound with a pyridine structure, 2-(2-pyridyl) thioacetamide, for its acid inhibition and ulcer treatment properties. Subsequently, by introducing a benzimidazole group, the lead compound known as timoprazole—a precursor to omeprazole—was obtained. Through structural optimization involving the introduction of a fluorinated alkoxy group in the pyridine ring, lansoprazole was derived. In comparison to omeprazole, lansoprazole exhibits a 40% increase in oral bioavailability, superior acid inhibition, ulcer healing promotion, and anti-Hp effects. Additionally, it demonstrates gastric mucosal protection associated with the activation of capsaicin-sensitive sensory neurons and the release of nitric oxide (NO) [32].

TABLE 22.1 Proton pump inhibitors on the market.

	Drug name	Chemical structure	Originator	Country	Launch date
First-generation	Omeprazole		Astra AB	Sweden	1988
	Lansoprazole		Takeda	Japan	1991
	Pantoprazole		Byk-Gulden	South Africa	1994
Second-generation	Rabeprazole		Eisai	Japan	1997
	Esomeprazole		AstraZeneca	Sweden	2000
	S-Pantoprazole		Emcure	India	2006
	Ilaprazole		Livzon	China	2008
	Dexlansoprazole		Takeda	America	2009

Pantoprazole is a "me-too" drug developed by German company Byk-Gulden (now a subsidiary of Takeda Pharmaceuticals) based on the structure of omeprazole. Comprising a pyridine ring substituted with two methoxy groups and a benzimidazole ring substituted with a difluoromethoxy group, pantoprazole made its initial debut in the South African market in 1994. Notably, it exhibits enhanced stability in both acidic and physiological environments compared to other PPIs. By irreversibly binding to Cys822 on the cytoplasmic side of the H^+, K^+-ATPase enzyme, this binding interaction remains unaffected by endogenous reducing agents, thereby resulting in a sustained and prolonged inhibition of gastric acid secretion [33].

Rabeprazole is a second-generation PPI developed by the Japanese pharmaceutical company Eisai Co., Ltd. It was first launched in Japan in 1997. By incorporating 3-methoxypropoxy and methyl substitutions on the pyridine ring, the electron cloud density is increased, resulting in a higher dissociation constant (pK_{a1}) compared to first-generation PPIs. As a result, rabeprazole can accumulate and act more quickly at higher pH environments within the gastric wall cells, providing a longer duration of action. Rabeprazole possesses multiple binding sites with the H^+, K^+-ATPase enzyme, including Cys321, Cys813, Cys822, and Cys892, forming disulfide bonds. This is in contrast to first-generation PPIs, which have fewer binding sites, thereby conferring a stronger inhibitory potency. Furthermore, rabeprazole undergoes primarily nonenzymatic metabolism in the body, converting to rabeprazole thioether, with only a small portion being metabolized by CYP2C19 and CYP3A4 to desmethyl-rabeprazole and rabeprazole sulfone. As a result, it is less affected by CYP2C19 genetic polymorphism and exhibits minimal drug-drug interactions [34].

Esomeprazole is the levo isomer of omeprazole, and it is a second-generation PPI developed by the British pharmaceutical company AstraZeneca. It was first launched in Sweden in 2000. In comparison to omeprazole, esomeprazole exhibits a reduced hepatic first-pass effect, resulting in increased oral bioavailability and relatively fewer drug-drug interactions [35].

Levopantoprazole is the levorotatory enantiomer of pantoprazole, developed by the Indian company Emcure. It was first launched in India in 2006. Levopantoprazole exhibits a higher potency and longer duration of action compared to the racemic form [36].

Ilaprazole, a second-generation PPI, was developed by Il-Yang Pharmaceutical Co., Ltd. in South Korea and introduced to the Chinese market by Livzon Pharmaceutical Group Inc. in 2008 [37]. Ilaprazole has a pyrrole substitution on the benzimidazole ring, with acid-inhibitory activity more than four times that of omeprazole. It is formulated as enteric-coated tablets with a recommended daily dosage range of only 5 − 10 mg. This medication exhibits an extended half-life, and its active compound undergoes minimal metabolism via the CYP2C19 enzyme, leading to negligible interindividual variations and minimal occurrence of adverse effects [38,39].

Dexlansoprazole is the dextrorotatory enantiomer of lansoprazole, developed by Takeda Pharmaceutical Company Limited in Japan and approved by the FDA in 2009 [40]. In the human body, the dextrorotatory enantiomer of lansoprazole exhibits a lower clearance rate compared to the levorotatory enantiomer. Dexlansoprazole is formulated as a controlled-release capsule with dual-drug delivery. The capsule contains enteric-coated granules that dissolve and are absorbed in different pH environments, approximately pH 5.5 in the proximal duodenum and pH 6.75 in the distal small intestine. This allows for peak plasma concentrations to be achieved at two separate intervals, approximately 1−2 hours and 4−5 hours after administration. Dexlansoprazole has an average residence time approximately twice as long as its racemic form and provides more sustained gastric acid suppression following a single oral dose.

2. Potassium-competitive acid blockers, also known as reversible PPIs (Table 22.2). These medications belong to the class of weakly basic substances. In acidic environments, they undergo protonation and accumulate at high concentrations in the gastric wall cells. Through hydrogen bonding and other molecular interactions, they competitively and reversibly inhibit the binding of K^+ to the H^+, K^+-ATPase enzyme, thereby impeding the process of hydrogen-potassium exchange and reducing gastric acid secretion. Compared to PPIs, these drugs exhibit chemical stability in acidic environments, have a long half-life, and achieve maximum efficacy upon initial administration, with rapid restoration of acid secretion after discontinuation. However, due to their reversible inhibitory mechanism, higher doses are required to achieve equivalent potency as PPs. Among the three potassium-competitive acid blockers currently available, vonoprazan, which is based on a pyrrole core, demonstrates the strongest acid suppression. After a single dose, it maintains a gastric pH above 4 for 87% of the 24-hour period. In controlled trials, a daily dose of 20 mg of vonoprazan has shown comparable rates of healing for GUs and DUs to that of 30 mg of lansoprazole.

TABLE 22.2 The potassium-competitive acid blockers currently available on the market.

Drug name	Chemical structure	Originator	Country	Launch date
Tegoprazan		CJ Health Care	Korea	2019
Vonoprazan		Takeda	Japan	2015
Revaprazan		Yuhan	Korea	2007

22.2 Why is omeprazole

22.2.1 Physiological functions and structural characteristics of proton pumps

The H^+, K^+-ATPase, also known as the proton pump, is a protein present in various organs of the human body, including the stomach, heart, kidneys, and pancreas. It is responsible for actively transporting hydrogen ions against the electrochemical gradient across biological membranes. The term "proton pump" specifically refers to the H^+, K^+-ATPase derived from gastric epithelial cells, as it was initially isolated from the gastric mucosa.

22.2.1.1 Molecular structure of proton pumps

The protein structure of the gastric H^+, K^+-ATPase consists of two components, namely the α subunit and the β subunit (Fig. 22.3). The α subunit comprises approximately 1033–1034 amino acid residues and is responsible for catalytic and acid secretion functions. On the other hand, the β subunit consists of 291 amino acid residues and plays a role in stabilizing the protein and assisting in acid secretion.

The gastric H^+, K^+-ATPase is composed of three regions: the cytoplasmic region, the transmembrane region, and the extracellular region. The α subunit is mainly located in the cytoplasmic and transmembrane regions. The cytoplasmic domain consists of functional domains, including the catalytic domain (A), the nucleotide-binding domain (N), and the phosphorylation domain (P). In the transmembrane region, it undergoes folding and traverses the lipid bilayer ten times, forming ten transmembrane helices (TM1-TM10). TM2, TM4, TM5, and TM6 together construct crucial cation-binding sites. During the acid secretion process, the shape of these binding sites changes with the rearrangement of TM helices, allowing them to bind with H^+ ions from the cytoplasm or K^+ ions from the extracellular space. TM1, TM2, TM3, and TM4 serve as "gates" that can expose or shield the cation-binding sites through the movement of the peptide chain, thereby controlling the passage of H^+ and K^+ [41]. The β subunit is primarily located in the extracellular domain and spans the membrane only once. It contains 6–10 glycosylation sites and 3 disulfide bonds in the extracellular region, which play important roles in the intracellular distribution, transport, and activity expression of H^+, K^+-ATPase. The N-terminal of the β subunit is situated in the cytoplasmic domain and can restrict the conformation of the phosphorylation domain of the α subunit, ensuring the stability of the conformation during the acid secretion process of H^+, K^+-ATPase.

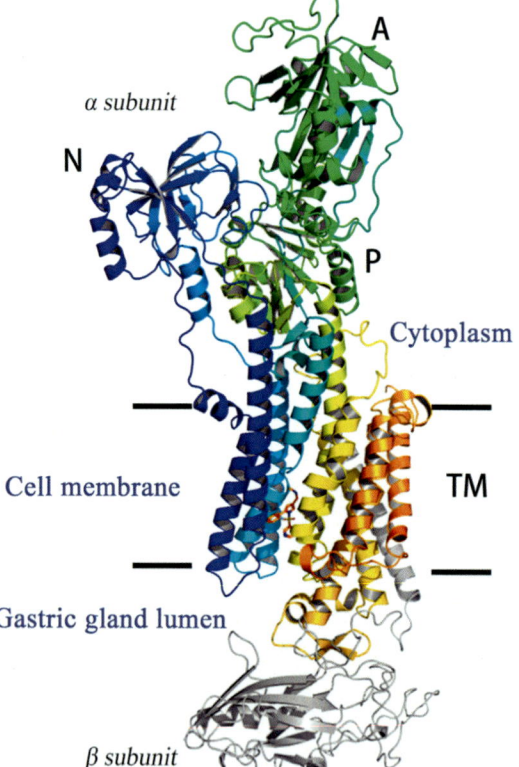

FIGURE 22.3 Protein structure of H^+, K^+-ATPase.

22.2.1.2 Mechanism of acid secretion by proton pumps

The gastric H^+, K^+-ATPase belongs to the P2-type ATPase protein family. The ion exchange process is powered by ATP and achieved through conformational changes between E_1 and E_2 states, characterized by phosphorylation and dephosphorylation (Fig. 22.4). In the E_1 conformation, the cation-binding site opens toward the cytoplasm, while in the E_2 conformation, it opens toward the extracellular space. In cells with sufficient ATP supply, the activated H^+, K^+-ATPase initially binds to intracellular hydrogen ions in the E_1 conformation. ATP coordinates with the phosphorylation domain's magnesium ion, resulting in the (H^+) E_1ATP form. Within the conserved DKTG sequence in the phosphorylation domain, an aspartic acid residue attacks ATP, causing the γ-phosphate bond to break, resulting in phosphorylation of the aspartic acid residue. After the reaction, ADP dissociates, yielding the (H^+) E_1P form. Protein structure rearranges exposing cation-binding sites into secretory canaliculi where hydrogen ions are actively transported against their concentration gradient resulting in the formation of E_2P form. Once hydrogen ions are depleted, potassium ions bind to the extracellular surface of the cytoplasm, leading to the closure of the cation-binding site. This process is accompanied by the rotation of the catalytic domain, exposing the phosphorylation site. The phosphorylated aspartic acid residue undergoes hydrolysis, releasing inorganic phosphate (Pi), resulting in the (K^+) E_2 form. Finally, the E_2 conformation transitions back to the E_1 conformation, allowing potassium to be pumped into the cytoplasm, completing one cycle [42]. Recent studies on the protein crystal structure of H^+, K^+-ATPase have revealed the existence of an E_2P-type proton pump complexed with ADP. This suggests that ADP generated after high-energy phosphate bond cleavage may not directly dissociate, and the precise mechanism behind this phenomenon remains to be elucidated [43,44].

In the gastric parietal cells, the gastric H^+, K^+-ATPase primarily expresses within two distinctive membrane systems. One is a tubular structure formed by the invagination and folding of the apical plasma membrane, known as the secretory canaliculus, which is lined with numerous microvilli supported by actin filaments and associated proteins. The other is a tubular or vesicular membrane structure with a smooth surface found in the cytoplasm, referred to as the tubulovesicular system.

During the resting state, proton pumps are stored in tubular vesicles, which are distributed throughout the cytoplasm. The cytoplasm contains numerous tubular vesicles. The microvilli are formed by the radial aggregation of fibrous actin proteins of varying lengths. In the resting state, the microfilaments protrude approximately 0.5 μm into the lumen and extend approximately 1 μm into the cytoplasm. The microvilli on secretory ducts are sparse and appear shorter and thicker in morphology.

Upon stimulation by neurotransmitters or endocrine substances, tubular vesicles are recruited to move toward the secretory canaliculus and fuse with the apical plasma membrane. This leads to a decrease in the number of tubular vesicles in the cytoplasm, while the activated proton pumps become embedded in the secretory canaliculus. As membrane components are replenished, the microfilaments within the microvilli extend toward the lumen, resulting in elongated microvilli and an increased membrane surface area of the secretory canaliculus. This allows for a greater number of proton pumps to be accommodated, enhancing acid secretion capacity. When stimulation ceases, gastric acid secretion stops and proton pumps are restored within the cytoplasm through endocytosis as tubular vesicles. The microfilaments disassemble, causing the collapse of the microvilli, which gradually recover through reorganization after approximately 60–90 minutes (Fig. 22.5) [45–48].

22.2.2 The development process of omeprazole

22.2.2.1 Initiation: investigation of local anesthetic agents

In 1967, Astra Hässle, a Swedish pharmaceutical company (one of the predecessors of AstraZeneca), established a gastrointestinal research department dedicated to developing antiacid secretory drugs for the treatment of PUs. At that time, it

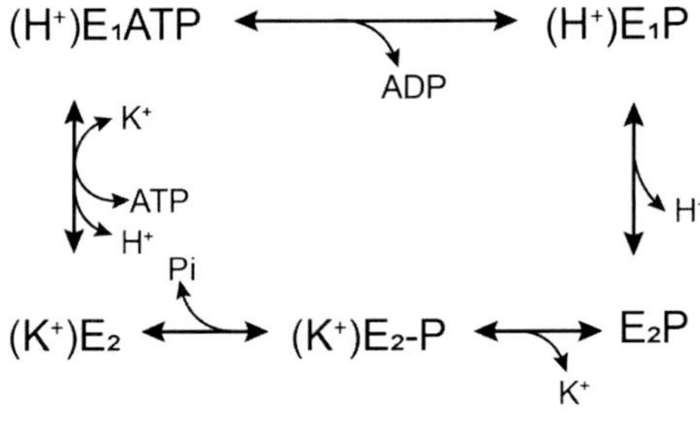

FIGURE 22.4 Conformational cycle of H^+, K^+-ATPase.

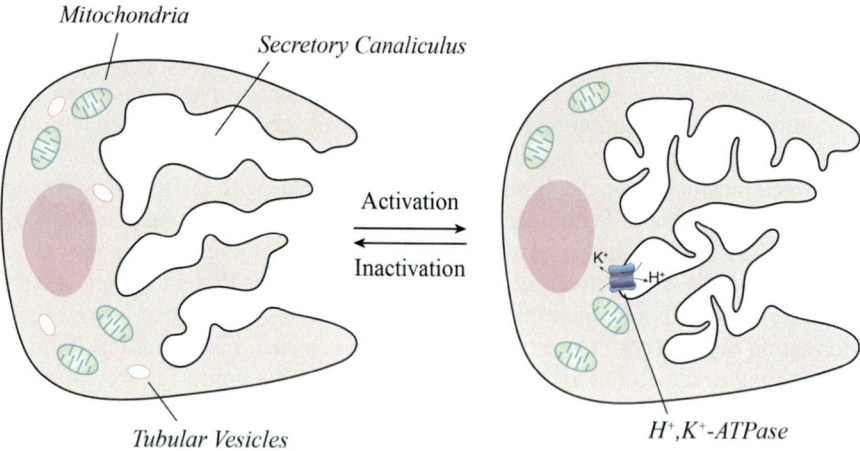

FIGURE 22.5 Acid secretion process in gastric parietal cells.

was known that gastrin, secreted by the gastric antral G cells, stimulates gastric acid secretion. Animal experimental studies showed that local anesthesia of the gastric antrum could block gastrin release. Therefore, the initial design of the project aimed to synthesize a local anesthetic drug that, when taken orally, would anesthetize the gastric antrum and inhibit gastric acid secretion. Existing local anesthetics were rendered ineffective in the stomach due to protonation. Consequently, Astra selected lidocaine, an existing local anesthetic available on the market, as the lead compound and employed rats with pyloric ligation as a pharmacological screening model to develop nonalkaline compounds exhibiting comparable local anesthetic effects to lidocaine. However, toxicological experiments have demonstrated that compounds exhibiting local anesthetic effects are more prone to induce toxicity. Therefore, considering safety concerns, scientists redirected their attention toward the selection of compounds devoid of local anesthetic effects while exhibiting acid suppression activity for further investigation. Among them, the aminomethylbenzoic ester compound H81/75 showed the most potential (Fig. 22.6). H81/75 lacked local anesthetic effects but demonstrated good acid suppression activity in rats and dogs. However, human trials conducted in 1971–1972 proved its ineffectiveness in humans. Thus, the development of acid suppression drugs based on the mechanism of local anesthesia was deemed a failure.

22.2.2.2 New starting point: 2-(2-pyridyl) thioacetamide

After experiencing previous setbacks, researchers made improvements to the project in two aspects: optimizing the toxicology-pharmacology experimental process and screening potential compounds. The optimized pharmacology-toxicology experimental process involves conducting acute toxicity tests on synthesized compounds in rats and dogs, calculating the median lethal dose (LD50) of the compound when administered orally to test animals. A higher LD50 value indicates lower toxicity of the compound. Once the compounds were confirmed to be nontoxic, they were administered via duodenal route to experimental dogs fitted with gastric fistulas to evaluate their in vivo activity. Evidently, the researchers learned from the previous failure and prioritized safety considerations.

In 1972, researchers discovered a compound called CMN131 (Fig. 22.7) at the Hungarian Pharmacology Conference, which exhibited inhibitory effects on gastric acid secretion. Developed by Laboratoires Servier in France, CMN131 demonstrated excellent gastric acid suppression effects in both rats and dogs. In acute toxicity tests, the LD50 for oral administration in rats was found to be 570 mg/kg. However, due to the detection of hepatotoxicity in long-term toxicity studies, further research on CMN131 has been terminated [49,50]. The researchers postulated that the toxic nature of CMN131 stemmed from the thioamide moiety within its structure. Consequently, they embarked on synthesizing thioether compounds substituted with sulfur heterocycles or imidazolines as a means to eliminate the toxic source of the molecule (Fig. 22.7).

The research team successfully synthesized a series of sulfur heterocycles, including H116/18, in 1972. However, these compounds did not exhibit any activity in the in vivo experiments conducted on dogs, rendering the modification plan unsuccessful. On the other hand, the initial lead compound, H77/67, which was a thioether compound substituted with an imidazoline moiety, not only passed the preliminary acute toxicity tests but also demonstrated efficacy in canine studies. Encouraged by these results, the researchers proceeded with structural optimization of the imidazoline ring.

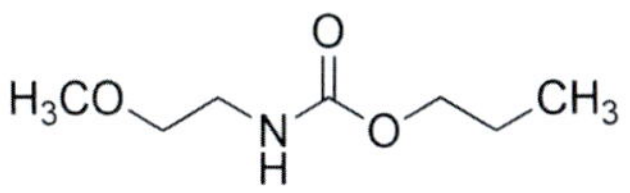

FIGURE 22.6 Compound H81/75.

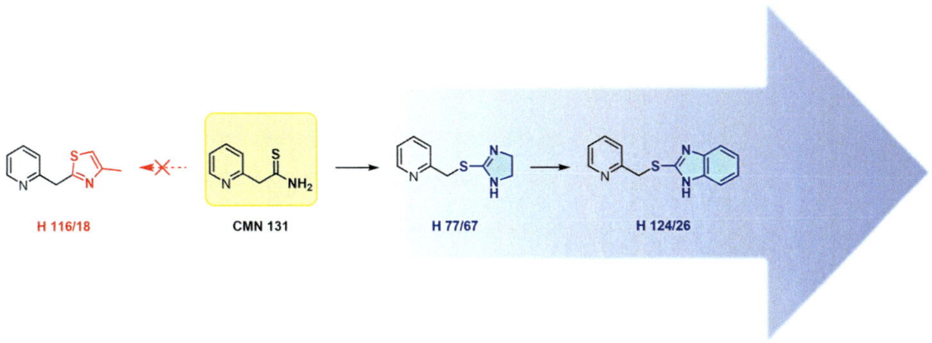

FIGURE 22.7 Modification strategies for compound CMN131.

22.2.2.3 Patent controversy: the birth of timoprazole

In June 1973, researchers synthesized a benzimidazole compound, H124/26 (Fig. 22.7), based on the work of H77/67. In animal experiments conducted in October of the same year, H124/26 exhibited the most potent gastric acid inhibitory activity among the compounds synthesized at that time, thus establishing it as a novel lead compound.

During the period of 1974, the research team conducted a systematic structure-activity relationship study centered around H124/26. By employing the principles of bioelectronic substitution strategy, a series of structural modifications were performed on three components of H124/26, namely the pyridine ring, the sulfur-containing linker, and the benzimidazole ring. However, the outcome was quite dramatic as none of the newly synthesized compounds exhibited superior activity to that of H124/26 (Table 22.3).

In the same year, through literature research, Astra Hässle discovered that compound H124/26 was covered by a patent from a Hungarian company for the treatment of tuberculosis. However, Astra Hässle failed to reach an agreement with the patent holder regarding the ownership of the patent for H124/26. Therefore, how can they overcome the patent barrier imposed by the other party? The pharmacology research department provided a solution: researchers isolated two metabolites of H124/26 from experimental dogs, namely thiol and sulfoxide forms. Among them, the sulfoxide form, H83/69 (Fig. 22.9), exhibited superior acid inhibition activity compared to H124/26 and also fell outside the scope of the opposing patent.

Therefore, H83/69, commonly known as timoprazole, emerged as the novel lead compound for subsequent investigations.

22.2.2.4 Full of twists and turns: safety evaluation of candidate drugs

In long-term toxicity tests on rats, two adverse reactions were observed with the use of timoprazole: a prevalent occurrence of thyroid enlargement and a rare incidence of thymus atrophy. The former is linked to the inhibitory effect of timoprazole on iodine uptake [51], while the latter may be attributed to the disruptive impact of timoprazole on the immune system. Finding a solution to mitigate the inhibitory effect of timoprazole on iodine uptake has emerged as another formidable challenge confronting the research and development team.

The research and development team chose to explore the use of antithyroid drugs that can inhibit iodine absorption as a starting point, actively searching the literature to seek ideas. Thiourea-based antithyroid drugs can block the synthesis of thyroid hormones by inhibiting iodine uptake. During the study of structure-activity relationships of thiourea compounds, researchers found that some mercapto-benzimidazole compounds lost their activity after introducing substituents, no longer affecting iodine uptake. Therefore, researchers attempted to introduce corresponding substituents on the timoprazole ring system to eliminate its impact on the thyroid and thymus. Specific data regarding this particular aspect of the work has not been publicly disclosed. It is known that substitution on the pyridine and benzimidazole rings, within a $\log P$ range of $0-0.2$, effectively mitigates the inhibitory impact of benzimidazole compounds on iodine uptake (with the $\log P$ value of the tested compounds falling within the range of $0-3$).

TABLE 22.3 Structure-activity relationship study based on H124/26.

A	Activity	B	Activity	C	Activity
4-methylthiazole	n.d.[a]	—CH₂—	++	2-methylthiazole	n.d.
3-methylpyrazole	++	—CH₂CH₂—	[b]	2-methylthiazoline	++
2-methylpiperidine	n.d.	—CH=CH—	+	2-methyloxazoline	+
3-methylpyridazine	n.d.	—C(OH)=CH—	+	2-methylimidazole	++
4-methylpyridine	n.d.	—CH₂NH—	+	2-methylbenzoxazole	++
2-methylpyridine N-oxide	+	—CH=N—	n.d.	2-methylbenzothiazole	+
2-methylbenzimidazole	n.d.	—CH₂O—	n.d.	2-methylbenzimidazole	+++
2-methylquinoline	+	—CH₂S—	+++	2-methyl-azabenzimidazole	++
2-methylpyridine	+++[c]	—SCH₂—	++	2-methyl-purine	+

Note: Detailed data was not provided in the original literature.
[a] Indicates no activity detected.
[b] Stimulates gastric acid secretion.
[c] Exhibits the most potent acid inhibition activity.

Compound H83/88 (Fig. 22.8) is the first safe and effective active compound derived from the modification of timoprazole, which did not cause thyroid enlargement or thymic atrophy in rats. Its acid inhibition activity is comparable to that of timoprazole; however, necrotizing vasculitis was found in organs such as the small intestine of tested dogs, suggesting an allergic reaction in the animals. This result nearly pushed the project to the brink of termination once again. After researchers summarized their findings, they discovered that necrotizing vasculitis was also observed in tested dogs during the development process of β receptor blockers in another department of the company. Therefore, it is speculated that this allergic reaction may not be caused by the tested compound itself. Analysis suggests that before experiments, laboratory dogs are uniformly dewormed and this allergic reaction may be caused by remnants of deworming drugs or intestinal parasites.

Based on the above speculation, the researchers proceeded in two directions. On one hand, they repeated the experiments with H83/88 using laboratory dogs in the United States that were free from parasitic infections. On the other hand, they selected compound H149/94 (Fig. 22.9) with stronger acid inhibition activity as a new candidate drug, and continued to advance the project.

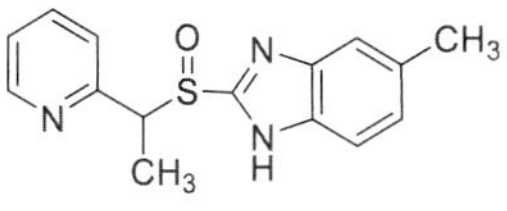

FIGURE 22.8 Compound H83/88.

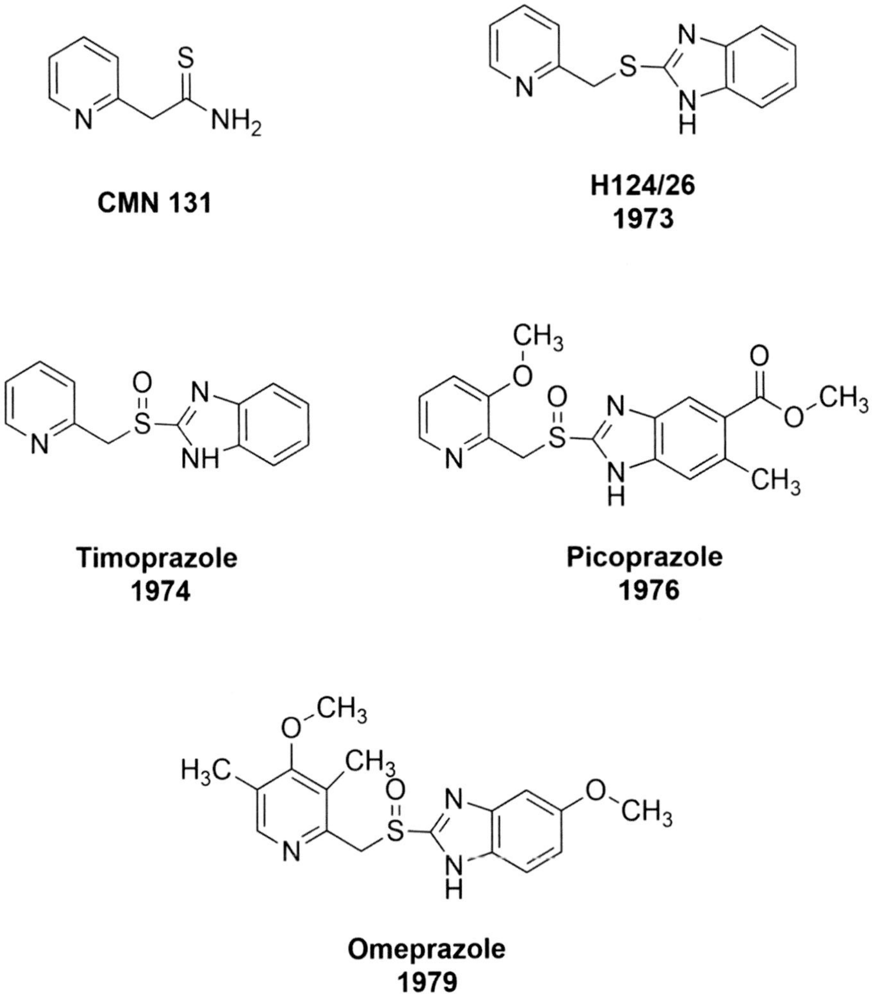

FIGURE 22.9 Key compounds in the development of omeprazole.

CMN 131

H124/26
1973

Timoprazole
1974

Picoprazole
1976

Omeprazole
1979

H149/94, also known as picoprazole, was the most potent among the substituted benzimidazole compounds developed at that time. No adverse reactions in the thyroid and thymus were observed in experimental animals. However, during a long-term toxicity study conducted in 1978, necrotizing vasculitis was again observed in the small intestines of dogs administered with picoprazole, leading to a temporary suspension of the project. Fortunately, a member of the scientific committee discovered, after studying the control group of experimental animals, that one-third of the untreated experimental dogs also showed varying degrees of necrotizing vasculitis. The research findings of Vera Stejskal, an immunologist from the toxicology department, also indicated that this allergic reaction was triggered by intestinal parasites. Upon investigation, it was confirmed that one male dog carried parasites and infected other individuals. Despite undergoing deworming treatment, susceptible test dogs still experienced hypersensitivity reactions due to remnants of intestinal parasite debris. Additionally, no necrotizing vasculitis was observed during the second phase of the toxicity study on H83/88 conducted in the United States.

Therefore, a second round of toxicity testing was conducted on picoprazole, excluding individuals prone to hypersensitivity reactions among the experimental dogs. The results indicated no significant adverse reactions associated with picoprazole, thus paving the way for its progression into clinical trials.

22.2.2.5 Novel drug discovery: identification of drug target

Because the discovery of timoprazole, research on its target and other active compounds in the same series has never ceased. Experimental results have shown that timoprazole does not act on the known H_2 receptors, acetylcholine receptors, or gastrin receptors at that time. However, timoprazole can inhibit gastric acid secretion induced by histamine and dibutyryl cyclic adenosine monophosphate (cAMP), with the gastric acid release process induced by dibutyryl cAMP being unaffected by H_2 receptor antagonists or CMN131. This suggests that the target of timoprazole and other active compounds in the same series is novel and unknown.

In 1977, during an academic conference in Uppsala, Sweden, focused on gastric ion transport, George Sachs presented his research findings regarding the gastric proton pump. He successfully isolated vesicles containing the proton pump from the stomach and also observed antibody expression levels in various organs using crude preparations derived from parietal cell acid-secreting membranes. This observation indicated not only the presence of the in the stomach but also its existence in other organs such as the thymus and pancreas. Consequently, this discovery sparked speculation among attendees about timoprazole's target being the proton pump while providing a plausible explanation for timoprazole's effects on both the thyroid and thymus. However, when benzimidazole compounds were tested in Sachs' laboratory using vesicles containing the proton pump, no activity was observed. Subsequent extensive research has confirmed that benzimidazole compounds are indeed inhibitors of the proton pump but necessitate activation within an acidic environment. Therefore, their activity can only be demonstrated when vesicles containing the proton pump are cocultured with benzimidazole compounds in an acidic solution.

22.2.2.6 Rescued from desperation: the launch of omeprazole

The experiments have shown that lead compounds based on timoprazole can selectively accumulate within the secretory canaliculi of gastric epithelial cells. The inhibitory capacity of these compounds on gastric acid secretion increases as the dissociation constant (pK_a) falls within a higher range. Building upon this discovery, researchers have further conducted structure-activity relationship studies on a series of timoprazole derivatives with the aim of increasing the pK_a values of the pyridine and benzimidazole rings (Table 22.4).

In 1979, researchers synthesized a compound, H168/68, known as omeprazole, with 3,5-methyl substitution and 4-methoxy substitution on the pyridine ring, as well as 5-methoxy substitution on the benzimidazole ring. Among compounds within the same series, omeprazole demonstrates an increased presence of electron-donating groups on its pyridine ring, resulting in a higher pK_a value for the pyridine ring and greater $-lgED_{50}$ values. Consequently, it possesses superior efficacy in inhibiting gastric acid secretion.

Omeprazole exhibits a pyridine ring pK_a that is one unit higher than that of timoprazole, resulting in greater accumulation within parietal cells. Moreover, in neutral environments, omeprazole demonstrates higher stability compared to ester-substituted picoprazole. Extensive in vitro and in vivo studies conducted in rats, dogs, and human tissue have consistently demonstrated omeprazole as the most potent compound in inhibiting gastric acid secretion. Importantly, omeprazole exerts

TABLE 22.4 Structure-activity relationship study based on dissociation constants.

R_1	R_2	ΔpK_a (the pyridine ring)	$-lgED^{a}_{50}$ (gastric acid inhibition)
H	5-methoxy	0	n.d.
4-methyl	5-methoxy	+0.76	5.2
3,5-dimethyl	5-methoxy	+0.94	5.6
4,5-dimethyl	5-methoxy	+1.23	5.3
5-methyl, 4-methoxy	5-methoxy	+1.82	5.9
3,5-dimethyl-4-methoxy	5-methoxy	+2.29	6.6

[a]The activity data mentioned above is derived from in vivo studies conducted using canines as a model.

its inhibitory effects without interfering with iodine uptake, inducing thymic atrophy or necrotizing vasculitis. Furthermore, preliminary safety evaluations have not revealed any additional adverse reactions associated with omeprazole.

In 1980, Astra Hässle submitted an investigational new drug application for omeprazole.

In 1982, omeprazole officially entered the clinical trial phase and presented exciting clinical trial results at that year's World Congress of Gastroenterology—out of 26 DU patients who took a daily dose of 40 mg omeprazole for 4 weeks, 25 individuals experienced complete healing.

In 1984, during a toxicity study on rats, it was discovered that prolonged use of high doses of omeprazole could lead to the development of tumors. As a result, the clinical trial research on omeprazole was temporarily halted [52]. Carcinoid tumors are benign tumors that arise as a consequence of decreased gastric acidity caused by omeprazole administration. This reduction in acidity triggers a positive feedback mechanism that stimulates the release of gastrin, a hormone that not only promotes gastric acid secretion but also exerts trophic effects on ECL cells in the intestine. Excessive levels of gastrin can lead to abnormal proliferation of these cells, ultimately giving rise to carcinoid tumors. Fortunately, subsequent research reports demonstrated that long-term use of ranitidine and partial gastrectomy [53] (surgical treatment for PUs) also had the potential to induce carcinoid tumor formation. Considering that carcinoid tumors are benign and have a relatively low tendency for malignant transformation, the clinical trials of omeprazole were able to resume.

In 1988, omeprazole was launched in Sweden under the brand name Losec [54].

22.2.2.7 Subsequent development: precision treatment and commercial demand

The birth of omeprazole has achieved a new breakthrough in antiulcer drugs, and the discovery of a completely new mechanism of action has promoted the significant development of this class of drugs. Based on its research history, pharmacokinetic properties, and mode of action, there are currently 7 imitation PPIs available on the global market. Among them, esomeprazole, a next-generation PPI introduced by the original company, is the levorotatory isomer of omeprazole. Compared to omeprazole, esomeprazole exhibits reduced hepatic first-pass effect, increased oral bioavailability, and relatively fewer drug-drug interactions. The market launch of esomeprazole not only reflects the clinical value of precision treatment but also safeguards the commercial interests of the original drug. In April 2001, the worldwide patent for omeprazole expired, followed by the expiration of the US patent in October 2001. The competition from generic drugs had a significant impact on AstraZeneca, resulting in a decrease in global sales from $6.26 billion in 2000 to $5.578 billion in 2001 and further down to $4.623 billion in 2002. However, esomeprazole, the new drug, lived up to expectations, with global sales reaching $568 million in 2001 and increasing to $1.978 billion in 2002, effectively recapturing market share. This serves as a successful case in the patent strategy for innovative drugs.

22.2.3 The mechanism of action of omeprazole

In the radiographic experiment conducted on mice, omeprazole was found to selectively label the tubulovesicles and secretory membranes containing H^+, K^+-ATPase in parietal cells. Purification and electrophoretic analysis of the radiolabeled membrane structures revealed that omeprazole selectively binds to a 92 kDa protein, which is the catalytic subunit of H^+, K^+-ATPase. Based on these findings, it can be concluded that omeprazole exclusively binds to the H^+, K^+-ATPase located in the gastric mucosa and does not bind to enzymes in other locations.

Omeprazole is a prodrug that lacks inhibitory activity on its own. It exerts its inhibitory effects on H^+, K^+-ATPase only after acid activation, both in vitro and in vivo (Fig. 22.10). A compelling demonstration of this is that the

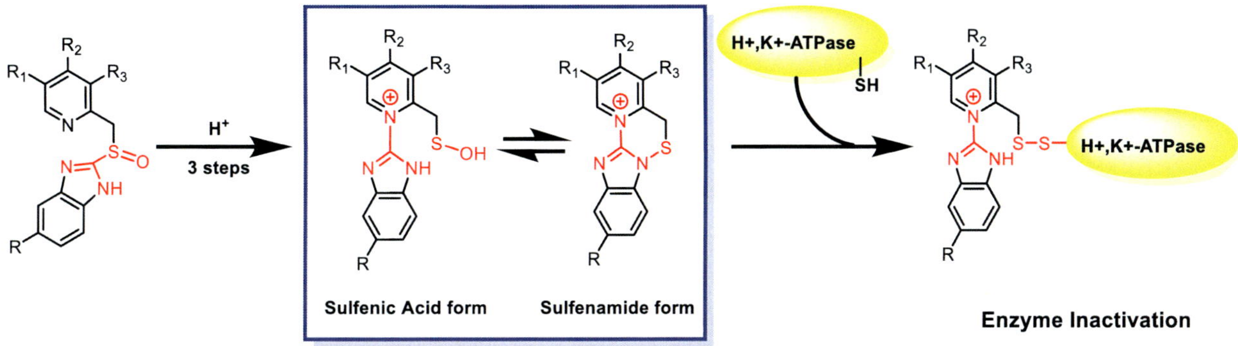

FIGURE 22.10 The mechanism of action of omeprazole.

administration of an H₂ receptor antagonist before omeprazole diminishes its activity. In vitro studies have revealed that omeprazole converts into an active intermediate, sulfenamide, and sulfonic acid forms in an acidic environment. This intermediate can form adducts with thiols (such as β-mercaptoethanol) through disulfide bond formation, suggesting that the inhibitory effect of omeprazole on H^+, K^+-ATPase may be achieved through covalent binding with cysteine residues containing thiol groups [49,53].

The cocultivation of H^+, K^+-ATPase with radiolabeled ATP labeled with ^{31}P and omeprazole labeled with ^{3}H revealed that for every 1 mole of ^{31}P binding site on the protein, there were 2 moles of ^{3}H binding, indicating a 2:1 ratio of omeprazole interaction with H^+, K^+-ATPase [4].

Therefore, the mechanism of action of omeprazole is as follows: the dissociation constant pK_1 of the pyridine ring in omeprazole is approximately 4, allowing it to undergo protonation in the acidic secretory canaliculi of gastric parietal cells and selectively accumulate within these cells. The dissociation constant pK_2 of the benzimidazole ring is approximately 0.79, and as the acidity increases, the nitrogen atom on the imidazole ring becomes protonated, thereby reducing the electron cloud density around the imidazole ring and further increasing the electrophilicity of the carbon atom at the 2-position. Subsequently, the nonprotonated nitrogen atom on the pyridine ring undergoes nucleophilic attack on the carbon atom at the 2-position of the imidazole ring (known as the Smiles rearrangement), leading to the formation of active molecules, including the sulfenic acid and sulfenamide forms [55]. These active metabolites covalently bind to cysteine residues containing thiol groups, specifically Cys813 in transmembrane regions 4~6 and Cys892 in transmembrane regions 7–8 of the H^+, K^+-ATPase, via disulfide bonds, thereby obstructing the entry of K^+ into the ion-binding site and preventing the conformational transition (i.e., from $E_2(K^+)$ to $(H^+) E_1ATP$) of the H^+, K^+-ATPase, ultimately achieving the inhibition of gastric acid secretion. The enzyme-inhibitor complex remains stable in an acidic environment, and acid secretion can be restored through the regeneration of proton pumps and the exchange of endogenous thiols such as glutathione and cysteine. However, the regeneration of proton pumps requires 60–92 hours, and the content of glutathione in the secretory canaliculi of parietal cells is minimal. Therefore, omeprazole's acid-suppressive effect is long-lasting and less influenced by blood drug concentrations.

22.3 Medicinal chemistry of omeprazole

22.3.1 The structural characteristics of omeprazole

Omeprazole, chemically known as 5-methoxy-2-[(4-methoxy-3,5-dimethyl-2-pyridinyl) methyl]-sulfinyl-1H-benzimidazole, is composed of three components: the pyridine ring, the benzimidazole ring, and the methylsulfinyl group. The protonation of the pyridine ring in acidic environments determines the selectivity of omeprazole. The involvement of the benzimidazole ring in the Smiles rearrangement is essential for the activity of omeprazole, while the methylsulfinyl group directly participates in covalent binding.

The dissociation constant pK_1 of the pyridine ring is approximately 4. When the surrounding environment has a pH value lower than 4, the pyridine ring undergoes protonation. This protonation allows the pyridine ring to exist predominantly in its ionic form, making it highly polar and unable to easily penetrate biological membranes. Within the body, the acidic secretory canaliculi of gastric parietal cells provide an environment with a pH of less than 4. Consequently, omeprazole exhibits selective accumulation within these secretory canaliculi of gastric parietal cells.

The activation process of omeprazole, specifically through the Smiles rearrangement, is driven by the nucleophilic attack of the unprotonated nitrogen on the 2-position of the benzimidazole ring. This ultimately leads to the formation of the active form, which consists of a sulfenic acid and a sulfinamide moiety within the spirocyclic intermediate. Sulfenic acid and sulfinamide exhibit stability in acidic environments, but their high polarity hinders their diffusion across biological membranes. They exhibit high reactivity with endogenous substances containing thiol groups and although they do not possess drug-like properties, they serve as ideal active intermediates.

22.3.2 The synthesis process of omeprazole

The structure of omeprazole can be divided into three components: a tetrasubstituted pyridine structure, a methoxy-substituted benzimidazole structure, and a sulfur-containing methylsulfinyl group. The synthesis process of omeprazole involves the key intermediate 5-methoxy-2-[(3,5-dimethyl-4-methoxy-2-pyridinyl) methylthio]-1H-benzimidazole (III) in thioether form. The synthesis process of omeprazole involves the formation of a thioether and the oxidation of the thioether. In the commonly used synthetic route for industrial production, the thioether structure (III) is obtained through a Williamson reaction between benzimidazole-2-thiol and pyridine halide under alkaline conditions, followed by oxidation to yield omeprazole.

22.3.2.1 The synthesis of the thioether

The thioether intermediate (III) can be synthesized through the condensation of 5-methoxy-1H-benzimidazole-2-thiol (I) and 2-chloromethyl-4-methoxy-3,5-dimethylpyridine hydrochloride (II).

22.3.2.1.1 Synthesis of compound I

The synthesis of compound I involves the following steps using 5-methoxy-1H-benzimidazole-2-thiol (I-1) as the starting material: firstly, I-1 undergoes an acetylation process to protect the amino group using acetic anhydride as the acylating reagent. Subsequently, a nitration reaction is carried out to introduce a nitro group at the 2-position of the benzene ring, resulting in the formation of 4-methoxy-2-nitroacetanilide (I-2). Under alkaline conditions, the amino group is deacetylated to obtain 4-methoxy-2-nitroaniline (I-3). Then, using stannous chloride as a reducing agent, the nitro group is reduced to yield 4-methoxy-1,2-phenylenediamine (I-4). In the final step, a cyclization reaction takes place in a mixture of carbon disulfide and potassium hydroxide in ethanol, leading to the formation of 5-methoxy-1H-benzimidazole-2-thiol (I). Alternatively, this step can also be directly performed using potassium ethoxide and sulfonyl chloride.

22.3.2.1.2 Synthesis of compound II

The synthesis of 2-chloromethyl-4-methoxy-3,5-dimethylpyridine hydrochloride (II) can proceed via two routes, using either 2,3,5-trimethylpyridine (II-1) or 3,5-dimethylpyridine (II-6) the starting materials.

Route 1: Starting with 2,3,5-trimethylpyridine (II-1), oxidation occurs with hydrogen peroxide as the oxidizing agent, forming 2,3,5-trimethylpyridine-N-oxide (II-2). A nitration reaction takes place in a mixed acid solution composed of nitric acid and concentrated sulfuric acid, introducing a nitro group at the 4-position of the pyridine ring, yielding 4-nitro-2,3,5-trimethylpyridine N-oxide (II-3). Subsequently, nucleophilic substitution occurs with sodium methoxide, where the nitro group is replaced by a methoxy group, resulting in the formation of 4-methoxy-2,3,5-trimethylpyridine N-oxide (II-4). Under the influence of acetic anhydride in the Boekelheide rearrangement reaction, 3,5-dimethyl-2-hydroxymethyl-4-methoxy-pyridine (II-5) is produced. Finally, using sulfonyl chloride as the chlorinating agent, 2-chloromethyl-4-methoxy-3,5-dimethylpyridine hydrochloride (II) is obtained. This synthetic route is widely employed in industrial production due to the ready availability of starting materials and reagents, mild reaction conditions, and high overall yield.

Route 2: The route described employs 3,5-dimethylpyridine (II-6) as the initial substrate, following a similar process to route 1. 3,5-dimethylpyridine (II-6) undergoes oxidation, nitration, and methoxy substitution, resulting in the formation of 4-methoxy-3,5-dimethylpyridine N-oxide (II-9). The Boekelheide rearrangement reaction takes place with dimethyl sulfate and ammonium persulfate, yielding 3,5-dimethyl-2-hydroxymethyl-4-methoxy-pyridine (II-5). Finally, through a chlorination reaction, compound (II) is generated. This synthetic route was previously employed in the early production of omeprazole. However, due to the use of highly toxic dimethyl sulfate and its relatively low yield, it has been replaced by route 1.

22.3.2.1.3 Synthesis of thioether compound III

The compound 5-methoxy-1H-benzimidazole-2-thiol (I) reacts with sodium hydroxide to form the sodium thiolate. The sodium thiolate then undergoes a Williamson reaction with 2-chloromethyl-4-methoxy-3,5-dimethylpyridine hydrochloride (II) to condense and produce 5-methoxy-2-[(3,5-dimethyl-4-methoxy-2-pyridinyl) methylthio]-1H-benzimidazole (III), which possesses a thioether moiety.

22.3.2.2 The oxidation of the thioether

The thioether compound III can be oxidized to a sulfoxide by using an oxidizing agent, such as *meta*-chloroperbenzoic acid. This reaction produces an achiral form of omeprazole. The sulfoxide structure of omeprazole is chiral, and its *S*-isomer, esomeprazole, is also a highly potent marketed drug. The synthesis process of esomeprazole primarily involves the asymmetric oxidation of the thioether compound III catalyzed by chiral catalysts. Further details on this process are beyond the scope of this discussion.

22.3.3 Structure-activity relationship of proton pump inhibitors

The molecular structure of benzimidazole PPIs can be roughly divided into three parts (Fig. 22.11): the substituted pyridine ring, the substituted benzimidazole ring, and the methyl sulfonyl linker.

22.3.3.1 The substituted pyridine ring

The most potent activity is observed with a substituent at the 2-position on the pyridine ring. The potency decreases when nitrogen oxide is introduced to the pyridine when using 4-pyridine, or single heterocycles such as thiazole, imidazole, and quinoline, as well as fused heterocycles such as quinoline and benzimidazole. The pK_a of the pyridine ring affects the degree of accumulation and onset speed of the drug in the gastric parietal cells. Introducing electron-donating groups can increase the electron density of the pyridine ring, which in turn elevates its pK_a. A higher pK_a facilitates faster and more concentrated drug accumulation in the gastric epithelial cells, reducing the onset time and enhancing the acid-suppressing potency. The introduction of electron-donating groups such as alkyl and alkoxy substituents at the 3-, 4-, and 5-positions on the pyridine ring is beneficial for augmenting activity. Conversely, substituents at the 6-position of the pyridine ring hinder the formation of spirocyclic intermediates due to steric hindrance.

22.3.3.2 The substituted benzimidazole ring

1*H*-1,3-benzimidazole is the most active and maintains some efficacy when substituted with dihydrothiazole, imidazole, or imidazopyridine heterocycles. During the reaction, the carbon atom at the 2-position of the benzimidazole ring undergoes nucleophilic attack by the unprotonated nitrogen atom on the pyridine ring, forming an active intermediate.

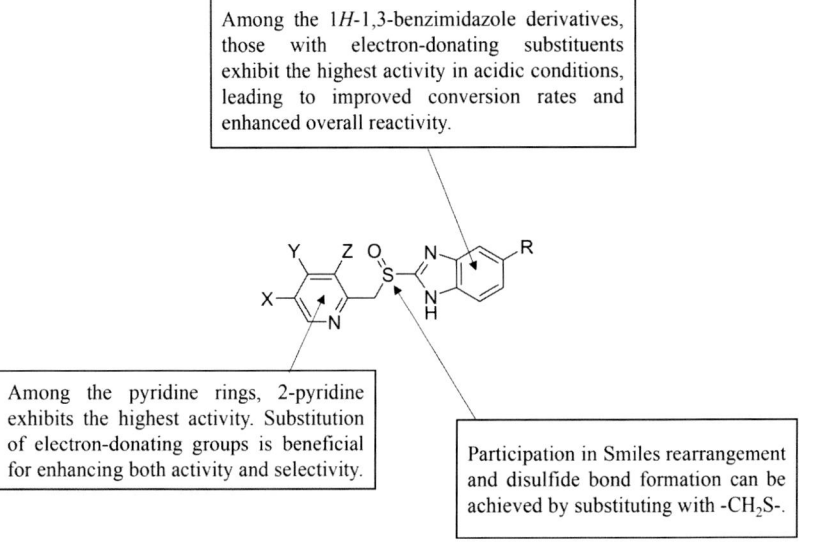

FIGURE 22.11 Structure-activity relationship of omeprazole.

Incorporating electron-withdrawing groups onto the benzimidazole ring indeed enhances the electrophilicity of the carbon atom at the 2-position, facilitating the Smiles rearrangement reaction. However, this modification may lead to premature consumption of the drug in the nonacidic environment before entering the gastric parietal cells, resulting in an overall decrease in effectiveness. On the other hand, electron-donating groups at the 6-position increase the pK_a of the nitrogen atom on the imidazole ring, making it more prone to protonation under acidic conditions. This further intensifies the electrophilicity of the carbon atom at the 2-position, enhancing the acid-catalyzed conversion rate and elevating the drug's potency.

22.3.3.3 The methyl sulfonyl linker

Activity can be sustained to some extent when the methyl sulfonyl linker in the PPI structure is replaced by -CH$_2$S-, -CH$_2$-, and -SCH$_2$- groups.

22.4 Clinical applications of omeprazole

22.4.1 The clinical indications and safety of omeprazole

22.4.1.1 The clinical indications of omeprazole

The clinical indications of omeprazole include:

22.4.1.1.1 Peptic ulcer

Omeprazole is typically prescribed at a standard dose of 20 mg/day to alleviate ulcer pain and promote healing. The treatment duration for DUs is typically 4–6 weeks, while GUs may require 6–8 weeks of treatment. In some cases, long-term maintenance therapy may be necessary to prevent ulcer recurrence. For patients with digestive ulcers who test positive for Hp infection, eradicating the bacteria should be prioritized. The eradication treatment can be administered concurrently with acid suppression therapy for a duration of 4 to 8 weeks or initiated after completing the acid suppression treatment. In cases of NSAID-related digestive ulcers, discontinuing the use of NSAIDs or opting for selective cyclooxygenase-2 inhibitors is recommended. For digestive ulcers associated with gastrinoma, the treatment involves using a double standard dose, administered twice daily [56].

22.4.1.1.2 *Helicobacter pylori* infection

Currently, the standard dosage of omeprazole combined with bismuth and two antibiotics, known as the "quadruple therapy," is considered the first-line treatment for Hp infection in China. The treatment duration is typically 10 or 14 days [57,58].

22.4.1.1.3 Nonsteroidal antiinflammatory drug-related gastrointestinal injury

The standard duration of omeprazole treatment is typically 4 to 8 weeks, prescribed for the management of gastrointestinal discomfort, GUs, and bleeding associated with NSAIDs. For patients requiring long-term NSAID use, omeprazole maintenance therapy is recommended to prevent gastrointestinal injury.

22.4.1.1.4 Gastroesophageal reflux disease

Gastroesophageal reflux disease (GERD) can be classified into reflux esophagitis, which refers to erosive esophagitis, and nonerosive reflux disease (NERD). Omeprazole is indicated for the treatment of erosive esophagitis, NERD characterized by excessive acid or acid sensitivity, gastroesophageal reflux disease with clearly defined extraesophageal symptoms, as well as the management of concurrent esophageal strictures and Barrett's esophagus. The recommended daily dosage of omeprazole is 20–60 mg, administered once daily, for a duration of 4–8 weeks [59–62].

22.4.1.1.5 Eosinophilic esophagitis

Eosinophilic esophagitis (EoE) is a chronic inflammation of the esophagus characterized by infiltration of eosinophilic granulocytes. Approximately 30%–50% of patients with EoE experience improvement in symptoms after treatment with PPI, which is referred to as PPI-responsive eosinophilic esophagitis [63,64].

22.4.1.1.6 Zollinger-Ellison syndrome

Zollinger-Ellison syndrome is a functional pancreatic neuroendocrine tumor characterized by elevated levels of gastrin in the bloodstream. Clinical manifestations primarily include a series of symptoms caused by high gastric acid levels, such as refractory PUs, gastroesophageal reflux disease, and diarrhea. The initial dosage of omeprazole for Zollinger-Ellison syndrome is 60 mg per dose, administered once daily, with dose adjustments made according to individual needs to control gastric acid secretion [65].

22.4.1.1.7 Prevention of stress ulcers

For critically ill patients, especially those on long-term mechanical ventilation and with coagulation disorders, intravenous administration of high-dose omeprazole is recommended as a prophylactic measure against stress ulcer development [66].

22.4.1.1.8 Functional dyspepsia

For patients presenting with abdominal pain and a burning sensation, standard-dose omeprazole is recommended for short-term treatment [67].

22.4.1.2 The safety of omeprazole

Omeprazole generally has a favorable safety profile. Common adverse reactions include headache, diarrhea, abdominal pain, nausea, and constipation, with an incidence rate of 1%−3%. These symptoms are usually mild and self-limiting. However, severe adverse reactions such as anaphylactic shock, lupus erythematosus, acute interstitial nephritis, and rhabdomyolysis are rare but possible. With the widespread use of omeprazole in recent years, drug-drug interactions and potential adverse reactions have also been a focus of concern. Coadministration of omeprazole with clopidogrel can impair the metabolism of the latter into its active form, reducing its therapeutic efficacy and increasing the risk of cardiovascular events. Omeprazole reduces gastric acidity, leading to decreased absorption of ketoconazole and itraconazole. It also inhibits certain cytochrome P450 enzymes, which can slow down the hepatic metabolism of drugs such as warfarin, diazepam, and phenytoin. Long-term treatment with omeprazole can maintain a higher gastric pH level, affecting the absorption of vitamin B_{12}, iron, and magnesium, resulting in vitamin B_{12} deficiency, iron-deficiency anemia, and hypomagnesemia. Omeprazole stimulates the release of gastrin via positive feedback regulation, leading to hypergastrinemia, which further contributes to gastric polyps and carcinoid tumors. It weakens the bactericidal effect against bacteria and pathogenic microorganisms, causing dysbiosis of the intestinal flora and increasing the risk of intestinal infections. The reduced gastric acidity promotes the proliferation of gastric bacteria, and when gastroesophageal reflux or therapeutic interventions occur, bacteria-containing gastric contents can invade the respiratory tract, triggering respiratory infections and increasing the incidence of community-acquired pneumonia [68−71].

22.4.2 Omeprazole and esomeprazole

After oral administration, omeprazole exhibits a significant first-pass effect, resulting in low oral bioavailability. Furthermore, there are notable variations in the pharmacokinetic properties and therapeutic effects of this medication among individuals. Consequently, in 1989, Astra initiated a novel acid-suppressing drug development project with the objective of identifying a compound that would possess lower hepatic clearance and higher oral bioavailability in comparison to omeprazole. Over the course of 1989−1994, more than 30 scientists synthesized hundreds of compounds, ultimately selecting four for preclinical research. Through a comprehensive evaluation of their pharmacokinetic properties, potency in suppressing acid, and safety, only one compound exhibited properties superior to omeprazole. This compound is known as esomeprazole, which is the *S*-isomer of omeprazole and is marketed as Nexium [53]. Esomeprazole demonstrates a reduced hepatic clearance compared to omeprazole, along with an increased oral bioavailability, resulting in a significant improvement in interindividual variability.

Omeprazole consists of a chiral sulfur atom, resulting in the presence of two enantiomers: *R*- and *S*-omeprazole. Both *R*- and *S*-omeprazole undergo protonation-induced rearrangement in acidic environments, leading to the formation of nonchiral sulfenic acid and sulfenamide, which share the same mechanism of action on the proton pump. Within the human body, however, due to the differential stereoselectivity of cytochrome P450 isozymes, *R*- and *S*-omeprazole exhibit distinct pharmacokinetic properties and pharmacological effects. Approximately 98% of *R*-omeprazole is metabolized by CYP2C19 to form 5-hydroxylated and 5′-demethylated products, while 2% is metabolized by CYP3A4 to yield a sulfone. On the other hand, *S*-omeprazole is metabolized by CYP2C19 (73%) and CYP3A4 (27%) (Fig. 22.12). The overall hepatic clearance rate of *S*-omeprazole in liver microsomes is significantly lower, approximately only one-third of the *R*-isomer (Fig. 22.13).

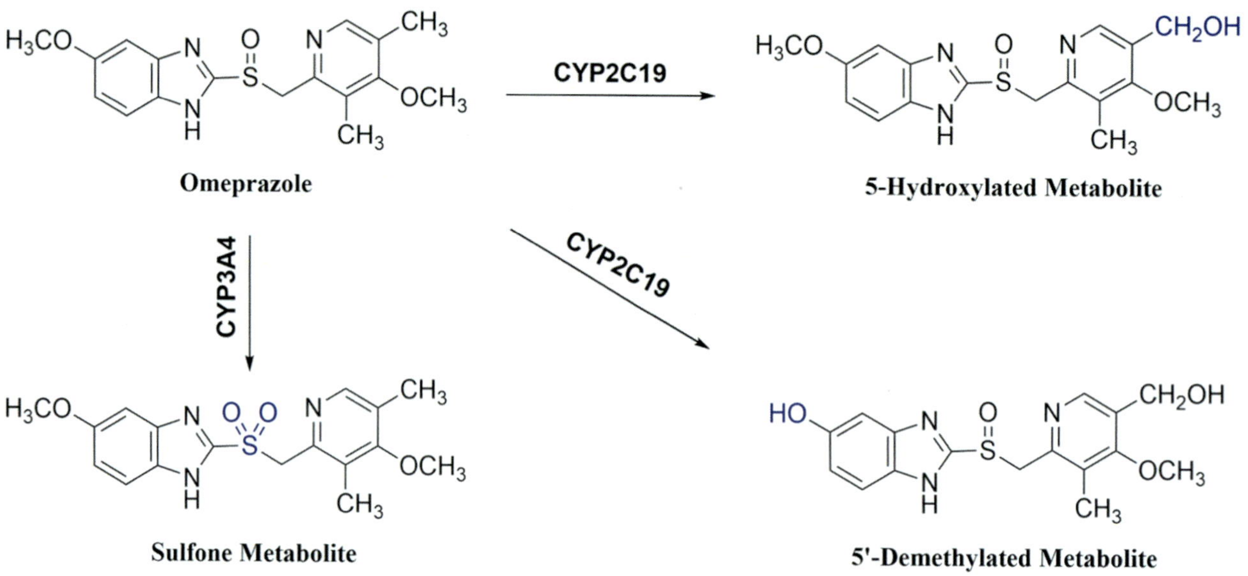

FIGURE 22.12 Metabolites of omeprazole.

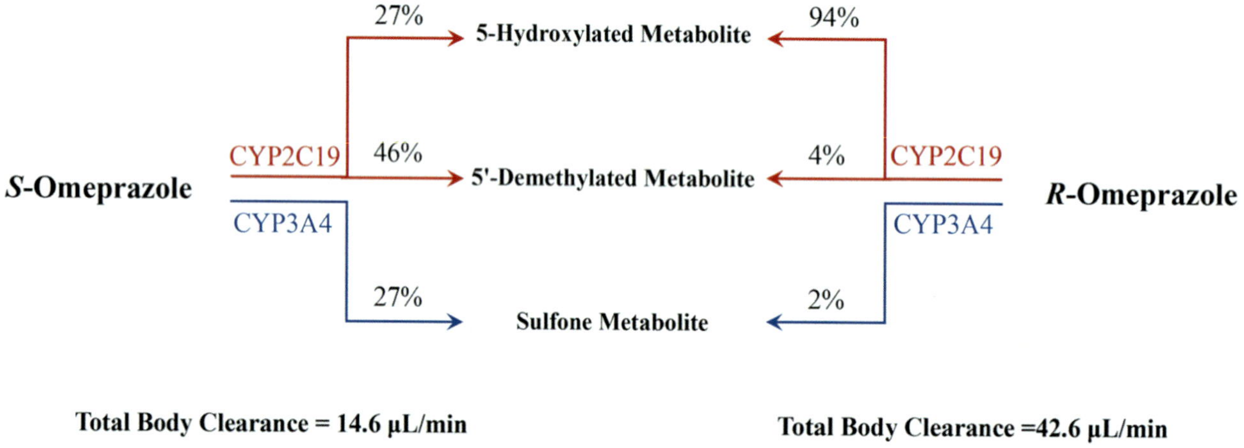

FIGURE 22.13 Metabolic differences of omeprazole and esomeprazole by P450 isoenzymes.

The cytochrome P450 enzyme CYP2C19 exhibits nucleotide polymorphism, which can be classified into poor metabolizer (PM), intermediate metabolizer, extensive metabolizer (EM), and ultrarapid metabolizer based on different alleles. As the names suggest, these variations significantly influence individual responses to omeprazole treatment. Clinical data has shown that for EMs, the steady-state blood drug concentration of S-omeprazole has an area under the concentration-time curve (AUC) that is twice that of the racemic mixture, whereas for R-omeprazole, the AUC is 4.5 times higher. In slow metabolizers, the AUC for S-omeprazole is only half that of R-omeprazole. The ratio of AUC between S-omeprazole and R-omeprazole in slow and EMs is 3 and 7.5, respectively, indicating that S-omeprazole exhibits less interindividual variability compared to the R-isomer [72]. The proportion of PMs with suboptimal performance of S-omeprazole is relatively small in the population, ranging from 1.2% to 3.8% in European Caucasians, approximately 23% in Asians, and 4% in African Americans [73].

Esomeprazole is currently employed in clinical practice for the treatment of acid-related disorders, including gastroesophageal reflux disease, Zollinger-Ellison syndrome, GUs, and DUs. It is also utilized in combination with antibiotics to aid in the management of Hp infection. Furthermore, it plays a role in the prevention and treatment of NSAID-induced GUs [74].

22.5 Summary and knowledge expansion

22.5.1 Chapter summary

This chapter provides an in-depth overview of the development process of omeprazole. The discovery of esomeprazole was limited by the technological capabilities of the time and relied on traditional methods of drug design, which depended on the intuition, experience, and chemical knowledge of the drug designers. Throughout this process, the research team encountered a series of challenges, including an unknown target, adverse reactions of lead compounds, patent disputes, and clinical setbacks, encompassing almost all possible issues that can arise during drug development. In response to these challenges, the development of omeprazole exemplifies some effective methods that may not be universally applicable but have proven successful. For compounds with unknown targets, direct in vivo activity testing can be conducted. In the case of adverse reactions of lead compounds, acute toxicity testing can be prioritized before activity screening. When the structure of a compound is protected by patents, attention can be directed toward its metabolites. Now standing in the era of rational drug design, we look back at this story where unexpected events coexisted with opportunities and hope to bring inspiration to readers.

22.5.2 Expansion of knowledge: the patent portfolio of omeprazole

Drugs, being a unique type of commodity, necessitate a development process that goes beyond merely focusing on their safety and therapeutic efficacy. Ensuring the protection of compound rights and expanding their commercial value becomes paramount when it comes to the successful development of a pharmaceutical product. AstraZeneca has executed a comprehensive patent strategy for omeprazole (trade name: Losec), aiming to maximize the protection of its patent rights and commercial value. This serves as an illustrative example of AstraZeneca's patent strategy in the United States.

22.5.2.1 Patent network strategy

Table 22.5 enumerates the Losec patents documented in the Orange Book of the United States, along with their respective expiration dates. AstraZeneca has strategically established a comprehensive patent network centered around

TABLE 22.5 The Losec patents documented in the Orange Book published by the FDA.

No.	Patent number	Patent type	Patent term
1	US4255431A	Compound	October 5, 2001
2	US4544750A	Intermediate	February 26, 2004
3	US4738974A	Alkali salt	October 19, 2007
4	US4636499A	Metabolite	November 30, 2005
5	US4786505A	Dosage form	October 20, 2007
6	US4853230A	Dosage form	October 20, 2007
7	US5093342A	Usage	August 2, 2010
8	US5386032A	Preparation method	July 31, 2012
9	US5599794A	Composition	August 4, 2014
10	US5629305A	Composition	August 4, 2014
11	US6147103A	Preparation method and composition	April 9, 2019
12	US6150380A	Crystal form	May 10, 2019
13	US6166213A	Preparation method and composition	April 9, 2019
14	US6191148B1	Preparation method and composition	April 9, 2019
15	US5690960A	Dosage form	November 25, 2014
16	US5900424A	Magnesium salt	May 4, 2016
17	US6428810B1	Dosage form	November 3, 2019

omeprazole compounds, including peripheral patents related to formulations and preparation methods. This strategic approach ensures the establishment of patent barriers for competitors and prolongs AstraZeneca's monopolistic position in the realms of patents and the market even after the expiration of the core patent. The patent protection coverage is extensive, encompassing various domains such as compounds, intermediates, formulations, preparation methods, combinations, crystal forms, and more, thereby averting potential breakthroughs by competitors in vulnerable aspects. Despite the gradual narrowing of rights protection as patents expire, this strategy has resulted in several years, and even up to an extended period of 18 years, of patent extension for critical knowledge assets. It has created valuable strategic opportunities for subsequent research and technology transfer. The following provides a specific overview.

The core patent of omeprazole is Patent No.1 filed on April 5, 1979. Through the approval of the patent term extension (PTE) system in the United States, it obtained a 2-year extension, extending the patent term to April 5, 2001. Later on, it received an additional 6-month pediatric exclusivity period for completing FDA-designated pediatric clinical trials, further extending the US patent to October 5, 2001. The PTE system aims to compensate for the patent term loss incurred during the drug approval process, caused by administrative review, for a particular active patent of a marketed drug. This system is implemented in both China and the United States. AstraZeneca has benefited from this system, not only gaining direct economic benefits from the 2-year patent extension but also strategically safeguarding the market share of their newly developed drug, esomeprazole (marketed as "Nexium"), which was launched in Sweden in 2000 and in the United States in 2001. Without the extension, even with the protection of peripheral patents, generic competition could have eroded omeprazole's market share, impacting the launch of esomeprazole. The pediatric exclusivity system is unique to the United States and aims to ensure the safety of medications for children. Patents 1−14 in Table 22.5 all enjoy a 6-month pediatric exclusivity period.

22.5.2.2 Product line extension strategy

The product line extension strategy involves making slight modifications to an existing drug to create a second-generation branded medication while applying for downstream patents to further strengthen the patent portfolio. AstraZeneca applied this strategy when they developed the *S*-isomer of omeprazole, known as esomeprazole, which was first launched in Sweden in 2000 and later in the United States in 2001. Despite clinical trial data indicating only a 3% improvement compared to omeprazole, AstraZeneca's successful marketing strategy enabled esomeprazole to successfully retain the market share of omeprazole [75].

AstraZeneca also pursued adjustments in dosage forms, salt forms, and dosage specifications to actively seek market exclusivity and expand the scope of patent protection. For example, in the U.S. market from 1989 to 1998, they launched omeprazole enteric capsules in three specifications: 10, 20, and 40 mg. In 2001, they introduced esomeprazole sodium enteric capsules in the 20 and 40 mg specifications. In 2005, esomeprazole sodium injection became available in the 20 and 40 mg specifications. Furthermore, in 2006, esomeprazole magnesium suspension was launched in the 20 and 40 mg specifications, followed by the introduction of esomeprazole magnesium oral suspension in the 2.5 and 5 mg specifications in 2011.

References

[1] Lanas A, Chan FKL. Peptic ulcer disease. Lancet 2017;390(10094):613−24.

[2] Marshall BJ, Warren JR. Unidentified curved bacilli in the stomach of patients with gastritis and peptic ulceration. Lancet 1984;1(8390):1311−15.

[3] Geibel JP, Wagner C. An update on acid secretion. Rev Physiol Biochem Pharmacol 2006;156:45−60.

[4] Sakai H, Fujii T, Takeguchi N. Proton-potassium (H + /K +) ATPases: properties and roles in health and diseases. In: Sigel A, Sigel H, Sigel RKO, editors. The alkali metal ions: their role for life. Cham: Springer International Publishing; 2016. p. 459−83.

[5] Schubert ML. Physiologic, pathophysiologic, and pharmacologic regulation of gastric acid secretion. Curr Opin Gastroenterol 2017;33(6):430−8.

[6] Gillen D, El-Omar EM, Wirz AA, et al. The acid response to gastrin distinguishes duodenal ulcer patients from *Helicobacter pylori*-infected healthy subjects. Gastroenterology 1998;114(1):50−7.

[7] Amano K. Numerical variation of parietal cells after vagotomy in cases of duodenal ulcer. Tohoku J Exp Med 1981;135(2):165−78.

[8] Yu LQ. Advances in research on *Helicobacter pylori*. Chin J Prev Control Chronic Dis 2010;18(02):218−19.

[9] Malfertheiner P, Chan FK, Mccoll KE. Peptic ulcer disease. Lancet 2009;374(9699):1449−61.

[10] Johnson KS, Ottemann KM. Colonization, localization, and inflammation: the roles of *H. pylori* chemotaxis in vivo. Curr Opin Microbiol 2018;41:51−7.

[11] Hu FL. Pathogenic factors of *Helicobacter pylori* and gastric mucosal barrier. Clin Medication J 2007;03:1−4.

[12] Lehours P, Ferrero RL. Review: helicobacter: inflammation, immunology, and vaccines. Helicobacter 2019;24(Suppl 1)e12644.

[13] Graham DY, Go MF, Lew GM, et al. *Helicobacter pylori* infection and exaggerated gastrin release. Effects of inflammation and progastrin processing. Scand J Gastroenterol 1993;28(8):690–4.
[14] Walker MM, Crabtree JE. *Helicobacter pylori* infection and the pathogenesis of duodenal ulceration. Ann N Y Acad Sci 1998;859:96–111.
[15] Zaki M, Coudron PE, Mccuen RW, et al. *H. pylori* acutely inhibits gastric secretion by activating CGRP sensory neurons coupled to stimulation of somatostatin and inhibition of histamine secretion. Am J Physiol Gastrointest Liver Physiol 2013;304(8):715–22.
[16] Olbe L, Hamlet A, Dalenback J, et al. A mechanism by which *Helicobacter pylori* infection of the antrum contributes to the development of duodenal ulcer. Gastroenterology 1996;110(5):1386–94.
[17] Waldum HL, Kleveland PM, Sordal OF. *Helicobacter pylori* and gastric acid: an intimate and reciprocal relationship. Ther Adv Gastroenterol 2016;9(6):836–44.
[18] El-Omar EM, Oien K, El-Nujumi A, et al. *Helicobacter pylori* infection and chronic gastric acid hyposecretion. Gastroenterology 1997;113(1):15–24.
[19] Naumann M, Sokolova O, Tegtmeyer N, et al. *Helicobacter pylori*: a paradigm pathogen for subverting host cell signal transmission. Trends Microbiol 2017;25(4):316–28.
[20] Kim N. Immunological reactions on *H. pylori* infection. In: Kim N, editor. Helicobacter pylori. Singapore: Springer Singapore; 2016. p. 35–52.
[21] Huang JQ, Sridhar S, Hunt RH. Role of *Helicobacter pylori* infection and non-steroidal anti-inflammatory drugs in peptic-ulcer disease: a meta-analysis. Lancet 2002;359(9300):14–22.
[22] Bjarnason I, Scarpignato C, Takeuchi K, et al. Determinants of the short-term gastric damage caused by NSAIDs in man. Aliment Pharmacol Ther 2007;26(1):95–106.
[23] Bjarnason I, Scarpignato C, Holmgren E, et al. Mechanisms of damage to the gastrointestinal tract from nonsteroidal anti-inflammatory drugs. Gastroenterology 2018;154(3):500–14.
[24] Bindu S, Mazumder S, Bandyopadhyay U. Non-steroidal anti-inflammatory drugs (NSAIDs) and organ damage: a current perspective. Biochem Pharmacol 2020;180(114147):1–21.
[25] Kanno T, Iijima K, Abe Y, et al. A multicenter prospective study on the prevalence of *Helicobacter pylori*-negative and nonsteroidal anti-inflammatory drugs-negative idiopathic peptic ulcers in Japan. J Gastroenterol Hepatol 2015;30(5):842–8.
[26] Chung WC, Jeon EJ, Kim DB, et al. Clinical characteristics of *Helicobacter pylori*-negative drug-negative peptic ulcer bleeding. World J Gastroenterol 2015;21(28):8636–43.
[27] Charpignon C, Lesgourgues B, Pariente A, et al. Peptic ulcer disease: one in five is related to neither *Helicobacter pylori* nor aspirin/NSAID intake. Aliment Pharmacol Ther 2013;38(8):946–54.
[28] Sbrozzi-Vanni A, Zullo A, Di Giulio E, et al. Low prevalence of idiopathic peptic ulcer disease: an Italian endoscopic survey. Dig Liver Dis 2010;42(11):773–6.
[29] Jang HJ, Choi MH, Shin WG, et al. Has peptic ulcer disease changed during the past ten years in Korea? A prospective multi-center study. Dig Dis Sci 2008;53(6):1527–31.
[30] Konturek SJ, Bielanski W, Plonka M, et al. *Helicobacter pylori*, non-steroidal anti-inflammatory drugs and smoking in risk pattern of gastroduodenal ulcers. Scand J Gastroenterol 2003;38(9):923–30.
[31] Chung C-S, Chiang T-H, Lee Y-C. A systematic approach for the diagnosis and treatment of idiopathic peptic ulcers. Korean J Intern Med 2015;30(5):559–70.
[32] Satoh H. Discovery of lansoprazole and its unique pharmacological properties independent from anti-secretory activity. Curr Pharm Des 2013;19(1):67–75.
[33] Bardou M, Martin J. Pantoprazole: from drug metabolism to clinical relevance. Expert Opin Drug Metab Toxicol 2008;4(4):471–83.
[34] Marelli S, Pace F. Rabeprazole for the treatment of acid-related disorders. Expert Rev Gastroenterol Hepatol 2012;6(4):423–35.
[35] Yuan H. Guiding principles for clinical application of proton pump inhibitors in hunan province (trial). Cent South Pharm 2016;14(07):673–83.
[36] Jiao HW, Sun LN, Li YQ, et al. Safety, pharmacokinetics, and pharmacodynamics of S-(-)-pantoprazole sodium injections after single and multiple intravenous doses in healthy Chinese subjects. Eur J Clin Pharmacol 2018;74(3):257–65.
[37] Ji XQ, Du JF, Chen G, et al. Efficacy of ilaprazole in the treatment of duodenal ulcers: a meta-analysis. World J Gastroenterol.2014;20(17):5119–23.
[38] Zhou LJ, Li JL, Zhang ZQ. Research progress of a new proton pump inhibitor- ilaprazole. Med Recapitulate 2012;18(10):1550–2.
[39] Hou XM, Wang XH, Yin X, et al. Physicochemical properties of ilaprazole sodium. Pharm Today 2013;23(03):132–134 + 141.
[40] Metz DC, Vakily M, Dixit T, et al. Review article: dual delayed release formulation of dexlansoprazole MR, a novel approach to overcome the limitations of conventional single release proton pump inhibitor therapy. Aliment Pharm Ther 2009;29(9):928–37.
[41] Abe K, Irie K, Nakanishi H, et al. Crystal structures of the gastric proton pump. Nature 2018;556(7700):214–18.
[42] Abe K, Tani K, Fujiyoshi Y. Systematic comparison of molecular conformations of H + , K + -ATPase reveals an important contribution of the A-M2 linker for the luminal gating. J Biol Chem 2014;289(44):30590–601.
[43] Dyla M, Kjaergaard M, Poulsen H, et al. Structure and mechanism of P-type ATPase ion pumps. Annu Rev Biochem 2020;89:583–603.
[44] Forte JG, Zhu L. Apical recycling of the gastric parietal cell H, K-ATPase. Annu Rev Physiol 2010;72:273–96.
[45] Peng GX, Li ZS, Tu ZX. Research progress of gastric proton pump. Foreign Med Sci (Sect Medgeography) 2005;02:83–5.
[46] Engevik AC, Kaji I, Goldenring JR. The physiology of the gastric parietal cell. Physiol Rev 2020;100(2):573–602.
[47] Li YM. Advances in cellular and molecular biology of gastric parietal cells and proton pumps. Foreign Med Sci (Sect Medgeography) 2002;03:140–2.
[48] Malen CE, Danree BH. New thiocarboxamides derivatives with specific gastric antisecretory properties. J Med Chem 1971;14(3):244–6.

[49] Lindberg P, Brändström A, Wallmark B, et al. Omeprazole: the first proton pump inhibitor. Med Res Rev 1990;10(1):1−54.
[50] Zhang ML, Sugawa H, Mori T. Inhibition of thyrocyte iodide uptake by H + K + ATPase inhibitor, timoprazole. Endocr J 1995;42(4):489−96.
[51] Larsson H, Carlsson E, Mattsson H, et al. Plasma gastrin and gastric enterochromaffinlike cell activation and proliferation. Studies with omeprazole and ranitidine in intact and antrectomized rats. Gastroenterology 1986;90(2):391−9.
[52] Mattsson H, Havu N, Bräutigam J, et al. Partial gastric corpectomy results in hypergastrinemia and development of gastric enterochromaffinlike-cell carcinoids in the rat. Gastroenterology 1991;100(2):311−19.
[53] Olbe L, Carlsson E, Lindberg P. A proton-pump inhibitor expedition: the case histories of omeprazole and esomeprazole. Nat Rev Drug Discov 2003;2(2):132−9.
[54] Sjöstrand SE, Olbe L, Fellenius E. The discovery and development of the proton pump inhibitor. In: Olbe L, editor. Proton pump inhibitors. Basel: Birkhäuser Basel; 1999. p. 3−20.
[55] Shin JM, Cho YM, Sachs G. Chemistry of covalent inhibition of the gastric (H + , K +)-ATPase by proton pump inhibitors. J Am Chem Soc 2004;126(25):7800−11.
[56] Yuan ZQ, Wang ZZ. Standardized diagnosis and treatment of peptic ulcer (2016, Xi'an). Chin J Digestion 2016;36(08):508−13.
[57] Chinese Society Of Gastroenterology, Chinese Study Group On Helicobacter pylori and peptic ulcer, Liu WZ, et al. Fifth Chinese national consensus report on the management of *Helicobacter pylori* infection. Chin J Intern Med 2017;56(07):532−45.
[58] Chi ZC. Update on prevention and treatment of *Helicobacter pylori* infection. World Chin J Digestol 2016;24(16):2454−62.
[59] Savarino V, Marabotto E, Zentilin P, et al. Proton pump inhibitors: use and misuse in the clinical setting. Expert Rev Clin Pharmacol 2018;11 (11):1123−34.
[60] Farrell B, Pottie K, Thompson W, et al. Deprescribing proton pump inhibitors: evidence-based clinical practice guideline. Can Fam Physician 2017;63(5):354−64.
[61] Chinese Society of Gastroenterology. Expert consensus opinion on gastroesophageal reflux disease in China in 2014. Chin J Gastroenterol, 2015, 20(03):155−168.
[62] Society of Gastroesophageal Reflux Disease, China International Exchange and Promotive Association for Medical and Health Care. Chinese consensus on multidisciplinary diagnosis and treatment of gastroesophageal reflux disease. Chin J Front Med Sci (Electronic Version), 2019, 11 (09):30−56.
[63] Guo CJ, Lin SR. Eosinophilic esophagitis. Chin J Pract Intern Med 2008;09:784−6.
[64] Li JS. ACG clinical guideline: diagnosis and treatment of eosinophilic esophagitis 2013 Chin J Gastroenterol Hepatol 2014;23(07):721−2.
[65] Expert Committee on Neuroendocrine Neoplasms, Chinese Society of Clinical Oncology. Chinese expert consensus on gastroenteropancreatic neuroendocrine tumors (2016 Edition). Chin Clin Oncol 2016; 21(10):927−946.
[66] Bai Y, Li YQ, Ren X, et al. Expert advice on prevention and treatment of stress ulcer (2018 Edition). Natl Med J China 2018;98(42):3392−5.
[67] Chen ZS. Consensus on diagnosis and treatment of functional dyspepsia with integrated traditional Chinese and western medicine (2010). Chin J Integr Traditional West Med 2011;31(11):1545−9.
[68] Mctavish D, Buckley MM, Heel RC. Omeprazole. An updated review of its pharmacology and therapeutic use in acid-related disorders. Drugs 1991;42(1):138−70.
[69] Vaezi MF, Yang YX, Howden CW. Complications of proton pump inhibitor therapy. Gastroenterology 2017;153(1):35−48.
[70] Shi XX, Zhen SB. Research progress on application safety of long-term proton pump inhibitor. Chin J N Drugs Clin Remedies 2016;35 (06):387−92.
[71] Liu F, Zhen SB. Focus on safety of proton pump inhibitors. Chin J N Drugs Clin Remedies 2012;31(09):493−8.
[72] Andersson T, Weidolf L. Stereoselective disposition of proton pump inhibitors. Clin Drug Investig 2008;28(5):263−79.
[73] Li XW, Zhen SB. Advances in *CYP2C*19 gene polymorphism and its impact on efficacy of proton pump inhibitor. Chin J N Drugs Clin Remedies 2013;32(10):775−9.
[74] Mckeage K, Blick SKA, Croxtall JD, et al. Esomeprazole: a review of its use in the management of gastric acid-related diseases in adults. Drugs 2008;68(11):1571−607.
[75] Sha YH, Li YD, Yang Y. Analysis of omeprazole intellectual property protection strategy. Chin J N Drugs 2013;22(06):624−8.

Chapter 23

The inhibitors of phosphodiesterase type 5A effectively treat erectile dysfunction

Lei Guo[1] and Hai-Bin Luo[2]

[1]School of Pharmaceutical Sciences, Sun Yat-Sen University, Guangzhou, P.R. China, [2]School of Pharmaceutical Sciences, Hainan University, Haikou, P.R. China

Chapter outline

- 23.1 The nitric oxide-cyclic guanosine monophosphate signaling pathway associated with penile erectile function   557
  - 23.1.1 Physiological mechanisms of penile erection   557
  - 23.1.2 Molecular biological mechanisms of priapism   558
  - 23.1.3 Phosphodiesterase protein structure and mechanism of action   558
- 23.2 Sildenafil for the management of male erectile dysfunction   559
  - 23.2.1 The discovery of sildenafil (UK-92480) and its structure-activity relationship study   562
  - 23.2.2 Unexpected findings of sildenafil in clinical trials: improvement in erectile dysfunction   565
- 23.3 The approval of second and third-generation highly selective phosphodiesterase type 5A inhibitors   565
  - 23.3.1 Second-generation selective phosphodiesterase type 5A inhibitor: vardenafil   565
  - 23.3.2 Tadalafil, a third-generation selective phosphodiesterase type 5A inhibitor   568
  - 23.3.3 Phosphodiesterase type 5A inhibitor activity, PK properties, and efficacy   572
- 23.4 Synthesis of selective phosphodiesterase type 5A inhibitors   576
  - 23.4.1 Synthesis of sildenafil citrate   576
  - 23.4.2 Synthesis of vardenafil hydrochloride   576
  - 23.4.3 Synthesis of tadalafil   577
- 23.5 Molecular mechanisms of phosphodiesterase type 5A inhibitors   578
  - 23.5.1 Protein structure of phosphodiesterase type 5A   578
  - 23.5.2 Molecular mechanisms of interaction between sildenafil or vardenafil and phosphodiesterase type 5A proteins   579
- 23.6 Summary and prospect   581
- References   582

23.1 The nitric oxide-cyclic guanosine monophosphate signaling pathway associated with penile erectile function

Erectile dysfunction (ED) refers to the inability of the penis to achieve and/or maintain a satisfactory erection for normal sexual intercourse over the past three months, resulting in impaired sexual function. Approximately 150 million men worldwide are affected by ED, with projections suggesting that this number will exceed 320 million by 2025 [1]. While not life-threatening, ED significantly impacts patients' quality of life, sexual relationships, and family stability and serves as an early indicator for various physical ailments.

23.1.1 Physiological mechanisms of penile erection

The occurrence of physiological priapism is a vascular response modulated by the nervous system, with both sympathetic and parasympathetic systems playing a role in regulating penile erection. Specifically, the parasympathetic system regulates penile erection by controlling the relaxation of blood vessels in the penis and smooth muscle within the corpus cavernosum. The normal stimulation nerve signal is transmitted from the hypothalamic erectile center to the corpus cavernosum nerve and then conveyed to the penile tissue through nonadrenergic and noncholinergic (NANC) nerves.

This process facilitates the release of bioactive factors from nerve terminals and endothelial cells, leading to the relaxation of the smooth muscle in the corpus cavernosum as well as congestion and expansion of this structure.

The enlarged penis simultaneously compresses the subtunica albuginea vein, thereby impeding blood return from the cavernous body and ultimately facilitating sufficient penile rigidity for sexual intercourse. Normal sexual psychological response, physiological structure, endocrine function, nerve function, and vascular function collectively form the foundation of penile erection; any abnormality in these aspects may result in ED [2]. The causes of ED can be categorized into two primary classifications: psychological and organic. Psychogenic ED is predominantly influenced by familial and social relationships, as well as traumatic experiences. On the other hand, organic ED encompasses a wide range of complex etiologies, including neurogenic factors (e.g., spinal cord injury and cavernous nerve injury), endocrine disorders (e.g., diabetes, hypogonadism, and hypercholesterolemia), vascular conditions (e.g., arteriosclerosis and venous leakage), drug-oriented aspects (e.g., antidepressants), systemic diseases (e.g., aging and cardiovascular diseases), and local lesions of the penis (e.g., peyronie's disease).

23.1.2 Molecular biological mechanisms of priapism

Sexual stimulation elicits activation of the sacral spinal parasympathetic center, transmitting signals to the corpus cavernosum. This stimulation induces the production of NANC neuronal nitric oxide synthase, leading to the release of nitric oxide (NO) in neurons within the corpus cavernosum. Concurrent sexual arousal triggers the release of acetylcholine (Ach), a neurotransmitter that stimulates inositol triphosphate (IP_3) expression in cavernosal endothelial cells' cytoplasm, resulting in an elevation of Ca^{2+} levels. When Ca^{2+} binds to calmodulin, it activates endothelial nitric oxide synthase, which facilitates the oxidation of *L*-arginine (*L*-Arg) to *L*-citrulline (*L*-Cit) and releases NO. The lipid-insoluble gas molecule NO possesses free radical properties, enabling it to rapidly diffuse across the cell membrane and exert its effects on neighboring target cells [3]. Upon diffusion into the corpus cavernosum and vascular smooth muscle cells, NO binds to Fe^{2+} at the active site of guanylate cyclase (GC), inducing a conformational change that enhances the catalytic activity of guanosine triphosphate (GTP) by this enzyme. The biological activity of cyclic guanosine monophosphate (cGMP), known as GTP, leads to an increase in cGMP levels. Acting as a second messenger, cGMP activates downstream cGMP-dependent protein kinase, which facilitates intracellular K^+ efflux, inhibits extracellular Ca^{2+} influx, and promotes Ca^{2+} uptake by the endoplasmic reticulum to reduce cytoplasmic Ca^{2+} concentration. Consequently, actin-myosin complex signaling is inhibited, resulting in smooth muscle cell relaxation and enhanced blood perfusion in penile arteries and cavernous sinus spaces compared to venous outflow, ultimately leading to erection (Fig. 23.1) [3].

In addition to the NO-cGMP pathway, other neurotransmitters (e.g., atrial natriuretic peptide and vasoactive intestinal polypeptide) or drugs (e.g., alprostadil) can activate the cyclic adenosine monophosphate (cAMP) signaling pathway and increase cAMP levels by binding to membrane receptors. This leads to ion channel phosphorylation, promoting intracellular K^+ efflux and inhibiting extracellular Ca^{2+} influx, resulting in smooth muscle relaxation and cavernous body hyperemia [3]. The resolution of erections depends on the expression levels of the second messengers, cAMP and cGMP. Phosphodiesterase (PDE), a protease that specifically hydrolyzes cAMP and cGMP into inactive 5′-AMP and 5′-GMP, respectively, regulates their expression levels. Therefore, effectively regulating PDE's catalytic hydrolysis activity can regulate the intracellular signaling of these second messengers.

23.1.3 Phosphodiesterase protein structure and mechanism of action

The PDE protease system has been discovered to be encoded by a total of 21 genes, with over 60 mRNA alternative splicing isoforms and nearly 100 PDE isoforms identified. Based on the amino acid sequence, substrate specificity, tissue distribution, regulatory properties, and homology of catalytic domains, the PDE enzyme family is classified into 11 distinct subfamilies. The PDE4/7/8 enzymes specifically catalyze the hydrolysis of cAMP, while the PDE5/6/9 specifically catalyze the hydrolysis of cGMP. Additionally, PDE1/2/3/10/11 can hydrolyze both cAMP and cGMP.

The PDE family typically exists as a dimer with monomers that share common structural components, including: (1) The N-terminal regulatory domain lacks sequence homology among the PDE subfamilies, yet it possesses potential functions in modulating protein catalytic activity or interacting with other cytokines; (2) The C-terminal domain, consisting of approximately 270 amino acids, exhibits a high degree of conservation, with sequence similarities ranging from 25% to 52% among different PDE subfamilies and from 65% to 80% among distinct isoforms within the same PDE subfamily. The primary role of this catalytic domain (CD) is to catalyze the hydrolysis of cAMP and cGMP [4,5]; (3) The function of the other C-terminal domain remains undetermined; however, it is capable of undergoing phosphorylation by other signaling factors to regulate the signaling pathway. For instance, in the case of the PDE5A protein (Fig. 23.2), theoretical

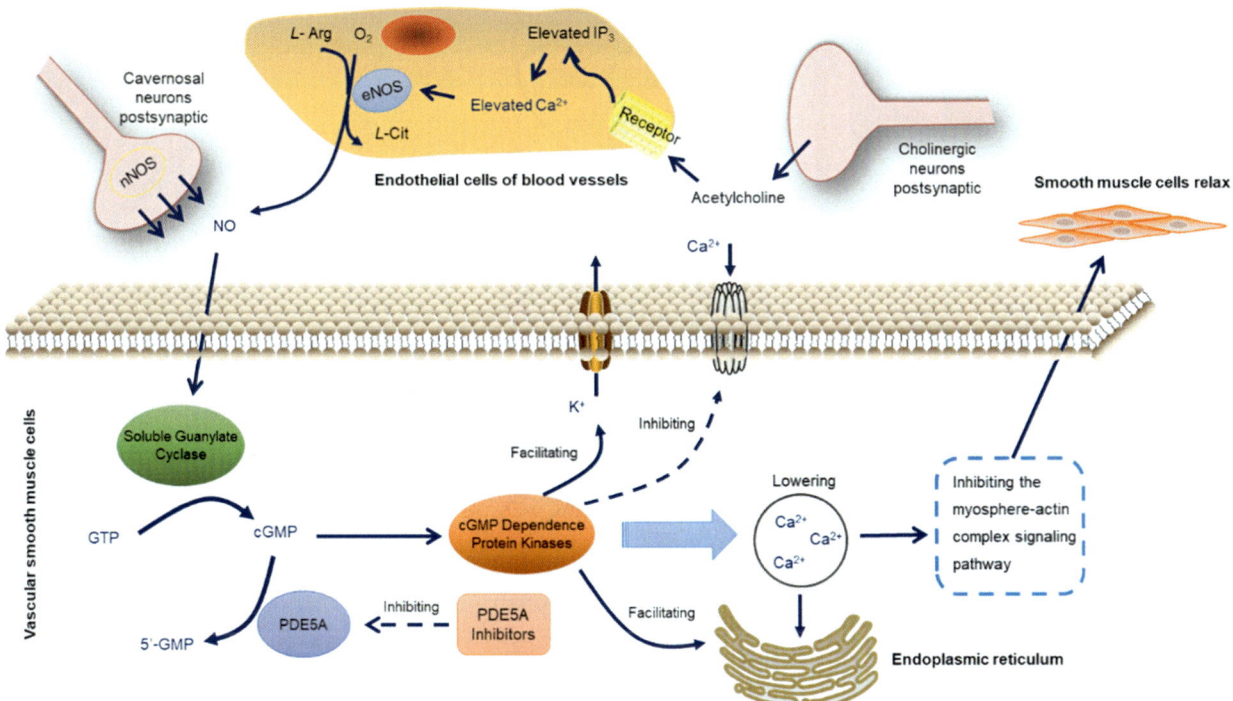

FIGURE 23.1 NO-cGMP signaling regulating vascular smooth muscle cell relaxation. *cGMP*, Cyclic guanosine monophosphate; *NO*, nitric oxide.

free energy calculations were compared with measured experimental values to speculate on the hydrolysis mechanism of cGMP. This hydrolysis was characterized as an S_N2-type reaction with a highly dissociated transition state, where the nucleophile was represented by a hydroxide ion positioned between two metal ions (Mg^{2+} and Zn^{2+}). First, the two metal ions function as anchoring agents, maintaining cGMP by forming chelation bonds with the phosphodiester group. Subsequently, the hydroxide ion acts as a nucleophile, attacking the positively charged phosphorus atom to form a transition state (TS) activation transition state. Finally, the phosphate ester bond at 3-position C of the sugar was cleaved to release the hydroxyl anion, which attracts a proton from His613 to yield the final product, GMP. All of these steps occur spontaneously in a single transition state and demonstrate a highly dissociated S_N2 hydrolysis mechanism. Therefore, the catalytic domain pocket of cAMP and cGMP catalyzed by PDE is also an ideally competitive binding target to PDE inhibitors [6].

In the PDE family, except for PDE6, which is specifically found in photoreceptor cells and the pineal gland, other subfamilies of PDEs have varying distributions across different tissues and cells. Notably, PDE5A is widely distributed throughout the human body, particularly in vascular myocytes, injured cardiomyocytes, lung tissues, brain tissue, platelets, kidney tissue, gastrointestinal tissues, and penile tissue (Fig. 23.3). These specific expression patterns and localizations are crucial for regulating physiological processes within specific tissues or cells [7]. Developing highly selective inhibitors targeting the PDE5A protein in these organs and tissues holds promise for intervening in both physiological and pathological processes associated with related diseases. Therefore, there is significant interest within the medical field regarding developing such inhibitors as well as their potential applications for treating various diseases. According to the Drug Discovery Intelligence database, six PDE5A inhibitors are currently available on the market, while another 20 are undergoing phase I or II clinical trials. Four representative examples of PDE5A inhibitors are listed in Table 23.1. Among them, sildenafil, the first selective PDE5A inhibitor developed by Pfizer Ltd., has achieved great success in the field of ED in men.

23.2 Sildenafil for the management of male erectile dysfunction

In March 1998, Pfizer's sildenafil citrate was approved by the Food and Drug Administration (FDA) as an orally administered, selective phosphodiesterase PDE5A inhibitor for the treatment of male ED, establishing it as one of the two groundbreaking advancements in andrology during the 1990s. Sildenafil, commercially known as Viagra, is a compound name derived from Vigor (representing vitality) and Niagra (referring to the world-renowned Niagara Falls),

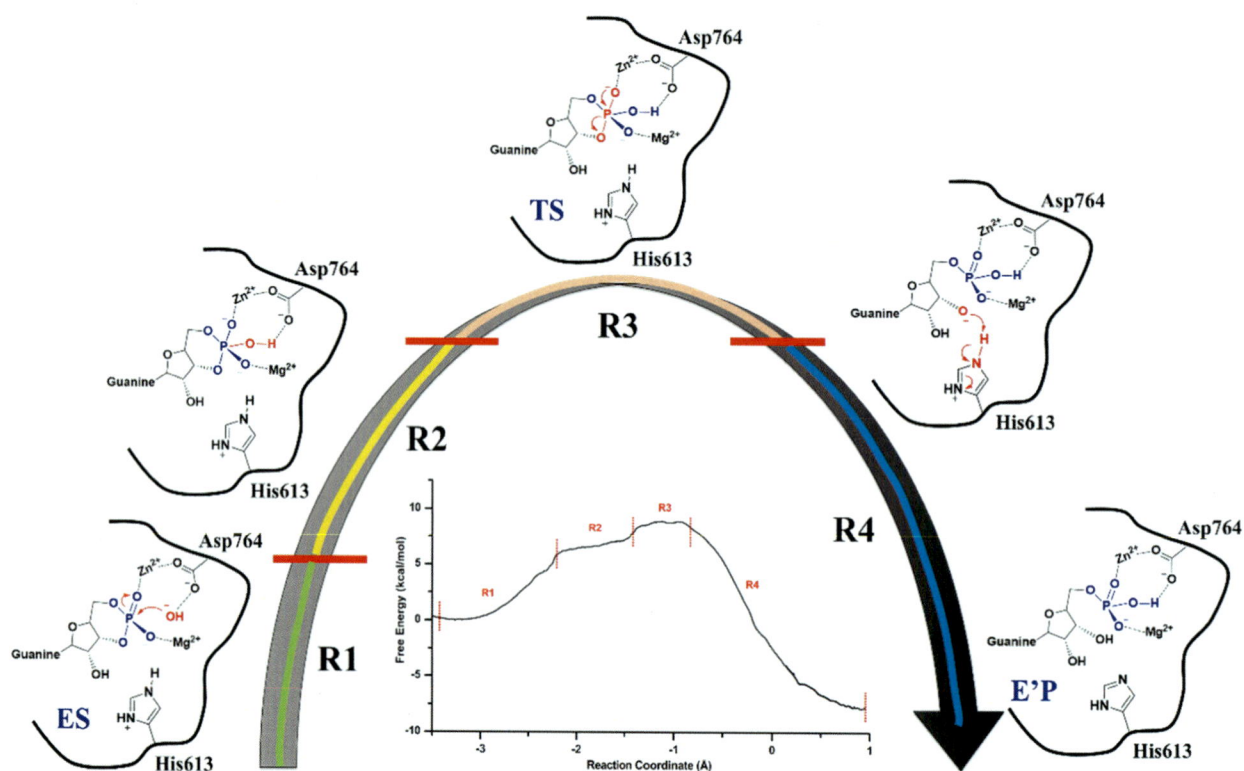

FIGURE 23.2 The proposed mechanism of cGMP hydrolysis in the catalytic domain pocket of PDE5A involving an S_N2 substitution reaction. *ES*, cGMP binding to PDE5A protein; *TS*, transition state; *E′P*, hydrolysate and PDE5A protein; *His613*, histidine at position 613; *Asp764*, aspartic acid at position 764; Mg^{2+}, magnesium ion; Zn^{2+}, zinc ion; *cGMP*, cyclic guanosine monophosphate; *PDE5A*, phosphodiesterase type 5A.

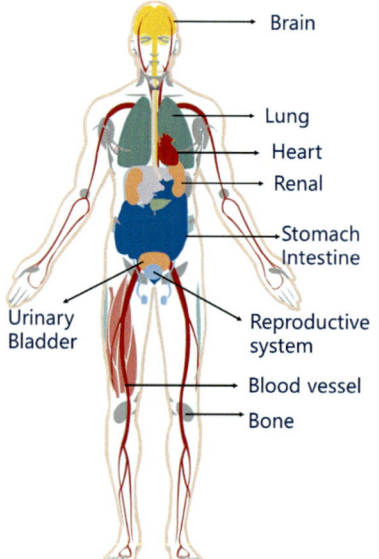

FIGURE 23.3 Schematic diagram of the distribution of PDE5A targets in human tissues and organs. *PDE5A*, Phosphodiesterase type 5A.

symbolizing an energetic cascade. Before entering the Chinese mainland market, this drug had already gained widespread attention and was named by the public as "Wei Ge," combining both transliteration and a connotation of appropriateness in men. However, due to the problem of a registered trademark, it was eventually selected as "Viagra," which was not well known to the public at that time, and landed in the domestic market of China. The successful

TABLE 23.1 Representative four marketed phosphodiesterase type 5A inhibitors.

Sildenafil 1998	Chemical name: 5-[2-Ethoxy-5-[(4-methyl-1-piperazinyl)sulfonyl]phenyl]-1-methyl-3-propyl-1,4-dihydro-7H-pyrazolo[4,3-d]pyrimidin-7-one
	CAS: 139755−83-2
	Molecular formula: $C_{22}H_{30}N_6O_4S$
	Molecular weight: 474.6 g/mol
	Product Name: Viagra
	Manufacturer: Pfizer Ltd.
Vardenafil hydrochloride 2003	Chemical name: 2-[2-Ethoxy-5-[(4-ethyl-1-piperazinyl)sulfonyl]phenyl]-5-methyl-7-propylimidazo[5,1-f][1,2,4] triazin-4(1H)-one
	CAS: 224785−91-5;
	Molecular formula: $C_{23}H_{33}ClN_6O_4S$
	Molecular weight: 525.1 g/mol
	Product Name: Levitra
	Manufacturer: Bayer Pharma AG
Tadalafil 2003	Chemical name: (6R, 12aR)-6-(1,3-Benzodioxol-5-yl)-2-methyl-2,3,6,7,12,12a-hexahydropyrazino[1′,2′-1,6]pyrido[3,4-b]indole-1,4-dione
	CAS: 171596-29-5
	Molecular formula: $C_{22}H_{19}N_3O$
	Molecular weight: 389.4 g/mol
	Product Name: Cialis
	Manufacturer: Lilly del Caribe, Inc.

(Continued)

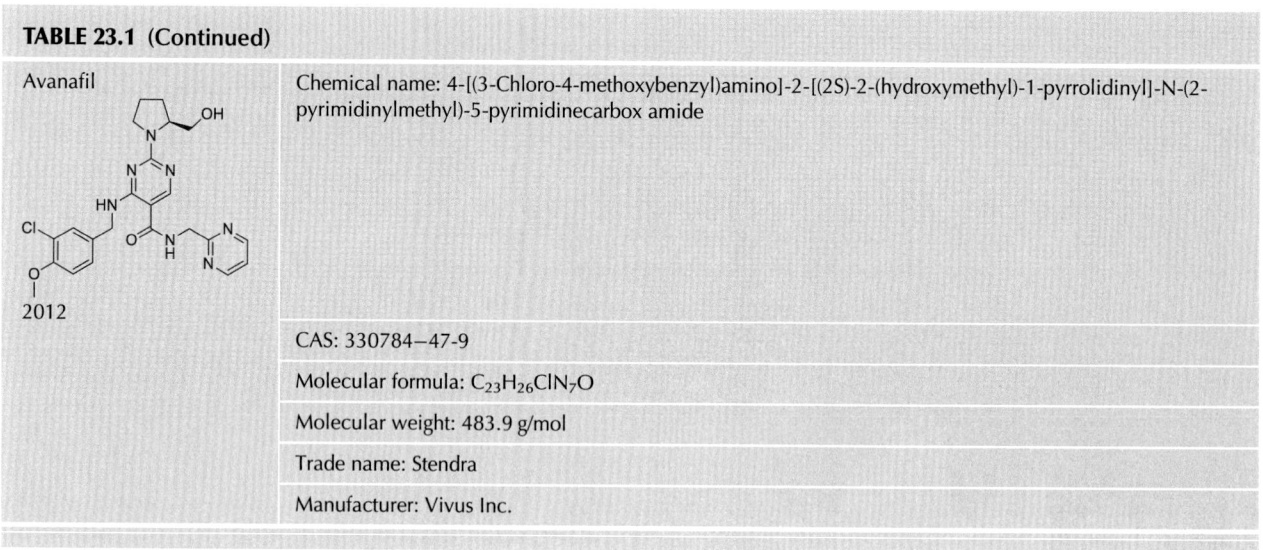

TABLE 23.1 (Continued)	
Avanafil 2012	Chemical name: 4-[(3-Chloro-4-methoxybenzyl)amino]-2-[(2S)-2-(hydroxymethyl)-1-pyrrolidinyl]-N-(2-pyrimidinylmethyl)-5-pyrimidinecarbox amide
	CAS: 330784–47-9
	Molecular formula: $C_{23}H_{26}ClN_7O$
	Molecular weight: 483.9 g/mol
	Trade name: Stendra
	Manufacturer: Vivus Inc.

marketing of sildenafil not only boosted Pfizer's reputation but also transformed the traditional perception of drug properties, shifting from simply treating diseases to enhancing the quality of human life. The company achieved profitable growth, with sales exceeding 1 billion US dollars in the second year on the market and surpassing 2 billion US dollars in 2012. Up to now, Viagra has been taken by over 2 billion men in 120 countries worldwide each year, making it a widely popular and successful blockbuster drug. The success of sildenafil greatly contributed to Pfizer's accumulation of over 20 billion dollars, providing a strong foundation for its rapid expansion and partly solidifying its leading position in the global pharmaceutical industry.

23.2.1 The discovery of sildenafil (UK-92480) and its structure-activity relationship study

In the 1980s, R. Furchgott and L. Ignarro et al. were awarded the Nobel Prize in Physiology and Medicine in 1998 for their groundbreaking research on the mechanism of action of NO gas molecules, which unraveled the mystery behind nitrate compounds' effectiveness in treating angina pectoris. The exogenous NO donor drug, nitroglycerin, undergoes hydrolysis catalyzed by mitochondrial acetaldehyde dehydrogenase to yield 1,2-dinitroglycerate and NO_2, which is subsequently converted to NO [8]. The gas molecule NO easily passes through cell membranes due to its lipid solubility and free radical nature. It activates GC and increases cGMP levels in vascular smooth muscle cells, leading to a decrease in intracellular Ca^{2+} concentration and relaxation of the muscles. Consequently, it reduces both preload and afterload on the heart, ultimately improving blood supply to the myocardium [9]. Furthermore, the NO generated from nitrates exhibits inhibitory effects on platelet aggregation and adhesion, thereby offering potential therapeutic benefits for angina pectoris management. However, these nitrates (such as nitroglycerin, a NO donor drug) are only efficacious for the short-term management of angina pectoris. Moreover, prolonged usage often leads to the development of drug tolerance among patients, rendering them inadequate for addressing the clinical demands associated with chronic angina pectoris. Therefore, researchers at Pfizer's European Research and Development Center initiated an investigation into novel methodologies for the treatment of various cardiovascular disorders, including chronic angina. Instead of augmenting NO supply, they explored the possibility of inducing relaxation in vascular smooth muscle to alleviate cardiac burden. At that time, five members of the PDE family had been reported, with PDE5A demonstrating superior selectivity toward cGMP hydrolysis. Notably, PDE5A exhibited predominant expression in vascular smooth muscle and platelets, suggesting that selective inhibition of PDE5A could potentially achieve the dual effects of vasodilation and antiplatelet aggregation, thereby serving as a promising long-term therapeutic approach for chronic angina treatment.

During that period, the availability of selective PDE5A inhibitors was limited, with zaprinast (Fig. 23.4) being the only reported antiallergic agent exhibiting weak inhibitory activity. Animal studies have demonstrated its modest vasodilator effect and weak affinity for the PDE5A protein, while also displaying some selectivity toward PDE1. To develop a more potent and selective compound, Pfizer's pharmaceutical chemists synthesized a series of heterocyclic compounds substituted with 2-alkoxyphenyl groups, sharing a similar core backbone as zaprinast. Among them, a pyrazolo

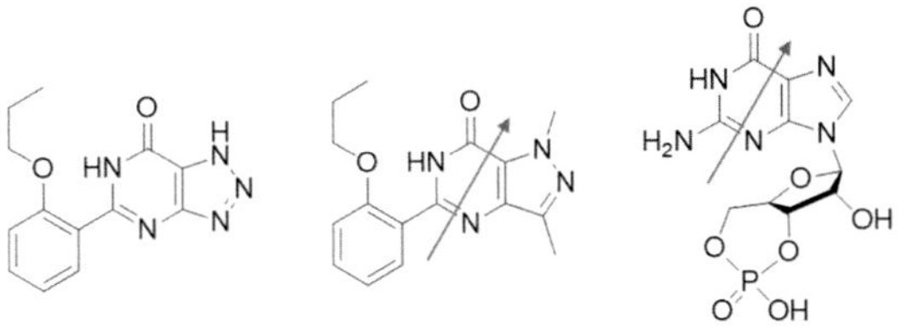

FIGURE 23.4 PDE inhibitory activity and structures of zaprinast 1 and pyrazolo[4,3-d]pyrimidin-7-one 2 compared to cGMP. Yellow arrows mean dipole moments. *cGMP*, Cyclic guanosine monophosphate; *PDE*, phosphodiesterase.

	IC$_{50}$ (nM)			Selectivity fold
	PDE1	PDE3	PDE5A	
zaprinast	9400	>100000	2000	4.7
2	3300	>100000	330	10

Selective fold = PDE1(IC$_{50}$)/PDE5A (IC$_{50}$), IC$_{50}$ is the concentration of inhibitor at which the activity level of PDE5A enzyme hydrolyzing cGMP is inhibited by 50% in vitro.

[4,3-d]pyrimidin-7-one compound derived from zaprinast was discovered to exhibit six times higher inhibitory activity against PDE5A compared to zaprinast itself, as evidenced by its IC$_{50}$ value. Furthermore, the selectivity toward PDE1 was enhanced by 10-fold (Fig. 23.4) [10]. However, due to the limited advancements in structural biology during that period, expressing and purifying PDE proteins *in vitro* was challenging, and there was a lack of crystal structure information on the PDE5A protein-small molecule complex to guide rational drug design. The backbone molecule was employed as a precursor compound for conducting a series of structural optimization and structure-activity relationship studies. Upon comparing the structure type, fragment size, and dipole moment of guanine (Fig. 23.4) between compounds 1 and 2 with the substrate of cGMP, it was suggested that either compound 1 or 2 could competitively target the PDE5A protein by mimicking cGMP. Therefore, the late modification strategy primarily focused on enhancing the cGMP structure by introducing a larger substituent at the 3-position of compound 1 to replace the space occupied by ribose in the cGMP structure. Additionally, considering the conformation of cGMP when bound to PDE's active center, it was considered to incorporate a polar substituent at the 5′-position of molecule 1's benzene ring as a replacement for the phosphate moiety (Table 23.2,).

After several rounds of structure optimization and activity testing, the structure-activity relationship of compounds with pyrazolo[4,3-d]pyrimidin-7-one structure was further clarified (Table 23.2), including: Compared with compound 2, compound 3, which replaced the methyl group at the 3-position of the backbone with the n-propyl group, compound 3 showed a 12-fold increased value IC$_{50}$ of inhibitory activity on PDE5A and nearly threefold increased selectivity on PDE1. After multiple rounds of structural optimization and activity testing, the structure-activity relationship of compounds containing pyrazolo[4,3-d]pyrimidin-7-one moiety was further elucidated (Table 23.2). Specifically, compound 3, replacing the methyl group at the 3-position of the backbone with an n-propyl group, exhibited a significant, approximately 12-fold increase in IC$_{50}$ value for inhibiting PDE5A activity when compared with compound 2. In the meantime, it demonstrated nearly threefold enhanced selectivity toward PDE1. Compound 4, with the deletion of the methyl group at the *N*1-position, exhibited a threefold decrease in IC$_{50}$ value for PDE5A inhibition compared with compound 3. Compound 5 was obtained by the elimination of the ethoxy group at the R$_2$ position of the 5-benzene ring, resulting in a significant decrease in its IC$_{50}$ value by a factor of 166 compared with compound 3. The IC$_{50}$ values for inhibitory activity against PDE5A were significantly reduced from compound 6 to compound 9 when the R group at the 5-position benzene ring was replaced with hydroxyl, cyclopropyl methoxyl, nitro, or tolesulfonamide.

The investigation into the structure-activity relationship of compound 10, combined with its analysis using single-crystal X-ray diffraction, revealed the formation of an intramolecular hydrogen bond between the oxygen atom of the ethoxy group and the N-H group located at position 6 of the pyrazolo[4,3-d]pyrimidin-7-one scaffold. The interaction effectively constrained the rotational movement of the benzene ring substituted at position 5 of the pyrazolo[4,3-d]pyrimidin-7-one, leading to a partial coplanarity between the benzene ring and the pyrazolopyrimidinone ring. As a result, this enhanced the activity of PDE5A inhibitors. In the field of medicinal chemistry, conformational restriction is a classical strategy for structural modification aimed at enhancing biological activity. This approach is frequently employed in the optimization of molecules with significant conformational flexibility, such as peptides. The binding free energy $\Delta G = (\Delta H - T\Delta S) < 0$ should generally be satisfied when the ligand binds to the target protein, with $\Delta S < 0$. This

TABLE 23.2 Structural-activity relationships of 3-propylpyrazolo[4,3-d]pyrimidin-7-one compounds.

Compounds	R_1	R_2	R_3	IC_{50} (nM)			Selectivity fold	LogP
				PDE1	PDE3	PDE5A		
3	Me	OEt	H	790	—	27	29	4.0
4	H	OEt	H	860	>10	82	10	—
5	Me	H	H	—	6300	4500	—	—
6	Me	OH	H	—	—	1000	—	—
7	Me	cyclopropyl-O-	H	—	47,000	960	—	—
8	Me	NO_2	H	—	—	4400	—	—
9	Me	$NHSO_2Me$	H	—	83,000	780	—	—
10 (UK-92480)	Me	OEt	$-SO_2$-N(piperazine)N-Me	260	65,000	3.6	72	2.7
11	Me	OEt	$-SO_2$-N(piperazine)N-CH$_2$CH$_2$OH	460	62,000	1.9	242	2.0
12	Me	OEt	$-SO_2$-N(piperazine)N-CONH$_2$	110	34,000	2.1	52	2.3
13	Me	OEt	$-SO_2$-N(piperazine)NH	390	>10	5.7	68	1.5

Notes: Selectivity fold = PDE(IC_{50})/PDE5A (IC_{50}), IC_{50} is the concentration of inhibitor when the activity level of PDE5A enzyme hydrolyzing cGMP is inhibited by 50% in vitro—means not determined. cGMP, Cyclic guanosine monophosphate; PDE5A, Phosphodiesterase type 5A.

indicates that the overall entropy of the complex decreases upon ligand-protein binding. It is crucial to overcome the energy consumed by conformational changes in degrees of freedom between the ligand and target protein during stable binding, and this portion of energy is compensated by nonbond interactions between the ligand and protein molecules. Mainly, this compensation energy comes from ΔH.

Conformational restriction of the small-molecule ligand can minimize the energy expenditure associated with changes in degrees of freedom. From a thermodynamic perspective, this reduction in ΔS corresponds to a decrease in entropy compensation provided by ΔH, resulting in a diminished ΔG value and enhanced binding affinity between the ligand and protein [11,12]. Considering the log$P$ value of 4.0 and the poor aqueous solubility of compound **3**, the researchers opted to introduce a hydrophilic moiety at the R_3 position to improve its solubility. Among various strategies for structural modification, the incorporation of sulfonyl amino groups emerged as a prevalent choice. The inhibitory activity of compounds **10–13** against PDE5A was significantly enhanced, with compounds **10** and **11** exhibiting the highest potency. Further investigations revealed that compound **11** had lower metabolic stability *in vivo* compared to compound **10**. As a result, the Pfizer research and development team ultimately selected compound **10** (UK-92480) as a promising candidate for further progression into clinical trials, eventually leading to its identification as sildenafil.

23.2.2 Unexpected findings of sildenafil in clinical trials: improvement in erectile dysfunction

The initial clinical studies revealed that sildenafil exhibited a comparatively reduced vasodilatory effect and a milder antihypertensive effect in comparison to nitroglycerin [13]. However, when combined with nitroglycerin, sildenafil demonstrated the potential to augment its antihypertensive impact and even induce an abrupt decrease in blood pressure, thereby introducing intricacy into the development of this medication. The half-life of sildenafil is relatively short, and its antihypertensive effect has a brief duration. Moreover, there is no apparent dose relationship observed. In terms of efficacy and pharmacokinetic properties, sildenafil does not offer any clear advantage over nitroglycerin, which is the primary medication for treating angina pectoris. Unfortunately, clinical trials to develop sildenafil for the treatment of cardiovascular disease were unsuccessful in 1993. However, the researchers have observed a negative effect in healthy young male volunteers who were given sildenafil or a placebo three times a day for 10 days. Specifically, some volunteers experienced an increased frequency or longer duration of penile erection after taking a relatively high dose of sildenafil compared to the placebo. The researchers then began to wonder if sildenafil, which was effective in helping healthy young men achieve priapism, could also be effective in middle-aged and older men with ED who had hypertension, heart disease, or diabetes. The prevailing belief among doctors at that time was that ED primarily had psychological causes, making it an extremely challenging medical condition to treat. Therefore, the development of an orally effective treatment for ED with the effectiveness of this drug would undoubtedly be a historic breakthrough.

After conducting multiple demonstrations and evaluations, as well as establishing a comprehensive clinical treatment evaluation plan, the researchers recruited 16 patients diagnosed with ED for the initial clinical pilot trial at the end of 1993. It can be inferred that the experimental findings exhibited highly promising outcomes since sildenafil effectively enhanced penile erectile function. Consequently, Pfizer conducted extensive, large-scale clinical trials until 1997, involving over 4500 subjects. The results demonstrated the efficacy of sildenafil in diverse populations of ED patients, with commonly observed dose-related adverse events including temporary headaches, flushing, indigestion, and visual disturbances. In March and September 1998, the US FDA and the European Agency for the Evaluation of Medicines (EMEA), respectively, approved sildenafil citrate for marketing as Viagra. A report in 2009 demonstrated that after more than a decade of clinical application, doctors and patients worldwide have widely recognized the efficacy and safety of sildenafil in treating ED. The effective rates of sildenafil at doses of 50 and 100 mg/person/time were found to be 77% and 84%, respectively. Overall, sildenafil exhibited a clinical efficacy rate of 80.8%. Furthermore, sildenafil has proven to be effective [14] in treating ED patients with various causes, degrees, and ages.

Although Pfizer marketed Viagra as a product of "fate and science," the discovery of this drug was not accidental. It resulted from a shift in creative thinking and research focus from angina to ED, as well as an improved understanding of the mechanisms behind erections. The introduction of sildenafil citrate into clinical practice has revolutionized the treatment of ED, relegating older techniques such as intracorporeal injection or penile prosthesis implantation to the brink of obsolescence (Table 23.3).

23.3 The approval of second and third-generation highly selective phosphodiesterase type 5A inhibitors

Due to its success in the market, sildenafil quickly revolutionized the field of ED treatment, raising public awareness and attention toward sexual health. It rapidly became the primary medication for treating ED. Following the discovery of sildenafil, other members of the PDE family (PDE7–11) were identified, which increased the demand for selectivity in PDE5A inhibitors. Furthermore, significant profits in the field of ED treatment motivated numerous pharmaceutical giants to pursue the development of PDE5A inhibitors. Apart from sildenafil, several other PDE5A inhibitors are currently available worldwide; among them, vardenafil, tadalafil, and avanafil have been approved by the US FDA as representative drugs (Fig. 23.5). Although these drugs share similar mechanisms of action and binding sites with PDE5A, they exhibit distinct pharmacokinetic properties, selectivity toward different PDE isoenzymes, and diverse binding modes with PDE5A.

23.3.1 Second-generation selective phosphodiesterase type 5A inhibitor: vardenafil

As a PDE5A inhibitor, sildenafil has gained widespread recognition for its remarkable and distinct therapeutic efficacy in treating ED during clinical trials. Consequently, several pharmaceutical companies have embarked on studying Pfizer's patent and endeavoring to overcome the hurdle of the original sildenafil patent through chemical structure modification. They aim to swiftly capture a significant share of the ED treatment market and achieve rapid development of

TABLE 23.3 The significant achievement in the development of phosphodiesterase type 5A inhibitor sildenafil.

Around 1986	Pfizer has set up a research and development team dedicated to developing selective PDE inhibitors for the treatment of cardiovascular-related diseases.
1989	The compound UK-92480 (later known as sildenafil) was initially synthesized, and later on, sildenafil citrate was identified during the development process.
1990	The study conducted by Louis Ignarro et al. revealed that the relaxation of corpus cavernosum smooth muscle could be achieved through the induction of NO and cGMP *via* electric field stimulation [15].
1991	The study of therapy for chronic angina began.
1991	In a preliminary clinical trial, administering a single dose of sildenafil citrate to healthy participants did not result in any significant impact on angina pectoris.
1991	The Clinical Study Reports 148–207 were the first to document the occurrence of penile erection as a side effect in healthy male subjects.
1991	Peter Ellis and Nick Terrett proposed that PDE5A inhibitors could be used to treat erectile dysfunction (ED) and improve sexual function.
1992	The subjects in Phase I and Phase II, who were healthy, received repeated treatment with sildenafil and experienced adverse effects on penile erection.
1992	In the initial phase 2 clinical study on angina pectoris, sildenafil citrate exhibited only a mild impact on hemodynamics.
Mid-1993	The clinical study for angina officially concluded that sildenafil was not effective.
Late 1993	The effectiveness of sildenafil was demonstrated in a small clinical pilot study conducted in Bristol, UK, with 16 patients suffering from erectile dysfunction who used an erection durometer.
Early 1994	The second pilot study further validated the effectiveness of a single dose of sildenafil in treating ED.
1994	Pfizer researchers discovered the presence of PDE5A protein in penile tissue and confirmed sildenafil's mechanism for treating erectile dysfunction by blocking PDE5A.
1994–97	The study involved twenty-one clinical trials with nearly 4,500 patients suffering from erectile dysfunction.
1997	Pfizer submitted Viagra to the FDA for priority review in treating erectile dysfunction (ED).
March 1998	The U.S. FDA has approved Viagra, the pioneering oral medication for treating ED.
1991–2000	Several research studies have highlighted the potential role of PDE5A in pulmonary vessels. Experimental models of pulmonary hypertension have examined the effects of zaprinast and other PDE5A inhibitors.
1998–2000	A small clinical trial, known as Pfizer study 1024, was conducted to assess the effectiveness of different doses of sildenafil in treating pulmonary hypertension.
In 2000	The successful long-term treatment of a patient with idiopathic pulmonary arterial hypertension (IPAH) using sildenafil was reported.
2002	A randomized phase III study of pulmonary arterial hypertension (PAH) (SUPER-1) was conducted.
June 2005	The US FDA has approved sildenafil, marketed as Revatio, for the treatment of pulmonary arterial hypertension (PAH).

PDE5A, Phosphodiesterase type 5A.

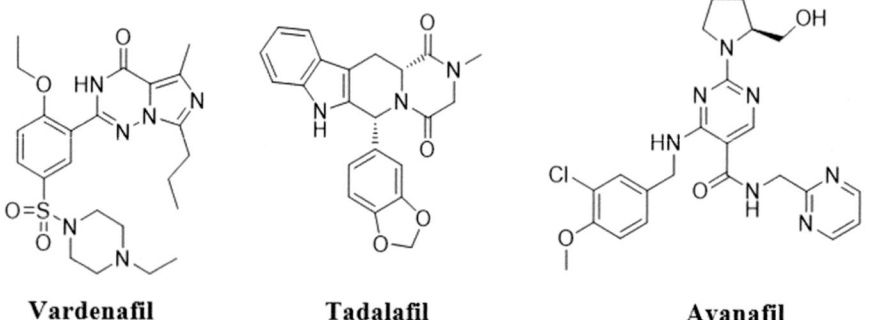

Vardenafil   **Tadalafil**   **Avanafil**

FIGURE 23.5 Subsequent PDE5A-selective inhibitors marketed drugs. *PDE5A*, Phosphodiesterase type 5A.

similar drugs. Vardenafil stands as an exemplary drug among these me-too medications, striving for rapid follow-up. According to the structure-activity relationship of sildenafil, the pyrazo-[4, 3-d]pyrimidine-7-one serves as a crucial core skeleton. The rapid discovery of novel PDE5A inhibitors while maintaining their shape, size, and dipole moment has become an essential objective for researchers at that time.

The research and development group of GlaxoSmithKline (GSK) Pharmaceutical Company utilized a scaffold hopping strategy to replace the N atom in the original pyrazo-[4, 3-d]pyrimidine-7-one backbone, resulting in new PDE5A inhibitors that are distinct from sildenafil. This strategy involves two directions, as illustrated in Fig. 23.6: 1) relocating the nitrogen atom from position a to position d; and 2) exchanging the N atom at position b with the C atom at position c. The screening results presented in Table 23.4 demonstrate that compounds (**14** and **15**) obtained from strategy 1

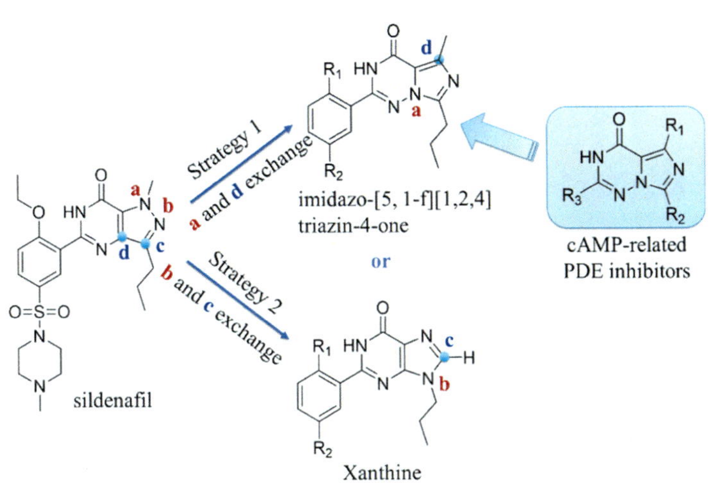

FIGURE 23.6 Discovery of vardenafil with imidazo-[5, 1-f][1,2,4] triazin-4-one as the dominant skeleton.

TABLE 23.4 The in vitro enzyme inhibition activity of phosphodiesterase type 5A inhibitors developed with strategies 1 and 2.

Strategies	Structure	R	Compounds	IC$_{50}$ (nmol/L)		Selectivity fold
				PDE1	PDE5A	
1	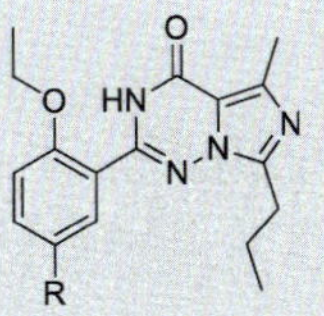	H	14	300	5	60
		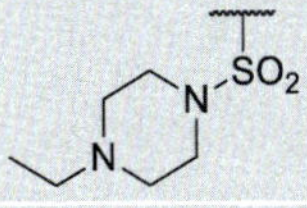 (piperazine-SO$_2$)	15 (BAY 38−9456)	180	0.7	257
2	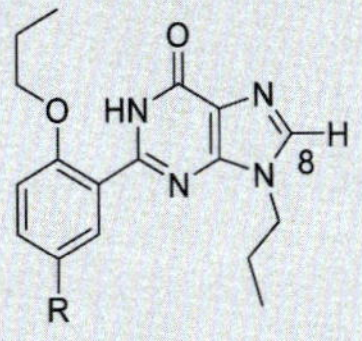	H	16	–	10	
		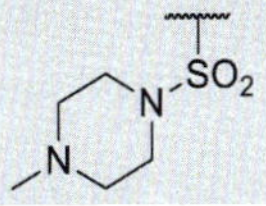 (piperazine-SO$_2$)	17		10	

Notes: Selective fold = PDE1(IC$_{50}$)/PDE5A (IC$_{50}$), IC$_{50}$ is the concentration of inhibitor at which the activity level of PDE5A enzyme hydrolyzing cGMP is inhibited by 50% in vitro. PDE5A, Phosphodiesterase type 5A.

exhibit superior inhibitory activity against PDE5A and selectivity against PDE1 compared to those (**16** and **17**) obtained from strategy 2. Moreover, the C-H bond located at the C-8 position in the hypoxanthine backbone obtained *via* strategy 2 is susceptible to oxidative metabolism within the human body. Therefore, researchers have chosen strategy 1 as their preferred direction for further optimization. The modified imidazo-[5, 1-f][1,2,4] triazin-4-one skeleton obtained from strategy 1 showed minimal changes in terms of shape, size, and dipole moment when compared to the original pyrazo-[4, 3-d]pyrimidine-7-one structure [16], thus maintaining its PDE5A inhibitory activity. Apparently, the molecular structure in question fell outside the scope of sildenafil's patent protection, and modifications made to other parts of the structure still followed sildenafil's main components. As a result, rapid replication occurred, leading to the prompt discovery of vardenafil, a selective PDE5A inhibitor later acquired by Bayer Pharmaceuticals. The successful replication of vardenafil has demonstrated the virtue of the scaffold hopping strategy as a traditional approach in medicinal chemistry. By replacing heteroatoms (N, O, S, etc.) with carbon atoms within the structural framework, new drug entities can be obtained that are beyond the protective scope of the original patent. This allows for the accelerated development of follow-on drugs based on existing medications. The swift market entry of vardenafil also serves as a prominent example of innovative me-too drug development.

23.3.2 Tadalafil, a third-generation selective phosphodiesterase type 5A inhibitor

In 2003, the approval of tadalafil (Cialis), also known as the "yellow pill," developed by GSK and subsequently transferred to Lilly-ICOS, posed a significant challenge for Pfizer researchers. By 2013, tadalafil had surpassed sildenafil's dominance in the field of ED treatment, with annual sales exceeding 2.22 billion US dollars, establishing its position as the leading medication in the ED market. Furthermore, by 2017, tadalafil's global market size had exceeded that of Viagra by nearly 1 billion US dollars. The research and development team of GSK published their discovery and optimization process of tadalafil in two consecutive research papers in J. Med Chem published by the American Chemical Society (Fig. 23.7) in 2003 [17,18]. Similar to sildenafil, in the early 1990s, the team embarked on developing an orally administered selective small-molecule PDE5A inhibitor for treating cardiovascular diseases such as hypertension and congestive heart failure. They discovered that β-carboline-based compounds could elevate cGMP levels in the rat cerebellum and dose-dependently alleviate the K^+-induced constriction of the rat aortic ring [19]. First, they tested the in vitro activity of β-carboline ethyl ester and demonstrated an IC_{50} value of 800 nM for inhibiting PDE5A [20]. Subsequently, they screened compounds with a similar structure from their in-house compound library and discovered compound **19** (GR30040X), which exhibited PDE5A inhibition with an IC_{50} value of 300 nmol/L. This value is close to that of the experimental control zaprinast (IC_{50} = 200 nmol/L) and also displayed selectivity for PDE1 to PDE4

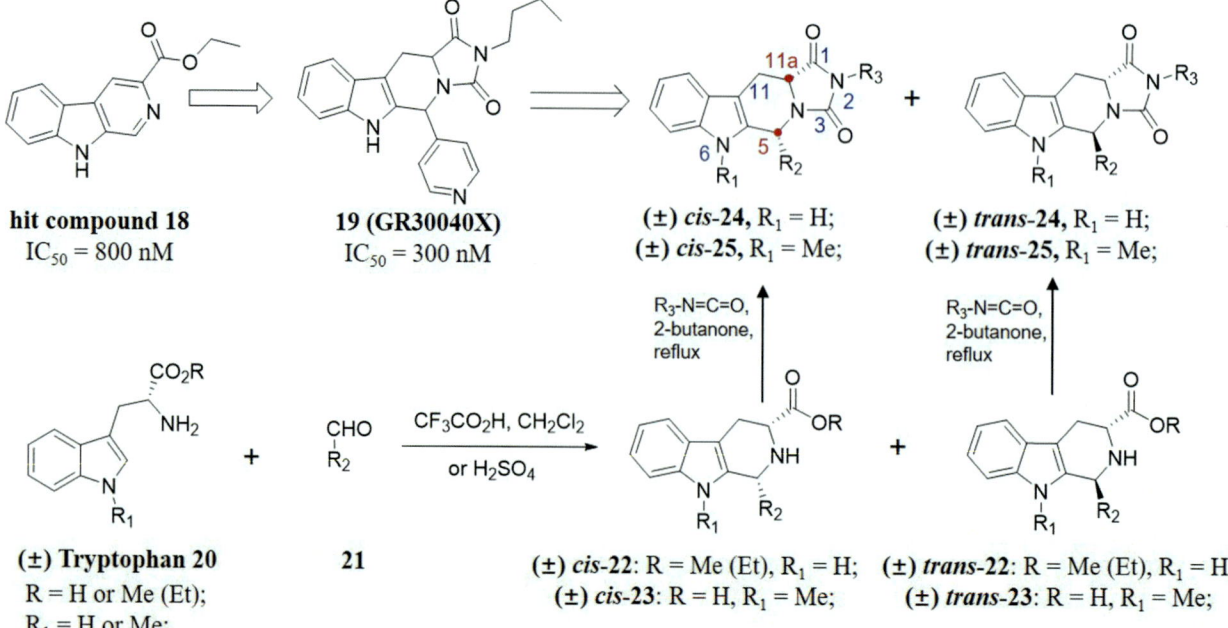

FIGURE 23.7 Synthesis of PDE5A inhibitors with the tetrahydro-β-carboline hydantoin structure. *PDE5A*, Phosphodiesterase type 5A.

comparable to zaprinast. Compound **19** possesses a tetrahydro-β-carboline hydantoin structure containing two chiral centers. The development of new drugs targeting PDE5A-selective inhibitors based on this structure can have completely independent intellectual property rights.

The racemic 1, 3-disubstituted tetrahydro-β-carboline derivatives **22** and **23** with *cis*- and *trans*-configurations were synthesized using a modified Pictet-Spengler reaction. Different aldehyde compounds **21** were used as starting materials, derived from either racemic tryptophan methyl ester (or ethyl ester) or N1-methyl tryptophan methyl ester (or ethyl ester). Subsequently, the obtained compounds **22** and **23** were reacted with various isocyanates to yield tetrahydro-β-carboline hydantoin derivatives **24** and **25** in both *cis*- and *trans*-configurations (Fig. 23.7). The tetrahydro-β-carboline hydantoin served as the basis for a series of targeted structural optimizations, with particular emphasis on R1, R2, and R3 moieties. However, elucidating the intricate structure-activity relationship poses challenges due to the presence of two chiral centers (Table 23.5).

The absolute configuration of chiral centers at positions 5 and 11a in compound **24** has not yet been determined, which is crucial to clarify to identify the compound with superior PDE5A inhibitory activity. In comparison to compound **19** structure and activity IC_{50} values, initial rounds of structure-activity relationship studies were conducted by substituting the pyridine at the 5 position using bioisosteres while keeping the R1 or R3 substitution intact in compounds **24** or **25**. The results revealed that the optimal substitution of R2 was a benzene ring with an IC_{50} value of 60 nmol/L (at this time, it still existed as a racemic *cis*-**24d** compound). Considering chemical synthesis, the benzene ring emerged as a readily accessible substituent, offering diverse substitution options that significantly enhanced structural diversity. Consequently, researchers have conducted further optimization of 5-C substitution on the benzene ring (Table 23.6).

By comparing the IC_{50} value of the compounds against PDE5A and the EC_{50} value of the compounds in increasing the cGMP concentration in rat aortic smooth muscle cells (RSMCS), the researchers found that: (1) The compound **24e**, bearing an electron-donating methoxy group at the para position of the benzene ring, exhibited superior performance compared to unsubstituted **24d**, compounds **24f**, and **24g** with electron-withdrawing chlorine atom substitution, or compound **24h** with cyanide substitution; (2) The substitution of 4′-methoxy group *trans*-**24e** is superior to the substitution of 2′-methoxy group *trans*-**24i**; (3) There was no significant difference between the *cis*- and *trans*- configurations of **24e** compound in inhibiting PDE5A activity. Additionally, when the substituent on R1 of the indole ring was a methyl group (**24** vs. **25**), there was a significant decrease in the IC_{50} value of PDE5A inhibitory activity for these compounds. This suggested that N-H at position 6 was possible to directly interact with amino acid residues within the catalytic domain pocket of PDE5A and should be preserved.

Based on the optimal compound **24e** obtained from this round of structure optimization, the 4′-methoxy substituent in the benzene ring at position C5 was fixed, and further investigation into the structure-activity relationship at position R3 was conducted in the third round (Table 23.7). When a hydrophobic group with varying spatial sizes was introduced as a substituent at R3, there were minimal changes observed in both IC_{50} and EC_{50} values of the compounds (from **24e** to **24n**), indicating that this site may be inserted into the hydrophobic pocket of the PDE5A protein with good tolerance for different space volumes. However, a basic group substituted at R3 significantly reduced inhibitory activity against

TABLE 23.5 The PDE5A inhibitory potency of C-5 Aromatic or heterocyclic derivatives.

Compd.	R$_2$	PDE5A IC$_{50}$ (μM)
19	4-pyridinyl	0.30
cis-**24a**	3-pyridinyl	0.09
cis-**24b**	3-thienyl	0.03
cis-**24c**	3-furanyl	0.10
cis-**24d**	phenyl	0.06

IC$_{50}$ error range ± 25%. *PDE5A*, Phosphodiesterase type 5A.

TABLE 23.6 Phosphodiesterase type 5A inhibition and cellular activity of substituted phenyl analogs.

Compd.	R'	PDE5A IC$_{50}$ (μM)[a]	RSMC EC$_{50}$ (μM)[a]
cis-24d	H	0.060	5
trans-24d	H	0.020	2
cis-24e	4'-OMe	0.008	0.7
trans-24e	4'-OMe	0.005	1
cis-24f	3'-Cl	0.050	4
trans-24f	3'-Cl	0.050	>10
cis-24g	4'-Cl	0.050	>10
trans-24g	4'-Cl	0.020	1.5
cis-24h	4'-CN	0.9	nd[b]
trans-24h	4'-CN	0.3	nd[b]
trans-24i	2'-OMe	1	nd[b]
cis-25	4'-OMe	>10	nd[b]
trans-25	4'-OMe	2	nd[b]

PDE5A, Phosphodiesterase type 5A.
[a]IC$_{50}$ or EC$_{50}$ error range ±25%;
[b]Uncertain.

PDE5A (from **24o** to **24r**), suggesting that it was not suitable to improve the water solubility by introducing a hydrophilic basic group into the R3 position.

Although the compounds represented by **24e** (*cis-* and *trans-*) exhibited favorable *in vitro* activity and selectivity toward the PDE family, the animal efficacy of ***trans*-24e** was unsatisfactory. In comparison to intravenous administration, oral administration of **24e** did not demonstrate a significant antihypertensive effect, indicating poor oral bioavailability (oral bioavailability refers to the ratio of the amount of orally administered medication that is absorbed by the gastrointestinal tract, passes through the liver, and enters the bloodstream compared to directly administering it into the bloodstream) of the tetrahydro-β-carboline hydantoins represented by **24e**. Therefore, improving the oral bioavailability of such structural compounds becomes a subsequent challenge to address.

Based on the structural modification of the hydantoin fragment in the most active optimized compound (*cis-/trans-*)-**24e**, researchers conducted a fourth round of structural modification to discover a single stereoisomer compound that exhibits equivalent IC$_{50}$ and EC$_{50}$ activity while significantly improving oral bioavailability. The research findings demonstrated a significant contribution of the two carbonyl groups within the hydantoin fragment to their activity (Fig. 23.8). Upon reduction, eliminating any carbonyl group led to a substantial decrease in both IC$_{50}$ and EC$_{50}$ values, as observed for

TABLE 23.7 Phosphodiesterase type 5A inhibition and cellular activity of N-substituted hydantoins.

Compd.	R$_3$	PDE5A IC$_{50}$ (μM)	RSMC EC$_{50}$ (μM)
cis-24e	**butyl**	**0.008**	**0.7**
trans-24e	**butyl**	**0.005**	**1**
trans-24j	hydrogen	0.020	3
cis-24k	methyl	0.010	1
cis-24l	ethyl	0.010	0.4
trans-24l	ethyl	0.007	1.5
cis-24m	benzyl	0.004	0.15
trans-24m	benzyl	0.018	>10
cis-24n	cyclohexyl	0.007	0.3
trans-24n	cyclohexyl	0.003	0.1
trans-24o	(3-pyridylmethyl)	0.020	5.5
trans-24p	(N,N-dimethylaminoethyl)	0.030	3.5
trans-24q	(2-(2-pyridyl)ethyl)	0.006	1.5
trans-24r	(2-(pyrrolidin-1-yl)ethyl)	0.100	10

Note: IC$_{50}$ or EC$_{50}$ error range ±25%. *PDE5A*, Phosphodiesterase type 5A.

cis-26~28. Hence, it is imperative to retain both carbonyl groups. Subsequently, fine-tuning the distance between these two carbonyls was achieved by replacing hydantoin with piperazinedione to investigate possible changes in activity. This modification did not significantly alter the activity of ***cis*-29a**.

Instead, the researchers conducted a fifth round of structure-activity studies to further investigate the relationship between the absolute configuration of the chiral center at position 6-C of **29a** and its inhibitory activity against PDE5A. Interestingly, it was observed that compounds **29a~g** with a six-membered piperazinedione backbone exhibited distinct PDE5A inhibitory activities compared to those possessing a five-membered hydantoin structure when introducing a chiral center at position 6-C in either *cis*- or *trans*-form (Table 23.8). The substituent contribution trend to PDE5A activity was as follows: 3′, 4′-OCH$_2$O > 4′-OMe > 4′-Me > 4′-Cl > 4′-CN > 3′-OMe, 4′-OMe. Compounds with cis-configuration exhibited significantly better activity than those with trans-configuration, such as ***cis*-29a** vs. ***trans*-29a** and ***cis*-29c** vs. ***trans*-29c**, among which the single configuration of ***cis*-29c** showed the best activity. When the R′ substituent was either 4′-OMe or 3′, 4′-OCH$_2$O, the resulting compounds (***cis*-29i**,***cis*-29m**, and ***cis*-29p**) retained their inhibitory activity when R3 was substituted with a hydrophobic group of different sizes (Table 23.8).

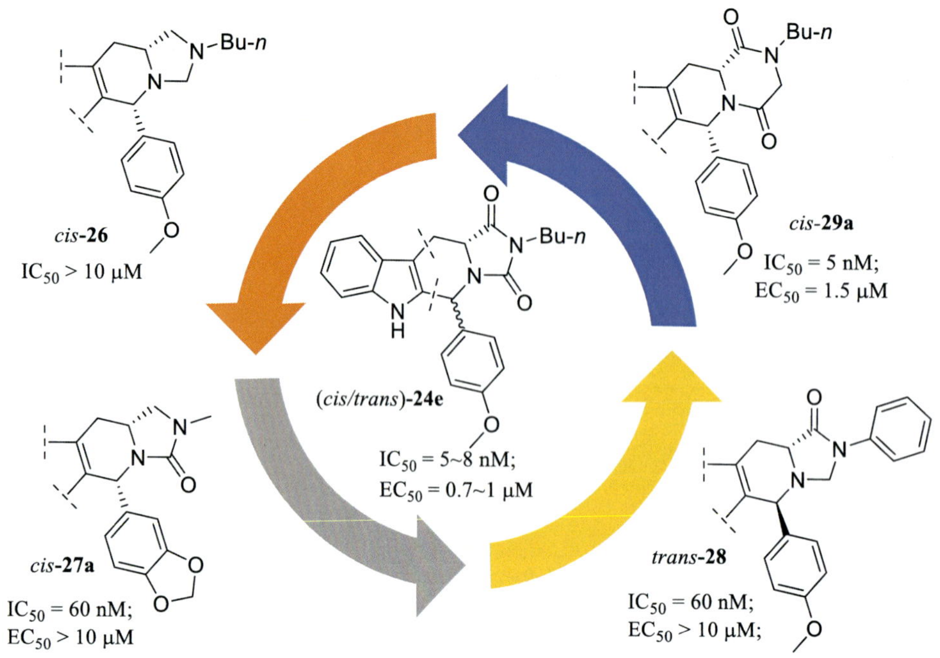

FIGURE 23.8 Modification of the hydantoin ring.

cis-**26**
IC$_{50}$ > 10 μM

cis-**27a**
IC$_{50}$ = 60 nM;
EC$_{50}$ > 10 μM

(*cis/trans*)-**24e**
IC$_{50}$ = 5~8 nM;
EC$_{50}$ = 0.7~1 μM

trans-**28**
IC$_{50}$ = 60 nM;
EC$_{50}$ > 10 μM;

cis-**29a**
IC$_{50}$ = 5 nM;
EC$_{50}$ = 1.5 μM

To further clarify the relationship between absolute stereoisomerism and the activity of *cis*-**29** series compounds, four diastereomeric isomers were synthesized using optically pure D-(-) tryptophan methyl ester and L-(+) tryptophan methyl ester as starting materials through a three-step process. The synthesized isomers included (6R, 12aR)-**30a**, (6R, 12aS)-**30b**, (6S, 12aS)-**30c**, and (6S, 12aR)-**30d**, respectively (Table 23.9). It is worth noting that the two diastereomers with the 6S configuration showed no PDE5A inhibitory activity; in contrast, there was an 18-fold difference in IC$_{50}$ values between the two diastereomers with the 6R configuration.

The absolute configuration of compound **30a** was determined as 6R, 12aR by X-ray single-crystal diffraction analysis. Utilizing this established configuration as the optimal skeletal structure, the activity of the R3 site was reconfirmed and found to be consistent with expectations. Notably, compound **30a** exhibited a selectivity of over 2000-fold for PDE1~PDE4 and more than 500-fold for PDE6. Additionally, pharmacokinetic studies in rats demonstrated excellent stability with a slow plasma clearance rate and remarkable oral bioavailability, reaching up to 63%. As a result, compound **30a** (GF196960) initially emerged as a promising clinical candidate for hypertension and congestive heart failure indications. Since the success of sildenafil as a PDE5A inhibitor for treating ED, Lilly-ICOS Company has decided to advance GF196960 into clinical trials for ED treatment. Subsequently, it received FDA approval in 2003 under the brand name Cialis.

23.3.3 Phosphodiesterase type 5A inhibitor activity, PK properties, and efficacy

According to the literature data, the IC$_{50}$ values of three representative PDE5A inhibitors available on the market were in the nanomolar range (nmol/L), indicating their high inhibitory activity (Table 23.10). However, different PDE5A inhibitors exhibited different PDE subtype selectivity. Sildenafil and vardenafil showed poor selectivity toward PDE6 protein, with only a 16−21-fold selectivity. On the other hand, tadalafil demonstrated higher selectivity toward the PDE6 but lower selectivity toward PDE11, with a 25-fold selectivity. Since various PDE isoforms are widely distributed in different tissues and organs within the human body, the lack of selectivity toward other PDE isoforms implies potential high inhibitory activity on those proteins (IC$_{50}$ < 1 μmol/L is generally considered indicative of high inhibitory activity), thereby increasing the likelihood of adverse reactions during clinical practice. In addition to the adverse effects associated with the inhibition of PDE5A targets (such as headache, dizziness, facial flushing, nausea, vomiting, dyspepsia, nasal congestion, and epistaxis), sildenafil (or vardenafil) can also induce visual dysfunction by inhibiting PDE6 in retinal tissue. Furthermore, tadalafil is frequently reported to cause muscle pain and joint pain, which may be attributed to the inhibition of PDE11 [21].

TABLE 23.8 PDE5 inhibition and cellular activity: structural-activity relationship on the phenyl ring at C-6 position.

Compd.	R'	R3	PDE5A IC$_{50}$ (μM)[a]	RSMC EC$_{50}$ (μM)[a]
cis-24e	4'-OMe	–	0.008	0.7
trans-24e	4'-OMe	–	0.005	1
cis-29a	**4'-OMe**	**n-butyl**	**0.005**	**1.5**
trans-29a	4'-OMe	n-butyl	0.070	>10
cis-29b	H	n-butyl	0.091	>10
cis-29c	**3',4'-OCH$_2$O**	**n-butyl**	**0.005**	**0.6**
trans-29c	3',4'-OCH$_2$O	n-butyl	0.138	3.5
cis-29d	4'-CN	n-butyl	0.758	nd[b]
cis-29e	4'-Cl	n-butyl	0.015	>10
cis-29f	4'-Me	n-butyl	0.026	0.35
cis-29g	3'-OMe, 4'-OMe	n-butyl	62%[c]	nd[b]
cis-29h	3',4'-OCH$_2$O	H	0.005	1.5
cis-29i	**3',4'-OCH$_2$O**	**methyl**	**0.005**	**0.6**
cis-29j	4'-OMe	methyl	0.012	0.6
cis-29k	4'-OMe	ethyl	0.005	0.5
cis-29l	3',4'-OCH$_2$O	cyclohexyl	0.041	0.2
cis-29m	3',4'-OCH$_2$O	i-propyl	0.009	0.5
cis-29n	4'-OMe	cyclopropylmethyl	0.005	0.3
cis-29o	4'-Me	cyclopropylmethyl	0.006	0.5
cis-29p	3',4'-OCH$_2$O	benzyl	0.006	0.5

[a] IC$_{50}$ or EC$_{50}$ error range ± 25%.
[b] Uncertain.
[c] The rate of inhibition of enzyme activity by the inhibitor at a concentration of 10 μM.

Pharmacokinetic studies (Table 23.11) demonstrated rapid absorption of oral sildenafil, with maximal plasma concentration (c_{max}) achieved within approximately one hour when administered in the fasting state at doses ranging from 25 to 100 mg/kg. The intestinal first-pass effect arises from partial degradation of the drug by digestive juices or intestinal enzymes during gastrointestinal absorption, while the hepatic first-pass effect results from partial metabolism of the drug by intrahepatic drug enzymes after entering the liver, potentially leading to decreased blood concentrations. The absolute oral bioavailability in humans is only 40%, and the mean half-life ($t_{1/2}$) of oral administration is approximately four hours. The area under the concentration-time curve (AUC) increases proportionally with different doses ranging from 25 to 200 mg/kg, indicating simple linear pharmacokinetics. The recommended clinical starting dose is 50 mg/kg.

TABLE 23.9 PDE5 inhibition and cellular activity: structural-activity relationship on the piperazinedione ring.

Compd.	R′	R₃	PDE5A IC$_{50}$ (μM)	RSMC EC$_{50}$ (μM)
30a (GF196960)	3′,4′-OCH$_2$O	Methyl	0.005	0.15
30b	3′,4′-OCH$_2$O	Methyl	0.090	–
30c	3′,4′-OCH$_2$O	Methyl	> 10	–
30d	3′,4′-OCH$_2$O	Methyl	6	–
31	3′,4′-OCH$_2$O	n-butyl	0.003	1
32	3′,4′-OCH$_2$O	i-propyl	0.008	0.15
33	4-OCH$_3$	cyclopentyl	0.017	0.2
34	3′,4′-OCH$_2$O	H	0.011	0.3

Note: The error range of IC$_{50}$ or EC$_{50}$ was ± 25%. PDE5A, Phosphodiesterase type 5A.

TABLE 23.10 Summary of phosphodiesterase selectivity of representative marketed phosphodiesterase type 5A inhibitors.

PDEs Family	Sildenafil	Vardenafil	Tadalafil
PDE1	375	1012	10,500
PDE2	39,375	273,810	> 25,000
PDE3	16,250	26,190	> 25,000
PDE4	3125	14,286	14,750
PDE5A	**1 (3.7)**	**1 (0.7)**	**1 (1.8)**
PDE6	16	21	550
PDE7	13,750	17,857	> 25,000
PDE8	> 62,500	1,000,000	> 25,000
PDE9	2250	16,667	> 25,000
PDE10	17,857	17,857	8750
PDE11	5952	5952	25

Note: Inhibitor PDE subtype selectivity fold was based on the respective PDE5A inhibitory activity IC$_{50}$. The values in parentheses are the inhibitor concentration (IC$_{50}$) in nmol/L when the activity level of PDE5A enzyme hydrolyzing cGMP was inhibited by 50% in vitro. PDE, Phosphodiesterase; PDE5A, phosphodiesterase type 5A.

TABLE 23.11 Pharmacokinetic properties of representative marketed phosphodiesterase type 5A inhibitors.

PDE5A Inhibitors	T_{max} (h)	$t_{1/2}$ (h)	c_{max} (ng/mL)	AUC (ng·h/mL)	F (%)	P450 isoenzymes CYP
Sildenafil (100 mg)	0.95	3.98	514	1670	40	3A4 (main), 2C9
Vardenafil (20 mg)	0.66	3.9	20.9	74.5	15	3A4 (main), 3A5, 2C9
Tadalafil (20 mg)	2	17.5	378	8066	—	3A4

T_{max}: ime of peak exposure to plasma concentration; $t_{1/2}$: mean half-life of oral administration; c_{max}: maximum plasma concentration; AUC: area under the concentration-time curve; F: absolute oral bioavailability; — indicates not determined. PDE5A, Phosphodiesterase type 5A.

Coadministration with a high-fat diet delays peak T_{max} by an average of 60 minutes and reduces c_{max} by an average of 29%. Hepatic elimination plays a predominant role for this drug, with its N-demethyl metabolite being primarily metabolized by hepatic cytochrome P450, such as isoenzymes CYP3A4 (major) and CYP2C9 (minor). The inhibitory activity of the N-demethyl metabolite towards PDE5A was found to be approximately 50% of that exhibited by the parent drug. Metabolism and material balance studies using radiolabeled sildenafil revealed a plasma protein binding rate of around 96% for ^{14}C-labeled sildenafil; excretion occurs mainly through urine ($\sim 13\%$) and feces ($\sim 80\%$) [14].

Vardenafil exhibited superior *in vitro* PDE5A inhibitory activity compared to sildenafil and demonstrated a faster onset of action *in vivo* (shorter time to peak plasma concentration, T_{max}), with plasma concentrations reaching c_{max} within approximately 40 minutes. However, the c_{max} and the AUC of vardenafil were not as high as those of sildenafil (Table 23.11). When administered with a high-fat diet, its absorption rate was also reduced, resulting in a prolonged peak time (T_{max}) of 60 minutes on average and an average decrease of 20% in c_{max}. Additionally, vardenafil exhibited a plasma protein binding rate of approximately 95%. Its metabolism primarily occurred through the liver enzyme P450 isoenzyme CYP3A4, with a minor contribution from CYP3A5 and CYP2C9 isoenzymes. The plasma elimination half-life of vardenafil was approximately 4 hours. Due to poor absorption and a significant first-pass effect, the average absolute bioavailability of vardenafil in humans was only about 15%. Following oral administration, vardenafil was predominantly excreted as metabolites in feces (91%–95%), with a smaller proportion eliminated *via* urine (2%–6%).

The oral absorption of tadalafil was rapid, albeit comparatively slower than the above two PDE5A inhibitors. The average maximum observed plasma concentration (c_{max}) of tadalafil was achieved within a range of 2–8 hours, varying among individuals. Food intake and administration time did not affect the rate and extent of absorption. In healthy subjects, the average half-life of oral administration of tadalafil was determined to be 17.5 hours when the c_{max} occurred at 2 hours. Estimating the absolute bioavailability of tadalafil in humans is challenging due to significant interindividual differences in pharmacokinetics; however, animal studies have demonstrated superior oral bioavailability for tadalafil compared to sildenafil or vardenafil. As an ED medication, the recommended clinical starting dose for tadalafil is 10 mg, with onset occurring approximately 30 minutes after oral administration and lasting up to 36 hours. For pulmonary artery hypertension treatment (refer to Section 23.6), a once-daily oral dosage of 40 mg is sufficient for achieving steady-state plasma concentrations within five days. Tadalafil exhibits a plasma protein binding rate of approximately 94% and undergoes hepatic metabolism primarily *via* the cytochrome P450 isoenzyme CYP3A4. Glucuronic acid methylcatechol serves as the major metabolite without any clinical activity and is excreted from the body through urine (approximately 36%) and feces (approximately 61%).

Sildenafil and vardenafil exhibit a shorter T_{max} and a faster onset of ED improvement. As an on-demand PDE5A inhibitor, sildenafil significantly enhances erectile quality, sexual satisfaction, self-esteem, and self-confidence in ED patients. However, for the treatment of pulmonary arterial hypertension (see Section 23.6), both sildenafil and vardenafil have a rapid metabolic rate in the body and a short duration of drug action, necessitating thrice-daily dosing to maintain optimal drug concentration. Given the progressive nature of PAH and its high mortality rates, patients with PAH need lifelong medication. Multiple daily doses pose challenges to patient compliance. Tadalafil demonstrates high oral bioavailability, a slow half-life of plasma clearance, and a more stable metabolism. Its delayed onset time for treating ED symptoms requires oral administration in advance. Although tadalafil has a longer duration of action compared to sildenafil or vardenafil with immediate onset effects on ED symptoms, clinical follow-up surveys report lower levels of satisfaction. Nevertheless, tadalafil surpasses sildenafil or vardenafil in long-term efficacy for chronic PAH treatment. Administration of a single oral dose of tadalafil at 40 mg per day ensures effective maintenance of drug concentration within the body while achieving steady-state plasma concentration within five days; hence, it is widely recommended for clinical management of PAH. Therefore, the selection of an appropriate therapeutic agent based on the pharmacodynamic characteristics determined by its chemical structure is crucial from a clinical diagnosis and treatment perspective—a consensus advocated by current clinical guidelines.

23.4 Synthesis of selective phosphodiesterase type 5A inhibitors

23.4.1 Synthesis of sildenafil citrate

The active pharmaceutical ingredient sildenafil citrate was synthesized using a similar method to the original patented synthesis route (Fig. 23.9) [22]. The starting materials, nitropyrazole compound **M-1** and o-ethoxybenzoic acid **M-3**, were utilized, and intermediates **M-2** and **M-4** were obtained through Pd/C hydrogenation reduction, chlorosulfonation, and sulfonylation reactions, respectively. Equimolar amounts of **M-2** and **M-4** were condensed to obtain the key intermediate, **M-5**. After optimizing these three steps, the total yield of **M-5** synthesis reached up to 96%. In the presence of a strong base, an intramolecular ring-closing reaction occurred in **M-5**, leading to the formation of sildenafil 10 [23] with a separation yield of 95%. The crude sildenafil citrate was ultimately synthesized in the presence of citric acid, followed by reflux refining with activated carbon and ethanol, resulting in the production of the final bulk form of sildenafil citrate. This synthesis process involves a limited number of reaction steps that are easy to operate with simple follow-up treatment procedures while achieving relatively high yields at each step. By effectively controlling the quality of key intermediate sildenafil, high-purity raw materials for sildenafil citrate can be prepared stably and efficiently with a single impurity content of less than 0.05%.

23.4.2 Synthesis of vardenafil hydrochloride

Several synthesis methods of vardenafil have been reported in the literature, among which the process synthesis method described in Nowakowski et al.'s patent is the most commonly used (Fig. 23.10). In this route, 2-ethoxybenzonitrile **M-6** serves as the starting material, and **M-7** is obtained through an addition reaction with hydroxylammonium hydrochloride. Pd/C reduction and hydrazine hydrolysis are employed to obtain **M-8**, followed by a two-step cyclization reaction to yield **M-13**. The final product, vardenafil 15, was synthesized by sulfonation, chlorination, and amination. The overall yield of this 8-step process is 25.8%. However, there are several drawbacks associated with this synthesis route: first, it requires pressurized equipment for hydrogen catalysis using Pd/C, resulting in high costs; second, posttreatment involving Pd/C can lead to fire hazards that affect product quality and limit industrial production; third, when synthesizing the key intermediate **M-12** using a one-pot method, numerous by-products are generated and reproducibility of product purity cannot be guaranteed. This original route has been optimized and improved as follows: utilizing 2-ethoxybenzonitrile **M-6** (blue route) as the starting material for synthesizing 2-ethoxybenzimine ethyl ester M15 *via* a Pinner reaction. Subsequently, vardenafil 15 is obtained through six steps, including hydrolysis, two-step cyclization, chlorosulfonation, and amination, with a total yield of 31.6% [24]. This optimized process route offers several

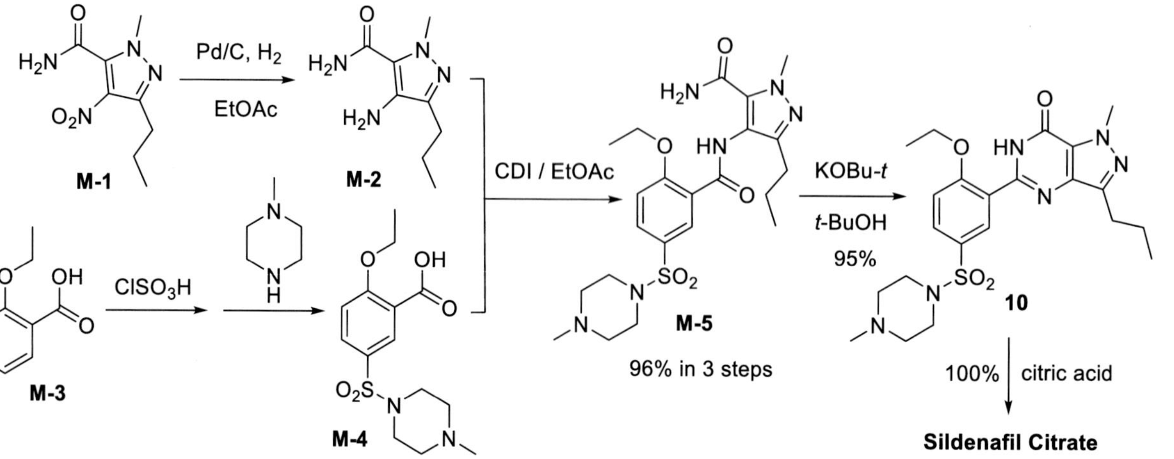

FIGURE 23.9 Synthesis route of the sildenafil citrate.

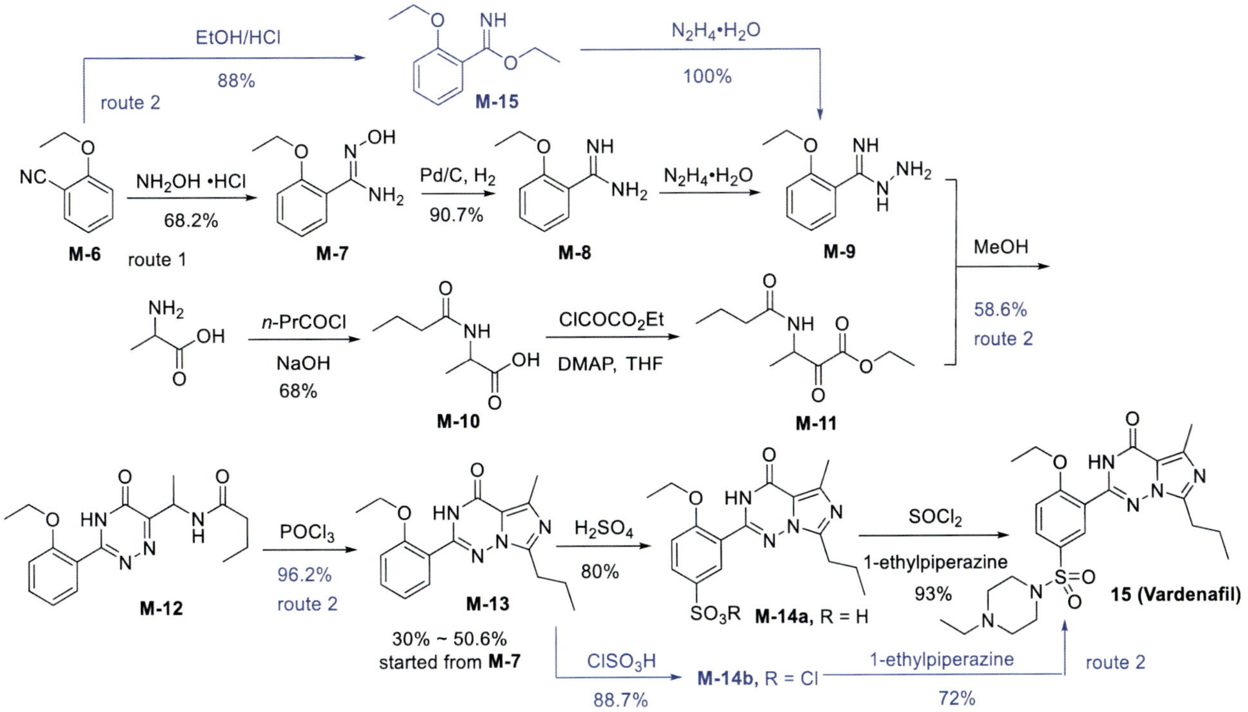

FIGURE 23.10 Synthetic process route of vardenafil.

advantages, such as a shorter route, reduced cost due to inexpensive raw materials, mild reaction conditions, fewer side reactions, simple posttreatment procedures, a higher total yield (25.8%) compared to existing patents reported in the literature, and superior product purity exceeding 99.6%, with less than 0.1% single impurity content meeting Chinese Pharmacopoeia's quality requirements [25].

23.4.3 Synthesis of tadalafil

The initial synthesis pathway of tadalafil was reported by Daugan et al. [26]. The Pictet-Spengler reaction (P-S reaction) was utilized to synthesize chiral tetrahydro-β-carbolines. D-tryptophan methyl ester was reacted with piperonal in methylene chloride using trifluoroacetic acid as a catalyst. After 5 days at 4°C, two different tetrahydrocarboline isomers (cis- and trans-) were obtained. The pure cis-tetrahydrocarboline structure (1R, 3R)-**M-17** was isolated using column chromatography and then reacted with chloroacetyl chloride in a basic medium of triethylamine in dichloromethane to form (1R, 3R)-**M-18**. This intermediate was further reacted with methylamine in methanol at 50°C for 16 hours, resulting in the synthesis of tadalafil with an overall yield of 25%. The synthesis of tadalafil in this route was successful; however, certain limitations were encountered, including prolonged reaction time, complex posttreatment procedures, and issues with reagent corrosion. Subsequent improvements have been made to enhance the process efficiency, resulting in high-purity tadalafil with a total yield of 56%, as shown in Fig. 23.11 [27].

The Pictet-Spengler reaction between D-tryptophan methyl ester hydrochloride and piperonal plays a crucial role in the synthesis of tadalafil during this preparation process. Additionally, the synthesis process involves crystallization-induced asymmetric transformation (CIAT). Isopropanol serves as the solvent for the P-S reaction. In the reaction, an equilibrium state is established between equal amounts of M-17 cis-product and trans-product. The trans isomer (1S, 3R)-**M-17** readily dissolves in isopropanol due to its excellent solubility, while the cis isomer (1R, 3R)-**M-17** remains almost insoluble even under reflux conditions. As a result, it directly precipitates within the reaction system. On the other hand, (1S, 3R)-**M-17** completely dissolves in isopropanol. Consequently, through the CIAT process in isopropanol, trans-tetrahydrocarbines (1S, 3R)-**M-17** gradually convert into cis-tetrahydrocarbines (1R, 3R)-**M-17** and continuously precipitate from the reaction solution (Fig. 23.12) [28]. Ultimately, this process route enables selective high-yield synthesis of the target intermediate cis-(1R, 3R)-**M-17**.

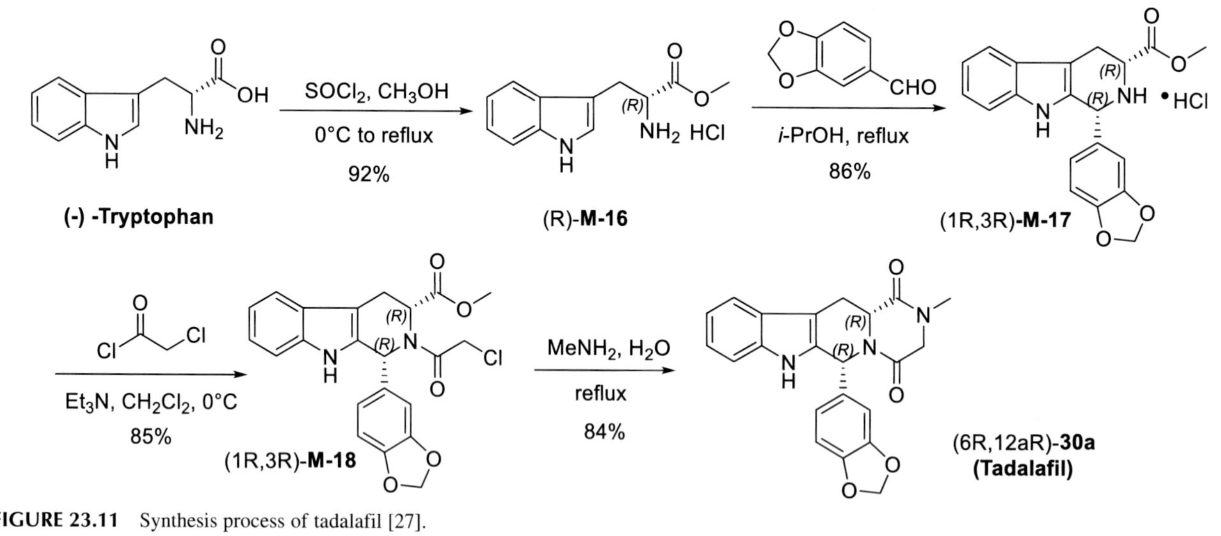

FIGURE 23.11 Synthesis process of tadalafil [27].

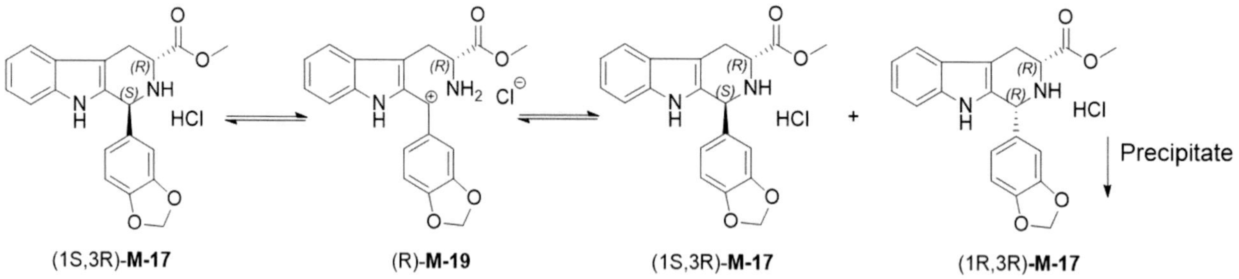

FIGURE 23.12 Mechanism of the CIAT process of the key intermediate *cis*-(1R, 3R)-**M-17**. *CIAT*, Crystallization-induced asymmetric transformation [29].

23.5 Molecular mechanisms of phosphodiesterase type 5A inhibitors

23.5.1 Protein structure of phosphodiesterase type 5A

Among the family of cyclic adenosine phosphodiesterases, only one isoform of PDE5, known as PDE5A, has been identified in humans. PDE5A consists of three isoenzymes (PDE5A1, PDE5A2, and PDE5A3) and functions as a cGMP-specific hydrolase due to its strong intracellular selectivity for cGMP (with a K value ranging from 2.9 to 6.2 μM) [30], surpassing its affinity for cAMP (with a Km value of 290 μM).

The N-terminal regulatory domain of PDE5A1, PDE5A2, and PDE5A3 comprises two individual GAF domains (a small-molecule-binding-domain (SMBD) identified in > 7400 protein), namely GAF-A and GAF-B. Comparative analysis of the amino acid sequences across different PDE subfamilies revealed substantial variations in this region attributed to differential mRNA splicing sites; however, the GAF domain within PDE5A exhibits a 33% sequence identity (Fig. 23.13) [29]. The GAF-A domain of PDE5A binds to cGMP and activates its catalytic activity [31]. However, the binding of cGMP to GAF-A can be inhibited by GAF-B, which also sequesters the phosphorylation site of the PDE5A protein. Additionally, PDE5A dimerization is facilitated by a 46-amino-acid R region near the N-terminus of GAF-B [32]. The conserved C-terminal domain contains the catalytic domain of cGMP, which facilitates the hydrolysis of cGMP through the cooperative participation of metal ions (Mg^{2+} and Zn^{2+}) (Fig. 23.2). Additionally, it serves as a competitive binding site for PDE5A inhibitors and their substrates [6].

Before the publication of the cocrystal structure of the PDE5A protein with small molecules, Turko et al. attempted site-directed mutagenesis to introduce mutations in 23 relatively conserved amino acids located within the catalytic domain of PDE5A [4]. By evaluating the inhibitory activity of Zaprinast against PDE5A, the amino acid residues that play an important role in the catalytic domain pocket for substrate binding were predicted, among which: (1) His653 and Asp764 are crucial for the catalytic activity of PDE5A; (2) His613, His617, His653, Asp654, His657, Glu682, Asp724, and Asp764 may contribute to the catalytic activity by forming a metal-binding pocket; (3) Tyr612 and

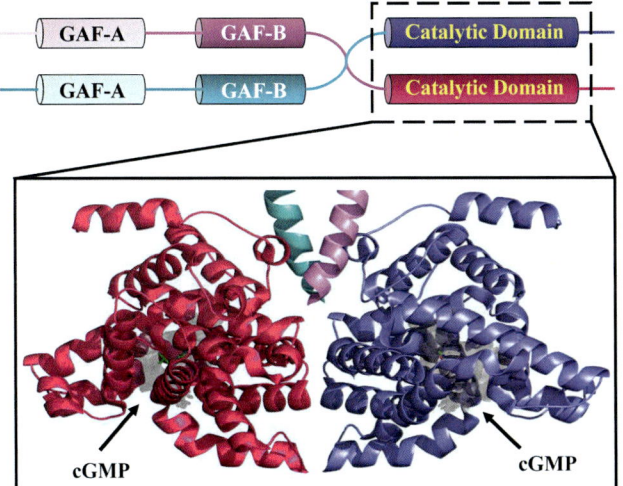

FIGURE 23.13 Schematic diagram of the PDE5A (or PDE6C) dimer (above), and a snapshot of the cryo-electron microscopy crystal structure of the catalytic domain at the C-terminus of full-length PDE5A (or PDE6C) dimer (PDB: 3JAB). *PDE5A*, Phosphodiesterase type 5A.

Glu785 play a key role in binding the substrate cGMP; (4) Although Zaprinast occupies the same site as the substrate binding site, their respective amino acid residues involved in binding are different. Subsequently, Turko et al. performed site-directed mutagenesis on the catalytic domain of PDE5A to evaluate sildenafil and its analogs. The results revealed a close correlation between the change in IC_{50} value and the alteration in cGMP affinity. This suggests that the interaction between sildenafil and the catalytic domain is similar to that of the substrate cGMP [33]. Notably, Tyr612, His617, His653, and Asp764 were identified as crucial amino acid residues involved in the interaction between sildenafil and PDE5A. However, these four amino acids are highly conserved within the PDE family. How can inhibitors like sildenafil achieve both high PDE5A inhibitory activity and selectivity toward other isoforms within the PDE family?

23.5.2 Molecular mechanisms of interaction between sildenafil or vardenafil and phosphodiesterase type 5A proteins

Although UK-92480 (sildenafil) is a selective PDE5A protein that was discovered earlier, the molecular interaction between this compound and the PDE5A protein remains unclear. Therefore, extensive studies have been conducted to elucidate the precise molecular interaction between these two entities. Given that sildenafil competitively binds to PDE5A inhibitors by mimicking cGMP, scientists have focused their attention on the catalytic active site of the PDE5A protein. This particular domain is situated at the center of the C-terminal helical domain and features a pocket with a depth of approximately 10 Å. The pocket has a narrow opening and an expansive internal space of around 330 $Å^3$ in volume. The catalytic domain pocket can be further divided into four distinct regions: metal-binding site (M site), core Q pocket (Q pocket), hydrophobic pocket (H pocket), and lid-covered region (L region) [34] (Fig. 23.14).

The cocrystal structure information of sildenafil and the PDE5A protein was initially elucidated by Sung et al. in 2003 [34]. The core Q pocket, located within the catalytic domain, accommodates the pyrazolopyrimidinone structure of sildenafil, which includes four highly conserved amino acids: Gln817, Phe820, Val782, and Tyr612 (Fig. 23.15). The structure of sildenafil showed: (1) The lactam group (N-H at position 6 and C=O at position 7) forms a strong bidentate hydrogen bond with Gln817, resembling the purine base of cGMP (N-H at position 1 and C=O at position 6). However, this structure differs from the pyrimidine base of cAMP (N=C at position 1 and N-2H at position 6). This structural dissimilarity contributes to its potent inhibitory activity against PDE5A as well as its selectivity. (2) The nitrogen atom at position 2 in the pyrazole ring establishes a hydrogen bond with a water molecule that is immobilized by Tyr612 and another Zn^{2+}-coordinated water molecule. Simultaneously, the pyrazole interacts with side chains formed by amino acid residues Val782, Leu785, Tyr612, and Phe820; the π-π interaction with Phe820 is particularly crucial. (3) Ethoxyphenyl inserts into hydrophobic pocket H, composed of residues Phe786, Ala783, Leu804, and Val782—distinctive among other PDEs. Furthermore, the hydrophilic sulfonyl amino group is positioned toward the entrance of the catalytically active pocket. The binding site for 4-methylpiperazine is located at the end of the loop adjacent to the catalytic active site and consists of residues Tyr664, Met816, Ala823, and Gly819 within the unique L region specific to PDE5A. This region acts as a flexible gate that regulates the entry and exit of small molecules into the core pocket Q. Therefore, sildenafil's high selectivity against the PDE5A family arises not only from its strong

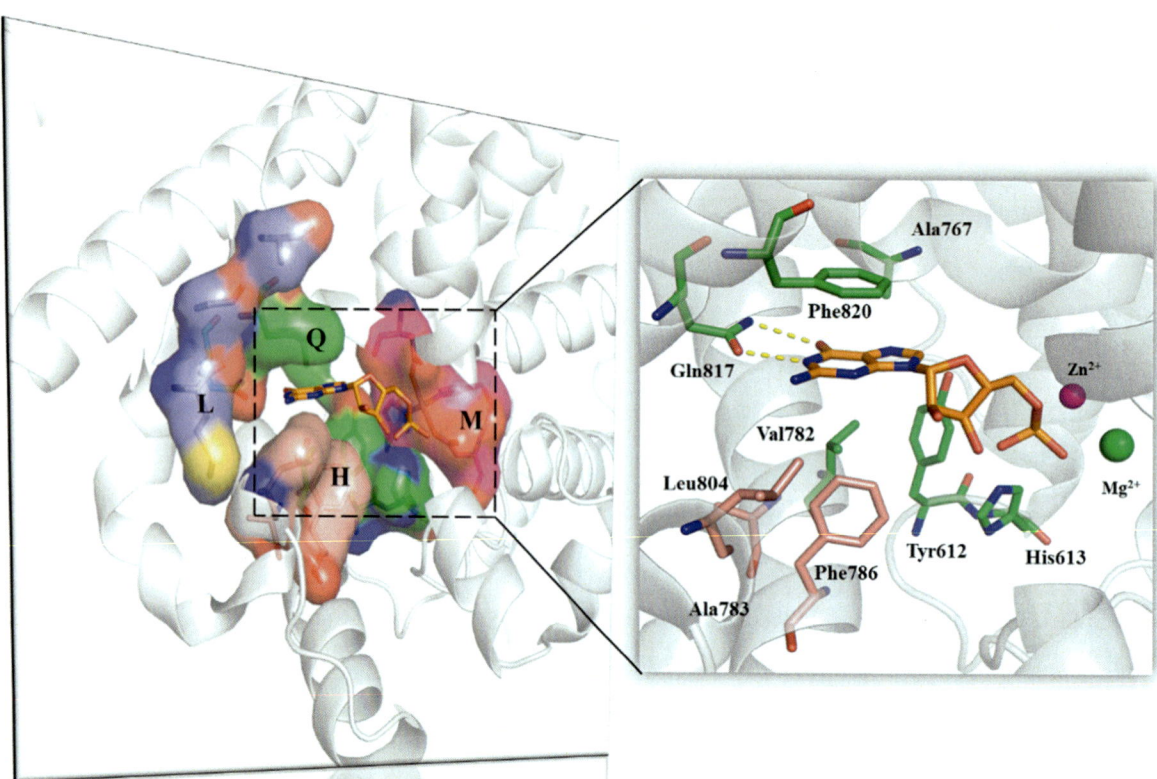

FIGURE 23.14 Crystal structure of PDE5A-GMP complex (PDB ID:1T9S) [35], the catalytic pocket is divided into M site (pink), Q pocket (green), L region (blue-purple), and H pocket (cherry pink), yellow dashed line: H bond. *PDE5A*, Phosphodiesterase type 5A; *GMP*, guanosine monophosphate.

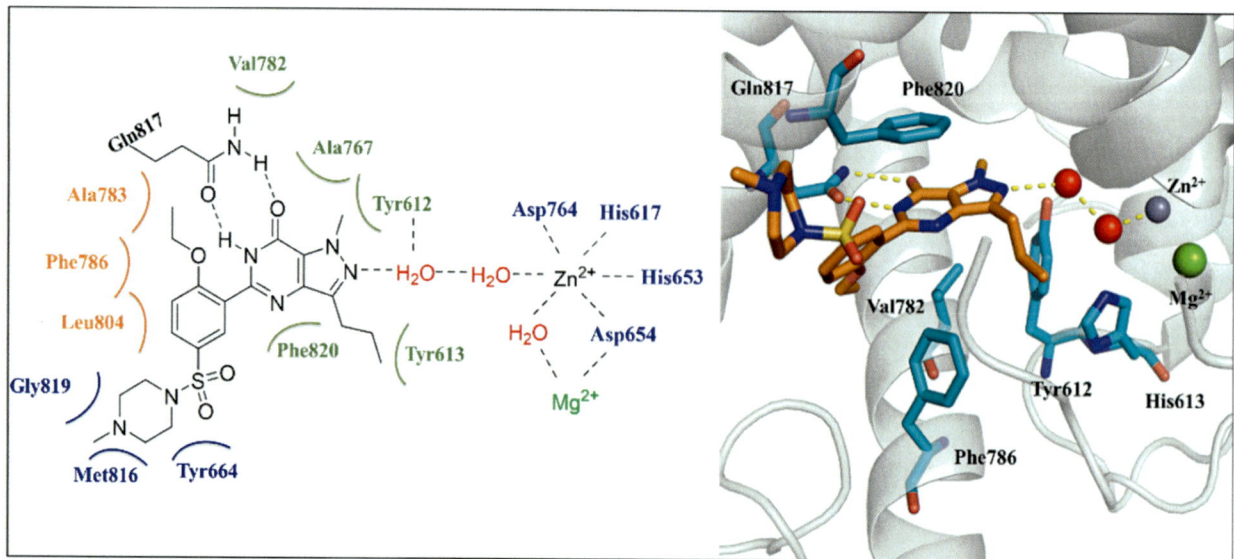

FIGURE 23.15 Molecular binding pattern of PDE5A-sildenafil complex (PDB ID: 1DUT). *PDE5A*, Phosphodiesterase type 5A.

interaction with conserved amino acid residues in the catalytic domain pocket but also from its distinct interaction with nonconserved amino acid residues. Cocrystallization analysis confirmed that vardenafil exhibits a similar binding mode to sildenafil (Fig. 23.16) [34], except for minimal interactions between vardenafil's 4-ethylpiperazine ring and PDE5A protein, thus demonstrating an identical mechanism of action.

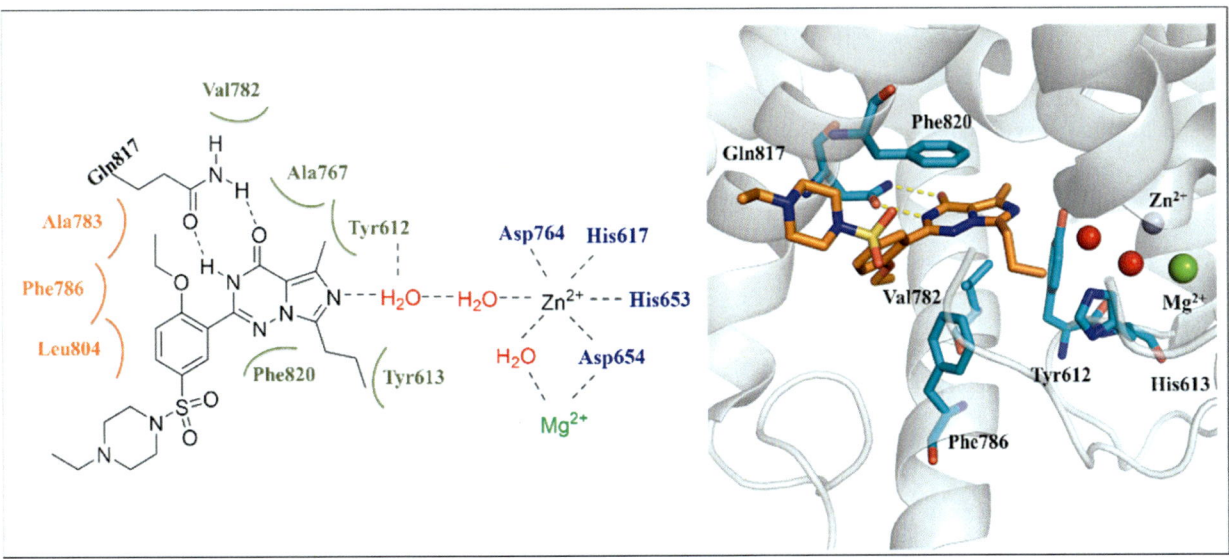

FIGURE 23.16 Molecular binding pattern of PDE5A-vardenafil complex (PDB ID: 1UHO). *PDE5A*, Phosphodiesterase type 5A.

23.6 Summary and prospect

The research and development of sildenafil began in the 1980s with the initial aim of targeting cardiovascular diseases like angina pectoris and coronary heart disease. However, the results of clinical phase I trials did not meet expectations, leading to the termination of further studies. Nevertheless, an unexpected discovery during these trials—an "adverse effect erection"—revived interest in sildenafil, ultimately making it the first oral drug for clinical treatment of ED. Currently, PDE5A inhibitors such as sildenafil, vardenafil, and tadalafil have gained global acceptance for the treatment of ED caused by various etiologies due to their well-established efficacy and safety profiles. Since its approval for ED therapy in 1998, researchers have continued to explore the potential benefits of sildenafil for cardiovascular and circulatory disorders. Phosphodiesterase PDE5A, a key protease in the pulmonary artery that regulates vasoconstriction, has been extensively studied in animal experiments, demonstrating that sildenafil-mediated inhibition of PDE5A activity can effectively suppress or delay hypoxia-induced acute elevation of pulmonary artery pressure and mitigate pulmonary vascular remodeling. In 1998, Sanchez et al. discovered an upregulation of PDE5A gene expression in the lungs of patients with PAH. Pfizer initiated a pioneering small-scale clinical trial to explore intravenous treatment for PAH, aiming to broaden its therapeutic indications. During this study period, over 80 PAH patients experienced significant reductions in both their pulmonary artery pressure and pulmonary circulatory resistance. Between 1998 and 2002, numerous basic studies have reported the efficacy of oral sildenafil in treating pulmonary hypertension.

Following that period from 2002 to 2005, several randomized controlled trials showcased the substantial influence of sildenafil in reducing symptoms of different types of PAH, such as idiopathic PAH, congenital heart disease-associated PAH, respiratory system disorder-related PAH, chronic thromboembolic PHA, and persistent neonatal PAH. The 12-week SUPER-1 trial, a large-scale, randomized, controlled, multicenter phase III clinical study, demonstrated the efficacy of sildenafil in enhancing exercise tolerance and improving pulmonary hemodynamic parameters among patients with PAH. Furthermore, long-term administration of sildenafil was found to sustain and enhance the 6-minute walk distance as well as improve heart function classification [36]. Consequently, in 2005, both the FDA and EMEA-approved sildenafil under the trade name Revatio for treating PAH. The recommended initial dosage is 20 mg, taken three times daily. Since then, this well-established treatment for ED has gained a broader understanding within medical circles and expanded its clinical applications to include pulmonary vascular disorders, bringing renewed hope to numerous patients with PAH.

With the increasing clinical application of sildenafil, several clinical trials have reported that PAH patients treated with a reduced dose of 20 mg twice a day may experience deterioration, while an increase in dosage leads to improvement. However, larger clinical trials have demonstrated that the optimal treatment dose for PAH using sildenafil should be 50 mg three times a day, which contradicts the recommended initial dose of 20 mg. Therefore, it is crucial to individualize and adjust the dosage of sildenafil based on therapeutic effects and adverse reactions when treating PAH. Sildenafil shows significant potential for improving the clinical symptoms of patients with PAH from various causes;

however, confirming its long-term benefits requires extensive multicenter trials involving larger groups of people. Moreover, it is crucial to fully recognize the side effects and drug interactions of sildenafil, especially when used together with other medications for pulmonary hypertension. Additionally, meticulous verification of its precise effectiveness is still necessary.

With the emergence of new indications for sildenafil in treating PAH, other PDE5A inhibitors quickly followed up in this therapeutic field. In June 2009, the FDA approved oral tadalafil at a daily dose of 40 mg, marketed as Adcirca, for managing patients with World Health Organization Class 1 pulmonary hypertension. Additionally, in June 2009, the FDA authorized a disintegrated oral vardenafil tablet containing 10 mg from GSK and Merck under the brand name Staxyn. Subsequently, in February 2020, China's National Medical Products Administration approved sildenafil (trade name: Rivanto) for treating adult patients with pulmonary arterial hypertension to improve their exercise capacity and delay clinical deterioration. The most recent Chinese guidelines on diagnosing and treating pulmonary arterial hypertension (2021 Edition) explicitly recommend these three PDE5A inhibitors as they significantly improve exercise tolerance and hemodynamics among Chinese PAH patients. Reflecting on the research progress of sildenafil over the past two decades, researchers are amazed by its unexpected effectiveness. Sildenafil, the pioneering oral medication with a significant impact on treating ED and PAH, undoubtedly provides immense benefits to the majority of patients. However, people's understanding of PDE5A inhibitors like sildenafil and tadalafil remains insufficient, particularly in the field of PAH treatment. Given their relatively short period of use, further investigation and exploration are essential. In the lengthy process of developing new drugs, pharmaceutical scientists need to possess not only the qualities of persevering scientists but also the abilities of intelligent analysis and perceptive insight. The discovery of sildenafil's "adverse reaction erection" during the development of antianginal drugs paved the way for the successful introduction of oral ED medications over two decades ago. Ongoing comprehension of sildenafil's efficacy is crucial, as it has a significant impact on pulmonary hypertension. This representative case of sildenafil highlights how new drug discovery is an incessant exploration process driven by knowledge acquisition. Pharmaceutical science remains a semiempirical scientific discipline that necessitates continual experimentation to identify and elucidate novel phenomena while striving toward unraveling the nature of things.

References

[1] Mckinlay JB. The worldwide prevalence and epidemiology of erectile dysfunction. Int J Impot Res 2000;(Suppl 4):S6–11.
[2] Liu JH, Luan Y. Molecular biological studies of erectile dysfunction: An update. Natl J Androl 2015;21(02): 99-106.
[3] Lue TF. Erectile dysfunction. N Engl J Med 2000;342(24):1802–13.
[4] Turko IV, Francis SF, Corbin JD. Potential roles of conserved amino acids in the catalytic domain of the cGMP-binding cGMP-specific phosphodiesterase. J Biol Chem 1998;273(11):6460–6.
[5] Lugnier C. Cyclic nucleotide phosphodiesterase (PDE) superfamily: a new target for the development of specific therapeutic agents. Pharmacol Ther 2006;109(3):366–98.
[6] Li Z, Wu Y, Feng L-J, et al. Ab Initio QM/MM study shows a highly dissociated SN2 hydrolysis mechanism for the cGMP-specific phosphodiesterase-5. J Chem Theory Comput 2014;10(12):5448–57.
[7] Maurice DH, Ke H, Ahmad F, et al. Advances in targeting cyclic nucleotide phosphodiesterases. Nat Rev Drug Discov 2014;13(4):290–314.
[8] Ignarro LJ. After 130 years, the molecular mechanism of action of nitroglycerin is revealed. Proc Natl Acad Sci U S A 2002;99(12):7816–27.
[9] Hare JM, Colucci WS. Role of nitric oxide in the regulation of myocardial function. Prog Cardiovasc Dis 1995;38(2):155–66.
[10] Terrett NK, Bell AS, Brown D, et al. Sildenafil (VIAGRATM), a potent and selective inhibitor of type 5 cGMP phosphodiesterase with utility for the treatment of male erectile dysfunction. Bioorg Med Chem Lett 1996;6(15):1819–24.
[11] Williams DH, Stephens E, O'Brien DP, et al. Understanding noncovalent interactions: ligand binding energy and catalytic efficiency from ligand-induced reductions in motion within receptors and enzymes. Angew Chem Int Ed Engl 2004;43(48):6596–616.
[12] Sheng CQ, Li J. Structural optimization of drugs: design strategies and empirical rules. Beijing: Chemical Industry Press; 2017. p. 9.
[13] Jackson G, Benjamin N, Jackson N, et al. Effects of sildenafil citrate on human hemodynamics. Am J Cardiol 1999;83(5A):13C–20C.
[14] Zhang K, Zhu JC. A decade's evidence review of sildenafil citrate. Natl J Androl 2009;15(01): 3-6.
[15] Ignarro LJ, Bush PA, Buga GM, et al. Nitric oxide and cyclic GMP formation upon electrical field stimulation cause relaxation of corpus cavernosum smooth muscle. Biochem Biophys Res Commun 1990;170(2):843–50.
[16] Haning H, Niewöhner U, Schenke T, et al. Imidazo[5,1-f]1, 2, 4triazin-4(3H)-ones, a new class of potent PDE 5 inhibitors. Bioorg Med Chem Lett 2002;12(6):865–8.
[17] Daugan A, Grondin P, Ruault C, et al. The discovery of tadalafil: a novel and highly selective PDE5 inhibitor. 1: 5,6,11,11a-tetrahydro-1H-imidazo[1',5':1,6]pyrido[3,4-b]indole-1,3(2H)-dione analogues. J Med Chem 2003;46(21):4525–32.
[18] Daugan A, Grondin P, Ruault C, et al. The discovery of tadalafil: a novel and highly selective PDE5 inhibitor. 2: 2,3,6,7,12,12a-hexahydropyrazino[1',2':1,6]pyrido[3,4-b]indole-1,4-dione analogues. J Med Chem 2003;46(21):4533–42 9.

[19] Elgoyhen B, Lorenzo PS, Tellez-IñóN MT, et al. Relaxant effects of beta-carbolines on rat aortic rings. J Pharmacol Exp Ther 1992;261(2):534–9.
[20] Koe BK, Lebel LA. Contrasting effects of ethyl beta-carboline-3-carboxylate (beta CCE) and diazepam on cerebellar cyclic GMP content and antagonism of both effects by Ro 15-1788, a specific benzodiazepine receptor blocker. Eur J Pharmacol 1983;90(1):97–102.
[21] Chen L, Jia JM, Zhong W, et al. Comparative study on adverse drug reactions of three phosphodiesterase-5 inhibitors (sildenafil, vardenafil and tadalafil). Eval Anal Drug Use Hospitals China 2009;09:711–14.
[22] Bell A.S., Brown D., Terrett N.K. Pyrazolopyrimidinone antianginal agents. EP, EP0463756B1. 1996.
[23] Dunn PJ. Synthesis of commercial phosphodiesterase(V) inhibitors. Org Process Res Dev 2005;9(1):88–97.
[24] Mao Y, Tian G, Liu Z, et al. An improved synthetic route for preparative process of vardenafil. Org Process Res Dev 2009;13(6):1206–8.
[25] Liu ZZ, Li Z-L, Lü P, et al. Process improvement on the synthesis of vardenafil. Chin J Synth Chem 2016;24(12):1094–7.
[26] Daugan C.M. Tetracyclic derivatives, process of preparation and use. US, US6025494 A, 2000.
[27] Yao SB, Cai MD, Lu XY, et al. Study on the synthesis of tadalafil. Fine Chem Intermed 2010;40(06):39–42.
[28] Shi X-X, Liu S-L, Xu W, et al. Highly stereoselective Pictet–Spengler reaction of d-tryptophan methyl ester with piperonal: convenient syntheses of Cialis (Tadalafil), 12a-epi-Cialis, and their deuterated analogues. Tetrah Asym 2008;19(4):435–42.
[29] Jansen C, Kooistra AJ, Kanev GK, et al. PDEStrIAn: a phosphodiesterase structure and ligand interaction annotated database as a tool for structure-based drug design. J Med Chem 2016;59(15):7029–65.
[30] Bender AT, Beavo JA. Cyclic nucleotide phosphodiesterases: molecular regulation to clinical use. Pharmacol Rev 2006;58(3):488–520.
[31] Rybalkin SD, Rybalkina IG, Shimizu-Albergine M, et al. PDE5 is converted to an activated state upon cGMP binding to the GAF A domain. EMBO J 2003;22(3):469–78.
[32] Blount MA, Zoraghi R, Ke H, et al. A 46-amino acid segment in phosphodiesterase-5 GAF-B domain provides for high vardenafil potency over sildenafil and tadalafil and is involved in phosphodiesterase-5 dimerization. Mol Pharmacol 2006;70(5):1822–31.
[33] Turko IV, Ballard SA, Francis SH, et al. Inhibition of cyclic GMP-binding cyclic GMP-specific phosphodiesterase (type 5) by sildenafil and related compounds. Mol Pharmacol 1999;56(1):124–30.
[34] Sung B-J, Yeon Hwang K, Ho Jeon Y, et al. Structure of the catalytic domain of human phosphodiesterase 5 with bound drug molecules. Nature 2003;425(6953):98–102.
[35] Zhang KYJ, Card GL, Suzuki Y, et al. A glutamine switch mechanism for nucleotide selectivity by phosphodiesterases. Mol Cell 2004;15(2):279–86.
[36] Galiè N, Ghofrani HA, Torbicki A, et al. Sildenafil citrate therapy for pulmonary arterial hypertension. N Engl J Med 2005;353(20):2148–57.

Chapter 24

GABA$_A$ receptor agonists: discovery of the general anesthetic propofol and its analogs

Bowen Ke[1] and Wei Zheng[2]

[1]*Department of Anesthesiology, Laboratory of Anesthesia and Critical Care Medicine, National-Local Joint Engineering Research Centre of Translational Medicine of Anesthesiology, West China Hospital, Sichuan University, Chengdu, P.R. China,* [2]*Haisco Pharmaceutical Group Co. Ltd., Chengdu, P.R. China*

Chapter outline

24.1 Introduction to anesthesia	585
24.2 Common drugs in clinical anesthesia	586
24.2.1 Inhalation anesthetics	586
24.2.2 Intravenous anesthetics	587
24.2.3 Local anesthetics	587
24.3 Medicinal chemistry of the general intravenous anesthetic propofol and its analogs	588
24.3.1 The GABA$_A$ receptor and the GABAergic system: the first step to decipher the general anesthesia	589
24.3.2 GABA$_A$ receptor agonists: finding a way to general anesthesia	593
24.3.3 The story of propofol: the unexpected birth of the king	595
24.3.4 Phenolic compounds: a new starting point	596
24.3.5 Optimization of the candidate: a process of constant tradeoffs	600
24.3.6 Propofol analogs: the emergence of ciprofol and fospropofol disodium	603
24.3.7 Pharmaceutical manufacturing technology: the key link to realize industrial production	611
24.3.8 Clinical application and metabolism of propofol in vivo	615
References	616

24.1 Introduction to anesthesia

Through more than a century of development, modern surgery has delved deep into various organs of the human body, enabling complex surgical procedures such as resection and reconstruction. The safe and successful completion of modern surgical procedures relies on three critical factors: infection control, hemorrhage management, and pain elimination. Anesthesia serves as the key to alleviating pain during surgery and, together with other techniques, forms the cornerstone of modern surgical science. Up to the present, anesthesia relieves the suffering of billions of patients every year. However, describing anesthesia is by no means an easy task. This chapter focuses on the definition and development process of general anesthesia drugs. Although there are significant pharmacological differences among various anesthetic agents, all forms of general anesthesia share a common feature: the ability to induce reversible loss of consciousness at low drug concentrations while causing loss of response at higher drug concentrations. Therefore, anesthesia is often described as a state of "loss of motor function, analgesia, amnesia, and muscle relaxation." While the definition of anesthesia is established, its mechanisms remain controversial. Despite the widespread clinical use of anesthetic drugs, our understanding of the molecular and neural network mechanisms underlying their anesthetic effects is still incomplete. The key mechanisms of anesthesia drugs, particularly general anesthetics, have yet to be fully elucidated. As one of the most crucial categories of drugs in medicine, the ambiguity surrounding the mechanism of anesthesia not only hinders the rational use of existing drugs but also impedes the research and development of new generations of anesthetic agents.

In 2005, on the occasion of the 125th anniversary of the journal Science, the elucidation of the mechanisms of general anesthesia drugs was listed among the 125 most challenging scientific questions in the world [1].

Since the beginning of the 21st century, the definition of anesthesia and the application of anesthetic drugs have greatly expanded. With the introduction of the concept of enhanced recovery after surgery, the application of anesthetic drugs has extended beyond simple surgical procedures to the entire perioperative period. As a result of this shift, the definition of anesthetic drugs has gradually expanded from traditional general and local anesthetics to include sedatives, analgesics, muscle relaxants, and myorelaxant antagonists—encompassing a broader range of anesthesia-related medications. Furthermore, new requirements have been proposed regarding the effectiveness, safety, controllability, and synergistic interactions among different drugs.

24.2 Common drugs in clinical anesthesia

Currently, the anesthetic drugs commonly used in clinical practice can be broadly classified into 3 categories: inhalation anesthetics, intravenous anesthetics, and local anesthetics. Inhalation anesthetics and intravenous anesthetics are primarily employed for general anesthesia, while local anesthetics are mainly used for local infiltration and regional nerve blockade anesthesia. These anesthetic drugs find extensive application in various conditions, including intraoperative anesthesia in the operating room (for surgical procedures), anesthesia outside the operating room (for interventions, endoscopy, oral procedures, medical aesthetics, etc.), pain management (for painless labor, postoperative analgesia, chronic pain, etc.), as well as sedation-hypnosis (for ICU sedation, sleep disorder treatment, etc.). This chapter primarily focuses on the discovery and development of intravenous general anesthetic propofol and its analogs, which are currently the most widely used in clinical practice.

24.2.1 Inhalation anesthetics

On October 16, 1846, William Morton, an American dentist, successfully performed the world's first general anesthesia using ether on a patient in the dome hall of the Massachusetts General Hospital, affiliated with Harvard Medical School (Fig. 24.1). Subsequently, general anesthesia rapidly gained acceptance in the medical community and became widely used. This event marked a turning point in surgery, shifting from a brutal and cruel "torture" to a safe, scientific, and alleviating therapeutic process, thus heralding the beginning of modern surgical science. In his book "The 100: A Ranking of the Most Influential Persons in History," American author Michael. H. Hart ranked the discoverer of ether anesthesia as the 37th most influential person, stating, "In history, few inventions have received such high praise and caused such significant changes in human conditions as anesthesia."

After ether was widely used for general anesthesia, a series of gas molecules with diverse chemical structures and pharmacological effects was subsequently discovered (Fig. 24.2), including volatile anesthetics such as potent halogenated ethers (such as sevoflurane) and alkanes (halothane), as well as gas anesthetics (such as nitrous oxide). Gas anesthetics, represented by nitrous oxide, had a short induction period, good analgesic effects, and rapid recovery after cessation of administration, but their anesthetic potency was relatively weak, making them suitable for minor procedures such as tooth extraction. In the 1950s, halothane was found and confirmed to have advantages such as low flammability, good induction

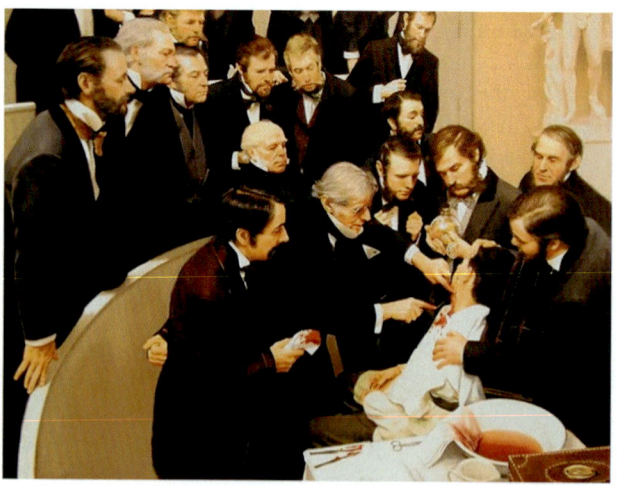

FIGURE 24.1 William Morton successfully performed the first human anesthesia using ether. *"Ether Day 1846" by Warren and Lucia Prosperi (2001).*

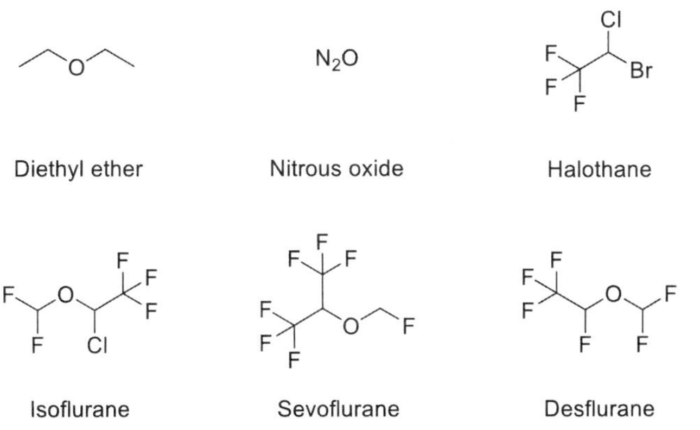

FIGURE 24.2 Chemical structure of partial inhalation anesthetics.

Diethyl ether   Nitrous oxide   Halothane

Isoflurane   Sevoflurane   Desflurane

tolerance, and rapid onset of action [2]. Subsequently, Terrell found another fluorinated gas, isoflurane, which was officially introduced for clinical anesthesia in 1981. Three years later, the anesthetic effects of sevoflurane were reported, and its physicochemical and pharmacological toxicological properties were comprehensively evaluated [3]. Even now, sevoflurane remains the most widely used inhalation anesthetic in clinical practice. In addition, other volatile inhalation anesthetics such as desflurane also play a significant role in general anesthesia management.

24.2.2 Intravenous anesthetics

Although inhalation anesthesia offers the advantages of convenient administration and controllable depth of anesthesia, further improvements are needed to address the drawbacks associated with it, such as operating room contamination, patient agitation during the recovery period, the risk of malignant hyperthermia, and the high cost of anesthesia equipment. To overcome the limitations of inhalation anesthesia, researchers have developed intravenous general anesthetics to meet the practical demands in clinical situations (hereinafter called intravenous anesthetics). Currently, intravenous anesthetics are widely employed for anesthesia induction, maintenance, and sedation in various scenarios.

Barbiturate compounds were discovered in the early 20th century. The introduction of thiopental sodium, a water-soluble barbiturate, in 1934 marked the official application of intravenous anesthetics in clinical practice (Fig. 24.3). Benzodiazepine drugs are primarily used for their anxiolytic, amnesic, or sedative effects. The first water-soluble benzodiazepine, midazolam, remains the most widely used sedative-anesthetic in the field of anesthesia due to its short half-life, potent anterograde amnesia, and lack of irritant effects [4]. The phencyclidine derivative, ketamine, exhibits strong analgesic and amnesic effects while presenting a distinct state of anesthesia and analgesia. Since ketamine has a mild effect on respiration, this feature becomes an advantage for its clinical application [5]. Etomidate, an imidazole derivative, is widely employed due to its stable hemodynamics, minimal respiratory depression, and desirable pharmacokinetic properties. However, the occurrence of myoclonus and prolonged suppression of adrenal cortical function during its use significantly limit its clinical application. Nevertheless, its favorable cardiovascular effects continue to attract the attention of anesthesiologists. Propofol, an alkylphenol derivative, currently stands as the most commonly used intravenous anesthetic in clinical practice. This compound possesses high lipid solubility and is primarily utilized for general anesthesia induction and maintenance, as well as for sedation in and out of the operating room.

24.2.3 Local anesthetics

Local anesthetics can block voltage-gated sodium channels, thereby inhibiting the generation and conduction of nerve impulses along axons. Based on this mechanism, local anesthetics do not act on the central nervous system and can reversibly block the occurrence and conduction of local sensory nerve impulses while maintaining the patient's consciousness, resulting in the reversible disappearance of local pain perception. In 1855, the Austrian chemist Neumann extracted and purified a compound from coca leaves, which was the first isolated monomeric compound with local anesthetic properties known as cocaine. However, due to its hallucinogenic and addictive properties, cocaine was eventually classified as a controlled substance by multiple countries.

Existing local anesthetics can be divided into two major categories: amino esters and amino amides. In 1905, the amino ester local anesthetic procaine was introduced for clinical use in surface anesthesia, infiltration anesthesia, and subarachnoid anesthesia. Procaine has a rapid onset of action and a duration of local anesthesia of 30–45 minutes, making it a short-acting

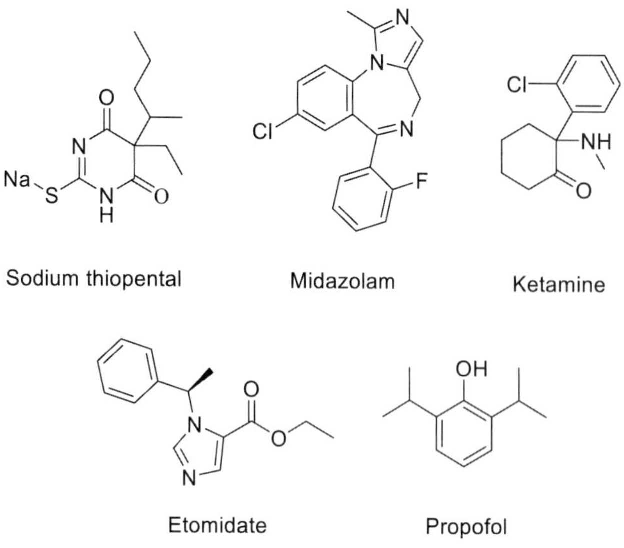

FIGURE 24.3 Chemical structures of partial intravenous anesthetics.

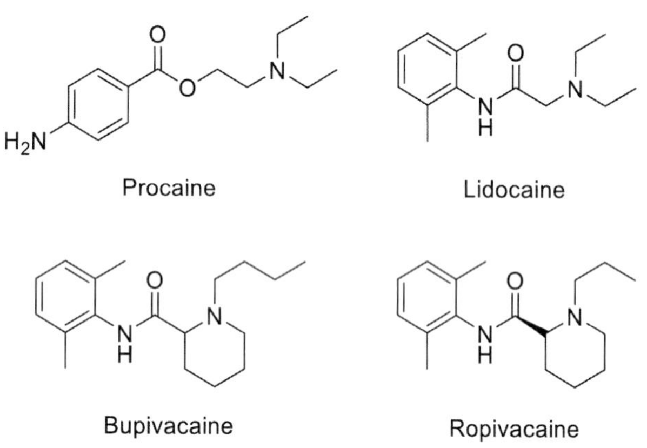

Sodium thiopental   Midazolam   Ketamine

Etomidate   Propofol

FIGURE 24.4 Chemical structures of partial local anesthetics.

Procaine   Lidocaine

Bupivacaine   Ropivacaine

local anesthetic. Compared to procaine, the amino amide local anesthetic lidocaine (Fig. 24.4) has higher potency and a longer duration of local anesthesia, typically producing an anesthetic effect of 60–90 minutes. It is commonly used for infiltration anesthesia and peripheral nerve blockade. In 1963, the long-acting local anesthetic bupivacaine entered clinical practice, with a duration of anesthesia that can be two to three times longer than lidocaine. However, bupivacaine has a significant blocking effect on β-receptors and can cause hypotension and bradycardia at high doses [6]. Another long-acting local anesthetic, ropivacaine, effectively blocks sensory nerves at low concentrations but has minimal effect on motor nerves, demonstrating a certain degree of motor-sensory separation [7]. Ester-type local anesthetics are primarily metabolized by plasma esterase, while amide-type local anesthetics are mainly metabolized by hepatic cytochrome P450 enzymes, which exhibit higher toxicity. Currently, the development of local anesthetics is mainly focused on prolonging the duration of action, improving safety, and achieving specific sensory nerve blockade.

24.3 Medicinal chemistry of the general intravenous anesthetic propofol and its analogs

Reviewing the progress of human society over the past centuries, the development of modern pharmaceuticals undoubtedly stands out as one of the most significant and impactful endeavors. Whether it is the discovery of antibiotics or the introduction of anticancer drugs, these advancements have undeniably contributed to the social progress of humanity. While the discovery of new drugs involves numerous complex and challenging tasks, like most intricate endeavors, pharmaceutical research can be simplified into several components. Taking the development of anesthetic drugs as an example, it first requires an understanding of the mechanisms underlying reversible loss of consciousness in the human body, elucidating the relevant targets of anesthesia such as ion channels, and establishing a close connection between these targets and the anesthetic state. Subsequently, it involves identifying lead compounds from millions of chemical entities that can interact with the targets and exert anesthetic effects. Once lead compounds with the desired effects are obtained, further structural optimization is pursued, aiming to screen for drug-candidate compounds that do not produce significant adverse reactions and do not interfere with vital life functions such as circulation and respiration.

In addition, it is necessary to evaluate whether the physicochemical and metabolic properties of the anesthetic candidate compounds can meet the administration methods (inhalation and intravenous injection) and clinical application scenarios (rapid onset and short half-life) of an anesthetic drug. Once candidate compounds are determined, the new drug development stage will begin. At this stage, candidate compounds will undergo rigorous pharmaceutical and clinical trials to obtain complete production and storage information, animal pharmacodynamics, toxicity, and clinical Phase I/II/III study data. Ultimately, according to the complete preclinical and clinical trial research results, as well as follow-up studies after marketing (known as clinical trial research Phase IV), we can truly determine which new anesthetic drugs will finally gain acceptance by patients and physicians and be favored for production and sales by enterprises.

While the above stages and steps are similar to the process of most new drug discovery, not every stage and step can be carried out smoothly as described. For example, in history, many drugs have been discovered accidentally during scientific research or other activities. In addition, some drugs have gone through a rigorous research and development process, but the development steps are not set in stone, and some drugs may not have their biological mechanisms of therapeutic action or some major adverse reactions truly elucidated until after marketing. Therefore, new drug development will not be completely rigid about the time and space order of modern new drug development described above. This chapter will use the discovery and development process of propofol and its analogs as the background to introduce and discuss the key work, including the role of $GABA_A$ receptors in general anesthesia, the discovery and development of $GABA_A$ receptor agonists, the discovery of propofol lead compounds, the optimization of propofol and its analogs, and production process research, to scientifically interpret general anesthetics from an objective perspective.

24.3.1 The $GABA_A$ receptor and the GABAergic system: the first step to decipher the general anesthesia

The development of new drugs often begins with a profound understanding of the disease. In this process, it is necessary to comprehend and delineate the clinical needs that require urgent solutions and identify the targets that may be closely associated with these clinical needs. However, the selection of appropriate targets or determining which stage of the disease (or indication) the novel drug development should focus on is not always clear from the outset. This ambiguity is one of the significant reasons why drug development entails substantial risks. For instance, due to limited knowledge regarding the pathogenesis of Alzheimer's disease and the absence of well-defined targets, the ongoing efforts to develop therapeutic drugs for Alzheimer's disease have encountered consecutive failures. Another example is general anesthesia. Although millions of patients worldwide undergo safe and reversible loss of consciousness, enabling surgical procedures with the aid of general anesthetics, the mechanism of these drugs has not been fully elucidated to date. General anesthesia, being one of the oldest and most perplexing pharmacological enigmas, still harbors numerous puzzles that remain unsolved. For example, how do molecules with such extensive structural diversity, ranging from simple inert gas molecules to complex small-molecule compounds, achieve the same anesthetic pharmacological effect? Is there a common mechanism that can explain the transition from conscious to unconscious states within a minuscule range of molecular concentration changes? These questions are closely intertwined with the development of anesthetic drugs but are highly contentious, reflecting the immense challenges and difficulties faced in the current pursuit of anesthetic drug development.

In the decades following the successful implementation of the first human anesthesia using ether, the field of anesthesia has both perplexed and inspired those who have endeavored to comprehend and elucidate its mechanisms. The initial understanding of anesthesia was marred by erroneous and absurd notions. At that time, it was believed that anesthetics were derived from lipids extracted from the brain, leading to the occurrence of anesthesia. However, coincidentally, the first significant theory regarding the mechanism of anesthetic action was also closely associated with lipids. Meyer and Overton were the pioneers who initially observed a positive correlation between the potency of anesthetics and their oil/water partition coefficients, as depicted in Fig. 24.5 [8]. Once the role of lipids in the structure of cell membranes was understood, this correlation implied that the site of action of general anesthetics is concentrated within the lipid bilayer of neuronal cell membranes. Over the following decades, the lipid-based nonspecific theory of anesthesia dominated the field. This theory suggested that anesthetics primarily induce anesthesia by increasing the fluidity of

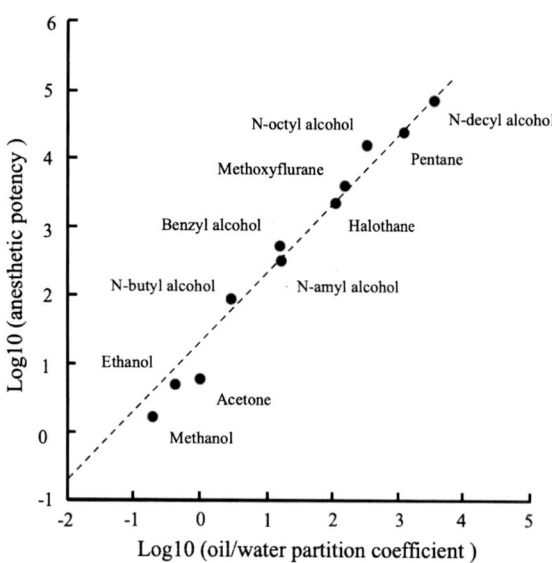

FIGURE 24.5 The correlation between anesthetic potency and the oil/water partition coefficient [8].

the lipid bilayer of neuronal cell membranes, which triggers lipid phase transitions. These transitions result in changes in the size or permeability of the lipid bilayer, thereby producing anesthesia. However, this theory has significant shortcomings that prevent it from being fully explanatory. For example, it is difficult to explain why the changes in the lipid bilayer of cell membranes are minimal at the effective concentrations of anesthetics. Furthermore, why is it not possible to achieve general anesthesia by manipulating the lipid bilayer using physical methods such as temperature changes?

With the rapid advancements in neuroscience and molecular biology, there have been new developments in our understanding of the nature of the anesthetic state. In the 1980s, the groundbreaking discoveries by Franks and Lieb propelled the shift in the mechanism of anesthesia from a lipid-centered theory to a protein-centered theory. For instance, the diminishing anesthetic effects of a homologous series of long-chain alcohols led to the abandonment of the traditional theory that anesthesia is solely produced by the disruptive effect of "nonspecific" mechanisms on the lipid bilayer. Further research revealed that the optical isomeric selectivity of anesthetic compounds reinforced the conclusion that anesthesia is associated with protein targets. The emerging viewpoint suggests that general anesthesia may arise from the specific interactions between drugs and hydrophobic regions of certain protein targets within neurons. Pharmacologists have systematically studied various ion channels, receptors, enzymes, and other protein targets implicated in anesthesia, including two-pore potassium channels (such as TASK1), N-methyl-D-aspartate (NMDA) receptors, glutamate receptors, and hyperpolarization-activated cyclic nucleotide-gated channels, among others. Among these targets, γ-aminobutyric acid (GABA) receptors are undoubtedly considered the most significant [9].

GABA receptors can be classified into $GABA_A$ receptors and $GABA_B$ receptors based on their structural and functional differences. $GABA_A$ receptor is a ligand-gated chloride ion channel receptor, which, upon binding with GABA, facilitates the opening of the channel and inhibits neuronal excitability by promoting the inward flow of chloride ions. On the other hand, the latter belongs to the C class of G-protein coupled receptors and, upon binding with GABA, exerts its physiological effects by recruiting G-proteins to mediate downstream signaling pathways [10]. Both types of GABA receptors play crucial roles in the regulation of the GABAergic system and are closely associated with the development of various neurological disorders such as anxiety disorders, epilepsy, and insomnia. Among them, the $GABA_A$ receptor is considered to be the primary target for general anesthesia (Fig. 24.6).

With the advancement of structural biology, scientists have gained deeper insights into the binding modes between general anesthetics and $GABA_A$ receptors (Fig. 24.7). It is increasingly recognized that the diverse pharmacological characteristics of anesthetics acting on $GABA_A$ receptors are closely associated with their binding sites at different locations. The binding site for the endogenous neurotransmitter GABA on the $GABA_A$ receptor is located on two or more extracellular interfaces, primarily within the region between the β2 and α1 subunits [11]. The $GABA_A$ receptor interacts through cation-π interactions with β2 subunit residue Y205, establishes electrostatic interactions with β2 subunit residues Y97 and E155, forms a salt bridge between the carboxyl group of GABA and α1 subunit residue R67, and engages in hydrogen bonding with β2 subunit residue T202. These interactions contribute to enhancing the binding affinity of GABA [11]. Additionally, the binding of general anesthetics to the $GABA_A$ receptor stabilizes the extracellular domain

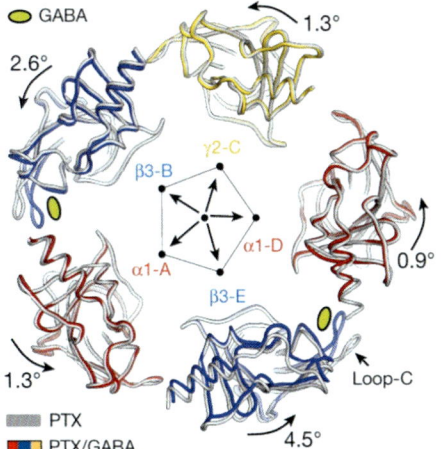

FIGURE 24.6 The crystal structure of endogenous GABA bound to the GABA$_A$ receptor [11]. *GABA*, γ-Aminobutyric acid.

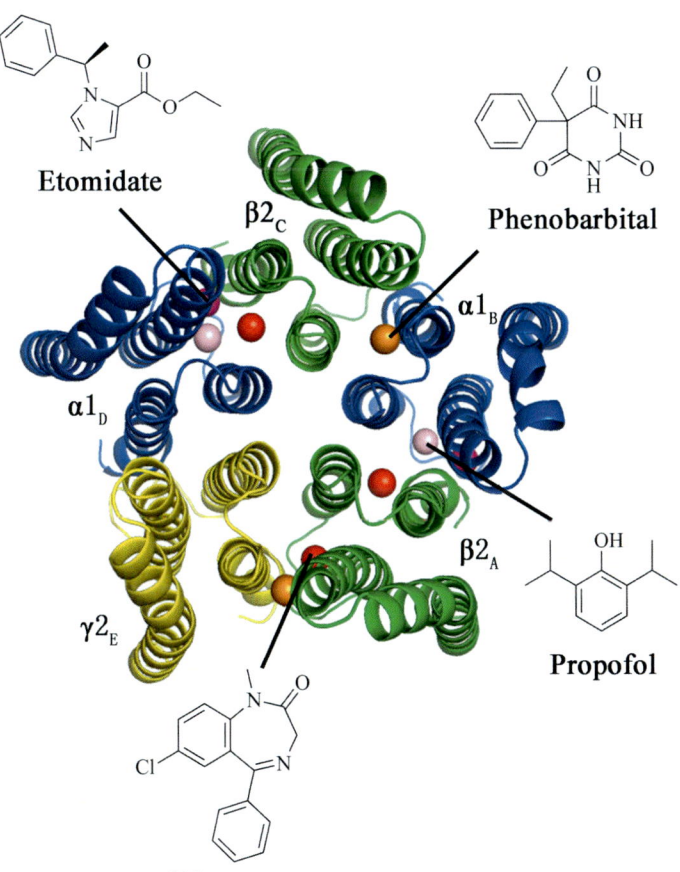

FIGURE 24.7 General anesthetics bind to different sites on the GABA$_A$ receptor [12].

interaction between GABA and the receptor. The binding sites of anesthetics to the receptor exhibit certain similarities. Specifically, propofol, etomidate, and benzodiazepines all target two equivalent sites at the interface between the β and α subunits within the transmembrane region of the GABA$_A$ receptor [12]. Furthermore, benzodiazepines can also bind to two additional sites located at the interface between the extracellular domains of the α and γ subunits and the transmembrane interface between the γ and β subunits of the receptor. Specifically, the interface between the extracellular domains of the α and γ subunits is closely associated with the specific antagonism of flumazenil by benzodiazepines.

Similarly, phenobarbital, like benzodiazepines, binds to the transmembrane interface between the γ and β subunits as well as between the α and β subunits of the GABA$_A$ receptor. The complexity of the binding between GABA$_A$ receptors and anesthetics, as well as the different subtypes of GABA$_A$ receptors, collectively determine the various pharmacological characteristics of anesthesia. For example, the sedative effects produced by benzodiazepines are associated with GABA$_A$ receptors containing the α1 subunit, while their anxiolytic effects involve the participation of GABA$_A$ receptors containing the α2 subunit in the limbic system [13].

The most general anesthetics and some partial anesthetics primarily exert their anesthesia effects through the GABA$_A$ receptor. For instance, intravenous anesthetics or sedatives such as propofol, etomidate, thiopental, and midazolam mainly act as positive allosteric modulators of the GABA$_A$ receptor [14]. They directly or indirectly interact with the GABA$_A$ receptor, enhancing the effects of GABA or directly triggering the opening of Cl$^-$ ion channels, thereby reducing neuronal excitability. However, this mechanism does not explain all phenomena. In fact, inhalation anesthetics have inhibitory effects on excitatory receptors such as nicotinic acetylcholine receptors and NMDA receptors, as well as voltage-gated Na$^+$ and Ca^{2+} channels [15,16]. Special molecules, such as ketamine, are also present in intravenous anesthetics and exert anesthetic effects by inhibiting NMDA receptors on glutamatergic neurons. Studying the GABA$_A$ receptor alone is insufficient to gain a systematic and accurate understanding of general anesthesia within the complex neural network. To comprehensively grasp the mechanism of general anesthesia, researchers have explored the GABAergic system, with the GABA$_A$ receptor as the core, at different levels ranging from the micro to the macro, as illustrated in Fig. 24.8. GABAergic neurons are a class of inhibitory neurons widely distributed across various brain regions. They release GABA after excitation, which acts on GABA receptors on the postsynaptic membrane, thereby reducing the excitability of secondary neurons. During the process of general anesthesia, there is a disruption of the delicate balance between inhibitory and excitatory neurons in key neural clusters. For example, the preoptic hypothalamic

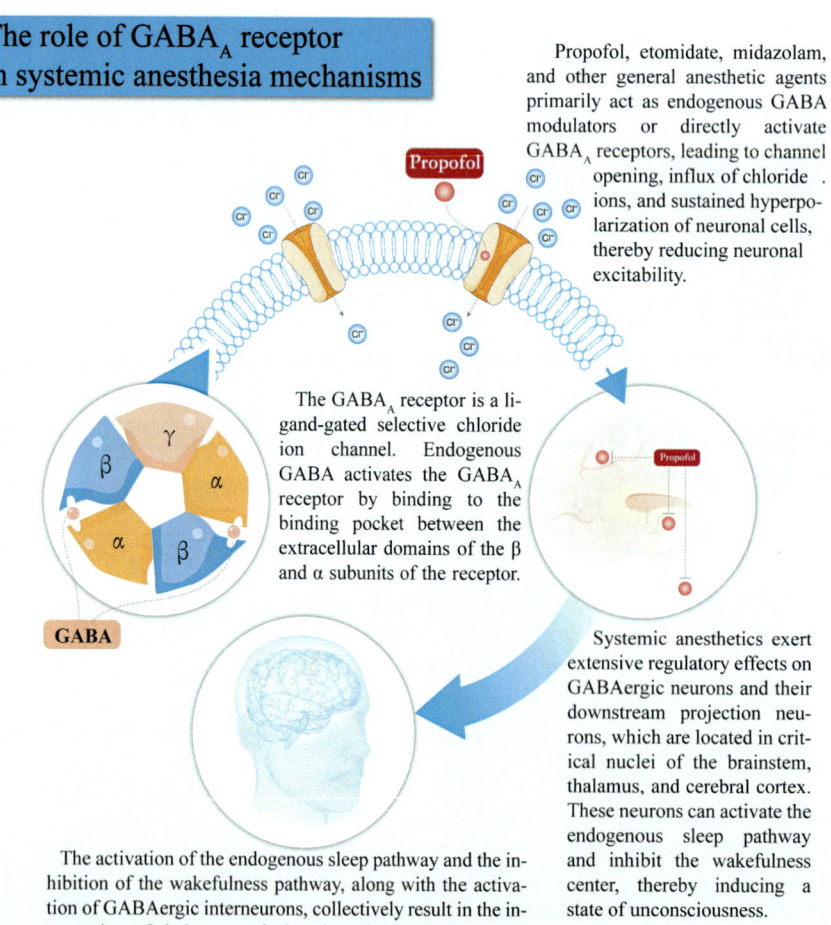

FIGURE 24.8 The role of GABA$_A$ receptor in systemic anesthesia mechanisms.

area (VLOP) and tuberomammillary nucleus are important nuclei in the endogenous sleep-wake pathway, which are believed to be involved in the activation of the sleep pathway and the inhibition of the wakefulness pathway closely related to general anesthesia [17]. Studies utilizing models of the frontal-parietal-cortical network have analyzed that general anesthetics disrupt the transmission of information between the thalamus and the cortex by acting on the GABAergic interneurons, leading to the loss of consciousness mediated by general anesthetics. The mechanisms of general anesthesia, as explained through the endogenous sleep-wake pathway and frontal-parietal-cortical network model, are still in the early stages of research. Further exploratory studies are needed to fully understand this complex phenomenon of general anesthesia involving the interactions within the neural network.

24.3.2 GABA$_A$ receptor agonists: finding a way to general anesthesia

The search for general anesthetics can be traced back to the 17th century. In 1656, Percival Christopher Wren and Daniel Johann Major performed the first intravenous anesthesia of animals by injecting red wine and ale into dogs with the help of a goose feather rod and balloon. For a long time, alcohol has been one of the few narcotic substances known to man. Modern high-throughput screening and computer simulation techniques provide powerful methods for finding lead compounds, but they have their own limitations. Although increasing evidence points to GABA$_A$ receptors as a possible key target in general anesthesia, the crystal structure of GABA$_A$ receptors was not resolved until the 21st century. As a transmembrane protein, GABA$_A$ receptor must bind to the nerve cell membrane under physiological conditions, and the dimensional structure of its protein cannot exist in isolation. In other words, the crystal structure of the GABA$_A$ receptor obtained by the scientists is the result under laboratory conditions and may not match the true conformation of the receptor that plays the anesthetic role under physiological conditions. As a transmembrane protein, the GABA$_A$ receptor membrane structure is highly hydrophobic, and it is difficult to achieve high-throughput drug screening. Therefore, whether it is a gap in information or a limitation in technology, scientists have to resort to other methods in the early stage to find anesthetic lead compounds.

In the absence of other obvious clues, starting with endogenous ligands to find lead compounds is a feasible strategy (Fig. 24.9). As the main inhibitory neurotransmitter, GABA can act specifically on GABA receptors and exert a variety of biological activities. Although this molecule naturally has high affinity and specificity for binding to its receptor, it cannot be used directly as an anesthetic drug because of its high hydropathy, which makes it unable to penetrate the blood—brain barrier (BBB). Naturally, structural modification of the GABA to obtain better physicochemical properties, especially a more suitable hydrophilic-lipophilic balance, has become an important idea for the development of anesthetic drugs. The first reported GABA analog capable of penetrating the BBB was baclofen (Fig. 24.9), chemically synthesized in 1962. Baclofen was obtained by adding a benzene ring structure containing a para halogen to the β-position of the GABA carbonyl group. The introduction of the aromatic structure greatly improved the lipid solubility of the compound, giving it the ability to penetrate the BBB and enter the central nervous system. However, baclofen also has many defects, such as a short half-life and low selectivity. Phenibut, a GABA derivative with a similar structure, also has similar psychopharmacological activity. Phenibut entered clinical trials in the 1960s but was eventually used more for sedation and anxiety, as well as for its cognitive-improving pharmacological activity. γ-hydroxybutyric acid (GHB), another GABA analog, has also attracted attention. In 1964, Laborit proposed the use of GHB for general anesthesia and psychiatric treatment first. When administered orally or intravenously, GHB can quickly cross the BBB and induce

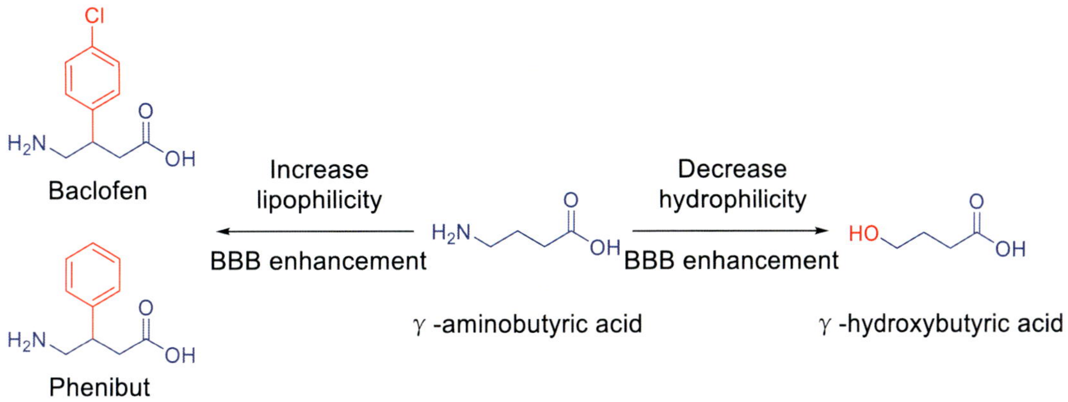

FIGURE 24.9 The discovery of GABA analogs. *GABA*, γ-Aminobutyric acid

a sleep-like state. However, when GHB is used for anesthetic induction, the incidence of adverse reactions such as myoclonic seizures and vomiting is very high, and the euphoria and relaxation lead to a large number of abuses, making it once a notorious drug listed in controlled products in many countries.

It is not easy to find the lead structures from endogenous molecules. The discovery of barbital derivatives was the result of an ongoing search for other active molecules for anesthesia while studying GABA analogs (Fig. 24.10). Unlike acting on GABA receptors directly, barbital derivatives exert the activity by prolonging the action of endogenous ligands on $GABA_A$ receptor (enhancing synaptic GABA transmission). In the early 20th century, Adolf von Baeyer first synthesized barbituric acid. Although this compound is difficult to penetrate the BBB due to its insufficient lipophilicity, its novel chemical structure has become the basic skeleton of all subsequent barbital derivatives with central nervous activity. Pharmaceutical chemists at Bayer have made extensive modifications and derivations of this skeleton and found that the lipophilic derivative barbital (5, 5-diethyl barbituric acid) has high activity in inducing sleep in animals. The action time of barbital derivatives is closely related to the metabolic rate of the substitutions on the C-5 position. Phenobarbital (5-ethyl-5-phenyl-barbituric acid) was obtained by replacing an ethyl group in barbital with a phenyl group. Saturated alkyl and phenyl groups are not easily metabolized in the body and have a long action time. Therefore, barbital and phenobarbital were quickly developed as long-acting (4–12 hours) sedative and hypnotic drugs. In the further structural modification, medium-acting and short-acting sedative and hypnotic drugs, cyclobarbital (2–8 hours) and pentobarbital (1–4 hours), were found. The substituents of them were unsaturated alkane or alkane-containing branched chains, and their metabolism was accelerated. The great success of barbital has led to the synthesis of more than 2,500 derivatives. Among them, the water-soluble sodium salt of lipophilic barbituric acid, pentothal sodium, was used in general anesthesia, which is hailed as an important milestone in the development of general anesthesia drugs, and the marketing of pentothal sodium also marked the opening of the era of modern intravenous anesthesia. Pentothal sodium became the first choice for intravenous anesthesia at that time because of its rapid effect, short duration of action, and weak excitatory effect.

The disadvantages of barbital derivatives are also very obvious. The compounds have strong inhibition on the cardiovascular and respiratory center, often leading to adverse effects such as excitement before anesthetic inhibition, high incidence of tremor, and delayed recovery. As a result, scientists continued to search for other nonbarbital narcotic drugs that target $GABA_A$ receptors. The pharmaceutical company Hoffton-La Roche first synthesized the 1, 4-benzodiazepine derivatives and found chlordiazepoxide to have sedative and hypnotic activity (Fig. 24.11). Compared with barbital derivatives, chlordiazepoxide has fewer adverse effects and a wider safety range, but its sedation depth is insufficient to achieve anesthesia. The narcotic activity of benzodiazepine derivatives is related to the GABA neurotransmitter. The α-subunit of $GABA_A$ has benzodiazepine-specific binding site, also known as benzodiazepine receptors. When benzodiazepine derivatives bind to the receptor at this site, they can increase the opening frequency of chloride ion channels and affinity between the receptor and GABA, thereby enhancing the effect of endogenous GABA.

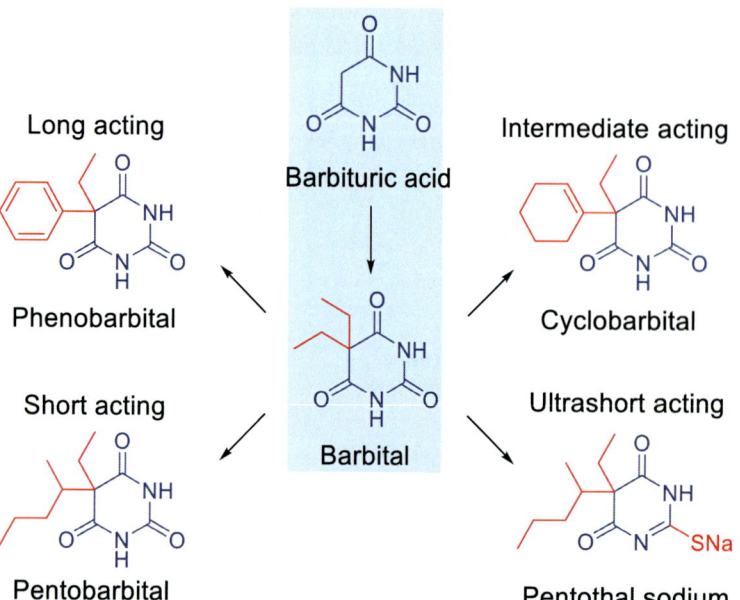

FIGURE 24.10 The discovery of barbiturates.

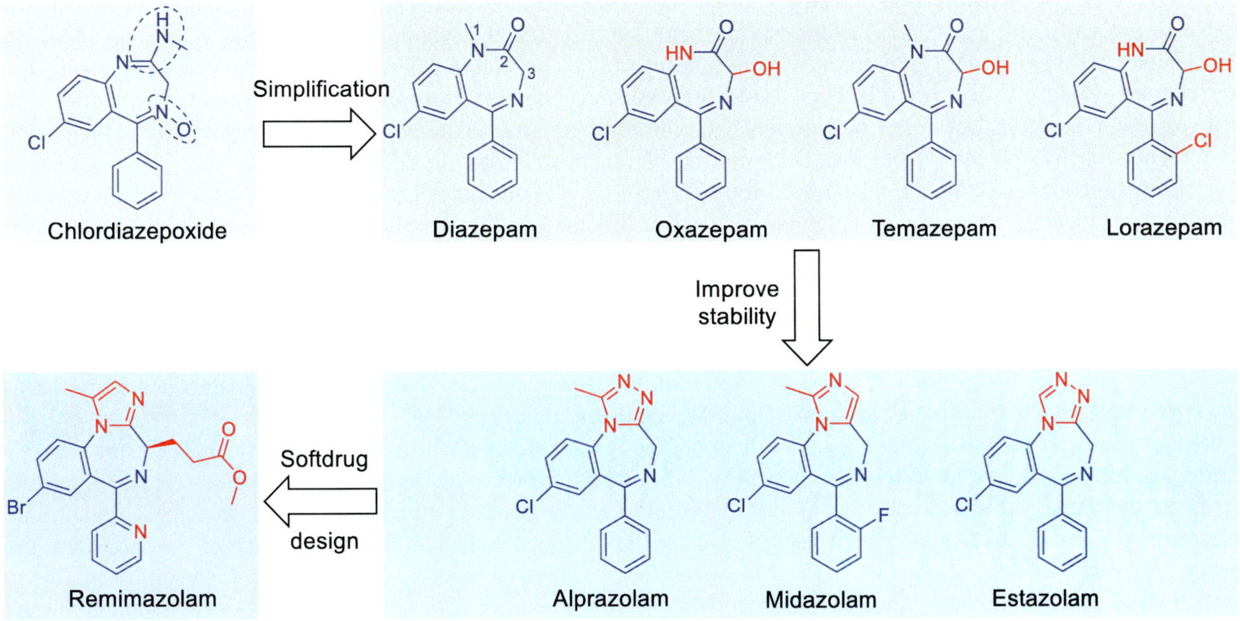

FIGURE 24.11 The discovery of benzodiazepines.

By studying the structure-activity relationship, the researchers found that the nitrogen oxidation structure and the amidine structure of the skeleton are not necessary for maintaining activity. Therefore, pharmaceutical chemists "subtracted" the structure of chlordiazepoxide to obtain diazepam. Diazepam is 3–10 times more active than chlordiazepoxide and has fewer adverse effects. The chemical synthesis is simpler and more convenient. Its 7-membered iminolactam ring is considered to be the key structure to maintain its activity. The discovery of diazepam established the important role of benzodiazepines in sedation and hypnosis. Diazepam is mainly metabolized in the liver, including N_1-demethylation, C_3-oxidation, and ring-opening. It was found that the metabolites of diazepam still had sedative and hypnotic activity, which led to the discovery of new drugs such as oxazepam and temazepam. To improve the metabolic stability, the researchers carried out further structural optimization of diazepam. A series of benzodiazepine drugs with the suffix azolam (-azolam) has been obtained by merging the benzodiazepine ring with N-atom five-membered heterocyclic ring (triazole, methyl-triazole, etc.), of which midazolam is one of the representatives. These molecules have stronger anesthetic pharmacological activities, and the newly formed ring significantly also improves the metabolic stability of the molecular. To better meet the complex application scenarios of clinical surgery, according to the soft drug strategy, GSK Pharmaceutical company introduced a readily hydrolyzable side chain on the 7-membered heterocyclic core and designed a new generation of short-acting $GABA_A$ receptor agonist—remimazolam. Remimazolam, developed by Paion AG, combines the safety of midazolam and the effectiveness of propofol, with rapid onset and rapid metabolism. Remimazolam is metabolized by tissue esterase, and the metabolites are inactive. It can be antagonized by flumazenil and has a high safety. In 2012, Chinese Yichang Humanwell Pharmaceutical Co., Ltd. entered into a cooperation with Paion to obtain the development rights of remimazolam in China. Remimazolam was marketed in China in 2020 for painless diagnostic sedation, general anesthesia, and ICU sedation. Remimazolam toluene sulfonate, developed by Jiangsu Hengrui Medicine Co., Ltd, was also approved in 2019 for sedation during routine gastroscopy.

24.3.3 The story of propofol: the unexpected birth of the king

John Baird Glen, the inventor of propofol (Fig. 24.3), was born on a farm on the Isle of Arran, Scotland. Motivated by his love of science, Glen chose to study veterinary medicine at the University of Glasgow and received a Graduate Diploma in Veterinary Anesthesia from the Royal Veterinary College. After graduation, Glenn worked mainly on the surgical anesthesia of various animals. At that time, anesthesia in animals was usually administered with acepromazine, followed by induction of anesthesia with sodium thiopental. After endotracheal intubation, maintenance was completed by inhalation of anesthetic gas. Such a protocol was cumbersome and risky. With an emphasis on the safety of anesthesia, Janssen Pharmaceutical Company first proposed the concept of diazepam analgesia, by using haloperidol and fentan (Janssen), fluorosulfone and fentanyl (British Crown Chemical), and methyltriazine and etorphine (Reckitt) to narcotize animals. However, the combination of multiple drugs led to the frequent occurrence of nerve excitation, and it was still unable to replace traditional general anesthesia in major surgery. In 1972 Glenn joined Imperial Chemical Industries (ICI, which later merged with Astra to form AstraZeneca) with a keen interest in drug development and experience as a veterinarian, where he was primarily responsible for screening compounds supplied by pharmaceutical chemists for their anesthetic/analgesic activities. ICI promoted the discovery of halothane as an anesthetic gas drug, which laid a solid foundation for the subsequent discovery and development of propofol. After ICI decided to enter the track of developing general anesthetics, it experienced the failure of several new anesthetic research projects, including water-soluble derivatives of etomidate and ketamine, propylene (Epontol and Bayer), and steroid composition (Althesin and Glaxo). Most of these failures were related to the physicochemical properties of the compounds. For example, alfaxalone and alfadolone in althesin had to be solubilized using polyoxyethylene castor oil (Cremophor EL) due to poor water solubility, resulting in frequent adverse reactions in animal experiments. After careful evaluation of the above compounds, ICI company realized that these poor physicochemical properties would bring insurmountable difficulties to the subsequent development of the project. Therefore, the researchers decided to take a new approach and look for lead compound structures with new skeletons from the compound library.

Researchers first selected a number series of lipophilic compounds with obvious differences in skeletons from the existing compound library for screening (generally, compounds with diverse structures will be selected in the initial screening stage to discover new active molecules with different skeletons as much as possible). In some original molecules designed and synthesized for antibiosis, they found that the molecules with phenol structure showed interesting anesthetic effects. On May 23, 1973, scientists observed the anesthetic activity of 2, 6-diisopropyl phenol (propofol) for the first time. After more than a year of pharmacodynamic verification in a variety of animal models including mouse, rat, cat, rabbit, and pig, these compounds were fortunately proved to have safe and good systemic anesthetic activity. Among them, propofol showed the characteristics of short induction time, fast recovery time, and good muscle relaxation effect, which made it have a high clinical development value. However, due to the poor water solubility of propofol, people still used polyoxyethylene castor oil as a cosolvent in the early development of the preparation, which caused adverse reactions such as pain and anaphylaxis at the injection site, and once reached the verge of terminating the development. But Glenn insisted that these adverse reactions may be from polyoxyethylene castor oil, rather than the compound itself. With his unremitting efforts and persistence, ICI company finally developed an improved formulation containing 10% soybean oil and 1.2% purified egg phospholipids, which greatly reduced the discomfort of clinical use and successfully promoted the smooth progress of its clinical trials.

Propofol fat emulsion (trade name: diprivan) was first marketed in the United Kingdom in 1986 and approved by the FDA in the United States in 1989. In 2016, propofol was added to the list of "essential medicines" by the World Health Organization. The birth of propofol changed the treatment concept of the entire anesthesia discipline, and general intravenous anesthesia has since become the "ace weapon" of anesthesiologists. As a powerful sedative, propofol can not only induce and maintain general anesthesia but can also be used in a short operation. In the over 30 years since its marketing, no general anesthetic has challenged its position in anesthesiology and clinical application. In 2018, Glenn was awarded the Lasker Medical Research Award for his contribution to the invention of propofol. Glenn's work was highly praised in the award citation: "He selected propofol from many compounds, devoted his life to the development of a fat emulsion of propofol, and promoted his company (AstraZeneca) to study propofol target-controlled infusion, making it the most widely used anesthetic drug and a boon to patients and anesthesiologists." To provide a true picture of the development of propofol, portions of this section were taken from two memoir articles by Dr. Glenn [18,19]. In the following content, we will give a comprehensive introduction to the development of propofol and its analogs.

24.3.4 Phenolic compounds: a new starting point

Medicinal chemistry is a highly challenging semiempirical discipline. Developing new drugs always begins with searching for a lead compound possessing the desired activity, regardless of whether the target is well-defined, and this process is not easy. In fact, it is very challenging to find a lead compound from millions of existing compounds, or from new compounds that are not yet known (requiring new design and synthesis methods). But sometimes, fortunately, lead compounds with drug-like properties also have similarities. For example, Lipinski's rule of five provides some guidance by analyzing molecular weight (less than 500), lipophilicity ($logP$ value less than 5), hydrogen bond donors (less than 5) and acceptors (less than 10), rotatable bonds (less than 10), etc., which can help medicinal chemists narrow down the screening range in the discovery of oral small-molecule drugs from a vast compound library. Another tricky problem in finding lead compounds is that compounds acting on the same target may have very different structures. In fact, the search for new drug lead compounds is endless, so it can never be certain which one is the best or which one is the last. For example, etomidate and midazolam are both $GABA_A$ receptor agonists, but it is hard to see any common features from their structures; thiopental sodium and sevoflurane have almost no similarities in their physical and chemical properties or molecular structures. From the above content, it can be seen that the chemical structures of $GABA_A$ agonists have high diversity, which brings great difficulty to finding new lead compound structures but obviously also provides opportunities for discovering better lead compounds or drugs.

It can be seen that both the failure of GABA derivatives and the success of barbiturates and benzodiazepines have accumulated valuable experience for the development of anesthetic drugs, and also strengthened the confidence of medicinal chemists to find new lead structures. In the 1960s, thiopental sodium was still the gold standard for clinical induction of anesthesia, so the scientists at ICI hoped to find a compound that could reproduce the good quality of general anesthesia of thiopental sodium but with faster metabolism. To achieve this goal, it was necessary to solve: (1) The new compound could meet the requirement of intravenous injection and have a rapid onset, smooth induction of anesthesia, and no obvious neuroexcitatory effect; (2) Simultaneously, the new compound had to metabolize faster than thiopental sodium and lose its anesthetic activity in a short time, so that it could maintain general anesthesia by repeated injection or continuous infusion. In fact, meeting the characteristics of a perfect general anesthetic was somewhat contradictory: on one hand, the drug needed to have a certain degree of water solubility to meet the requirement of intravenous injection; on the other hand, to quickly penetrate the BBB and enter the brain, the compound had to have high lipophilicity and low molecular weight. These contradictory properties led to the frustration of ICI scientists in the early stage of research and development.

However, persistent perseverance made ICI's scientists eventually become fortunate. After encountering numerous obstacles in other research directions, they decided to select a series of molecules originally intended for antibacterial uses from the existing compound library and test them for anesthetic activity, unexpectedly obtaining surprising progress. Among the selected lipophilic compounds, the first ones observed to have anesthetic activity were phenol and monosubstituted phenol derivatives. This was also the first time that it was discovered that phenolic compounds had anesthetic activity (Table 24.1). Although the anesthetic activity of this class of lead compounds was not high, the discovery of new structures was enough to encourage the researchers. In mice, phenol 1 showed weak anesthetic activity (ED_{50} = 70 mg/kg). Its para-alkyl monosubstituted compound 2 increased its potency by nearly twice (ED_{50} = 30−40 mg/kg) in vivo. However, it was not comparable to other existing anesthetics, such as etomidate with an ED_{50} of 1−1.5 mg/kg. Another bad news was that the safety of the para-substituted phenol 2 derivatives did not improve with the increase in potency, and the therapeutic index was equivalent to that of phenol, both less than 2. A slight consolation was that although the potency of the ortho-monosubstituted compound 4 did not further increase significantly, its safety was improved to some extent. Additionally, it was found that these compounds also had various defects, such as 2-(1-methylbutyl) phenol 3, which could cause obvious

TABLE 24.1 Structure-activity relationship of phenol, ortho-substituted, and para-monosubstituted alkyl phenol derivatives.

$R_2 = R_4 = R_5 = H$

ID	R_1	R_3	ED_{50} (mg/kg)	LD_{50} (mg/kg)	TI
1	H	H	70	100	1.4
2	$CH(CH_3)_2$	H	30−40	100−120	2.5−4
3	$CH(CH_3)C_2H_5$	H	30−40	60−80	1.5−2.7
4	$CH(CH_3)$-n-C_3H_7	H	20−30	100	3.3−5
5	H	$CH(CH_3)_2$	30−40	40−60	1−2
6	H	$CH(CH_3)C_2H_5$	−	40−60	−

respiratory depression at effective doses, and the muscle relaxation effect produced was also weak. Nevertheless, scientists first confirmed that phenolic compounds had general anesthetic activity, providing a new molecular skeleton for the development of future anesthetic drugs.

Because of the disadvantages of phenolic compounds, such as low activity, poor selectivity, and high toxicity, they cannot be directly used as candidate compounds for drug development. In the process of iterative optimization of rationally designed lead compounds, the primary task of medicinal chemists is to improve the activity, specificity, and duration of action of the lead compounds as much as possible. Generally, there are some experiences that can be utilized in the optimization of lead compounds. For example, introducing or reducing hydrophobic or hydrophilic groups to change the lipophilicity and polarity of the compounds, introducing steric hindrance groups to maintain a specific conformation, employing bioisostere of specific groups, and designing groups that are easy to decompose or modify in biological environments to achieve rapid release (prodrugs) or rapid metabolism (soft drugs). Therefore, how to reduce the adverse reactions of phenolic compounds became the first key problem to be solved. Improving the activity and selectivity of lead compounds, as well as increasing the therapeutic index of compounds, is a reasonable direction.

Table 24.2 presents a series of multisubstituted alkyl phenol compounds designed by ICI's medicinal chemists, including di- and tri-substituted derivatives. In this optimization process, the researchers mainly investigated the effect of different substitution sites on the anesthetic activity and safety of the compounds, but the progress was not smooth. The researchers quickly discovered that after the para-position of phenol was substituted, the activity and safety of both di- and tri-substituted compounds did not improve as expected. Especially when there was one or more large steric hindrance bulky substituents, the activity of the compounds was significantly affected. For example, compound 8 exhibited a sharp decrease in ED_{50} from 30–40 to 80 mg/kg when a tert-butyl group was introduced at the ortho position. When two ortho-positions of compound 17 were simultaneously introduced with tert-butyl groups, the anesthetic activity was further reduced (ED_{50} = 80–100 mg/kg). Encouragingly, increased steric hindrance of the substituents did not necessarily result in decreased activity. After introducing substituents of appropriate size (such as isopropyl group), the derivatives obtained more satisfactory results: derivatives with medium steric hindrance groups (such as compounds 12, 14, and 16) could maintain high anesthetic activity (ED_{50} = 20–30 mg/kg) while obtaining higher safety (therapeutic index greater than 4).

TABLE 24.2 Structure-activity relationship of multisubstituted para-alkylated phenol derivatives.

$R_2 = R_4 = H$

ID	R_1	R_3	R_5	ED_{50} (mg/kg)	LD_{50} (mg/kg)	TI
7	CH_3	CH_3	H	30–40	100–120	2.5–4
8	CH_3	$C(CH_3)_3$	H	80	180–200	2.24–2.5
9	$C(CH_3)_3$	CH_3	H	30	100–120[a]	3.3–4
10	$CH(CH_3)_2$	C_2H_5	H	40	120	3
11	$CH(CH_3)_2$	$CH(CH_3)_2$	H	40–60	120	2–3
12	$CH(CH_3)C_2H_5$	$CH(CH_3)C_2H_5$	H	20–30	120	4–6
13	$C(CH_3)_3$	$C(CH_3)_3$	H	40–60	100–120	1.7–3
14	$CH(CH_3)_2$	CH_3	$CH(CH_3)_2$	20	80–100[a,b]	4–5
15	$CH(CH_3)_2$	C_2H_5	$CH(CH_3)_2$	20	80–100	4–5
16	$CH(CH_3)C_2H_5$	CH_3	$CH(CH_3)C_2H_5$	30	140	4.7
17	$C(CH_3)_3$	CH_3	$C(CH_3)_3$	80–100	180–200[a]	1.8–2.5

[a]Delayed mortality occurred.
[b]Severe pulmonary damage occurred 3 days after the injection of 20 mg/kg in rabbits.

However, another result observed in animal experiments aroused the researchers' high alert: although the dose administered was much lower than the half-lethal dose measured by acute toxicity, most para-methyl substituted compounds showed delayed death of animals on the 5th to 7th day after administration. The researchers speculated that, because the para-position was occupied by a substituent, the compounds were difficult to metabolize through a similar pathway as other phenolic series compounds (that is, they were converted to hydroquinone intermediates by phase I metabolism and then conjugated with glucuronic acid by phase II metabolism) (Fig. 24.27), and these compounds might undergo different metabolic pathways, involving the production of toxic intermediates such as para-quinone methides [20]. Although the researchers did not extensively investigate an in-depth study on this abnormal metabolism, the safety risks suggested by the experimental results cast a shadow over the development of para-substituted derivatives.

Similarly, the results of analyzing compounds with meta-substitution modifications were not satisfactory, and the anesthetic activity and safety of the di-, tri-, or even tetra-substituted compounds did not achieve significant improvement (Table 24.3). Among them, compound 20 (3, 6-diisopropyl-2-methylphenol) was outstanding in terms of ED_{50} data (20 mg/kg), but obvious neurological excitement reactions were observed in experimental animals at a lower dose (20 mg/kg), indicating that the compound possessed considerable central nervous system toxicity and posed a safety risk.

However, the ortho-substituted compounds did not disappoint the researchers. Compared with other series of compounds, although the 2,6-dialkyl phenol derivatives in Table 24.4 did not have outstanding anesthetic activity (ED_{50} = 15−40 mg/kg), their therapeutic index was better than other series. Although compared with 2,4-dialkyl phenol derivatives (such as compound 12) or 2,4,6-trialkyl phenol derivatives (such as compounds 15 and 16), the 2,6-dialkyl phenol series derivatives did not show obvious advantages in terms of key data such as ED_{50} or LD_{50}, this series of derivatives did not show the phenomenon of delayed death of animals similar to para-substituted derivatives in animal experiments, suggesting that the metabolites of this series of compounds had higher safety. This feature is very critical for anesthetics that need to be administered continuously for a long time. The potential toxicity of the metabolites of para-substituted derivatives is a risk that has to be carefully considered. After careful analysis, the researchers finally decided to abandon the para-substituted derivatives and look for candidate compounds from the 2,6-dialkyl phenol derivatives. Of course, this series of compounds also had obvious shortcomings: although the duration of anesthesia was prolonged with the increase of alkyl chain length of substituents, most compounds had too short anesthesia time (< 5 minutes). Additionally, the slow induction speed of anesthesia was also an issue that cannot be ignored, and it also implied that the compounds could not quickly and effectively penetrate the BBB. Fortunately, compound 26 (2,6-diethylphenol) in this series unexpectedly stood out. Although 26 did not induce anesthesia quickly (10−15 seconds onset), it showed the highest efficacy (ED_{50} = 15−20 mg/kg) while ensuring safety (therapeutic index = 5−6.7), and therefore received high attention from researchers.

TABLE 24.3 Structure-activity relationship of phenol meta-alkyl multisubstituted derivatives.

$R_3 = H$

ID	R_1	R_2	R_4	R_5	ED_{50} (mg/kg)	LD_{50} (mg/kg)
18	CH_3	H	$CH(CH_3)_2$	H	30−40	80−100
19	$CH(CH_3)_2$	H	CH_3	H	30	100
20	CH_3	$CH(CH_3)_2$	H	$CH(CH_3)_2$	20	100
21	$CH(CH_3)_2$	CH_3	H	$CH(CH_3)_2$	40	100−120
22	n-C_4H_9	CH_3	H	$CH(CH_3)_2$	50	150
23	$CH(CH_3)_2$	CH_3	CH_3	$CH(CH_3)_2$	120	160−180
24	C_2H_5	CH_3	CH_3	C_2H_5	60−80	160

TABLE 24.4 Structure-activity relationship of 2,6-dialkyl phenol derivatives.

$R_2 = R_3 = R_4 = H$

ID	R₁	R₅	Onset time	Duration time	ED₅₀	TI
24	CH_3	CH_3	I	B	20–30	2.7–4
26	C_2H_5	C_2H_5	S	B	15–20	5–6.7
27	C_2H_5	n-C_3H_7	VS	B	20–40	2.5–5
28	n-C_3H_7	n-C_3H_7	I	B	20–30	3.3–5
29	n-C_3H_7	n-C_4H_9	VS	B	20–40	2.5–6

I, Immediate, < 10 s; *S*, slow, 10–15 s; *VS*, very slow, > 15 s; *B*, brief, < 5 min; *M*, moderate, 5–10 min; *L*, long, > 10 min.

24.3.5 Optimization of the candidate: a process of constant tradeoffs

In the process of new drug development, pharmaceutical chemists are like walking on a tightrope. They must carefully adjust and evaluate the various properties of the compound and sometimes have to circumvent the obstacles of patent protection. After obtaining compound 26, scientists focused on the structure-activity relationship study of 2, 6-disubstituted derivatives, hoping to use this as a breakthrough to obtain drug candidates with drug properties. Theoretically, as long as the influences of the structural changes on biological activities, physical and chemical properties, and in vivo metabolism can be summarized, the corresponding structure-activity relationship can be established and the best compound can be inferred. However, in fact, a comprehensive understanding of the structure-activity relationship is much more difficult than imagined. For example, a ligand needs to bind (such as hydrogen bonding, hydrophobic interaction, and even covalent binding) at the appropriate site of the receptor to regulate the dominant conformation of the target and play its biological functions. Therefore, it is not easy to consider and discover the influences of the subtle differences in the structures of ligands on the flexible structural changes of complex biological macromolecules. Moreover, the molecular structure of a drug requires pharmaceutical chemists to pay attention to its physicochemical properties, such as solubility, lipid solubility, and total polar surface area, and to study and summarize the influence of the pharmacokinetic properties of the molecule, such as absorption, distribution, metabolism, and excretion. In many cases, people will find that the study of the structure-activity relationship is like a jigsaw puzzle, which does not require the researchers to fully understand every detail. In fact, there is no way to fully understand. As a result, medicinal chemists often paint a picture of a molecule from fragmented information, and their experience plays a decisive role.

Table 24.5 shows the further derivative strategy of ICI's pharmaceutical chemists based on compound 26. When the total number of substituent carbon units was 7 (compounds 34–36), the potency reached the maximum value. However, when the total number of substituent carbon units reached or exceeded 8, the anesthesia induction was slow and the anesthesia time was prolonged at high doses (compounds 37–39), suggesting that the compounds accumulated in the body. Although these compounds were eliminated due to the shortcomings of slow induction of anesthesia, weak central excitation, and muscle relaxation, the efficacy and safety data also further strengthened the confidence of investigators to continue to search for candidate compounds based on this skeleton. It is worth mentioning that researchers at that time also designed and synthesized several cyclohexyl-substituted phenol derivatives for structural diversity. The cycloalkyl substitution appeared to affect the anesthetic activity of the compounds, but the results gave the researchers incomplete information, so that they did not go on to design more cyclo-substituted compounds for testing. The authors of this chapter speculate that the researchers at that time did not realize that different ring structures could have a large impact on their anesthetic activities and might even have completely different effects, which also laid the foreshadowing of the development of a new generation of ciprofol.

In view of the discovery history of propofol, derivatives of 2, 6-dialkylphenol are the most interesting series (Table 24.6). The compounds in this series were generally highly active and had good safety ($LD_{50}/ED_{50} \geq 5$). As the

TABLE 24.5 Structure-activity relationship of 2-*n*-alkyl-6-*sec*-alkylphenols.

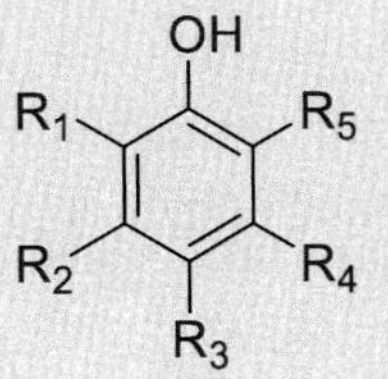

$R_2 = R_3 = R_4 = H$

ID	R1	R5	$\sum C$	Onset time	Duration time	ED50	TI
30	CH$_3$	CH(CH$_3$)$_2$	4	I	B	20–30	2.7–4
31	C$_2$H$_5$	CH(CH$_3$)$_2$	5	I	B	15–20	3–5.3
32	C$_2$H$_5$	CH(CH$_3$)C$_2$H$_5$	6	I	B	10–15	5.3–8
33	*n*-C$_3$H$_7$	CH(CH$_3$)$_2$	6	I	B	20–30	2.7–4
34	C$_2$H$_5$	CH(CH$_3$)-*n*-C$_3$H$_7$	7	I	B	10–20	5–12
35	*n*-C$_3$H$_7$	CH(CH$_3$)C$_2$H$_5$	7	S	B	10–20	6–12
36	*n*-C$_4$H$_9$	CH(CH$_3$)$_2$	7	I	B	20	5
37	CH$_3$	CH(CH$_3$)-*n*-C$_5$H$_{11}$	8	VS	L	15–20	5–6.7
38	*n*-C$_4$H$_9$	CH(CH$_3$)C$_2$H$_5$	8	VS	M	20–30	4–6
39	*n*-C$_3$H$_7$	CH(CH$_3$)-*n*-C$_4$H$_9$	9	VS	M	50	2.8

I, Immediate, < 10 s; *S*, slow, 10–15 s; *VS*, very slow, > 15 s; *B*, brief, < 5 min; *M*, moderate, 5–10 min; *L*, long, > 10 min.

TABLE 24.6 Structure-activity relationship of 2,6-Di-*sec*-alkylphenols.

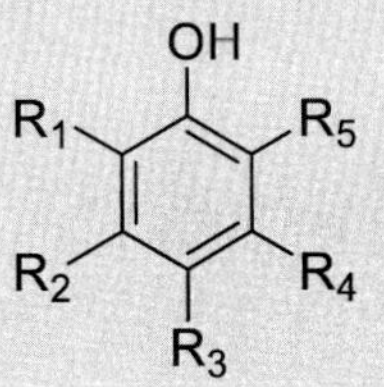

$R_2 = R_3 = R_4 = H$

ID	R$_1$	R$_5$	$\sum^C$	Onset time	Duration time	ED$_{50}$	TI
40	CH(CH$_3$)$_2$	-*n*-C$_3$H$_5$	6	I	B	20–30	4–7
41	CH(CH$_3$)$_2$	CH(CH$_3$)$_2$	6	I	B	5–10	5–10
42	CH(CH$_3$)$_2$	CH(CH$_3$)C$_2$H$_5$	7	I	B	5–10	5–10
43	CH(CH$_3$)C$_2$H$_5$	-*n*-C$_3$H$_5$	7	S	B	20–40	3–7
44	CH(CH$_3$)$_2$	CH(CH$_3$)-*n*-C$_3$H$_7$	8	S	L	10–15	5.3–8
45	CH(CH$_3$)C$_2$H$_5$	CH(CH$_3$)C$_2$H$_5$	8	S	M	5–10	6–12
46	CH(CH$_3$)$_2$	CH(CH$_3$)-*n*-C$_4$H$_9$	9	S	L	10–15	6.7–12
47	CH(CH$_3$)-*n*-C$_3$H$_7$	CH(CH$_3$)-*n*-C$_3$H$_7$	10	VS	L	15–20	8–12

I, Immediate, < 10 s; *S*, slow, 10–15 s; *VS*, very slow, > 15 s; *B*, brief, < 5 min; *M*, moderate, 5–10 min; *L*, long, > 10 min.

chain length of the substituent increased, the anesthetic activity changed. When the number of substituent carbon units was between 6 and 8, the activity reached the maximum. When the number of carbon units was greater than or equal to 9, the anesthetic activity of the compound tended to be stable. When the number of carbon units was less than or equal to 7, the induction speed of anesthesia was faster, and the induction speed changed slower when the number of carbon units continued to increase. When the number of substituent carbon units was greater than or equal to 8, the lipophilicity of the molecule was increased, the duration of anesthesia was correspondingly prolonged, and significant accumulation was observed at high doses. Although the total number of substituent carbon atoms was greater than 8, 2, 6-di-tert-butylphenol had no anesthetic activity, which may be due to the large steric hindrance of ortho-groups affecting its affinity with the $GABA_A$ receptor. In addition to showing good anesthetic activity and safety, analgesic effects were also observed. Similar to other phenol derivatives, these compounds typically had lower therapeutic indices in rabbits than in mice and induced frequent nerve excitation with less muscle relaxation. One of the few exceptions was compound 41 (2, 6-diisopropylphenol), which not only produced smooth and rapid induction and fast recovery from anesthesia but also had good muscle relaxation and a short duration of anesthesia. Among many candidates, compound 41 was finally selected by ICI as a drug-candidate compound due to its high activity, low toxicity, and good drug-like properties, which was also the famous new generation of intravenous anesthetic propofol [20]. Fig. 24.12 visually summarizes the discovery of propofol.

The action of propofol on the $GABA_A$ receptor is primarily focused on indirect and direct effects (Fig. 24.13). In the presence of GABA, propofol binds to the $GABA_A$ receptor and allosterically enhances the action of GABA, prolonging the inhibitory postsynaptic currents mediated by the $GABA_A$ receptor and altering the receptor's inactivation and desensitization properties. In the absence of GABA, high concentrations of propofol can directly activate the $GABA_A$ receptor. The crystal structure of the complex reveals that the binding site of propofol with the $GABA_A$ receptor is located at the β-α subunit interface, which is similar to the binding site of benzodiazepine-like drugs and is considered to be closely associated with both the indirect and direct effects of drugs on the $GABA_A$ receptor. In terms of binding mode, the two isopropyl groups of propofol, one pointing toward the channel axis and the other toward the lipid layer, while the hydrophobic group of the latter interacts with the αP233, which produces M1π-helix. The isopropyl group near the channel points toward β15, forming further van der Waals contacts. The benzene ring in the structure of propofol is parallel to the cell membrane's normal, and its hydroxyl group extends and forms a hydrogen bond with the carbonyl oxygen of the isoleucine at position α228, which is a determinant of the anesthetic potency of propofol.

Additionally, researchers have employed computational methods such as molecular docking, molecular dynamics simulations, and umbrella sampling to further understand the regulation of propofol on the $GABA_A$ receptor. By calculating the MM/GBSA binding free energy and the potential of mean force (PMF), the researchers effectively simulated the difference of the free energy barriers for ion permeation in the open state (bound to GABA or propofol) and closed state (cryo-EM structure PDB ID: 6HUJ) of the $GABA_A$ receptor. The left image in Fig. 24.14 illustrates the M2 helical structure in the central ion channel of the $GABA_A$ receptor and the calculated PMF for chloride ion passage through the channel from top to bottom. In the PMF curve, researchers observed that propofol, upon binding to the predicted site on the $GABA_A$ receptor, significantly decreases the energy barrier for chloride ion passage through the ion channel (Fig. 24.14, right). This further explains how propofol leads to the opening of the receptor's ion channel, causing inward Cl-flow and subsequently reducing neuronal excitability.

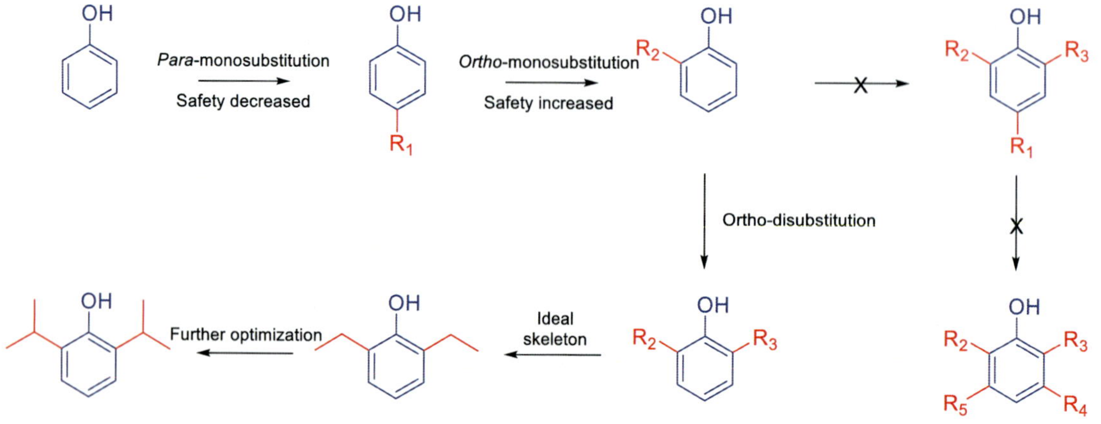

FIGURE 24.12 The discovery of propofol.

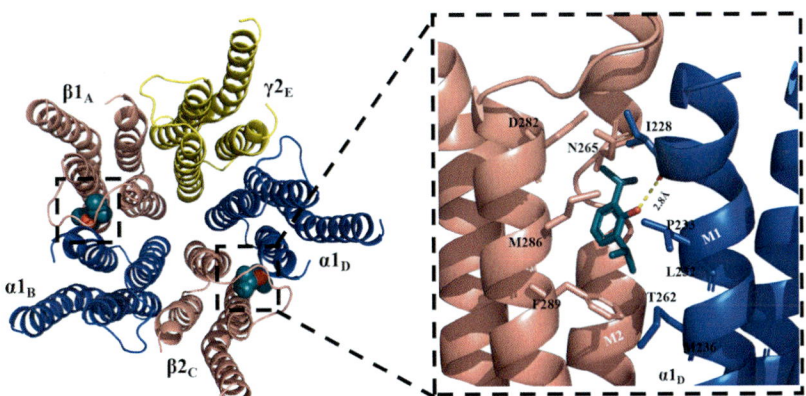

FIGURE 24.13 Crystal structure of propofol and GABA$_A$ receptor complex [12].

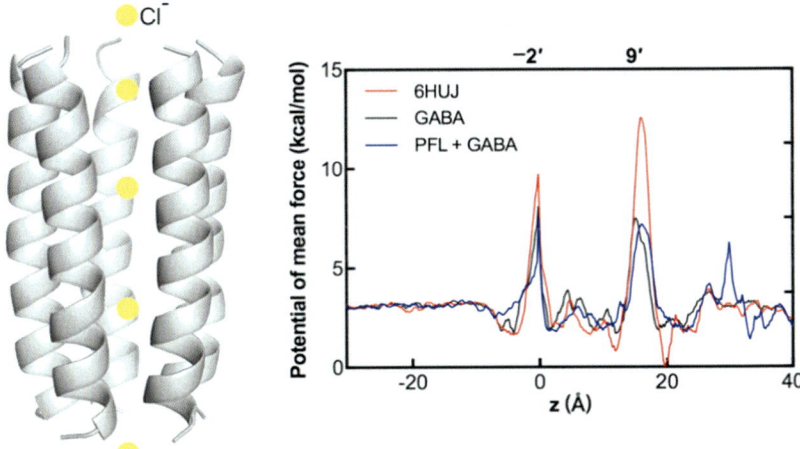

FIGURE 24.14 The energy barrier of propofol-bound GABA$_A$ receptors to chloride by umbrella sampling.

24.3.6 Propofol analogs: the emergence of ciprofol and fospropofol disodium

As one of the foremost intravenous anesthetic agents in clinical practice, propofol is not devoid of noteworthy adverse reactions. During administration, propofol's local vascular irritation-induced pain is specifically termed "injection pain." Statistically, 28%−90% of patients undergoing propofol administration experience injection pain. This phenomenon can heighten patients' tension and anxiety, disrupt the smooth induction of anesthesia, diminish patient comfort, and reduce overall satisfaction with the anesthesia process. Furthermore, propofol induces a rapid decrease in systolic, diastolic, and mean arterial blood pressure, causing pronounced hemodynamic fluctuations. Owing to propofol-induced respiratory depression, auxiliary ventilation measures are often required to maintain adequate oxygen saturation, rendering the procedure more intricate. Additionally, when propofol is administered as a lipid emulsion for continuous infusion, it can potentially result in hyperlipidemia. Hence, current research in medicinal chemistry on propofol primarily focuses on preserving its clinical merits while mitigating its adverse effects. These objects encompass: (1) reducing the drug concentration in the aqueous phase of lipid emulsion to alleviate injection pain; (2) enhancing drug potency to address issues related to excessive lipid infusion during continuous administration; (3) augmenting the therapeutic index to minimize its impact on the circulatory and respiratory systems; (4) improving the compound's water solubility.

In seeking compounds superior to propofol while preserving its existing attributes, it is evidently a formidable challenge. Researchers at Haisco Pharmaceutical Group have chosen to design multiple series of candidate compounds based on the established principles of classical medicinal chemistry, building upon the existing scaffold of propofol (Table 24.7) [21,22]. Employing the classic loss of righting reflex (LORR) model in mice, these molecules have been evaluated across various parameters, including the time to LORR (onset time), duration of LORR (anesthesia maintenance time), walking time (time to return to consciousness), and post-administration adverse reactions, with the aim of assessing both their efficacy and safety. It is hoped that this approach will uncover candidate compounds that exhibit high efficacy, low toxicity, and significant clinical advantages.

TABLE 24.7 Compounds of the benzocyclobutene series.

Propofol ED_{50} = 11.7 mg/kg → m-methyl propofol ED_{50} = 40 mg/kg →

Compound	R_1	R_2	R_3	R_4	ED_{50} (mg/kg)	Safety index
48	i-Pr	Me	H	H	16.3	5.2
49	i-Pr	Et	H	H	14.3	2.4
50	i-Pr	▲	H	H	18.5	3.6
51	i-Pr	OH	H	H	24.5	ND
52	i-Pr	=O	H	H	36.9	ND
53	Br	Me	H	H	39.0	ND
54	i-Pr	Me	OH	H	27.5	ND
55	i-Pr	Me	OMe	H	5.8	3.8
56	i-Pr	Me	OEt	H	6.0	3.7
57	i-Pr	Me	Oi-Pr	H	ND	ND
58	i-Pr	Me	O~~O~	H	ND	ND
59	i-Pr	Et	OMe	H	10.0	5.8
60	i-Bu	Me	OMe	H	5.0	ND
61	Et	Me	OMe	H	16.2	>5
62	i-Pr	Me	OMe	Br	42.5	ND
63	i-Pr	Me	CN	H	7.7	7.4
64	i-Pr	Me	N_3	H	9.4	5.9

Researchers initially noted that the meta-position of the phenol ring might be a more suitable modification site. For instance, *meta*-methyl propofol demonstrates a favorable safety profile (therapeutic index 2.5−3.0) while retaining some degree of anesthetic activity. By fusing the *meta*-methyl group in the structure of *meta*-methyl propofol with the *ortho*-isopropyl group, a series of fused bicyclic compounds containing benzocyclobutene can naturally be derived (Table 24.7). Similar structures can be found in many marketed drugs or candidate new drugs undergoing clinical trials, such as Ivabradine, Sibutramine, Butorphanol, Carboplatin, and Apalutamide. This suggests that the cyclobutene structure possesses adequate in vivo stability. Furthermore, compared to direct substitution modification on the benzene ring, this approach not only reduces the molecular weight of compounds but also enhances the rigidity of the scaffold while introducing chiral centers. Based on the aforementioned design strategy, certain benzocyclobutene compounds were subsequently synthesized for investigating novel structure-activity relationships.

After a comprehensive assessment of the compounds' ED_{50} values and safety indices, researchers selected compounds **48** and **63**, which exhibited good activity and high safety, for chiral separation. These compounds were then tested for their individual enantiomers for their anesthetic activity. The results showed that compound **48a** (ED_{50} = 16.0 mg/kg) and **63b** (ED_{50} = 8.2 mg/kg) exhibited anesthetic activity at animal level that was not inferior to propofol, with a certain advantage in terms of safety compared to propofol (Table 24.8). Unfortunately, when compound **48a** and **63b** were evaluated for dose-response relationships in large animal models, especially beagle dogs, severe adverse effects were observed, including iris congestion, a significant increase in heart rate, and respiratory frequency. Results from $GABA_A$ receptor binding assays showed that **48a** and **63b** exhibited relatively weak binding to $GABA_A$ receptors (at a test concentration of 10 μM, the inhibition rates were only 33% and 19%, respectively). It was speculated that the anesthetic activity exhibited by these two compounds might not be solely attributable to their activation of the $GABA_A$ receptors. Despite additional structural modifications and functional group optimizations, which failed to significantly enhance the anesthetic activity and safety of the benzocyclobutene series compounds, researchers were compelled to abandon further exploration of this compound series. Consequently, they embarked on a fresh search for new candidate compounds.

In 2008 Pharmacofore Corporation, leveraging the symmetrical structure characteristics of propofol, unveiled a propofol derivative, PF-0713 (a compound with 2*R*,6*R*-diisobutyl-substituted phenol). This derivative exhibited a significant enhancement in anesthetic activity (ED_{50} = 2.69 mg/kg) in comparison to propofol (ED_{50} = 11.7 mg/kg) (Fig. 24.15) [23]. Inspired by this outcome, researchers at Haisco embarked on another attempt to incorporate rigid structures into the compound's architecture, with the aim of facilitating BBB penetration. Given the suboptimal results from previous benzocyclobutene design strategy, researchers refrained from extensive modifications to the phenyl ring and instead of focused on optimizing the side chain. Additionally, mindful of the potential detrimental effects of excessive steric hindrance on the compound's activity (e.g., as observed with the *tert*-butyl substitution leading to reduced anesthetic activity), researchers prudently opted a smaller cyclopropyl groups with reduced steric hindrance. The introduction of cyclopropyl disrupted the inherent symmetry of the propofol molecule, introducing new chiral centers. This design strategy further reduced the lipophilicity of the compounds. During this screening process, researchers fortuitously identified multiple highly active candidate compounds, including compounds **66** (ED_{50} = 4.5 mg/kg), **67** (ED_{50} = 3.6 mg/kg), and **71** (ED_{50} = 3.7 mg/kg). All these compounds exhibited a distinct advantage over propofol (Table 24.9).

TABLE 24.8 The optimization of benzocyclobutene series compounds.

Compound		Onset time (s)	Duration time (s)	ED_{50}	Safety index
(2,6-diisopropylphenol, propofol)	Propofol	<10	303.2 ± 97.8	11.7	2.7
(isopropyl-OH-benzocyclobutene)	Racemate	<10	319.7 ± 158.4	16.3 ± 1.4	5.2 ± 1.7
	48a (*R*)	<10	373.5 ± 98.2	16.0 ± 5.9	5.4 ± 0.3
	48b (*S*)	<10	332.1 ± 198.5	18.3 ± 2.2	4.1 ± 0.6
(isopropyl-OH-CN-benzocyclobutene)	Racemate	<10	340.8 ± 180.0	7.7 ± 0.1	7.4 ± 0.5
	63a (*S*)	<10	521.4 ± 180.6	14.3 ± 0.1	3.7 ± 0.2
	63b (*R*)	13.8 ± 4.2	364.8 ± 110.4	8.2 ± 1.7	9.1 ± 1.9

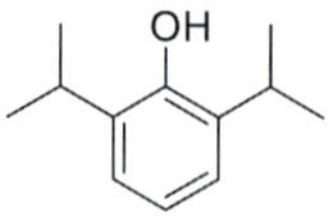

Propofol
ED$_{50}$ = 11.7 mg/kg
LD$_{50}$ = 31.3 mg/kg

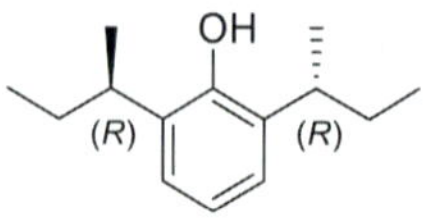

65 (PF-0713)
ED$_{50}$ = 2.69 mg/kg
LD$_{50}$ = 23.8 mg/kg

FIGURE 24.15 Propofol and compound **65** with 2,6-diisobutyl substitution.

TABLE 24.9 2,6-Diisubstituted phenolic compounds.

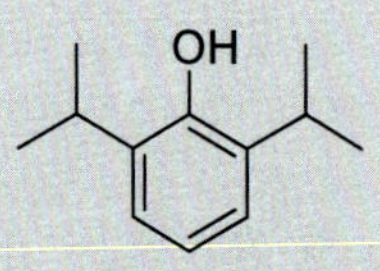

Propofol
ED$_{50}$ = 11.7 mg/kg
LD$_{50}$ = 31.3 mg/kg

chirality / steric hindrance

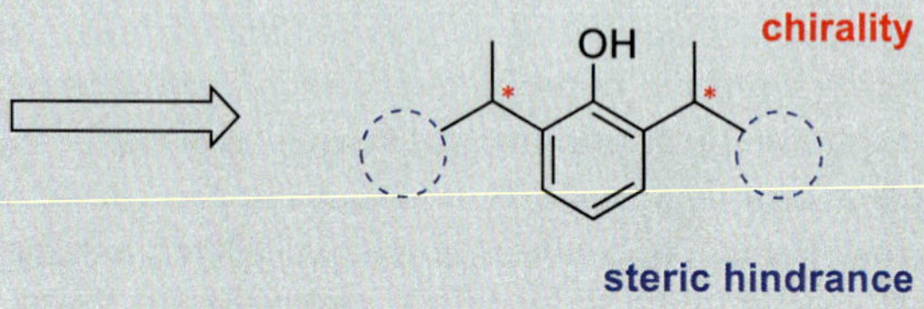

Compound	Structure	ED$_{50}$ (mg/kg)	LD$_{50}$ (mg/kg)	clogP
Propofol	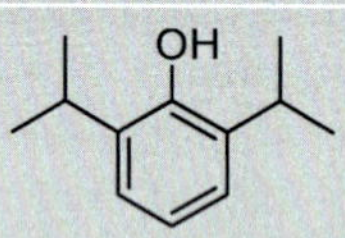	11.7	31.3	3.929
66	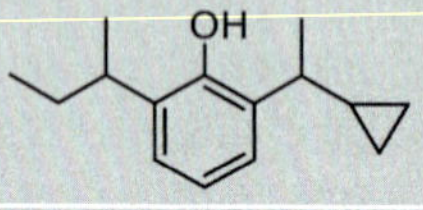	4.5	38.1	4.902
67	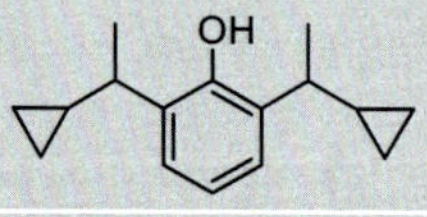	3.6	>15.0	4.817
68	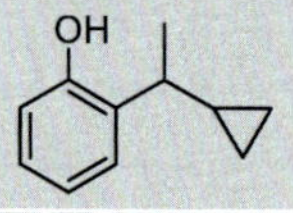	14.0	64.8	3.146
69	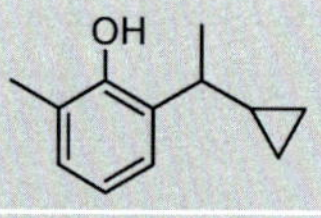	7.4	54.9	3.595
70	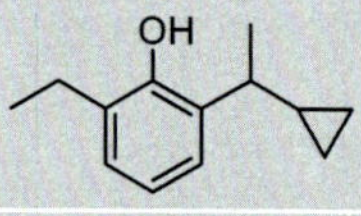	7.7	57.1	3.974
71	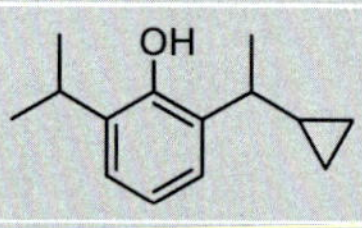	3.7	22.7	4.373
72	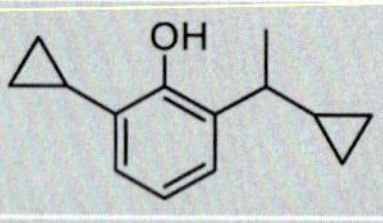	14.6	80.0	3.889

(Continued)

TABLE 24.9 (Continued)

No.	Structure			
73		10.5	40.0	NA
74		7.4	67.0	NA
75		6.2	53.2	NA
76		7.1	40.0	4.932
77		19.9	115.0	5.491
78		30.1	>100.0	NA
79		9.0	74.7	5.346
80		NA	NA	5.745
81		9.8	98.2	5.261

In the study of 2,6-diisubstituted phenolic compound, it was observed that due to their relatively small molecular weight, even subtle structural alterations in the compact side chains could exert a substantial impact on pharmacological efficacy and the oil-water partition coefficient. Consequently, the introduction of cyclopropyl group not only significantly enhanced the drug's activity but also increased the oil-water partition coefficient, in concurrence with the steric hindrance effect of the side chain functional group. The fine-tuning of spatial arrangements often plays a pivotal role in the binding affinity of a drug with its target, and the molecular partition coefficient can be a critical indicator of whether the molecule can effectively reduce the incidence of injection pain. Therefore, the introduction of a tricyclic ring system contributed to the feasibility of drug development from multiple perspectives. Researchers further proceeded to optically separate the enantiomers and racemate of chiral compounds **66**, **67**, and **71** and evaluated these compounds in vitro and in vivo (Fig. 24.16). The results indicated that the target binding activity and in vivo efficacy were superior for the *R* configuration in comparison to their corresponding *S* configuration and the racemic compounds. Moreover, all of these were superior to propofol (Table 24.10).

Researchers selected compounds **66** (*R,R*), **67** (*R,R*), and **71** (*R*) for pharmacokinetic studies in rats. The results showed that **71** (*R*) exhibited superior pharmacokinetic parameters, including a higher drug peak concentration (C_{max}), longer half-life

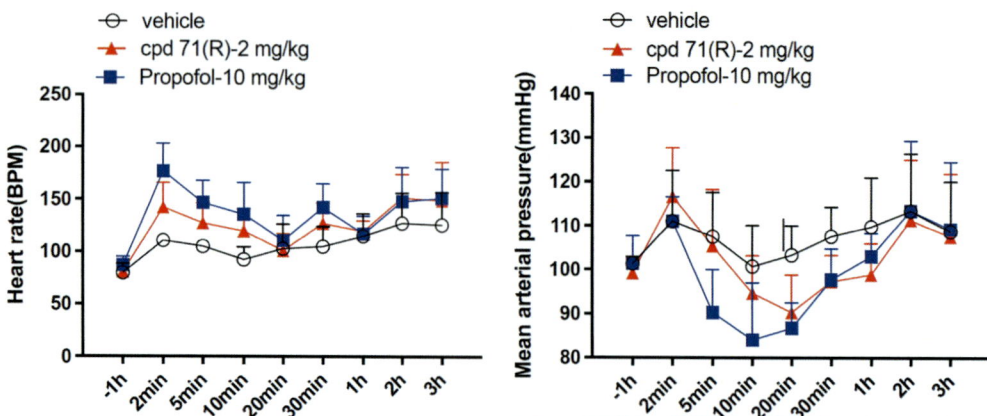

FIGURE 24.16 The impact of compound **71** (R) on cardiovascular function in telemetry beagle dogs.

TABLE 24.10 The separation of 2,6-diisubstituted phenolic compounds.

Compound	Structure	Configuration	ED$_{50}$ (mg/kg)	LD$_{50}$ (mg/kg)
Propofol		–	11.7	31.3
66		Mix	4.5	38.1
		R,R	2.0	14.3
		R,S	10.1	65.4
		S,R	1.3	8.3
		S,S	5.3	36.8
67		mix	3.6	>15.0
		R,R	1.5	~6.3
		R,S	5.9	43.6
		S,S	19.5	149.0
71		mix	3.7	22.7
		R	1.5	9.9
		S	7.9	50.0

($t_{1/2}$), and lower clearance rate (CL). Clinical investigations have indicated significant hemodynamics effects of propofol. To further validate whether **71** (R) had a superior ability to maintain blood pressure, the researchers employed classical animal models. These evaluations included: (1) Testing the effect of **71** (R) and propofol on the circulatory system in telemetry rat models: At comparable anesthesia durations, **71** (R) at a low dose (2 mg/kg) exhibited similar effects on mean arterial pressure (MAP) as propofol (8 mg/kg). At a high dose (4 mg/kg), **71** (R) had a better blood pressure reduction compared to propofol (16 mg/kg), with reductions of approximately 20% and 30%, respectively. (2) Evaluating the impact of **71** (R) and propofol on cardiovascular function using telemetry beagle dog models: The results indicated that when maintaining the equivalent anesthetic potency, **71** (R) slightly outperformed propofol in terms of MAP reduction (10% vs. 20%).

The researchers also conducted separate tests on **71** (R) and propofol to assess their effects on GABA$_A$ receptor-mediated currents and their impact on primary mouse neuronal cells. The results demonstrated that **71** (R) (EC$_{50}$ = 1.1 μM) had a stronger activation effect on the GABA$_A$ receptor compared to propofol (EC$_{50}$ = 5.3 μM). Furthermore, the ratio of propofol's IC$_{50}$ for neuronal viability to its EC$_{50}$ for GABA$_A$ activation was lower than that of

71 (*R*), suggesting that **71** (*R*) had a better safety profile. Due to its higher lipophilicity, the free drug concentration of **71** (*R*) in the lipid emulsion aqueous phase (0.30 mg/mL) was significantly lower than that of propofol (12.58 mg/mL), indicating a potentially lower incidence of clinical injection pain. In an overall assessment of early drug properties, **71** (*R*) emerged as the preferred candidate compound among numerous candidates, thanks to its superior target binding ability, higher anesthetic potency, and a certain degree of safety advantage. Ultimately, it was selected for the successful development of the next-generation intravenous anesthetic, Ciprofol (Fig. 24.17).

In order to further investigate the possible binding modes of compound 71 (R) and the differences in activity between chiral compounds, researchers conducted molecular simulations of ciprofol and its derivatives using the GABA$_A$ receptor structure in Glide XP precision mode. The docking results indicate that the binding sites and modes of ciprofol and its chiral isomers are consistent with the cryo-electron microscopy structure of propofol. The phenolic hydroxyl group forms a hydrogen bond with the amino acid residue Ile228 of the GABA$_A$ receptor, while the alkyl side chains on both sides occupy the hydrophobic binding pockets in the upper left and lower right corners of the binding site (Fig. 24.13). The docking scores for propofol, ciprofol, and its chiral isomers were −6.674, −7.027 and −6.915, respectively (lower scores indicate stronger theoretical binding ability). The ranking of the docking results also aligns with the ED$_{50}$ results of these compounds: propofol has the highest ED$_{50}$ (11.7 mg/kg), ciprofol has the lowest ED$_{50}$ (1.5 mg/kg), and the chiral isomers are intermediate (7.9 mg/kg). Referring to the binding conformation of propofol, the researchers analyzed the preferred conformations of ciprofol and its chiral isomers, and found that ciprofol exhibits a high degree of similarity in molecular conformation to propofol. Moreover, the cyclopropyl moiety better fills the spatial cavity of the binding pocket, providing an explanation for the higher efficacy of ciprofol compared to propofol.

Subsequently, the researchers conducted molecular dynamics simulations to verify the docking of the three compounds. The results show that the binding modes of the three molecules exhibit good conformational stability during a 100 ns simulation, with RMSD values of 2.35 ± 0.54 Å, 1.23 ± 0.36 Å, and 2.61 ± 0.48 Å, respectively. The hydrogen bond lengths are 2.83 ± 0.16 Å, 3.11 ± 0.28 Å, and 2.90 ± 0.23 Å (Fig. 24.18). Among them, ciprofol exhibits the most stable conformation, but its hydrogen bond length is longer, indicating a weaker hydrogen bond interaction compared to propofol. Generally, shorter hydrogen bonds indicate stronger binding affinity and greater conformational stability. Why does ciprofol show the opposite trend? It is speculated that this may be closely related to the phospholipid bilayer where the GABA$_A$ receptor is situated. The binding site of this class of compounds is located in the transmembrane region of the protein, in the middle of the phospholipid bilayer. Therefore, hydrophobic small molecules often have the opportunity to bind. Consequently, the importance of hydroxyl group hydrogen bonds in the binding mode of this class of compounds is relatively weakened, and intermolecular hydrophobic interactions become the key driving forces of binding. In

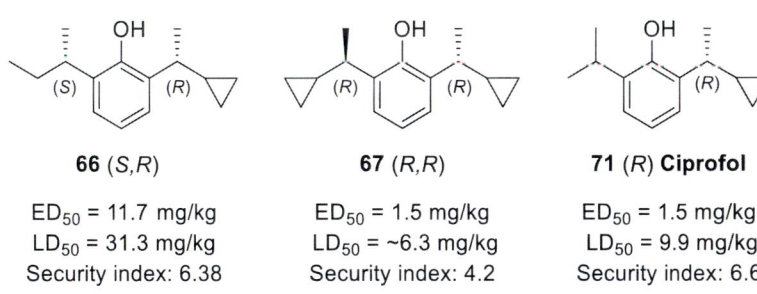

FIGURE 24.17 Candidates from the 2,6-diisubstituted phenolic compound series: **66, 67**, and Ciprofol.

66 (*S,R*)
ED$_{50}$ = 11.7 mg/kg
LD$_{50}$ = 31.3 mg/kg
Security index: 6.38

67 (*R,R*)
ED$_{50}$ = 1.5 mg/kg
LD$_{50}$ = ~6.3 mg/kg
Security index: 4.2

71 (*R*) **Ciprofol**
ED$_{50}$ = 1.5 mg/kg
LD$_{50}$ = 9.9 mg/kg
Security index: 6.6

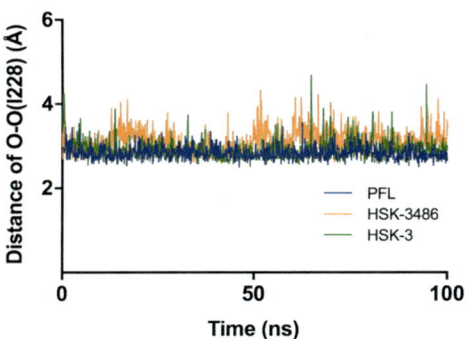

FIGURE 24.18 Hydrogen bond between phenol hydroxyl group and GABA$_A$ receptor residue Ile228 in propofol, ciprofol and their chiral isomers in 100 ns molecular dynamics simulation.

comparison to propofol, the larger cyclopropyl structure of ciprofol better occupies the gap between the receptor and the phospholipid bilayer, resulting in enhanced conformational stability and binding ability. However, despite having an additional cyclopropyl group, why do the chiral isomers of ciprofol exhibit lower activity than ciprofol itself? The possible reason is that the cyclopropyl moiety of the chiral isomers must be oriented inward, but due to the limited space inside, the overall binding conformation of the molecule is slightly more tilted, resulting in relatively poorer conformational stability and slightly weaker binding ability. MM/GBSA binding free energy calculations reveal that in the absence of the phospholipid bilayer, the binding free energies of the three compounds are -26.5 ± 4.9 kcal/mol, -24.0 ± 6.4 kcal/mol, and -22.2 ± 4.9 kcal/mol, respectively. However, when the phospholipid bilayer is included, the corresponding binding free energy results become -32.6 ± 2.1 kcal/mol, -37.4 ± 2.3 kcal/mol, and -34.8 ± 1.0 kcal/mol (Table 24.11). Only when the phospholipid bilayer is included, the conclusions from the free energy calculations align organically with the structures, providing a comprehensive explanation for the differences in binding affinity and binding conformation between ciprofol and propofol, along with their underlying physical and chemical reasons.

Although efforts have been made to optimize the properties of propofol and etomidate, their water solubility issues have not been effectively solved. To meet the requirements for intravenous administration, all clinically used formulations are lipid emulsions of the oil-in-water type. However, the clinical use of lipid emulsions often leads to various adverse events, such as injection pain, bacterial infection, and propofol infusion syndrome (hyperlipidemia resulting from prolonged infusion). Achieving a balance between water solubility and permeability for propofol and its analogs presents a significant challenge for medicinal chemists. While it is common to balance these properties in the early stages of drug development, optimal equilibrium is often difficult to achieve. This is particularly true when it comes to structural modifications of drug molecules, as it is challenging to simultaneously benefit both their biological activity and pharmacokinetic properties. Therefore, to address the water solubility issue of propofol while maintaining its anesthetic activity, medicinal chemists have once again attempted structural modifications using a prodrug strategy.

Most of the prodrug designs for propofol are based on hydroxy-phenol chemical modifications. A common approach to enhancing the water solubility of the compound is to introduce highly charged chemical groups, such as phosphates esters or water-soluble amino acids. Some researchers have attempted to transform propofol into a prodrug by introducing amino acid fragments, but unexpected cardiac toxicity was observed, and satisfactory improvement was not achieved. LusedraTM, approved by the US FDA in 2008, was the first propofol prodrug for clinical use, with the active ingredient fospropofol sodium (Fig. 24.19) [24]. Fospropofol sodium, developed by Yichang Humanwell Healthcare in China, also submitted an NDA to the original CFDA in 2018. Fospropofol sodium is a water-soluble phosphate ester prodrug, which greatly improves the compound's water solubility by introducing a phosphate ester into the chemical structure of propofol, and exhibits excellent drug stability in aqueous formulations. Once administered intravenously, fospropofol sodium rapidly releases propofol under the action of alkaline phosphatase. Compared to propofol, fospropofol sodium has a longer elimination half-life, larger distribution volume, and higher plasma clearance rate. Phase II and III clinical trial results have demonstrated that fospropofol sodium leads to faster recovery and higher patient satisfaction when used for sedation.

As a prodrug of propofol, the safety of its metabolites cannot be ignored. The enzymatic breakdown of fospropofol sodium in the body releases a molecule of formaldehyde, which may lead to the accumulation of formic acid. Additionally, there have been reported that the inorganic phosphate salts produced after the metabolism of the drug may cause mild to moderate perineal sensory abnormalities and itching a few minutes after injection. Nevertheless, the success of fospropofol sodium remains a remarkable example of prodrug design to improve the unfavorable physicochemical properties of the parent drug propofol, reducing adverse events to some extent, improving drug safety, and demonstrating the ability of medicinal chemists to achieve molecular optimization through simple structural modifications.

TABLE 24.11 MM/GBSA calculations of propofol, ciprofol and their chiral isomers with GABA$_A$ receptors.

Compound	ED$_{50}$ (mg/kg)	Ligand RMSD (Å)	MM/GBSA binding free energy (kcal/mol)	
			With phospholipid bilayer	Without phospholipid bilayer
Propofol	11.7	2.35 ± 0.54	−32.6 ± 2.1	−26.5 ± 4.9
Ciprofol	1.5	1.23 ± 0.36	−37.4 ± 2.3	−24.0 ± 6.4
Ciprofol chiral isomers	7.9	2.61 ± 0.48	−34.8 ± 1.0	−22.2 ± 4.9

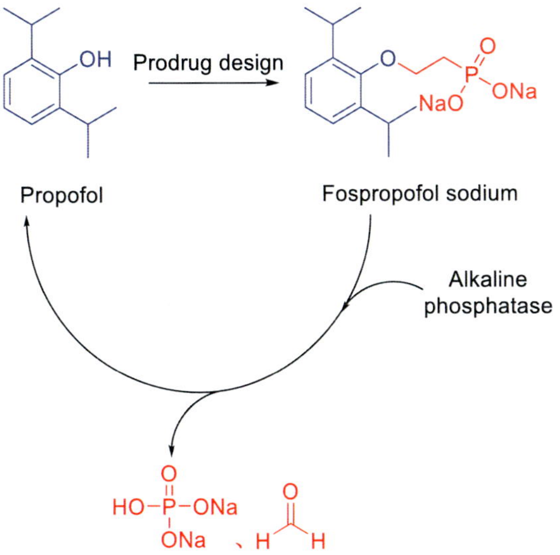

FIGURE 24.19 Prodrug design of fospropofol sodium.

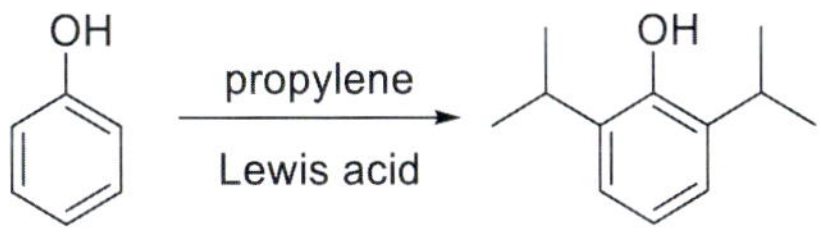

FIGURE 24.20 Industrial synthesis method 1 of propofol.

24.3.7 Pharmaceutical manufacturing technology: the key link to realize industrial production

The development process of a new drug typically goes through multiple synthetic routes. At different stages of new drug development, the requirements for synthetic routes and processes are also different. During the early compound screening stage, the work primarily focuses on medicinal chemistry, and the goal is to quickly synthesize as many compounds as possible for biological testing, screen out active compounds through evaluation, and establish a clear structure-efficacy relationship. At this stage, the demand for compounds is generally in the milligram to hundred milligram range, and there are no high requirements for synthesis conditions, purification methods, or yields. Obtaining compounds with a certain level of purity is sufficient. However, in the later stages of compound development, it is necessary to conduct systematic research on production processes, quality control and stability, and there are clear requirements and standards for the synthesis routes, synthesis methods, purification methods and production environments. The development process of a new drug requires more attention to controllability in terms of quality, yield, safety, and cost, as well as the convenience of production operations. In this stage, the supply of compounds needs to be aligned with the requirements of clinical research, generally at kilogram scale or above, and the production conditions and environment must comply with good manufacturing practice (GMP) requirements or meet GMP conditions. With the gradual advancement of clinical research, drug development is gradually transitioning from the preparation of clinical samples to the preparation of commercial production. The scale of preparation often needs to reach tens of kilograms or even metric tons. There are extremely high requirements for synthesis routes and process conditions. For example, the purification process generally adopts convenient methods such as recrystallization or vacuum distillation to avoid using column chromatography, which is associated with high contamination, complex operations, and a large amount of waste. The main mode of administration of propofol and ciprofol is intravenous emulsion injection. As injectable products, they need to meet strict relevant substance restrictions (e.g., the United States Pharmacopoeia and the European Pharmacopoeia), which also puts higher requirements on the synthesis and production process of the active pharmaceutical ingredient (API).

The conventional production process of propofol, synthesized through the Friedel-Crafts alkylation reaction using propylene gas and phenol, has been widely employed and has garnered a series of patents (Fig. 24.20). In this production process, a Lewis acid catalyst is utilized to facilitate the synthetic reaction. Upon completion of the reaction, crude product separation and purification are typically achieved through high vacuum distillation to meet the various requirements for the API. However, this traditional synthetic process exhibits notable drawbacks: (1) the Friedel-Crafts alkylation reaction requires high temperature and pressure, which pose certain safety hazards; (2) more importantly, the alkylation reaction also generates two major byproducts, namely 2,4-diisopropylphenol and 2,4,6-triisopropylphenol. In the final API, the content of all these impurities must be controlled at 0.05% or lower. Consequently, this process imposes extremely high demands on the operations, separation, and purification of production. Therefore, in the subsequent process improvements, researchers developed an in situ synthesis method of propylene using isopropanol and strong acid (aluminum sulfate silicate catalyst) to avoid the direct use of propylene gas.

Another method for synthesizing propofol involves initial alkylation of para-substituted phenol followed by removal of the para-substituent under alkaline conditions (Fig. 24.21). This method primarily utilizes 4-chlorophenol or 4-hydroxybenzoic acid as starting materials, and isopropanol is used instead of propylene gas for the alkylation reaction in the presence of sulfuric acid. Although high-purity propofol still needs to be purified by high vacuum distillation, this synthesis process offers two distinct advantages: (1) due to the occupation of the para-position by the substituent (4-Cl, 4-OH), it avoids the generation of alkylated byproducts, including 2,4-diisopropylphenol and 2,4,6-triisopropylphenol; (2) the intermediates after the alkylation reaction can undergo purification steps, allowing for the use of higher purity starting materials in the subsequent reaction. The above improvements can effectively avoid the production of major impurities in API and improve the stability of the production process, and the quality of propofol products through the final vacuum distillation operation can be significantly improved. However, this route also has limitations: both steps of the reactions are involved in the acid-base neutralization process (concentrated sulfuric acid requires neutralization with sodium hydroxide after the alkylation reaction, and sodium hydroxide needs to be neutralized with hydrochloric acid after the removal of the para-substituent), and the industrial-scale acid-base neutralization process is accompanied by high heat release, which presents certain operational safety risks. The researchers then optimized this process route, after the Friedel-Craft reaction and para-substituent removal reaction, the reaction liquid was directly put into water to separate the intermediate and the crude propofol through toluene extraction, avoiding the problem of heat release during the neutralization process. Subsequently, researchers optimized this process. Briefly, after the Friedel-Crafts alkylation and para-substituent removal reactions, the reaction mixture was directly transferred into water and then was extracted with toluene to separate the intermediate and crude propofol, avoiding the problem of heat release in the neutralization process, which was not only ensured the yield but also simplified the synthesis route with improved operation safety [25].

The synthesis of ciprofol as an API presents greater challenges due to its asymmetric skeletal structure and chiral center. To meet the early requirements of medicinal chemistry research, scientists at Hesco Pharmaceutical group initially designed two routes. Fig. 24.22 illustrates the first synthesis route, which involves chiral separation of ciprofol

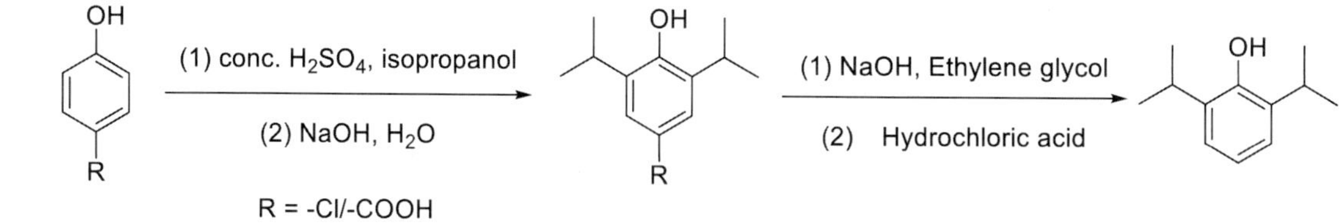

FIGURE 24.21 Industrial synthesis method 2 of propofol.

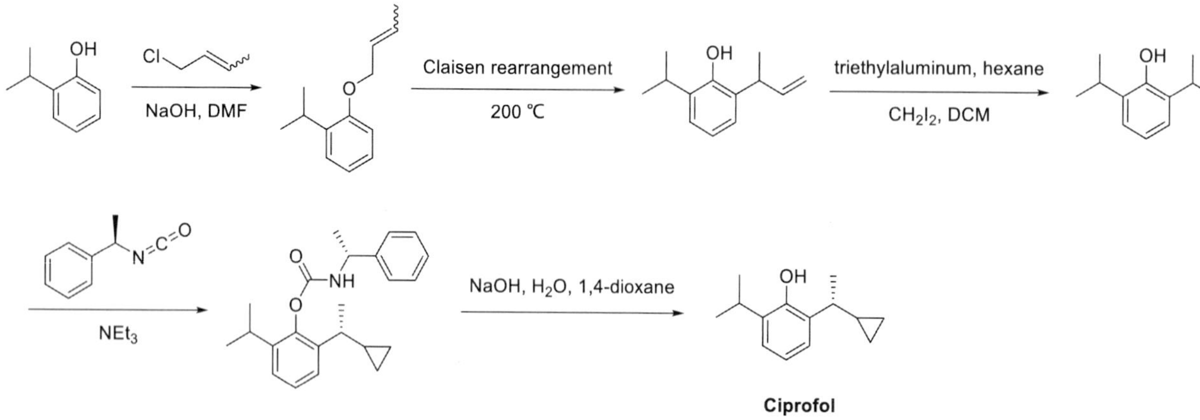

FIGURE 24.22 Chemical synthesis method 1 of ciprofol.

after successfully obtaining the racemate of ciprofol. Although this route allows for small-scale synthesis in the laboratory, the intermediates and compounds need to be purified by multiple-column chromatography, resulting in a lower overall yield, which is not favorable for the rapid acquisition of candidate compounds with a certain number.

In order to address the challenge of rapid purification of the target compound, researchers have designed a second synthesis route for ciprofol (Fig. 24.23). This route begins with 2-isopropylphenol as the initial raw material, which undergoes a substitution reaction with NBS and reacts with a Weber amide compound under the participation of butyllithium to obtain a carbonyl compound. Subsequently, the intermediate undergoes an addition reaction with Grignard reagent, removing the benzyl protecting group and in situ eliminating the hydroxyl group to obtain the racemate of ciprofol. The racemate undergoes a condensation reaction with R-(+)-phenylethyl isocyanate, followed by chiral separation and dissociation to obtain 99% ciprofol with a 99% enantiomer excess (ee). This route involves multiple synthetic steps and intricate operations, and still maintains a relatively low overall yield (approximately 2% only). Additionally, the process requires the use of n-butyllithium or Grignard reagent, which has demanding control requirements and is unsuitable for large-scale production of the API.

Based on the results of the pharmaceutical chemistry synthesis route, the researchers have continuously developed and designed three synthetic routes for the industrial synthesis of ciprofol. The first industrial synthesis route: bromophenol as the raw material undergoes coupling to obtain a cyclopropyl olefin intermediate. The intermediate is hydrogenated to obtain the racemate of ciprofol, which is coupled with R-(+)-phenylethyl isocyanate, followed by chiral separation, resulting in 99% ee of ciprofol (Fig. 24.24). This synthesis route is relatively concise and operationally

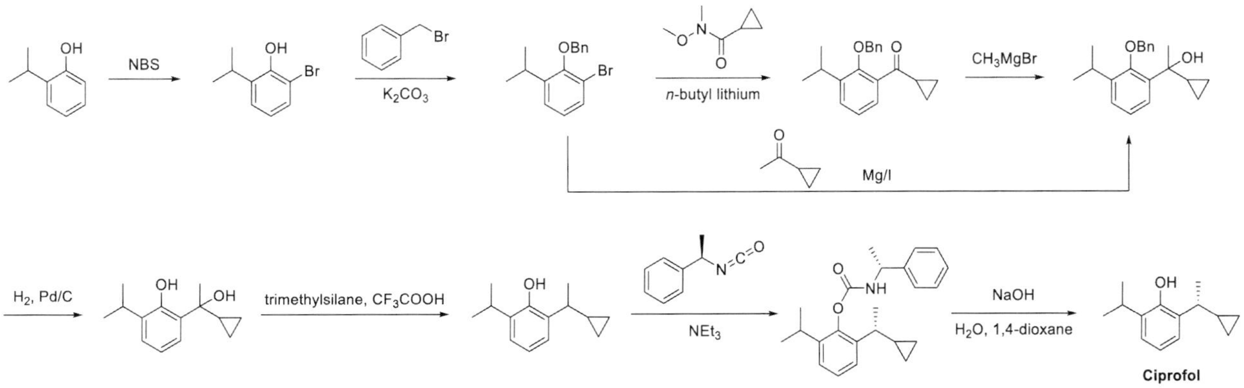

FIGURE 24.23 Chemical synthesis method 2 of ciprofol.

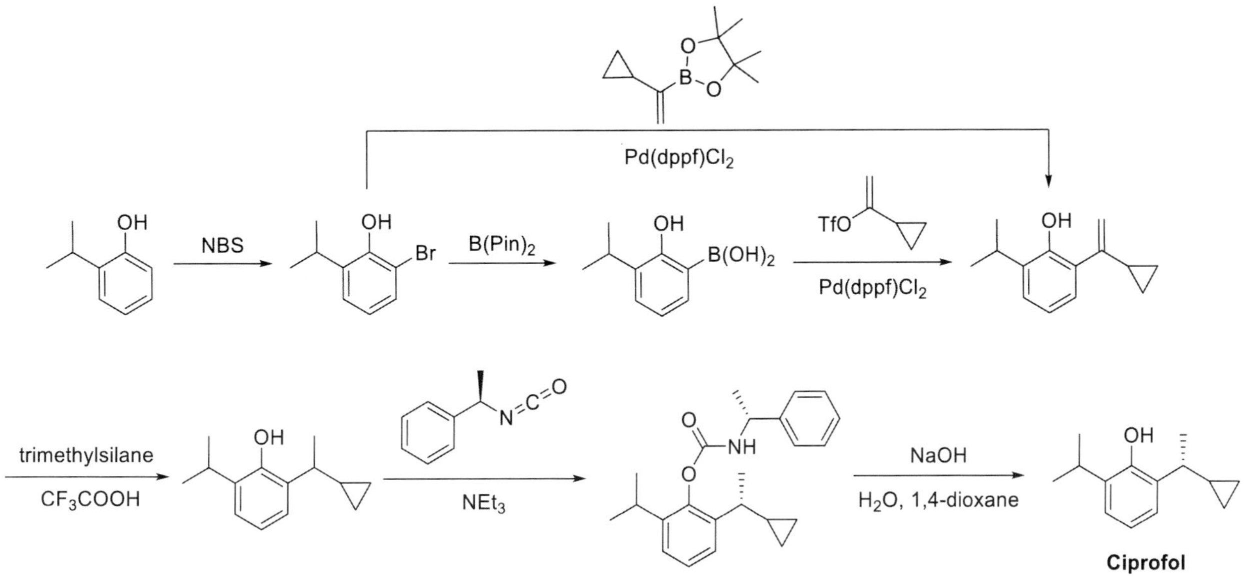

FIGURE 24.24 Industrial synthesis method 1 of ciprofol.

straightforward. However, the availability of cyclopropyl olefin intermediate is limited, and its stability is poor, making it difficult to store for an extended period. Therefore, it still poses challenges for industrial applications.

The second route for the industrial synthesis of ciprofol deviates from the previous approach (Fig. 24.25). This method involves the initial preparation of an intermediate with a carboxyl side chain, which performs chiral separation with cinchonidine salt to yield a 99% ee carboxylic compound. The carboxyl group of this compound is subsequently reduced, followed by oxidation and reaction with a Wittig reagent to obtain an olefin intermediate. The olefin intermediate is then subjected to the Simmons-Smith reaction and removed protective group from hydroxyl group, resulting in a 99% ee of ciprofol. However, this synthesis route is lengthier and involves intricate reaction operations and postprocessing conditions, and it requires the use of various special reagents, such as titanium tetrachloride, sodium borohydride, boron trifluoride etherate, and Wittig reagents, limiting the industrial applicability of this synthesis route.

In the developed third industrial synthesis of ciprofol (Fig. 24.26), 2-isopropylphenol is employed as the initial raw material, followed by nucleophilic substitution reaction, Claisen rearrangement reaction, and Simmons-Smith reaction to obtain the racemate of ciprofol. Subsequently, it is coupled with R-(+)-phenylethyl isocyanate, and subsequently subjected to chiral separation and hydrolysis reactions to release the crude product. Finally, Wiped-Film molecular distillation is employed to obtain ciprofol with a 99% ee. The synthesis route has various advantages that make it suitable for industrial applications, such as classic reactions in each step, easy availability of raw materials, simple process operation, moderate length of synthesis steps, and mild process conditions. Through continuous optimization of process conditions, this route ensures the preparation of samples for clinical phase I, phase II, and phase III trials and validates the production batches before market launch, with a potential improvement in overall yield to approximately 24% and positive economic benefits.

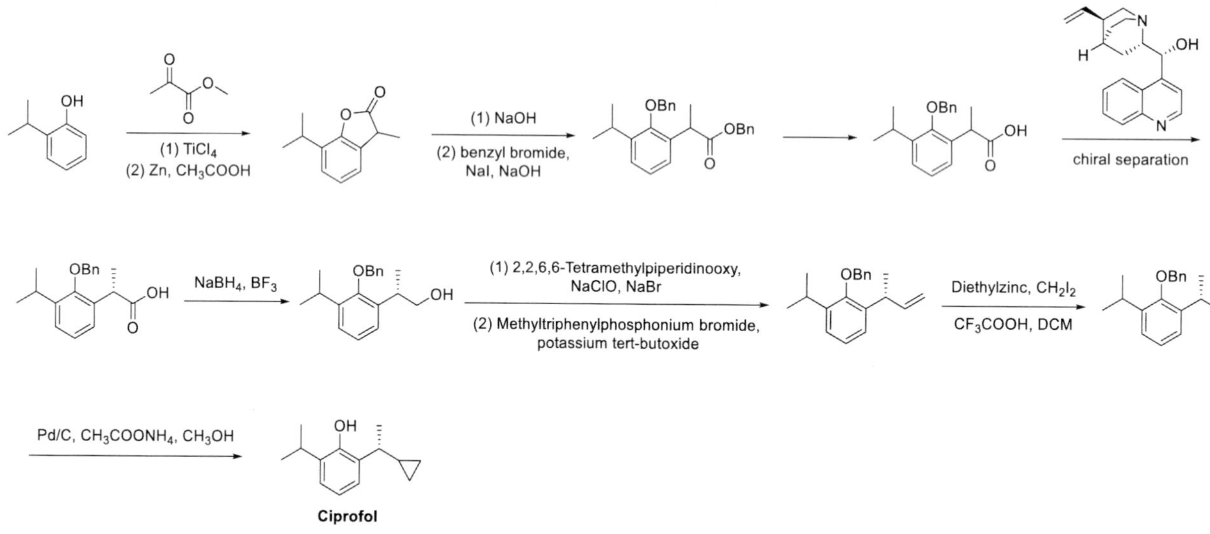

FIGURE 24.25 Industrial synthesis method 2 of ciprofol.

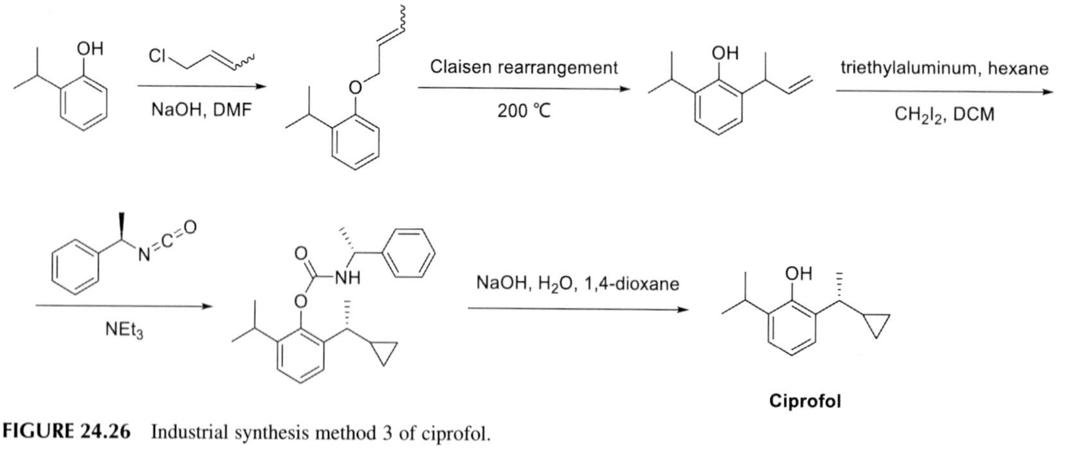

FIGURE 24.26 Industrial synthesis method 3 of ciprofol.

In short, the development of novel drug synthesis routes and process optimization is an ongoing endeavor that spans the entire lifecycle of a product. It is necessary to continuously introduce innovative methods and technologies to enhance the stability of the process and product quality, reduce quality risks, and ensure patient safety in medication administration. Furthermore, it becomes possible to improve the overall yield of the manufacturing process, reduce environmental pollution, and minimize production costs by continuously optimizing production processes.

24.3.8 Clinical application and metabolism of propofol in vivo

Propofol ($C_{12}H_{18}O$) is an alkyl phenolic compound with a molecular weight of 178 and is colorless or light-yellow oily liquid at room temperature. Melting point: 19°C, boiling point: 246°C, relative density: 0.962 g/mL. Propofol is insoluble in water, but soluble in most organic solvents, and easily soluble in n-hexane and methanol. Due to its phenolic hydroxyl group, propofol exhibits certain acidity and reducibility and can chelate with many metal ions. There are many different formulations of propofol products on the market, and the most widely used formulations are 1% propofol, 10% soybean oil, 1.2% purified lecithin, 2.24% glycerin, and sodium hydroxide to regulate pH. In order to prevent microbial growth, it is also necessary to add edetate sodium (EDTA).

Since approved for clinical use in the 1970s, propofol has become the most commonly used intravenous anesthetic. Propofol can be used for both induction and maintenance of anesthesia, and the usual induction dose is 1.0–2.5 mg/kg. Its usage and dosage are shown in Table 24.12. There are many factors affecting the induced dose of propofol, mainly including age, fat removal weight, and blood volume [26]. For elderly patients, with cardiovascular diseases, or obesity, the dosage of propofol should be calculated according to the patient's age, comorbidities and ideal body weight, and the infusion speed should be adjusted according to individual needs and different surgical stimuli, while the patient's vital signs such as heart rate and blood pressure should be closely monitored. When propofol is combined with benzodiazepines and opioids, it can play a synergistic role, and the required infusion speed and drug concentration are reduced [27,28]. With the development of medical technology and health services, there is an increasing demand for painless technology outside the operating room. Including gastroduodenoscopy, tracheoscopy, hysteroscopy and other operations, the use of anesthetic drugs allows patients to complete the corresponding examination in the unconscious, painless process, with a safe and rapid recovery. More and more clinicians and patients pay attention to it. Propofol has the characteristics of fast onset, exact effect, little respiratory irritation, quick recovery, and less postoperative discomfort. It is an ideal anesthetic drug outside operation [29].

However, propofol also has some clinical application problems. Its suppression of the circulatory system and respiratory system is particularly obvious. The incidence of apnea caused by the induced dose is 24%–30%, and the time can be as long as 30 seconds, and if combined with opioids, it can significantly increase the incidence of apnea. Propofol also reduces myocardial contractile force and cardiac output, and meanwhile significantly dilates peripheral blood vessels. It also reduces peripheral resistance, leading to a reduction in systolic blood pressure by 24%–40% during induction and maintenance. Therefore, propofol should be used by experienced doctors in places with complete monitoring and rescue measures while paying close attention to the circulation and breathing of patients, and timely symptomatic treatment [30]. The adverse effects of propofol also include local irritation symptoms, such as injection pain, phlebitis. Because of the use of lipid emulsion as a solvent, when used for long-term infusion, especially in the intensive care unit, propofol can cause lipid metabolism abnormalities. The occurrence of propofol infusion syndrome has also been reported [31]. In addition, propofol may increase the concentration of dopamine in the nucleus accumbens, so that patients may feel euphoric. So, propofol may have a certain degree of addiction. In recent years, there have been many reports on the adverse social effects and even criminal cases brought about by the abuse of propofol, suggesting that we should pay attention to the management of propofol.

TABLE 24.12 Intravenous use and dosage of propofol.

General anesthesia induction	1–2.5 mg/kg, intravenous infusion, the dose was adjusted according to age, weight, and circulation status
General anesthesia maintenance	50–150 μg/(kg·min), intravenous infusion, complex opioids and muscle relaxants are required
Sedation	50–75 μg/(kg·min), intravenous infusion

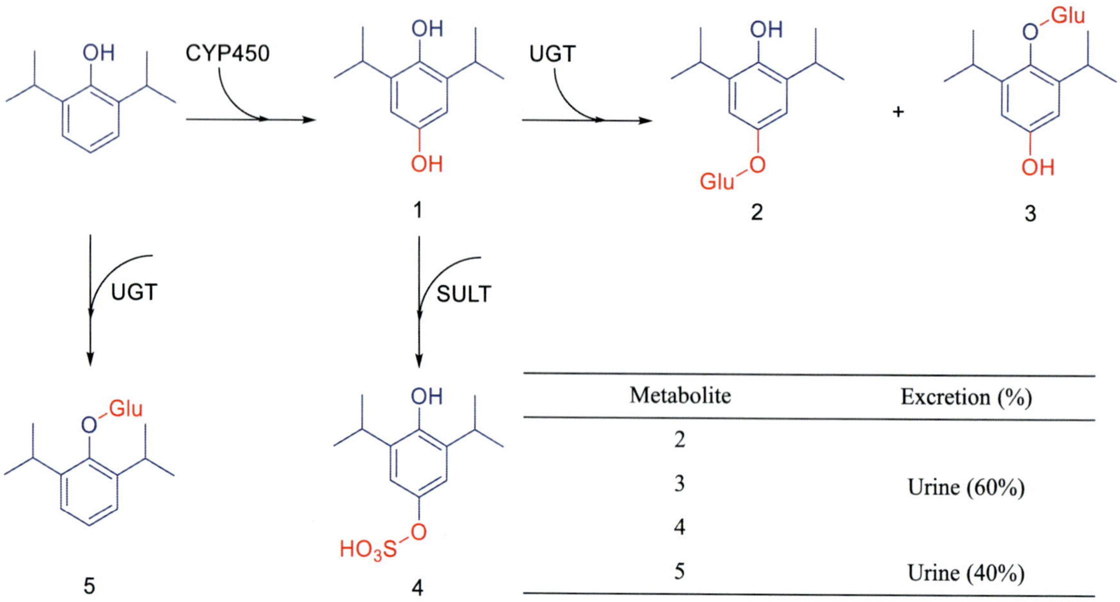

FIGURE 24.27 Metabolic pathway of propofol in vivo.

Metabolite	Excretion (%)
2	
3	Urine (60%)
4	
5	Urine (40%)

Propofol is injected intravenously and oxidized to 1, 4-diisopropyl hydroquinone by cytochrome P450 enzyme (CYP450) in the liver. Propofol and 1, 4-diisopropyl hydroquinone can be combined with glucuronic acid to form propofo-1-glucuronic acid, hydroquinone-1-glucuronic acid, and hydroquinone-4-glucuronic acid under the action of glucuronyltransferase (UGT), which are excreted by the kidney. 1, 4-diisopropyl hydroquinone can be further metabolized to propofol sulfate by sulfotransferase (SULT) (Fig. 24.27). Less than 1% of propofol metabolites were excreted from urine and only 2% were excreted from feces. In fact, the clearance rate of propofol was extremely high (1.5−2.2 L/min), exceeding hepatic blood flow, indicating a possible extra-hepatic metabolic pathway. Propofol metabolism can be directly confirmed in patients who receive liver transplantation and are in the anhepatic stage. Further research results show that the kidney and lung are also important metabolic sites of propofol [32,33].

In practical clinical use, propofol is often used in combination with benzodiazepines and opioids to optimize the anesthesia regimen (i.e., to cause loss of consciousness and block the response to nose-harming stimuli). However, propofol has obvious inhibition on CYP450 enzyme system, so it will affect the metabolism of drugs dependent on this enzyme and reduce the clearance rate of drugs [34]. In addition, propofol has the effect of inhibiting hemodynamics, which can affect the pharmacokinetic performance of another drug. So, it is necessary to adjust the dosage of drugs. Here, we mainly introduce several common propofol - benzodiazepines and opioid interactions [35,36]:

1. Midazolam: Midazolam has an effect on the pharmacokinetics of propofol, which can increase the blood concentration of propofol and reduce the clearance rate, which is mainly due to the influence of the combination of the two drugs on hemodynamics. Accordingly, propofol also has an impact on the pharmacokinetics of midazolam, and when the blood concentration of propofol reaches the level of sedation, the blood concentration of midazolam will also increase by 27%.
2. Afentanil: Afentanil has been shown to increase the blood concentration of propofol by reducing the clearance of propofol. Propofol increased the blood concentration of afentanil by reducing the elimination of afentanil and rapid and slow distribution clearance.
3. Remifentanil: Propofol can reduce the clearance rate of remifentanil distribution by 41%, eliminate the clearance rate by 15%, and increase its blood concentration.

References

[1] Miller G. What is the biological basis of consciousness. Science 2005;309(5731):79.
[2] Suckling CW. Some chemical and physical factors in the development of fluothane. Br J Anaesth 1957;29(10):466−72.
[3] Wallin RF, Regan BM, Napoli MD, Stern IJ. Sevoflurane - new inhalational anesthetic agent. Anesthesia Analgesia 1975;54(6):758−66.
[4] Kanto JH. Midazolam - the 1st water-soluble benzodiazepine pharmacology, pharmacokinetics and efficacy in insomnia and anesthesia. Pharmacotherapy 1985;5(3):138−55.

[5] White PF, Way WL, Trevor AJ. Ketamine - its pharmacology and therapeutic uses. Anesthesiology 1982;56(2):119−36.
[6] Rosen MA, Thigpen JW, Shnider SM, Foutz SE, Levinson G, Koike M. Bupivacaine-induced cardiotoxicity in hypoxic and acidotic sheep. Anesthesia Analgesia 1985;64(11):1089−96.
[7] Simpson D, Curran MP, Oldfield V, Keating GM. Ropivacaine - a review of its use in regional anaesthesia and acute pain management. Drugs 2005;65(18):2675−717.
[8] Franks NP. Molecular targets underlying general anaesthesia. Br J Pharmacol 2006;147:72−81.
[9] Hemmings HC, Akabas MH, Goldstein PA, Trudell JR, Orser BA, Harrison NL. Emerging molecular mechanisms of general anesthetic action. Trends Pharmacol Sci 2005;26(10):503−10.
[10] Evenseth LSM, Gabrielsen M, Sylte I. The GABA(B) receptor-structure, ligand binding and drug development. Molecules 2020;25(13).
[11] Masiulis S, Desai R, Uchanski T, Martin IS, Laverty D, Karia D, et al. GABA(A) receptor signalling mechanisms revealed by structural pharmacology. Nature 2019;565(7740):454−9.
[12] Kim JJ, Gharpure A, Teng J, Zhuang Y, Howard RJ, Zhu S, et al. Shared structural mechanisms of general anaesthetics and benzodiazepines. Nature 2020;585(7824):303−8.
[13] Castellano D, Shepard RD, Lu W. Looking for novelty in an "old" receptor: recent advances toward our understanding of GABA(A)Rs and their implications in receptor pharmacology. Front Neurosci 2021;14.
[14] Antkowiak B, Rammes G. GABA(A) receptor-targeted drug development - new perspectives in perioperative anesthesia. Exp Opin Drug Discov 2019;14(7):683−99.
[15] Herold KF, Nau C, Wei O, Hemmings Jr. HC. Isoflurane inhibits the tetrodotoxin-resistant voltage-gated sodium channel Na(v)1.8. Anesthesiology 2009;111(3):591−9.
[16] Violet JM, Downie DL, Nakisa RC, Lieb WR, Franks NP. Differential sensitivities of mammalian neuronal and muscle nicotinic acetylcholine receptors to general anesthetics. Anesthesiology 1997;86(4):866−74.
[17] Hemmings IIC, Jr.;, Riegelhaupt PM, Kelz MB, Solt K, Eckenhoff RG, et al. Towards a comprehensive understanding of anesthetic mechanisms of action: a decade of discovery. Trends Pharmacol Sci 2019;40(7):464−81.
[18] Glen JB. Balancing tricks and mini-pigs: steps along the road to propofol. Cell 2018;175(1):22−6.
[19] Glen JB. Try, try, and try again: personal reflections on the development of propofol. Br J Anaesth 2019;123(1):3−9.
[20] James R, Glen JB. Synthesis, biological evaluation, and preliminary structure-activity considerations of a series of alkylphenols as intravenous anesthetic agents. J Med Chem 1980;23(12):1350−7.
[21] Zhang C, Li F, Yu Y, Huang A, He P, Lei M, et al. Design, synthesis, and evaluation of a series of novel benzocyclobutene derivatives as general anesthetics. J Med Chem 2017;60(9):3618−25.
[22] Qin L, Ren L, Wan S, Liu G, Luo X, Liu Z, et al. Design, synthesis, and evaluation of novel 2,6-disubstituted phenol derivatives as general anesthetics. J Med Chem 2017;60(9):3606−17.
[23] Sneyd JR, Rigby-Jones AE. New drugs and technologies, intravenous anaesthesia is on the move (again). Br J Anaesth 2010;105(3):246−54.
[24] Hughes B. 2008 FDA drug approvals. Nat Rev Drug Discov 2009;8(2):93−6.
[25] Pramanik C, Kotharkar S, Patil P, Gotrane D, More Y, Borhade A, et al. Commercial manufacturing of propofol: simplifying the isolation process and control on related substances. Org Process Res Develop 2014;18(1):152−6.
[26] Kazama T, Morita K, Ikeda T, Kurita T, Sato S. Comparison of predicted induction dose with predetermined physiologic characteristics of patients and with pharmacokinetic models incorporating those characteristics as covariates. Anesthesiology 2003;98(2):299−305.
[27] Lichtenbelt BJ, Olofsen E, Dahan A, van Kleef JW, Struys MMRF, Vuyk J. Propofol reduces the distribution and clearance of midazolam. Anesthesia Analgesia 2010;110(6):1597−606.
[28] Lichtenbelt BJ, Mertens M, Vuyk J. Strategies to optimise propofol-opioid anaesthesia. Clin Pharmacokinet 2004;43(9):577−93.
[29] Smith I, White PF, Nathanson M, Gouldson R. Propofol - an update on its clinical use. Anesthesiology 1994;81(4):1005−43.
[30] Larsen R, Rathgeber J, Bagdahn A, Lange H, Rieke H. Effects of propofol on cardiovascular dynamics and coronary blood flow in geriatric patients. A comparison with etomidate. Anaesthesia 1988;43(Suppl):25−31.
[31] Fodale V, La Monaca E. Propofol infusion syndrome - an overview of a perplexing disease. Drug Saf 2008;31(4):293−303.
[32] Takizawa D, Sato E, Hiraoka H, Tomioka A, Yamamoto K, Horiuchi R, et al. Changes in apparent systemic clearance of propofol during transplantation of living related donor liver. Br J Anaesth 2005;95(5):643−7.
[33] Takizawa D, Hiraoka H, Goto F, Yamamoto K, Horiuchi R. Human kidneys play an important role in the elimination of propofol. Anesthesiology 2005;102(2):327−30.
[34] Chen TL, Ueng TH, Chen SH, Lee PH, Fan SZ, Liu CC. Human cytochrome-P450 monooxygenase system is suppressed by propofol. Br J Anaesth 1995;74(5):558−62.
[35] Vuyk J, Lichtenbelt BJ, Olofsen E, van Kleef JW, Dahan A. Mixed-effects modeling of the influence of midazolam on propofol pharmacokinetics. Anesthesia Analgesia 2009;108(5):1522−30.
[36] Mertens MJ, Vuyk J, Olofsen E, Bovill JG, Burm AGL. Propofol alters the pharmacokinetics of alfentanil in healthy male volunteers. Anesthesiology 2001;94(6):949−57.

Chapter 25

The discovery of risperidone: a case of multiple target antipsychotic drug

Zhiyu Li and Xiaoke Guo
China Pharmaceutical University, Nanjing, Jiangsu Province, P.R. China

Chapter outline

25.1 Antipsychotic drugs	619
25.1.1 Classical antipsychotic drugs	619
25.1.2 Atypical antipsychotic drugs	620
25.1.3 Multiple target drug design	621
25.2 Medicinal chemistry of risperidone	623
25.2.1 The pharmacological basis of risperidone	623
25.2.2 Discovery of risperidone	624
25.2.3 The synthesis of risperidone	626
25.3 Characteristics of risperidone's effects	627
25.3.1 Pharmacological characteristics of risperidone	627
25.3.2 Pharmacokinetics of risperidone	629
25.3.3 Drug-drug Interaction of risperidone and others	629
25.3.4 Progress of risperidone	630
25.3.5 Conclusion and perspective	631
References	631

25.1 Antipsychotic drugs

The human mind is engaged in intricate activities, and psychiatric or neurological disorders can arise from various factors, presenting as diverse conditions like schizophrenia, anxiety, depression, and mania. Projections and statistics from the World Health Organization indicate that about one-fourth of the global population will grapple with mental or neurological disorders at some juncture in their lives. In China, the estimated incidence of mental illness is approximately 17%. In the current epoch of profound global socioeconomic transformations, mental illness has ascended to become the third most prevalent health challenge facing humanity, surpassed solely by cardiovascular diseases and cancer.

25.1.1 Classical antipsychotic drugs

The etiology of mental illnesses is inherently intricate, and multiple hypotheses exist regarding the mechanisms of the action of drugs. In the early stages, a prevailing theory suggested that schizophrenia might be linked to dysfunctions in the dopaminergic system, where an excess of dopamine (DA), hypersensitivity of DA receptors, or hyperfunctioning dopaminergic neurons could precipitate psychotic symptoms. Consequently, early antipsychotic drugs primarily focused on the blockade of DA receptors. DA is unevenly distributed in the brain, with the majority located in the striatum, substantia nigra, and pallidum. Various pathways for DA in the brain exist (Fig. 25.1), including the mesolimbic and mesocortical pathways, integral to behaviors such as cognition, emotion, and affect. In patients with schizophrenia, dysfunction in both of these pathways is commonly observed, accompanied by an increased expression of DA receptors in the brain. As a result, antipsychotic drugs achieve therapeutic effects by concurrently blocking DA D_2 receptors in these two pathways. The tuberoinfundibular pathway, which regulates the endocrine function of the anterior pituitary, constitutes the third pathway. Another significant pathway is the nigrostriatal pathway, which belongs to the extrapyramidal system and is crucial for maintaining coordinated movement. The diminished function of this pathway can lead to Parkinson's disease, while hyperfunction can result in hyperkinetic disorders. Classical antipsychotic drugs function as DA receptor antagonists, blocking DA receptors in the mesolimbic and mesocortical systems, thereby reducing DA function and exerting an antipsychotic effect. However, they can also inhibit

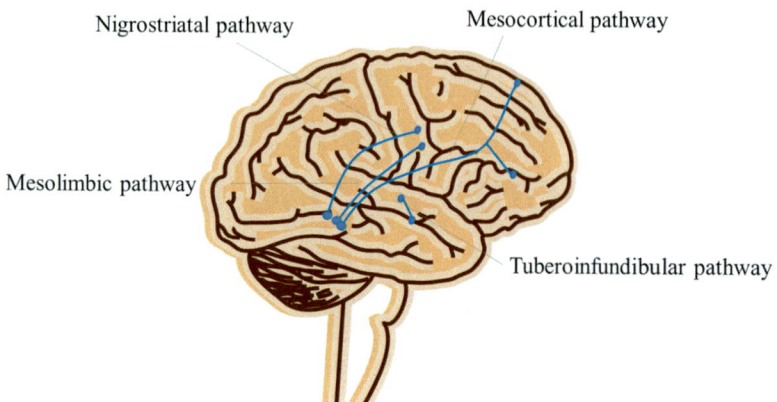

FIGURE 25.1 Dopamine pathways in the brain.

the dopaminergic system in the nigrostriatal pathway, inducing adverse reactions in the extrapyramidal system, such as dystonia, parkinsonism, akathisia, and tardive dyskinesia [1].

The predominant early-discovered drugs were D_2 receptor antagonists, recognized as classical antipsychotics. Based on their structural characteristics, they fall into five categories (see Table 25.1): (1) phenothiazines, exemplified by chlorpromazine; (2) thioxanthenes, exemplified by chlorprothixene; (3) butyrophenones, exemplified by flupentixol; (4) benzamides, exemplified by sulpiride; and (5) dibenzodiazepines, exemplified by clozapine. Classical antipsychotics commonly elicit extrapyramidal side effects, with an incidence rate ranging from 25% to 60%. This is attributed to the inhibition of the DA neurotransmitter system in the limbic system and cortex, resulting in antipsychotic effects. However, inhibition of the DA neurotransmitter system in the substantial nigrostriatal pathway can lead to extrapyramidal side effects and endocrine changes [1,2].

It is noteworthy that despite targeting DA receptors, these drugs exhibit certain limitations in adhering strictly to the DA theory. Notably, certain medications demonstrate significant antipsychotic effects despite having relatively weak interactions with D_2 receptors. This phenomenon suggests that specific antipsychotic drugs may possess multitarget properties.

With the progress in psychopharmacology, extensive investigations have been undertaken by researchers into the mechanisms underlying adverse drug reactions, particularly emphasizing extrapyramidal side effects and tardive dyskinesia. It is now widely acknowledged that schizophrenia correlates with an overactive central DA neurotransmission system. The distinction between the antipsychotic effect and extrapyramidal side effects lies in the fact that the former is achieved through the inhibition of the DA neurotransmission system in the limbic system and cerebral cortex, whereas the latter stems from the inhibition of the nigrostriatal DA neurotransmission system. Among the benzamide antipsychotic drugs, sulpiride stands out for its minimal extrapyramidal side effects, owing to its specific antagonism of DA D_2 receptors. This results in selective inhibition of neuronal cells in the limbic system, with lesser influence on the striatum and substantia nigra. Additionally, research has unveiled that chlorprothixene can selectively inhibit DA neurotransmission, acting specifically on dopaminergic neurons in the mesocortex, and is associated with fewer extrapyramidal side effects and a minimal occurrence of tardive dyskinesia. This observation indicates the potential separation of the antipsychotic effect from extrapyramidal side effects, providing a theoretical foundation for the development of atypical antipsychotic drugs. Researchers have initiated exploration of alternative drug targets beyond DA, with a current emphasis on serotonin (5-HT) receptors, particularly the 5-HT_2 receptor. Serotonin, being the most abundant neurotransmitter in the nervous system, governs numerous brain functions and is closely linked to emotional regulation. Presently, seven subtypes of 5-HT receptors have been identified, spanning from 5-HT_1 to 5-HT_7. Antagonists of the 5-HT_2 receptor can enhance DA release in the nigrostriatal pathway, thereby reinstating dopaminergic regulation of motor function. Leveraging this understanding, the design of a drug that simultaneously antagonizes both D_2 receptors and 5-HT_2 receptors would mitigate extrapyramidal side effects through the interaction of these two neurotransmitter systems. Consequently, scientists are actively engaged in developing novel atypical antipsychotic drugs based on this integrated approach [1–3].

25.1.2 Atypical antipsychotic drugs

Atypical antipsychotic drugs constitute a class of medications renowned for their significant therapeutic efficacy in alleviating symptoms of psychosis, concurrently enhancing cognitive function, and demonstrating minimal or negligible

TABLE 25.1 Classification of classical antipsychotic drugs and representative examples.

Structure classification	Drug names	Structural formulas
Phenothiazines	Chlorpromazine	
Thioxanthenes	Chlorprothixene	
Butyrophenones	Flupentixol	
Benzamides	Sulpiride	
Dibenzodiazepines	Clozapine	

extrapyramidal adverse reactions. A pivotal breakthrough in the realm of nonclassical antipsychotics was the unveiling of clozapine, a benzodiazepine-class atypical antipsychotic drug. The current understanding of the mechanisms of action for atypical antipsychotic drugs can be broadly classified into the following categories:

1. Dual antagonism of serotonin (5-HT_{2A}) and DA (D_2) receptors.
2. Dual antagonism of DA D_2 and D_3 receptors.
3. Dual action involving DA D_1 receptor stimulation and D_2 receptor antagonism.
4. The hypothesis of multiple receptor interactions.

25.1.3 Multiple target drug design

Multiple target drug design confers several advantages over single target drugs, particularly within the realms of medicinal chemistry and biology: (1) It offers superior therapeutic efficacy. Complex diseases, such as malignant tumors and neurodegenerative disorders, involve intricate pathological mechanisms and processes arising from the interplay of multiple factors.

While single-target drugs can only modulate a specific step in disease progression, multitarget drugs can concurrently act on various pathological pathways, eliciting synergistic effects and thereby enhancing the therapeutic outcome. (2) Multitarget drugs tend to manifest fewer adverse reactions. Biological drug targets typically engage in multiple signaling pathways and possess diverse biological functions. The excessive inhibition or activation of a specific target can impact nontarget pathways, leading to the occurrence of adverse reactions. In contrast, multitarget drugs can balance different pathological factors associated with the same disease. By exerting their pharmacological effects through the coordinated inhibition of multiple targets with relatively weak affinity, they avoid intense inhibition or activation of a single biological target, thereby minimizing the likelihood of adverse reactions. (3) Multitarget drugs are less susceptible to drug resistance. Organisms function as intricate biological network systems, and prolonged use of single-target drugs can activate compensatory signaling pathways or counteracting protective mechanisms, resulting in decreased drug sensitivity and the emergence of drug resistance. Multitarget drugs can mitigate the development of drug resistance by simultaneously intervening in compensatory signaling pathways. The rational design of multitarget drug molecules primarily involves combining pharmacophores to achieve the aforementioned objectives, with common strategies being pharmacophore-coupling and pharmacophore-merging. The coupling pharmacophore approach, while broadly applicable, often results in multitarget drug molecules with relatively large molecular weights, potentially negatively impacting solubility and oral absorption. This method has found utility in the early stages of drug development. For instance, the classic antibacterial drug Sultamicillin (Fig. 25.2A) exemplifies a multitarget antibacterial drug that combines the semisynthetic antibiotic Ampicillin with the β-lactamase inhibitor Sulbactam using a methylene linker. Conversely, the pharmacophore-merging approach leverages the structural similarity of ligands or ligand binding sites associated with different targets of the same disease. This approach offers the advantage of obtaining multitarget drugs with relatively smaller molecular weights, favorable physicochemical properties, and desirable pharmacokinetic characteristics, thereby enhancing the likelihood of successful drug development. However, its applicability is confined to situations where ligands or ligand binding sites of different targets exhibit structural similarity, and these targets typically share functional similarities. This limitation makes it challenging to modulate various pathological aspects of complex diseases and achieve optimal therapeutic effects. In recent years, the application of multitarget drug design has gained widespread traction, particularly in the development of anticancer drugs. A notable example is Sorafenib (Fig. 25.2B), an oral anticancer drug FDA-approved in 2005. Sorafenib exhibits a multifaceted mechanism, inhibiting the activity of VEGFR, PDGFR, FLT3, and KIT receptor tyrosine kinases while also serving as a potent inhibitor of Raf kinases. On one hand, sorafenib impedes c-Raf kinase activity and downstream signaling, disrupting the phosphorylation processes of mitogen-activated extracellular signal-regulated kinase (MEK) and extracellular regulated protein kinase (ERK) and reducing the levels of ERK phosphorylation, thereby exerting antiproliferative effects. On the other hand, sorafenib binds to VEGFR-2, VEGFR-3, and PDGFR-β, inhibiting the autophosphorylation of tyrosine kinase receptors and demonstrating antiangiogenic activity. Sorafenib stands as a highly successful illustration of a multitarget anticancer drug.

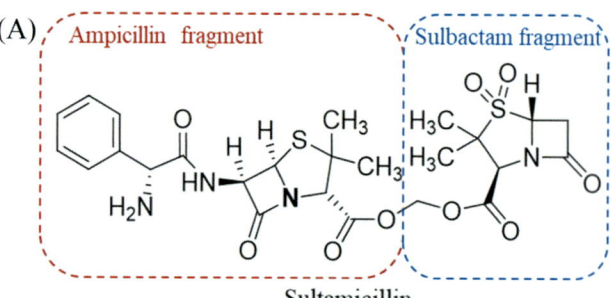

FIGURE 25.2 (A) The structural formula of the multitarget drug Sultamicillin. (B) The structural formula of the multitarget drug Sorafenib.

25.2 Medicinal chemistry of risperidone

Risperidone (Fig. 25.3), categorized as a second-generation, nonclassical antipsychotic drug, was introduced to the Chinese market in 1997 and is presently listed in the national essential medicines catalog.

25.2.1 The pharmacological basis of risperidone

In 1967, Dr. Paul A. Janssen, along with his team at Janssen Pharmaceuticals in Belgium, pioneered the development of the iconic antipsychotic medication Haloperidol (Fig. 25.4). Following approval by the FDA, haloperidol emerged as the most effective treatment for schizophrenia at that time.

The origin of haloperidol can be traced back to research on piperidine derivatives (Fig. 25.5). Initially, Dr. Janssen directed efforts toward developing a novel class of anesthetics. However, substituting the methyl group on the nitrogen atom of piperidine with a propionyl group unexpectedly resulted in decreased analgesic activity but exhibited antipsychotic effects akin to chlorpromazine (Table 25.1). Through structure-activity relationship studies, it was discerned that extending the propyl group to butyl eliminated the morphine-like activity of the butyrophenones while enhancing the antipsychotic effect. Consequently, a class of antipsychotic drugs with a butyrophenone structure was developed, and optimal efficacy was achieved when a fluorine atom substituted the para position on the phenyl ring of the butyrophenone fragment, leading to the synthesis of haloperidol (originally designated as R1625). Notably, its distinguishing feature lies in its stronger antipsychotic action compared to phenothiazines like chlorpromazine, while also finding utility as an anxiolytic agent [4].

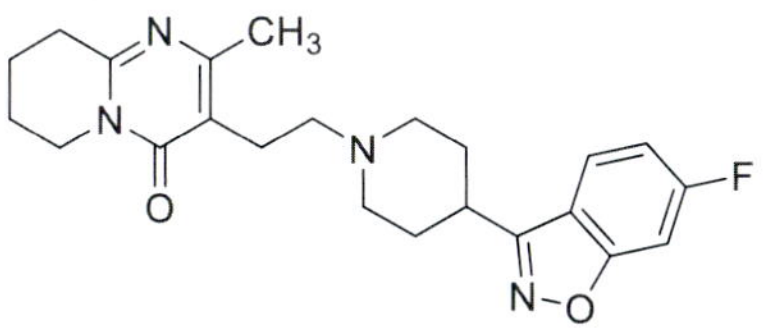

FIGURE 25.3 Chemical structure of risperidone.

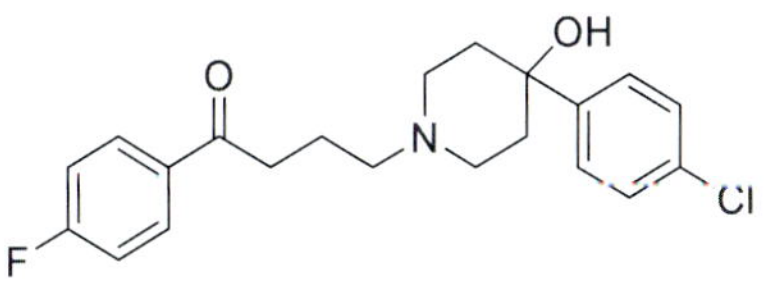

FIGURE 25.4 Chemical structure of haloperidol.

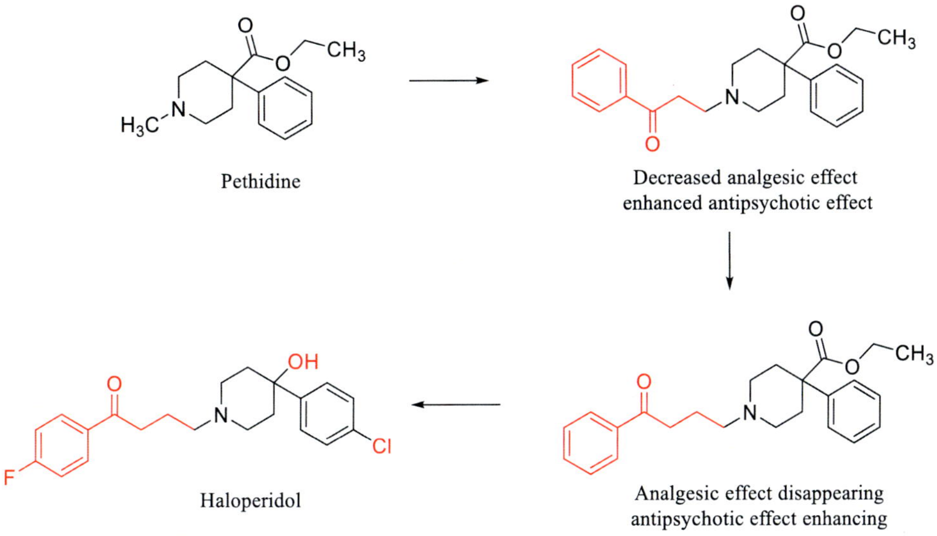

FIGURE 25.5 The discovery of haloperidol.

Following the clinical application of haloperidol, notable extrapyramidal side effects and teratogenic effects were observed. This spurred scientists to explore new antipsychotic drugs aimed at mitigating extrapyramidal side effects. At this juncture, substantial advancements had occurred in the field of psychopharmacology, with two drug evaluation models laying the foundation for the discovery of multitarget drugs:

1. The drug discrimination (DD) model [4]

    Behavioral pharmacologists employ animal models for DD, a scientific approach to studying the "subjective" effects of different drugs. In essence, rats are placed in a box with two buttons to acquire food. Button 1 is linked to the administration of physiological saline, while button 2 is associated with the administration of the training drug. Through multiple training sessions, rats can subjectively distinguish the training drug from physiological saline and appropriately select the button to obtain food. When assessing a drug, the correct response rate of rats in choosing button 1 or 2 after the administration of the test drug is utilized to determine whether the test drug exhibits a more potent effect compared to the training drug. This method, enabling the test animal to discriminate the subjective experience induced by one drug treatment from another, is known as DD.

2. The lysergic acid diethylamide (LSD) model [4,5]

    Before the 1970s, the standard animal model for investigating schizophrenia involved the use of amphetamines or other catecholamine-releasing agents to induce positive symptoms of schizophrenia in rodents. Despite LSD's ability to induce similar psychiatric symptoms, it was employed as a pharmacological model because it failed to induce behaviors associated with subjective consciousness in animals. However, through DD analysis of LSD, it was revealed that antipsychotic drugs, including the DA receptor antagonist Haloperidol, could suppress rat behavior but were unable to counteract LSD's discriminative effects. Further analysis suggested that LSD might exert its effects through the DA and serotonin (5-HT) systems in the brain. Subsequent investigations demonstrated that 5-HT receptor antagonists could indeed counteract LSD, although this counteraction was only partial. This implies that the psychotic symptoms induced by LSD necessitate the synergistic pharmacological actions of both DA receptor antagonists and 5-HT receptor antagonists, highlighting the involvement of 5-HT receptors in the pathological basis of psychosis. The evolution of these two animal models in psychopharmacology and the insights gained from data analysis spurred scientists at Janssen Pharmaceuticals to explore compounds with the capability to simultaneously antagonize both DA and serotonin (5-HT) receptors. This endeavor laid the foundation for the discovery of risperidone.

25.2.2 Discovery of risperidone

Upon realizing that their compounds, including haloperidol, were unable to entirely counteract the activity of LSD, scientists at Janssen Pharmaceuticals initiated a screening process for additional 5-HT receptor antagonists and DA receptor antagonists to identify novel lead compounds.

In 1985, they discovered ritanserin (R55667; Fig. 25.6), a highly selective 5-HT$_{2A}$ antagonist. Ritanserin exhibited the capacity to alleviate negative symptoms of schizophrenia and certain extrapyramidal reactions, but it still fell short of complete antagonism of LSD effects. Subsequently, medicinal chemists engaged in optimization efforts based on ritanserin. Initially, they explored replacing the thizolopyrididinone in ritanserin with its bioisostere pyridopyrimidinone, as well as substituting the side chain with the para-fluorobenzoyl fragment present in haloperidol. This led to the development of pirenperone, the first pure LSD antagonist that simultaneously antagonizes both DA and 5-HT receptors. However, pirenperone's pharmacokinetic properties in the human body were not satisfactory. Continuing their efforts, in 1985, the research team conducted structural optimization based on pirenperone, resulting in the long-acting dual antagonist, risperidone (R64766), a benzisoxazole derivative. Risperidone not only completely antagonizes LSD but also exhibits no stimulant activity resembling LSD (Fig. 25.6). [5,6]

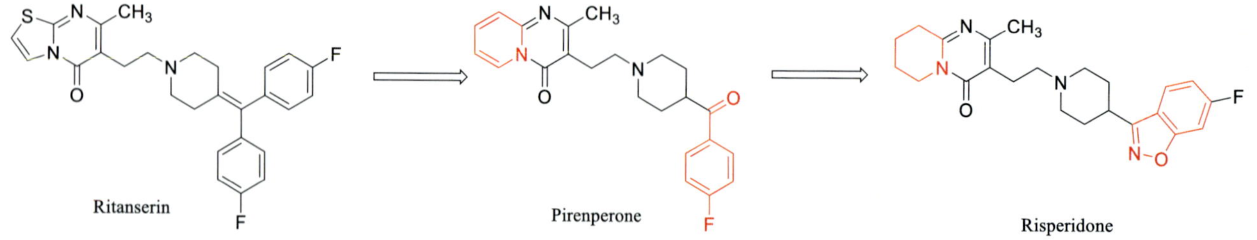

FIGURE 25.6 The discovery of Risperidone.

Fortunately, through structural analysis of pirenperone and risperidone, it can be deduced that these are dual-acting small-molecule inhibitors created by combining the pharmacophore moiety of ritanserin (depicted in Fig. 25.7; highlighted in yellow) with the pharmacophore moiety of haloperidol (highlighted in blue) within a single molecule. Consequently, risperidone is commonly regarded as a drug molecule designed through the principle of fragment merging, demonstrating characteristics of a multitarget drug. The successful design of risperidone also involves further medicinal chemistry optimization, including the refinement of the blue-colored moiety, to enhance the druggability of the new molecule.

In the *in vitro* receptor binding studies of risperidone, haloperidol, and ritanserin (Table 25.2), it was observed that both risperidone and ritanserin exhibit high binding affinity to the 5-HT$_2$ receptor, with Ki values of 0.16 and 0.30 nM, respectively. Additionally, risperidone, akin to haloperidol, demonstrates a high affinity for the D$_2$ receptor, with K$_i$ values of 3.13 and 1.55 nM, respectively. Risperidone also displays higher affinity for the α1-adrenergic receptor (K_i = 0.8 nM), histamine H$_1$ receptor (K_i = 2.23 nM), and α$_2$-adrenergic receptor (K_i = 7.54 nM) compared to ritanserin and haloperidol. Furthermore, the binding of risperidone to these receptors exhibits a rapid binding rate and a slow dissociation rate, resulting in stable antagonism of receptor activity [7–9].

The distinctive aspect of this design is the role of risperidone as a highly selective 5-HT$_2$/D$_2$ dual receptor balanced antagonist, demonstrating elevated efficacy with minimal extrapyramidal side effects. While its antagonistic effect on LSD is comparable to that of ritanserin, risperidone has superior pharmacokinetic properties. Consequently, it emerged as the first marketed multitarget antipsychotic drug, gaining approval in the United Kingdom in 1992, the United States in 1993, and China in 1997.

Combination principles are frequently employed strategies in drug design, primarily involving the fusion of pharmacophore structures from two different drugs into a single molecule or the harmonious integration of their pharmacophoric moieties within a molecule, the latter termed a hybrid molecule. The resulting molecule may inherit properties from both drugs, augmenting pharmacological effects while minimizing their respective adverse reactions. Alternatively, it may capitalize on the strengths of both drugs to complement each other, achieving therapeutic outcomes synergistically.

When designing drug molecules, medicinal chemists predominantly employ two combination methods: overlapping and linking (Fig. 25.8). The former involves leveraging the shared portion of the pharmacophoric moieties from both molecules, while the latter simply connects the pharmacophoric moieties of two molecules. A classic example of the combination principle is the nonsteroidal antiinflammatory drug Benorilate (Fig. 25.9). To reduce the acidity of aspirin and mitigate its gastrointestinal adverse effects, aspirin, an nonsteroidal anti-inflammatory drug (NSAID), was linked to paracetamol, an antipyretic analgesic drug, through an ester bond. This design minimizes gastric irritation upon oral administration. In the body, benorilate undergoes decomposition to regenerate the original two parent drugs, combining the antiinflammatory properties of aspirin with the antipyretic analgesic properties of paracetamol. This results in a synergistic antipyretic and analgesic effect, with benorilate exhibiting fewer adverse reactions and being suitable for use in the elderly and children.

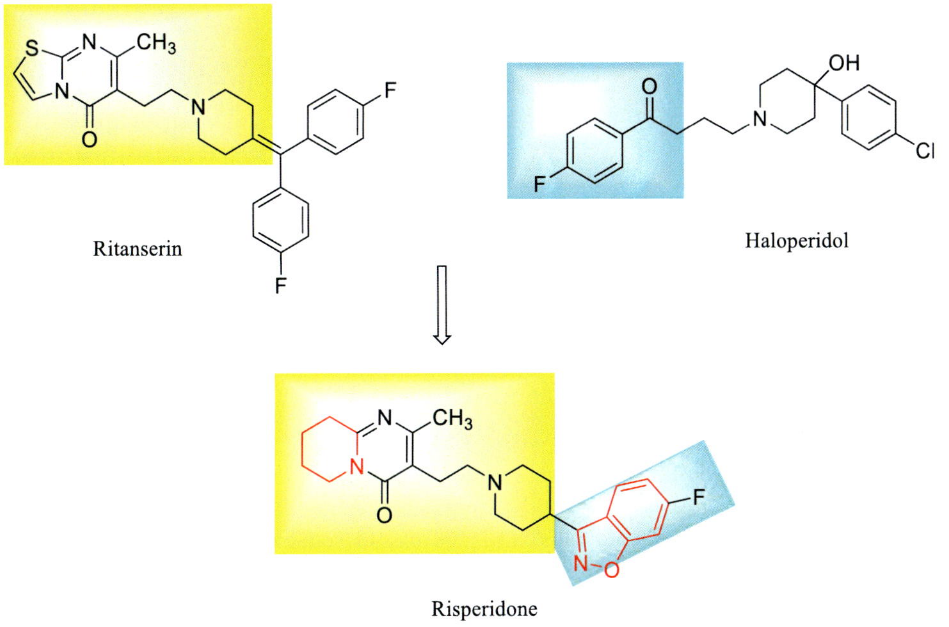

FIGURE 25.7 The design of risperidone.

TABLE 25.2 Affinity of risperidone, haloperidol, and ritanserin for 5-HT and DA receptor subtypes [K_i (nM)] [7].

Receptor/Drug	Risperidone	Haloperidol	Ritanserin
5-HT$_2$	0.16	25	0.30
5-HT$_{1A}$	253	3080	1370
D$_2$	3.1	1.5	30
D$_1$	534	255	718
α$_1$	0.81	10.9	35.7
α$_2$	7.54	\	56.4
H$_1$	2.33	593	11.8

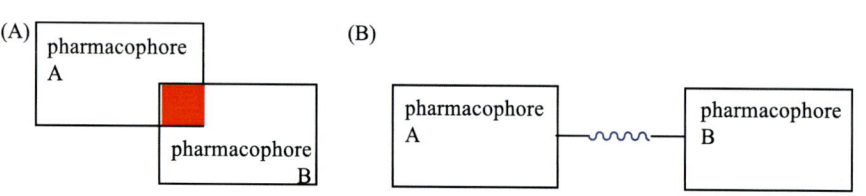

FIGURE 25.8 Combination methods of combination principle.

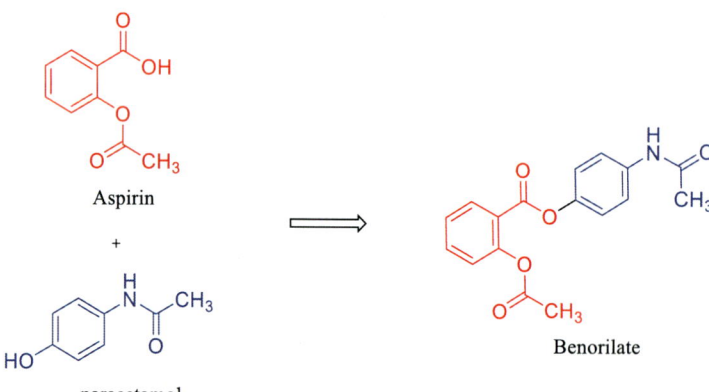

FIGURE 25.9 Benorilate: a design utilizing the combination principle.

25.2.3 The synthesis of risperidone

Physical and chemical properties of risperidone (Fig. 25.10):

Chemical name: 3-[2-[4-(6-fluoro-1,2-benzisoxazol-3-yl)-1-piperidinyl]ethyl]-6,7,8,9-tetrahydro-2-methyl-4H-pyrido[1,2-a]pyrimidin-4-one.

Physical and chemical properties: white crystalline powder; m.p.: 170.0°C; solubility (25°C): 44.74 mg/L.

Industrial synthetic routes of risperidone [10–12]:

There are multiple industrial synthetic routes for the production of risperidone, and in this chapter, two routes (Fig. 25.11) will be briefly introduced:

Route A: Starting from 2-aminopyridine, the compound undergoes cyclization with methyl acetoacetate, followed by reduction, cross-coupling, and Brown hydroboration to yield 2-(2-methyl-4-oxo-6,7,8,9-tetrahydro-4H-pyrido[1,2-a]pyrimidin-3-yl)acetaldehyde. Subsequently, the compound is subjected to reductive amination with (2,4-difluorophenyl)(pyridin-4-yl)methanone, followed by oximation and cyclization to obtain Risperidone.

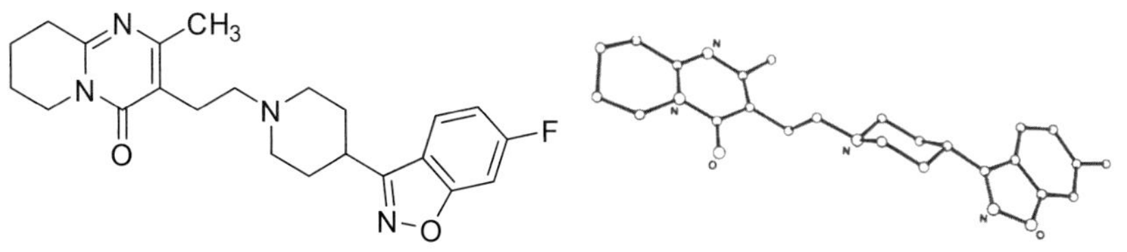

FIGURE 25.10 Structure of Risperidone (left); perspective view of Risperidone based on X-ray analysis (right).

Route B: Starting from 4-piperidinemethanoic acid, the compound undergoes amino protection and chlorination to yield 1-ethoxymethoxycarbonyl-4-piperidinemethanoyl chloride. This intermediate is then subjected to Friedel-Crafts acylation with 1,3-difluorobenzene, followed by deprotection, oximation, cyclization, and salt formation to obtain Risperidone hydrochloride, specifically 6-fluoro-3-(4-piperidinyl)-1,2-benzisoxazole hydrochloride. This compound is then condensed with 3-(2-chloroethyl)-6,7,8,9-tetrahydro-2-methyl-4H-pyrido[1,2-a]pyrimidin-4-one under alkaline catalysis to produce Risperidone.

25.3 Characteristics of risperidone's effects

25.3.1 Pharmacological characteristics of risperidone

25.3.1.1 Pharmacological mechanism of risperidone

Risperidone is a multitarget antipsychotic agent (Table 25.1) characterized by high affinity for $5\text{-}HT_{2A}$ and D_2 receptors. It also binds to $\alpha 1$ adrenergic receptors with lower affinity for histamine H_1 and α_2 adrenergic receptors, while showing no binding affinity to cholinergic receptors [7,8,12].

Notably, risperidone exhibits a low incidence of extrapyramidal side effects. It maintains an optimal $D_2/5\text{-}HT_{2A}$ antagonism ratio, with 20 times greater affinity for $5\text{-}HT_{2A}$ receptors than for D_2 receptors, and demonstrates a clear dose-response relationship. In comparison to traditional antipsychotic medications, risperidone is associated with fewer anticholinergic side effects, minimal weight gain, and a lower potential for inducing diabetes.

1. Mesolimbic pathway: Inhibiting postsynaptic D_2 receptors → amelioration of positive symptoms.
2. Mesocortical pathway: Blocking $5\text{-}HT_{2A}$ receptors → enhances DA function → amelioration of negative symptoms → increases $5\text{-}HT_{1A}$ excitability → improves both emotional and negative symptoms.
3. Nigrostriatal pathway: Blocking $5\text{-}HT_{2A}$ receptors → enhances DA function → reducing extrapyramidal side effects.

As a potent D_2 receptor antagonist, risperidone proves effective in ameliorating symptoms in patients with schizophrenia. Its balanced antagonistic effects on the central nervous system's $5\text{-}HT_{2A}$ and D_2 receptors contribute to a reduction in the occurrence of extrapyramidal side effects. Consequently, risperidone is not only effective in treating the positive symptoms of schizophrenia, such as hallucinations, delusions, disorganized thinking, hostility, and suspicion, but also addresses negative symptoms, including blunted affect and diminished speech, as well as affective symptoms like depression, guilt, and anxiety.

In patients with chronic schizophrenia, the administration of risperidone at a dosage of 5–10 mg/day has been shown to restore sleep patterns and improve sleep efficiency, with more pronounced improvements compared to haloperidol. Following multiple doses over a 4-week period, risperidone significantly and sustainably increases serum prolactin levels in individuals with schizophrenia.

25.3.1.2 Indications of risperidone [13,14]

1. Schizophrenia
   Risperidone is employed in the management of various psychiatric conditions, including first-episode psychosis, chronic schizophrenia, and treatment-resistant schizophrenia. It demonstrates notable efficacy in alleviating both positive and negative symptoms associated with schizophrenia.
2. Affective disorder
   Risperidone is utilized for major depressive disorder, severe impulsivity, and rapid cycling disorders.

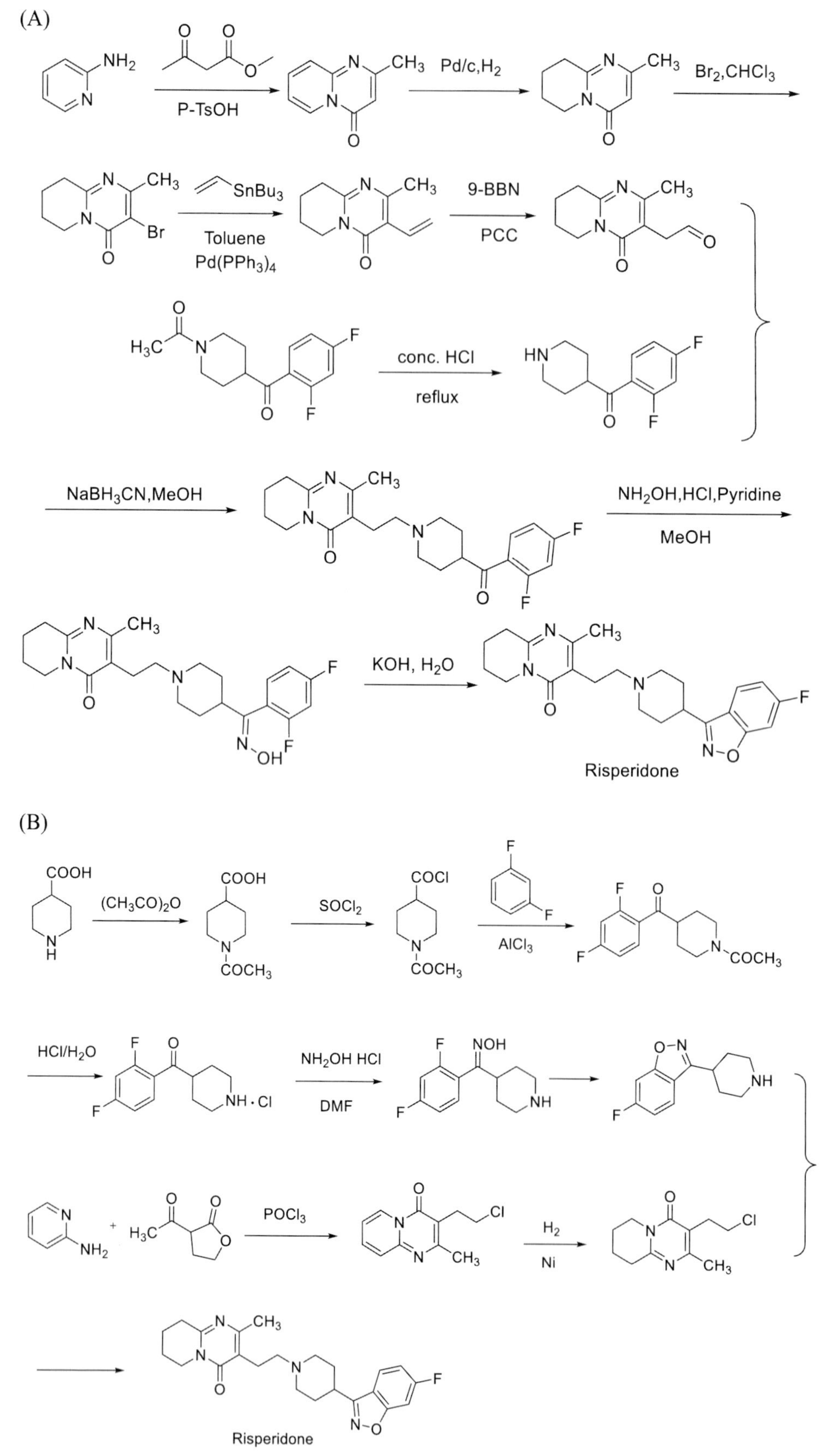

628 Medicinal Chemistry and Drug Development

FIGURE 25.11 Industrial synthesis routes of risperidone.

3. Obsessive compulsive disorder
    Risperidone is indicated for the treatment of refractory obsessive-compulsive disorder, particularly in patients presenting with schizotypal obsessive symptoms.
4. Tardive dyskinesia
5. Others
    Additionally, it is prescribed for Tourette syndrome and behavioral disturbances associated with mental retardation.

25.3.1.3 Adverse effects of risperidone

Risperidone has a relatively low toxicity compared to classical antipsychotic drugs and a lower incidence of extrapyramidal side effects [14–16].

1. At doses below 6 mg/day, extrapyramidal side effects are minimal. However, as the dosage increases, the risk of extrapyramidal side effects becomes greater and is alleviated by reducing the dosage. There have been no reports of delayed-onset movement disorders associated with this medication.
2. Adverse reactions: menstrual disorders, drowsiness, fatigue, insomnia, salivation, and headache. Few difficulty in concentrating and mild memory impairment, while large doses will produce gait instability.
3. Risperidone can produce dose-dependent orthostatic hypotension and compensatory reflex heart rate acceleration due to antagonism of adrenergic α1 receptors, thus cardiovascular patients should be used with caution.

25.3.2 Pharmacokinetics of risperidone [13,17]

Oral absorption of Risperidone is complete, with an oral bioavailability ranging from 66% to 82%. Peak blood concentrations are achieved 1–2 hours after administration and remain unaffected by food intake, allowing for convenient dosing with meals and promoting patient compliance. Risperidone undergoes extensive metabolic pathways (Fig. 25.12), including hydroxylation, oxidation, and N-dealkylation. The primary hepatic metabolism of risperidone is catalyzed by P450 enzymes, leading to the formation of its major metabolite, paliperidone, which possesses 70% of the antipsychotic activity of risperidone.

Widely distributed throughout the body, risperidone and its metabolites exhibit approximately 90% plasma protein binding and have an apparent volume of distribution of 1.2 L/kg. The major route of elimination for risperidone is renal excretion, with approximately 70% excreted in the urine and 15% in the feces within one week of administration. The plasma elimination half-life ($t_{1/2}\beta$) of risperidone and its active metabolite, paliperidone, is 2.8 and 20.5 hours, respectively, while the $t_{1/2}\beta$ of the active fraction is approximately 24 hours. In poor metabolizers, the $t_{1/2}\beta$ of risperidone is prolonged to approximately 16 hours, while the $t_{1/2}\beta$ of the active fraction remains unchanged. Renal impairment leads to a decrease in the renal clearance of risperidone.

Despite the generation of a new chiral center, paliperidone, the active metabolite of risperidone, exhibits a longer duration of action compared to risperidone. Consequently, it has been further developed as a new drug and is marketed as a racemic mixture.

25.3.3 Drug-drug Interaction of risperidone and others

Risperidone primarily undergoes hepatic metabolism *via* the enzyme CYP2D6, leading to the formation of paliperidone. CYP3A4 also participates in partial metabolism. Consequently, drugs that induce or inhibit CYP2D6 and CYP3A4 can influence the plasma concentration of risperidone. For example, antidepressant medications such as paroxetine and fluoxetine exert inhibitory effects on CYP2D6, impeding the metabolism of risperidone into paliperidone and consequently increasing the plasma concentration of risperidone. Conversely, the antiepileptic drug carbamazepine induces CYP2D6, accelerating the metabolism of risperidone [18].

Other examples of drug interactions are as follows:

1. Concomitant use of tricyclic antidepressants may lead to orthostatic hypotension and should be used with caution.
2. Coadministration of trihexyphenidyl with risperidone can reduce and alleviate extrapyramidal adverse reactions.
3. Combining risperidone with antihypertensive drugs can enhance the antihypertensive effect.
4. Concurrent use of risperidone with antihistamine drugs may result in excessive sedation.
5. Combining risperidone with antibiotics such as chloramphenicol, ciprofloxacin, and erythromycin, which possess enzyme-inhibitory effects, can inhibit drug-metabolizing enzymes. This leads to an enhanced effect, prolonged

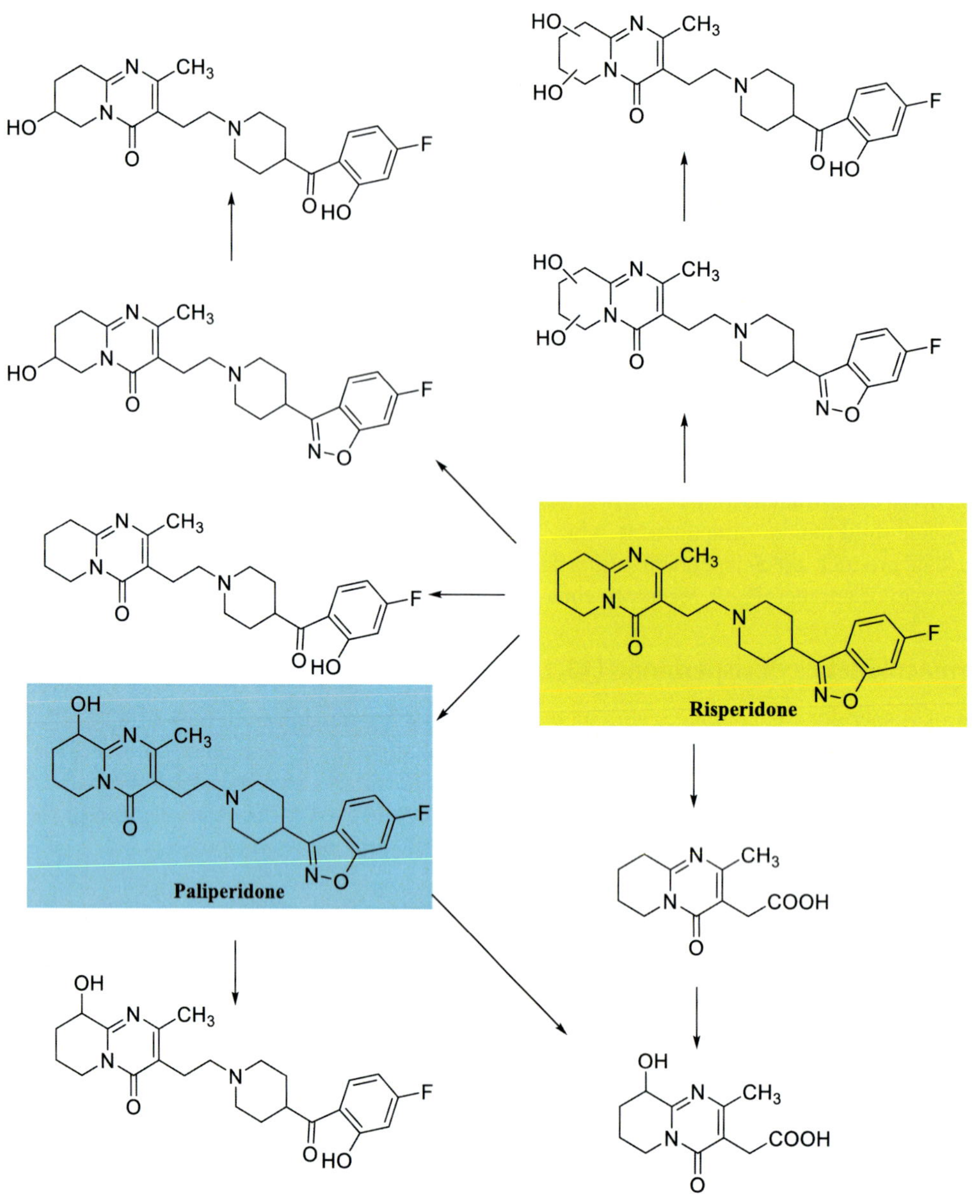

FIGURE 25.12 Metabolism of risperidone.

action, and even accumulation of risperidone. Therefore, the dosage of risperidone should be appropriately reduced when used in combination with these medications.
6. Drugs like rifampicin and prednisone, which exhibit enzyme-inducing effects, can enhance the metabolism of risperidone, reducing its plasma concentration. On the other hand, discontinuation of these drugs may increase the plasma concentration of risperidone and cause symptoms of toxicity.
7. Certain β-blockers can increase the plasma concentration of risperidone, potentially leading to an increased risk of adverse reactions.

25.3.4 Progress of risperidone

Risperidone, as a first-line medication for antipsychotic treatment, stands as a classic example in the realm of antipsychotic drugs and has been on the market for nearly three decades. Janssen Pharmaceuticals has established a "textbook-like" paradigm in the evolution of risperidone. Given the limited patent lifespan of pharmaceuticals, pharmaceutical enterprises employ various strategies to extend product lifecycles.

In 1992, risperidone tablets were first introduced in the United Kingdom for the treatment of schizophrenia. Subsequently, in 1996, a rapid-acting formulation was developed, followed by the creation of a long-acting formulation, risperidone microspheres, in 2002. This formulation, administered once every two weeks, currently stands as the sole long-acting injectable suitable for both schizophrenia and bipolar disorder. In 2006, the indications for risperidone were expanded in the United States to include the treatment of irritability symptoms associated with autism spectrum disorder in children and adolescents aged 5–16. These symptoms encompass aggression toward others, deliberate self-harm, irritable mood, and rapid mood changes.

In the same year, the oral sustained-release formulation of risperidone's metabolite, paliperidone, the only oral formulation approved for schizoaffective disorder worldwide, was launched. In 2009, the long-acting formulation of paliperidone, paliperidone palmitate, a suspension-type injectable with a release cycle of four weeks, was introduced. Furthermore, in 2015, an ultra-long-acting formulation of paliperidone was released, which is still the only antipsychotic medication requiring administration only four times a year.

In 2018, the monthly subcutaneous injection of risperidone was introduced for the treatment of adult schizophrenia. As of the present, the development of risperidone continues, and we eagerly anticipate the emergence of novel formulations or combination drugs of risperidone that will further benefit the treatment of psychiatric disorders.

25.3.5 Conclusion and perspective

The discovery of risperidone unfolded through a series of opportunities and intricate coincidences, leveraging Janssen Pharmaceuticals' extensive development experience in the central nervous system drugs field, coupled with advancements in new technologies and methodologies like DD, behavioral pharmacology, and the LSD model. The exploration and discovery of Risperidone were steered by the collaborative efforts of the medicinal chemistry research team, entailing a significant amount of foundational research and divergent multitarget thinking. This characteristic serves as an inspiration to readers of this book, underscoring the pivotal importance of diverse thinking in the realm of drug development.

References

[1] You Q. Medicinal chemistry. 4th ed Beijing: Chemical Industry Press; 2021. p. 123−54.
[2] Gerlach J. New antipsychotics: classification, efficacy, and adverse effects. Schizophrenia Bull 1991;17(2):289−309.
[3] Ni W, Zhou H, Xiang G, et al. Advances in research on atypical antipsychotic drugs. Med Pharm Guide 2010;29(3):342−6.
[4] Francis CC. Discovering Risperidone: the LSD model of psychopathology. Nat Rev 2003;2:315−19.
[5] Meert TF, Haes P, Janssen PA. Risperidone (R64766), a potent and complete LSD antagonist in drug discrimination by rats. Psychopharmacology 1989;97:206−12.
[6] Janssen PA, Niemegeers CJ, Awouters F, et al. Pharmacology of Risperidone (R64766), a new antipsychotic with serotonin-S_2 and dopamine-D_2 antagonistic properties. J Pharmacol Exp Therap 1988;244(2):685−93.
[7] LeysenN JE, Gommeren W, Eens A, et al. Biochemical profile of Risperidone, a new antipsychotic. J Pharmacol Exp Therap 1988;247(2):661−70.
[8] Susan G, Andrew F. Risperidone-a review of its pharmacology and therapeutic potential in the treatment of schizophrenia. Drugs 1994;48(2):253−73.
[9] Megens AA, Awouters FH, Niemegeers CJ. Differential effects of the new antipsychotic Risperidone on large and small motor movements in rats: a comparison with haloperidol. Psychopharmacology 1988;95:492−6.
[10] Kim DM, Kang MS, Kim JS, et al. An efficient synthesis of Risperidone via stille reaction: antipsychotic, 5-HT_2, and dopamine-D_2-antagonist. Arch Pharmacal Res 2005;28(9):1019−22.
[11] Guan Y, Yu X, Wang X. Synthesis of the antipsychotic drug Risperidone. Chem Prod Technol 2008;15(1):17−19.
[12] Lu X, Pan L, Tang C, et al. Synthesis of Risperidone. Chin J Med Chem 2007;17(2):89−91.
[13] Cardoni AA. Risperidone: review and assessment of its role in the treatment of schizophrenia. Ann Pharmacother 1995;29:610−18.
[14] Zhao L. Clinical application of Risperidone. Chin Med Rehabil 2001;(1):20−1.
[15] Li H, Gu N. New antipsychotic drug: Risperidone. Shanghai Arch Psych 1997;(1):49−52.
[16] Gu N. Risperidone - a new antipsychotic drug. Chin J N Drugs Clin Remedies 1992;11(5):314−15.
[17] Qin H. Comparison of the new antipsychotic drugs Risperidone and Alizapride. J Prim Med Forum 2006;10(9):426−7.
[18] Chen F, Qin H, Dong W. Drug interactions of Risperidone. J Clin Psych 2005;15(6):373−4.

Chapter 26

A case study on the first-in-class antirenal anemia drug roxadustat

Xiaojin Zhang and Qidong You
China Pharmaceutical University, Nanjing, P.R China

Chapter outline

26.1 Renal anemia and its pathogenesis	633	
26.1.1 Introduction to renal anemia	633	
26.1.2 Proteolytic degradation and degron	633	
26.1.3 Hypoxia-inducible factor and prolyl hydroxylase	634	
26.2 Medications for the treatment of renal anemia	636	
26.2.1 Commonly used drugs for renal anemia treatment	636	
26.2.2 Prolyl hydroxylase inhibitors	638	
26.3 Development process of roxadustat	639	
26.3.1 Structure and mechanism of prolyl hydroxylase	639	
26.3.2 Identification and optimization of hit compounds	643	
26.3.3 Lead discovery and optimization of prolyl hydroxylase domain inhibitors	643	
26.3.4 Clinical research on roxadustat	645	
26.3.5 Synthetic process of roxadustat	647	
26.4 Conclusion	648	
References	648	

26.1 Renal anemia and its pathogenesis

26.1.1 Introduction to renal anemia

Chronic kidney disease (CKD) is a chronic and progressive condition characterized by significant renal disorders that pose a threat to human health. The prevalence of CKD in China is approximately 11%, while in America and Europe, it ranges from 10% to 15% [1]. During the course of CKD, various complications arise, among which renal anemia is highly prevalent and profoundly impacts the patient's survival and quality of life. Furthermore, it contributes significantly to the increased incidence and mortality of cardiovascular diseases. The kidneys not only serve as vital metabolic organs but also play a crucial role in the production and secretion of erythropoietin (EPO) in adults. Therefore, when a patient's renal function declines or becomes impaired, the functionality of renal fibroblasts responsible for EPO production is compromised, leading to a severe deficiency in endogenous EPO production [2].

EPO is a glycoprotein consisting of 165 amino acids and plays a critical role in human erythropoiesis. The primitive bone marrow stem cells undergo a series of differentiations, eventually transforming into erythrocytic burst-forming units. These units further differentiate into erythroid colonies and proerythroblasts, progressing through early, intermediate, and late stages of erythroblast maturation until they become reticulocytes. After nuclear extrusion, they mature into circulating red blood cells. Stimulation of EPO is necessary during the transition from burst-forming units of erythroid colonies to proerythroblasts to ensure proper differentiation of erythroid progenitor cells and to prevent apoptosis (Fig. 26.1) [2]. Consequently, CKD patients experience severe anemia due to inadequate EPO secretion, a condition commonly known as renal anemia.

26.1.2 Proteolytic degradation and degron

As the foremost executors of biological functions, proteins hold significant importance in maintaining normal life activities. However, under certain physiological and pathological conditions, proteins can exhibit structural anomalies, such

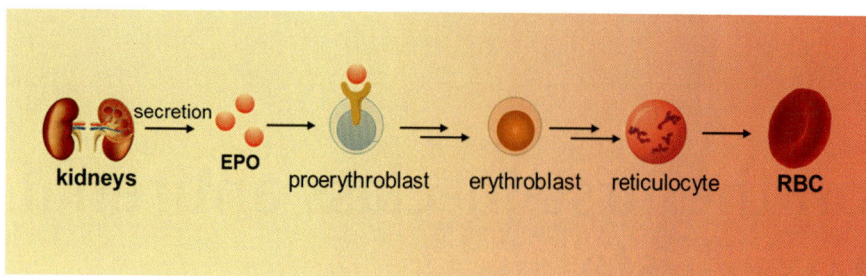

FIGURE 26.1 The secretion of EPO by the kidneys is crucial in the process of erythropoiesis.

as misfolding, which impairs their functionality and disrupts normal organism activities. A noteworthy example of this is the prion virus, where misfolded prion proteins continuously infect functional proteins within the organism, ultimately leading to the complete loss of their functionality and the demise of the host. Additionally, excessive activation of normal proteins can also have adverse physiological effects. Therefore, living organisms have evolved specific protein degradation systems to ensure the timely elimination of misfolded and functionally impaired proteins, as well as excessively activated normal proteins, to maintain the biological environment's homeostasis. Among eukaryotic organisms, including humans, two primary protein degradation systems exist: the ubiquitin-proteasome degradation system and the autophagy-lysosome degradation system. Of the two systems, the ubiquitin-proteasome degradation system holds greater significance, as it accounts for 80%—90% of protein degradation in eukaryotes [3].

The ubiquitin-proteasome system is composed of a series of interconnected enzymes and proteasomes. Functionally, these enzymes can be categorized into two groups: E3-E2 ubiquitin ligases and deubiquitinating enzymes. In the process of protein degradation, the ubiquitin ligases recognize the "degradation signal" on the target protein, leading to its ubiquitination. The ubiquitinated protein is then recognized by the proteasome and broken down into short peptides consisting of less than 10 amino acid residues. Therefore, the precise recognition and selective degradation of specific targets are crucial and closely related to the degradation signal, referred to as "degron." In certain proteins that undergo degradation regulation, specific amino acid residues may exist at the N- or C-terminus, which can undergo posttranslational modifications catalyzed by relevant enzymes in the organism. These modified amino acid sites can act as recognition motifs, referred to as "recognin" for the protein degradation system, enabling precise identification. These amino acids on the target protein are referred to as degrons. Different degradation pathways are defined based on different degrons. Eukaryotes primarily utilize pathways such as the proline (Pro) degron pathway, arginine (Arg) degron pathway, formylmethionine (fMet) degron pathway, and others [4]. The specific amino acid residues corresponding to the respective degrons require specific posttranslational modifications, such as hydroxylation or acetylation, in order to be accurately recognized by specific E3-E2 ligases, known as recognition motifs. Subsequently, they are labeled with ubiquitin for degradation and transported to the cellular protein clearance factory—the proteasome, where the proteins are hydrolyzed into amino acid fragments (Fig. 26.2).

26.1.3 Hypoxia-inducible factor and prolyl hydroxylase

Due to renal cell injury, patients with CKD may experience insufficient secretion of EPO, which plays a crucial role in the human hematopoietic system. The precise regulation of EPO expression in the body is a topic of interest. The human body regulates EPO expression by monitoring oxygen levels, a crucial element necessary for our survival, which we continuously inhale. However, the correlation between oxygen and EPO expression is not direct. The body has evolved a unique system referred to as the cellular oxygen-sensing pathway, which acts as a "bridge" between oxygen and EPO expression. Upon delving deeper into the study of this system, scientists have discovered that its function extends beyond the mere regulation of EPO. It consists of several components, with the hypoxia-inducible factor (HIF) being the most crucial element. As a transcription regulatory factor, HIF has a crucial role in entering the cell nucleus and binding to specific DNA sequences. This binding promotes the transcription of relevant genes, leading to an increase in the expression level of specific proteins that regulate corresponding physiological functions, including the earlier-mentioned EPO gene. It is worth noting that there are three distinct subtypes of HIFs: HIF-1, HIF-2, and HIF-3. Functionally, HIF-1 primarily regulates the body's energy metabolism in response to hypoxia, while HIF-2 is involved in red blood cells and blood vessel formation. HIF-3, on the other hand, serves as a negative feedback regulator of the other two subtypes [5]. Structurally, HIF is a heterodimeric protein consisting of two different subunits, namely HIF-α and HIF-β. The transcriptionally active form of HIF is the HIF-α/β heterodimer, which is formed through the

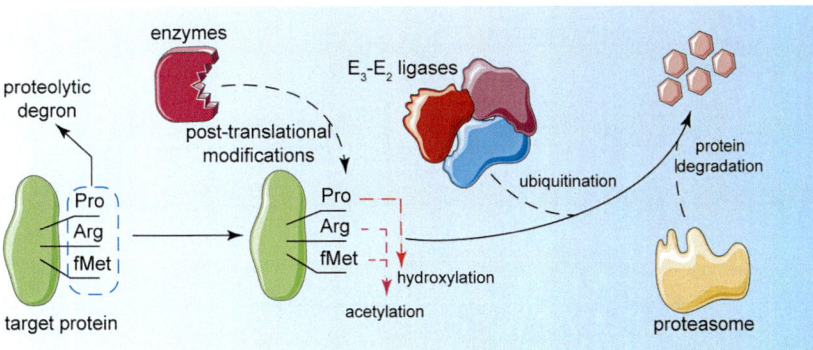

FIGURE 26.2 Illustration of proteolytic degron and protein degradation process.

dimerization of these two subunits. This heterodimer can bind to DNA and exert its transcriptional activity. The HIF-β subunit, also known as aryl hydrocarbon receptor nuclear translocator (ARNT), is constitutively expressed and its cellular concentration remains unaltered by oxygen levels. On the other hand, the HIF-α subunit is regulated by cellular oxygen concentration, allowing it to sensitively perceive changes in oxygen levels within the cells. Consequently, it adjusts the cellular HIF-α concentration accordingly, thereby modulating the overall transcriptional activity of HIF. This modulation subsequently affects the expression of downstream functional proteins involved in various signaling pathways, enabling the body to adapt to hypoxic environments. Therefore, HIF-α serves as the key subunit responsible for regulating HIF activity [5].

From the perspective of the protein's three-dimensional structure, the HIF-α subunit belongs to the basic-helix-loop-helix (bHLH)-PAS (Per/ARNT/Sim, PAS) superfamily (Fig. 26.3). The HIF-1α protein consists of 826 amino acid residues, whereas the HIF-2α protein contains 870 amino acid residues. Both HIF-1α and HIF-2α possess bHLH, PAS-A, and PAS-B domains at the N-terminus, exhibiting a high degree of homology. These domains facilitate the dimerization of HIF-α with HIF-β subunits and their binding to hypoxia response elements (HREs) on the target gene. Additionally, both subunits have conserved oxygen-dependent degradation domains and two transcription activation domains (TAD), including N-TAD and C-TAD, at the C-terminus [6].

As a fundamental regulatory component of the oxygen-sensing pathway in organisms, HIF itself is susceptible to modulation by various factors, highlighting the remarkable evolutionary adaptation of biomacromolecules in living organisms. Upon closer examination, if HIF malfunctions while regulating other downstream proteins, it often leads to more severe consequences. For example, the aberrant expression of HIF-2α can trigger the development of clear cell renal cell carcinoma. Therefore, the regulation of HIF itself is of paramount importance, especially regarding the "degron" mentioned earlier. Under normoxic conditions, specific proline residues (Pro402 and Pro564 for the HIF-1α subunit; Pro405 and Pro531 for the HIF-2α subunit) (Fig. 26.3) within the HIF-α sequence act as the "degrons" and undergo hydroxylation mediated by an oxygen-dependent enzyme, namely prolyl hydroxylase domain (PHD). The hydroxylated HIF-α subunit is precisely recognized and bound by the von Hippel-Lindau (VHL) tumor suppressor protein. The VHL protein recruits an E3 ubiquitin ligase complex, leading to the ubiquitination of the HIF-α subunit. Ultimately, HIF-1α is degraded by the proteasome system, resulting in the loss of its ability to regulate downstream target genes (Figs. 26.3 and 26.4).

Under hypoxic conditions, the hydroxylation activity of PHD enzymes is inhibited, allowing HIF-α to evade recognition by VHL and proteasomal degradation. Consequently, it can form a heterodimer with HIF-β and translocate into the nucleus as an active transcriptional HIF dimer. This dimer then binds to specific HRE sequences on target genes, such as the *EPO* gene, promoting their transcription and enabling the organism to adapt to a hypoxic state [6]. In the regulatory process of HIF, PHD enzymes play a crucial role by linking oxygen levels to the expression level and transcriptional activity of HIF. PHD enzymes belong to the family of Fe^{2+}, oxygen, and 2-oxoglutarate (2OG) dependent hydroxylases [7]. In humans, there are three main subtypes of PHD enzymes: PHD1, PHD2, and PHD3. Although highly conserved in protein sequence and hydroxylation capacity, these subtypes exhibit variations in their expression patterns within the organism. Among the three subtypes, PHD2 is widely expressed in the body and plays a critical role in the hydroxylation regulation of HIF, particularly in the kidneys and liver. Therefore, PHD2 is the primary subtype responsible for the functional regulation of HIF in the body, making it a crucial target for the development of novel drugs related to cellular oxygen-sensing pathways [8].

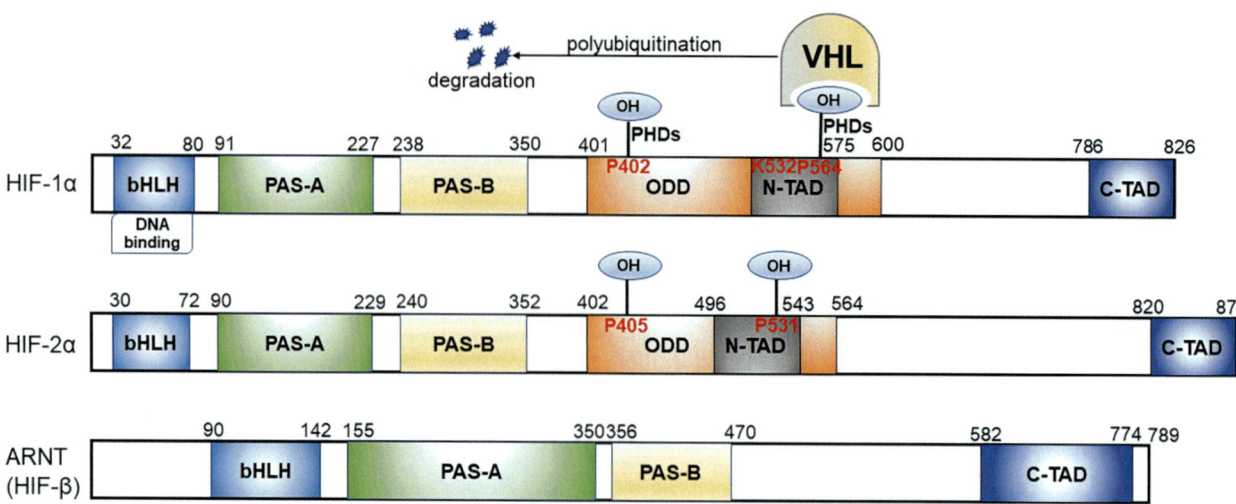

FIGURE 26.3 The structural domains of HIF-α and HIF-β subunits and the oxygen-dependent degradation regulatory sites.

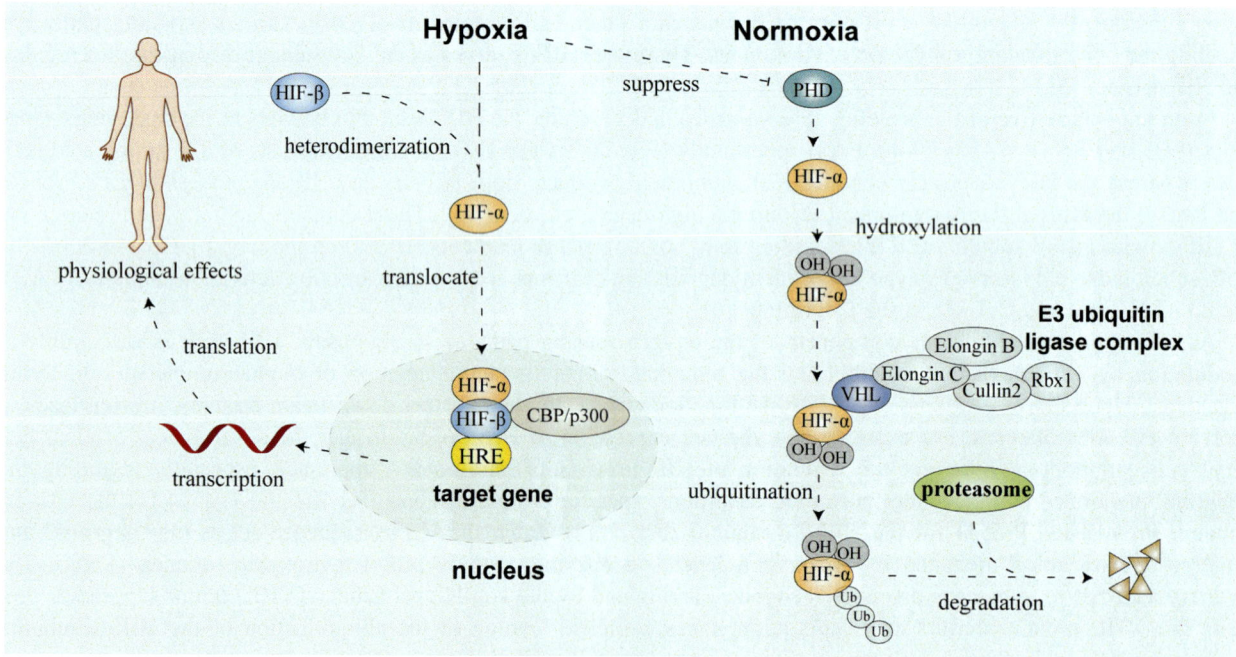

FIGURE 26.4 The mechanism of the PHD-HIF-VHL oxygen-sensing pathway.

26.2 Medications for the treatment of renal anemia

26.2.1 Commonly used drugs for renal anemia treatment

Until the mechanism of renal anemia is fully elucidated, the treatment strategy has primarily relied on observing the phenotypic manifestations or symptoms. During this period, the therapy for renal anemia did not differ significantly from the treatment approaches used for other forms of anemia, such as blood transfusion therapy. This "palliative" approach provided limited improvement for patients with renal anemia and often led to serious adverse reactions such as infections and hypersensitivity responses [9]. This dilemma was partially alleviated with the advent of recombinant human erythropoietin (rhEPO). rhEPO, similar to endogenous EPO, possesses identical physiological functions, activating EPO receptors and downstream signaling pathways to promote RBC production. In 1987, the first commercialized rhEPO, epoetin-α, was introduced, and subsequently, rhEPO underwent three generations of development [10]. Significant emphasis was placed on structural modifications of rhEPO through glycosylation, polyethylene glycosylation (PEGylation), dimerization, and other methods to achieve prolonged half-life and improved bioavailability within the human body. Currently, multiple bioequivalent forms of EPO have been marketed (Table 26.1). The emergence of rhEPO and its bioequivalent forms has been a groundbreaking development, providing the first clinical alternative to RBC transfusion therapy and becoming the primary treatment strategy for renal anemia patients over the past 30 years.

Epogen (epoetin alfa) is a pioneering rhEPO that shares an identical structure with endogenous EPO. Developed and introduced to the market by Amgen in 1989, it marked a significant milestone in the field. Neorecormon (epoetin beta), another member of the first generation of erythropoiesis-stimulating agents (ESAs), is a glycosylated derivative of epoetin alfa. These ESAs are characterized by a relatively short half-life of 6−9 hours within the human body, necessitating administration 1 to 3 times per week. However, despite the need for frequent administration, ensuring patient compliance with the prescribed regimen remains a challenge [11].

Darbepoetin alfa (Aranesp, Amgen) is a second-generation ESA that was introduced to the market in 2001. In comparison to endogenous EPO, darbepoetin alfa features two additional N-linked glycosylated side chains, which extend its half-life to 25 hours within the human body [12]. Although the affinity of darbepoetin alfa for receptors has slightly decreased, its overall bioavailability has improved, enabling once-weekly or biweekly administration. Other glycosylated modifications of rhEPO include AMG 205 and AMG 114, with AMG 114 currently undergoing phase II/III clinical studies [13].

The third generation of ESAs is characterized by their prolonged half-life achieved through the process of PEGylation, which involves the attachment of PEG to EPO. This modification transforms them into persistent EPO receptor agonists. One example of such a modified agent is methoxy PEG-epoetin beta, marketed as Mircera by Roche, which was introduced to the market in 2007 [14]. Mircera has a half-life of 130−140 hours in the human body, enabling dosing intervals of every 2 weeks or once a month. Other PEG-modified agents include PEG-darbepoetin and Hematide.

Although rhEPO and its biologics have become commonly used medications for the treatment of renal anemia, their clinical use still faces some persistent issues. rhEPO, being a biomacromolecule, must be administered *via* intravenous or subcutaneous injection, which prevents oral administration and significantly reduces patient compliance. As a result, many renal anemia patients who have not yet undergone dialysis are deprived of effective treatment. Furthermore, patients often exhibit individual variability, with some individuals having higher hemoglobin levels or being more sensitive to exogenous rhEPO, which makes them susceptible to severe cardiovascular adverse events associated with the treatment. Additionally, exogenous EPO supplementation inhibits the absorption of iron ions, necessitating the combination of EPO injections with iron agents. Studies have indicated that long-term use of such rhEPO drugs can lead to severe degradation of the patient's hematopoietic function, accompanied by the occurrence of multiple adverse reactions such as iron deficiency, tolerance issues, and uncontrollable hypertension. With the increased dosages of rhEPO-like biopharmaceuticals, the mortality rate and incidence of cardiovascular diseases among CKD patients have also risen. The 2012 guidelines on clinical pharmacotherapy for renal anemia published by the Global Renal Outcome Improvement Organization highlighted the significance of proper iron supplementation during the treatment of renal anemia with rhEPO-like medications. The recommendation considers factors such as the patient's hemoglobin levels, clinical condition, and the necessity to monitor blood pressure fluctuations [15].

According to research on the pathophysiological and physiological mechanisms of renal anemia, researchers have developed several small-molecule therapeutic agents that target various molecular pathways. These medications encompass inhibitors of the transcription factor GATA [16], hematopoietic stem cell phosphatase [17], and PHD [18]. Notably, orally administered small-molecule inhibitors of PHD have gained considerable attention as a prominent field of research in the development of novel therapeutic strategies for renal anemia, demonstrating remarkable progress.

TABLE 26.1 Currently marketed rhEPO and its biosimilars.

Drug name	Research institution	Year of launch
Epoetinalfa (Epogen; Procrit)	Amgen/Ortho-McNeil	1989
Epoetin beta (NeoRecormon)	Chugai/Roche	1990
EPIAO	3SBio	1998
rhEPO alfa (Eporon)	Dong-A/Lion	1999
Darbepoetin alfa (Aranesp)	Amgen	2001
Methoxy polyethylene glycol-epoetin-beta (Mircera)	Roche	2007

26.2.2 Prolyl hydroxylase inhibitors

As previously mentioned, HIF-α is a crucial transcription factor that regulates *EPO* gene expression in the kidneys and liver. PHD enzymes, primarily PHD2, control the degradation of HIF-α in the body. Inhibition of PHD activity stabilizes HIF-α, promoting *EPO* gene expression and increasing endogenous EPO levels [19]. Moreover, increasing endogenous HIF-α levels stimulate the expression of membrane iron transport proteins (ferroportin), transferrin, and transferrin receptors. It also inhibits hepcidin expression, promoting iron absorption and utilization. This synergistic approach promotes erythrocyte production, facilitates their maturation, and alleviates anemia symptoms. Hence, small-molecule PHD inhibitors regulate the increase in endogenous EPO and iron metabolism, mimicking the body's physiological regulatory mechanisms and effectively correcting renal anemia [20] (Fig. 26.5). Compared to the administration of exogenous biological drugs such as rhEPO and its analogs, PHD inhibitors have advantages such as oral administration, no need for additional iron supplementation, endogenous regulation, and improved safety profiles.

Let us now shift our focus to the PHD enzyme itself. As previously mentioned, PHD enzymes are a type of dioxygenase that rely on O_2, 2OG, and Fe(II) for their catalytic activity. Any disruption to these factors results in changes to their catalytic activity. Additionally, apart from oxygen, the catalytic activity of PHDs can be inhibited if Fe(II) ions are competitively substituted by other divalent ions or if their concentration decreases due to chelation by iron chelators [21]. Moreover, if the endogenous cofactor 2OG of PHD enzymes is competitively inhibited and unable to bind to proteins, the hydroxylation catalytic activity of PHDs is almost completely lost. Based on the modulation of PHD enzyme activity, PHD2 inhibitors can be broadly classified into two types. The first type includes iron chelators such as cobalt, copper, and nickel, as well as compounds such as deferoxamine and 3,4-dihydroxybenzoic acid. The second type consists of analogs of the endogenous cofactor 2OG. Research has demonstrated that although PHD inhibitors of the iron chelator type can stabilize HIF, their use is associated with significant off-target effects due to the widespread

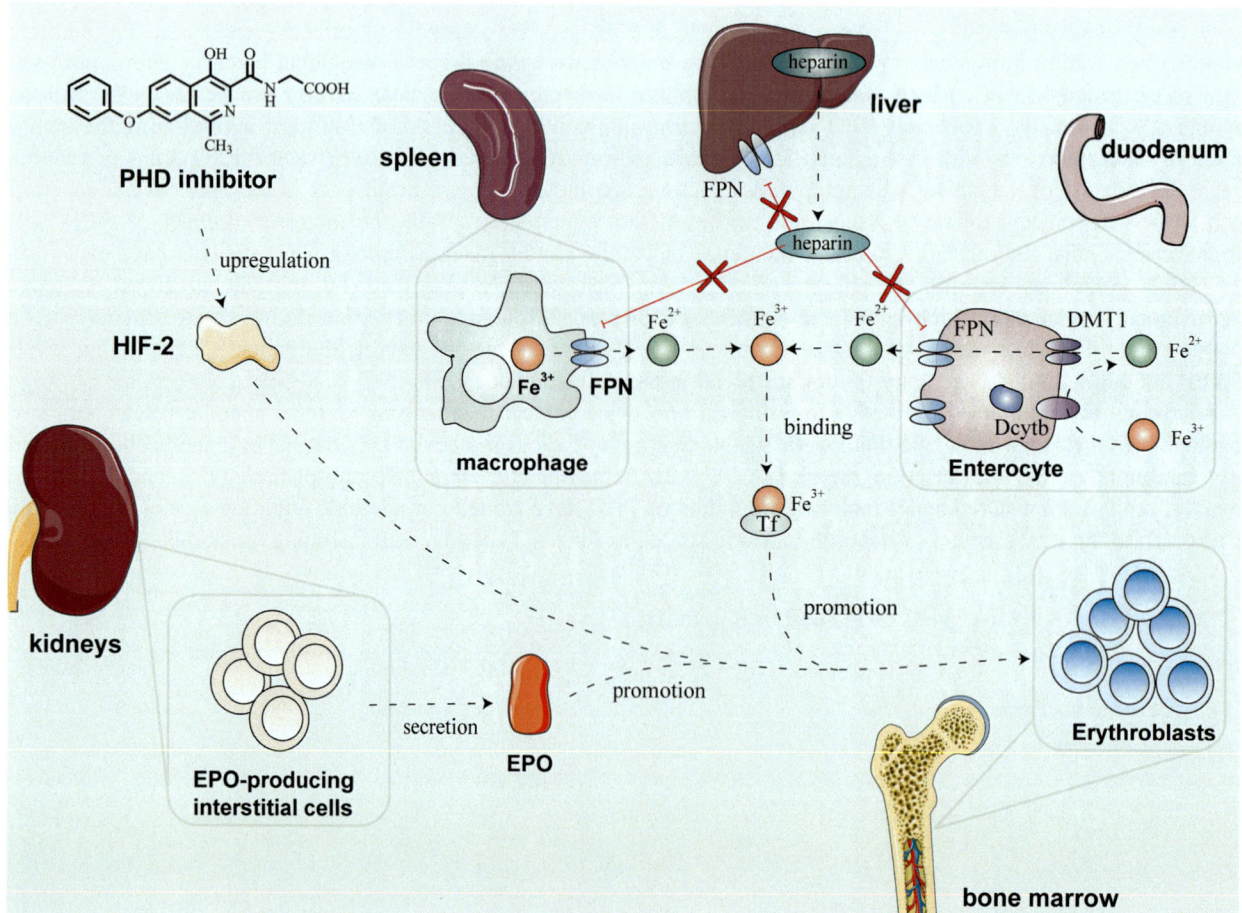

FIGURE 26.5 The mechanism of anemia treatment by endogenously regulated HIF pathway through PHD inhibition.

distribution of ferrous ions in the human body. Crucial proteins in the human body, such as peroxidases, catalases, and monoamine oxidases, all contain ferrous ions. It can be envisioned that the use of iron chelators would result in notable off-target effects and, consequently, a range of safety concerns. Therefore, such molecules have not advanced further in clinical applications [21]. Conversely, PHD-targeting inhibitors that are analogs of the endogenous cofactor 2OG have significantly enhanced both their effectiveness and safety, rendering them suitable for drug development. Consequently, they have garnered increased attention from the academic community and pharmaceutical companies.

Numerous PHD inhibitors with diverse structural types have been reported, with some of them already available in the market or progressing through different stages of clinical trials (Table 26.2). FG-2216, originally developed by FibroGen, emerged as the pioneering PHD inhibitor to enter clinical trials, commencing phase I studies in 1995. However, its progression was halted in 2007 due to an outbreak of fulminant liver failure. Despite receiving FDA reapproval for clinical trial research in 2011, FG-2216 has remained in a stagnant state at phase II, with no further information being disclosed. FG-4592 (generic name: roxadustat) is a derivative of FG-2212, developed by FibroGen as well. It gained recognition as the pioneering small-molecule PHD inhibitor drug and was introduced to the market in China in December 2018. Roxadustat is utilized for treating anemia resulting from CKD in patients undergoing dialysis, marking a significant advancement in the treatment of renal anemia [22].

Soon after the approval of roxadustat, on June 29, 2020, AKB-6548 (generic name: vadadustat), developed by Akebia Corporation of the United States, and GSK-1278863 (generic name: daprodustat), developed by GlaxoSmithKline (GSK) of the United Kingdom, received marketing approval in Japan for the treatment of renal anemia associated with CKD [23,24]. Subsequently, in September 2020, JTZ-951 (generic name: enarodustat), developed by Japan Tobacco, also received marketing approval in Japan. In January 2021, BAY-85-3934 (generic name: molidustat), developed by Bayer, was also approved for marketing in Japan. On March 7, 2022, ZYAN-1 (generic name: desidustat), developed by Zydus Cadila received marketing approval in India.

In addition, several PHD inhibitors originally developed by Chinese research institutions are currently undergoing clinical trials. One notable example is DDO-3055, a novel oral PHD inhibitor jointly developed by China Pharmaceutical University and Hengrui Medicine [25,26]. DDO-3055 was derived from an innovative design that utilized a structure-based drug design strategy, developed by Professor You's research group at China Pharmaceutical University. It features a unique structure with a 5-alkynyl pyridinylformylglycine scaffold. On April 15, 2019, DDO-3055 tablets received clinical approval for the treatment of anemia caused by CKD, including both dialysis and nondialysis patients. Studies have indicated that DDO-3055 exhibits a more pronounced erythropoiesis-promoting effect compared to roxadustat, reaching levels close to normal, and it may also possess superior safety profiles.

26.3 Development process of roxadustat

26.3.1 Structure and mechanism of prolyl hydroxylase

With the continuous advancement of medicinal chemistry, drug development has evolved from the initial "trial and error" and "luck-based" approaches to today's rational drug design. During the development of drugs targeting specific targets, the 3D structure of the target serves as the foundation for innovative drug molecule design. The advent and ongoing innovation of technologies such as X-ray crystallography, cryo-electron microscopy, and molecular simulation have enabled the observation of interactions between biomacromolecules and drug molecules. These advancements have further refined the rational drug design process, transitioning from a coarse, static approach to a more refined and dynamic one. It is evident that the development of drugs targeting PHD aligns with the principles of rational drug design.

From a structural perspective, the PHD subtypes demonstrate a significant level of homology. Among these subtypes, extensive research has been conducted on PHD2, which is closely linked to anemia treatment. PHD2 is composed of 426 amino acid residues and has a molecular weight of 46 kDa. Its structure primarily consists of two essential domains: the *N*-terminal catalytic functional domain and the *C*-terminal domain. The *N*-terminal catalytic functional domain is a zinc finger domain, while the *C*-terminal domain functions as a crucial 2OG-dependent dioxygenase [7]. Structural biology studies have revealed that the *C*-terminal domain of PHD2 contains an active catalytic pocket, which binds to metal ions (Fe^{2+}) and 2OG, both closely associated with hydroxylation functionality (Fig. 26.6) [27].

When PHD2 binds to its hydroxylated substrate, HIF-α, the critical proline residue of HIF-α (such as Pro564 residue in HIF-1α) approaches spatially to the 2OG substrate, facilitating the hydroxylation reaction (Fig. 26.7A). The catalytic pocket of PHD2 consists of amino acid residues, including His313, Asp315, His374, and Arg383, along with 2OG and Fe^{2+}. Within this pocket, the two oxygen atoms in the adjacent carbonyl and carboxyl groups of 2OG can chelate with Fe^{2+} ions, forming a stable octahedral coordination structure centered around the position of the Fe^{2+} ion. This

TABLE 26.2 PHD inhibitors that have been approved or are in clinical trials.

Development code/generic name	Research institution[a]	Development status	Structures
FG-2216/IOX3	FibroGen	Termination in Phase II	
FG-4592 Roxadustat	FibroGen Astra Zeneca Astellas Pharma	Approved 2018.12	
AKB-6548 Vadadustat	Akebia Vifor Mitsubishi Tanabe	Approved 2020.6	
GSK-1278863 Daprodustat	GlaxoSmithKline	Approved 2020.6	
JTZ-951 Enarodustat	Japan Tobacco Salubris	Approved 2020.9	
Bay-85−3934 Molidustat	Bayer	Approved 2021.01	
ZYAN-1 Desidustat	Zydus Cadila China Medical System	Approved 2022.03	
DDO-3055	China Pharmaceutical University Hengrui Medicine	Phase I	

[a]The first institution is the originator of the drug.

structure includes a water molecule and three key amino acid residues: His313, His374, and Asp315. The water molecule can be replaced by an oxygen molecule, enabling the catalytic hydroxylation reaction to occur. Additionally, the carboxyl groups at both ends of 2OG engage in electrostatic interactions with Arg383 and form hydrogen bonds with Tyr303 through a water molecule (Fig. 26.7B) [28]. Although the binding mode of the endogenous substrate 2OG to

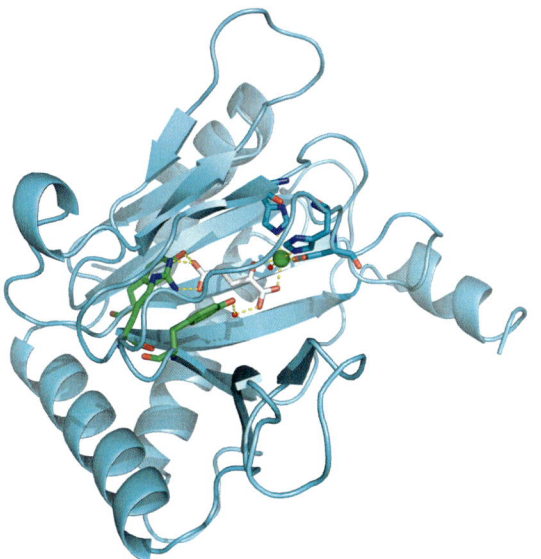

FIGURE 26.6 The crystal structure of PHD2 in complex with its endogenous ligands, 2OG and Fe^{2+} (PDB ID: 3OUJ) [27].

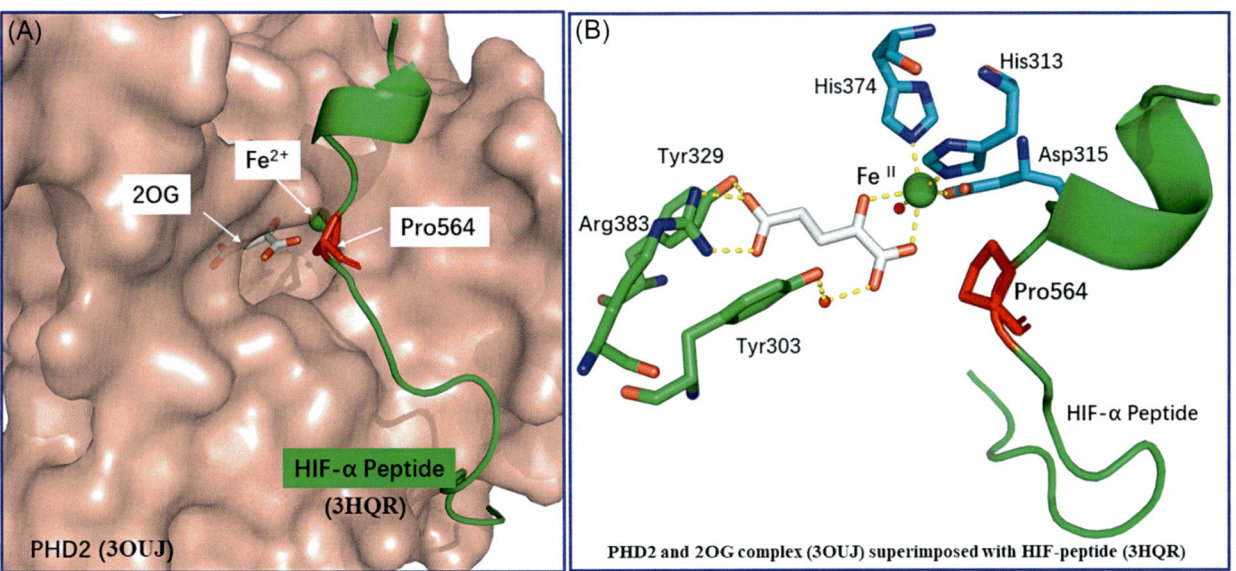

FIGURE 26.7 (A) the schematic diagram of the catalytic pocket of PHD2 in complex with the HIF peptide. The crystal structure of PHD2 (PDB ID: 3OUJ) [27]; (B) the overlay of PHD2 protein with the hydroxylated substrate HIF-α peptide (PDB ID: 3HQR) [28].

the protein has been structurally elucidated, it is crucial to explore the dynamic process of PHD catalyzing HIF hydroxylation to provide more precise guidance for medicinal chemists in drug design.

Fortunately, researchers have elucidated the precise hydroxylation mechanism of HIF-α by the PHD2 enzyme. As shown in Fig. 26.8, the catalytic cycle begins at state (A). Initially, an oxygen molecule replaces a water molecule at a specific position and coordinates with the Fe^{2+} ion. Subsequently, the π-π bond within the oxygen molecule is broken, transitioning the cycle to state (B). In the next stage, two possible transition states can occur. One involves the attack of the carbonyl group of 2OG by one of the unbound oxygen atoms in state (B), while the Fe^{2+} ion undergoes oxidation from divalent to tetravalent. This results in the formation of an oxygen bridge with 2OG, referred to as state (C)-1. Due to the instability of the newly formed oxygen bridge, the oxygen single bond, which remains after the cleavage of the oxygen molecule's π-π bond, further undergoes cleavage, leading to the decarboxylation of 2OG. The other transition state involves the direct decarboxylation of state (B), producing a pentacyclic intermediate known as state (C)-2. Both transition states proceed to state (D), where one oxygen atom from the oxygen molecule is transferred to the framework of 2OG, while the other oxygen atom directly binds

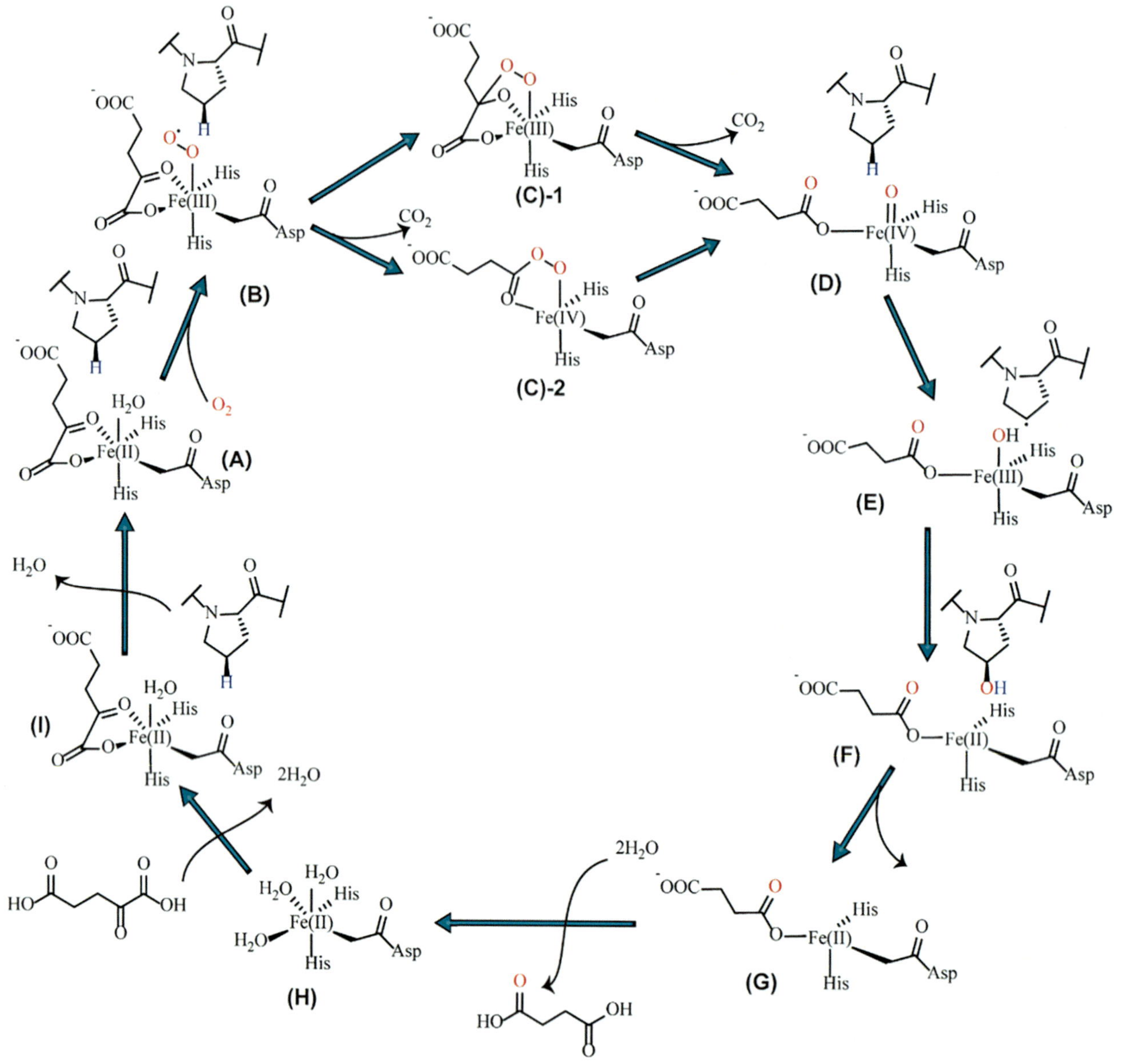

FIGURE 26.8 The catalytic cycle mechanism of HIF-α hydroxylation by the PHD2 enzyme.

to the tetravalent iron ion, resulting in an intermediate with significant oxidative potential. When the HIF-α substrate, binds to PHD2, the crucial proline residue of the HIF-α peptide is close to the newly activated oxygen atom. At this stage, the activated oxygen atom selectively removes a hydrogen atom from the 3α position of the proline residue, converting it into a hydroxyl group, while the tetravalent iron ion is reduced to trivalent iron in the state (E). Subsequently, the hydroxyl group is transferred to the proline residue ring, completing the hydroxylation process, while the iron ion is further reduced to divalent iron, corresponding to state (F). After state (G), the hydroxylated proline residue dissociates from the complex, allowing a water molecule to return to its original position, and 2OG is converted into succinate, which is released from the system. Two water molecules temporarily coordinate with the Fe^{2+} ion, replacing 2OG, and the entire catalytic cycle enters the state (H). Then, a new molecule of 2OG occupies the two binding sites previously occupied by water molecules, forming the octahedral ferrous ion cage together with the remaining water molecule and the amino acid residue in the pocket, representing the state (I). This state awaits the reoccupation of the water molecule binding site by the proline residue of the subsequent HIF-α peptide segment, marking the completion of a full catalytic cycle [29].

The investigation of the structural and biochemical aspects of PHD, along with the exploration of its catalytic mechanism, has provided a solid foundation for the subsequent development of highly specific and potent PHD inhibitors.

26.3.2 Identification and optimization of hit compounds

PHD inhibitors are designed to mimic the structure of the endogenous substrate 2OG (**1**). Currently, the structural origins for the majority of reported PHD inhibitors can be attributed to *N*-oxalylglycine (NOG) (**2**) [30], and its precursor, dimethyl oxalylglycine (DMOG) (**3**) (Fig. 26.9). In comparison to the endogenous ligand 2OG (**1**) of PHD enzymes, NOG replaces the C-3 carbon atom of 2OG with a nitrogen atom while maintaining the remaining structure identical to 2OG. It still retains the essential segments necessary for chelating with ferrous ions and forming a salt bridge with Arg383, enabling it to competitively bind to the PHD protein. However, it is unable to achieve hydroxylation cycling of HIF-α peptide as efficiently as 2OG, thereby inhibiting PHD activity. DMOG, as the precursor of NOG, exhibits superior membrane permeability compared to NOG, resulting in enhanced cellular activity. Both NOG and DMOG serve as important tool molecules for the development and evaluation of PHD inhibitors. Subsequent selective PHD inhibitors are derived from modifications and optimizations based on the structure of NOG. The initial structural modifications focus on NOG itself, where researchers have discovered that introducing methyl groups into its main chain can enhance its activity [31]. However, these NOG derivatives are molecules in relatively small sizes with weak binding affinities to PHD and they exhibit apparent promiscuity in interacting with other 2OG enzymes.

In recent years, significant progress has been made in the field of structural biology, leading to enhanced insights into the catalytic mechanisms of PHD enzymes. Consequently, the strategies for developing selective inhibitors targeting PHD have gained clarity and precision. FibroGen, a prominent pharmaceutical company and research team, has established itself as a frontrunner in the development of these selective inhibitors targeting PHD enzymes. Although specific details regarding the early stages of FibroGen's flagship drug, roxadustat, have not been publicly disclosed, valuable insights can be derived from relevant patents and the analysis of reported structures. The resources provided offer insights into the lead optimization and discovery process of roxadustat.

FibroGen has undertaken structural modifications and optimizations of NOG, which involve the exploration of new metal-chelating moieties. A series of compounds designed and screened by FibroGen, taking inspiration from previously reported PHD inhibitors such as 1,10-phenanthroline, derivatives of 8-hydroxyquinoline, isoquinoline, and pyridine-like small molecules. In order to enhance the activity of the compounds and address the limitations of the hit compound NOG, which include its low molecular weight, limited binding interactions with the target protein, and weak chelation ability, FibroGen employed a strategy of incorporating various metal chelating fragments while designing selective PHD inhibitors. Following this approach, FibroGen synthesized a hit compound **4** (FG-2179, Fig. 26.9), which features a picotinoylglycine scaffold. The nitrogen atom in the pyridine and the nitrogen atom in the amide group of **4** can form strong chelation with Fe^{2+} in the catalytic pocket of PHD2. Compound **4** demonstrated enhanced inhibitory activity toward the PHD2 enzyme compared to NOG and DMOG [32].

26.3.3 Lead discovery and optimization of prolyl hydroxylase domain inhibitors

Researchers aim to obtain lead compounds that exhibit higher selectivity, improved activity, and potential for further development through structural modifications and derivatization of the scaffold based on compound **4**. Despite significant alterations in the structure of **4** compared to the initial tool molecule **2**, its relatively low molecular weight, essential chelating fragments, and relatively simple core still offer potential for additional chemical exploration. The modifications have primarily focused on the pyridine core, resulting in the synthesis of a series of new compounds by

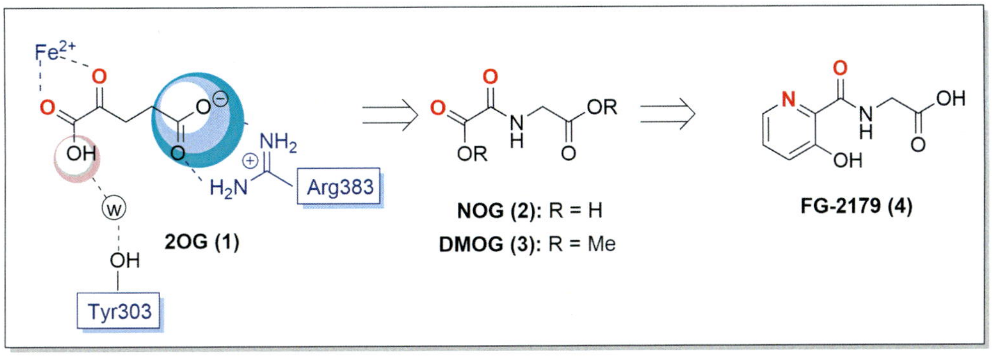

FIGURE 26.9 Discovery of hit compound FG-2179 with a picotinoylglycine scaffold.

introducing aromatic rings at various positions of the pyridine ring. Compound **5**, which features an isoquinoline core (Fig. 26.10A), demonstrates further enhancement in activity compared to compound **4**. Consequently, compound **5** has been formally designated as the lead compound for subsequent optimization. Further investigations have elucidated the mechanism underlying the increased activity of isoquinoline-based compounds. In 2006, the Schofield research group at the University of Oxford resolved and reported the crystal structure of the iodinated analog **6** of compound **5** bound to the PHD2 protein. This represents the first crystal complex structure between a nonNOG inhibitor and the PHD2 protein, thus establishing the structural biology foundation for understanding the structure-activity relationships of PHD2 inhibitors and facilitating their further design and optimization [33]. The crystal structure reveals that the oxygen atom in the amide of compound **6** and the nitrogen atom in the isoquinoline form a stable bidentate chelation with the iron ion in the catalytic center of the PHD2 protein. The carboxyl group forms an ionic bond and hydrogen bond network with Arg383 and Tyr329, while the phenolic hydroxyl occupies a position previously occupied by a bound water molecule and forms a hydrogen bond with Tyr303. Notably, the phenyl ring fused with the pyridine ring in the structure of compound **5** extends outward from the catalytic pocket, potentially obstructing the binding of the HIF-α peptide containing the critical Pro564 residue to PHD2. This may be a crucial factor contributing to its enhanced activity in inhibiting PHD2 and blocking HIF-α hydroxylation (Fig. 26.10B and C) [33].

Researchers conducted a series of optimizations on the lead compound to enhance its pharmacological and pharmacokinetic properties, aiming to obtain a drug candidate for clinical development. Ultimately, they obtained the first compound to enter clinical studies, compound **7**, also known as FG-2216, by introducing a chlorine atom adjacent to the pyridine nitrogen atom in the quinoline core. During phase I clinical trials, FG-2216 demonstrated the ability to stabilize EPO expression and elevate hemoglobin levels in patients with CKD. However, a case of fulminant liver necrosis leading to death occurred during phase II clinical studies, which prompted researchers to terminate the clinical trial of FG-2216. Subsequent investigations suggested no direct association between this adverse reaction event and FG-2216 [34]. However, it has been recognized that due to the relatively small molecular size of FG-2216, it has the potential to bind to the catalytic pocket of other 2OG-dependent oxygenases, such as epigenetic histone demethylases (KDMs), leading to unintended inhibitory effects on these enzymes. This lack of selectivity may have contributed to the occurrence of adverse reactions. The downfall of FG-2216 compelled its original research company, FibroGen, to make improvements to this compound series. Fortunately, FibroGen adopted different medicinal chemistry strategies for the

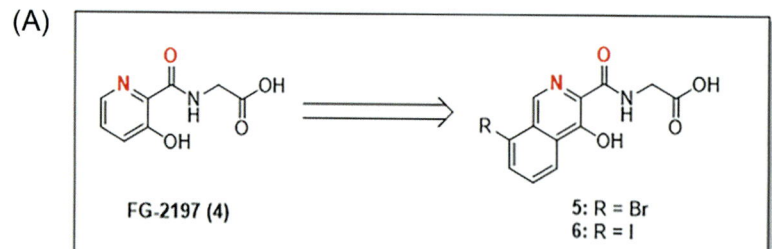

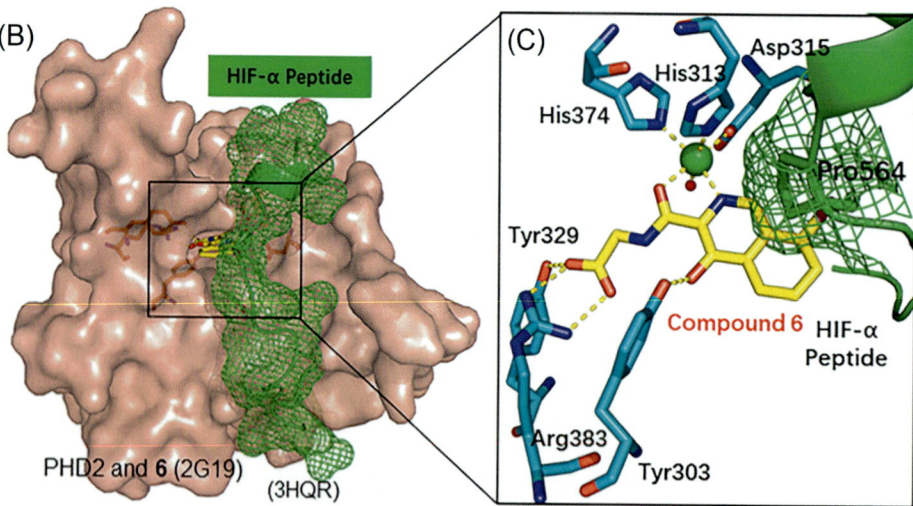

FIGURE 26.10 Structure optimization and lead discovery based on the picotinoylglycine hit compound FG-2179. (A) Discovery of the isoquinolinecarboxylglycine lead compound; (B, C) crystal structures of PHD2 in complex with **6** (PDB ID: 2G19) and superimposed analysis with the HIF-α peptide substrate (PDB ID: 3HQR).

same batch of FG-2216 and subsequent follow-up compounds. These strategies included introducing bulkier substituents with steric hindrance, bioisosteric replacement of the phenyl ring fused with the pyridine ring, and bioisosteric substitution or heteroatom replacement of the pyridine ring. These modifications aimed to prevent the clinical failure of FG-2216 and facilitate the rapid development of alternative candidates for clinical trials. Among them, the most significant medicinal chemistry strategy involved the synthesis of compound **8** (FG-4592) [35], a compound structurally similar to FG-2216, as well as thieno[2,3-*d*]pyrimidine derivative **9**, pyrrolo[2,3-*d*]pyrimidine derivative **10** [36], thiazolo[5,4-*d*]pyrimidine derivative **11** [37], pyrrolo[2,3-*b*]quinoxaline derivative **12** [38], and coumarin derivative **13** (Fig. 26.11) [39]. In vitro assays revealed that FG-4592 exhibited comparable activity to FG-2216, but the introduction of an isocoumarin phenoxyl substituent further enhanced its binding affinity and selectivity toward PHD2. FibroGen designated FG-4592 as a backup candidate for FG-2216, thus advancing it into the clinical trial phase once again.

26.3.4 Clinical research on roxadustat

26.3.4.1 Pharmacodynamics and pharmacokinetics of roxadustat

In terms of pharmacodynamics, roxadustat competitively binds reversibly to the 2OG cosubstrate binding pocket of PHD proteins, thereby inhibiting PHD activity. This inhibition results in the stabilization of HIF-α in patients with CKD, leading to an upregulation of the transcription level of the downstream *EPO* gene. Consequently, this physiological regulation of EPO production leads to a temporary increase in EPO levels within the patient's body, improving hematopoiesis and alleviating anemia. Additionally, the stabilization of HIF-α inhibits the secretion of heparin in patients, preventing the degradation of iron absorption and transport-related proteins. As a result, the patient's iron metabolism is enhanced, promoting the synthesis of endogenous hemoglobin. The synergistic effect of roxadustat in stimulating EPO production further reverses the symptoms of anemia in patients [40]. Early preclinical studies have demonstrated a dose-dependent increase in hemoglobin concentration in rats treated with roxadustat. Clinical studies using the structurally related compound FG-2216, which resembles roxadustat, have shown that EPO levels in patients can be increased up to fivefold within 12 hours after oral administration at a dose of 20 mg/kg. This indicates that roxadustat can maintain a significant pharmacological effect over an extended period.

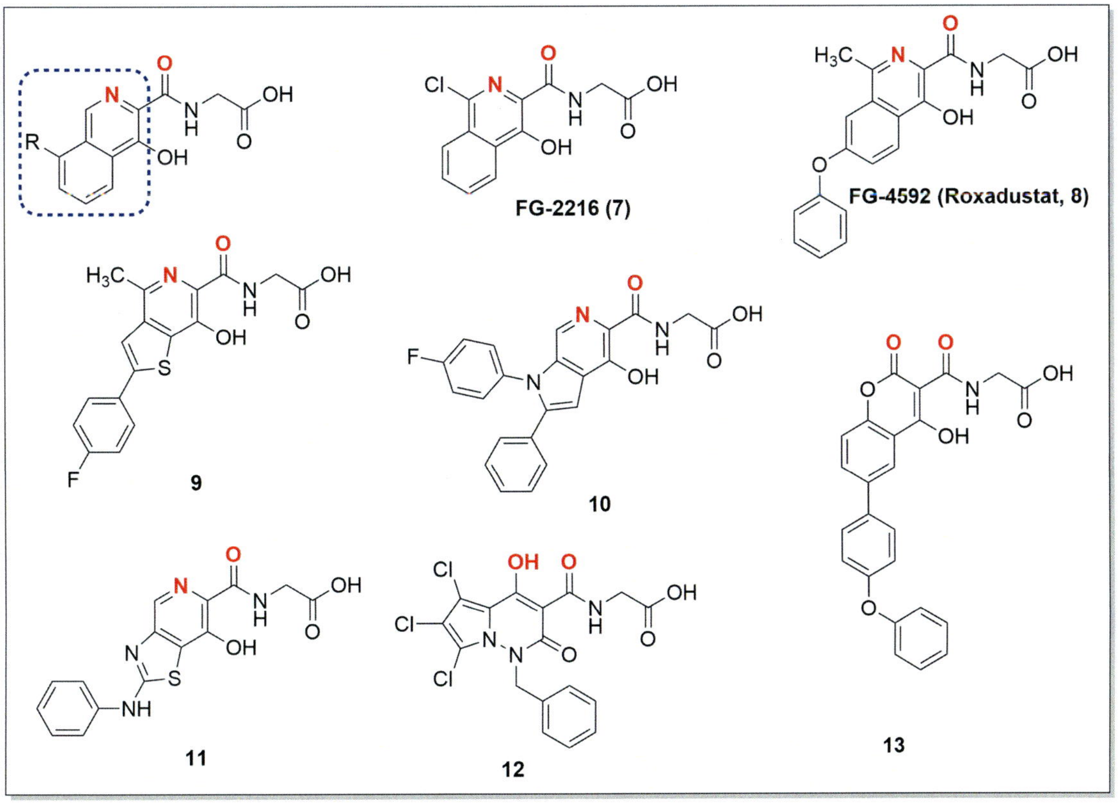

FIGURE 26.11 Structures of roxadustat and related structurally diverse analogs.

The pharmacokinetics of roxadustat were evaluated in a study involving Caucasian (European) and Japanese (Asian) subjects who received various doses of the drug. No abnormalities in blood drug concentration or area under the curve were observed in these subjects. Similarly, a pharmacokinetic study conducted on Chinese subjects, involving both single and multiple doses of roxadustat, did not reveal any abnormalities in its pharmacokinetic properties. These studies also indicated that there was no evidence of drug accumulation, suggesting that roxadustat does not exhibit species-specific differences in its pharmacokinetic properties [40]. Additionally, several drug interaction studies involving medications such as warfarin and omeprazole did not show any significant interactions with roxadustat [41,42]. Furthermore, the pharmacokinetic characteristics of roxadustat in patients with moderate hepatic impairment were found to be similar to those in healthy subjects [43].

The pharmacodynamic efficacy and pharmacokinetic stability of roxadustat make it a promising candidate as an oral therapy for renal anemia. However, further rigorous assessment of its efficacy and safety in clinical settings is still required to determine whether roxadustat can truly become a safe and effective antianemia drug.

26.3.4.2 Phase II and phase III clinical trials of roxadustat

FibroGen, the parent company responsible for the original research of roxadustat, engaged in a series of partnerships with AstraZeneca and Astellas. Roxadustat underwent multiple clinical trial studies, targeting diverse populations across different regions worldwide. The primary countries included Japan, the United States, and China.

A randomized, double-blind, multicenter clinical phase II study (NCT01964196), conducted in Japan over 24 weeks, investigated the efficacy of roxadustat in nondialysis-dependent patients with CKD. The study demonstrated a significant improvement in hemoglobin levels among participants receiving roxadustat compared to those in the placebo group. The recruitment criteria for the roxadustat clinical trials included the following aspects: (1) participants aged between 18 and 80 years, (2) stage 3 or 4 CKD patients with an estimated glomerular filtration rate not exceeding 89 mL/min/1.73 m^2 as assessed by professional institutions, and (3) plasma ferritin level greater than 30 ng/mL, with plasma folate and vitamin B12 levels not lower than 4 ng/mL and 180 pg/mL, respectively. Once the inclusion criteria were met, the participants were divided into groups. The treatment group received roxadustat three times a week during the initial 6 weeks, followed by dose adjustments over the subsequent 18 weeks to maintain the desired hemoglobin levels. Ultimately, 83 participants completed this clinical trial. The results indicated that the mean increase in hemoglobin levels for the low, medium, and high-dose groups was 0.200 (0.160), 0.453 (0.256), and 0.570 (0.240), respectively, while the placebo control group exhibited a mean increase of −0.052 (0.142). The difference between the two groups was statistically significant ($P < .001$). Moreover, compared to the baseline hemoglobin levels, the concentrations increased by 1.10, 1.33, and 1.55 for the low, medium, and high-dose groups, respectively, whereas the untreated control group experienced a decrease of 0.17 [44]. In a randomized, double-blind, dose-safety study conducted in China (NCT01599507), the high-dose group did not show noteworthy adverse reactions compared to the low-dose group, indicating that high-dose roxadustat did not lead to significant adverse effects. Additionally, the administration group in this clinical trial exhibited a significant decrease in heparin levels compared to the placebo group, suggesting that roxadustat can alleviate iron absorption obstruction in patients [45]. Subsequent phase III studies conducted in different regions, including a randomized, double-blind, placebo-controlled phase III study in China (NCT02652819) and a larger-scale randomized, double-blind, placebo-controlled phase III study conducted globally (NCT01750190), demonstrated that roxadustat significantly increased patients' hemoglobin levels compared to the placebo group [46].

The investigational drug roxadustat underwent a series of phase II and phase III clinical studies to assess its advantages and disadvantages compared to conventional rhEPO therapy for the treatment of renal anemia. In a randomized, double-blind phase II clinical study conducted in China (NCT01596855), with first-generation rhEPO (epoetin alfa) as a positive reference, roxadustat showed no significant inferiority in the treatment of patients with end-stage kidney disease receiving hemodialysis. Furthermore, it resulted in a significant reduction of heparin levels in these patients [47]. Likewise, in a global, randomized, open-label phase II clinical study (NCT01147666), roxadustat demonstrated good efficacy and tolerability compared to epoetin alfa. In this study, participants received rhEPO therapy for the initial 4 weeks of treatment, and then some participants switched to roxadustat, with no significant decrease in hemoglobin levels observed in subsequent testing compared to the initial levels [47]. In subsequent larger-scale phase III clinical trials, roxadustat conducted several noninferiority trials using rhEPO therapy as the reference. A 24-week, randomized, double-blind clinical study conducted in Japan (NCT02952092), involving patients with CKD undergoing hemodialysis, showed no significant difference in its ability to improve and maintain hemoglobin levels compared to second-generation rhEPO (earbepoetin alfa). In another global phase III clinical study (NCT02273726), roxadustat demonstrated an increase in patients' hemoglobin levels of 0.39 g/L during the 28–52 week treatment period, compared to no significant decrease observed with epoetin alfa [48].

Roxadustat has exhibited favorable pharmacological properties, as well as favorable pharmacokinetic properties related to absorption, distribution, metabolism, and excretion. It has also demonstrated safety in clinical research. In 2018, roxadustat received approval from the National Medical Products Administration (NMPA) in China for the treatment of renal anemia in CKD patients undergoing dialysis [22]. In 2019, it was approved by the Ministry of Health, labor, and welfare in Japan for the treatment of anemia in CKD patients undergoing dialysis [49]. During the same year, FibroGen submitted a New Drug Application to the U.S. Food and Drug Administration (FDA) for roxadustat, with indications similar to those in China and Japan [50]. Subsequently, both the NMPA and the Ministry of Health, labor, and welfare approved roxadustat for the treatment of anemia in nondialysis CKD patients [51,52]. Currently, roxadustat is still undergoing clinical research for chemotherapy-induced anemia and myelodysplastic syndrome-associated anemia [53].

26.3.5 Synthetic process of roxadustat

To date, the synthetic methods of roxadustat have been disclosed by FibroGen, the original research company, in two patents. In the first patent (WO2004108681), researchers utilized 4-phenoxyphthalic acid as the starting material. They successfully synthesized roxadustat through a series of eight sequential reactions, including cyclization, isomerization, bromination, hydrolysis, protection and methylation, deprotection, condensation, and deprotection (Route 1) [54]. However, this route, outlined in the initial laboratory preparation method, possesses certain limitations. First, the pathway involves multiple complex protection and deprotection steps, resulting in a cumbersome synthesis process. Second, the utilization of reactive alkali metal sodium and organometallic lithium reagents poses challenges for achieving large-scale industrial production.

Synthetic Route 1. *Reagents and conditions:* (a) glycine, DCM; then MeOH, H$_2$SO$_4$; (b) Na, BuOH; (c) POBr$_3$, NaHCO$_3$; (d) NaOH; (e) 1) PhCH$_2$Br, K$_2$CO$_3$, 2) CH$_3$I, BuLi; (f) KOH; (g) Benzyl glycinate hydrochloride, Et$_3$N, *i*BuOCOCl; (h) H$_2$, Pd/C.

To meet the substantial demand for candidate drugs in clinical trials, FibroGen researchers have made substantial optimizations to the synthetic route of roxadustat, intending to achieve industrial-scale production. In an alternative patented route [55], the researchers utilized 5-bromophthalide as the starting material and implemented a series of steps, including substitution, ring opening, hydrolysis, and cyclization, to create the crucial intermediate 4-hydroxy-7-

phenoxyisoquinoline-3-carboxylic acid ester. This intermediate, when reacted with tetramethyldiaminomethane, underwent substitution and reduction reactions to introduce a methyl group onto the parent scaffold. Subsequently, the intermediate underwent a condensation reaction to give the desired product, roxadustat (Route 2). Compared to the original route, this method entirely avoids complicated protection and deprotection steps and eliminates the use of certain hazardous reagents. Consequently, this synthetic route is more suitable for industrial-scale production.

Synthetic Route 2. *Reagents and conditions:* (a) phenol, K_2CO_3, acetylacetone, CuBr, DCM; (b) $B(OMe)_3$, $(Ph)_3PCl_2$, $SOCl_2$, toluence, reflux; (c) CH_3OH; (d) K_2CO_3, KI, Ts-Gly-OMe; (e) 1) CH_3ONa; 2) AcOH, H_2O; (f) tetramethyldiaminomethane, AcOH; (g) Ac_2O; then morpholine; (h) H_2, Pd-C, Na_2CO_3; (i) glycine, CH_3ONa; then AcOH.

26.4 Conclusion

Renal anemia is a significant complication of CKD, imposing a persistent economic and lifestyle burden on affected individuals. Although the introduction of rhEPO injections has reduced the need for blood transfusions in most patients, its therapeutic efficacy and patient compliance still require improvement. Recent advancements in understanding the PHD-HIF-EPO hypoxia signaling pathway have shed light on the pathogenesis of renal anemia. Building upon this knowledge, the development of PHD inhibitors, such as the first-in-class drug roxadustat, has shown promising results in triggering endogenous physiological regulation and reversing renal anemia. This approach represents a paradigm shift toward targeted development of physiologically compatible drugs that modulate intrinsic pathways, offering new avenues for the treatment of renal anemia.

References

[1] Jha V, Garcia-Garcia G, Iseki K, et al. Chronic kidney disease: global dimension and perspectives. Lancet 2013;382(9888):260−72.
[2] Koury MJ, Haase VH. Anaemia in kidney disease: harnessing hypoxia responses for therapy. Nat Rev Nephrol 2015;11(7):394−410.
[3] Kwon YT, Ciechanover A. The ubiquitin code in the ubiquitin-proteasome system and autophagy. Trends Biochem Sci 2017;42(11):873−86.
[4] Varshavsky A. N-degron and C-degron pathways of protein degradation. Proc Natl Acad Sci USA 2019;116(2):358−66.
[5] Li Z, You Q, Zhang X. Small-molecule modulators of the hypoxia-inducible factor pathway: development and therapeutic applications. J Med Chem 2019;62(12):5725−49.

[6] Schofield CJ, Ratcliffe PJ. Oxygen sensing by HIF hydroxylases. Nat Rev Mol Cell Biol 2004;5(5):343−54.
[7] Bruick RK, Mcknight SL. A conserved family of prolyl-4-hydroxylases that modify HIF. Science 2001;294(5545):1337−40.
[8] Watts ER, Walmsley SR. Inflammation and hypoxia: HIF and PHD isoform selectivity. Trends Mol Med 2019;25(1):33−46.
[9] Collister D, Rigatto C, Tangri N. Anemia management in chronic kidney disease and dialysis: a narrative review. Curr Opin Nephrol Hypertens 2017;26(3):214−18.
[10] Kalantar-Zadeh K. History of erythropoiesis-stimulating agents, the development of biosimilars, and the future of anemia treatment in nephrology. Am J Nephrol 2017;45(3):235−47.
[11] Hayat A, Haria D, Salifu MO. Erythropoietin stimulating agents in the management of anemia of chronic kidney disease. Patient Prefer Adher 2008;2:195−200.
[12] Walker RG. Erythropoietin stimulating agents and epoetin alfa revisited: what's really relevant? Clin J Am Soc Nephro 2008;3:935−7.
[13] Sinclair AM. Erythropoiesis stimulating agents: approaches to modulate activity. Biologics 2013;7:161−74.
[14] Jurado Garcia JM, Torres Sanchez E, Olmos Hidalgo D, et al. Erythropoietin pharmacology. Clin Transl Oncol 2007;9:715−22.
[15] Zadrazil J, Horak P. Pathophysiology of anemia in chronic kidney diseases: a review. Biomed Pap Med Fac Univ Palacky Olomouc Czech Repub 2015;159(2):197−202.
[16] Nakano Y, Imagawa S, Matsumoto K, et al. Oral administration of K-11706 inhibits GATA binding activity, enhances hypoxia-inducible factor 1 binding activity, and restores indicators in an in vivo mouse model of anemia of chronic disease. Blood 2004;104(13):4300−7.
[17] Klingmüller U, Lorenz U, Cantley LC, et al. Specific recruitment of SH-PTP1 to the erythropoietin receptor causes inactivation of JAK2 and termination of proliferative signals. Cell 1995;80(5):729−38.
[18] Sugahara M, Tanaka T, Nangaku M. Prolyl hydroxylase domain inhibitors as a novel therapeutic approach against anemia in chronic kidney disease. Kidney Int 2017;92(2):306−12.
[19] Semenza GL. Regulation of oxygen homeostasis by hypoxia-inducible factor 1. Physiology 2009;24:97−106.
[20] Franke K, Kalucka J, Mamlouk S, et al. HIF-1alpha is a protective factor in conditional PHD2-deficient mice suffering from severe HIF-2alphainduced excessive erythropoiesis. Blood 2013;121:1436−45.
[21] Joharapurkar AA, Pandya VB, Patel VJ, et al. Prolyl hydroxylase inhibitors: a breakthrough in the therapy of anemia associated with chronic diseases. J Med Chem 2018;61(16):6964−82.
[22] Web Sites: https://fibrogen.gcs-web.com/news-releases/news-release-details/roxadustat-approved-china-treatment-anemia-chronic-kidney. (accessed Sep 08, 2020).
[23] Web Sites: https://ir.akebia.com/news-releases/news-release-details/akebia-therapeutics-announces-approval-vadadustat-japan (accessed Sep 08, 2020).
[24] Web Sites: https://www.gsk.com/en-gb/media/press-releases/gsk-submits-first-regulatory-application-for-daprodustat-in-japan-for-patients-with-renal-anaemia-due-to-chronic-kidney-disease (accessed Sep 08, 2020).
[25] Zhang X, Lei Y, Hu T, et al. Discovery of clinical candidate (5-(3-(4-Chlorophenoxy)prop-1-yn-1-yl)-3-hydroxypicolinoyl)glycine, an orally bioavailable prolyl hydroxylase inhibitor for the treatment of anemia. J Med Chem 2020;63(17):10045−60.
[26] You Q., Zhang X., Lei Y., et al. Alkynyl pyridine prolyl hydroxylase inhibitor, and preparation method and medical use thereof. EP3360862A1, 2018.
[27] Rosen MD, Venkatesan H, Peltier HM, et al. Benzimidazole-2-pyrazole HIF prolyl 4-hydroxylase inhibitors as oral erythropoietin secretagogues. ACS Med Chem Lett 2010;1(9):526−9.
[28] Chowdhury R, Mcdonough MA, Mecinović J, et al. Structural basis for binding of hypoxia-inducible factor to the oxygen-sensing prolyl hydroxylases. Structure 2009;17(7):981−9.
[29] Islam MS, Leissing TM, Chowdhury R, et al. 2-Oxoglutarate-dependent oxygenases. Annu Rev Biochem 2018;87:585−620.
[30] Cunliffe CJ, Franklin TJ, Hales NJ, et al. Novel inhibitors of prolyl 4-hydroxylase. 3. Inhibition by the substrate analogue N-oxaloglycine and its derivatives. J Med Chem 1992;35(14):2652−8.
[31] Rose NR, McDonough MA, King ON, et al. Inhibition of 2-oxoglutarate dependent oxygenases. Chem Soc Rev 2011;40(8):4364−97.
[32] Ivan M, Haberberger T, Gervasi DC, et al. Biochemical purification and pharmacological inhibition of a mammalian prolyl hydroxylase acting on hypoxia-inducible factor. Proc Natl Acad Sci USA 2002;99(21):13459−64.
[33] Mcdonough MA, Li V, Flashman E, et al. Cellular oxygen sensing: crystal structure of hypoxia-inducible factor prolyl hydroxylase (PHD2). Proc Natl Acad Sci USA 2006;103(26):9814−19.
[34] Rabinowitz MH. Inhibition of hypoxia-inducible factor prolyl hydroxylase domain oxygen sensors: tricking the body into mounting orchestrated survival and repair responses. J Med Chem 2013;56(23):9369−402.
[35] Guenzler-Pukall V, Wang Q, Langsetmo PI, et al. Methods for reducing blood pressure. WO2009058403A1, 2009.
[36] Klaus SJ, Neff TB. Hypoxia inducible factor (HIF) hydroxylase inhibitors for the treatment of anemia. US20060276477A1, 2006.
[37] Deng S, Wu M, Turtle ED, et al. Preparation of pyrrolopyridines and thiazolopyridines, particularly N-[(4-hydroxy-1H-pyrrolo[2,3-c]-pyridin-5-yl)carbonyl]glycine and N-(7-hydroxythiazolo[4,5-c]-pyridin-6-yl)carbonyl]glycine derivatives, as hypoxia inducible factor hydroxylase modulators. WO2007115315A2, 2007.
[38] Zhou X, Arend MP, Wu M, et al. Preparation of isothiazole-pyridine derivatives as modulators of HIF (hypoxia inducible factor) activity. WO2009089547A1, 2009.
[39] Ho W, Wright L, Deng S, et al. Chromen-3-ylamide derivatives as hypoxia inducible factor hydroxylase inhibitors useful in the treatment of diseases and preparation thereof. WO2009100250A1 2009.
[40] Dhillon S. Roxadustat: first global approval. Drugs 2019;79:563−72.

[41] Groenendaal-Van de Meent D, Den Adel M, Rijnders S, et al. The hypoxia-inducible factor prolyl-hydroxylase inhibitor roxadustat (FG-4592) and warfarin in healthy volunteers: a pharmacokinetic and pharmacodynamic drug-drug interaction study. Clin Ther 2016;38(4):918–28.

[42] Groenendaal-Van de Meent D, Den Adel M, Van Dijk J, et al. Effect of multiple doses of omeprazole on the pharmacokinetics, safety, and tolerability of roxadustat in healthy subjects. Eur J Drug Metab Pharmacokinet 2018;43(6):685–92.

[43] Groenendaal-Van de Meent D, Adel MD, Noukens J, et al. Effect of moderate hepatic impairment on the pharmacokinetics and pharmacodynamics of roxadustat, an oral hypoxia-inducible factor prolyl hydroxylase inhibitor. Clin Drug Investig 2016;36(9):743–51.

[44] Akizawa T, Iwasaki M, Otsuka T, et al. Roxadustat treatment of chronic kidney disease-associated anemia in Japanese patients not on dialysis: a phase 2, randomized, double-blind, placebo-controlled trial. Adv Ther 2019;36(6):1438–54.

[45] Chen N, Qian J, Chen J, et al. Phase 2 studies of oral hypoxia-inducible factor prolyl hydroxylase inhibitor FG-4592 for treatment of anemia in China. Nephrol Dial Transpl 2017;32(8):1373–86.

[46] Chen N, Hao C, Peng X, et al. Roxadustat for anemia in patients with kidney disease not receiving dialysis. N Engl J Med 2019;381(11):1001–10.

[47] Provenzano R, Besarab A, Wright S, et al. Roxadustat (FG-4592) versus epoetin alfa for anemia in patients receiving maintenance hemodialysis: a phase 2, randomized, 6- to 19-week, open-label, active-comparator, dose-ranging, safety and exploratory efficacy study. Am J Kidney Dis 2016;67(6):912–24.

[48] Web Sites: https://fibrogen.gcs-web.com/news-releases/news-release-details/asn-kidney-week-2018-data-presented-two-japanese-phase-3-studies (accessed June 03, 2020).

[49] Web Sites: https://www.astellas.com/en/news/15096 (accessed June 03, 2020).

[50] Web Sites: https://fibrogen.gcs-web.com/news-releases/news-release-details/fibrogen-submits-new-drug-application-us-fda-roxadustat-patients (accessed June 03, 2020).

[51] Web Sites: https://fibrogen.gcs-web.com/news-releases/news-release-details/roxadustat-approved-china-treatment-anemia-chronic-kidney (accessed June 03, 2020).

[52] Web Sites: https://www.astellas.com/en/news/15546 (accessed June 03, 2020).

[53] Web Sites: https://fibrogen.gcs-web.com/news-releases/news-release-details/fibrogen-announces-initiation-phase-2-clinical-trial-roxadustat (accessed June 03, 2020).

[54] Volkmar G, Eric D, Michael P, et al. Novel nitrogen-containing heteroaryl compounds and methods of use thereof. WO2004108681, 2004.

[55] Claudia W, Jung M, Michael D, et al. Crystalline forms of a prolyl hydroxylase inhibitor. WO2014014835, 2014.

Chapter 27

Function, pharmaceutical, and pharmacological research and development of natural tetracyclic dipyranocoumarin (+)-calanolide A and its analogs

Tao Ma[1], Purong Zheng[2], Xueyuan Li[3], Xiaoqiao Hong[4] and Gang Liu[4]

[1]School of Chinese Materia Medica, Beijing University of Chinese Medicine, Beijing, P.R. China, [2]Ningbo Combireg Pharmaceutical Technology Co. Ltd., Ningbo, Zhejiang, P.R. China, [3]Institute of Basic Medical Sciences, Chinese Academy of Medical Sciences, Beijing, P.R. China, [4]School of Pharmaceutical Sciences, Tsinghua University, Beijing, P.R. China

Chapter outline

27.1 Discovery and structural diversity of natural tetracyclic dipyranocoumarins	651
27.2 Natural nonnucleoside reverse transcriptase inhibitors	654
27.2.1 Anti-HIV-1 activity of calanolides	654
27.2.2 Anti-HIV-1 activity of inophyllums	656
27.2.3 Anti-HIV-1 activity of cordatolides	657
27.2.4 Investigation of 1 in clinical trial	657
27.3 Anti-HIV-1 activity of improved calanolides	658
27.3.1 Total synthesis of (±)-1	658
27.3.2 Enantioselective total synthesis of optical 1	659
27.3.3 Other representative calanolide analogs	659
27.4 (+)-Calanolide A and its derivatives inhibit replicating and non-replicating *Mycobacterium tuberculosis*	666
27.4.1 Natural product 1 as an anti-*Mycobacterium tuberculosis* compound	666
27.4.2 Preliminary structural modifications	667
27.4.3 The discovered and optimized tetrahydropyranocoumarins derived from the nitrofuran moiety exhibit potent activity against both R-*Mycobacterium tuberculosis* and NR-*Mycobacterium tuberculosis*	668
27.4.4 Mechanism of antibacterial activity of tetrahydrobenzopyran nitrofuran derivatives	670
27.5 Fluorescent activity of nitrofuran derivatives: a revelatory outcome	672
27.5.1 Relationship between structure and molecular fluorescence activity	672
27.5.2 How do nitrofuran compounds interact with Rv2466c and mycothiol (160)	674
27.5.3 The action of mycothiol (MSH, 160)	675
27.5.4 Utilization of compound 125 as an innovative fluorescent diagnostic reagent for drug sensitivity testing in tuberculosis diagnosis	677
27.5.5 Implementing single-cell diagnostic technology for nitrofuran compounds	678
27.6 Summary and outlook	683
References	685
Further reading	687

27.1 Discovery and structural diversity of natural tetracyclic dipyranocoumarins

Coumarins are well-known natural products with a broad range of biological activities [1–3]. In 1992, researchers from the National Cancer Institute (NCI) in the United States isolated a novel dipyranocoumarin (+)-calanolide A (1, Table 27.1) from the Malaysian rainforest plant *Calophyllum lanigerum* [4], and subsequently others isolated (+)-inophyllum B (3) from *Calophyllum inophyllum* in 1993 [6]. Both compounds represented a new type of natural nonnucleoside reverse transcriptase inhibitor (NNRTI) for human immunodeficiency virus (HIV)-1. Scientists were then interested in plants of the genus *Calophyllum* and other naturally occurring pyranocoumarins and anticipated isolating

TABLE 27.1 Chemical structures of naturally occurring *Calophyllum* dipyranocoumarins.

Scaffolds	Representative compounds
	1: R = n-C$_3$H$_7$, R$_1$ = OH, R$_2$ = H, (+)-calanolide A [4] 2: R = n-C$_3$H$_7$, R$_2$ = OH, R$_1$ = H, (+)-calanolide B [4,5] 3: R = C$_6$H$_5$, R$_1$ = OH, R$_2$ = H, (+)-inophyllum B [5–7] 4: R = C$_6$H$_5$, R$_2$ = OH, R$_1$ = H, (+)-inophyllum P [5,6] 5: R = CH$_3$, R$_1$ = OH, R$_2$ = H, (+)-cordatolide A [8,9] 6: R = CH$_3$, R$_2$ = OH, R$_1$ = H, (+)-cordatolide B [8,9] 7: R = n-C$_3$H$_7$, R$_1$ = OCH$_3$, R$_2$ = H, (+)-12-methoxy calanolide A [4] 8: R = n-C$_3$H$_7$, R$_1$ = OAc, R$_2$ = H, (+)-12-acetoxy calanolide A [4] 9: R = n-C$_3$H$_7$, R$_2$ = OCH$_3$, R$_1$ = H, (+)-12-methoxy calanolide B [4] 10: R = CH$_3$, R$_2$ = OCH$_3$, R$_1$ = H, (+)-12-methoxy cordatolide B [9]
	11: R = C$_6$H$_5$, R$_1$ = R$_3$ = CH$_3$, R$_2$ = R$_4$ = H, (+)-inophyllum C [5–7,10] 12: R = C$_6$H$_5$, R$_2$ = R$_3$ = CH$_3$, R$_1$ = R$_4$ = H, (+)-inophyllum E [5–7,10] 13: R = C$_6$H$_5$, R$_2$ = R$_4$ = CH$_3$, R$_1$ = R$_3$ = H, (−)-soulattrolone [11]
	14: R = n-C$_3$H$_7$, R$_2$ = R$_4$ = CH$_3$, R$_1$ = R$_3$ = R$_6$ = H, R$_5$ = OH, (−)-calanolide F [12] 15: R = n-C$_3$H$_7$, R$_2$ = R$_3$ = CH$_3$, R$_1$ = R$_4$ = R$_6$ = H, R$_5$ = OH, (−)-calanolide B (costatolide) [13,14] 16: R = C$_6$H$_5$, R$_2$ = R$_3$ = CH$_3$, R$_1$ = R$_4$ = R$_6$ = H, R$_5$ = OH, (−)-inophyllum P (soulattrolide) [15] 17: R = C$_6$H$_5$, R$_1$ = R$_3$ = CH$_3$, R$_2$ = R$_4$ = R$_6$ = H, R$_5$ = OH, (+)-inophyllum A [6,16] 18: R = C$_6$H$_5$, R$_1$ = R$_3$ = CH$_3$, R$_2$ = R$_4$ = R$_5$ = H, R$_6$ = OH, (+)-inophyllum D [6,7]
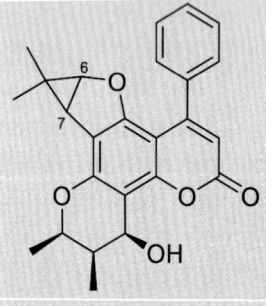	19: 6α, 7α: (+)-inophyllum G-1 [6] 20: 6β, 7β: (−)-inophyllum G-2 [6]
	21: R = n-C$_3$H$_7$, (+)-pseudocalanolide C [4,12,17,18] 22: R = CH$_3$, (+)-pseudocordatolide C [12] 23: R = C$_6$H$_5$, 6,7-gem dimethyl, trans-tomentolide A [19]
	24: R = n-C$_3$H$_7$, R$_1$ = CH$_3$, R$_2$ = H, tomentolide B [19] 25: R = n-C$_3$H$_7$, R$_2$ = CH$_3$, R$_1$ = H, (+)-pseudocalanolide D [4,12,17]

(Continued)

TABLE 27.1 (Continued)

Scaffolds	Representative compounds
	26: R = n-C$_3$H$_7$, (+)-calanolide E [20] 27: R = CH$_3$, (+)-cordatolide E [12]
	28: R$_1$ = CH$_3$, R$_2$ = H, calophyllic acid [6] 29: R$_1$ = H, R$_2$ = CH$_3$, isocalophyllic acid [6]
	30: oblongulide [8,9]
	31: 12-oxocalanolide A [21]
	32: (−)-dihydrocalanolide B [22]

more of them from *Calophyllum* species. According to the ring varieties, these compounds are structurally divided into three skeletons, including (1) tetracyclic dipyranocoumarins in which the ring D contains a gem-dimethyl group, such as 1, (+)-calanolide B (2), 3 and (+)-cordatolide A (5); (2) tetracyclic dipyranocoumarins with reversed D and C pyran rings, namely, the gem-dimethyl group is present in ring C, as seen in the (+)-pseudocalanolide C (21) and (+)-pseudocalanolide D (25); and (3) tricyclic pyranocoumarins, i.e., (+)-calanolide E (26) and (+)-cordatolide E (27), in which ring C is open. Individual members of the groups vary with respect to the C_4 substituent of the lactone ring (ring B), where *n*-propyl (calanolides), phenyl (inophyllums), and methyl groups (cordatolides) are encountered, which are the most representative in terms of their anti-HIV-1 activity. [Note: Starting in the 1950s, NCI initiated a large-scale screening and isolation program for active components or constituents of natural products supported by the government and donors. This program was later expanded to include screening in the fields of nonnatural small molecular compounds and biologics, primarily targeting cancer and HIV-1, and established many relevant high-throughput cell-based screening assays. The global screening program for 60 human cancer cell lines from 9 types of cancer continues today and has discovered renowned anticancer drugs such as paclitaxel, romidepsin, eribulin, sipuleucel-T (vaccine), and ddi-nutuximab (Ch14.18). If interested, readers could refer to the NCI Development Therapeutics Program (DTP).].

27.2 Natural nonnucleoside reverse transcriptase inhibitors

27.2.1 Anti-HIV-1 activity of calanolides

27.2.1.1 Anti-HIV-1 activity in cell culture assay

Natural compound 1 effectively inhibits HIV-1 replication with an EC_{50} value of 0.1 μmol/L and a cytotoxicity IC_{50} value of 20 μmol/L, thus giving a therapeutic index (IC_{50}/EC_{50}) value of 200 [4]. Compound 1 is inactive against HIV-2 and the simian immunodeficiency virus (SIV). Subsequent studies indicate that 1 belongs to the NNRTI of HIV-1 [23–26]. Flavin et al. first reported the anti-HIV-1 activity of racemic ($\pm$)-1 and resolved 1 and (−)-1 against both laboratory strains and clinical isolates of HIV-1, as shown in Table 27.2 [21]. The cytotoxicity of ($\pm$)-1, 1, and (−)-1 in different cell lines was approximately the same. Among them, 1 exhibited the most potent anti-HIV-1 activity [4]. Interestingly, both the azidothymidine (AZT)-resistant (AZT, the first nucleoside reverse transcriptase inhibitor anti-HIV-1 drug, azidothymidine) strain G910−6 and the pyridinone-resistant strain A17 were also effectively inhibited by ($\pm$)-1 and 1 [4,21,22]. Compound 1 was more active than ($\pm$)-1 against the AZT-resistant strain G910−6, with EC_{50} values of 0.027 and 0.108 μmol/L, respectively, indicating (+)-1 is the optimal configuration.

Stereoisomers of 1, such as 15 and its dihydro analog 32, were also determined to be NNRTIs that possessed similar antiviral properties to 1. In fresh human cells, 15 and 32 were highly effective against low-passage clinical virus strains, including representative strains of the various HIV-1 clades [26a]. Especially 1, 15, and 32 were highly active against viral isolates with the Y181C mutation (Y and C stand for tyrosine and cysteine, respectively) in the HIV-1 reverse transcriptase (RT) (Table 27.3). Y181C is a highly frequent mutation in both laboratory and clinical viral isolates that is associated with high-level resistance to most other NNRTIs, such as nevirapine (NVP), pyridinone, E-BPTU, UC38, and diphenylsulfone [26a,b]. Therefore, the discovery of this unique biological property of tetracyclic dipyranocoumarin compounds sparked great interest in the development of the first natural anti-HIV-1 drug.

The synthetic intermediate [($\pm$)-12-oxo-1, (31)] is disclosed to also exhibit anti-HIV-1 activity with one less chiral carbon center than 1 [27]. This feature suggests that 31 would be an attractive candidate for drug development because its preparation was comparably convenient. Therefore, ($\pm$)-31, (+)-31, and (−)-31 were synthesized and evaluated for their antiviral activities against HIV-1, SIV, and HIV-2 using CEM-SS cells infected with various laboratory virus strains and clinical isolates of viruses [28]. The results (Table 27.4) indicated that these 12-oxo-calanolides were active against both HIV-1 and SIV but inactive against HIV-2.

Compounds 1, 15, and 32 were then tested for their additive or synergistic anti-HIV activities with a variety of mechanistically diverse HIV inhibitors such as AZT, zidovudine (ZDV), lamivudine (3TC), dideoxycytidine (ddC), dideoxyinosine (ddI) that are nucleoside reverse transcriptase inhibitors, NVP (NNRTI), indinavir (IDV), saquinavir (SQV), ritonavir (RTV), and nelfinavir (NFV), which are protease inhibitors (Table 27.5) [29]. The highly synergistic effects (synergy volumes greater than 100 $\mu mol/L^2$%) were observed when the compounds were combined with the ZDV and 3TC, the PIs NFV, SQV, and RTV, and the thiocarboxanilide. For instance, 1 exhibits a highly synergistic effect on ZDV and 3TC, RTV, and thiocarboxanilide, with additive effects on ddC, IDV, and SQV. Compound 15, on the other hand, exhibited synergistic effects with ZDV, 3TC, ddC, ddI, thiocarboxanilide, SQV, RTV, and NFV, with a synergy volume of 525 $\mu mol/L^2$% when combined with ddC, demonstrating the strongest synergistic therapeutic efficacy on cell assay. Compound 32 showed a synergistic effect between ZDV and thiocarboxanilide.

TABLE 27.2 Anti-HIV-1 activity of (±)-1, (+)-1, and (−)-1.

Strain/cell line		(±)-1	(+)-1	(−)-1	AZT[e]	ddC[e]
III$_B$/MT2	EC$_{50}$ (μmol/L)	0.108	0.053		0.029	0.900
	IC$_{50}$ (μmol/L)	6.86	14.80	7.31	51.64	83.80
	TI[d]	64	279		1780	93
RF$_{11}$/CEM	EC$_{50}$ (μmol/L)	0.486	0.267		0.023	0.189
	IC$_{50}$ (μmol/L)	22.81	22.96	18.70	301.60	47.34
	TI[d]	47	86		13113	250
G910–6[b]/MT2	EC$_{50}$ (μmol/L)	0.108	0.027			0.994
	IC$_{50}$ (μmol/L)	7.42	7.17	6.16	131.71	212.10
	TI[d]	69	266			213
H112–2[a]/MT2	EC$_{50}$ (μmol/L)	0.135	0.107		0.037	1.562
	IC$_{50}$ (μmol/L)	6.53	7.15	6.21	119.84	258.97
	TI[d]	48	67		3236	166
A17[c]/MT2	EC$_{50}$ (μmol/L)	0.297	0.427		0.014	0.331
	IC$_{50}$ (μmol/L)	6.94	6.99	5.89	83.44	134.93
	TI[d]	23	16		5960	4.0

[Note: The therapeutic index (TI) often refers to the ratio between the median lethal dose (LD$_{50}$) and the 50% effective dose (ED$_{50}$), or it can sometimes indicate the ratio between the 50% maximal inhibitory concentration (IC$_{50}$) in host cells and the 50% inhibitory concentration (EC$_{50}$) against the virus, using a host cell-based viral replication model. Specifically, the ED$_{50}$ represents the dosage that can elicit a 50% maximum response or induce a positive reaction in 50% of experimental subjects. On the other hand, the LD$_{50}$ signifies the dosage that results in the death of half the tested animals, serving as a toxicological indicator. Furthermore, the IC$_{50}$ corresponds to the half maximal inhibitory concentration, which is used to measure or indicate the inhibitory effects of compounds on cellular biological or biochemical functions, primarily in vitro inhibitory assays. Conversely, in vivo experiments refer to studies conducted within a living organism, such as using cells as hosts for viruses or animals as disease models. The EC$_{50}$ value obtained from host cell experiments represents the concentration that can induce a 50% maximum effect. Consequently, the therapeutic index (TI) derived from host cell experiments can be expressed as the ratio of IC$_{50}$ to EC$_{50}$. It is important to note that while a smaller ED$_{50}$ (EC$_{50}$) value and a larger LD$_{50}$ (IC$_{50}$) value suggest a potentially safer drug, the therapeutic index does not necessarily reflect the actual safety profile of a medication].
[a]*Pre-AZT treatment isolate.*
[b]*Post-AZT treatment isolate.*
[c]*Pyridinone-resistant isolate.*
[d]*TI = IC$_{50}$/EC$_{50}$.*
[e]*AZT and ddC are the positive control drugs.*

Furthermore, 1, 15, and 32 were evaluated in different host cell lines, such as CEM-SS, H9, MT2, AA5, and V937, infected with both laboratory-derived and clinical strains of HIV-1, HIV-2, and SIV [26a]. The anti-HIV-1 EC$_{50}$ values ranged from 0.08 to 0.5 μmol/L, 0.06 to 1.4 μmol/L, and 0.1 to 8.8 μmol/L for 1, 15, and 32, respectively, but no compound exhibited activity against HIV-2 or SIV.

27.2.1.2 Anti-HIV-1 activity of novel tetracyclic dipyranocoumarins in a mouse hollow fiber model

Compound 1 represents a novel class of HIV-1-specific NNRTIs with several attractive properties, including (1) 1 displays activity against a wide range of HIV-1 strains in both established and freshly prepared human cells, including fresh peripheral blood leukocytes and macrophages, and activity against all laboratory and clinical isolates of HIV-1; (2) 1 has a unique sensitivity profile to drug-resistant virus isolates, especially to the Y181C mutant virus; (3) 1-induced resistant mutation site (T139I) is completely different from all the drug-resistant sites induced by other marketing drugs or developing drug candidates, made 1 being unable to pose a risk of cross-resistance when used in combination with other drugs; (4) 1 exerts a unique additive or synergistic efficacy in combination with other antiretroviral agents; (5) the ideal lipophilic characteristics enables 1 to effectively gradually distribute into brain and lymph nodes in rats after oral or intravenous injection. Therefore, an evaluation of 1 in an assay of antiviral efficacy using a hollow fiber model in a SCID mouse was conducted by administering 200 mg/kg orally once a day or 150 mg/kg twice a day [30]. It was found to significantly

TABLE 27.3 Activities of calanolides against viral resistant to HIV-1-specific inhibitors.

Drug to which isolates are resistant (mutation)	EC_{50} (μmol/L)[a]				
	1	15	32	Nevirapine[a]	AZT[a]
IIIB (control)	0.1	0.2	0.2	0.01	0.05
UC10-costatolide (K103N)	>27	>270	>20	ND[b]	0.003
Oxathiin carboxanilide (L100I)	>27	>270	>20	0.1	0.04
Thiazolobenzimidazole (V108I)	24.0	4.4	3.5	0.3	0.04
TIBO-R82150 (A98G-V108I)	22.0	1.6	5.1	0.6	0.05
Calanolide A (T139I)	>27	4.5	>20	0.01	0.01
Diphenylsulfone (Y181C)	0.08	0.08	<0.01	5.9	0.01
Nevirapine (Y181C)	<0.01	<0.01	0.09	>38	0.03
Pyridinone (Y181C-L103N)	0.12	0.8	0.8	>38	0.01
E-BPTU (Y181C)	0.1	<0.08	<0.06	1.9	0.03
3TC(M184V)	0.3	1.3	1.0	0.01	0.02
UC38(Y181C)	0.2	<0.03	0.1	1.9	0.01
Costatolide (Y188H)	>27	>27	>27	ND[b]	0.004
HEPT (P236L)	0.6	1.1	0.2	0.02	0.01

[a]Nevirapine (NNRTI) and AZT (NRTI) are the positive control compounds.
[b]ND, not determined.

TABLE 27.4 Antiviral activity of (±)-, (+)-, and (−)-12-oxo-1 (31) against CEM-SS cells infected with various viruses.

Virus	EC_{50} (μmol/L)				
	(±)-31	(+)-31	(−)-31	ddC[a]	1
HIV-1(R_F)	0.4	0.9	3.41	0.05	0.27
HIV-1(SK1)	0.17	0.17	0.27	0.05	0.14
HIV-1(III_B)	0.51	1.0	1.88	0.02	0.17
SIV(Delta)	1.24	1.66	6.12	0.19	Inactive
HIV-2(ROD)	5.57	15.90	ND[b]	0.03	Inactive

[a]ddC was used as a positive control drug.
[b]ND, not determined.

reduce the viral loading in animals by two orders of magnitude, and a synergistic effect between compound 1 and AZT was also observed. These results prompted researchers to conduct a phase I clinical trial, as outlined below.

27.2.2 Anti-HIV-1 activity of inophyllums

As discussed in Table 27.1, a series of inophyllum compounds were also isolated, including 3, 4, 11, 12, 17–20, 28, and 29 [6]. Among them, 3 and 4 showed their EC_{50} values of 38 and 130 nmol/L, respectively, while the IC_{50} values for HIV-1 in cell culture were 1.4 and 1.6 μmol/L, respectively. Both 3 and 4 possess the *trans*-$C_{10,11}$-dimethyl chromanone ring, which differs from the stereochemistry of the hydroxyl group at the C_{12} position. The substitutions of the C_{12}-

TABLE 27.5 Effects of calanolides in combination with inhibitors of HIV-1 replication.[a]

Drugs	MOA	Synergy volume ($\mu mol/L^2\%$)[b]		
		1	15	32
Resobene	B/F	12 ± 2	10 ± 1	4 ± 2
ZDV	NRTI	136 ± 15	223 ± 29	111 ± 8
3TC	NRTI	129 ± 18	156 ± 29	25 ± 3
ddC	NRTI	74 ± 7	525 ± 49	67 ± 8
ddI	NRTI	95 ± 10	152 ± 12	37 ± 6
Nevirapine	NNRTI	42 ± 21	39 ± 10	67 ± 21
UC10	NNRTI	12 ± 3	30 ± 2	50 ± 9
Thiocarboxanilide	NNRTI	123 ± 10	152 ± 12	143 ± 12
Ritonavir	PI	112 ± 8	182 ± 15	ND
Indinavir	PI	12 ± 1	20 ± 1	ND
Saquinavir	PI	95 ± 15	120 ± 12	ND
Nelfinavir	PI	49 ± 15	120 ± 12	ND

Mechanism of action (MOA): B/F, virus attachment and cell-cell fusion inhibitor; PI, protease inhibitor; ND, not defined.
[a]Data were analyzed using MacSynergy II at the 95% confidence interval and average synergy/antagonism values are presented.
[b]Within the concentration ranges used, no evidence of synergistic toxicity was detected for any of these combinations in anti-HIV assays.

position significantly decrease its activity against HIV-1, such that 11 (10 μmol/L against HIV-1 RT) and 12 (10 μmol/L against HIV-1 RT) were much less active, and the closely related 18 (11 μmol/L against HIV-1 RT) and 17 (30 μmol/L against HIV-1 RT) having the cis-10,11-dimethylchromanol ring were also less active. Furthermore, 16, which has a similar structure to 15, is a potent inhibitor with an IC_{50} value of 0.34 μmol/L for HIV-1 RT [31]. No appreciable activity was observed toward HIV-2 RT or avian myeloblastosis virus reverse transcriptase. The absolute configuration of 16 (10S, 11R, and 12S) and other structurally related HIV-1 inhibitors was also evaluated, but not as a disclosed activity [32].

27.2.3 Anti-HIV-1 activity of cordatolides

Compounds 5 and 6 (Table 27.1) were isolated from *Calophyllum cordato-oblongum* [8,9] and inhibited HIV-1 RT with IC_{50} values of 12.3 and 19.0 μmol/L, respectively [32]. Although 5 has the same stereochemistry, its ability to inhibit HIV-1 RT was much lower than that of 1 and 3. Thus, the substituents located at the C_4-position are important for antiviral activity, indicating that the *n*-propyl group in 1 is optimal.

27.2.4 Investigation of 1 in clinical trial

The safety and pharmacokinetics were initially examined in four successive single-dose cohorts (200, 400, 600, and 800 mg) of healthy, HIV-negative volunteers in a phase I trial, with a minimum of 47 subjects treated with 1 [33]. Dizziness, taste perversion, headache, eructation, and nausea were the most frequently observed adverse events. The calculation of the terminal-phase half-life ($T_{1/2}$) was approximately 20 hours for the 800-mg dose group. Compound 1 could be rapidly absorbed following administration, with time to maximum concentration of drug in plasma (T_{max}) values ranging from 2.4 to 5.2 hours after dosing, depending on the dose. Plasma levels of 1 were quite variable among patients at all doses; however, both the maximal concentration in plasma (C_{max}), and the area under the plasma concentration-time curve (AUC) increased proportionately in relation to the dose. Based on the data, the plasma drug concentration in females is higher than that in males, but the data after body weight standardization shows that there is no significant difference between females and males. Interestingly, the measured human plasma concentration of 1 is higher than the one predicted by animal data, implying that 1 was more efficiently absorbed in humans.

In a continuing clinical study, the safety and pharmacokinetics of multiple escalating doses of 1 were investigated in the same 47 healthy, HIV-seronegative individuals [34]. All adverse events observed in the study were mild to moderate in intensity and were transient. The most common adverse events were headaches, dizziness, nausea, and taste perversion (oily aftertaste). No dose-related adverse events were observed. In all cohorts examined, the administration of 1 produced highly variable plasma levels and absorption profiles. No accumulation of the parent compound was observed over the 5-day treatment course, and the AUC value on day 5 was approximately one-half of the value on the first day of dosing. After continuous administrations of 600 and 800 mg twice daily for 5 days, the mean elimination half-life was 15.5 and 35.2 hours, respectively. These pharmacokinetic properties, along with the benign safety observations and unique in vitro antiresistance profiles, highly advanced further clinical investigations of 1 as an anti-HIV-1 agent derived from a natural product.

Until recently, 1 was the only natural product evaluated in clinical trials, potentially for patients with acquired immune deficiency syndrome (AIDS). Unfortunately, it was stopped after the phase I trial in health donors due to the difficulty of the synthesis process on a large scale at that time, which failed to provide enough compounds in a timely manner, and other excellent new anti-AIDS drugs were continuously approved for marketing, which eventually made the 1 lose the advantage and necessity of further clinical investigations.

27.3 Anti-HIV-1 activity of improved calanolides

27.3.1 Total synthesis of (±)-1

After the identification of 1 in 1992, the total synthesis of the racemic compound (Fig. 27.1) was soon reported by Chenera et al. in 1993 [35]. Using phloroglucinol as the starting material, the coumarin intermediate (33) was synthesized with a Pechmann condensation reaction. Classical Friedel-Crafts acylation in the presence of tigloyl chloride and ring closure in the presence of K_2CO_3 afforded the ring D with relatively equal ratios of cis- and trans-isomers (35). The chromene compound was then condensed with 3-chloro-3-methyl-1-butyne to produce ring C; 10,11-trans-chromanone (36) was readily separated from the cis-version (37) through column chromatography. Finally, (±)-1 was obtained by the Luche reduction of 36 under the catalysis of $CeCl_3$, which promoted the formation of the cis-configuration between C_{10}-methyl and C_{12}-hydroxy groups with a total yield of 15%.

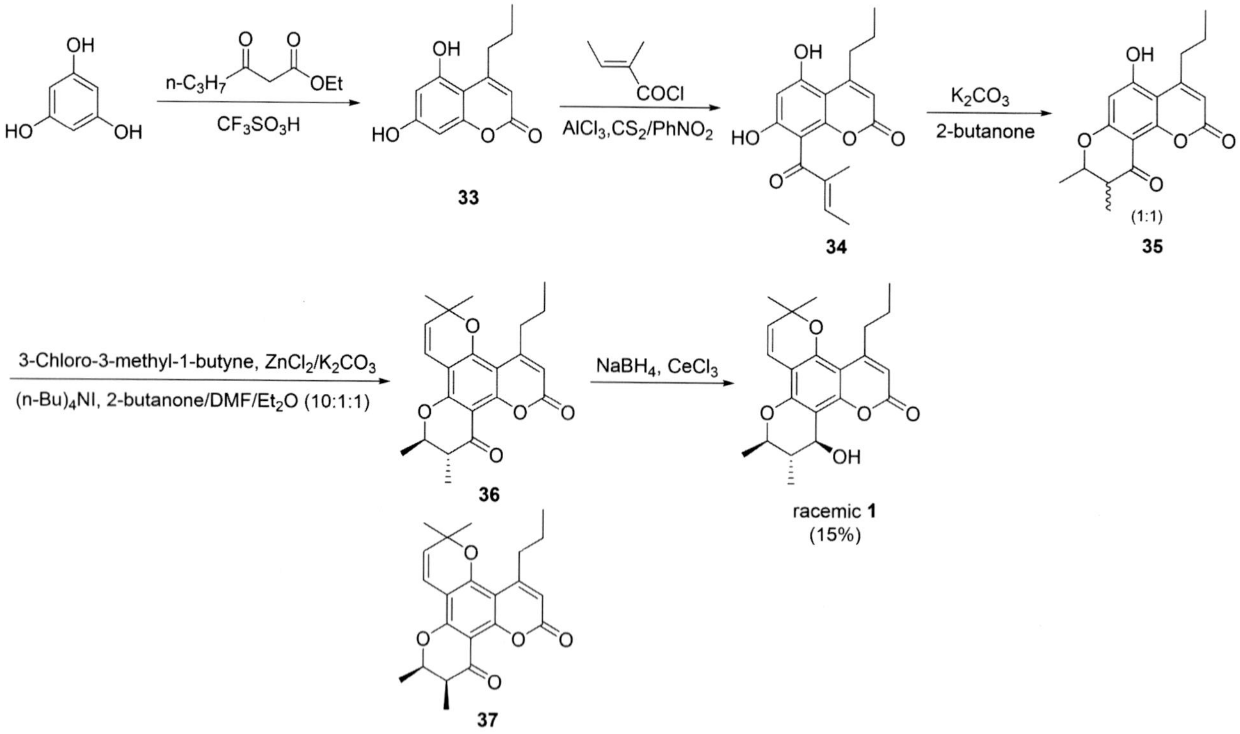

FIGURE 27.1 The synthetic route of racemic 1 reported by Chenera et al.

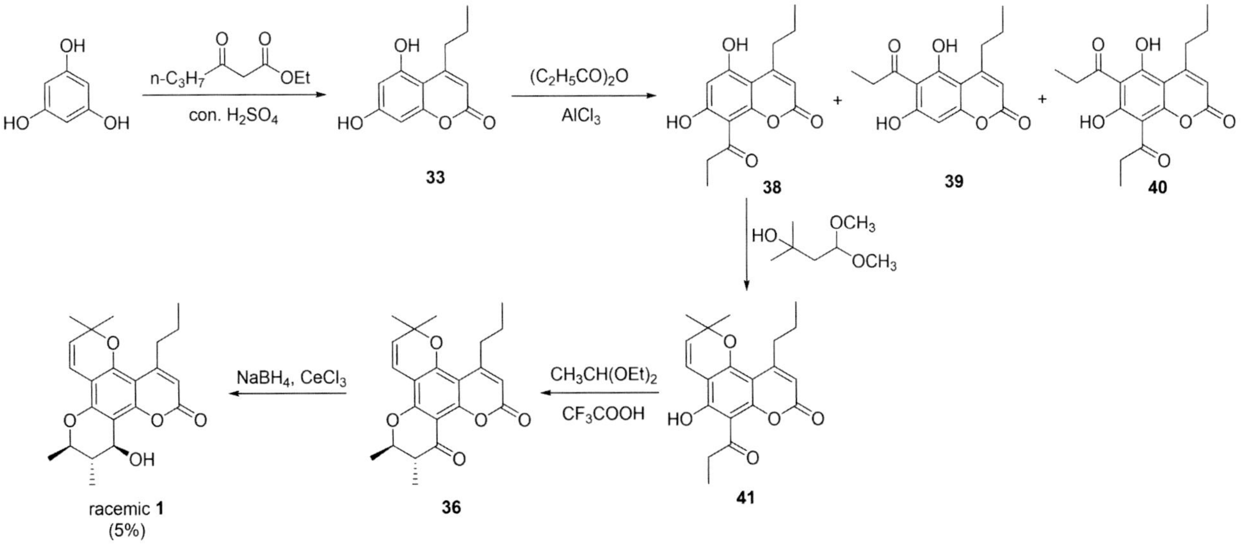

FIGURE 27.2 The synthetic route of racemic 1 reported by Kucherenko et al.

Starting with coumarin 33, another synthetic route (Fig. 27.2) was reported by Kucherenko et al. [36]. When the coumarin was reacted with propionic anhydride, C_6-acylation (39), C_8-acylation (38), and $C_{6,8}$-diacylation (40) were equally identified. After separation using silica gel column chromatography, the desired 38 was then condensed with 4,4-dimethoxy-2-methyl-butan2-ol to form ring C. The treatment of 41 with acetaldehyde diethyl acetal in the presence of trifluoroacetic acid and pyridine formed the racemic chromanone 36 with the desired stereochemical arrangement. Through a Luche reduction, compound ($\pm$)-1 was finally produced with a total yield of only 5%.

27.3.2 Enantioselective total synthesis of optical 1

The synthesis of optical 1 was achieved through an asymmetric catalysis approach. In 1995, Deshpande et al. first reported the asymmetric synthesis of optical 1 and 2 (Fig. 27.3) [37]. Starting with coumarin (33), C_8-formylation (42) was followed by a regioselective Vilsmeier reaction. As in Fig. 27.1, ring C was subsequently constructed by condensation with 3-chloro-3-methyl-1-butyne. The chiral centers in the chroman system were introduced using (Z)-crotyldiisopinocampheyl-borane, and then a mercury (II) acetate-assisted cyclization of the resulting O-alkenyl phenol was implemented to produce the required trans, trans-Me-Me-OH substituted chroman (benzo[b]pyran ring). After enantioselective 2 was prepared, optical 1 was gained by the conversion of 2 using a modified Mitsunobu reaction (PMe₃, diethyl azodicarboxylate, and chloroacetic acid), and the resulting ester was saponified with ammonium hydroxide in methanol. The total yield was 18%.

In 1998, Trost et al. reported another synthetic route (Fig. 27.4) to produce 1 and 15 using a similar strategy to the previous route, in which the chirality in chromans was introduced in a catalytic reaction [38]. In this route, the asymmetric preparation of alkylated products of phenol (compound 48) is the key step. This route achieved a palladium-catalyzed olefin alkylation reaction. Chiral hydroxyl compound 50 (93:7, diastereomeric ratio) was obtained by selectively borohydride benzopyran (chromone) (compound 49) using 9-BBN chemistry. The hydroxyl group of 50 is oxidized by the Dess Martin reagent to gain chiral aldehydes, which are then stabilized and cyclized under a Lewis acid (ZnCl₂) catalysis to offer thermally unstable ent-15 (10:1, diastereomeric ratio). The latter can be converted into optical compound 1 under Mitsunobu conversion conditions with a total yield of 9%.

27.3.3 Other representative calanolide analogs

Galinis et al. reported the catalytic reduction of the $\triangle^{7,8}$-olefinic bonds in 1 and 15 (32 and 58), as well as the chemical modifications of the C_{12}-hydroxyl group (51−57 and 61) and C_{12}-carbon (31, 60, and 62) (Fig. 27.5) [39]. All these compounds did not exceed anti-HIV-1 activity.

Zembower et al. prepared a series of racemic structural analogs of ($\pm$)-1 in Fig. 27.6, which focused on the modification of the trans-10,11-dimethyldihydropyran-12-ol ring (ring D) [27]. The results indicated that the substitution of

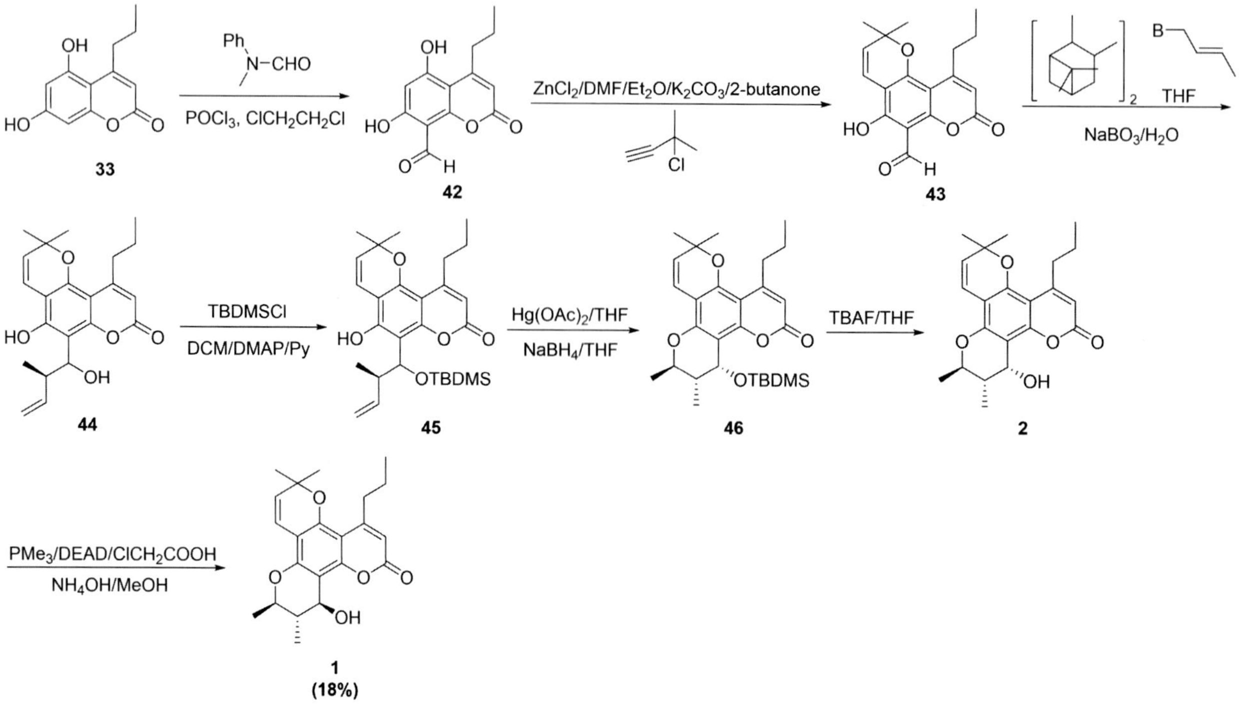

FIGURE 27.3 The chiral synthesis of 1 and 2.

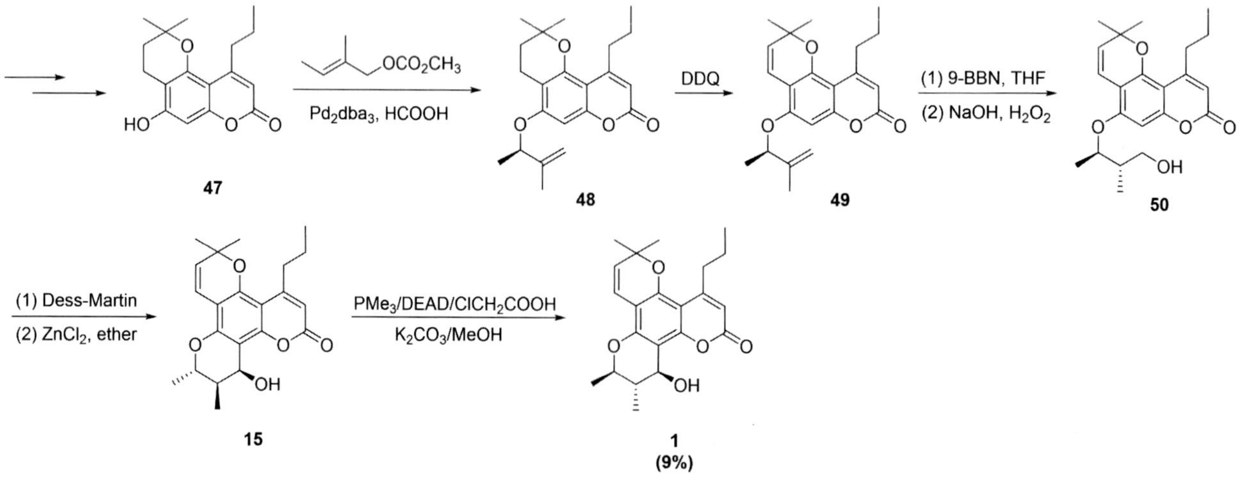

FIGURE 27.4 The chiral synthesis of 15 and 1.

the 10-methyl group with an ethyl chain (64) induced a fourfold reduction in potency compared to (±)-1. Substitution of the 10-methyl group with an isopropyl moiety (65) eliminated the anti-HIV activity. These compounds represent the first ketone derivatives in the calanolides to exhibit anti-HIV activity. Analogs showing anti-HIV activity in the CEM-SS cytoprotection assay were further confirmed to be inhibitors of HIV-1 reverse transcriptase.

Sharma et al. envisaged that the replacement of the oxygen atom in the coumarin ring (C_1-position) of 1 with the nitrogen atom would produce quinolinone with a calanolide skeleton, namely 77 (aza-1) in Fig. 27.7. The EC_{50} value of 77 (0.12 μmol/L) was lower than (±)-1 (0.27 μmol/L). The IC_{50} values of 77 and (±)-1 were 15 and 23 μmol/L, respectively, giving a similar TI value [40,41].

The research group of the authors of this chapter has synthesized and evaluated many diverse analogs containing the tetracyclic dipyranocoumarin backbone of calanolides in the past more than 20 years [42]. The earliest results indicated

51 52 53 54 55 32 56

57 58 59 60 61 31 62

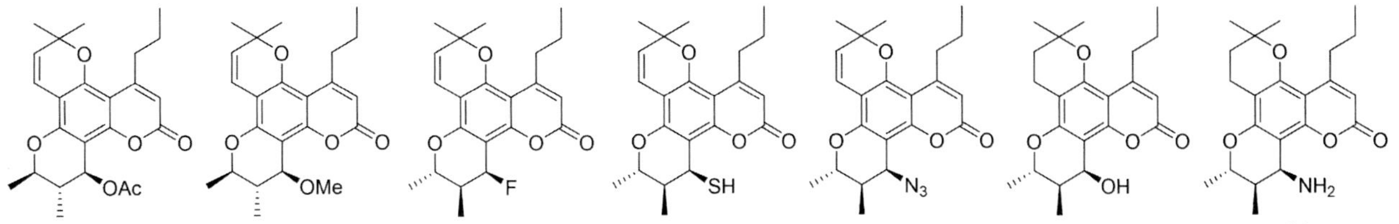

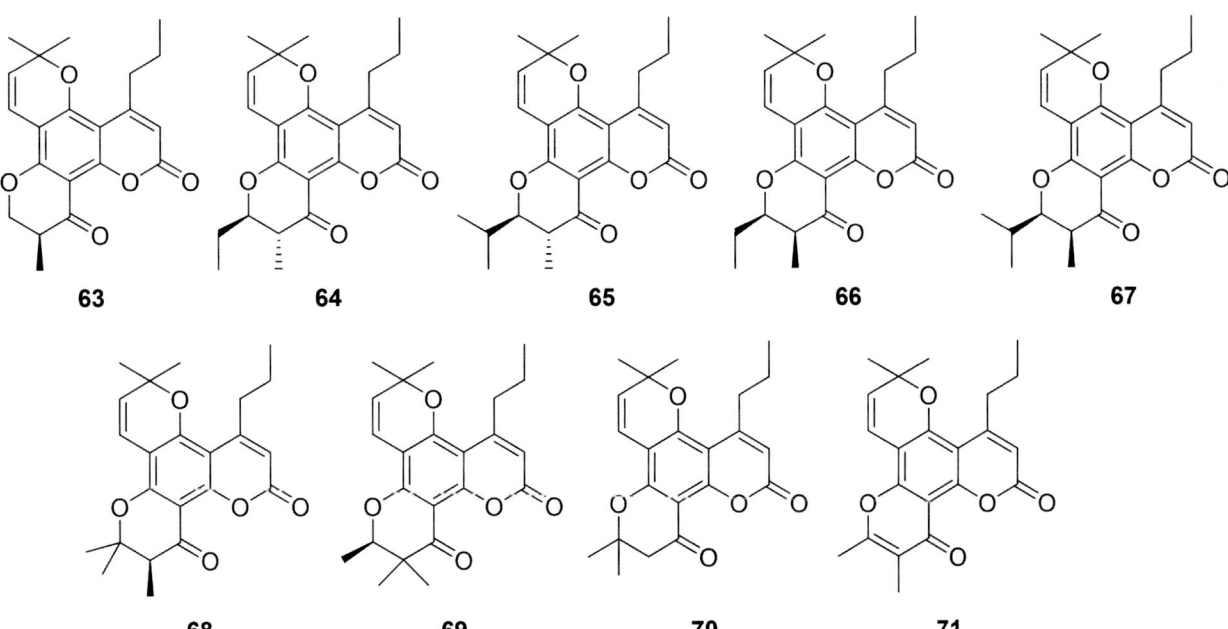

FIGURE 27.5 The modified analogs reported by Galinis et al.

63 64 65 66 67

68 69 70 71

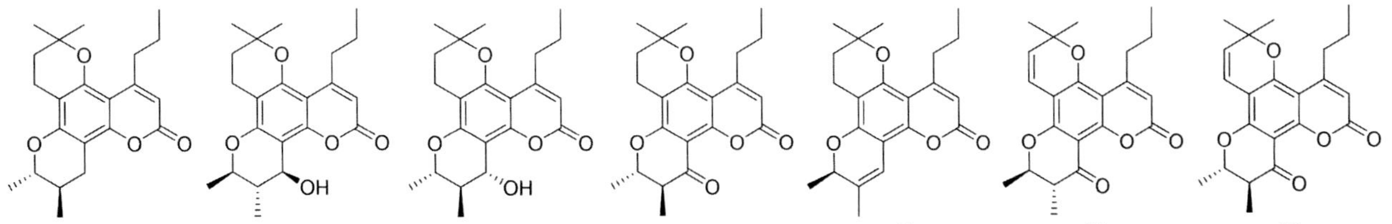

FIGURE 27.6 Representative calanolide analogs displaying the C_{12}-keto moiety reported by Zembower et al.

that (±)-11-demethyl-1 (78, $EC_{50}=0.31$ μmol/L) exhibited similar potencies as (±)-1, whereas 6,6,11-demethyl-1 (79) displayed diminished activity. According to the results, the presence of two methyl groups at the C_6 position might be necessary for the antiviral activity. As a result, the first lead compound in our lab, 78, was identified [43,44]. The racemic versions of the three main *Calophyllum* coumarins, 1, 3, and their 11-demethyl analogs (78, 80, and 81) were then chemically resolved into their corresponding optically active enantiomers through the synthesis of their (−)-menthol acetylated derivatives, respectively (Figs. 27.8 and 27.9). Their inhibitory activities against HIV-1 were tested in vitro, and it was concluded that 1 was the most potent compound with the lowest cytotoxicity [45].

A further investigation of the template of 1, (±)-11-demethyl-12-oxo 1 (82), which contains two fewer chiral carbon centers at the C_{11}- and C_{12}-positions than the precursor 1, exhibited comparably inhibitory activity ($EC_{50}=0.11$ μmol/L) and an improved therapeutic index ($TI=818$) against HIV-1 in vitro. A chemical library involving more than 200 compounds was then designed and prepared that could introduce nine different substituent-diversity points into its core structure (Fig. 27.10). The evaluations of their anti-HIV-1 activity in vitro provided complete structure-activity relationships (SARs). A new compound (10-bromomethyl-11-demethyl-12-oxo 1, 83) that displayed a much higher

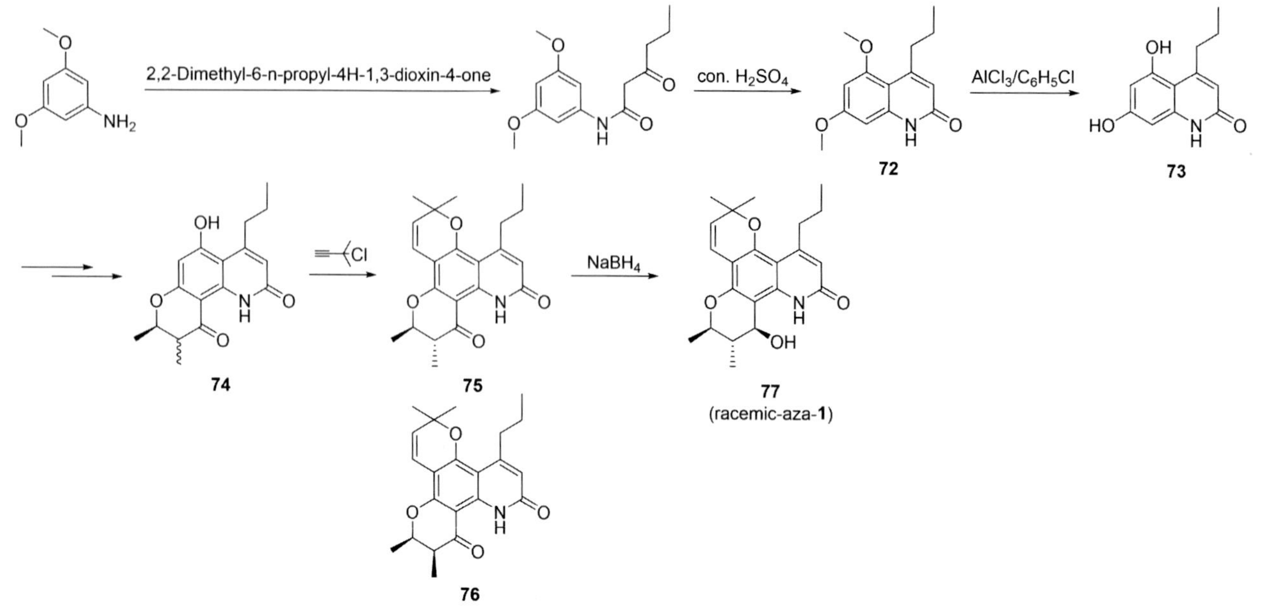

FIGURE 27.7 The synthetic route of 77 reported by Sharma et al.

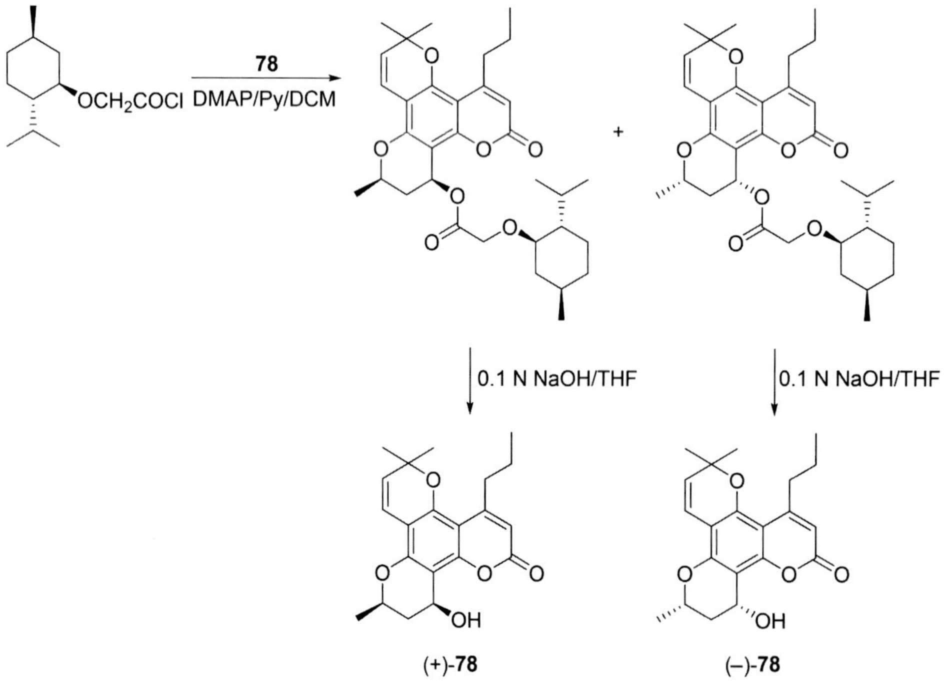

FIGURE 27.8 Chemical resolution of racemic calanolides, with analog 78 as an example.

inhibitory potency and wider therapeutic index (EC_{50} = 2.85 nmol/L, TI > 10,626) than 1, was discovered. This finding provided an important clue that modifications of the C ring at the C_{10} position could be conducted to obtain drug candidates with better activity against HIV-1 and an improved selectivity index (Fig. 27.11) [46].

Encouraged by the results described above, our continuous implementation of bioisostere to replace bromo methylene provided more detailed conclusions regarding the next round of SARs focusing on the C_{10} position in ring C [47]. At this point, the evaluation focuses on druggability profiles, covering various aspects such as chemical synthesis processes, crystal form studies, quality and quantitative control, formulations, comprehensive safety evaluations, and activity and pharmacokinetic parameter improvement in animals. A novel candidate, 10-chloromethyl-11-demethyl-12-oxo 1

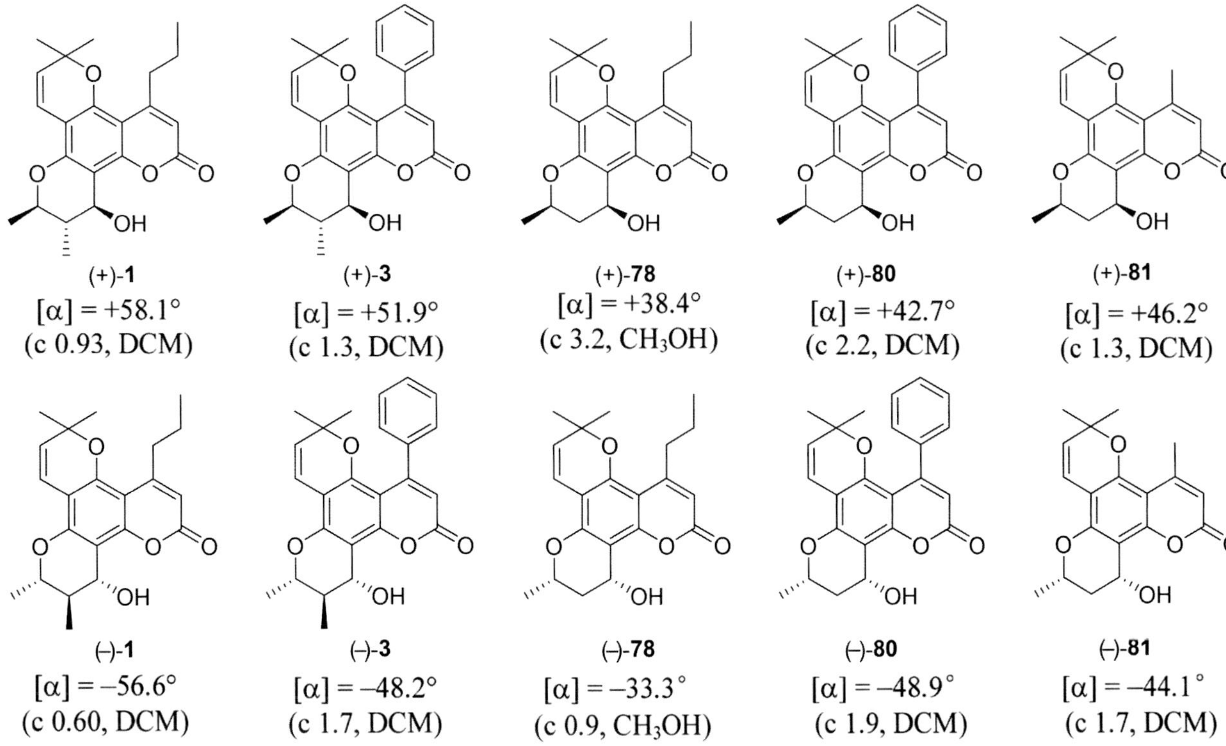

FIGURE 27.9 The optically active calanolide analogs produced through chemical resolution.

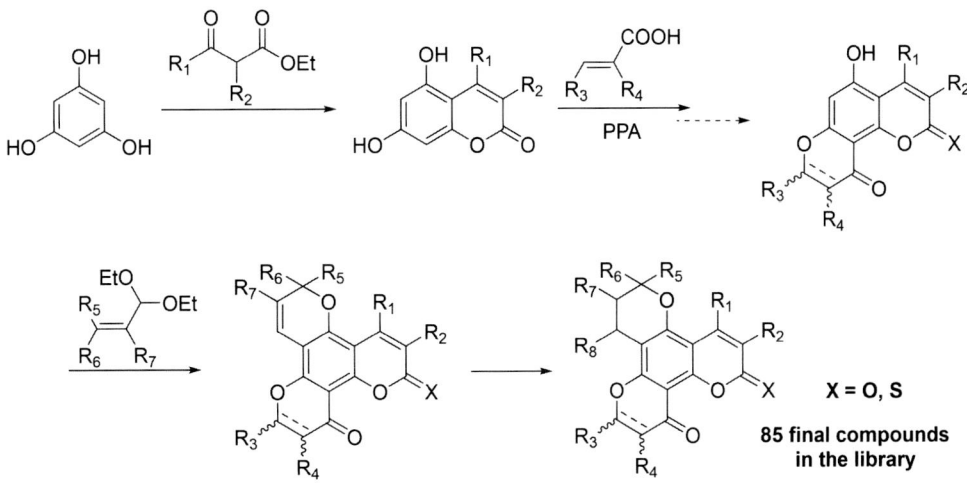

FIGURE 27.10 The synthetic strategy used to construct a chemical library based on the scaffold of 82.

(84, generic name F18), was finally determined to display optimal druggable profiles, with 60% oral bioavailability in rats and C_{max} = 0.336 μg/mL (T_{max} = 8 hours). The oral single dose was tolerated in mice (>2.4 g/kg), and no long-term treatment toxicity was observed in rats. In particular, the F18 exhibited highly efficient inhibition of wild-type HIV-1 and Y181C mutant HIV-1 at an EC_{50} = 7.4 nmol/L and 0.46 nmol/L, respectively.

F18 showed a highly efficient inhibition of the live wild-type HIV-1 NL4−3 virus (subtype B, X4) at an EC_{50} = 63 nmol/L in the PBMC-based assay, and a twofold higher value than NVP (EC_{50} = 25 nmol/L). Additionally, F18 displayed broad antiviral activities against various isolated HIV-1 strains in the clinic. As with natural compound 1, F18 did not inhibit SIV either.

664 Medicinal Chemistry and Drug Development

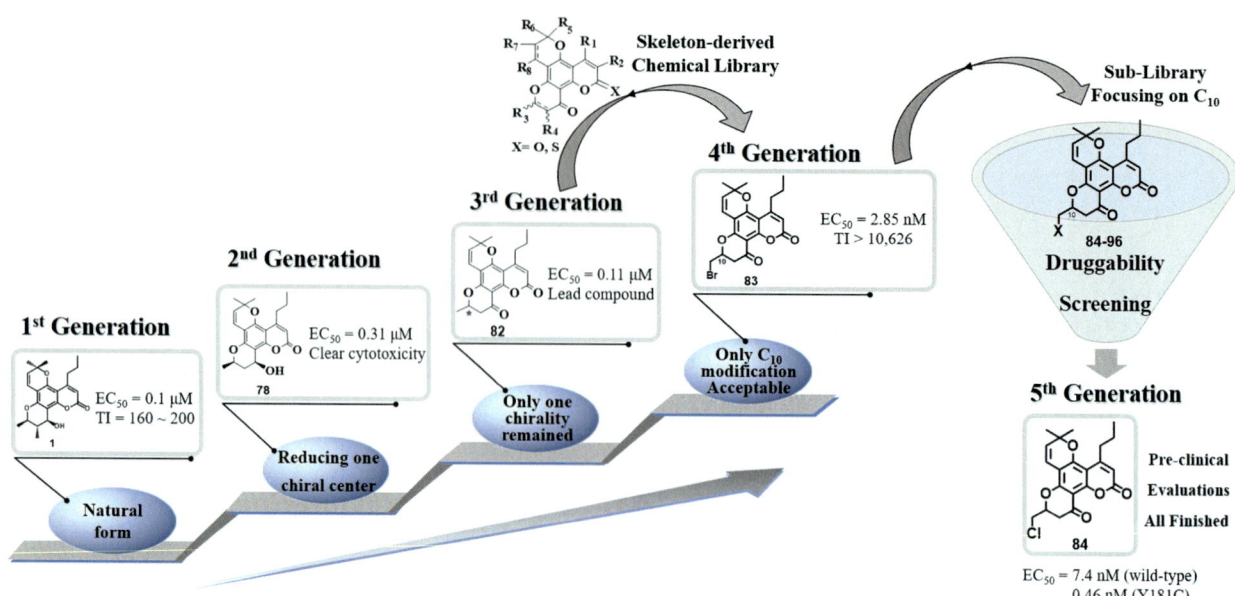

FIGURE 27.11 Evolution of active calanolide analogs and identification of drug candidate 84 (F18).

The virus-resistant strains induced by F18 in vitro under drug-pressure screening mainly produced the L100I mutation rather than the T139I mutation induced by natural 1, which is also different from the resistance mutation sites of other clinically used NNRTIs. Therefore, F18 has different resistance characteristics compared to other NNRTIs. Y181C, the most prevalent mutation induced by NVP in the clinic, was highly sensitive to F18, with an $EC_{50} = 1.0$ nmol/L, suggesting that the interaction between F18 and the NNRTI binding pocket may differ from NVP. According to the in silico docking analysis, the mutation of tyrosine 181 to cysteine results in the rotation of F18 in the binding pocket and the formation of a new hydrogen bond between the chlorine residue of F18 and cysteine 181 of RT, therefore improving the antiviral activity of F18 against the Y181C mutant. However, the Y181 mutation abolished the binding of NVP to RT due to a lack of π-π interactions. Additionally, F18 also exhibited excellent antiviral activity in inhibiting other clinically prevalent mutations, such as V106A, G190A, or the multiple mutation K103N/Y181C/G190A [48].

Since combination therapy with at least three antiretrovirals (ARVs) has become the gold standard for HIV-1 treatment, drug-drug interactions should be a key issue to be considered in drug development. F18 does not exert antagonistic effects on the other 8 ARVs (AZT/ddI/d4T/3TC/NVP/EFV/NFV/RAL) when used in two-drug combinations to treat both wild-type and drug-resistant viruses. Interestingly, F18 exerts strongly synergistic effects with NVP, AZT, and 3TC against NVP-, AZT-, and 3TC-resistant viruses, respectively. Overall, F18 is an ideal ARV candidate for treating HIV-1-infected patients [49].

The enantio-separation of racemic ($\pm$)-F18 into (R)-F18 and (S)-F18 was achieved with a chiral stationary phase using high-performance liquid chromatography (HPLC), and their absolute configurations were determined by measuring their electronic circular dichroism spectra, combined with modern quantum-chemical calculations (Fig. 27.12) [50]. Further investigations revealed that (R)-F18 was more potent than (S)-F18 against the virus; for the wild-type HIV-1 virus strain (pNL4-3 WT), the activity was about 7.4 times higher (refer to the first row of data in Table 27.6). The activity of (R)-F18 against other single- and double-resistant site virus strains was also stronger than (S)-F18 but ineffective against the three resistant sites (V106A/G190A/F227L) virus strains.

The large-scale industrial synthesis route of ($\pm$)-F18 was optimized, and the route shown in Fig. 27.13 was established for the preparation of ($\pm$)-F18 at the kg level. This route adopts the same method as the synthesis of a chemical library to build rings B and C and then utilizes the classic Friedel Crafts acylation reaction to finally establish the D ring under Lewis acid ($AlCl_3$) catalysis and alkaline conditions.

The metabolic profile and the results of associated biochemical studies of ($\pm$)-F18 in vitro and in vivo were reported by our collaborators [51]. Through studies, twenty-three metabolites of F18 were detected after incubation by human liver microsomes. The metabolism of F18 involved C_4-propyl chain oxidation, 10-chloromethyl oxidative de-chlorination, and 12-carbonyl reduction. Three other metabolites (99, 101, and 102, Fig. 27.14) were also detected in rat blood after the oral administration of F18. The oxidative metabolism of F18 was mainly catalyzed by cytochrome P450 3A4 in human microsomes; therefore, attention should be paid when used in combination with CYP450 3A4 inhibitor drugs in the clinic.

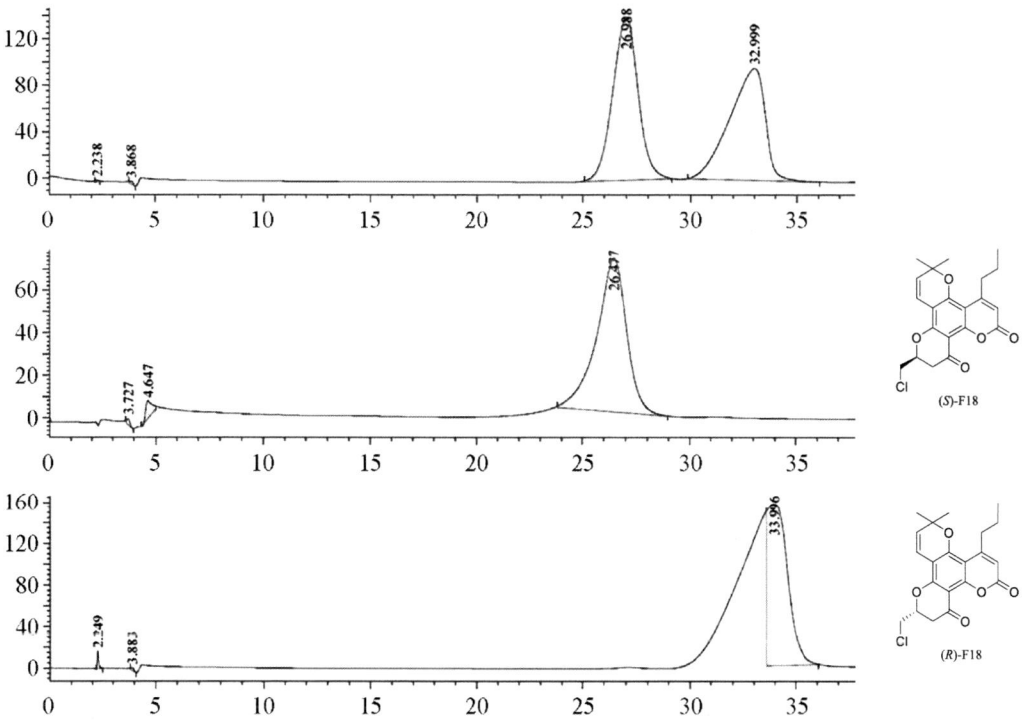

FIGURE 27.12 Chemical structures of (R)-F18 (bottom panel) and (S)-F18 (middle panel) and chromatograms of enantiomers (top panel).

TABLE 27.6 In vitro antiviral activity of (±)-F18, (S)-F18, and (R)-F18 against the NNRTI-resistant HIV-1 pseudo-virus in the GHOST (3)-CCR5 cell line.

Virus	EC$_{50}$ (95%CI) [μmol/L]		
	(±)-F18	(S)-F18	(R)-F18
pNL4–3 WT	0.027 (0.0193–0.0372)	0.126 (0.0845–0.1876)	0.017 (0.0112–0.0249)
L100I	0.932 (0.6683–1.2990)	1.178 (0.3938–3.5240)	0.702 (0.4249–1.1600)
K101E	0.259 (0.1220–0.5478)	2.816 (0.5352–14.810)	0.293 (0.1977–0.4333)
K103N	0.576 (0.3786–0.8753)	1.228 (0.6127–2.4630)	0.565 (0.4052–0.7888)
V106A	0.045 (0.0311–0.0646)	0.120 (0.0727–0.1978)	0.082 (0.0599–0.1110)
T139I	0.131 (0.1042–0.3325)	0.415 (0.1134–20.170)	0.079 (0.0688–0.1534)
T139R	1.188 (0.7470–1.3574)	3.413 (3.0786–3.7529)	0.616 (0.4659–0.8148)
V179D	0.019 (0.0143–0.0260)	0.068 (0.0606–0.0922)	0.016 (0.0124–0.0200)
Y181C	0.001 (0.0009–0.0013)	0.006 (0.0042–0.0076)	0.001 (0.0004–0.0007)
Y188H	>6	>6	>6
Y188L	>6	>6	>6
G190A	0.534 (0.3902–0.7299)	1.127 (0.6862–1.8490)	0.352 (0.2373–0.5212)
P225H	0.474 (0.3820–0.5871)	2.387 (1.4430–3.9480)	0.256 (0.1594–0.4127)
K103N/P225H	0.008 (0.0045–0.0138)	0.014 (0.0093–0.0206)	0.007 (0.0051–0.0093)
K103N/Y181C	>6	>6	>6
K103N/Y181C/G190A	0.092 (0.0645–0.1304)	0.075 (0.0480–0.1185)	0.138 (0.0764–0.2493)
V106A/F227L	0.658 (0.2779–1.5560)	1.430 (0.4908–4.1670)	0.565 (0.4777–0.6671)
V106A/G190A/F227L	>6	>6	>6

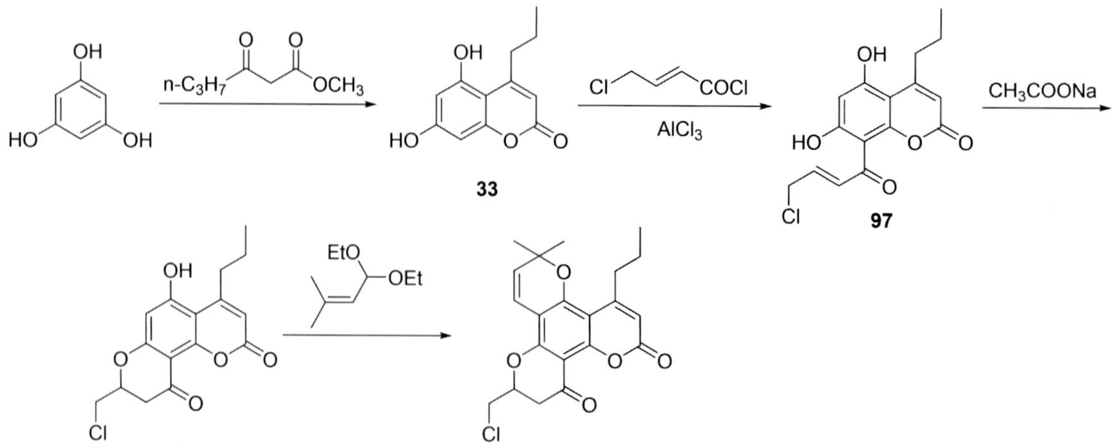

FIGURE 27.13 Synthetic route for the large-scale synthesis of (±)-F18.

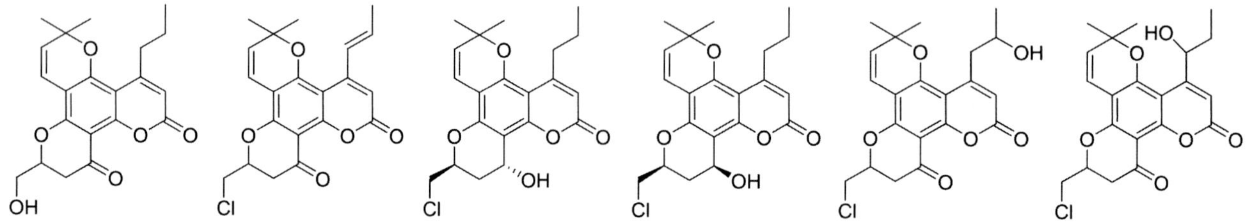

FIGURE 27.14 The structures of main metabolites of F18 in vivo.

27.4 (+)-Calanolide A and its derivatives inhibit replicating and non-replicating *Mycobacterium tuberculosis*

27.4.1 Natural product 1 as an anti-*Mycobacterium tuberculosis* compound

In 2004, it was alternatively found that 1 could inhibit the proliferation of the Mycobacterium tuberculosis (*Mtb*) H37RV strain (Fig. 27.15), employing the BACTEC 460 radioactive isotope technology [52]. Among the tested tetracyclic bis-pyran coumarin natural products, the minimum inhibitory concentration (MIC) range, inhibiting 99% of bacterial growth, fell between 3.1 and 6.3 μg/mL. The cytotoxicity of compounds against VERO cells exhibited an IC_{50} value ranging from 6.6 to 10 μg/mL. Of note, 1 exhibited a relatively favorable selective index (IC_{50}/MIC value) of 2.46. Further modified analogs of 1 were synthesized to increase their antimicrobial activity while reducing cytotoxicity. Nevertheless, the outcomes of these modifications were not deemed satisfactory [53].

Starting with compound 1, researchers proceeded with the SAR studies. It has been confirmed that the 12-OH tetrahydropyran at ring D is an integral component for maintaining antimicrobial activity. When it is 12-ketone at ring D, the antimicrobial activity against the H37Rv strain was missed almost completely, which is showcased by compounds 36, 37, and 106 (Fig. 27.15). Researchers further explored diverse substitutions for the D-ring, aiming to identify new active compounds. Surprisingly, compounds obtained by replacing the D-ring of 1 with a nitrofuran ring demonstrated high inhibitory activity against *Mtb* (such as 123, depicted in Fig. 27.18 below). Attractively, it displayed effectiveness against both replicating H37Rv strain (R-*Mtb*) and nonreplicating *Mtb* (non-replicating (NR)-*Mtb*) (Note: NR-*Mtb* refers to the latent Mycobacterium tuberculosis, which exhibits very slow metabolism and strong drug resistance), and therefore, these compounds represent a novel class of compounds for an anti-*Mtb* activity that will be discussed in detail in the third part of this section.

In another aspect, compound 1 also seems promising for further studies. It can inhibit a wide variety of drug-resistant strains of *Mtb*, including isoniazid (INH), rifampin, streptomycin, and ethambutol (EMB), with MIC values ranging from 8.0 to 16.0 μg/mL. The following interesting finding was that 1 exhibited good inhibitory activity against

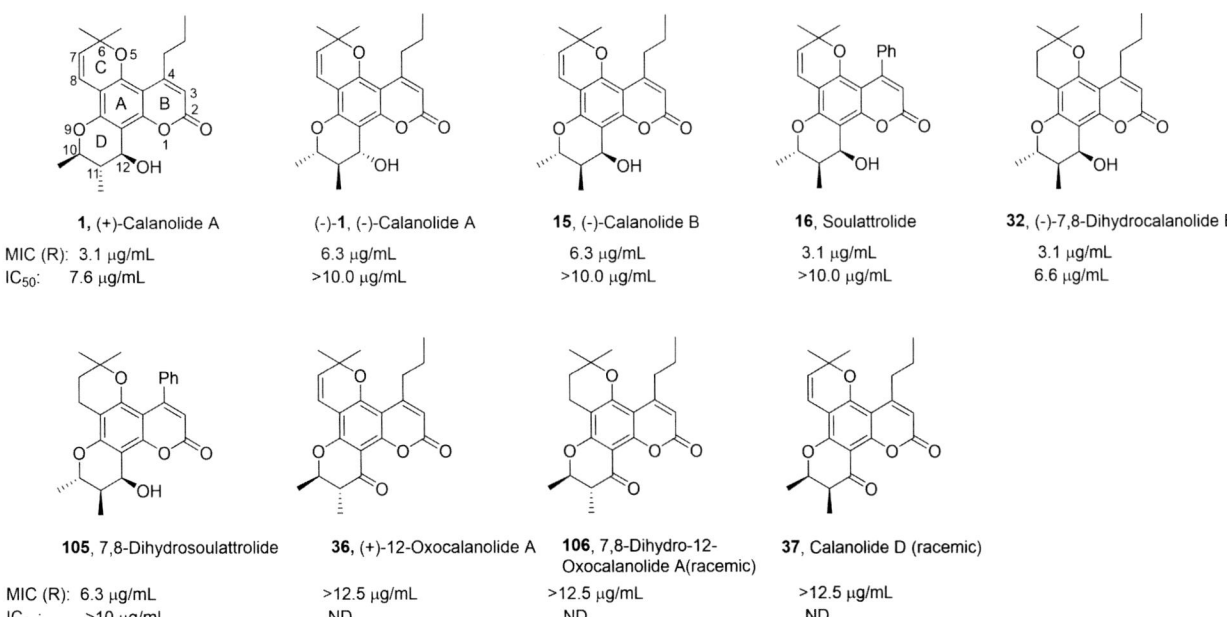

FIGURE 27.15 Antimicrobial activity of natural 1 and other tetracyclic pyranocoumarins (*Mtb* strain: H37Rv).

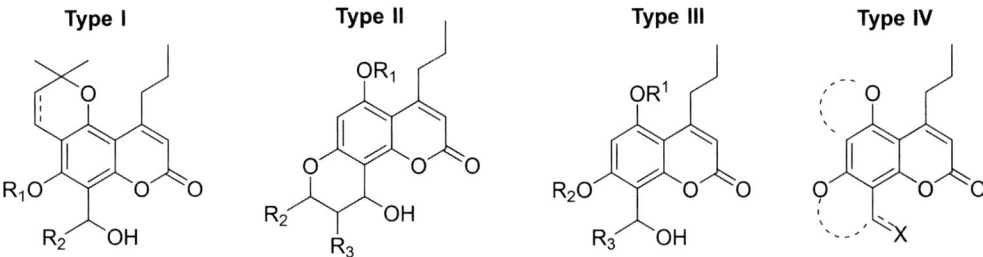

FIGURE 27.16 The preliminary four-type modifications.

intracellular bacteria in three macrophage-based screening assays, including J774, MM6, and bone marrow-derived murine macrophages, with MIC values ranging from 1.0 to 2.0 μg/mL, indicating that these compounds can readily penetrate host macrophage membranes and effectively destroy intracellular *Mtb*. These preliminary results are meaningful because *Mtb* infections in the human body are primarily found within macrophages, especially in lung macrophages, but in a latent state. This type of compound can likely shorten the clinical treatment period for tuberculosis (TB) patients by inhibiting both replicating and latent *Mtb*. In the meantime, compound 1 was disclosed to affect the ribonucleic acid (RNA) and deoxyribonucleic acid (DNA) synthesis of *Mtb*. The mechanism of action is believed to be like that of the first-line antituberculosis drug, rifampin, which is considered a DNA-dependent RNA polymerase inhibitor [52]. (Note: Generally, experiments conducted using cells, tissues, organs, etc., taken from living organisms are referred to as ex vivo experiments. The Latin term "in vivo" means "within the living," referring to inside a living organism; "in vitro" means "within the glass," referring to inside a glass container; and "ex vivo" means "out of the living," referring to outside a living organism.).

27.4.2 Preliminary structural modifications [53]

Through conducting SAR studies, four-type modifications, as depicted in Fig. 27.16, were designed and investigated with a primary focus on simplifying the natural molecule structure. Fig. 27.17 illustrates that all compounds essentially lost their inhibitory activity against *Mtb*. Notably, compound 111, which replaced the 12-OH group of 1 with -NH_2, also displayed a loss of activity, implying that an amine moiety was not tolerable at the C_{12} position in respect of anti-*Mtb* activity.

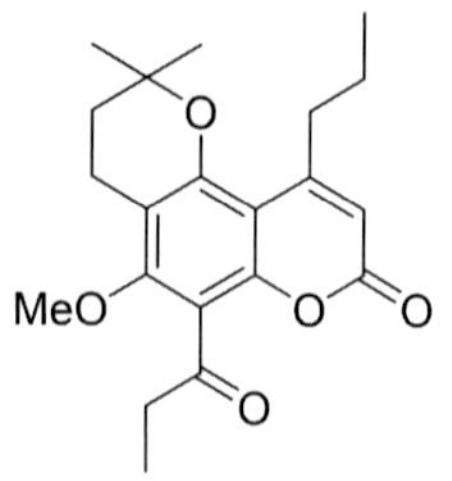

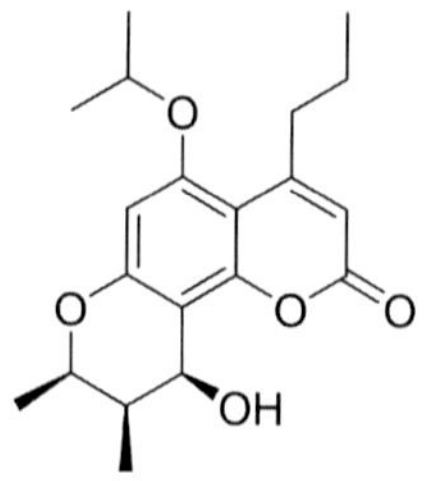

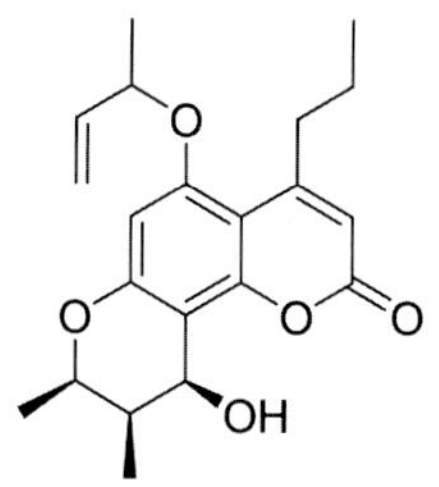

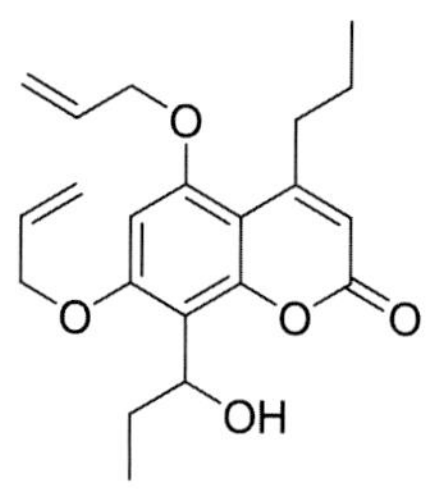

668 Medicinal Chemistry and Drug Development

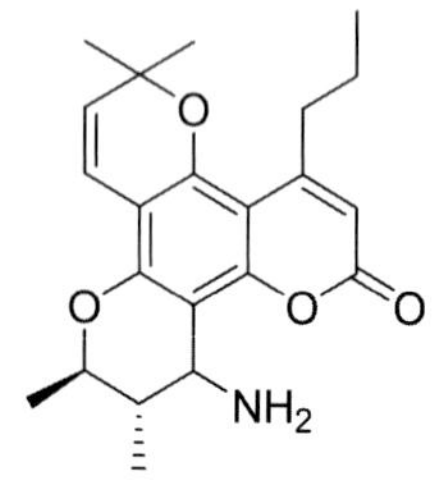

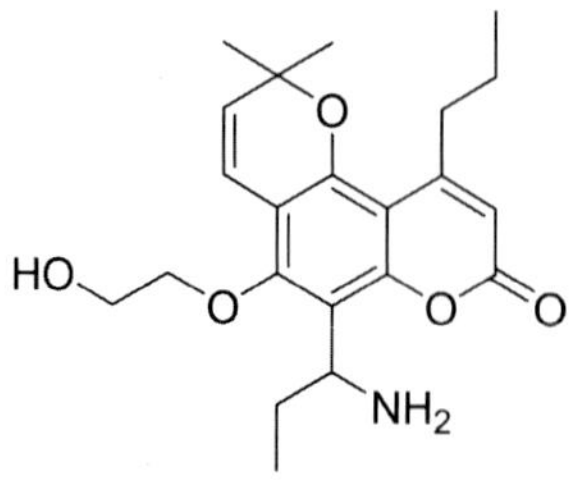

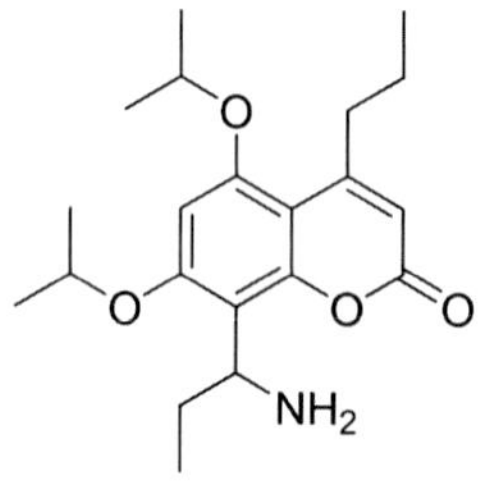

FIGURE 27.17 The evaluated compounds for the preliminary SAR studies.

27.4.3 The discovered and optimized tetrahydropyranocoumarins derived from the nitrofuran moiety exhibit potent activity against both R-*Mycobacterium tuberculosis* and NR-*Mycobacterium tuberculosis* [54]

The presence of NR-*Mtb* (latent TB) along with the emergence of drug-resistant TB have become great challenges to tackle, and have some public health issues. In response to this need, Professor Carl F. Nathan et al. at Cornell University's Medical College have developed a high-throughput screening assay under a B2 level laboratory that is capable of simultaneously reporting anti-R-*Mtb* and anti-NR-*Mtb* activities. It built into an advantage of the model by leveraging the inactivated strain, mc26220 Δ panCD Δ lysA. mc26220 Δ panCD Δ lysA lack of infectivity; however, it can be extensively utilized in B2-level bio-laboratories. The tetrahydropyranocoumarins synthesized by the authors of this chapter were tested readily with this assay. The results showed the compounds depicted in Fig. 27.18 displayed promising inhibitory activity against R-*Mtb* and NR-*Mtb*. The analogs without a D-ring and the analogs substituted at the C_9-position gained a moderate inhibitory activity range (MIC_{90} = 2.0−23 µg/mL, 114−121). Compounds featured a "3-oxo-furan" on the D-ring, also exhibiting moderate anti-R-*Mtb* activity (MIC_{90} = 6.3 µg/mL, 122). Surprisingly, a group of compounds with a D-ring replaced by 2-nitrofuran (123) demonstrated strong inhibitory activity against both R-*Mtb* (MIC_{90} = 0.31 µg/mL) and NR-*Mtb* (MIC_{90} = 0.625 µg/mL). Further evaluation of the cytotoxicity in HepG2 liver cells revealed an IC_{50} value of 2.5 µg/mL, resulting in a selectivity index of 4−8. For the synthesis of these compounds, please refer to Ref. [55].

The researchers proceed with the thorough SARs of 123. The elaboration based on 123 includes: (1) systematic incorporation of various substituents (124x) at different positions (Fig. 27.19); (2) saturated the C = C double bonds in ring B and C (125 and 126); (3) 3-hydroxy-2-nitro-dihydrofuran (127); (4) opening of ring C (128x); (5) removal of the nitro group (130); (6) varying the linkage between the nitrofuran moiety and the coumarin scaffold (129, 131, and 132). Notably, compound 128a exhibited a remarkable improvement in activity with a 16-fold increase, achieving an MIC value of 0.08 µg/mL. Its activity against NR-*Mtb* also increased, with a MIC value of 0.2 µg/mL. The compound displayed an IC_{50} value of 10 µg/mL in HepG2 liver cells, resulting in an increased selectivity index of 50−125 (Fig. 27.20).

Further studies of the SARs, as shown in Fig. 27.20, revealed that 3-hydroxy-2-nitro-dihydrofurans (133a and 133b) presented similar antimycobacterial activity, but they also displayed higher cytotoxicity. Compounds with substitutions at the C_5 position (134 and 135) and compounds with fused B-ring structures (136 and 137) maintained certain antimicrobial activity but failed to improve the selectivity index as well. Compounds obtained through other modifications of the nitrofuran structure showed a significant decrease in antimicrobial activity (138−144) [54,55], implicating that the nitrofuran moiety is crucial for antimicrobial activity.

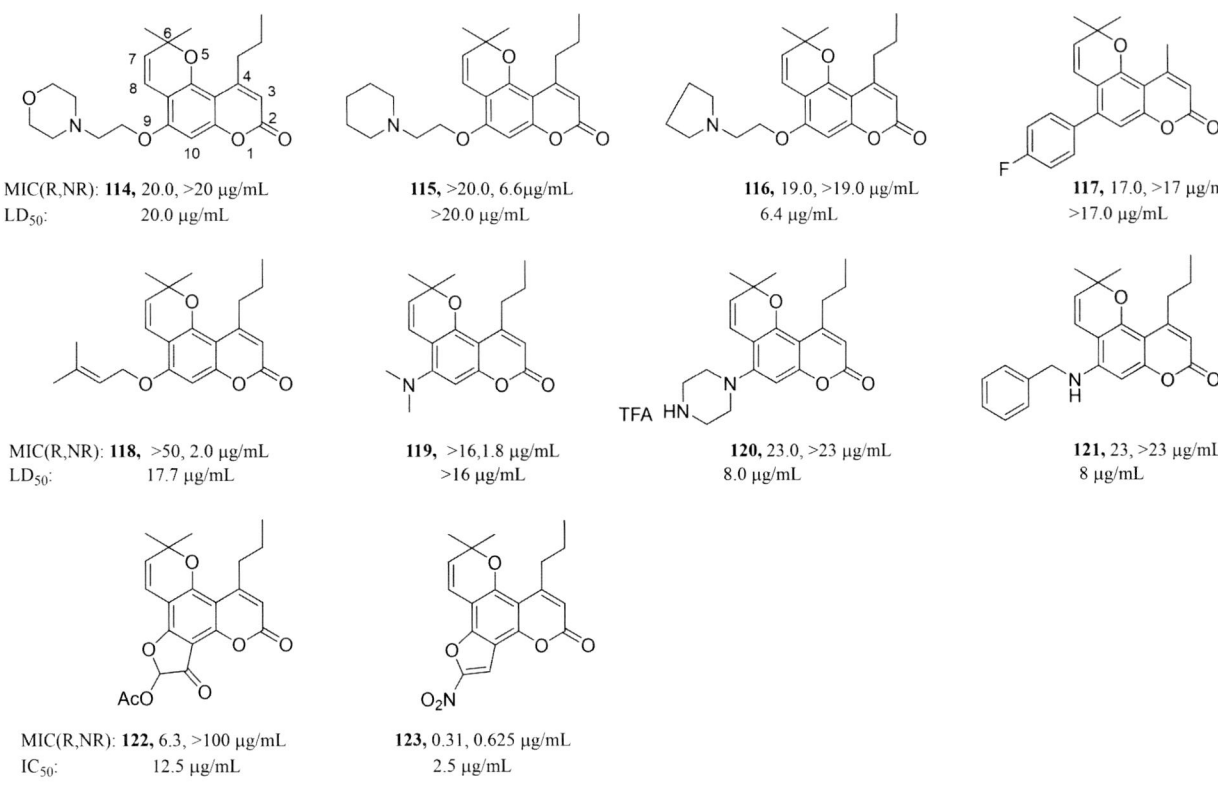

FIGURE 27.18 The antimicrobial activity of compound 123, a 2-nitrofuran derivative, was first discovered.

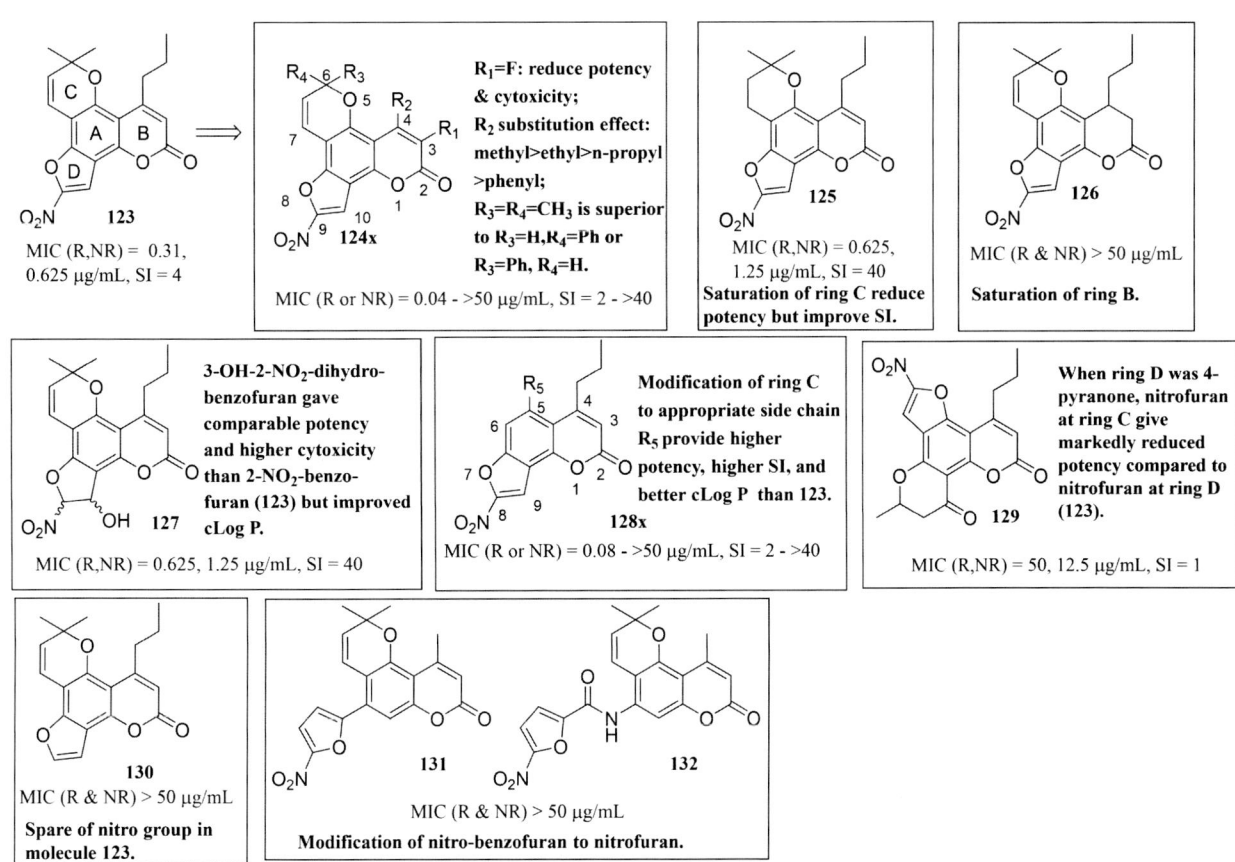

FIGURE 27.19 The structural optimization of compound 123 and its corresponding SARs.

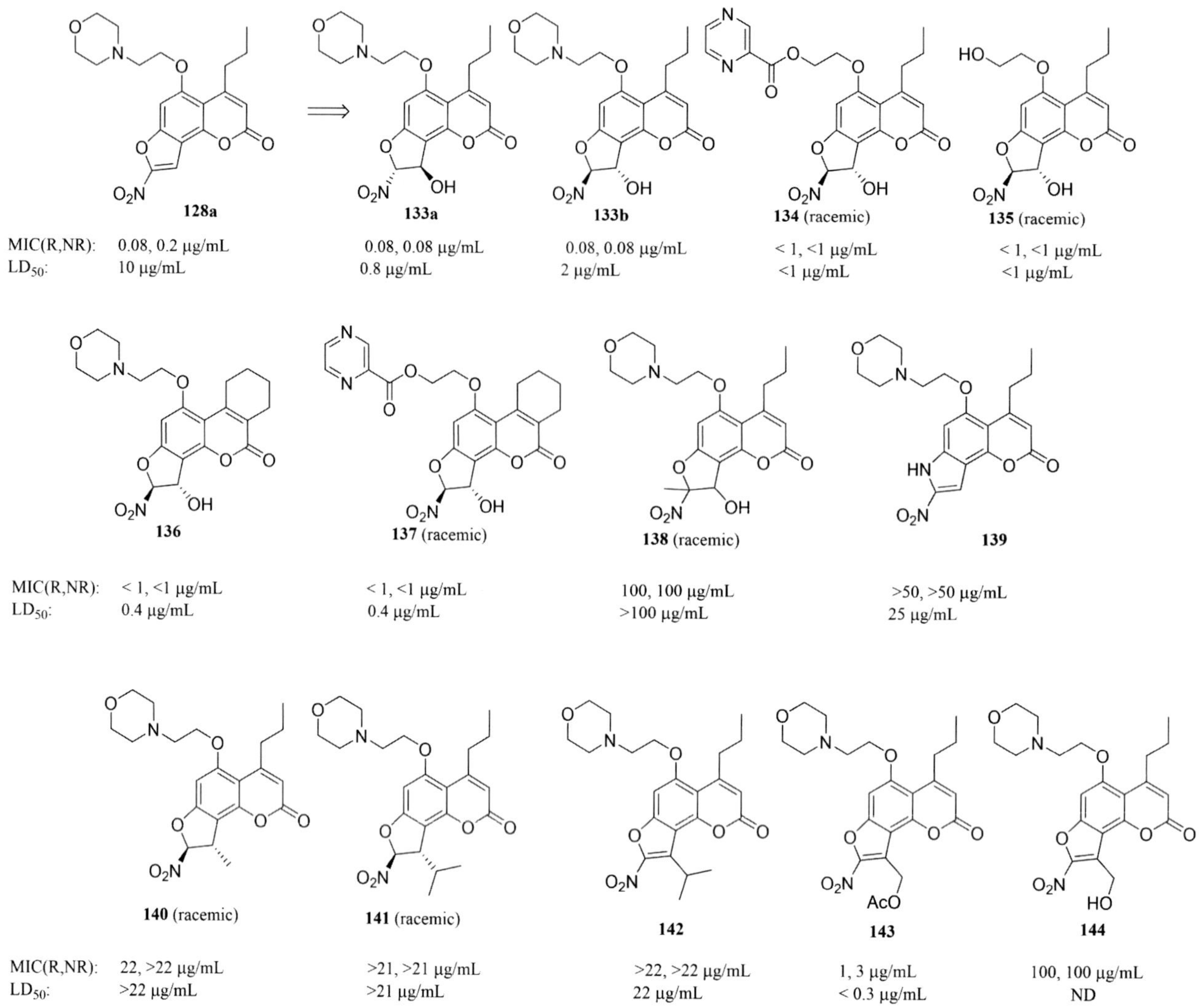

FIGURE 27.20 Antimicrobial activity of nitrofuran-based tetracyclic coumarin derivatives.

The compounds 123 and 125 demonstrated meaningful results by inhibiting the wild-type strain of *Mtb* in human macrophages. They were able to reduce bacterial growth by an average logarithmic value of 2−4 (2−4 log10) at a concentration of 1.0 μg/mL. Furthermore, at a testing concentration of 25 μg/mL, they did not show any inhibitory activity against *Escherichia coli*, *Staphylococcus aureus*, *Pseudomonas aeruginosa*, and *Candida albicans*, indicating a favorable anti-*Mtb* selectivity. Unfortunately, further investigations indicated that both compounds 123 and 128a exhibited genotoxicity that was believed to be caused by the α,β-unsaturated structure of the nitrofuran, which acts as a Michael acceptor in a nonspecific manner with potential reactive species in the body, including donors such as amino groups, thiol groups, and glutathione on proteins. This nonspecific addition reaction may lead to unpredictable safety issues, eventually necessitating the termination of the development steps for such compounds.

27.4.4 Mechanism of antibacterial activity of tetrahydrobenzopyran nitrofuran derivatives

The intriguing anti-*Mtb* activities sparked the interest of researchers to explore the antibacterial mechanism of tetrahydrobenzopyran nitrofuran coumarins (NFCs). Researchers generated multiple bacterial clones resistant to compound 125 using Mycobacterium bovis and Bacillus calmette-Guérin (BCG) as model bacteria. The analysis of these resistant clones through whole-genome sequencing revealed that rv2466c, a nitroreductase code gene, was the only mutated gene among the 18 clones that interestingly remained sensitive to other anti-TB drugs. (Note: due to the heterogeneity of bacterial populations under experimental conditions, multiple resistant clones can emerge under drug pressure (such as by giving certain drug concentrations), including clones with mutations at the same or different resistant sites.). Further experiments confirmed that BCG with the rv2466c gene knocked out exhibited resistance to compound 125; however, when the wild-type rv2466c gene was complemented into the resistant clone (W181C mutation), the bacteria regained sensitivity to compound 125. Overexpression of the wild-type rv2466c gene also increased the sensitivity of the new strain to compound 125 by 2–4 times. These results strongly indicated that the Rv2466c protein, encoded by the rv2466c gene, is the target of NFC compounds.

The hypothesis is then that the antibacterial activity of 125 is achieved through the reduction of its nitro group, leading to the release of reactive oxygen species. Subsequently, wild-type *M. smegmatis (M. smeg)* and *M. smeg* strains with rv2466c gene mutations were coincubated with compound 125. The bacterial lysates were analyzed using HPLC-mass spectrometry (HPLC-Ms) to detect changes in the concentration of 125. In the lysate of wild-type *M. smeg*, a new ultraviolet absorption peak was detected, and its molecular weight matched the chemical structure of the fully reduced product, 125-NH_2 (125b) (Fig. 27.21A). This was accompanied by a decrease in the ultraviolet absorption peak of compound 125 over time and an increase in the ultraviolet absorption peak of the reduced product. In contrast, this observation was not detectable in the lysate of the mutant strain. Through the synthesized reference compounds, the researchers ultimately confirmed that compound 125 was indeed reduced to the corresponding amino compound 125b in the lysate of the wild-type bacteria, with some detecting much less 125a, 125c, and 125d by liquid chromatography (LC)-Ms analysis (Fig. 27.21).

Reduction of compound 125 by *Mtb* happened in the presence of nitroreductase (Rv2466c) and was believed to require cofactors, given that the reduction of compound 125 solely occurred within the lysate of bacteria rather than under a pure recombinant Rv2466c enzyme environment. Literature suggests that the majority of known nitroreductases rely on deazaflavins or flavin-based cofactors, such as flavin adenine dinucleotide or flavin mononucleotide [56]. However, experimental studies proved that Rv2466c does not rely on these typical cofactors to facilitate its reduction of 125. Subsequent studies involved the fractionation of the bacterial lysate from wild-type *M. smegs via* size exclusion spin column chromatography, followed by coincubation with 125. Finally, researchers identified a low molecular weight auxiliary factor, namely mycothiol (mycothiol (MSH), 160), which was able to effectively assist Rv2466c undergoing reduction, which is a small thiol compound secreted by streptomycetes. The chemical structure of mycothiol can be referred to Fig. 27.22 [57].

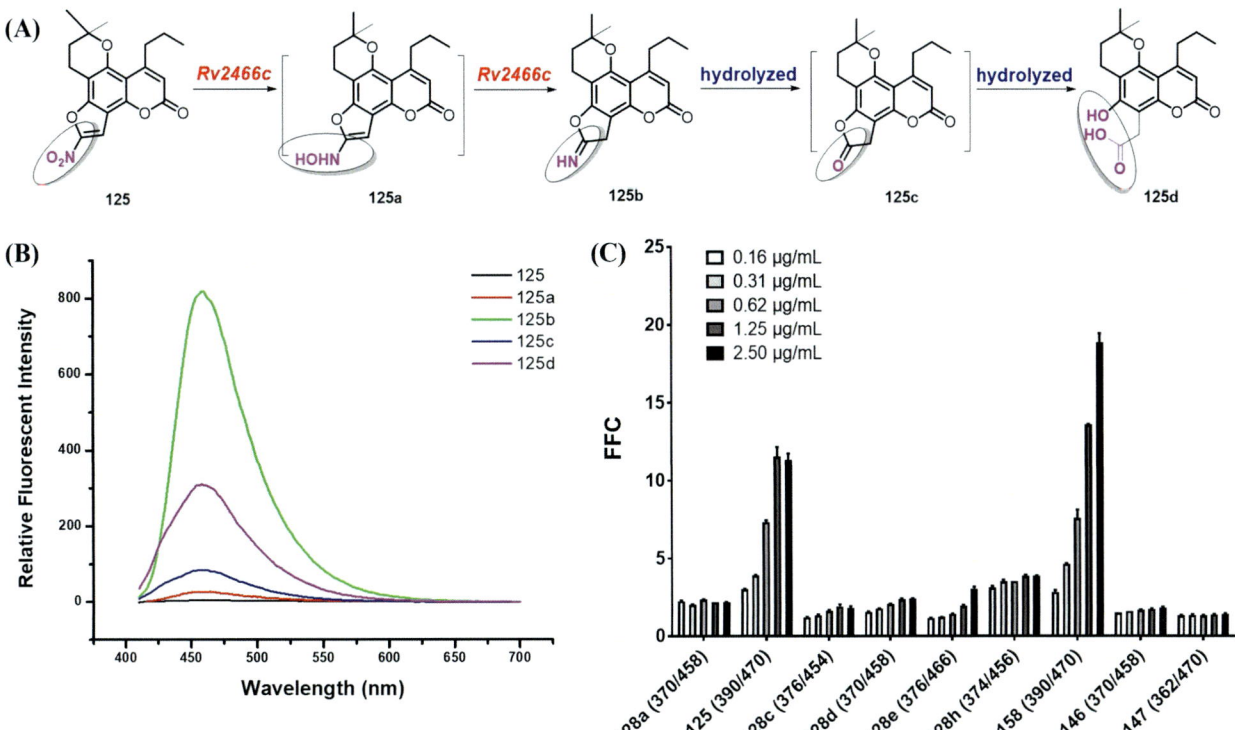

FIGURE 27.21 (A) HPLC-Ms analysis of the reduction products of compound 125 in the bacterial lysate of *M. smeg*. (B) Fluorescence emission spectra and intensity of these reduced and hydrolysis species. (C) When exposed to wild-type BCG bacteria, notable fluorescence changes (FFC), as well as the corresponding excitation and emission wavelengths, can be detected in the extracellular environment for compounds 125 and 158.

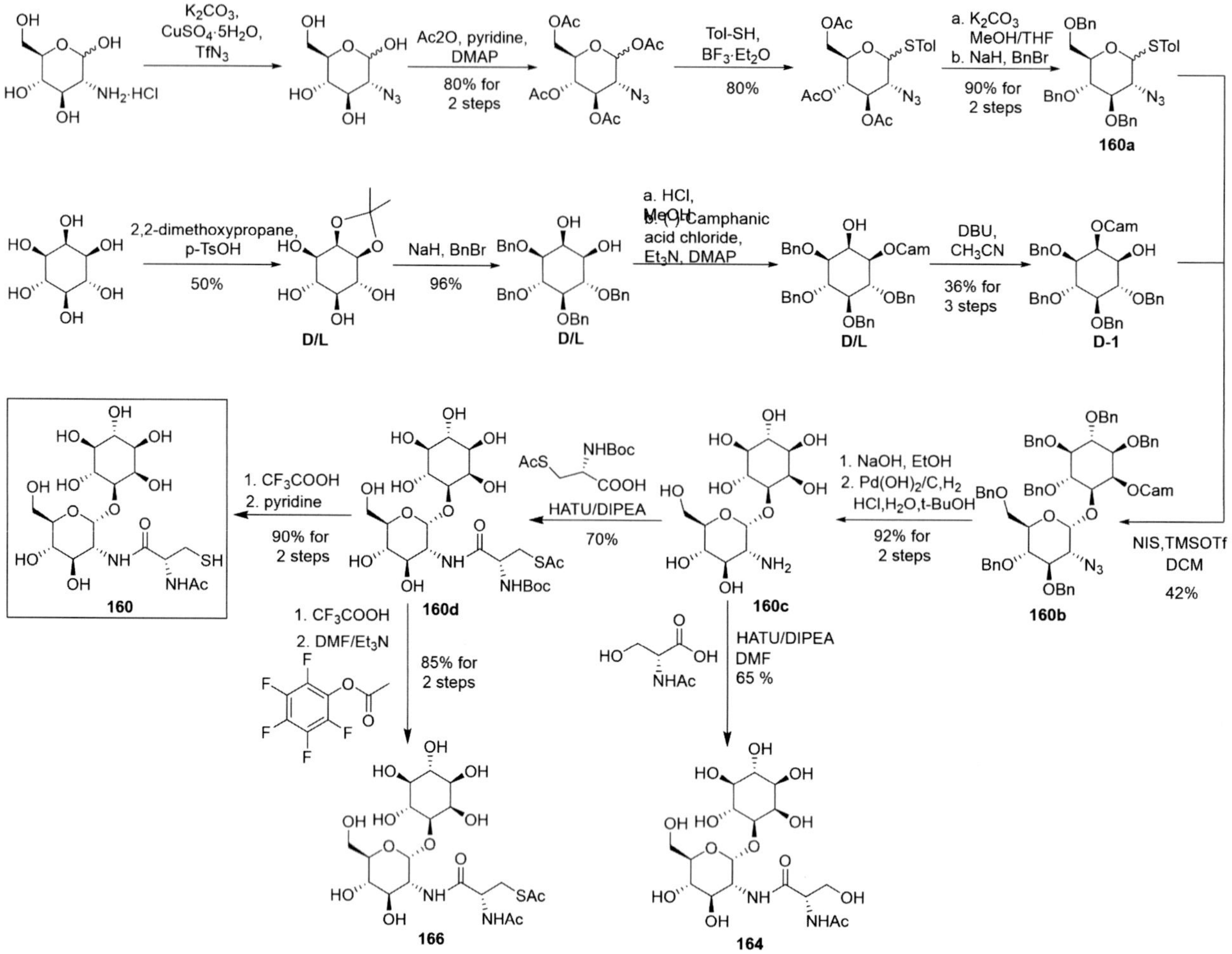

FIGURE 27.22 Synthetic route for MSH and its derivatives (compounds 164 and 166).

27.5 Fluorescent activity of nitrofuran derivatives: a revelatory outcome

27.5.1 Relationship between structure and molecular fluorescence activity

When a push electron-containing heteroatom substitutes for the C_7 position in a coumarin molecule, it is commonly referred to as a fluorophore [58]. NFC molecules possess the core structure of coumarin (A/B rings) with an oxygen heteroatom at the C_7 position (furan structure). At this point, researchers began to recognize that NFC molecules may also exhibit fluorescent properties. However, the strong electron-withdrawing nitro group may quench the fluorescence activity of NFC molecules due to its photo-induced electron transfer (PET) effect. Conversely, reduced molecules, such as keeping an amino group in compound 125b, may serve as an electron-donating group and diminish the nitro's PET, which could reopen the fluorescence from a quenched state (off). When a fluorescent molecule is excited, electrons in the highest occupied molecular orbital (HOMO) transition to the lowest unoccupied molecular orbital (LUMO), and subsequent fluorescence occurs as electrons in the LUMO transition back to the HOMO. Intramolecular charge transfer refers to the charge transfer within a molecule due to uneven distribution. In the case of coumarin molecules, an electron-donating group at the C_7 position, such as -OH or -NH_2, can induce intramolecular charge transfer from the C_7 position to the C_3 position, resulting in fluorescence. The nitro group of NFCs precisely prevents this charge transfer process due to its PET effect, leading to fluorescence quenching. Based on the above consideration, NFC molecules might be promising for the fluorescence diagnostic reagents for *Mtb*, as displayed in Fig. 27.23, with their dual anti-R-*Mtb* and anti-NR-*Mtb* activities. Researchers then coincubated the NFC molecules in Fig. 27.23 with recombinant Rv2466c and MSH in vitro and attempted to observe the changes in fluorescence (fluorescent fold change, FFC). For those molecules exhibiting strong fluorescence activity, they were further cocultured in a dose-dependent manner with BCG, and the FFC was calculated (Fig. 27.21C). Researchers were delighted to find that compounds 125 and 158 demonstrated significant fluorescence off-to-on activity [59]. Through synthesis, they obtained potential reduction products of compound 125 and

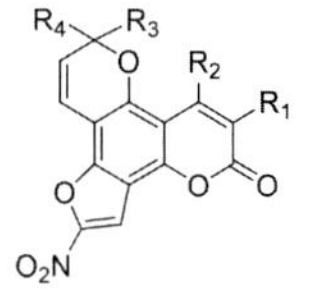

FIGURE 27.23 Molecule structures of compounds with fluorescence activity in the presence of recombinant Rv2466c and MSH that evaluated for anti-R-*Mtb* and NR-*Mtb* activity.

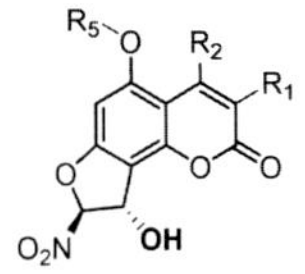

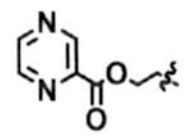

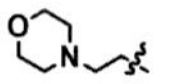

124x

Compounds	R₁	R₂	R₃	R₄
124a	H	methyl	H	H
124b	H	n-propyl	Ph	H
124c	H	morpholinyl	H	H

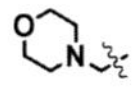

Compounds	R₅	R₂	R₁
133b	morpholinyl	n-propyl	H
134	pyrazine-carbonyloxy	n-propyl	H
146	morpholinyl	cyclopentyl	
147	morpholinyl	cyclohexyl	

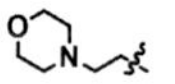

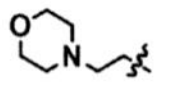

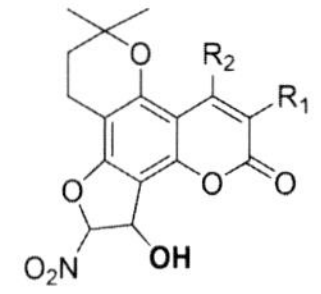

Compounds	R₁	R₂
148	H	n-propyl
149		cyclohexyl
150		cyclopentyl
151	F	methyl

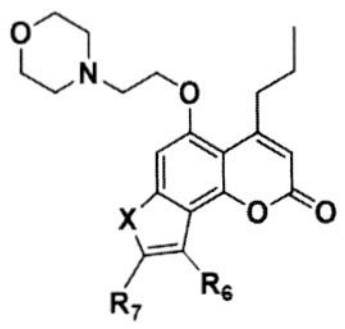

Compounds	X	R₆	R₇
139	NH	H	NO₂
142	O	isopropyl	NO₂
143	O	AcO-CH₂	NO₂
153	O	H	CN

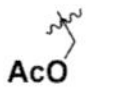

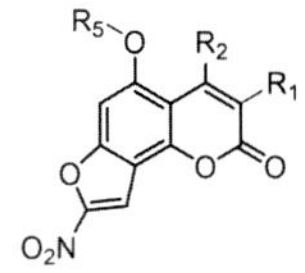

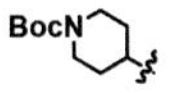

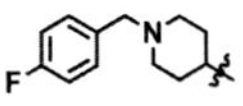

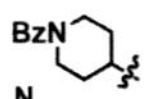

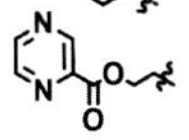

Compounds	R₅	R₂	R₁
145	H	n-propyl	H
128a	morpholinyl	n-propyl	H
128b	methyl	n-propyl	H
128c	TFA⁺H₂N-piperidinyl	n-propyl	H
128d	BocN-piperidinyl	n-propyl	H
128e	F-benzyl-piperidinyl	n-propyl	H
128f	BzN-piperidinyl	n-propyl	H
128g	pyrazine-carbonyloxy	n-propyl	H
128h	HO-	n-propyl	H
128i	morpholinyl	cyclopentyl	
128j	morpholinyl	cyclohexyl	
128k	-Ac	methyl	H
128l	methyl	methyl	H

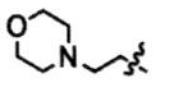

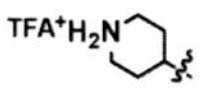

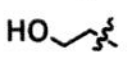

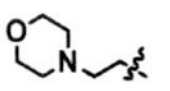

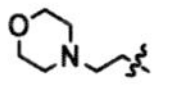

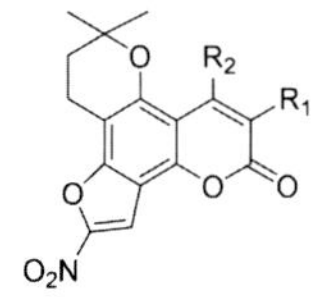

Compounds	R₁	R₂
125	H	n-propyl
152	F	methyl

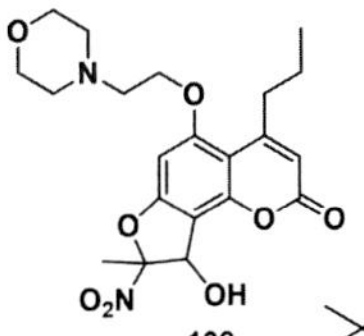

138   154   155   156   157   158   159

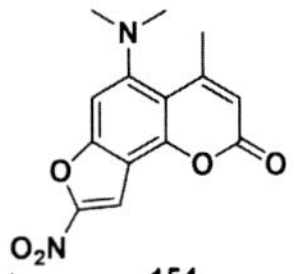

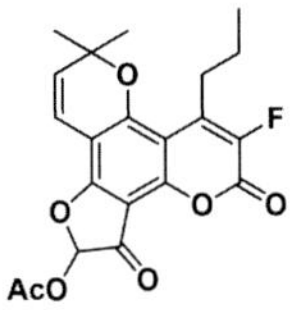

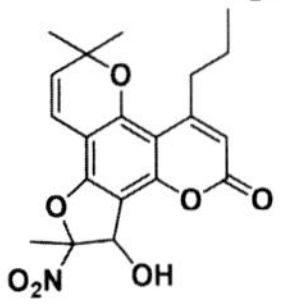

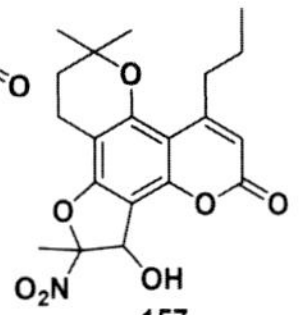

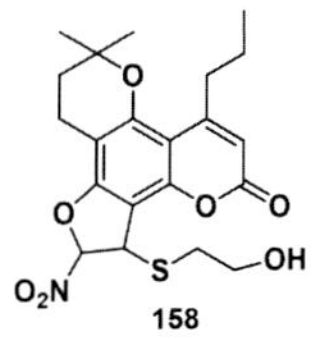

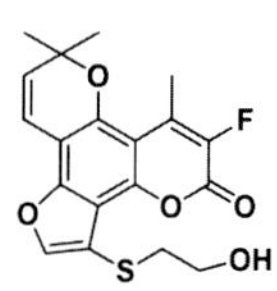

secondary hydrolysis products in the bacterial culture system, namely compounds 125a to 125d (Fig. 27.21A). The results demonstrated that 125b (compound 125-NH$_2$) was the primary fluorescent product, with a 220-fold increase in fluorescence intensity after reduction at the enzyme level. Since compound 159 itself had no fluorescence activity under Rv2466c and MSH reductive conditions, researchers believed that the 158 molecule might be fluorescently functionalized after thioether was hydrolyzed to 125 in the medium, thereby exhibiting fluorescence activity as a prodrug.

27.5.2 How do nitrofuran compounds interact with Rv2466c and mycothiol (160)

Previous experiments proved that the reduction of NFC-like compounds by Rv2466c requires the assistance of a cofactor, mycothiol (MSH). However, understanding the intricacies of their interactions has become a new point of interest for researchers. Employing computer-assisted docking methods, researchers conducted docking simulations of 28 NFC compounds with Rv2466c, employing a modified noncovalent approach (Schrodinger, Inc.: Maestro v10.7, 2016) (Fig. 27.24A) [59]. The predictions revealed that Rv2466c might interact with 11 amino acid residues of Rv2466c, including P20, W21, N51, R54, Y61, H104, T153, R200, Q205, D150, and V151. Subsequently, 11 predicted mutant Rv2466c proteins were generated and prepared, and the compound 128c, chosen for its good solubility, was used as a tool molecule to study the potential interactions due to the fact that Rv2466c can also reduce it to the corresponding 128c-NH$_2$. Fluorescence functional experiments (Fig. 27.24B) and differential scanning fluorimetry (DSF; Fig. 27.24C) were conducted, revealing that residues W21, N51, and Y61 played crucial roles in forming the stable ternary complex Rv2466c-MSH-NFC (RvMN). These residues were found to be actively involved in the interaction with compound 128c (Fig. 27.24B, C, and D) [59]. The DSF results of other mutated proteins were not presented, and readers interested in further details are encouraged to refer to the literature [59]. DSF is a method for evaluating the thermal stability of proteins by detecting the fluorescence dye binding signal during a slow temperature increase. When the protein structure collapses,

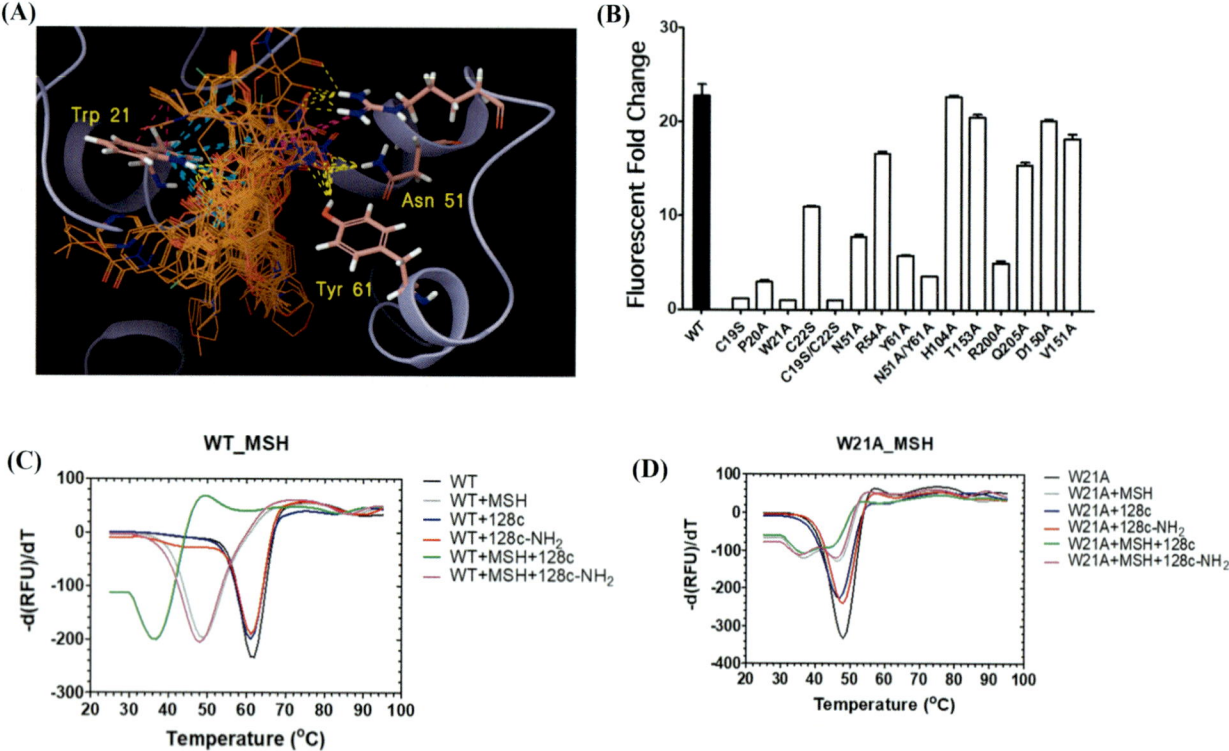

FIGURE 27.24 Utilizing a modified noncovalent approach (Schrodinger, Inc: Maestro v10.7, 2016) and functional experiments to predict potential interactions between NFC compounds and Rv2466c (PDBcode:4NXI). (A) Overlay results of docking 28 compounds binding; (B) Fluorescence changes of compound 128c under the influence of various mutant forms of Rv2466c protein assisted by MSH; (C) DSF studying the temperature changes of wild-type Rv2466c in the presence of 128c and its reduced product 128c-NH$_2$; (D) Temperature changes of the W21A mutant form of Rv2466c in the presence of 128c and its reduced product 128c-NH$_2$.

the temperature at which the folded and unfolded protein states are in dynamic equilibrium ($\Delta G = 0$) is known as the protein denaturation temperature (T_m). Generally, the more stable a protein is, the higher its Tm value; however, some time there will be inverse results. This method offers advantages such as accurate data, high throughput, minimal protein sample loss, and a wide range of temperature changes for the compound. As shown in Fig. 27.24C, MSH caused a $-13°C$ shift in ΔT_m for the nonmutated wild-type Rv2466c, and compound 128 (not compound 128c) further changed the Tm value of the wild-type Rv2466c by $-12°C$, whereas the W21A mutant did not (Fig. 27.24D). This result suggests that the reduced compound 128c dissociates from the Rv2466c-MSH-NFC (RvMN) ternary complex.

27.5.3 The action of mycothiol (MSH, 160)

27.5.3.1 Synthesis of 160 and its derivatives

Actinomycetes secretes a low-molecular-weight thiol compound, mycothiol (MSH, compound 160), and employs it for self-defense against oxidative stress or resistance to antibiotics. As previously noted, the reduction of NFC compounds by Rv2466c killing *Mtb* relies on the assistance of 160. Its chemical structure consists of three parts, namely the D-*myo*-inositol moiety, amino glucosamine moiety, and cysteine moiety. The chemical synthesis of 160 presents challenges, including the need for an effective D-*myo*-inositol receptor protection strategy, the requirement for robust α-selective chemistry for the stereoselective preparation of α-glycosidic bonds, and the necessity for an appropriate purification method after the GlcN-Ins portion is connected to the side-chain cysteine moiety. In response, the researchers in this chapter have developed a method capable of stabilizing the synthesis of 160 on a large scale (Fig. 27.22) [60]. This approach was employed to investigate the contributions of each component of 160 to the reduction activity of Rv2466c.

As depicted in Fig. 27.22, while synthesizing 160b, derivatives featuring a β-configuration were also derived from 161 (designated as compound 161c). Similarly, through the condensation of 161a with diverse alcohols, compounds 162 and 165 were generated, enabling the substitution of the inositol fragment in the molecule with cyclohexane and ethoxy groups, respectively.

Concerning 163, which lacks the D-*myo*-inositol moiety, its synthesis involved the condensation of intermediate 163d with *N*-Boc-*S*-acetyl-L-cysteine. Subsequent steps included deprotection using trifluoroacetic acid and pyridine-induced acetyl group migration (as illustrated in Fig. 27.25). The dimer of 163 (designated as 167) was obtained through iodine oxidation. Additionally, the derivative 168 was synthesized through the condensation of MSH-3d with *N*-Ac-L-serine.

The objectives of designing analogs of 160 are as follows: Compound 161 is intended to understand the impact of the absolute configuration between inositol and sugar on activity. Compounds 162 and 163 were aimed at elucidating the contribution of hydroxyl groups on inositol and inositol itself to activity. Compounds 164, 166, and 167 were to understand whether the thiol group of cysteine is involved in the formation of disulfide bonds with Rv2466c. Compound 165 was to explore whether a smaller number of hydroxyl groups could mimic the role of inositol's multiple hydroxyl groups. Compound 168 is a competitive molecule with a thiol group based on the observed active effects of compound 163 (Fig. 27.26).

27.5.3.2 Structure activity relationships of compound 160 and its derivatives

DSF experiments confirmed that 163, lacking the inositol moiety, exhibited the same ΔTm value as 160 ($-12°C$, Fig. 27.27), indicating that the 163 moiety alone is sufficient to assist Rv2466c in the reduction of NFCs. This result provides a simplified tool molecule for later investigations into the mechanism of Rv2446c.

The mechanism proposed by the researchers for the reduction of NFC compounds by Rv2466c includes the following steps (Fig. 27.28): In the first step, the 163 portion of MSH (the non-myo-inositol part) initially binds to Rv2466c. In the second step, the thiol group of 163 exchanges with the C_{19}-SH of Rv2466c in its reduced state, forming a new disulfide protein-MSH conjugate (Rv2466c-S19-SM). This step then releases two hydrogen atoms while leading it to adopt an active conformation or inducing a relaxed conformation. The third step involves the recruitment of 128c by the protein, leading it to interact with amino acid residues, i.e., W21, N51, and Y61 of Rv2466c, and form a stable ternary complex, RvMN. Herein, the nitro group of 128c forms hydrogen bonds with N51 and Y61 of Rv2466c, while W21 of Rv2466c engages in π-π interactions with the coumarin ring (A/B ring). In the fourth step, the nitro group of RvMN is reduced to a fluorescent amino compound, 128c-NH_2, by the two hydrogen atoms generated during the formation of the disulfide bond between 163 and Rv2466c. Finally, 128c-NH_2 dissociates from the RvMN ternary complex after losing interactions with N51 and Y61, emitting coumarin fluorescence upon excitation by 370 nm light.

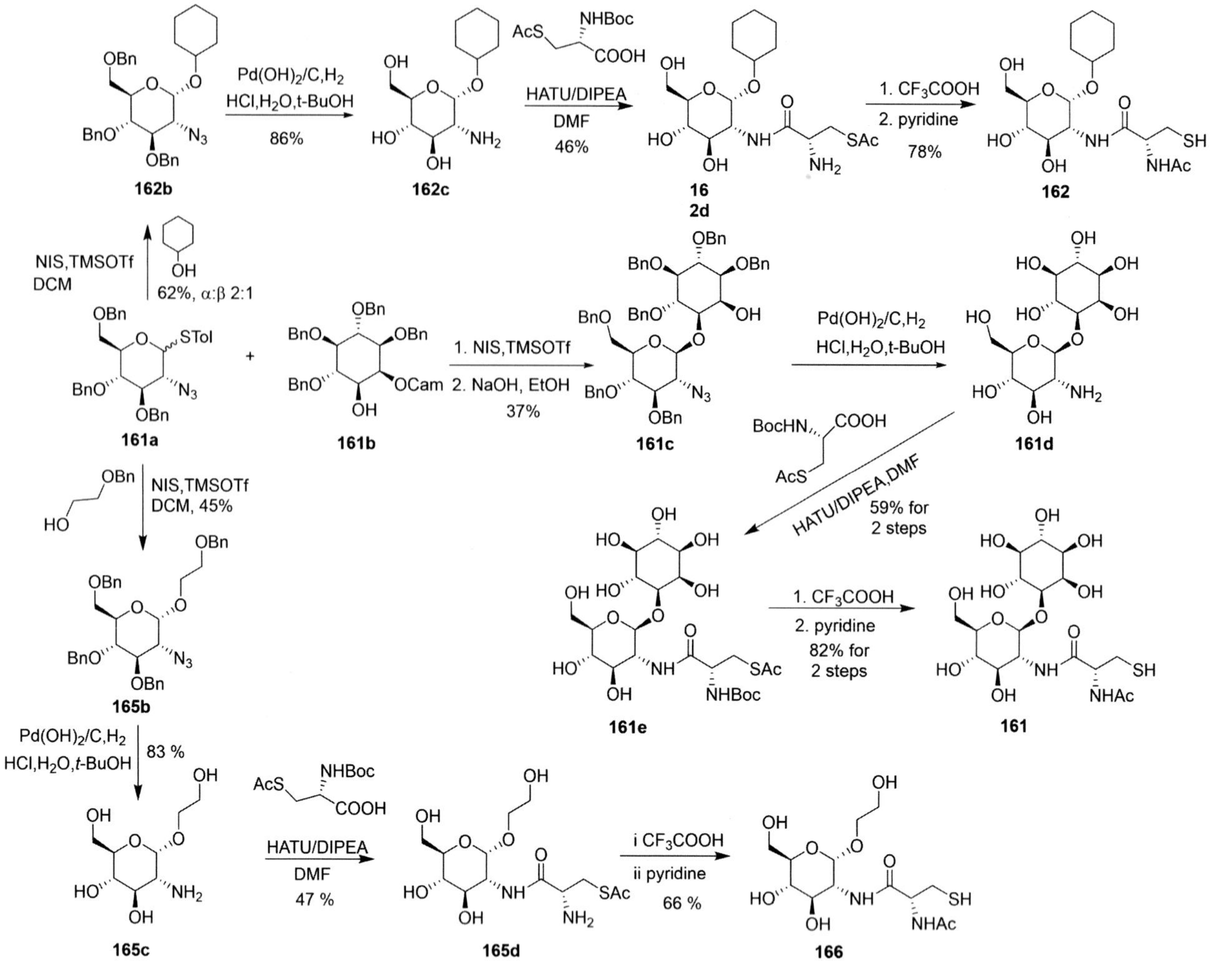

FIGURE 27.25 Synthesis of MSH derivatives (compounds 161, 162, and 165).

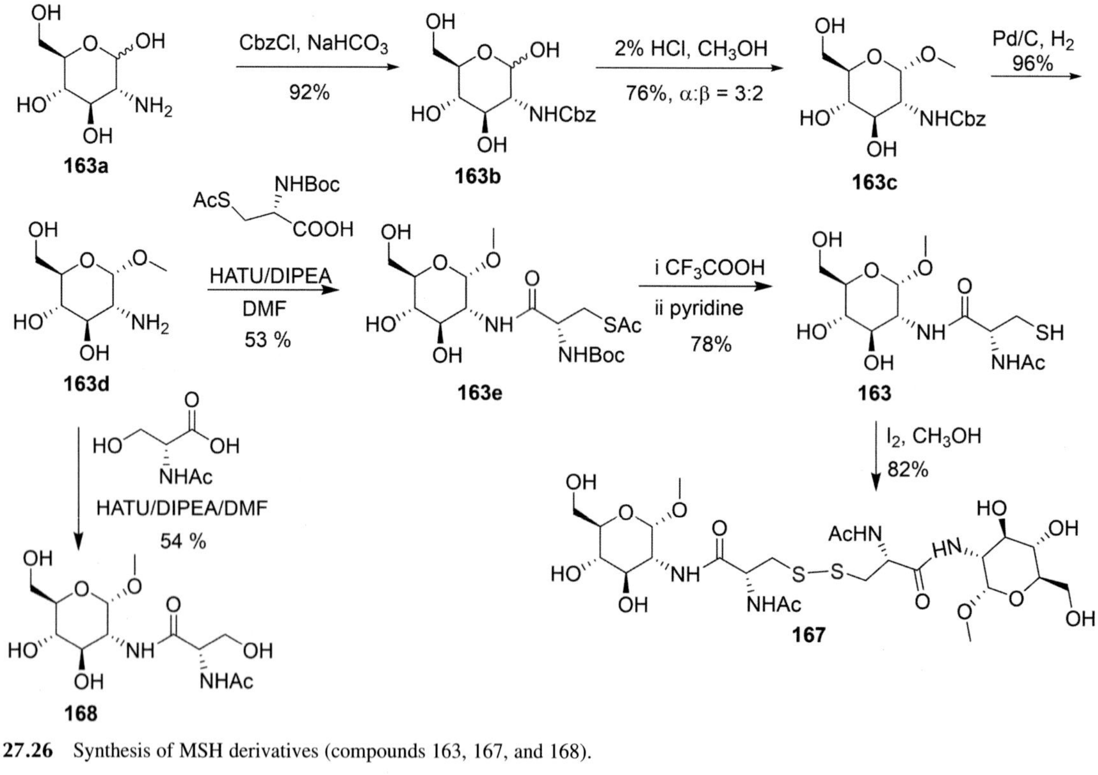

FIGURE 27.26 Synthesis of MSH derivatives (compounds 163, 167, and 168).

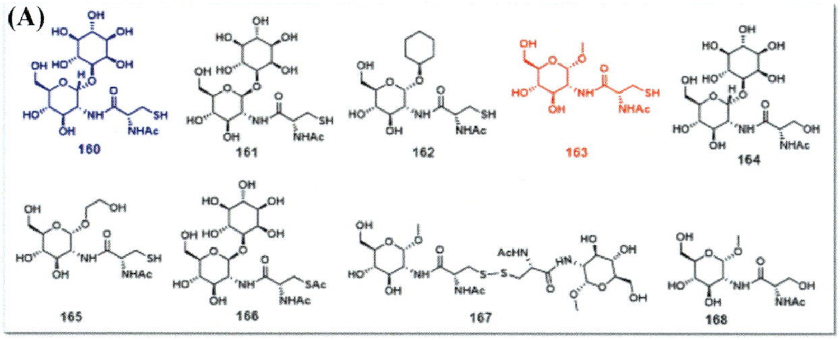

(B)	ΔT_m (°C) to Ctrl-	
	Without 128c	With 128c
160	-12	-24
161	-19	-24
162	0, -19	-23
163	0, -12	-23
164	0	0
165	-21	-24
166	0, -21	-26
167	-23	-26
168	0	0

FIGURE 27.27 Compound 160 assists Rv2466c in the reduction of NFC molecular compound 128c. (A) 8 designed MSH analogs; (B) the DSF study results of 8 MSH analogs.

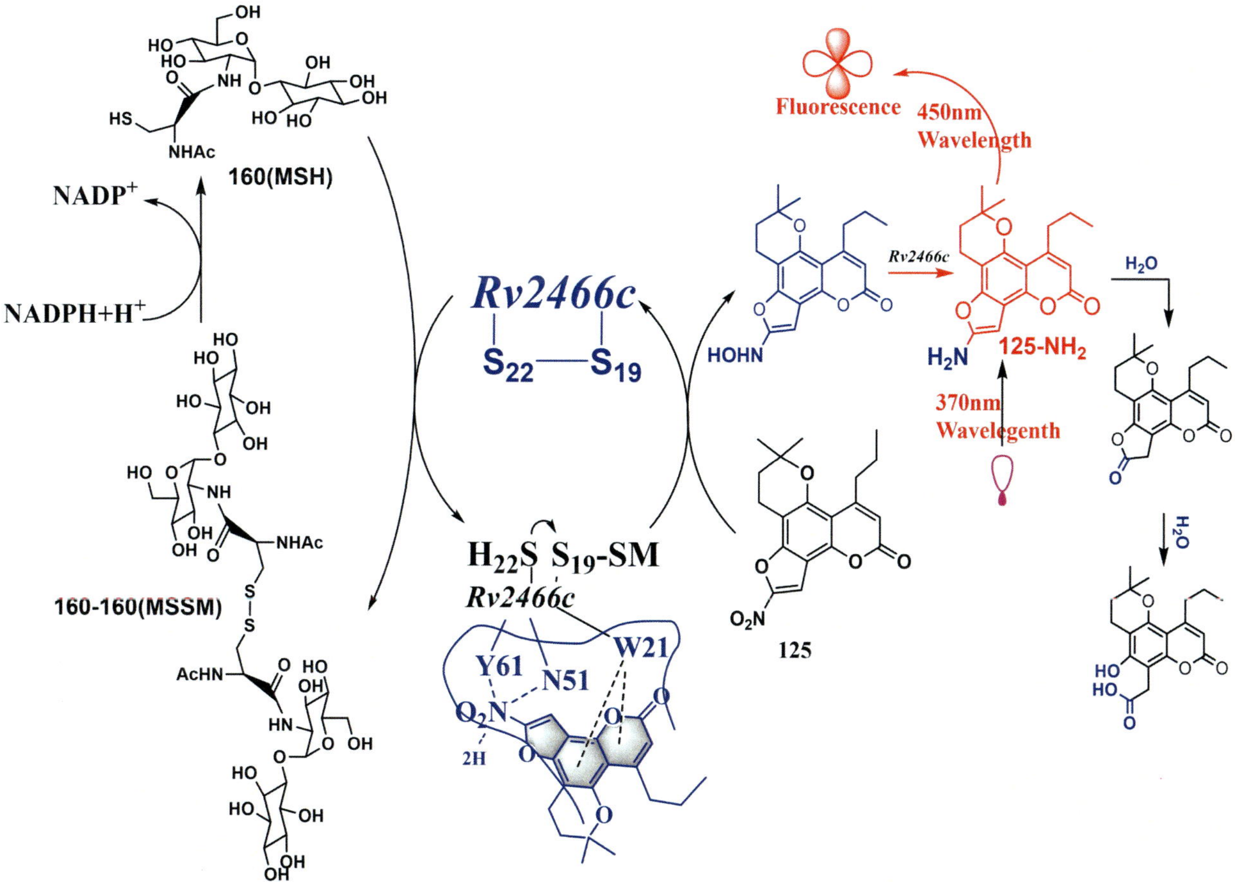

FIGURE 27.28 Mechanism of reduction of NFC 125 by Rv2466c.

27.5.4 Utilization of compound 125 as an innovative fluorescent diagnostic reagent for drug sensitivity testing in tuberculosis diagnosis [59]

Considering the possibility of residual drugs exhibiting fluorescence after clinical treatment, researchers conducted further comparative experiments involving clinically used drugs and nitro-containing drug candidates currently undergoing clinical trials. These nitro-containing compounds include PA-824, metronidazole, BTZ-04329, and IMMLG-6944, none of which demonstrated fluorescence in the presence of Rv2466c or BCG. In addition, as anticipated, clinically used drugs without nitro groups, such as rifampicin (RIF), INH, and pyrazinamide, also showed no significant fluorescence changes before and after treatment. Moreover, at the tested concentrations, compound 125 did not exhibit noticeable fluorescence changes for gram-positive bacteria like *S. aureus* or gram-negative bacteria such as *P. aeruginosa, E. coli*, and others.

The correlation between the bacterial load and the fluorescence intensity changes in the detection pattern of BCG by compound 125 is notable. However, clinical isolates, including two drug-sensitive strains, three multidrug-resistant strains (MDR-TB strains), and three extensively drug-resistant strains (XDR-TB strains), exhibit varying sensitivities to compound 125. The sensitivity for detecting clinical isolates of *Mtb* ranges between 1.5×10^4 and 1.2×10^6 cells/mL, with a detection threshold set at 1.559 (the fold change in fluorescence before and after). These results encourage further exploration of drug sensitivity experiments on clinical sputum samples.

In vitro antimicrobial susceptibility testing refers to experiments conducted outside of the body to determine the inhibitory or bactericidal capabilities of drugs. The BD BACTEC MGIT 960 method (MGIT 960) is an automated, nonradiative, and noninvasive testing technology for rapid culture and sensitivity experiments on *Mtb* clinical sputum samples. This technology utilizes oxygen-sensitive sensors to detect the residual oxygen content in bacterial culture tubes, providing a fully automated process for reporting positive results. When the bacterial culture reaches a certain density and depletes the oxygen in the culture tube to the sensor's detection threshold, the system automatically reports a positive result. Typically, the concentration of bacteria in the culture tube at the time of a positive result is around 10^6 cells/mL. The MGIT-960 apparatus can simultaneously monitor 960 culture tubes. Researchers directly assessed the drug resistance of bacteria cultured in the MGIT 960 system to first-line drugs, including RIF, INH, and EMB. Each group selected 22 samples, with the MIC for the RIF group ranging from 0.125 to 2.0 μg/mL. Six RIF-resistant patients (MIC ≥ 4 μg/mL) were identified, resulting in a resistance rate of 27.3%. This rate is consistent with the resistance rate (28.11%, $n = 6724$) recorded in clinical tests at the Capital Medical University Chest Hospital over the past 3 years (2014–2016). For the INH group, the MIC of the 22 samples ranged from 0.8 to >6.4 μg/mL. The resistance proportions for both INH and EMB at $10 > 320$ μg/mL were both 22.7%. In contrast, the hospital's clinical test statistics for the past 3 years indicated an INH resistance rate of 35.5% ($n = 6724$) and an EMB resistance rate of 16.8% ($n = 6724$). These differences are considered due to the increased sensitivity and accuracy of the new fluorescence method.

Due to its faster characteristics, coupled with the rapid culture technology of MGIT 960, this fluorescence method can determine the drug-resistant types and values of newly diagnosed patients within a week. Therefore, it can be conveniently applied to drug susceptibility testing in the clinical diagnosis of tuberculosis.

27.5.5 Implementing single-cell diagnostic technology for nitrofuran compounds

In a previous observation, researchers noted that when utilizing the enzyme-linked immunosorbent assay (ELISA) method to detect fluorescence in *Mtb* bacterial culture, only compounds 125 and 158 exhibited detectable fluorescence outside the bacterial cells (in the culture medium). Analysis suggested that only the reduction products of these compounds could be excreted outside the bacterial cells. Conversely, the corresponding reduced-NH_2 products (fluorescence) of other molecules might be "anchored" inside the cells, thus hindering the detection of fluorescence in the culture medium. To validate this hypothesis, researchers used the soluble compound 128c for verification. Excitingly, under wide-field fluorescence microscopy, single fluorescent bacteria could be clearly observed (Fig. 27.29). However, a new challenge emerged as this molecule exhibited poor fluorescence selectivity for other bacterial species.

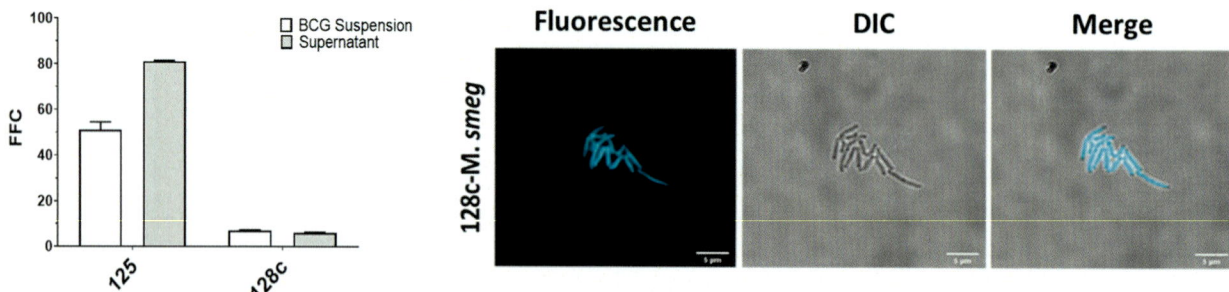

FIGURE 27.29 ELISA detection and single-cell imaging of *M. smeg* labeled with Compound 128c. (A) Fluorescence detected by the ELISA method in the supernatant and suspension after incubation of BCG with the compound. (B) Single-cell imaging of *M. smeg* labeled with 128c.

Researchers continued their investigation by utilizing the unique composition of actinomycete cell walls, specifically trehalose, as a guiding molecule. They connected compound 128c to trehalose in various ways (compounds 169−173, Fig. 27.30) and ultimately found that compound 173 could selectively provide fluorescence for single *Mtb* cells (Fig. 27.31). To further enhance the fluorescence activity of 173, modifications were made based on 125 and 128c. This section focused on enhancing fluorescence activity through the removal of nonessential structures, the addition of conjugated groups, reinforcement of the main structure rigidity, and enhancement of the ICT effect. The SARs are

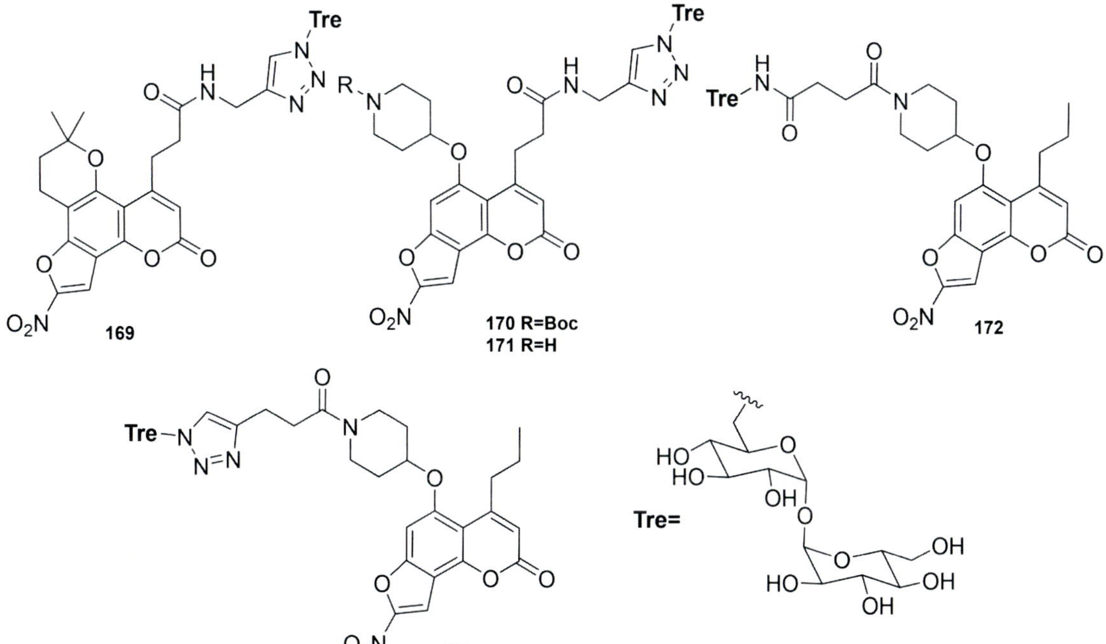

FIGURE 27.30 Conjugates of the novel tuberculosis fluorescence probe molecule NFC with trehalose (Tre) [61].

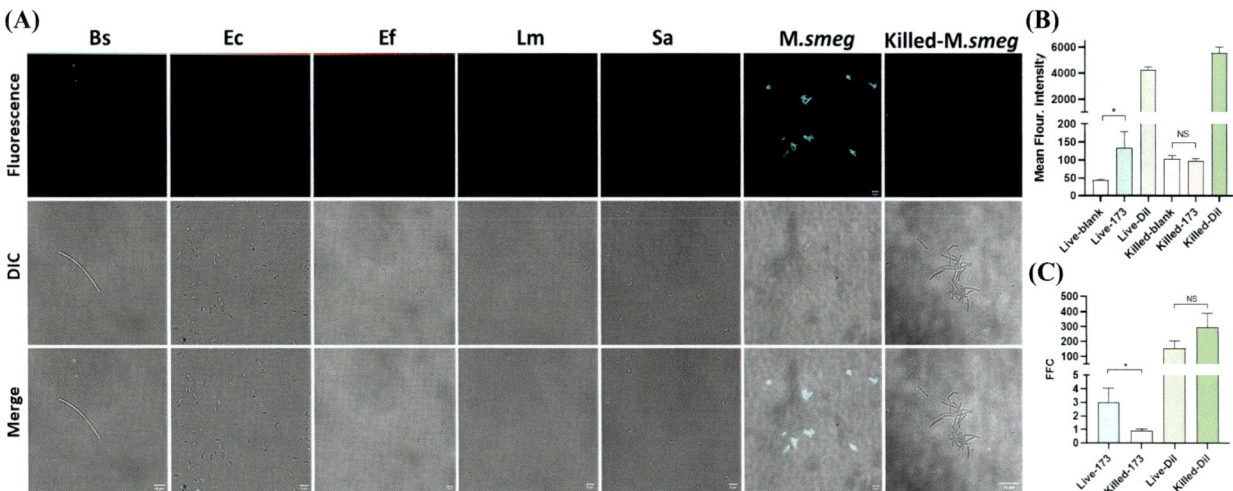

FIGURE 27.31 Fluorescent-specific labeling of bacteria by compound 173. (A) Fluorescence imaging of various bacteria after incubation with compound 173, including *Bacillus subtilis* (Bs), *E. coli* (Ec), *Enterococcus faecalis* (Ff), *Listeria monocytogenes* (Lm), *S. aureus* (Sa), *Mycobacterium smegmatis* (*M. smeg*), and heat-killed *M. smegmatis* (killed-*M. smeg*); blue represents bacteria labeled with 173, DIC is the bright-field image captured by differential interference contrast microscopy, and Merge is the overlap of fluorescence and DIC images; (B) Flow cytometric analysis of the average fluorescence intensity for *M. smeg* and killed-*M. smeg*; (C) Ratio change in fluorescence intensity values before and after labeling with compound 173.

summarized in Fig. 27.32. The oxygen atom in the nitrofuran ring is highly conservative, and various modifications can be made at the low-conservative C_5 position. Optimal activity is observed when the C_4 position is a propyl group. Introducing ethyl, phenyl, and phenol structures at the C_3 position enhances fluorescence activity. Subsequently, compound 174, with a C_3-position vinyl group, was synthesized. Compound 174 exhibited superior fluorescence activity compared to 173 and had a larger Stokes shift (Fig. 27.33).

This is the first to develop a diagnostic method of Mtb upon a specific nitroreductase as a fluorescent off-to-on switch relaying on a coumarin pharmacophore (or herein called fluorophore). The authors of this chapter are interested in the nitroreductase-base diagnosis of Mtb because of its expression in both active and NR-Mtb, making it an ideal enzyme switch for fluorescent probes to label live mycobacteria, even those under latent conditions. Coumarin fluorophore generally emits fluorescence ranging from 450 to 500 nm. Nevertheless, it is important to note that a common challenge exists in the form of fluorescent background interference within a similar visible light range from coumarin fluorophores when dealing with clinical samples. The researchers of this chapter want to improve it with a red fluorescence of clinically practicable diagnosis, and a cyanine fluorophore was selected. Nevertheless, the same strategy was employed by the designation of 175 (Fig. 27.34). Compound 175 consists of a cyanine-based fluorescent dye, a nitrobenzyl group, and a trehalose moiety. The limit of detection of 175 was determined to be 3.5×10^2 colony-forming units (CFU) for M. smeg and 4.3×10^2 CFU for laboratory Mtb strains H37Rv, respectively (Fig. 27.35).

Compound 175 exhibited a fluorescence turn-on response (E_x/E_m = 561 nm/586 nm) by a new specific nitroreductase, Rv3368c, and thus generated strong red fluorescence in single Mtb (Fig. 27.36), specifically colorized phagocytosed Mtb, and rapidly tracked the process of Mtb infection (Fig. 27.37). In addition, 175 detected Mtb in the sputum of patients with TB with remarkable specificity and sensitivity (Fig. 27.38). Of note, nitroreductase Rv3368c was successfully identified by the synthesis of biotinylated 175 offering a pulldown probe of 176 (Fig. 27.34). The NCBI search results for Rv3368c homologs demonstrated that Rv3368c was conserved in the Mycobacteriaceae [62].

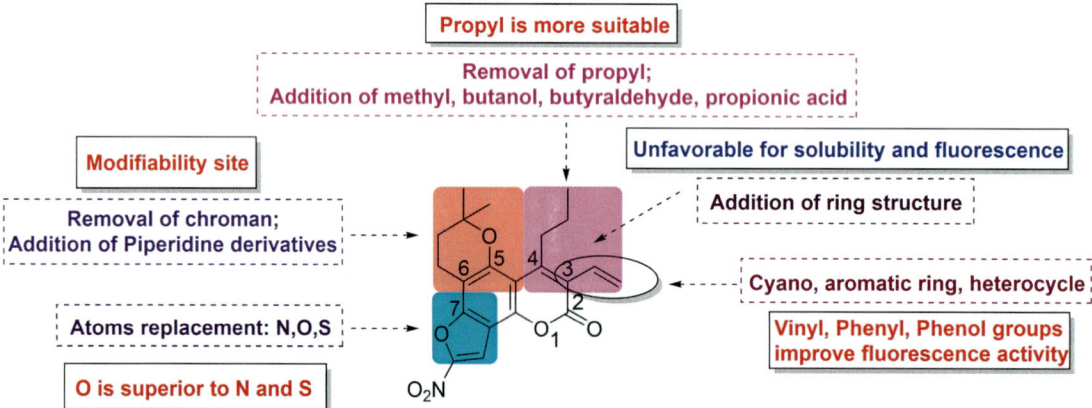

FIGURE 27.32 Structure-fluorescence activity relationship of NFC compounds.

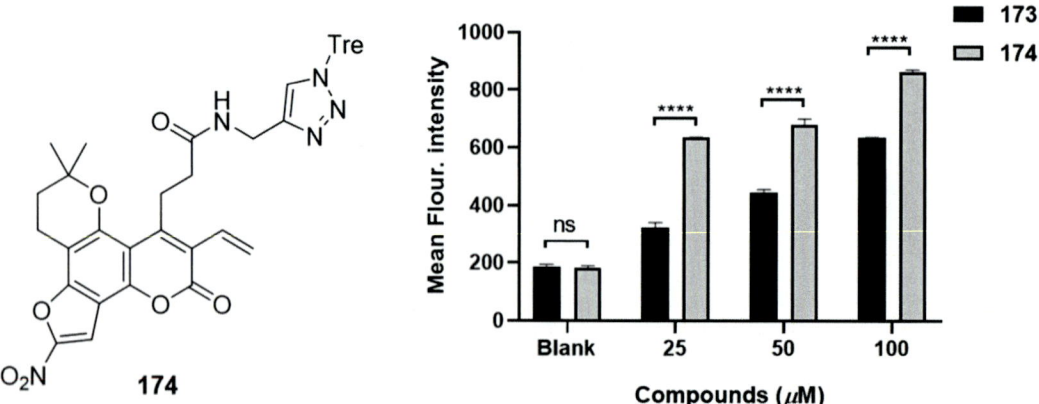

FIGURE 27.33 Structure and Fluorescence Activity of Compound 174.

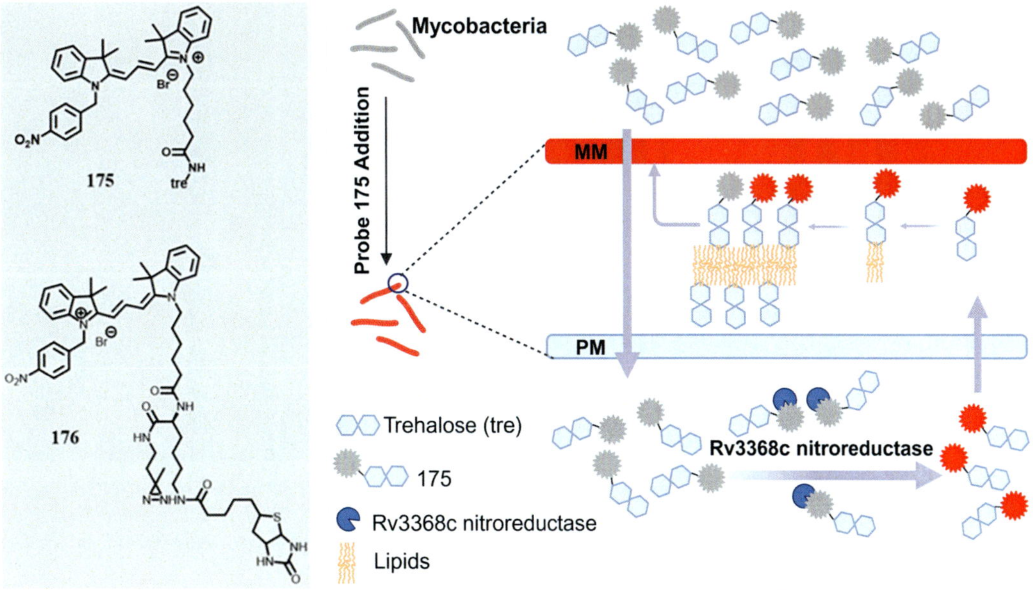

FIGURE 27.34 Structures of probes 175, 176, and the schematic illustration depicting the mechanism by which probe 175 is specifically reduced by a nitroreductase Rv3368c, generates its fluorescence, and is incorporated into the mycomembrane of mycobacteria.

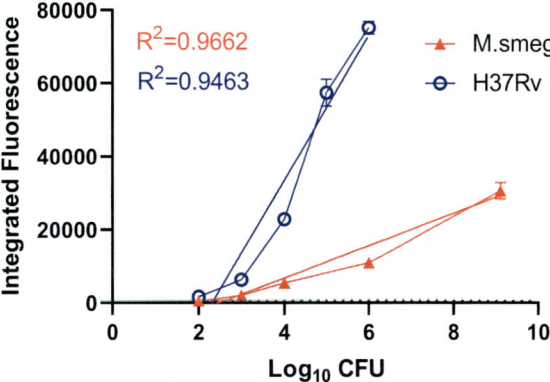

FIGURE 27.35 Correlation of integrated fluorescence and the number of *M. smeg* or H37Rv in culture medium. *M. smeg* or H37Rv were imaged after incubation with 175 (1 μM) for 1 h. Horizontal lines show the mean integrated fluorescence of control samples lacking *M. smeg* or H37Rv. ImageJ was used to calculate the integrated fluorescence.

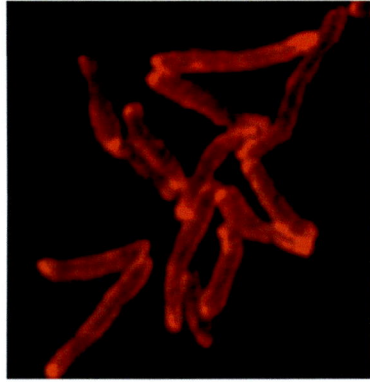

FIGURE 27.36 Imaging of *M. smeg* with 175. Freshly cultured *M. smeg* were treated with 175 (1.0 μM) for 1 h.

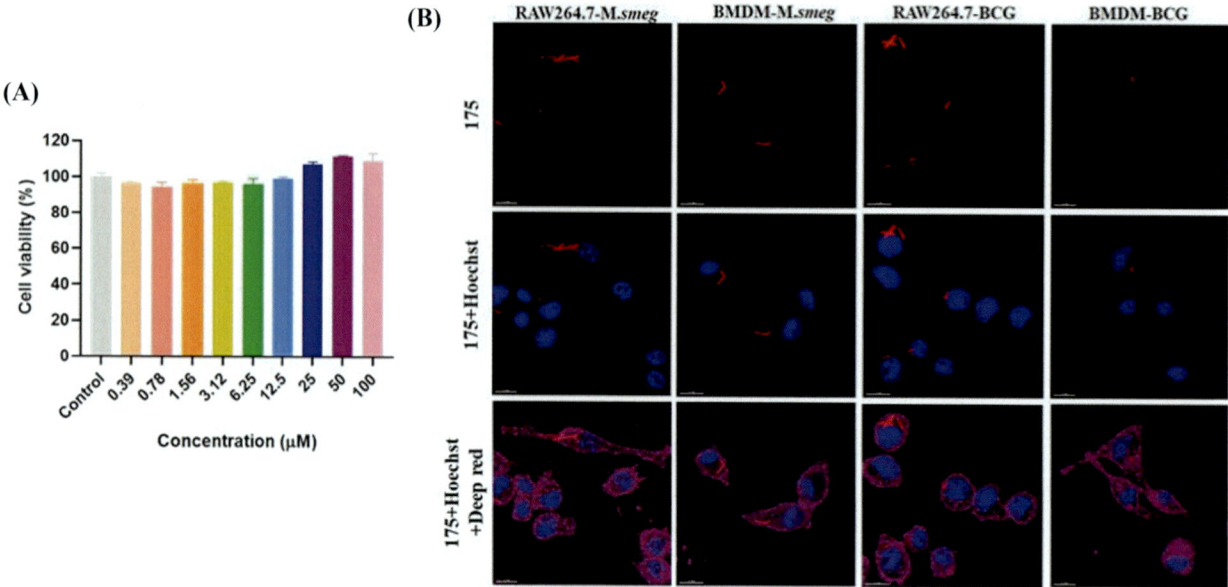

FIGURE 27.37 Imaging phagocytosed *Mtb*. Freshly cultured (A) Cell viability of probe 175 was determined by the MTT assay. (B) *M. smeg* or BCG were incubated with macrophages at a 10-to-1 ratio in a complete medium for 4 h, respectively. The macrophages were washed three times with PBS, followed by incubation with 175 (1 μM) for 1 h. Then macrophages were treated with a nuclear dye (Hoechst 33342) and a cell membrane dye (CellMask Deep Red Plasma Membrane Stains) according to the manufacturer's protocol.

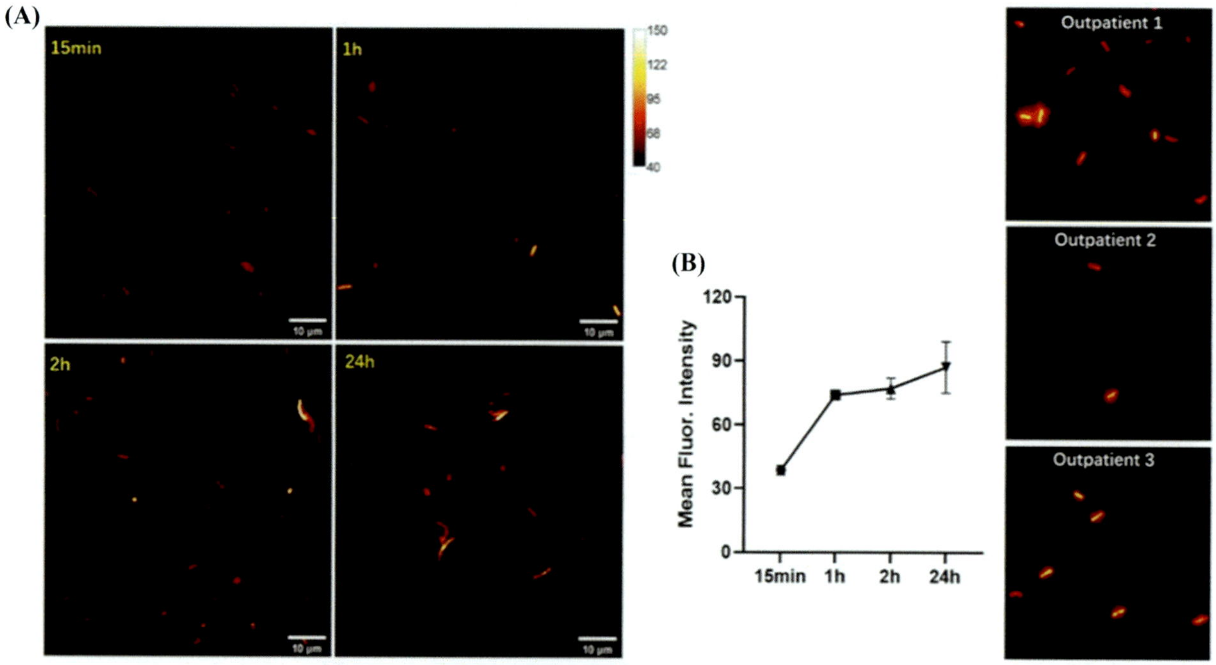

	Culture-positive patients (n = 92)		Sensitivity (95% CI)	Healthy donors (n = 96)		Specificity (95% CI)
	+	−		+	−	
AO	84	8	91.3% (85.5%–97.1%)	3	93	96.9% (94.4%–100.3%)
175	79	13	85.9% (78.8%–93.0%)	1	95	99.0% (96.9%–101.0%)

FIGURE 27.38 Diagnosing *Mtb* in patients with TB using 175. (A) The imaging of sputum samples of TB-positive outpatients treated with 10 μM of 175 for 15 min, 1 h, 2 h, and 24 h. (B) The mean fluorescence intensity (Mean Fluor. Intensity) of the images in Fig. 27.38A was calculated by ImageJ. (C) The sensitivity and specificity of auramine O (AO) and 175.

Function, pharmaceutical, and pharmacological research and development **Chapter | 27** 683

27.6 Summary and outlook

This chapter narrates the fascinating metamorphosis of the natural product molecule (+)-calanolide A (1) and the researchers' continuous efforts in the face of many challenges, as depicted in Fig. 27.39. The unwavering dedication and curiosity that led to the raising of new challenges have been pivotal factors in the transformative journey of this natural molecule. (+)-Calanolide A was initially identified as an HIV-1 NNRTI in 1992, showcasing distinctive

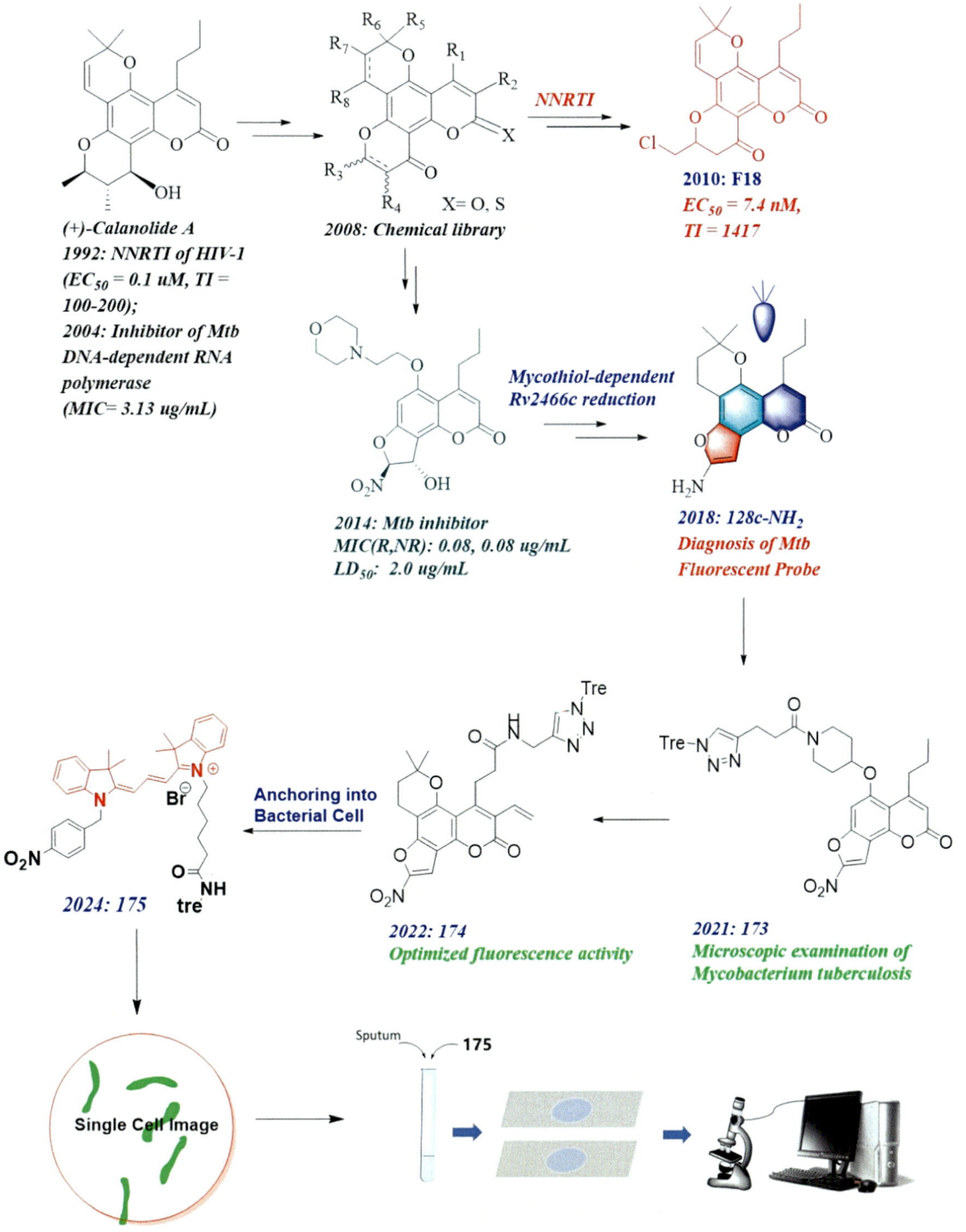

FIGURE 27.39 Key events in the functional transformation of the (+)-calanolide A molecule.

molecular features with significant biological and pharmacological implications. It stands out as the sole natural candidate for anti-HIV drug development that has undergone clinical trial Phase I investigation. However, as a candidate for anti-HIV drugs, whether it is the natural compound (+)-calanolide A itself or its more drug-like derivative (F18) obtained through optimization, further progress in clinical trial investigation and development has been halted. This is attributed to the challenges in synthetic process preparation and competition with other meaningful molecules.

The second turning point in the study of this class of molecules occurred in 2004, when (+)-calanolide A was rediscovered to possess anti-*Mtb* activity with a mechanism distinct from clinically used anti-TB drugs. This inspired researchers to initially explore the possibility of the development of a molecule with dual inhibitory activity against both HIV-1 and *Mtb*. At that time, it was already known that approximately 50% of AIDS patients die from recurrent TB (latent *Mtb* tends to reactivate in immunocompromised individuals, such as AIDS patients). However, after careful evaluation, it was deemed that developing such dual-activity inhibitors posed obvious risks. This is because viruses and bacteria often exhibit substantial differences in sensitivity to drugs, making it easy to induce alternative new drug resistance in vivo. Particularly, the unique characteristics of wild-type *Mtb*, such as its special lipophilic cell wall, insensitivity to pH, and the ability to hide within host cells, make it more prone to developing resistance. Therefore, considering various factors and in collaboration with their research partners, the authors of this chapter ultimately made the strategic decision to channel their efforts exclusively into the development of molecules specifically targeting *Mtb*.

Until now, clinical treatment of TB still relies primarily on chemotherapy, but the treatment period is quite long; for instance, at least 6 therapeutic months even for those TB patients who are sensitive to the first-line drugs, and drug resistance often develops rapidly. One reason is the pressure from host cells, often causing *Mtb* to transition into a very slow replicating and metabolic state. In addition, individual differences in drug pharmacokinetics, are also often leading to variations in effective drug distribution at the patient's lesion site, and contributing to drug resistance in some patients. When the drug treatment is incomplete or not timely, *Mtb* can replicate again.

There is no feasible technology to directly detect whether *Mtb* is in a replicating or a latent state without symptoms after treatment. Key questions such as whether latent *Mtb* will develop into a replicating state and/or when it might happen cannot be answered, making it very challenging to implement precise clinical treatment. As a result, the treatment period must be prolonged. As a result, international public health organizations often focus on and support research addressing such critical global medical and health issues. The Bill and Melinda Gates Foundation has played a crucial role in supporting this project. The research team of the chapter's authors, along with their collaborators, including Professor Carl F. Nathan from Weill Cornell Medicine, aimed at drug discovery by simultaneously combating replicating R-*Mtb* and NR-*Mtb*. However, the development of anti-TB drugs based on (+)-calanolide A failed again due to the drug-like properties of the molecules, namely the genotoxicity of NFC molecules. Despite this, researchers hold a strong interest in the distinctively high activity and bacteriostatic selectivity of this class of molecules. After approximately 7 years of research, they ultimately discovered that the molecules can be reduced by a novel nitroreductase, Rv2466c, with the assistance of a low-molecular-weight thiol compound, MSH, secreted by mycobacteria. The released reactive oxygen species is believed to exert a bactericidal effect, and the interaction between the tripartite complex RvMN (NFC-Rv2466c-MSH) was essentially elucidated. At this point, researchers realized that NFC molecules possess the basic molecular framework characteristics of the fluorescent probe coumarin. There is potential for their fluorescence to be "off to on" by bacteria. As a result, they developed a novel fluorescence diagnostic reagent for TB drug susceptibility testing.

At this point, researchers continued to contemplate the newly observed phenomenon: why did some NFC molecules, reducible by Rv2466c in vitro, not exhibit fluorescence changes in the bacterial culture medium while others did? They speculated that the reduced fluorescent molecules might be "anchored" and retained inside the bacteria. This led them to explore whether bacteria themselves could be fluorescently labeled. With various advanced technological platforms at Tsinghua University, they had excellent experimental conditions to test this hypothesis. In this attempt, researchers discovered fluorescent bacteria at the single-cell level, leading to the development of a method for the single-cell diagnosis of *Mtb*. It is crucial to emphasize that single-cell diagnostic technology holds broad potential applications. It not only significantly enhances the sensitivity of clinical bacteriology microscopic examination, simplifying the operational steps of clinical bacteriology microscopic diagnosis and reducing the exposure of laboratory technicians, but it also has the potential to contribute to understanding the interactions between host cells and infected *Mtb*, establishing new host cell-based diagnostic technologies, discovering new drug targets, and laying the foundation for developing new anti-TB drugs. Currently, the fluorescence technology based on nitroreductase for single-cell *Mtb* detection has been moved to an efficient and practical fluorophore, the cyan-dye technology.

Finally, this chapter showcases a drug development case starting with a natural lead compound. The research began with an understanding of the impact of reducing chiral centers in natural product molecules on their anti-HIV-1 activity.

It involved the construction of diverse chemical libraries, the establishment of high-throughput screening assays based on new cellular functions, detailed SAR studies, investigations into the molecular action of mechanisms, and application-oriented research driven by new mechanisms. From the perspective of medicinal chemistry, establishing compound diversity, including molecular scaffold diversity, diversity of substituents, and stereochemical diversity, is crucial. This case also involves considerations of STRs and structure-metabolism relationships (SMTs) during the lead optimization phase, as well as chemical process optimization. The chapter illustrates to the readers the most critical factors in medicinal chemistry: the driving force of interest, application orientation, and the significance of long-term perseverance. Through the relentless efforts of generation after generation of researchers, the natural product (+)-calanolide A has been endowed with the best prospect for application, truly embodying the magnificent transformation of a natural molecule through medicinal chemistry research.

References

[1] Vlietinck AJ, Bruyne TD, Apers S, et al. Plant-derived leading compounds for chemotherapy of HIV infection. Planta Medica 1998;64(2):97−109.
[2] Yang SS, Cragg GM, Newman DJ, et al. Natural product-based anti-HIV drug discovery and development facilitated by the NCI developmental therapeutics program. J Nat Prod 2001;64(2):265−77.
[3] Song A, Zhang J, Lam KS. Synthesis and reaction of 7-fluoro-4-methyl-6-nitro-2-oxo-2*H*-1-benzopyran-3-carboxylic acid: a novel scaffold for combinatorial synthesis of coumarins. J Com Chem 2004;6(1):112−20.
[4] Kashman Y, Gustafson KR, Fuller RW, et al. The calanolides, a novel HIV-inhibitory class of coumarin derivatives from the tropical rainforest tree, *Calopyllum Lanigerum*. J Med Chem 1992;35(15):2735−43.
[5] Spino C, Dodier M, Sotheeswaran S. Anti-HIV coumarins from *Calophyllum* seed oil. Bioorg Med Chem Lett 1998;8(24):3475−8.
[6] Patil AD, Freyer AJ, Eggleston DS, et al. The inophyllums, novel inhibitor of HIV-1 RT isolated from the Malaysian tree, *Calophyllum inophyllum* Linn. J Med Chem 1993;36(26):4131−8.
[7] Kawazu K, Ohigashi H, Mitsui T. The piscicidal constituents of *Calophyllum inophyllum* Linn. Tetrahedron Lett 1968;9(19):2383−5.
[8] Dharmaratne HRW, Sotheeswaran S, Balasubramaniam S, et al. Triterpenoids and coumarins from the leaves of *Calophyllum cordato-oblongum*. Phytochemistry 1985;24(7):1553−6.
[9] Dharmaratne HRW, Sajeevani JRDM, Marasinghe GPK, et al. Distribution of pyranocoumarins in *Calophyllum cordato-oblongum*. Phytochemistry 1998;49(4):995−8.
[10] Cao SG, Sim KY, Pereira J, et al. Courmains from *Calophyllum teysmannii*. Phytochemistry 1998;47(5):773−7.
[11] Gustafson KR, Bokesch HR, Fuller RW, et al. Calanone, a novel coumarin from *Calophyllum teysmannii*. Tetrahedron Lett 1994;35(32):5821−4.
[12] Mckee TC, Fuller RW, Covington CD, et al. New pyranocoumarins isolated from *Calophyllum lanigerum* and *Calophyllum teysmannii*. J Nat Prod 1996;59(8):754−8.
[13] Fuller RW, Bokesch HR, Gustafson KR, et al. HIV-inhibitory coumarins from latex of the tropical rainforest tree *Calophyllum teysmannii* var. inophylloide. Bioorg Med Chem Lett 1994;4(16):1961−4.
[14] Stout GH, Stevens KL. The structures of costatolide. J Org Chem 1964;29(12):3604−9.
[15] Bandara BMR, Dharmaratne HRW, Sotheeswaran S, et al. Two chemically distinct groups of *Calophyllum* species from Sri Lanka. Phytochemistry 1986;25(2):425−8.
[16] Gunasekera SP, Jayatilake GS, Selliah SS, et al. Chemical investigation of Ceylonese plants. Part 27. extractives of *Calophyllum cuneifolium* Thw. and *Calophyllum soulattri* Burm. f. (Guttiferae). J Chem Soc Perkin Trans 1 1977;13:1505−11.
[17] Mckee TC, Cardellina JH, Dreyer GB, et al. The pseudocalanolides: structure revision of calanolides C and D. J Nat Prod 1995;58(6):916−20.
[18] Dharmaratne HRW, Sotheeswaran S, Balasubramaniam S. Triterpenes and neoflavonoids of *Calophyllum lankaensis* and *Calophyllum thwaitesii*. Phytochemistry 1984;23(11):2601−3.
[19] Nigam SK, Mitraitra CR. Constituents of *Calophyllum Tomentosum* and *Calophyllum Apetalum* nuts: structure of a new 4-alkyl- and of two new 4-phenyl-coumarins. Tetrahedron Lett 1967;8(28):2633−6.
[20] Mckee TC, Covington CD, Fuller RW, et al. Pyranocoumarins from tropical species of genus *Calophyllum*: a chemotaxonomic study of extracts in NCI collection. J Nat Prod 1998;61(10):1252−6.
[21] Flavin MT, Rizzo JD, Khilevich A, et al. Synthesis, chromatographic resolution, and anti-HIV activity of (±)-calanolide A and its enantiomers. J Med Chem 1996;39(6):1303−13.
[22] Buckheitr WJR, Fliakas-Boltz V, Decker WD, et al. Comparative anti-HIV evaluation of diverse HIV-1-specific RT inhibitor-resistant virus isolates demonstrates the existence of distinct phenotypic subgroups. Antivir Res 1995;26(2):117−32.
[23] Boyer PL, Currens MJ, Mcmahon JB, et al. Analysis of nonnucleoside drug-resistant variants of HIV-1 reverse transcriptase. J Virol 1993;67(4):2412−20.
[24] Currens MJ, Gulakowski RJ, Mariner JM, et al. Antiviral activity and mechanism of action of calanolide A against the HIV-1. J Pharmacol Exp Ther 1996;279(2):645−51.

[25] Currens MJ, Mariner JM, McMahon, et al. Kinetic analysis of inhibition of HIV-1 reverse transcriptase by calanolide A. J Pharmacol Exp Ther 1996;279(2):652−61.
[26] (a) Buckheit Jr RW, White EL, Fliakas-Boltz V, et al. Unique anti-HIV activities of the nonnucleoside RT inhibitors calanolide A, costatolide, and dihydrocostatolide. Antimicrob. Agents Chemother. 1999;43(8):1827−34.
(b) Quan Y, Motakis D, Buckheit Jr RW, et al. Sensitivity and resistance to (+)-calanolide A of wild type and mutated forms of HIV-1 reverse transcriptase. Antivir. Ther. 1999;4(4):203−9.
[27] Zembower DE, Liao S, Flavin MT, et al. Structural analogues of the calanolide anti-HIV agents. Modification of the *trans*-10,11-dimethyldihydropyran-12-ol ring (ring C). J Med Chem 1997;40(6):1005−17.
[28] Xu ZQ, Buckheit Jr RW, Stup TL, et al. *In vitro* anti-HIV activity of the chromanone derivatives, 12-oxocalanolide A, a vovel NNRTI. Bioorg Med Chem Lett 1998;8(16):2179−84.
[29] Buckheit Jr RW, Russell JD, Xu ZQ, et al. ANTI-HIV-1 activity of calanolides used in combination with other mechanically diverse inhibitors of HIV-1 replication. Antivir Chem Chemother 2000;11(5):321−7.
[30] Xu ZQ, Hollingshead MG, Borgel S, et al. *In vivo* anti-HIV activity of (+)-calanolide A in the hollow fiber mouse model. Bioorg Med Chem Lett 1999;9(2):133−8.
[31] Pengsuparp T, Serit M, Hughes SH, et al. Specific inhibition of HIV-1 RT mediated by soulattrolide, a coumarin isolated from the latex of *Calophyllum teysmannii*. J Nat Prod 1996;59(9):839−42.
[32] Dharmaratne HRW, Wanigasekera WMAP, Mata-Greenwood E, et al. Inhibition of HIV-1 RT activity by cordatolides isolated from *Calophyllum cordato-oblongum*. Planta Med 1998;64(5):460−1.
[33] Creagh T, Ruckle JL, Tolbert DT, et al. Safety and pharmacokinetics of single doses of (+)-calanolide A, a novel, naturally occurring nonnucleoside RT inhibitor, in healthy, human immunodeficiency virus-negative human subjects. Antimicrob Agents Chemother 2001;45(5):1379−86.
[34] Eiznhamer DA, Creagh T, Ruckle JL, et al. Safety and pharmacokinetic profile of multiple escalating doses of (+)-calanolide A, a naturally occurring non-nucleoside reverse transcriptase inhibitor, in healthy HIV-negative volunteers. HIV Clin Trials 2002;3(6):435−50.
[35] Chenera B, West ML, Finkelstein JA, et al. Total synthesis of (±)-calanolide A, a non-nucleoside inhibitor of HIV-1 reverse transcriptase. J Org Chem 1993;58(21):5605−6.
[36] Kucherenko A, Flavin MT, Boulanger WA, et al. Novel approach for synthesis of (±)-calanolide A and its anti-HIV activity. Tetrahedron Lett 1995;36(31):5475−8.
[37] Deshpande PP, Tagliaferri F, Victory SF, et al. Synthesis of optically active calanolides A and B. J Org Chem 1995;60(10):2964−5.
[38] Trost BM, Toste FD. A catalytic enantioselective approach to chromans and chromanols. A total synthesis of (−)-calanolides A and B and the vitamin E nucleus. J Am Chem Soc 1998;120(35):9074−5.
[39] Galinis DL, Fuller RW, Mckee TC, et al. Structure-activity modifications of the HIV-1 inhibitors (+)-calanolide A and (−)-calanolide B. J Med Chem 1996;39(22):4507−10.
[40] Sharma GVM, Ilangovan A, Narayanan VL, et al. First synthesis of aza-calanolides − a new class of anti-HIV active compounds. Tetrahedron 2003;59(1):95−9.
[41] Gurjar M.K., Sharma G.V.M., Ilangovan A., et al. India patent application no. 1441/DEL/98; US Patent 6,191,279, 2001.
[42] Zhou CM, Wang L, Zhao ZZ. Synthesis of 11-demethyl and 6,6-demethyl calanolide A. Chin Chem Lett 1997;8(10):859−60.
[43] Wang L, Zhang XQ, Chen HS, et al. Improved synthesis and pharmacological evaluation of racemic 11-demethyl calanolide A. Yao Xue Xue Bao 2008;43(7):707−18.
[44] Peng ZG, Chen HS, Wang L, et al. Anti-HIV activities of HIV-1 RT inhibitor racemic 11-demethyl calanolide A. Yao Xue Xue Bao 2008;43(5):456−60.
[45] Ma T, Gao Q, Chen ZZ, et al. Chemical resolution of (±)-calanolide A, (±)-cordatolide A and their 11-demethyl analogues. Bioorg Med Chem Lett 2008;18(3):1079−83.
[46] Ma T, Liu L, Xue H, et al. Chemical library and structure-activity relationships of 11-demethyl-12-oxo calanolide A analogues as anti-HIV-1 agents. J Med Chem 2008;51(5):1432−46.
[47] Xue H, Lu XF, Zheng PR, et al. Highly suppressing wild-type HIV-1 and Y181C mutant HIV-1 strains by 10-chloromethyl-11-demethyl-12-oxo calanolide A with druggable profile. J Med Chem 2010;53(3):1397−401.
[48] Lu XF, Liu L, Zhang X, et al. F18, a novel small-molecule NNRTI, inhibits HIV-1 replication using distinct binding motifs as demonstrated by resistance selection and docking analysis. Antimicrob Agents Chemother 2011;56(1):341−51.
[49] Zhang LL, Xue H, Li L, et al. HPLC enantio-separation, absolute configuration determination and anti-HIV-1 activity of (±)-F18 enantiomers. Yao Xue Xue Bao 2015;50(6):733−7.
[50] Wu XM, Zhang QH, Guo JM, et al. Metabolism of F18, a derivative of calanolide A, in human liver microsomes and cytosol. Front Pharm 2017;8.
[51] Xu ZQ, Barrow WW, Suling WJ, et al. Anti-HIV natural product (+)-calanolide A is active against both drug-susceptible and drug-resistant strains of *Mycobacterium tuberculosis*. Bioorg Med Chem 2004;12(5):1199−207.
[52] Xu ZQ, Pupek K, Suling WJ, et al. Pyranocoumarin, a novel anti-TB pharmacophore: synthesis and biological evaluation against *Mycobacterium tuberculosis*. Bioorg Med Chem 2006;14(13):4610−26.
[53] Zheng PR, Somersan-Karakaya S, Lu SC, et al. Synthetic calanolides with bactericidal activity against replicating and non-replicating *Mycobacterium tuberculosis*. J Med Chem 2014;57(9):3755−72.
[54] Lu S, Zheng P, Liu G. Iodine (III)-mediated tandem oxidative cyclization for construction of 2-nitrobenzo[b]furans. J Org Chem 2012;77(17):7711−17.

[55] Liu ZJ, Guo XY, Liu G. N-oxide heterocycles and imidazoles replacing ring D of calanolides against *Mycobacterium tuberculosis*. Chin Chem Lett 2016;27(1):51−4.
[56] Roldan MD, Perez-Reinado E, Castillo F, et al. Reduction of polynitroaromatic compounds: the bacterial nitroreductases. FEMS Microbiol Rev 2008;32(3):474−500.
[57] Negri A, Javidnia P, Mu R, et al. Identification of a mycothiol-dependent nitro-oxidoreductase from *Mycobacterium tuberculosis*. ACS Infect Dis 2018;4(5):771−87.
[58] Grimm JB, Heckman LM, Lavis LD. The chemistry of small-molecule fluorogenic probes. Prog Mol Biol Transl Sci 2013;113:1−34.
[59] Mu R, Kong CC, Yu WJ, et al. Nitrooxidoreductase Rv2466c-dependent fluorescent probe for *Mycobacterium tuberculosis* diagnosis and drug susceptibility testing. ACS Infect Dis 2019;5(6):949−61.
[60] Liu ZJ, Wu YZ, Liu G. Efficient and convenient total synthesis of mycothiol on a large scale. J Chin Pharm Sci 2015;24(6):347−55.
[61] Li XY, Geng PF, Hong XQ, et al. Detecting *Mycobacterium tuberculosis* using a nitrofuranyl calanolide−trehalose probe based on nitroreductase Rv2466c. Chem Commun (Camb) 2021;57(97):13174−7.
[62] Hong XQ, Geng PF, et al. From bench to clinic: a nitroreductase Rv3368c-responsive cyanine-based probe for the specific detection of live *Mycobacterium tuberculosis*. Anal Chem 2024;96(4):1576−86.

Further reading

Albesa-Jove D, Comino N, Tersa M, et al. The redox state regulates the conformation of Rv2466c to activate the antitubercular prodrug TP053. J Biol Chem 2015;290(52):31077−89.

Jothivasan VK, Hamilton CJ. Mycothiol: synthesis, biosynthesis and biological functions of the major low molecular weight thiol in actinomycetes. Nat Prod Rep 2008;25(6):1091−117.

Chapter 28

Bisphosphonates: a targeted therapeutic medication for skeletal system

Shuai Han[1] and Yonghui Zhang[2]

[1]*WuXi AppTec Co., Ltd., Pudong New Area, Shanghai, P.R. China,* [2]*School of Pharmaceutical Sciences, Tsinghua University, Haidian District, Beijing, P.R. China*

Chapter outline

28.1 Unveiling the saga of bisphosphonates 689
    28.1.1 Pyrophosphate and hypophosphatasia 689
    28.1.2 Discovery of bisphosphonate compounds and their biological functions 691
    28.1.3 Historical progression of bisphosphonate drug development 691
28.2 Elucidating the mechanisms of action of bisphosphonate drugs 692
    28.2.1 Osteoporosis and bisphosphonates 692
    28.2.2 Isoprenoid biosynthesis pathway and farnesyl pyrophosphate synthase 693
    28.2.3 Molecular mechanisms of action of bisphosphonates on osteoclasts 694
28.3 Medicinal chemistry of nitrogen-containing bisphosphonates 696
    28.3.1 Farnesyl pyrophosphate synthase as the molecular target of nitrogen-containing bisphosphonates 696
    28.3.2 Structure-activity relationships of nitrogen-containing bisphosphonates 698
    28.3.3 Design and development of next-generation lipophilic bisphosphonate inhibitors 703
    28.3.4 In vivo distribution and metabolism of bisphosphonates 705
28.4 Novel applications of bisphosphonate inhibitors 706
    28.4.1 Bisphosphonate drugs and inhibitors in anticancer therapy 706
    28.4.2 Development of lipophilic bisphosphonate inhibitors as vaccine adjuvants 707
References 707

28.1 Unveiling the saga of bisphosphonates

28.1.1 Pyrophosphate and hypophosphatasia

Zoledronate, a widely employed antiosteoporotic agent (Fig. 28.1), stands as a prime example of bisphosphonate medications. A defining attribute of this class of drugs lies in their capacity for specific targeting of the skeletal system. Delving into the origins of their development, it becomes evident that the discovery of zoledronate did not stem directly from research dedicated to osteoporosis therapies. Rather, its genesis can be traced to biological investigations into the mechanisms of calcification, an unexpected outcome of scientific inquiry.

Calcification is a process characterized by the accumulation of calcium salts within body tissues. While physiological calcification is essential for normal bone formation, pathological calcification of soft tissues, including arteries, heart valves, lungs, and cartilage, can lead to various diseases [1,2]. Hydroxyapatite, the primary inorganic component of bone, is a common form of calcium deposit. Abnormal deposition of hydroxyapatite in soft tissues surrounding joints, such as tendons, can result in calcific tendinitis (hydroxyapatite deposition disease) [3]. Therefore, investigating and comprehending the mechanisms underlying calcification can contribute to the development of effective treatments and preventive strategies for these disorders. In 1962, Herbert Fleisch and colleagues discovered, through in vitro experiments, that inorganic pyrophosphate (PPi), a constituent of urine, acts as a calcification inhibitor (Fig. 28.2A), suppressing the deposition of hydroxyapatite [4]. Around the same time, a rare genetic bone disease known as hypophosphatasia was identified. This inherited disorder is characterized by defective bone and tooth mineralization due to

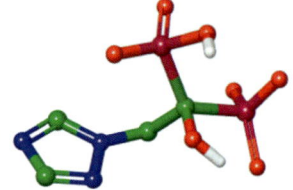

FIGURE 28.1 Zoledronate structural formula and 3D ball-and-stick model.

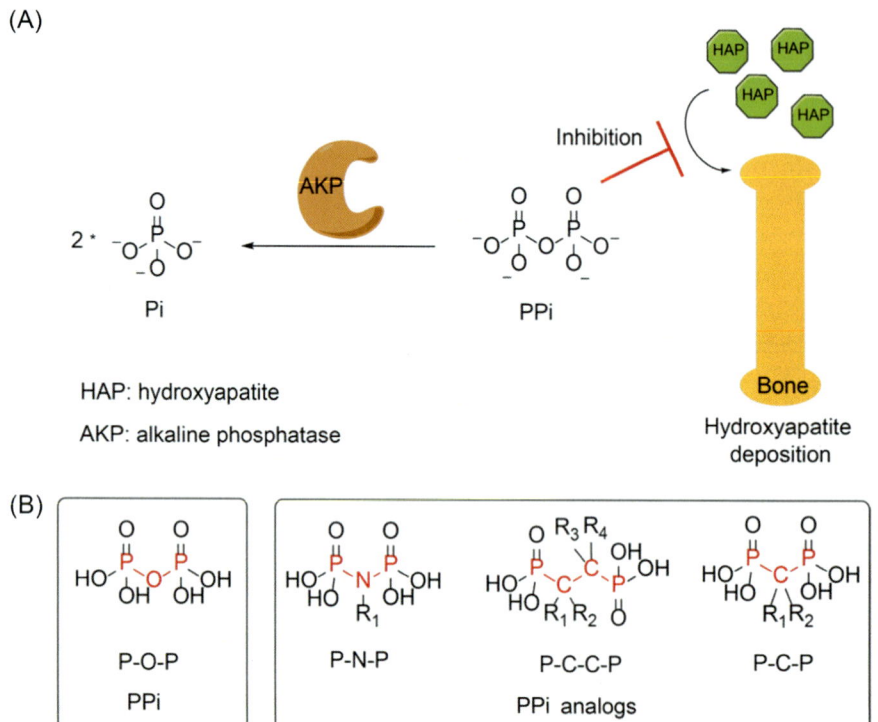

FIGURE 28.2 (A) Pyrophosphate inhibition of hydroxyapatite deposition. (B) Schematic representation of the structure of pyrophosphate and various skeletal analogs.

alkaline phosphatase deficiency [5]. Russell et al. observed that children with hypophosphatasia exhibited abnormally elevated levels of pyrophosphate in their plasma and urine [6]. Considering the recently discovered inhibitory effect of pyrophosphate on calcification, Russell and collaborators hypothesized that alkaline phosphatase, within the patients' bodies, acts as a natural regulator of pyrophosphate metabolism. They proposed that alkaline phosphatase facilitates the metabolic breakdown of pyrophosphate, thereby controlling its concentration and indirectly influencing the calcification process. Subsequent in vitro enzymatic experiments further substantiated this hypothesis. For instance, under physiological conditions (pH 7.4), alkaline phosphatase exhibits a high affinity for pyrophosphate and catalyzes its degradation.

Notably, the clinical manifestations of this rare disease, hypophosphatasia, in conjunction with various in vivo and in vitro experimental findings point toward a dual role of pyrophosphate in mineralization. While appropriate levels of pyrophosphate in the body prevent the calcification of soft tissues, excessively high levels can paradoxically lead to hypophosphatasia-like conditions characterized by defective mineralization of the skeletal.

The discovery of pyrophosphate's role in regulating calcification within the body prompted scientists to investigate its potential as a therapeutic agent to inhibit pathological calcification. However, experimental findings revealed that pyrophosphate exhibited efficacy in animal models of vascular, dermal, and renal ectopic calcification only when administered directly *via* intravenous injection [7]. Oral administration of pyrophosphate or other polyphosphate salts resulted in their degradation within the animals' gastrointestinal tracts, abolishing the desired therapeutic effects. Consequently, developing pyrophosphate analogs that retain the ability to inhibit calcification (preventing calcium salt deposition) while resisting degradation upon oral administration became a crucial goal in the development of antiosteoporosis drugs.

Based on the connectivity of phosphorus and oxygen atoms in the pyrophosphate structure (Fig. 28.2B), researchers initially classified its structural linkage type as P-O-P. Subsequently, analogs with P-N-P, P-C-C-P, and P-C-P skeletal types were developed. However, subsequent in vitro and in vivo animal studies demonstrated that only P-C-P compounds exhibited both the desired calcification inhibitory activity and favorable oral stability [8,9]. This novel class of P-C-P skeletal compounds, known as bisphosphonates, constitutes the focus of this chapter. Bisphosphonates are characterized by two acidic phosphonate "heads" (Fig. 28.2B), with the two phosphonate groups linked by a carbon atom. The remaining two valences of the carbon atom are occupied by various substituent groups that form the "tail," resulting in structurally diverse bisphosphonate compounds.

28.1.2 Discovery of bisphosphonate compounds and their biological functions

The discovery of bisphosphonates' exceptional ability to inhibit calcification and their oral stability stimulated further research into their biological activity. Pyrophosphate, a structural analog of bisphosphonates, demonstrated its capacity to inhibit the dissolution of hydroxyapatite crystals [10], suggesting a similar biological function for bisphosphonates [11]. The prevailing scientific view at the time posited that the solubility of bone minerals might influence their rate of removal (i.e., bone resorption). Bisphosphonates' modulation of the solubility properties of hydroxyapatite, the major inorganic component of bone, naturally drew attention to its potential effects on bone resorption. In 1969, Fleisch H., Russell R. G., and Francis M. D. published two pivotal back-to-back research articles in the same issue of Science. Their work elucidated bisphosphonate compounds' biological functions in vitro, demonstrating their inhibition of calcium phosphate crystal formation and pathological calcification in vivo [12], as well as their inhibition of hydroxyapatite dissolution and bone resorption in vitro and in vivo [13]. The same year, the first human data on bisphosphonate therapy in patients with osteopetrosis were published in the Lancet. This study laid the groundwork for the subsequent development of etidronate (Fig. 28.5), the first-generation bisphosphonate drug approved for clinical use in 1977.

Since their introduction into the pharmaceutical realm in 1969, bisphosphonates have been extensively studied in clinical applications, pharmacological mechanisms, and novel therapeutic areas, maintaining their prominence in the pharmaceutical landscape for half a century. Various experimental systems, including in vitro bone organ culture, normal animal bone resorption processes, and experimentally induced bone resorption [5], have consistently corroborated bisphosphonates' ability to suppress osteoclast-mediated bone resorption. Calcitriol, vitamin D, and retinoids can induce bone resorption, leading to the mobilization of skeletal calcium into the circulation, resulting in hypercalcemia [14]. The hypercalcemic rat model induced by retinoids provides an efficient screening system for bone resorption inhibitors. Ibandronate (Compound **11**) was discovered using this method. Zoledronate (Fig. 28.5) was identified through a hypercalcemia rat model induced by calcitriol, leading to its clinical evaluation and subsequent market approval. In numerous animal models of osteoporosis, bisphosphonates have consistently demonstrated promising effects in preventing bone deterioration.

Recent research has revealed that bisphosphonates possess not only traditional antiosteoporotic properties but also anticancer potential. For instance, zoledronate exhibits promising anticancer effects or clinical synergy in multiple myeloma and breast cancer [15,16]. In Kirsten Rat Sarcoma (KRAS)-mutant mouse lung adenocarcinoma models, the combination of lipophilic bisphosphonates and rapamycin exerts a potent synergistic anticancer effect [17]. Moreover, lipophilic bisphosphonates can serve as potent vaccine adjuvants, enhancing the immune response to vaccines [18]. These diverse applications and properties of bisphosphonates will be discussed in detail in Section 28.4.

28.1.3 Historical progression of bisphosphonate drug development

The development of bisphosphonate drugs dates back to 1966, but it was not until 1969, when scientists published research articles on their biological function in Science, that bisphosphonates gained significant attention in the pharmaceutical research community. The same year, the first clinical trial of a bisphosphonate drug, etidronate, was initiated, leading to its approval by the US Food and Drug Administration (FDA) in 1977 for the treatment of symptomatic Paget's disease of the bone. Etidronate, a first-generation bisphosphonate, paved the way for the successful development of more effective second- and third-generation bisphosphonates. In 1987, pamidronate (Fig. 28.5) received FDA approval in the United States for the prevention of bone loss and osteoporosis. In the late 1990s, risedronate (Fig. 28.12) was approved by the FDA for the treatment of osteoporosis and Paget's disease of the bone. Zoledronate, included in the World Health Organization's List of Essential Medicines, was approved by the FDA in the early 2000s for the treatment of osteoporosis, bone destruction caused by cancer, hypercalcemia, and Paget's disease of bone. Compared to first-generation bisphosphonates, these second- and third-generation drugs exhibited enhanced biological

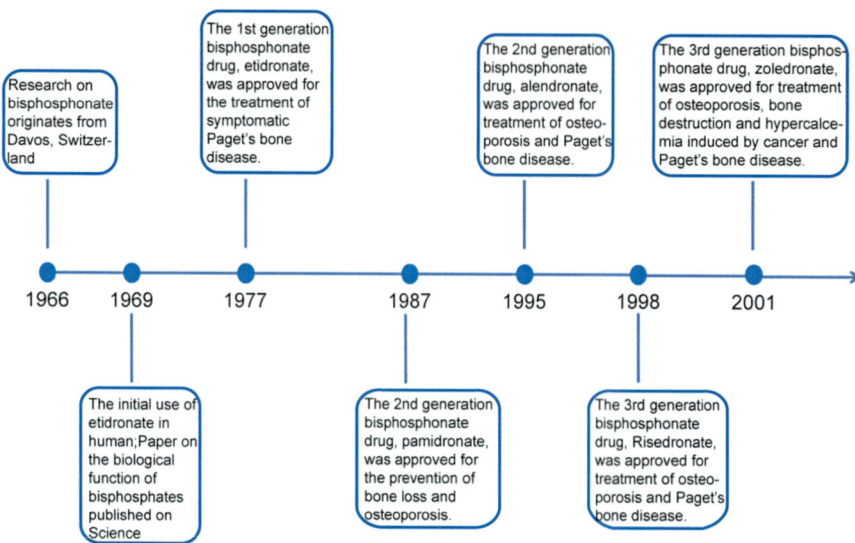

FIGURE 28.3 Historical timeline of key developments and market approvals of bisphosphonate drugs.

activity, with potency improvements ranging from 10- to 100-fold. The clinical trials of various bisphosphonate drugs have spanned 30–40 years. This extensive research has led to the establishment of well-defined clinical indications for bisphosphonate therapy, primarily including the treatment of osteoporosis, Paget's disease of bone, cancer-related hypercalcemia, and bone resorption-related diseases. Fig. 28.3 presents a timeline of the major developments and milestones in bisphosphonate drug research.

28.2 Elucidating the mechanisms of action of bisphosphonate drugs

28.2.1 Osteoporosis and bisphosphonates

Within the intricate framework of the human skeletal system, a delicate balance exists between the opposing processes of bone resorption and bone formation. Bone resorption involves the breakdown of bone tissue, liberating minerals into the bloodstream. This process is primarily mediated by specialized cells known as osteoclasts. Conversely, bone formation, orchestrated by osteoblasts, represents the anabolic counterpart, synthesizing the essential bone matrix components. When this tightly regulated equilibrium is disrupted, favoring excessive bone resorption over formation, conditions such as osteoporosis may arise [19]. Remarkably, bisphosphonates, a class of therapeutic agents, exhibit a pronounced affinity for skeletal tissues, surpassing that of other tissues. This remarkable selectivity stems from the strong interaction between the bisphosphonate moiety and hydroxyapatite, the principal mineral component of bone. As a result, upon entering the body, the majority of bisphosphonates accumulate within bone tissue. The remaining unbound fraction undergoes rapid elimination *via* renal excretion [20,21]. The unique biodistribution of bisphosphonates facilitates their intimate interaction with osteoclasts, the primary cellular mediators of bone resorption. Despite their inherent polarity, hindered by the presence of two negatively charged phosphate groups, bisphosphonates are remarkably internalized by osteoclasts [22]. Radiolabeled alendronate (Fig. 28.12), when administered to neonatal rats, demonstrated substantial adsorption onto osteoclast surfaces [21]. Furthermore, in experiments involving rabbit osteoclasts, fluorescently labeled alendronate analogs were rapidly internalized into intracellular vesicles [22].

Once internalized by osteoclasts, bisphosphonates exert their inhibitory effects on bone resorption through diverse mechanisms, encompassing the modulation of osteoclast recruitment, differentiation, and resorptive activity. Additionally, they induce osteoclast apoptosis and disrupt their cytoskeletal organization [5,23–29]. The selective targeting of osteoclasts and the potent suppression of bone resorption by bisphosphonates underpin their therapeutic efficacy in the management of osteoporosis. Mechanistic studies at the molecular level have revealed that the potent antiresorptive effects of nitrogen-containing bisphosphonates are attributed to their remarkable inhibitory action on the protein target, farnesyl pyrophosphate synthase (FPPS). FPPS, a key metabolic enzyme in the mevalonate (MVA)biosynthetic pathway, governs the production of essential downstream metabolites, including cholesterol and farnesyl pyrophosphate (FPP).

28.2.2 Isoprenoid biosynthesis pathway and farnesyl pyrophosphate synthase

Terpenes, also known as isoprenoids, constitute the largest class of natural products (∼60%), showcasing nature's remarkable chemical diversity [30]. Their biosynthesis is governed by the intricate isoprenoid biosynthetic pathway, found across various life forms, encompassing eukaryotes (plants, animals, and fungi) and prokaryotes (bacteria and archaea). This comprehensive pathway comprises two branches: the upstream MVA or non-MVA also named Methylerythritol 4-phosphate (MEP) pathway pathways, followed by the downstream terpene biosynthetic pathway [31,32]. Terpenes and isoprenoids perform diverse and essential biological functions. For instance, carotenoids, serving as accessory pigments to chlorophyll, facilitate photosynthesis in plants. Phytohormones, such as abscisic acid and gibberellins, regulate plant growth and development. Sterols, integral components of cell membranes in eukaryotes and bacteria, contribute to membrane fluidity and integrity. Quinones, crucial electron carriers, participate in the electron transport chain within cells. Protein prenylation, a type of posttranslational modification, plays a pivotal role in protein subcellular localization and regulation [31,32]. As depicted in Fig. 28.4, the biosynthesis of terpenoid structures originates from two five-carbon precursors: isopentenyl pyrophosphate (IPP) and dimethylallyl pyrophosphate (DMAPP). Depending on the organism, these precursors are synthesized via either the MVA pathway (predominant in higher eukaryotes and archaea) or the MEP pathway (predominant in bacteria, plants, and apicomplexan protists) [32]. Subsequently, under the catalysis of various enzymes, these five-carbon precursors undergo condensation reactions, giving rise to pyrophosphate derivatives of varying carbon chain lengths, including the ten-carbon geranyl pyrophosphate (GPP), the fifteen-carbon FPP, and the twenty-carbon geranylgeranyl pyrophosphate (GGPP). These pyrophosphate derivatives serve as intermediates for the further biosynthesis of downstream products, such as cholesterol, coenzyme Q10, and diterpenes [32].

As illustrated in Fig. 28.4, FPPS, a pivotal enzyme in this pathway, catalyzes the initial condensation reaction between DMAPP and IPP, liberating a molecule of PPi to yield the ten-carbon intermediate GPP. Subsequently, FPPS further catalyzes the reaction between IPP and GPP, resulting in the formation of the fifteen-carbon product FPP [32]. The synthesis of the twenty-carbon intermediate GGPP from IPP as the building block requires the enzymatic action of geranylgeranyl pyrophosphate synthase (GGPPS) [32]. Notably, the generated FPP and GGPP serve as posttranslational modification substrates for small GTPases, such as Rac, Ras, and Rho, facilitating their proper membrane localization and enabling them to execute their respective signal transduction functions [32,33]. Additionally, FPP undergoes a series of subsequent enzymatic transformations catalyzed by nineteen other enzymes, including squalene synthase, squalene epoxidase, and lanosterol demethylase, ultimately leading to the formation of cholesterol, a vital functional molecule in the human body [32]. Furthermore, other enzymatic reactions can yield essential metabolites such as coenzyme Q10, isoprenoid alcohols, and heme A [32,34]. Intriguingly, the five-carbon precursor IPP can interact with the butyrophilin subfamily 3 member A1 (BTN3A1) receptor, thereby activating Vγ9Vδ2 T cells [32,35,36].

Owing to the crucial role of FPPS in posttranslational protein modifications, nitrogen-containing bisphosphonates, such as alendronate, risedronate, and zoledronate, acting as its specific inhibitors, can modulate the proper localization

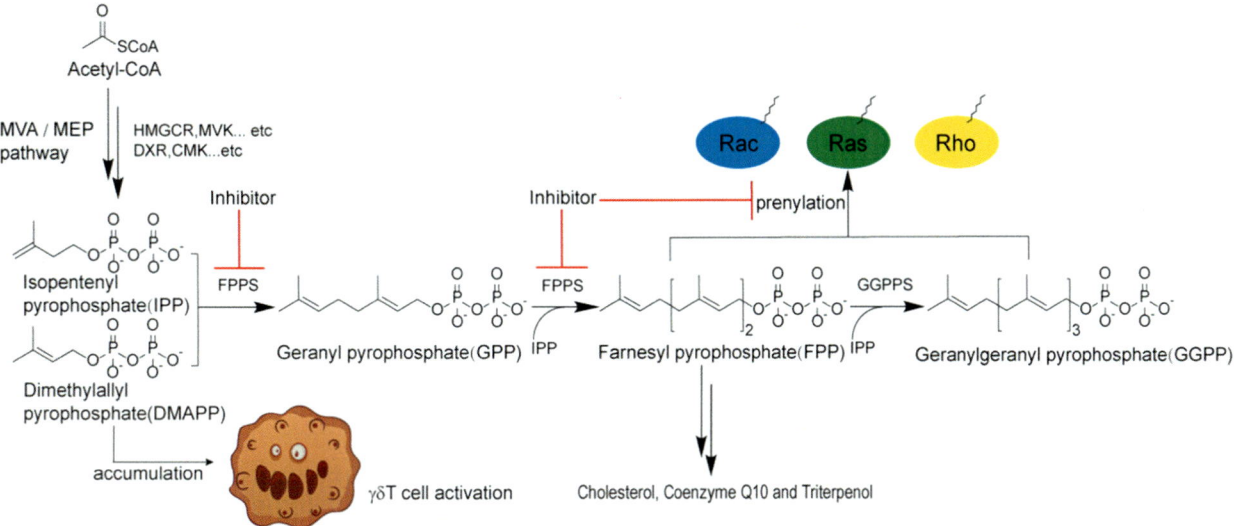

FIGURE 28.4 Schematic representation of the isoprenoid biosynthesis pathway.

of various small GTPases, including Rap, Rac, Rho, Rab, and Cdc42. This disruption of small GTPase localization leads to the disorganization of the cellular cytoskeleton, alterations in intracellular trafficking, and impairment of osteoclast integrin-mediated signaling pathways [37–39]. The remarkable affinity of nitrogen-containing bisphosphonates for osteoclasts in bone tissue [21], their selective internalization by osteoclasts, and their potent targeting of FPPS ultimately contribute to the favorable clinical outcomes observed with these drugs in the treatment of osteoporosis. Recent research has identified FPPS as a potential novel target for immunotherapy and antitumor strategies due to its central role in the MVA pathway. This aspect will be further explored in the subsequent fourth section.

28.2.3 Molecular mechanisms of action of bisphosphonates on osteoclasts

With regard to the mechanisms of action of bisphosphonate drugs, two distinct molecular pathways have been identified to date. Based on these two molecular mechanisms and the structural differences of the drug molecules, bisphosphonates can be further categorized into two primary types: nitrogen-containing bisphosphonates and nonnitrogen-containing bisphosphonates (Fig. 28.5). In the chronological order of their market introduction, first-generation bisphosphonates are exclusively nonnitrogen-containing, while second- and third-generation bisphosphonates are all nitrogen-containing. These two types of bisphosphonates exhibit entirely different molecular mechanisms of action.

The first-generation nitrogen-free bisphosphonates, such as clodronate, etidronate, and tiludronate, primarily disrupt normal osteoclast function by mimicking pyrophosphate, eventually leading to osteoclast apoptosis. In eukaryotic protein translation, transfer ribonucleic acid (RNA) (tRNA) is required for amino acid transport, and different tRNAs carry corresponding amino acids, participating in the elongation stage of protein translation and ultimately forming thousands of protein sequences. "Loading" amino acids onto their corresponding tRNAs requires two highly specific biochemical reactions: (1) amino acid activation, in which amino acids react with adenosine triphosphate (ATP) to form an activated amino acid-adenosine monophosphate (AMP) intermediate, releasing a molecule of inorganic PPi for subsequent loading steps; and (2) amino acid loading, in which the amino acid-AMP intermediate reacts with the corresponding tRNA to form the corresponding aminoacyl-tRNA [40]. The entire process is catalyzed by class II aminoacyl-tRNA synthetases (Fig. 28.6), where the first step is a reversible reaction in which pyrophosphate reacts with the amino acid-AMP intermediate, catalyzed by class II aminoacyl-tRNA synthetases, to form the amino acid and release an ATP molecule. However, the first-generation nitrogen-free bisphosphonates, due to their structural similarity to pyrophosphate and the fact that most molecules have relatively small side chain R substituents, can mimic the binding of pyrophosphate to the enzyme's active site, generating a class of nonhydrolyzable ATP analogs, AppCp (Fig. 28.6). These nucleotides are toxic to cells, interfering with various normal metabolic processes and subsequently inducing the apoptosis of target cells. Studies have shown that clodronate, etidronate, and tiludronate can all be metabolized to toxic AppCp-like metabolites in cells, while other nitrogen-containing bisphosphonates, such as alendronate, ibandronate, and pamidronate, do not exhibit the presence of AppCp-like toxic metabolites in cellular experiments [41]. Since bisphosphonates specifically accumulate in bone-related cells, especially osteoclasts, the AppCp-like toxic metabolites of first-generation bisphosphonates can easily accumulate to extremely high concentrations (>1 mM) [42] and affect multiple

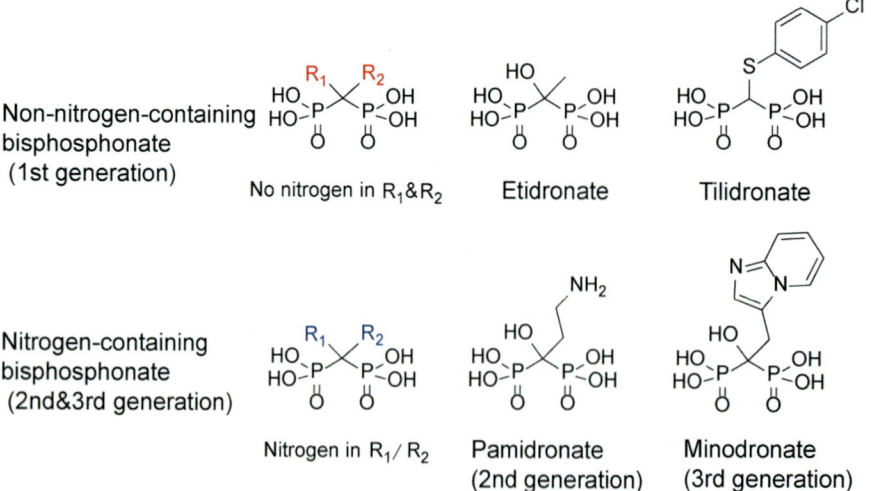

FIGURE 28.5 General structural formulae and representative molecular structures of the two types of bisphosphonates.

intracellular metabolic processes, such as mitochondrial membrane potential disruption and caspase-3 activation, ultimately leading to osteoclast apoptosis [43]. It is precisely because bisphosphonates specifically target bone, are internalized specifically by osteoclasts, and ultimately lead to osteoclast apoptosis that the purpose of treating osteoporosis is achieved.

Second- and third-generation nitrogen-containing bisphosphonates predominantly exert their effects by inhibiting FPPS in the MVA pathway. This inhibition prevents the isoprenylation of certain essential small G proteins, thereby disrupting the formation of the cytoskeleton, intracellular vesicle trafficking, and integrin-mediated signaling processes in osteoclasts, ultimately inducing apoptosis. FPPS, a magnesium-dependent metabolic enzyme, catalyzes the head-to-tail condensation of DMAPP and IPP, yielding the all-trans isoprenoid pyrophosphate products GPP and FPP, as depicted in Fig. 28.6. In this process, DMAPP undergoes deprotonation under the influence of Mg^{2+}, generating a carbocationic intermediate. Subsequently, the carbon-carbon double bond of IPP engages in a nucleophilic attack on this intermediate, leading to the elimination of a proton and the formation of the ten-carbon product GPP. Through a similar mechanism, FPPS catalyzes the condensation of another IPP molecule with GPP to generate the corresponding fifteen-carbon product FPP [32]. The basic nitrogen atom of nitrogen-containing bisphosphonates readily undergoes protonation, mimicking the carbocationic intermediate state (Fig. 28.7). During enzyme catalysis, it occupies the intermediate site of DMAPP [44], thereby inhibiting the enzyme's activity.

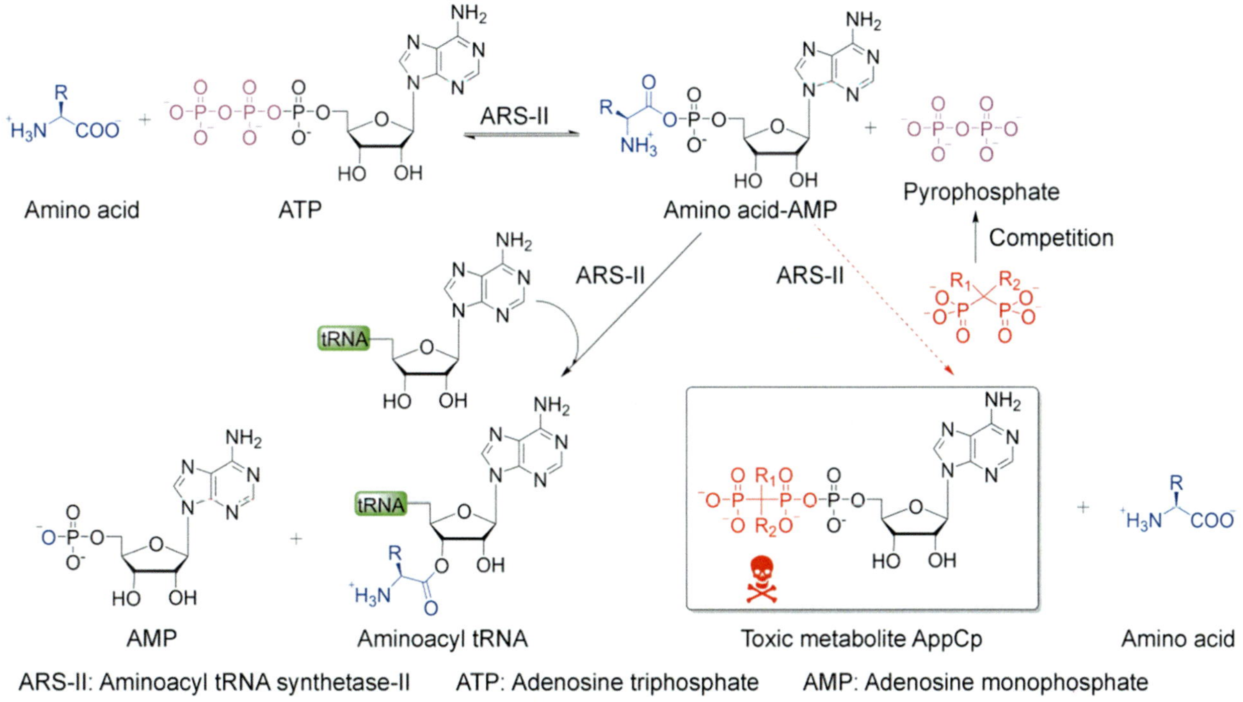

FIGURE 28.6 Molecular mechanism of cytotoxicity of first-generation nitrogen-free bisphosphonates.

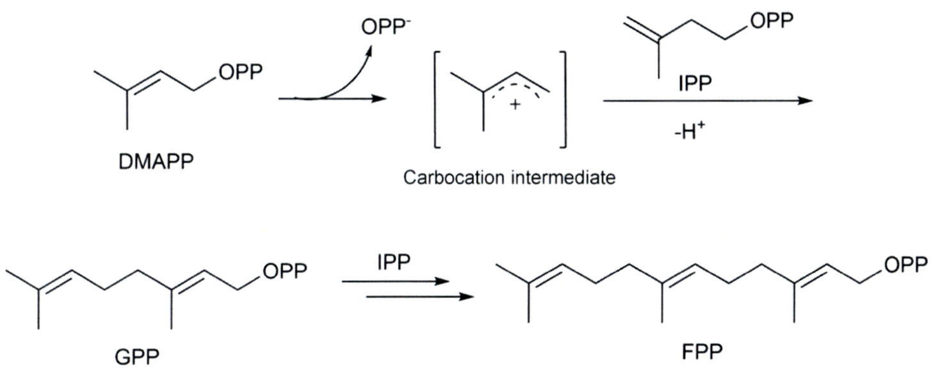

FIGURE 28.7 Schematic representation of the catalytic mechanism of FPPS. *FPPS*, Farnesyl pyrophosphate synthase.

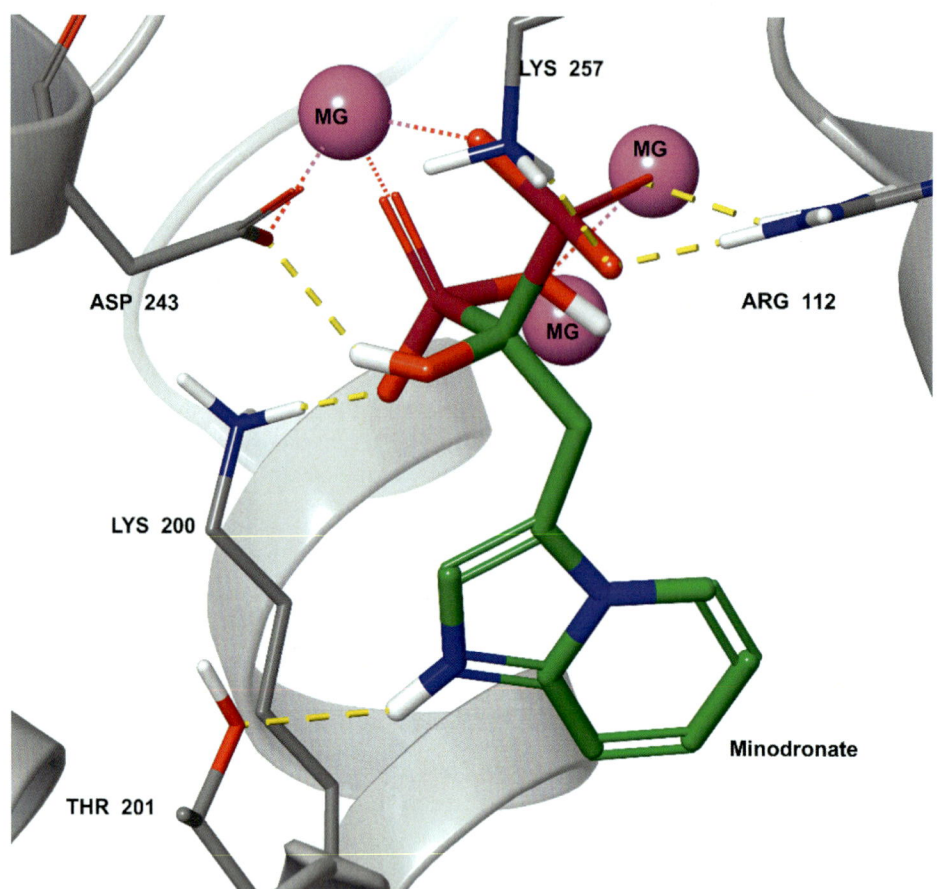

FIGURE 28.8 Binding mode of minodronic acid to FPPS (PDB ID: 3B7L). *FPPS*, Farnesyl pyrophosphate synthase.

Exemplified by minodronic acid, the binding mode of it to FPPS is shown in Fig. 28.8, in which the diphosphonate head group mimics the pyrophosphate moiety of the substrate DMAPP and chelates with three Mg^{2+} ions, forming an octahedral hexacoordinated chelation mode (for simplicity, water molecules and molecules not directly interacting with the diphosphonate in the coordination sphere are not shown).

In addition, salt bridge (ionic) interactions are formed with nearby basic amino acid residues Lys257, Arg112, and Lys200; a hydrogen bond interaction is formed between a protonated nitrogen atom on its imidazopyridine ring and Thr201. These interactions ultimately confer minodronic acid's potent inhibitory effect on FPPS at the enzymatic level (K_i = 3 nM).

28.3 Medicinal chemistry of nitrogen-containing bisphosphonates

28.3.1 Farnesyl pyrophosphate synthase as the molecular target of nitrogen-containing bisphosphonates

FPPS is an enzyme rich in α-helices, and its normal catalytic function is dependent on Mg^{2+}. Fig. 28.9 presents a cylindrical model of FPPS, where α-helices are represented as cylinders. This protein comprises 11 distinct α-helices connected by 10 loop regions. The cyan model represents the apo structure of FPPS from Staphylococcus aureus, while the magenta model depicts the complex crystal structure of FPPS from Escherichia coli bound to its substrates, IPP (yellow corey-pauling-koltun (CPK) model) and substrate analog S-DMAPP (modeled below the blue Mg^{2+} sphere). The superposition of the two states reveals that FPPS exists in at least two conformations: an open state in the absence of substrate (cyan) and a closed state upon binding of the two substrates (magenta). Upon substrate binding, α8-α11 undergoes significant conformational changes, collectively contracting inward to sequester the active site from the bulk solvent, thereby ensuring the efficient progression of the enzymatic reaction.

Comparative sequence analysis across species revealed that divergent FPPS protein sequences typically encompass two conserved DDXXD (D refers to Aspartic acid, X refers to any amino acids) sequences, as illustrated by the red CPK model in Fig. 28.10. This motif serves to chelate three Mg^{2+} ions, depicted as blue spheres in the figure, which

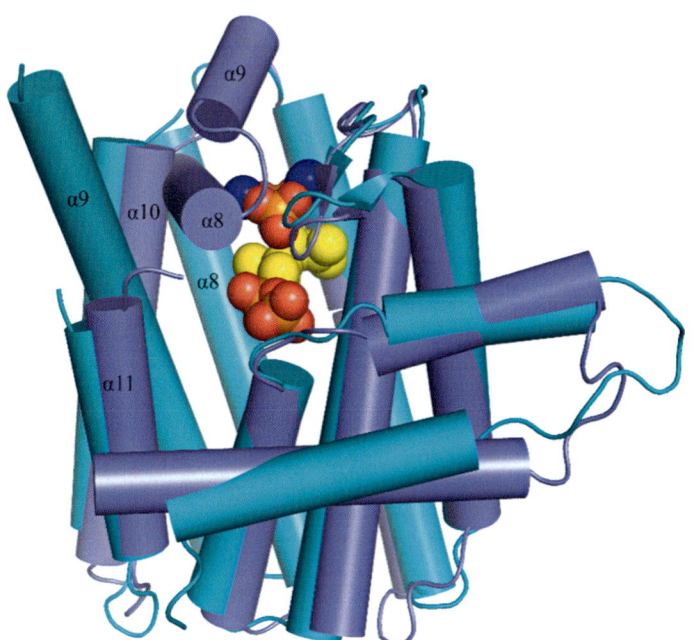

FIGURE 28.9 Cylindrical model depiction of the FPPS protein. *FPPS*, Farnesyl pyrophosphate synthase.

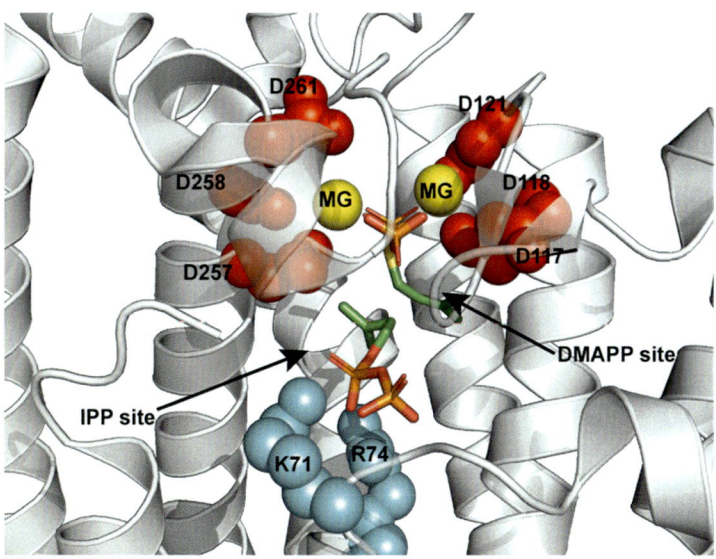

FIGURE 28.10 Crystallographic depiction of FPPS and schematic representation of its substrate binding pocket (PDB ID: 1ZW5 & 1RQI). *FPPS*, Farnesyl pyrophosphate synthase.

coordinate octahedrally with multiple surrounding aspartate residues and phosphate groups. This coordination facilitates the departure of DMAPP's pyrophosphate moiety, forming the key intermediate dimethylallyl carbocation, which undergoes a head-to-tail condensation reaction with the other substrate, IPP. Unlike DMAPP, IPP does not bind to Mg^{2+} *via* its pyrophosphate moiety but rather interacts with the protein through the basic amino acid residues Arg57 and Lys60, as depicted in Fig. 28.10. The precise mechanism by which FPPS catalyzes the condensation reaction between DMAPP and IPP has been extensively studied and elucidated: DMAPP initially binds to the protein, inducing a conformational change in FPPS from an open to a partially closed conformation, which remodels the shape of its active site, allowing the IPP binding pocket to fully form. Subsequently, IPP binding to the DMAPP-$3Mg^{2+}$-FPPS complex triggers a further conformational change, converting four amino acid residues (KRRK), K refers to Lysine, R refers to Arginine at the carbon terminus from a flexible, disordered state to an ordered state, thereby sealing off the entire reaction active site and inducing a fully closed conformation in the protein. Only in this fully closed conformation can the catalytic reaction proceed, accompanied by the release of PPi. FPPS then reverts to its original open conformation, the ten-carbon product GPP is displaced to the DMAPP site, and another molecule of IPP is loaded, enabling the next catalytic condensation to form the fifteen-carbon product FPP. Upon FPP release, FPPS once again adopts the open conformation, binds the next DMAPP molecule, and initiates another round of the catalytic cycle [32].

28.3.2 Structure-activity relationships of nitrogen-containing bisphosphonates

As previously mentioned, nitrogen-containing bisphosphonates, the predominant class of bisphosphonates currently used in clinical practice, have FPPS as their molecular target. Novel lipophilic bisphosphonates are also optimized from the second- and third-generation nitrogen-containing bisphosphonates. Therefore, this section primarily focuses on the molecular design and optimization of nitrogen-containing bisphosphonates, a class of inhibitors.

Typically, nitrogen-containing bisphosphonate drugs occupy the DMAPP substrate site of FPPS, displaying similar binding modes. Taking the complex crystal structure of zoledronic acid (ZOL) with FPPS (PDB ID: 2F8C) as an example, this section illustrates the nitrogen-containing bisphosphonates' binding mode with their target protein FPPS. Based on this, the principles of molecular design and optimization of nitrogen-containing bisphosphonates are explored. As depicted in Fig. 28.11, ZOL chelates with three Mg^{2+} ions, and its bisphosphonate group engages in ion-pair (salt bridge) interactions with the adjacent basic amino acid residues Arg112 and Lys200, also forming a hydrogen bond network with neighboring water molecules (not shown for simplicity in the schematic). Moreover, the nitrogen atom on the imidazole ring of ZOL readily undergoes protonation, mimicking the carbocation transition state in the FPPS-catalyzed process. Its suitable orientation allows ZOL to form two hydrogen bonds with Lys200 and Thr201, and the imidazole ring itself engages in cation-π interaction with the electropositive Lys200, further enhancing ZOL's binding affinity. It is evident from the binding mode and the structure-activity relationship of its derivatives that the position and orientation of the bisphosphonate group and the nitrogen-containing group are crucial for their activity. Modifications to the bisphosphonate group often lead to a significant decrease in activity, while changing the position of the nitrogen atom in the nitrogen-containing group can disrupt the hydrogen bond network it forms with Lys200 and Thr201, thereby affecting the activity.

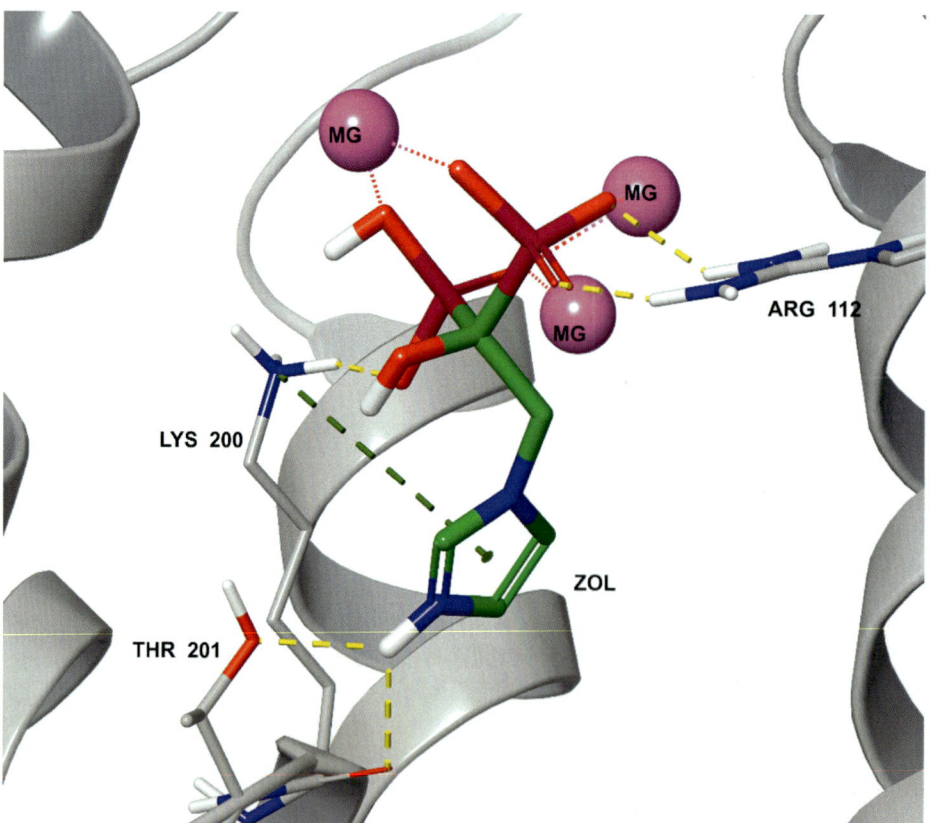

FIGURE 28.11 Binding mode of zoledronic acid with FPPS (PDB ID: 2F8C). *FPPS*, Farnesyl pyrophosphate synthase.

The structure of nitrogen-containing bisphosphonates can be represented by the general formula, as shown in Fig. 28.12, which contains three primary substructures: (1) the bisphosphonate group. As the principal functional group, the bisphosphonate group can form an octahedral coordination structure with the Mg^{2+} of FPPS, serving as a crucial pharmacophore for the affinity with the target FPPS and playing an irreplaceable role in maintaining the overall molecular activity and specific distribution within skeletal tissues. Substituting one of the phosphate groups of the bisphosphonate group with a sulfonic acid group or carboxylic acid group significantly decreases its FPPS inhibitory activity; replacing the bisphosphonate group with a monophosphate group also leads to a loss of activity. (2) The R_1 moiety. As one of the substituents on the connecting carbon atom between the two phosphate groups, the R_1 moiety can influence the affinity of the bisphosphonate with FPPS and also impact its affinity with skeletal tissues. Compared to R_1 being hydrogen, the presence of a hydroxyl group in R_1 enhances the affinity of the bisphosphonate for bones and its inhibitory activity against FPPS. Studies have found that the presence of the hydroxyl group also enhances the binding ability of the bisphosphonate to FPPS [45]. (3) The R_2 moiety. R_2 is a nitrogen-containing substituent that is essential for ensuring high affinity with FPPS. The nitrogen atom in R_2 typically exhibits alkalinity and is easily protonated under physiological conditions, which enables it to mimic the carbon cationic intermediate of FPPS catalytic reactions. Crystallographic studies of protein-molecule complexes have demonstrated that the nitrogen atom in R_2 forms an important hydrogen-bonding network with the main chain carbonyl groups of Thr201 and Lys200 in FPPS, playing a crucial role in maintaining its high activity. For instance, replacing the pyridine of alendronate with a phenyl ring leads to a 100-fold decrease in its activity.

Pamidronate, alendronate, and risedronate are all second-generation bisphosphonates, and most of these compounds are alkylamino-substituted derivatives, which exhibit significantly increased activity compared to the nitrogen-free first-generation bisphosphonates. ZOL, minodronic acid, and ibandronic acid belong to the third-generation bisphosphonate drugs, all of which have nitrogen-containing aromatic heterocyclic substituents, leading to significantly enhanced in vitro and in vivo activity compared to second-generation bisphosphonate drugs. Among them, ZOL is the most potent bisphosphonate drug in terms of in vivo activity (inhibiting bone resorption). In the marketed bisphosphonate drugs, the majority have a hydroxyl group as the R_1 substitution in their structure, and the presence of the hydroxyl group is related to their ability to enhance specific distribution in bone tissue. Table 28.1 shows the structure-activity relationships of the main nitrogen-containing second-generation bisphosphonate drugs and their derivatives. The optimization starting point for second-generation bisphosphonates is pamidronate (1). Based on the importance of the nitrogen atom in maintaining the activity of second-generation bisphosphonates, subsequent optimization has focused on finding derivatives with at least one nitrogen atom substitution. The distance between the methylene diphosphonate group of pamidronate and its terminal amino group is two carbon atoms; by adding an additional methylene group, alendronate is obtained, which results in eightfold

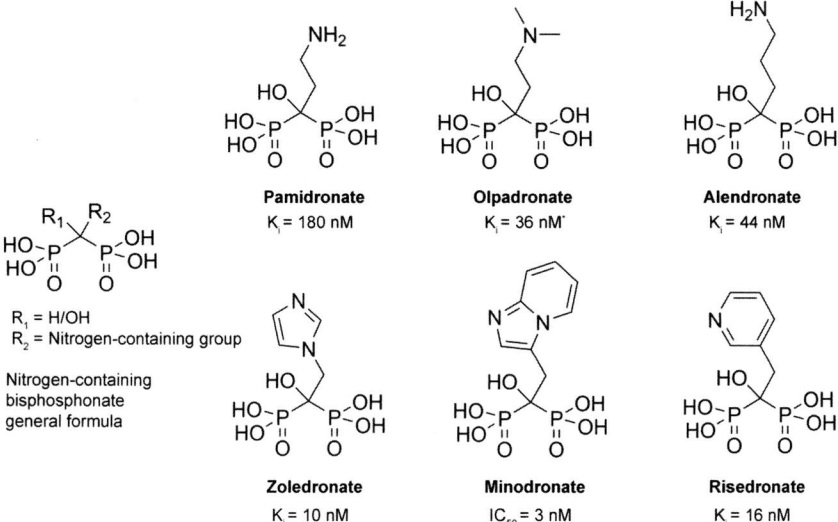

FIGURE 28.12 The general formula for the structure of nitrogen-containing bisphosphonates, as well as the structures and activity data of representative drugs (*no in vitro activity data, estimated from in vivo activity data relative to pamidronate).

TABLE 28.1 The structure-activity relationships of main nitrogen-containing second-generation bisphosphonate drugs and their derivatives.

Name	R_1	R_2	K_i/IC_{50}[a] (nM)	ED_{50}[b] (μg/kg)
1 (Pamidronate)	OH	–CH₂CH₂NH₂	180	61
2 (Alendronate)	OH	–(CH₂)₃NH₂	44	8
3	OH	–(CH₂)₄NH₂	194	20
4 (Neridronate)	OH	–(CH₂)₅NH₂	416	60
5	OH	–CH₂CH₂NH(CH₃)	–	~15
6 (Olpadronate)	OH	–CH₂CH₂N(CH₃)₂	36[c]	12
7	H	–CH₂CH₂N(CH₃)₂	–	100
8	NH₂	–CH₂CH₂N(CH₃)₂	–	>200
9	OH	–CH₂CH₂N(C₂H₅)₂	–	3
10	OH	–CH₂CH₂NHC(O)CH₃	–	>1000
11 (Ibandronate)	OH	–CH₂CH₂N(CH₃)(C₅H₁₁)	46	1.1
12	OH	–CH₂CH₂-pyrrolidinyl	–	10
13	OH	–CH₂CH₂-(3-phenyl-pyrrolidinyl)	–	70
14	OH	–CH₂CH₂-piperidinyl	–	5.6
15	OH	–CH₂CH₂-azepanyl	–	25
16	OH	–CH₂CH₂-azocanyl	–	>300

(Continued)

TABLE 28.1 (Continued)				
Name	R₁	R₂	K_i/IC_{50}^a (nM)	ED_{50}^b (μg/kg)
17	OH	piperidine (N-H, 2-position attachment)	–	50
18	OH	piperidine (3-position attachment, NH)	–	250
19	OH	piperidine (4-position attachment, NH)	–	~2500

^{a}Unless otherwise specified, all values are K_i values for FPPS.
^{b}ED50 is the subcutaneous dose of the compound that can alleviate 50% of the hypercalcemia induced by 1,25-dihydroxyvitamin D3 in TPTX rats (50% decrease in blood calcium concentration).
^{c}The K_i value here is estimated from the in vivo ED50 relative to the ED50 value of pamidronate.

and fourfold increases in in vivo and in vitro activity, respectively. Continuing to increase the chain length to four carbon atoms (compound **3**) and five carbon atoms (compound **4**, neridronate) weakens the in vivo and in vitro activity. Alkylating the terminal amino group also enhances the in vivo and in vitro activity; for example, compounds **5** and **6** (olpadronate) show an approximately fivefold increase in in vivo activity; after diethylation of the terminal amino group, compound **9** exhibits a 20-fold increase in activity; further lengthening the terminal alkyl group to five carbon atoms results in the formation of compound **11** (ibandronate), with further enhanced activity. Keeping the R₂ group unchanged and replacing the R₁ group with a hydrogen atom and an amino group, compounds **7** and **8** are obtained, with significantly reduced in vivo activity compared to **6** (olpadronate), indicating that the hydroxyl group in the R₁ group contributes the most to the activity. Acetylating the terminal amino group of pamidronate (**1**) to mask its charge results in a severe decrease in activity (compound **10**), demonstrating the crucial importance of protonated nitrogen atom substitutions for maintaining activity. Furthermore, by designing compounds **12–16** with cyclic alkyl substitutions of the terminal amino group, it is shown that compounds with five- to seven-membered ring substitutions (**12–15**) maintain high levels of activity, whereas further increasing the substitutions to an eight-membered ring in compound **16** leads to a significant decrease in activity. According to the results of this structure-activity relationship study, in combination with the binding mode of bisphosphonates to FPPS as mentioned earlier, it is evident that the nitrogen atom provides a significant expandable space in the binding pocket in a hydrophobic environment. This can be fully utilized to subsequently optimize the physicochemical properties of the compounds. Adjustment of the position and orientation of the basic nitrogen atoms yields compounds **17–19**, and the differences in their activity indicate that the orientation of the nitrogen atom also significantly influences the final activity of bisphosphonate molecules.

Table 28.2 presents the structure-activity relationships of ZOL and its related derivatives. In this section, the structure-activity relationships of third-generation nitrogen-containing bisphosphonates are explored using ZOL as a typical representative. After the successful development of second-generation bisphosphonates, researchers discovered that the R2 group can also be replaced by nitrogen-containing aromatic heterocycles, and the activity is usually higher after such substitution. For example, compound **20**, with an imidazole ring at the terminal end, has an in vivo activity of 5 μg/kg. Based on this, by methylating the NH hydrogen atom on the imidazole ring, compound **21** is obtained, with a further approximately eightfold increase in in vivo activity, which is consistent with the increase in in vitro activity. By changing the substitution site on the imidazole ring, while the in vitro activity of compound **22** is slightly weakened, the in vivo activity is improved by approximately 10-fold compared to compound **20**. Increasing the number of carbon atoms between the imidazole ring and the methylene diphosphonate significantly reduces the activity of compound **23**. By further substituting the imidazole ring with a methyl and a phenyl group based on **22**, compounds **24**, **25**, and **26** show decreased in vitro and in vivo activity, especially with a significant decrease in the activity of compound **25**. Therefore, the space that can be modified for the 22-series compounds is limited. Finally, by changing the substitution pattern of the imidazole ring, ZOL (ZOL, compound **27**) is obtained, which, although not exhibiting the best in vitro

TABLE 28.2 The structure-activity relationships of third-generation nitrogen-containing bisphosphonate zoledronic acid and its derivatives.

Name	R₁	R₂	K_i/IC_{50}[a] (nM)	ED_{50}[b] (μg/kg)
20	OH	2-imidazolyl-methyl (NH)	18[c]	5
21	OH	1-methyl-2-imidazolyl-methyl	2[c]	0.6
22	OH	4(5)-imidazolyl-methyl	30	0.3
23	OH	4(5)-imidazolyl-ethyl	67[c]	20
24	OH	2-methyl-4(5)-imidazolyl-methyl	51[c]	15
25	OH	2-phenyl-4(5)-imidazolyl-methyl	–	>3000
26	OH	5-methyl-4-imidazolyl-methyl	5.1[c]	1.5
27 (Zoledronate)	OH	1-imidazolyl-methyl	10	0.07
28	OH	2-methyl-1-imidazolyl-methyl	10[c]	3
29	OH	4,5-dimethyl-1-imidazolyl-methyl	–	1.5
30	OH	1-imidazolyl-ethyl	–	45

(Continued)

Name	R₁	R₂	K_i/IC_{50}^a (nM)	ED_{50}^b (μg/kg)
31	OH	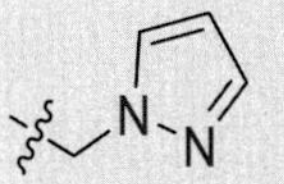 (CH₂-pyrazole)	–	>300
32	OH	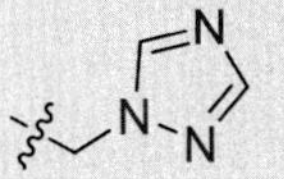 (CH₂-1,2,4-triazole)	–	600

[a]Unless otherwise specified, all values are K_i values for FPPS.
[b]ED50 is the subcutaneous dose of the compound that can alleviate 50% of the hypercalcemia induced by 1,25-dihydroxyvitamin D3 in TPTX rats (50% decrease in blood calcium concentration).
[c]This value represents the IC50.

enzymatic activity, has the best in vivo activity among bisphosphonate drugs currently, reaching 0.07 μg/kg. Further methylation on the imidazole ring produces compounds **28** and **29**, both of which show a decrease in in vivo activity of more than 10-fold compared to ZOL. Based on the binding mode of ZOL to FPPS, it is suggested that the methylation substitution may hinder the formation of the optimal binding conformation, weakening the binding affinity of the corresponding derivatives to FPPS. Increasing the distance between the imidazole ring and the methylene diphosphonate yields compound **30**, which also exhibits a significant decrease in in vivo activity. Changing the position of the key nitrogen atom of ZOL results in compound **31**, with a significant decrease in activity. Additionally, transforming one nitrogen atom on the imidazole ring into 1,2,4-triazole also leads to a significant decrease in activity. Based on the binding mode of ZOL, it can be inferred that the decreased alkalinity of the substitution in compound **32** prevents protonation under physiological conditions, weakening its binding affinity to FPPS, ultimately resulting in a significant decrease in in vivo activity.

28.3.3 Design and development of next-generation lipophilic bisphosphonate inhibitors

Due to the structural characteristics of bisphosphonate drugs, they easily adsorb into bone tissue. Additionally, nitrogen-containing bisphosphonate compounds exhibit high activity against FPPS. As a result, second- and third-generation bisphosphonate drugs generally demonstrate good in vivo activity in the treatment of osteoporosis. However, the highly polar nature of the bisphosphonate groups leads to poor lipid solubility, making it difficult for these drugs to penetrate and distribute into soft tissue cells. Hence, their clinical application is limited to bone-related diseases. Despite numerous research reports on the potential of FPPS as a target and some bisphosphonate compounds in the treatment of cancer and other diseases [15,16,46], their application in the treatment of soft tissue-related cancers has been unsatisfactory [46]. To address this issue, medicinal chemists have developed new lipophilic bisphosphonates (as depicted by the general structure shown in Table 28.3), primarily composed of three parts, namely the bisphosphonate head, the nitrogen-containing aromatic linker, and the lipophilic tail (often a hydrophobic long carbon chain). Compared to traditional nitrogen-containing bisphosphonates, this class of lipophilic bisphosphonates has a higher lipid-water partition coefficient (logP). This improved cell membrane permeability results in better activity in cell experiments and animal models [17,47]. The enhanced hydrophobicity also helps to weaken the affinity of bisphosphonates for bone tissue, thereby increasing their proportion of distribution in soft tissue.

As shown in Table 28.3, based on the structural types with the nitrogen-containing aromatic ring R₂, the most extensively researched derivatives currently belong to two major categories: those based on pyridine (**33–36**) and those based on imidazole (**38–42**). In the former group, when the carbon chain length of the lipophilic long carbon chain is seven, compound **33** exhibits higher enzymatic activity. However, as the carbon chain length is further increased to 11 and 13, the activity gradually decreases. When R₂ is substituted with adjacent aminopyridine (**36**) while maintaining a carbon chain length of 6, its activity is comparable to ZOL. Upon removal of the nitrogen atom from the pyridine ring, the compound completely loses its inhibitory activity against FPPS due to its inability to form a cationic center. Among the latter imidazole series derivatives, compounds with carbon chain lengths of 4–8 generally exhibit good FPPS enzymatic inhibition activity. However, when the chain length exceeds 10, the corresponding inhibitory activity significantly decreases, possibly due to the excessively long carbon chain causing collision effects with the highly conserved Phe98 and Phe99 in FPPS [48].

TABLE 28.3 The chemical structure and structure-activity relationships of lipophilic bisphosphonates.

Name	R₁	X₁	R₂	X₂	n	IC$_{50}$/K$_i^a$ (nM)
27 (Zoledronate)	–	–	–	–	–	100/1.3[b]
33	H	CH$_2$	3-pyridyl	O	6	1.3[c]
34	H	CH$_2$	3-pyridyl	O	10	50[c]
35	H	CH$_2$	3-pyridyl	O	12	1584[c]
36	H	NH	2,3-pyridyl	O	6	90
37	H	NH	phenyl	O	8	>30,000
38	OH	CH$_2$	imidazolyl	CH$_2$	0	80
39	OH	CH$_2$	imidazolyl	CH$_2$	3	30
40	OH	CH$_2$	imidazolyl	CH$_2$	5	44
41	OH	CH$_2$	imidazolyl	CH$_2$	7	36/1.0[b]
42	OH	CH$_2$	imidazolyl	CH$_2$	9	230

[a] Unless otherwise specified, all values are IC50 values for FPPS.
[b] The former represents the IC50 value, while the latter represents the K_i value. These values may differ from the data listed in Table 28.2 due to their source from different research groups.
[c] This value represents the Ki.

TABLE 28.4 A comparison of cellular activity between zoledronic acid and lipophilic bisphosphonates.

Name	AlogP [a]	Cancer cell growth inhibition EC_{50}			TNF-α EC_{50} [b] (μM)
		SF-268 (μM)	MCF-7 (μM)	NCI-H460 (μM)	
27 (Zoledronate)	−0.93	15.8	20	15.8	170
33	−0.17	1.0	2.5	0.5	–
34	1.07	0.1	0.2	0.06	–
35	1.67	0.013	0.4	0.005	–
38	−0.17	–	–	–	210
39	0.39	–	–	–	250
40	0.78	–	–	–	81
41	1.21	–	–	–	23
42	1.71	–	–	–	7.6

[a] The AlogP values were calculated using the online logP prediction website (http://www.vcclab.org/lab/alogps/).
[b] The EC50 value here serves as a measure of the ability to activate Vγ9Vδ2 T cells, and it partially reflects the activity of FPPS inhibitors at the cellular level.

In terms of enzymatic inhibition activity, compounds **33–35** are comparable or inferior to ZOL (**27**), but in the growth inhibition experiments of cancer cells SF-268, MCF-7, and NCI-H460, the inhibitory activity of ZOL is weaker than that of **33–35**. As shown in Table 28.4, as the carbon chain length increases, although their enzymatic inhibition activity against FPPS decreases, their ability to inhibit cancer cell growth becomes stronger, which is related to the increasing lipid solubility of compounds **33–35**. With the increasing value of molecular logP, the membrane permeability of the compounds also continuously increases, to some extent compensating for the loss in their enzymatic inhibition activity. Furthermore, the experimental data of compounds **38–42** on the activation of Vγ9Vδ2 T cells (Table 28.4, TNF-α EC50 represents the ability to activate Vγ9Vδ2 T cells) further illustrates the advantages of lipophilic bisphosphonates in cell permeability. Similarly, with the lengthening of the lipophilic carbon chain, their logP values continuously increase, and the membrane permeability also continuously strengthens. Coupled with their high enzymatic inhibition activity against FPPS, this leads to a continuously enhanced ability to activate Vγ9Vδ2 T cells. It is worth noting that while the improvement in the cellular activity of these lipophilic bisphosphonates relies on the increase in lipid solubility, the enhancement of cellular effects of some compounds is also related to their targeting of another pathway, the GGPPS target. For example, compound **41**, whose enzymatic inhibition activity at the Ki level is similar to ZOL, exhibits approximately 5–6 times greater activity in inhibiting cancer cell growth [17]. Besides a higher logP value, this is also due to its approximately ninefold higher inhibition activity against GGPPS compared to ZOL.

28.3.4 In vivo distribution and metabolism of bisphosphonates

After entering the human body, small-molecule drugs undergo processes of absorption, distribution, metabolism, and excretion, collectively referred to as the drug's ADME properties. These processes are the body's disposition of foreign drug molecules and have a significant impact on the ultimate therapeutic effect of the drug. The chemical structure of small molecules determines certain physicochemical properties, which not only influence their affinity with target molecules but also affect the ADME processes in the human body. However, due to its unique structure characterized by highly polar bisphosphonate groups, the ADME properties of bisphosphonate drugs can be considered distinct. Generally, bisphosphonates are not easily absorbed *via* oral administration, and after entering the body, they are selectively distributed to bone tissue. Due to their high polarity, they have difficulty entering the liver for metabolism by various hepatic enzymes and are almost entirely excreted in their molecular form through renal organs (urine).

The absorption rate of bisphosphonates into the human body after gastrointestinal absorption is low, leading to a correspondingly low oral bioavailability. Only half of the bisphosphonate drugs that enter the blood have a high affinity for bone tissue and are rapidly adsorbed onto the bones, while the remaining half is quickly excreted and disappears from the plasma. The retention time of bisphosphonates in the skeletal system depends on the affinity of the bisphosphonate molecule itself for the skeletal system, the strength of renal excretion function, bone turnover rate, and

TABLE 28.5 Metabolic data of representative third-generation bisphosphonate drugs in the human body.

	Etidronate	Pamidronate	Zoledronate
Half-life (h)	6.0 ± 0.7	2.2	0.23
oral bioavailability (%)	2.3 ± 1.1	0.1–1.2	1.0
Overall clearance rate (mL/min)	182 ± 21	181 ± 78	85 ± 33
Renal clearance rate (mL/min)	105 ± 14	79 ± 29	–
Volume of distribution (L)	98 ± 41	29.5	9.0 ± 2.2

available binding sites [49]. The elimination half-life of bisphosphonate drugs in the body varies from several days to several months, and in some individuals, the elimination half-life of certain bisphosphonate molecules can even be as long as 10 years. Therefore, although bisphosphonate drug molecules share similar distribution and metabolism characteristics, the specific metabolic characteristics can differ depending on the particular bisphosphonate drug used and the pathophysiological conditions of the patient. For example, the bone turnover rate differs between patients without osteoporosis and those with osteoporosis, leading to significant differences in the elimination half-life following the administration of bisphosphonates. In addition, according to Tc-99m imaging studies, the distribution of bisphosphonates in bone tissue differs among patients with different bone diseases; for instance, in patients with Paget's disease, the distribution of bisphosphonate molecules is concentrated in the lumbar vertebrae, while in patients with osteoporosis, they are evenly distributed within the bone tissue [49]. Table 28.5 presents the metabolic data of three representative bisphosphonates in the human body.

28.4 Novel applications of bisphosphonate inhibitors

28.4.1 Bisphosphonate drugs and inhibitors in anticancer therapy

For many years, bisphosphonate drugs have been limited in their application to bone-related diseases such as osteoporosis, Paget's disease, tumor-related hypercalcemia, and osteolysis. However, in recent years, with ongoing research in this field, whether in clinical research [15,16,46] or preclinical research [50], bisphosphonates, as a class of established drugs, have gradually demonstrated therapeutic potential in new disease areas.

In a clinical trial investigating the anticancer efficacy of ZOL [46], researchers found that adding ZOL acid to adjuvant endocrine therapy improved disease-free survival in premenopausal estrogen-responsive early-stage breast cancer patients. Compared to endocrine therapy alone, the addition of ZOL during endocrine therapy led to a 36% reduction in the risk of disease progression. A systematic review and metaanalysis of 15 clinical trials involving the use of ZOL in early-stage breast cancer (stages I–III) revealed that, as an adjuvant therapy, ZOL statistically significantly improved overall survival and reduced the risk of fractures compared to a placebo or nontreatment group [15]. In a clinical trial investigating whether ZOL can be applied to multiple myeloma [16], researchers recruited a total of 1960 patients for the trial and found that ZOL significantly increased progression-free survival by 12% (compared to clodronic acid) and extended the progression-free survival period by 2 months. Therefore, for patients newly diagnosed with multiple myeloma, researchers recommended immediate treatment with ZOL, which not only prevents skeletal-related events but also has potential advantages in antimyeloma treatment.

In addition, in preclinical studies related to various cancers, bisphosphonate drugs have demonstrated potential direct or indirect anticancer effects. It has been found that nitrogen-containing bisphosphonates possess the ability to inhibit cancer cell proliferation and induce apoptosis in breast cancer, prostate cancer, ovarian cancer, bladder cancer, liver cancer, osteosarcoma, leukemia, melanoma, and multiple myeloma cells [50]. As described in the second section, their main biological mechanism is achieved through the inhibition of FPPS, thereby interfering with the posttranslational modification of important small G proteins such as Ras and Rho. Furthermore, research has also revealed that nitrogen-containing bisphosphonate drugs accumulate IPP by inhibiting FPPS, which, under the action of aminoacyl-tRNA synthetase, forms ApppI, a toxic cellular metabolite, through binding with AMP, leading to direct induction of apoptosis by blocking mitochondrial adenylate nucleotide translocase [51]. ZOL can also reduce the adhesion of prostate cancer cells to the mineralized bone matrix by inhibiting the prenylation, especially geranylgeranylation, of G proteins, thus potentially contributing to the ability of bisphosphonates to inhibit cancer cell metastasis [52]. As mentioned earlier, nitrogen-containing bisphosphonates can also promote the accumulation of IPP by inhibiting FPPS, thereby activating Vγ9Vδ2 T cells. As major histocompatibility complex (MHC)-independent receptors recognizing tumor cells, γδ T cells are potent "cancer killers" and are expected to be an alternative αβ T-cell therapy for cancers resistant to γδ T-cell therapy [50].

In a mouse model of lung adenocarcinoma with KRAS mutation, researchers found that the use of the lipophilic bisphosphonate compound BPH-1222 (compound **41**) alone could block the prenylation of KRAS, but it also led to the accumulation of p62 and the activation of NF-B, resulting in a reduction in in vivo efficacy [17]. Furthermore, when used in combination with the autophagy inducer rapamycin, it prevented the NF-B activation induced by p62 accumulation, thereby inhibiting the in vivo proliferation of cancer cells. The combination of BPH-1222 and rapamycin produced a potent synergistic anticancer effect compared to the use of BPH-1222 or rapamycin alone.

28.4.2 Development of lipophilic bisphosphonate inhibitors as vaccine adjuvants

Adjuvants are nonspecific immunomodulators that, when used in conjunction with vaccines, can induce robust immune responses for preventing infectious diseases such as influenza or enhancing the efficacy of noninfectious disease vaccines such as cancer vaccines [18]. Researchers drew inspiration from a rare autoimmune deficiency disorder called MVA kinase deficiency and ultimately identified the MVA pathway, particularly HMG-CoA reductase, FPPS, and GGPPS, as novel targets for immunomodulation.

Reports have indicated that small-molecule adjuvants require sufficient local tissue retention and concentration to achieve optimal immunostimulatory effects [53]. However, nitrogen-containing bisphosphonate compounds such as ZOL have demonstrated weak tissue penetration capability and strong bone affinity, leading to rapid clearance upon injection into muscle tissue, thus failing to achieve potent adjuvant effects. Therefore, the use of lipophilic bisphosphonates can extend their retention time in muscle tissue to achieve immunostimulatory adjuvant effects. Studies have shown that in mouse models, TH-Z93 (compound **36**) and TH-Z145 (compound **37**, a selective GGPPS inhibitor), in combination with the antigen ovalbumin, produced potent adjuvant effects, significantly enhancing antibody titers and affinity. However, the coadministration of GGPP and TH-Z93 or TH-Z145 completely abolished the adjuvant effect, indicating that these two lipophilic bisphosphonates ultimately lead to reduced GGPP synthesis and the subsequent adjuvant effect by inhibiting FPPS and GGPPS. Subsequent research further confirmed that the lipophilic bisphosphonates TH-Z93 and TH-Z145, through blocking the synthesis of GGPP, disrupted the prenylation of small G protein Rab5 in antigen-presenting cells, inhibited endosome maturation, thereby extending antigen retention time, enhancing antigen presentation, and activating T cells.

Furthermore, in a highly pathogenic avian influenza mouse model, both TH-Z93 and TH-Z145 demonstrated strong protective effects. In a mouse model combined with anti-PD1 antibody therapy, the combination of TH-Z93 and TH-Z145 with PD1 antibody significantly improved the survival rates of TC-1-E7 tumor model mice compared to the use of PD1 antibody alone.

References

[1] Sergio B, Eileen G, Kristy C, et al. Nano-analytical electron microscopy reveals fundamental insights into human cardiovascular tissue calcification. Nat Mater 2013;12(6):576–83.
[2] Miller JD. Cardiovascular calcification: orbicular origins. Nat Mater 2013;12(6):476–8.
[3] Beckmann NM. Calcium apatite deposition disease: diagnosis and treatment. Radiol Res Pract 2016;2016:1–16.
[4] Fleisch H, Bisaz S. Isolation from urine of pyrophosphate, a calcification inhibitor. Am J Physiol 1962;203(4):671–5.
[5] Russell RG. Bisphosphonates: the first 40 years. Bone 2011;49(1):2–19.
[6] Russell R. Excretion of inorganic pyrophosphate in hypophosphatasia. Lancet 1965;2(7410):461–4.
[7] Schibler D, Russell RG, Fleisch H. Inhibition by pyrophosphate and polyphosphate of aortic calcification induced by Vitamin D3 in rats. Clin Sci 1968;35(2):363–72.
[8] Jung A, Bisaz S, Fleisch H. The binding of pyrophosphate and two diphosphonates by hydroxyapatite crystals. Calcif Tissue Res 1973;11(4):269–80.
[9] Fleisch HA, Russell RG, Bisaz S, et al. The inhibitory effect of phosphonates on the formation of calcium phosphate crystals in vitro and on aortic and kidney calcification in vivo. Eur J Clin Invest 1970;1(1):12–18.
[10] Fleisch H, Maerki J, Russell RG. Effect of pyrophosphate on dissolution of hydroxyapatite and its possible importance in calcium homeostasis. Proc Soc Exp Biol Med 1966;122(2):317–20.

[11] Russell RG, Muhlbauer RC, Bisaz S, et al. The influence of pyrophosphate, condensed phosphates, phosphonates and other phosphate compounds on the dissolution of hydroxyapatite in vitro and on bone resorption induced by parathyroid hormone in tissue culture and in thyroparathyroidecto-mised rats. Calcif Tissue Res 1970;6(3):83−196.

[12] Francis MD, Russell RG, Fleisch H. Diphosphonates inhibit formation of calcium phosphate crystals in vitro and pathological calcification in vivo. Science 1969;165(3899):1264−6.

[13] Fleisch H, Russell RG, Francis MD. Diphosphonates inhibit hydroxyapatite dissolution in vitro and bone resorption in tissue culture and in vivo. Science 1969;165(3899):1262−4.

[14] Teitelbaum SL. Bone resorption by osteoclasts. Science 2000;289(5484):1504−8.

[15] Valachis A, Nearchou A, Polyzos NP, et al. Adjuvant therapy with zoledronic acid in patients with breast cancer: a systematic review and meta-analysis. Oncologist 2013;18(4):353−61.

[16] Morgan GJ. First-line treatment with zoledronic acid as compared with clodronic acid in multiple myeloma (MRC Myeloma IX): a randomised controlled trial. Lancet 2010;376(9757):1989−99.

[17] Xia YF, Liu YL, Xie YH, et al. A combination therapy for KRAS-driven lung adenocarcinomas using lipophilic bisphosphonates and rapamycin. Sci Transl Med 2014;6(263) 263ra161.

[18] Xia Y, Xie Y, Yu Z, et al. The mevalonate pathway is a druggable target for vaccine adjuvant discovery. Cell 2018;175(4):1059−73 e1021.

[19] Kaur M, Nagpal M, Singh M. Osteoblast-n-osteoclast: making headway to osteoporosis treatment. Curr Drug Targets 2020;21(16):1640−51.

[20] Drake MT, Clarke BL, Khosla S. Bisphosphonates: mechanism of action and role in clinical practice. Mayo Clin Proc 2008;83(9):1032−45.

[21] Sato M, Grasser W, Endo N, et al. Bisphosphonate action. Alendronate localisation in rat bone and effects on osteoclast ultrastructure. J Clin Invest 1991;88(6):2095−105.

[22] Thompson K, Rogers MJ, Coxon FP, et al. Cytosolic entry of bisphosphonate drugs requires acidification of vesicles after fluid-phase endocytosis. Mol Pharmacol 2006;69(5):1624−32.

[23] Flanagan AM, Chambers TJ. Dichloromethylenebisphosphonate (Cl_2MBP) inhibits bone resorption through injury to osteoclasts that resorb Cl_2MBP-coated bone. Bone Min 1986;6(1):33−43.

[24] Ito M, Chokki M, Ogino Y, et al. Comparison of the cytotoxic effects of bisphosphnates in vitro and in vivo. Calcif Tissue Int 1998;63(2):143−7.

[25] Li BJ, Chau JF, Wang XY, et al. Bisphosphonates, specific inhibitors of osteoclast function and a class of drugs for osteoporosis therapy. J Cell Biochem 2011;112(5):1229−42.

[26] Breuil V, Cosman F, Stein L, et al. Human osteoclast formation and activity in vitro: effects of alendronate. J Bone Miner Res 1998;13(11):1721−9.

[27] Hughes DE, Cosman F, Stein L, et al. Bisphosphonates promote apoptosis in murine osteoclasts in vitro and in vivo. J Bone Miner Res 1995;10(10):1478−87.

[28] Selander KS, Mönkkönen J, Karhukorpi EK, et al. Characteristics of clodronate-induced apoptosis in osteoclasts and macrophages. Mol Pharmacol 1996;50(5):1127−38.

[29] Murakami H, Takahashi N, Sasaki T, et al. A possible mechanism of the specific action of bisphosphonates on osteoclasts: tiludronate preferentially affects polarized osteoclasts having ruffled borders. Bone 1995;17(2):137−44.

[30] Firn R. Nature's chemicals. The natural products that shaped our world. Illustrated edition. New York: Oxford University Press Inc.; 2010.

[31] Lange BM, Rujan T, Martin W, et al. Isoprenoid biosynthesis: the evolution of two ancient and distinct pathways across genomes. Proc Natl Acad Sci USA 2000;97(24):13172−7.

[32] Han S. Discovery, development and activity study of novel *Hs*FPPS non-bisphosphonate inhibitors. Beijing: Tsinghua University,; 2020.

[33] Ten K, Hordijk PL. Targeting and localized signalling by small GTPases. Biol Cell 2007;99(1):1−12.

[34] Zhang Y, Cao R, Yin F, et al. Lipophilic pyridinium bisphosphonates: potent gammadelta T cell stimulators. Angew Chem Int Ed 2010;49(6):1136−8.

[35] Sandstrom A, Peigne CM, Leger A, et al. The intracellular B30.2 domain of butyrophilin 3A1 binds phosphoantigens to mediate activation of human Vgamma9Vdelta2 T cells. Immunity 2014;40(4):490−500.

[36] Tanaka Y, Morita CT, Tanaka Y, et al. Natural and synthetic non-peptide antigens recognized by human gamma delta T cells. Nature 1995;375(6527):155−8.

[37] Luckman SP, Hughes DE, Coxon FP, et al. Nitrogen-containing bisphosphonates inhibit the mevalonate pathway and prevent post-translational prenylation of GTP-binding proteins, including Ras. J Bone Miner Res 1998;13(4):581−9.

[38] Dunford JE, Rogers MJ, Ebetino FH, et al. Inhibition of protein prenylation by bisphosphonates causes sustained activation of Rac, Cdc42, and Rho GTPases. J Bone Miner Res 2006;21(5):684−94.

[39] Rogers MJ, Crockett JC, Coxon FP, et al. Biochemical and molecular mechanisms of action of bisphosphonates. Bone 2011;49(1):34−41.

[40] Rogers MJ, Brown RJ, Hodkin V, et al. Bisphosphonates are incorporated into adenine nucleotides by human aminoacyl-tRNA synthetase enzymes. Biochem Biophys Res Commun 1996;224(3):863−9.

[41] Benford HL, Frith JC, Auriola S, et al. Farnesol and geranylgeraniol prevent activation of caspases by aminobisphosphonates: biochemical evidence for two distinct pharmacological classes of bisphosphonate drugs. Mol Pharmacol 1999;56(1):131−40.

[42] Mönkkönen H, Rogers MJ, Makkonen N, et al. The cellular uptake and metabolism of clodronate in RAW 264 macrophages. Pharm Res 2001;18(11):1550−5.

[43] Benford HL, Mcgowan NW, Helfrich MH, et al. Visualization of bisphosphonate-induced caspase-3 activity in apoptotic osteoclasts in vitro. Bone 2001;28(5):465−73.
[44] L KATHRYN, Guo K, Dunford JE, et al. The molecular mechanism of nitrogen-containing bisphosphonates as antiosteoporosis drugs. Proc Natl Acad Sci USA 2006;103(20):7829−34.
[45] Dunford JE, Kwaasi AA, Rogers MJ, et al. Structure−activity relationships among the nitrogen containing bisphosphonates in clinical use and other analogues: time-dependent inhibition of human farnesyl pyrophosphate synthase. J Med Chem 2008;51(7):2187−95.
[46] Gnant M, Mlineritsch B, Schippinger W, et al. Endocrine therapy plus zoledronic acid in premenopausal breast cancer. N Engl J Med 2009;360(7):679−91.
[47] Zhang YH, Cao R, Yin F, et al. Lipophilic bisphosphonates as dual farnesyl/geranylgeranyl diphosphate synthase inhibitors: an X-ray and NMR investigation. J Am Chem Soc 2009;131(14):5153−62.
[48] Zhang YH, Zhu W, Liu YL, et al. Chemo-immunotherapeutic antimalarials targeting isoprenoid biosynthesis. ACS Med Chem Lett 2013;4(4):423−7.
[49] Cremers M, Pillai GC, Papapoulos SE. Pharmacokinetics/pharmacodynamics of bisphosphonates: use for optimization of intermittent therapy for osteoporosis. Clin Pharmacokinetics 2005;44(6):551−70.
[50] Stresing V, Daubine F, Benzaid I, et al. Bisphosphonates in cancer therapy. Cancer Lett 2007;257(1):16−35.
[51] Mönkkönen H, Auriola S, Lehenkari P, et al. A new endogenous ATP analog (ApppI) inhibits the mitochondrial adenine nucleotide translocase (ANT) and is responsible for the apoptosis induced by nitrogen-containing bisphosphonates. Br J Pharmacol 2006;147(4):437−45.
[52] Coxon JP, Oades GM, Kirby RS, et al. Zoledronic acid induces apoptosis and inhibits adhesionto mineralized matrix in prostate cancer cells via inhibition of protein prenylation. BJU Int 2004;94(1):164−70.
[53] Wu H, Singh M, Miller AT, et al. Rational design of small molecules as vaccine adjuvants. Sci Transl Med 2014;6(263) 263ra160.

Chapter 29

Celecoxib targets cyclooxygenase in nonsteroidal antiinflammatory drugs

Yong Wang[1,2] and Ya-qiu Long[3]

[1]School of Medicine and Pharmacy, Key Laboratory of Marine Drugs, Chinese Ministry of Education, Ocean University of China, Shandong, P.R. China, [2]Laboratory for Marine Drugs and Bioproducts, Pilot National Laboratory for Marine Science and Technology, Qingdao, P.R. China, [3]College of Pharmaceutical Sciences, Soochow University, Suzhou, P.R. China

Chapter outline

29.1 Nonsteroidal antiinflammatory drugs and cyclooxygenase	711
29.1.1 Introduction to nonsteroidal antiinflammatory drugs	711
29.1.2 Mechanism of action of nonsteroidal antiinflammatory drugs	712
29.2 Selective cyclooxygenase-2 inhibitor celecoxib	715
29.2.1 Cyclooxygenase inhibitors	715
29.2.2 Cyclooxygenase-2 selective inhibitor celecoxib	716
29.3 Other representative coxib drugs	731
29.4 Summary and perspective	732
References	732

29.1 Nonsteroidal antiinflammatory drugs and cyclooxygenase

29.1.1 Introduction to nonsteroidal antiinflammatory drugs

Inflammation is a defensive response of the body to external infections, sometimes causing damage such as local redness, swelling, and pain. In clinical practice, there are two main categories of drugs for treating inflammation: glucocorticoid antiinflammatory drugs with a steroid structure and nonsteroidal antiinflammatory drugs (NSAIDs). Glucocorticoid antiinflammatory drugs effectively treat arthritis but can cause drug dependence and adrenal function degeneration in long-term treatment. Currently, NSAIDs are the most widely used therapeutic agents for their antiinflammatory, antipyretic, and analgesic effects, making them the first choice for treating fever, pain, rheumatic disorders, and other degenerative inflammatory joint diseases. The first historically significant NSAID was aspirin (also known as acetylsalicylic acid, compound A in Fig. 29.1), which has been used in clinics for over 100 years and is considered one of the most famous and legendary drugs worldwide. Even today, the global annual production of aspirin is approximately 50,000 tons, reflecting the value and significance of this drug [1].

Structure-activity relationship studies indicate that the acidic group (carboxyl group) of aspirin is essential and that reducing this acidity weakens its antiinflammatory activity. Further studies reveal that aspirin acts as a covalent inhibitor of prostaglandin cyclooxygenase (COX), as shown in Fig. 29.1. In 1971, Vane and other researchers successfully demonstrated for the first time that nonsteroidal antiinflammatory substances could block the biosynthesis of prostaglandins (PGs) [2]. The presence of PGs helps regulate various physiological and pathological functions. Therefore, COX has been identified as a therapeutic intervention target for NSAIDs.

Initially, it was widely believed that COX was a single enzyme present in cells, leading to the assumption that inhibition of COX would inevitably have dual effects [3,4]. In an attempt to eliminate or alleviate the gastrointestinal side effects and renal toxicity caused by aspirin-like antiinflammatory drugs, pharmacologists adopted a series of strategies, which included combining NSAIDs with gastrointestinal protective agents to counteract the side effects caused by NSAIDs and introducing nitric oxide-releasing groups into the structure of NSAIDs to reduce the occurrence of ulcers by dilating blood vessels [5]. It was not until 1991 that biologists discovered two isoforms of COX, namely COX-1 and

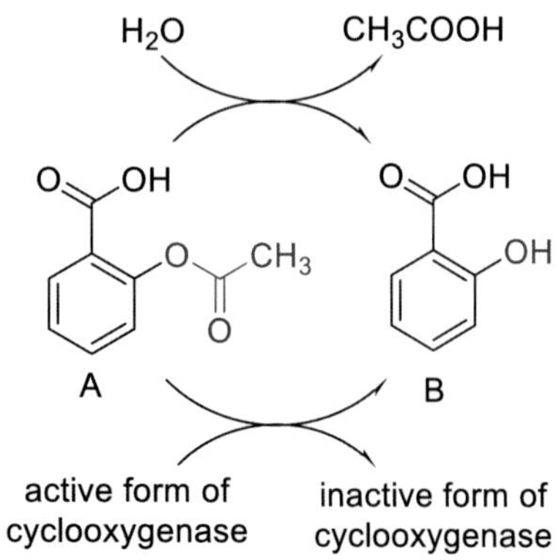

FIGURE 29.1 Mode of action of aspirin.

COX-2, which have different tissue distributions and physiological functions [5]. COX-1 is produced only under physiological conditions and can be used to synthesize transmitters such as PGs and thromboxanes (TXs). On the other hand, COX-2 is only produced under certain conditions, such as inflammation. Consequently, Vane proposed the hypothesis that selectively inhibiting COX-2 with NSAIDs could effectively treat inflammation while reducing the side effects caused by inhibiting COX-1.

According to the mechanism of action, the NSAIDs currently used clinically can be divided into four main classes (Fig. 29.2) [6]: (1) Those that completely inhibit COX activity without selectivity for COX-1 and COX-2, such as aspirin. These drugs have strong antiinflammatory and antirheumatic effects and are still the preferred drugs for rheumatoid arthritis, but they can cause gastrointestinal bleeding under long-term treatment. (2) Those that simultaneously inhibit COX-1 and COX-2 but tend to favor COX-2, such as celecoxib. They are primarily used to treat rheumatoid arthritis and osteoarthritis, with a lower incidence of ulcers and kidney toxicity. (3) Those that selectively inhibit COX-2, such as rofecoxib, reduce the side effects associated with COX-1 inhibition but increase the risk of heart attack and stroke. (4) Those with weak inhibitory activity against both COX-1 and COX-2, such as 5-aminosalicylic acid, are primarily used to treat ulcerative colitis.

29.1.2 Mechanism of action of nonsteroidal antiinflammatory drugs

29.1.2.1 Biological functions of prostaglandins

PGs are hormones that mediate local autocrine and paracrine signals, as illustrated in Fig. 29.3. Their biosynthesis involves three steps: (1) Phospholipase A2 catalyzes the release of arachidonic acid (AA) from the phospholipids of the cell membrane. (2) AA is biologically transformed by the dual functions of COX, resulting in the production of unstable prostaglandin G2 (PGG2). Through the catalysis of peroxidase, PGG2 is immediately converted into prostaglandin H2 (PGH2). (3) Through the action of specific synthases and isomerases, PGH2 is further converted into PGs, TX, prostaglandin E (including PGE1 and PGE2), etc [7].

PGs are involved in many physiological and pathological processes, which serve dual roles as protective physiological functions and potential causes of fever and inflammation. PGs exert their effects mainly by binding to four high-affinity G-protein-coupled receptors: prostaglandin E receptors for PGE2, prostaglandin I receptors for PGI2, prostaglandin D receptors for PGD2, and prostaglandin F receptors for PGF2α [8]. These receptors are associated with various signal transduction pathways. In the cardiovascular system, PGD2, PGE2, and PGI2 act as effective vasodilators, while TXA2 has vasoconstrictive properties and plays a crucial role in inducing platelet aggregation. In the respiratory system, PGF2α and TXA2 are bronchoconstrictors, while PGI2 and PGE2 are bronchodilators. In the gastrointestinal tract, PGE2, PGF2α, and PGI2 protect the gastric mucosa by reducing acid secretion, enhancing mucosal blood flow, stimulating mucus formation, and promoting bicarbonate secretion [3]. PGs also mediate the inflammatory response to tissue damage, with PGE2 typically causing symptoms like redness and fever due to vasodilation and tissue swelling from increased vascular permeability [9].

29.1.2.2 Cyclooxygenase

In the early 1990s, while studying the gene expression of the Rous sarcoma virus, Simmons and his colleagues discovered a new mRNA transcript encoding a protein with high sequence similarity to COX, indicating the presence of COX

(1)
diclofenac sodium
flurbiprofen
indometacin
(2)
celecoxib
meloxicam
(3)
rofexib
(4)
5-aminosalicylic acid
nabumetone
diflunisal

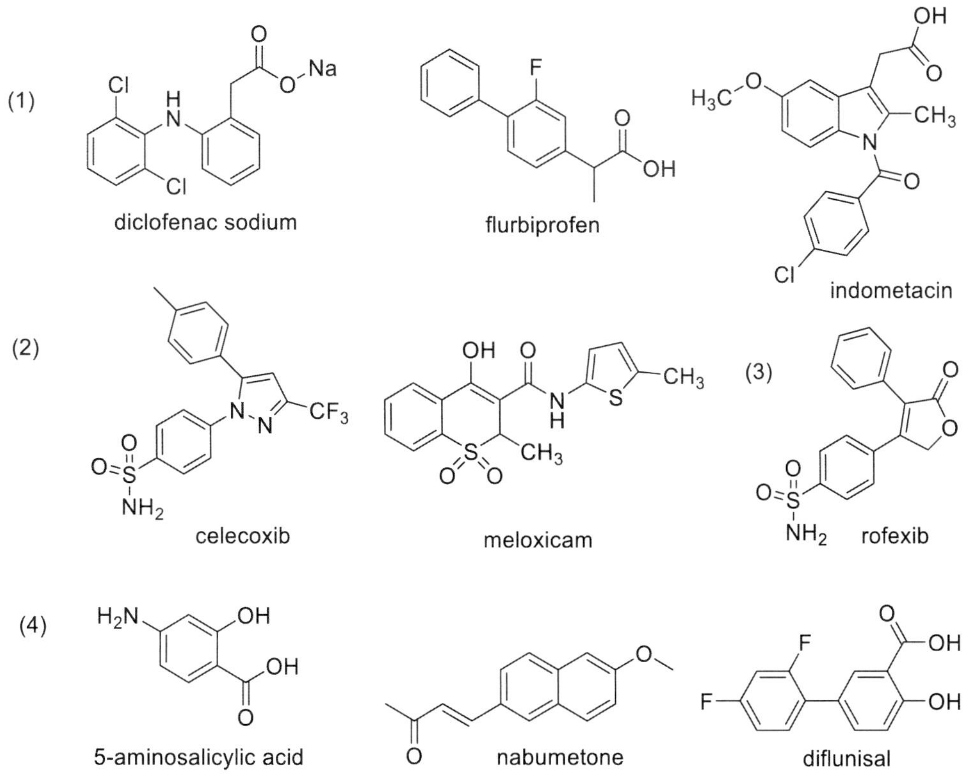

FIGURE 29.2 Typical NSAIDs that belong to different types of COX inhibitors.

membrane phospholipid
phospholipase A2
arachidonic acid
cyclooxygenase
prostaglandin G2
peroxidase
prostaglandin H2
prostaglandin I
prostaglandin E
thromboxane
prostaglandin D
prostaglandin

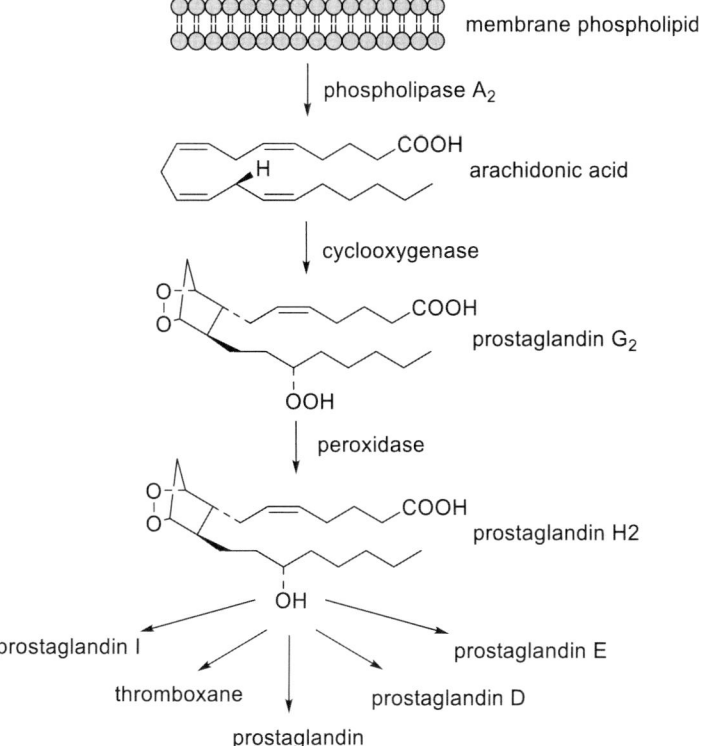

FIGURE 29.3 Synthesis of prostaglandin.

isoforms [10]. Subsequent findings in various cells, including mouse fibroblasts, rat mesangial cells, RAW264.7 cells, and rat alveolar macrophages, supported the existence of this isoform, although its physiological relevance remained unclear. Needleman's group ultimately confirmed that the COX induced during inflammation was the same enzyme Simmons had cloned and subsequently renamed. The original enzyme, isolated from seminal vesicles, was named COX-1. It was later discovered that COX-1 is almost ubiquitous, playing a "housekeeping" role in many tissues, including cell protection in the gastric mucosa, regulation of renal blood flow, and platelet aggregation. In contrast, the "inducible" form, the second subtype discovered and named COX-2, is an isoform of COX-1 [9]. Because the isoforms are independently expressed, the genes for these two enzymes are located on different chromosomes in humans, exhibiting distinct characteristics [5,11]. While COX-1 is expressed in many tissues, producing PGs that serve as "caretakers," COX-2 is not generally detected in most normal tissues. However, its expression can be rapidly induced by stimuli such as pro-inflammatory cytokines, lipopolysaccharides, mitogens, carcinogens, growth factors, hormones, and electrolyte imbalances, leading to increased synthesis of PGs in inflammatory and tumor tissues (Fig. 29.4). Therefore, the inducible isoform COX-2 is more closely linked to the physiological processes of inflammation and various cancers [12,13].

The sequences of the COX isoforms are highly homologous (65%), and their overall structure is highly conserved. The monomeric COX protein consists of three structural domains: (1) an N-terminal Epidermal Growth Factor-like domain; (2) a membrane-binding domain (MBD) of approximately 48 amino acids that anchors the protein to the lipid bilayer; (3) a C-terminal catalytic domain—a spherical structure with the COX active site capable of accommodating substrates or inhibitors. This domain also contains a heme cofactor for the peroxidase activity. The COX active site consists of a long hydrophobic channel that serves as the binding site for NSAIDs. This channel extends from the MBD to the catalytic domain. The AA binding site is located in the upper part of the channel, from Arg120 to close to Tyr385 [14]. Ser530, located in the middle of the channel, is the binding site for aspirin acetyl groups. In COX-2, three amino acids different from COX-1 (Val523, Val424, and Arg513) form a larger cavity that is more accessible for binding small-molecule drugs. Val523 in COX-2 can be exchanged with the corresponding isoleucine residue in the active site of COX-1, causing a structural change that restricts the side pocket of COX-1 and prevents drug molecules from entering. Therefore, the additional pocket in COX-2 (highlighted in the red line area) is a determinant of the selectivity of COX-2 inhibitors. Additionally, in the side pocket of COX-2, an arginine replaces the histidine found in COX-1. This arginine can interact with the polar portion of small-molecule drugs, enhancing their binding activity [15,16] (Fig. 29.5).

In 2002, the Simmons group identified and cloned a new form of COX in the dog's brain, distinct from both COX-1 and COX-2. This enzyme was highly sensitive to acetaminophen (paracetamol). This variant of COX-1, originating from the same gene, was named COX-3. It is produced by selective splicing of the COX-1 gene and accounts for approximately 5% of the total COX-1 content. The COX activity of COX-3 is about 80% lower than that of COX-1. A unique feature of COX-3, compared to COX-1 and COX-2, is its heightened sensitivity to acetaminophen [17]. Currently, acetaminophen and antipyrine have been demonstrated as selective COX-3 inhibitors, showing central antipyretic and analgesic effects in mouse models [17,18].

Research in COX pharmacology spans more than a century. With the continuous emergence of new biotechnological tools, the development of COX-2 selective inhibitors is no longer limited to traditional NSAIDs. These inhibitors have found new applications in the treatment of conditions such as colon cancer and Alzheimer's disease [19].

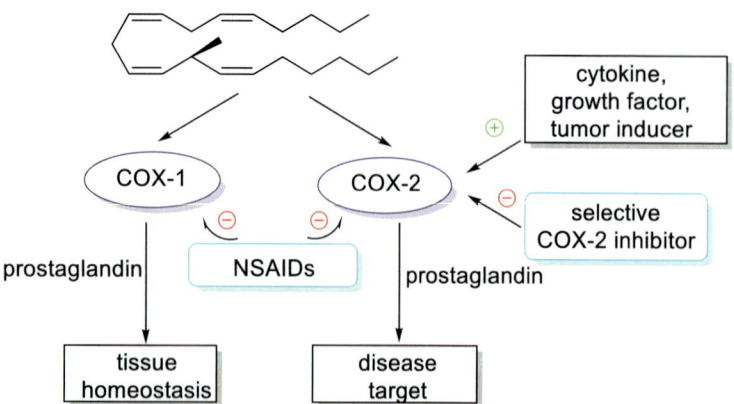

FIGURE 29.4 Schematic representation of the role of COX.

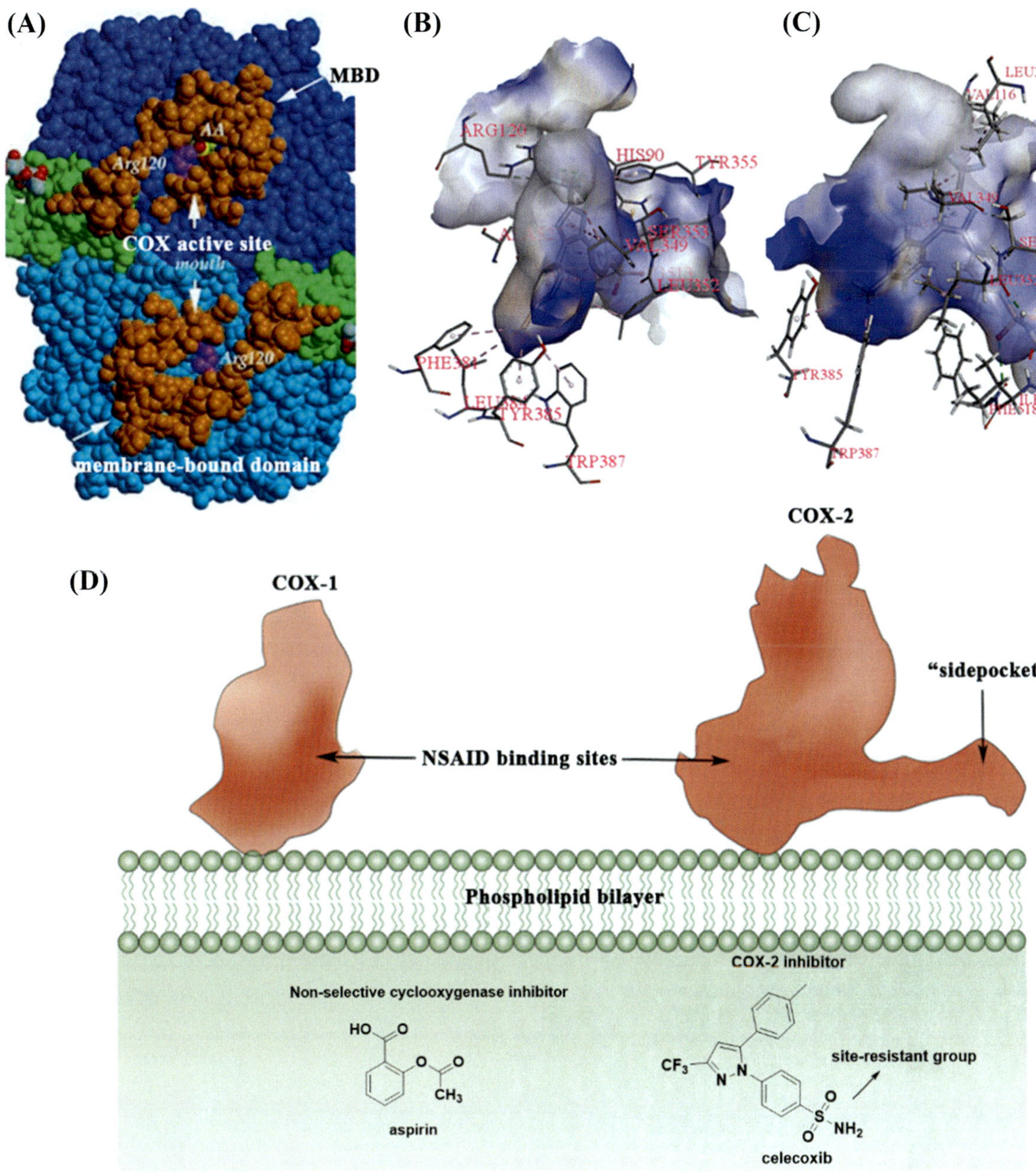

FIGURE 29.5 COX subtype characteristics. (A) Spatial modeling of COX-1; (B) Cocrystal of COX-2 inhibitors with COX-1 (PDB:1CX2); (C) Cocrystal of COX-2 inhibitors with COX-2 (PDB:3KK6); (D) Comparison of COX-1 and COX-2 binding sites.

29.2 Selective cyclooxygenase-2 inhibitor celecoxib

29.2.1 Cyclooxygenase inhibitors

COX activity originates from two different isoenzymes: COX-1 and COX-2. The differences in their protein structure and tissue distribution provide a theoretical basis for the development of selective antiinflammatory and analgesic drugs, particularly COX-2 selective inhibitors, which may reduce the risk of gastrointestinal side effects [19]. Therefore, the discovery of COX-2 greatly facilitated the development of NSAIDs. Within a decade of its discovery, two blockbuster antiinflammatory drugs, celecoxib and rofecoxib, were successively approved for the market. Interestingly, based on the understanding that COX-1 is involved in normal physiological functions and COX-2 is responsible for inflammatory responses, researchers initially sought highly selective and potent COX-2 inhibitors. This pursuit led to a binary development model, whereby the development of new drugs based on COX inhibitors falls into a "black or white" dichotomy.

In the mid-1990s, the crystal structures of COX-1 and COX-2 were successively solved, clearly demonstrating the binding modes of NSAIDs with COX enzymes. By analyzing the cocrystal of flurbiprofen with the COX protein [20], pharmacologists found that the unsubstituted benzene ring of flurbiprofen could form van der Waals forces with Tyr385 and Ser530, which are close to heme. Ser530 is critical for COX-1 activity and serves as the acetyl-binding site for aspirin. The carboxyl group of flurbiprofen can form hydrogen bonds and salt bridges with Arg120. In the crystal complex of the COX-2 protein binding to indomethacin, the benzene rings of indomethacin and flurbiprofen occupy similar positions. The chlorine atom on the benzene ring interacts with Leu384, altering the molecular conformation of the indomethacin side chain and allowing the indole ring to form van der Waals forces with Val349 and Ser353. Importantly, the oxygen atom of the indomethacin amide bond can form a hydrogen bond with the hydroxyl group of Ser530, thereby increasing the binding capacity of indomethacin to the protein. SC-558 inhibits COX-2 activity approximately 1900 times more than COX-1, with its central imidazole ring positioned similarly to flurbiprofen and indomethacin. The benzene ring with the attached bromine atom and the benzene ring with the attached sulfonylamide group are located in hydrophobic pockets on both sides of the active site, respectively. The sulfonylamide is close to the polar region on the surface of COX-2, interacting with His90, Gln192, and Arg513. This region is absent in COX-1, which explains the high selectivity of SC-558 for COX-2 [16] (Fig. 29.6).

In reviewing the reported COX inhibitors, it was found that COX-1 selective inhibitors can inhibit enzyme activity by various mechanisms, but most are competitive and reversible. On the other hand, COX-2 selective inhibitors exhibit time-dependent and irreversible inhibition, possibly due to the interaction of the sulfonylamide group with the COX-2 side pocket [21]. Early COX-2 selective inhibitors can be classified into two main categories (Fig. 29.7): (1) diaryl ether or aryl heterocyclic ether compounds (sulfonylamide class), represented by nimesulide, flosulide [15], NS-398 [22], and L-745337 [23]; (2) diaryl heterocyclic compounds, represented by DuP-697 [24], SC-57666 [25], SC-58125 [26], and celecoxib [27].

29.2.2 Cyclooxygenase-2 selective inhibitor celecoxib

29.2.2.1 Discovery of coxib lead compounds

In the early development of coxib drugs, both hit compounds and lead compounds were discovered and identified through phenotypic/functional screening. Phenotypic drug discovery is a method that involves screening with highly disease-relevant biological efficacy models. After discovering lead compounds, the mechanism of action of active molecules is studied, providing advantages in identifying new drug targets or mechanisms directly related to the disease. In 1990, researchers at DuPont Pharmaceuticals discovered the lead compound DuP-697 during the screening of antiinflammatory drugs using experimental animal models (Fig. 29.7) [24]. DuP-697 exhibited potent antiinflammatory

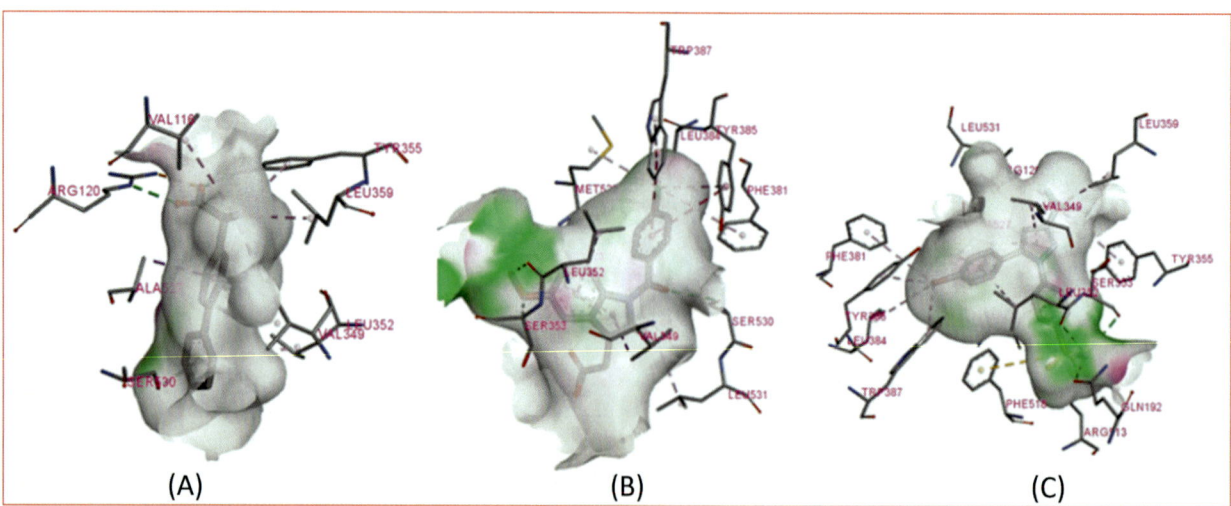

FIGURE 29.6 Binding mode of COX enzyme to NSAIDs. (A) cocrystal of flurbiprofen with COX-1 (PDB: 1EQH); (B) cocrystal of indomethacin with COX-2 (PDB: 4COX); (C) cocrystal of SC-558 with COX-2 (PDB: 6COX).

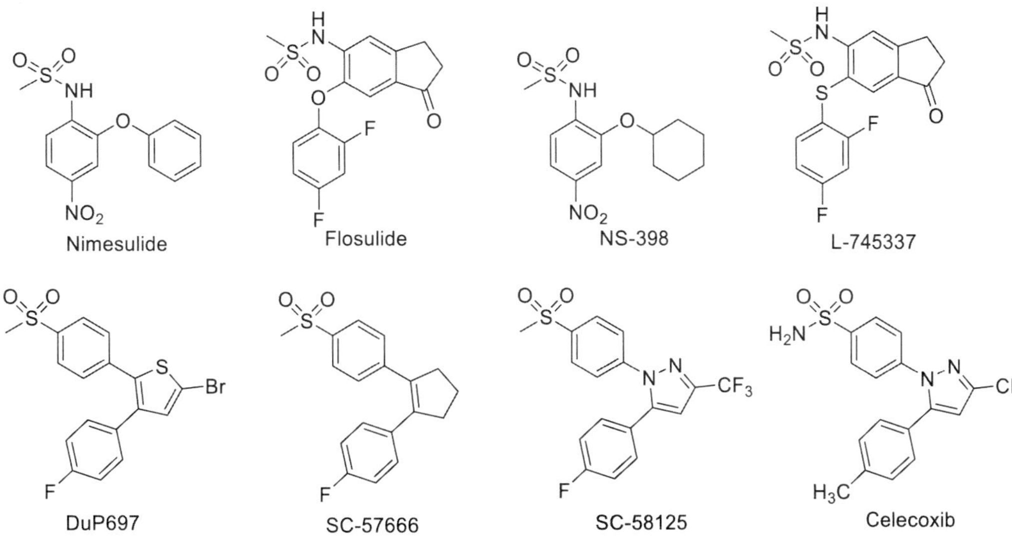

FIGURE 29.7 Early COX-2 inhibitors.

effects with minimal gastrointestinal ulcer side effects. Further in vitro enzymatic experiments revealed significant inhibitory activity of DuP-697 on prostaglandin synthesis in the rat brain (mainly COX-2), while its activity on COX in rat kidney tissue (mainly COX-1) was weaker. The IC_{50} values for human COX-2 and COX-1 were 10 and 800 nM, respectively, with inhibitory Ki values of 0.3 and 5.3 μmol/L. In vivo experiments confirmed its good antiinflammatory activity and gastrointestinal tolerability. However, clinical trials showed that its half-life ($t_{1/2}$ = 242 hours) was too long, potentially leading to cumulative toxicity in the human body, which prevented its further development. Nevertheless, DuP-697 and another clinical candidate, NS-398, are typical representatives of early coxib lead compounds, establishing the molecular structural foundation for subsequent development. Simultaneously, based on DuP-697, Monsanto Company developed sulfonamide-1,5-diaryl pyrazole COX-2 inhibitors, while Merck focused on the development of methyl sulfonylphenyl COX-2 inhibitors.

SC-57666 and SC-58125 (Fig. 29.7), belonging to the class of diaryl heterocyclic compounds, were developed by Seale Corporation (then a subsidiary of Monsanto) based on DuP-697. They utilized cyclopentene and pyrazole as the linker groups to connect the A and B aromatic rings. Using cyclopentene as the linker, Seale Corporation conducted extensive structure-activity relationship studies on the A and B rings. They found that a 4-methylsulfonyl group on the A ring significantly influenced activity and selectivity, whereas various aromatic ring substitutions at the 2-position of the B ring had no appreciable effect on activity. This led to the determination of the basic pharmacophore model, as shown in Fig. 29.8. Research revealed that when the C ring was a pyrazole or a five-membered lactone ring, the compound exhibited better activity and drug-like properties. It was also discovered that the spatial orientation of the two aromatic rings in these tricyclic inhibitors was crucial for COX inhibitory activity and selectivity; they needed to be located in adjacent positions to the central aromatic ring. Seale Corporation selected SC-58125 as a template for further structural modifications to discover safe and effective selective COX-2 inhibitors [27].

29.2.2.2 Structural optimization of coxib drugs

29.2.2.2.1 Optimization of the 4-sulfonylamino group in A-ring

Considering that the 4-methylsulfonylphenyl or 4-sulfonylaminophenyl groups at the 1-position of the pyrazole ring of SC-58125 were a key substituent for inhibiting COX-2 activity, researchers first investigated the 4-sulfonamide group in compound 1 and found that modifying the nitrogen atom by methylation or dimethylation (Table 29.1) resulted in a loss of COX inhibitory activity for compounds 2 and 3. Similarly, compound 4, which replaced the sulfonylamino group with a methylsulfonylamino group, also did not exhibit COX inhibitory activity. Subsequently, they applied the bioisostere principle to replace sulfonamide groups with nitro groups (compound 5) and trifluoroacetyl groups (compound 6), but these did not demonstrate ideal inhibitory activity. Therefore, substituting the 4-methylsulfonylphenyl or 4-sulfonylamino phenyl group at the 1-position of the pyrazole ring is crucial for maintaining effective COX-2 inhibitory activity. Furthermore, as shown in Fig. 29.5, sulfonamide groups occupy the lateral pockets of COX-2.

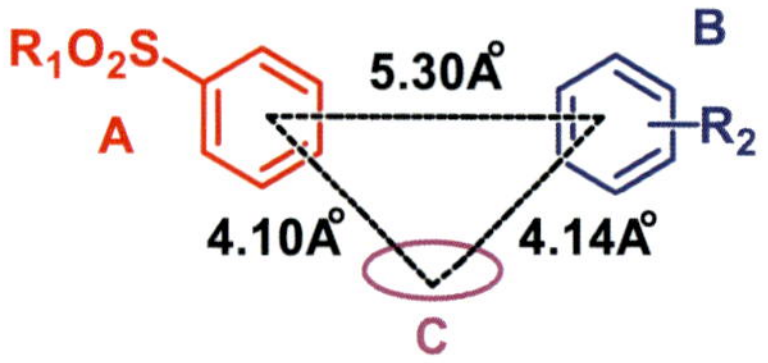

FIGURE 29.8 Pharmacophore model of COX-2 inhibitors.

TABLE 29.1 In vitro COX-1 and COX-2 inhibitory activity of 1,5-diarylpyrazole.

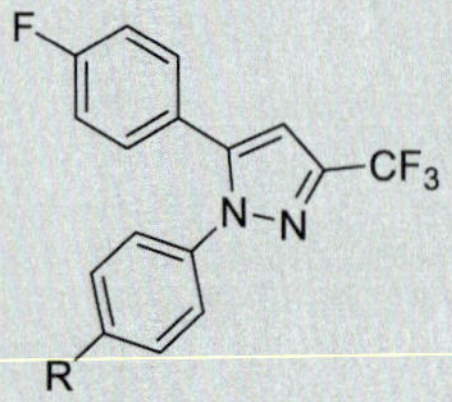

Compounds	R	IC$_{50}$ (μmol/L)	
		COX-1	COX-2
SC-58125	SO$_2$CH$_3$	>1 000	0.1
1	SO$_2$NH$_2$	25.5	0.041
2	SO$_2$NHCH$_3$	>100	>100
3	SO$_2$N(CH$_3$)$_2$	>100	>100
4	NHSO$_2$CH$_3$	>100	>100
5	NO$_2$	1.75	>100
6	COCF$_3$	>100	>100

29.2.2.2.2 Optimization of 3- and 4-position substituents of pyrazole ring

Previous structural investigations (Table 29.2) indicated that introducing trifluoromethyl and difluoromethyl groups at the 3-position of the pyrazole ring can improve both in vitro activity and selectivity, as seen in Compounds 7 and 8. By replacing the fluorine atom with a monofluoromethyl group, compound 9 showed no inhibitory activity against COX-1 and decreased inhibitory activity against COX-2 compared to compound 1. Removal of the trifluoromethyl group in compound 10 also leads to a total loss of inhibitory activity on both COX enzymes. The activity of compound 11, which was obtained by replacing trifluoromethyl with methyl groups and shares a similar spatial structure, also significantly decreased. Compounds 12 and 13 derived from single-substituted methyl groups exhibited good activity against COX-2 while showing no activity against COX-1. Interestingly, introducing larger aromatic substituents at the 5-position of the aromatic ring (compounds 14 and 15) exhibited good inhibitory activity, although selectivity was reduced. Replacing the hydrogen atom with a fluorine atom at the para position of the 5-position benzene ring and introducing cyano, carboxyl, and carboxyl derivatives at the 3-position of the pyrrole ring (compounds 17–21) resulted in no inhibitory activity, except for compound 21, which showed good activity with poor selectivity. Compound 22, obtained by replacing trifluoromethyl with an electron-donating methoxy group, lost its activity, indicating that an electron-withdrawing group at the pyrrole 3-position is essential for the inhibitory activity on COXs.

The different substituents at the 4-position of pyrazole have a significant impact on the COX inhibitory activity (data not listed). When substituted with halogens or methyl groups, compounds demonstrated good activity against COX but lacked selectivity. In terms of activity and selectivity, ethyl substitution seemed optimal. When the 4-position was unsubstituted, the compound exhibited ideal activity against COX-2. Considering that introducing a substituent at the 4-position will increase the difficulty of synthesis, no further exploration was conducted.

TABLE 29.2 In vitro COX-1 and COX-2 inhibitory activity of 1,5-diarylpyrazole.

Compounds	R	X	IC$_{50}$ (μmol/L)	
			COX-1	COX-2
7	CF$_3$	H	55.1	0.032
8	CHF$_2$	H	33.7	0.13
9	CH$_2$F	H	>100	0.20
10	H	F	>100	>100
11	CH$_3$	H	>100	62.8
12	CH$_2$OH	Cl	>100	0.83
13	CH$_2$CN	Cl	>100	0.12
14	CH$_2$OCH$_2$Ph	Cl	8.98	0.029
15	4-Methoxyphenyl	Cl	8.49	0.10
16	5-Chloro-2-thienyl	Cl	>100	0.052
17	CN	F	>100	0.34
18	CO$_2$H	F	>100	>100
19	CO$_2$Me	F	>100	>100
20	CONH$_2$	F	>100	>100
21	CONH(3-chlorophenyl)	F	1.92	0.056
22	OMe	H	>100	>100

29.2.2.2.3 Optimization of B-ring substituents

The aryl substituent at the 5-position exhibited great flexibility in maintaining COX-2 inhibitory activity. Considering that the para position of the benzene ring is easily metabolized by oxidation, systematic structural modifications were carried out on this position to achieve compounds with improved physicochemical properties, such as water solubility, logP, and pKa, and to reduce susceptibility to oxidative metabolism (Table 29.3). In the case of retaining the trifluoromethyl group at the pyrazole 3-position, different halogen substitutions at various positions on the benzene ring resulted in compounds 23–26, all showing good COX-2 selective inhibitory activity, with compound 26 being the most optimal. Replacing the trifluoromethyl group of compound 26 with a difluoromethyl group resulted in compound 27, which exhibited reduced COX selectivity. The introduction of electron-withdrawing groups such as trifluoromethyl, nitro, and cyano (compounds 28–30) led to a significant decrease in the activity. Introducing a methoxy group at the para position of the 5-position benzene ring with trifluoromethyl or difluoromethyl at the pyrrole 3-position resulted in improved activity for compounds 32 and 33 compared to compound 1. Unfortunately, the selectivity of these two compounds against COX decreased. To further enhance selectivity, introducing halogen atoms at the *m*-position of the 5-position benzene ring resulted in compounds 36 and 37. These compounds maintained inhibitory activity against COX and restored selectivity. Apart from introducing a methoxy group at the 5-position benzene ring to give good activity and selectivity, the introduction of a methyl group (compounds 33–35) achieved similar effects, significantly improving both inhibitory activity and selectivity compared to earlier compounds (Table 29.4).

TABLE 29.3 In vitro COX-1 and COX-2 inhibitory activity of 1,5-diarylpyrazole.

Compounds	R¹	R²	IC$_{50}$ (μmol/L)	
			COX-1	COX-2
1	4-F	CF$_3$	25.5	0.041
23	2-F	CF$_3$	29.5	0.058
24	3-F	CF$_3$	>100	7.73
25	2-Cl	CF$_3$	31.3	0.056
26	4-Cl	CF$_3$	17.8	0.01
27	4-Cl	CHF$_2$	5.7	0.01
28	4-CF$_3$	CF$_3$	>100	8.23
29	4-NO$_2$	CF$_3$	>100	2.63
30	4-CN	CHF$_2$	>100	29.7
31	4-OCH$_3$	CF$_3$	2.58	0.008
32	4-OCH$_3$	CHF$_2$	0.083	0.015
33	2-CH$_3$	CF$_3$	33.9	0.069
34	4-CH$_3$	CF$_3$	15.0	0.04
35	4-CH$_3$	CHF$_2$	12.5	0.013

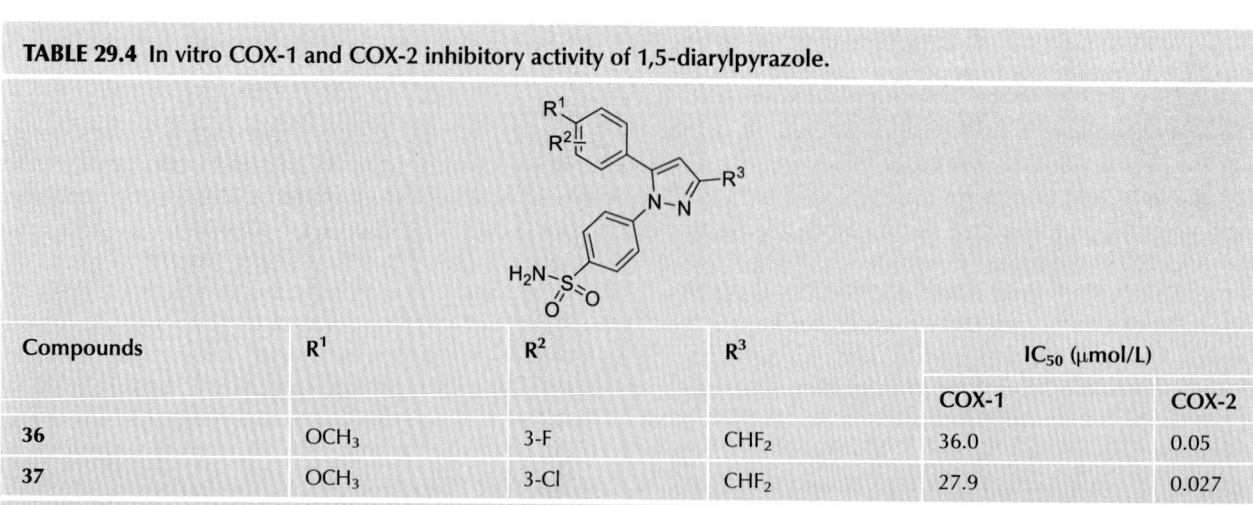

TABLE 29.4 In vitro COX-1 and COX-2 inhibitory activity of 1,5-diarylpyrazole.

Compounds	R¹	R²	R³	IC$_{50}$ (μmol/L)	
				COX-1	COX-2
36	OCH$_3$	3-F	CHF$_2$	36.0	0.05
37	OCH$_3$	3-Cl	CHF$_2$	27.9	0.027

TABLE 29.5 In vitro COX-1 and COX-2 inhibitory activity of 1,5-diarylpyrazole.

Compounds	R^1	R^2	IC$_{50}$ (µmol/L)	
			COX-1	COX-2
34	4-CH$_3$	CF$_3$	15.0	0.04
38	4-CH$_2$CH$_3$	CF$_3$	29.0	0.86
31	4-OCH$_3$	CF$_3$	2.58	0.008
39	4-OCH$_2$CH$_3$	CF$_3$	28.2	0.64

To further explore the impact of methyl (Compound 34) and methoxy (Compound 31) groups at the para position of the 5-position benzene ring on activity (Table 29.5), researchers investigated their homologous ethyl and ethoxy groups. It was found that elongating the substituent led to decreased inhibitory activity of the compounds against COX. Compared to compound 34, which has a 4-methyl group, compound 38 with a 4-ethyl group showed approximately 20 times less COX-2 inhibitory activity, and compound 39 with a 4-ethoxy group exhibited about 80 times less activity compared to compound 31 with a 4-methoxy group. In summary, introducing an electron-donating group, either methyl or methoxy, at the para position of the 5-position benzene ring not only further enhanced the inhibitory activity of compounds against COX but also played a crucial role in the selective inhibition between the two isoforms of the enzyme.

Researchers further investigated the impact of substituting the 5-position aromatic ring on inhibitory activity. When pyridine replaced the benzene ring, compounds 40–42 exhibited significantly reduced inhibition against COX. However, when using thiophene, compounds 43 and 44 exhibited excellent inhibitory activity against both COX-1 and COX-2, comparable to that of compounds 34 and 31. Nevertheless, these two compounds were not extensively studied subsequently, likely due to the poor pharmacological characteristics of the thiophene ring. Subsequent substitutions with furan, benzofuran, benzothiophene, and cyclohexene resulted in compounds 45–48, all exhibiting good inhibitory activity against COX-2 and selectivity against COX-1. As mentioned earlier, it was found that the *p*-position of the 5-position benzene ring was favorable for maintaining activity when substituted with methyl or methoxy. Therefore, the researchers cyclized the 4- and 5-positions of the benzene ring to obtain compounds 49–52. Except for compound 52, all other compounds maintained good COX-1/2 inhibitory activity (Table 29.6). The comprehensive structure-activity relationships of compounds 23–52 further indicated that having an aromatic ring at the 5-position of the pyrazole was favorable for maintaining activity, and having methyl or methoxy at the *p*-position of the aromatic ring was more advantageous for improving selectivity.

29.2.2.3 Selection of celecoxib as a candidate drug

In summary, compounds with para-sulfonamide phenyl substitutione exhibited excellent COX-2 inhibitory activity among COX-2 inhibitors. The substituent at the 3-position of the pyrazole ring had a significant impact on the activity, with trifluoromethyl and difluoromethyl substitutions showing optimal activity and selectivity. Additionally, substitutions on the 5-position of the benzene ring in the pyrazole play a crucial role in the in vitro activity and selectivity of these compounds. Compounds 26, 27, 31, 34, 35, and 36 were selected for in vitro ADME (absorption, distribution, metabolism, and excretion) studies, and the results showed that although compound 26 has good COX-2 inhibitory activity and selectivity, its plasma half-life in rats can still reach 117 hours, which may bring additional metabolic burden to the human body. However, replacing the chlorine atom at the para position of the 5-position benzene ring in compound 26 with methyl or methoxy groups (compounds 31 and 34) reduced the plasma half-life to 3–6 hours.

TABLE 29.6 In vitro COX-1 and COX-2 inhibitory activity of 5-arylpyrazole.

Compounds	R¹	R²	IC$_{50}$ (μmol/L) COX-1	IC$_{50}$ (μmol/L) COX-2
40	2-pyridyl	CF$_3$	93.3	45.6
41	3-pyridyl	CF$_3$	>100	45.0
42	4-pyridyl	CF$_3$	209	64.7
43	5-bromo-2-thienyl	CF$_3$	2.91	0.012
44	5-chloro-2-thienyl	CF$_3$	4.69	0.026
45	5-methyl-2-furyl	CHF$_2$	>100	3.29
46	3-benzothienyl	CF$_3$	70.7	0.35
47	2-benzofuryl	CF$_3$	>100	0.89
48	1-cyclohexenyl	CF$_3$	>100	0.084
49	(indanyl)	CF$_3$	15.5	0.031
41	(dihydrobenzothienyl)	CF$_3$	12.9	0.23
50	(dihydrobenzofuryl)	CF$_3$	1.21	0.021
51	(benzodioxolyl)	CHF$_2$	1.92	0.024
52	(methyl-benzodioxolyl)	CF$_3$	674	0.052

Replacing the trifluoromethyl group in compound 34 with a difluoromethyl group (compound 35) resulted in a half-life of 3.3 hours, similar to that of compound 34 at 3.5 hours. The half-life of 3-fluoro-4-methoxy derivative 36 was 3.5 hours, which was almost the same as 34 and 35 (Table 29.7).

Various in vivo pharmacological studies and preliminary safety assessments, including the rat carrageenan-induced paw edema model, rat adjuvant-induced arthritis model, and rat carrageenan-induced hyperalgesia model, along with gastrointestinal toxicity tests conducted 5 hours postadministration, indicated that most pyrazole compounds exhibited good antiinflammatory activity comparable to traditional NSAIDs (Table 29.8). However, unlike traditional NSAIDs, most compounds did not show adverse reactions, particularly gastrointestinal damage, at a dose of 200 mg/kg.

Overall, compound 34 (celecoxib) demonstrated the best in vivo and in vitro antiinflammatory activity, pharmacokinetic characteristics, and low toxicity. As shown in Table 29.8, celecoxib exhibited antiinflammatory efficacy

TABLE 29.7 Pharmacokinetic data of selected pyrazole compounds in rats.

Compounds	Dose (mg/kg)	Administration route	Plasma half-life (h)
26	20	oral	117
31	10	oral	5.6
27	10	i.v.	4.5
34	10	i.v.	3.5
36	10	i.v.	3.5
35	10	oral	3.3

TABLE 29.8 In vivo pharmacodynamic evaluation of selected pyrazole compounds.

Compounds	ED$_{50}$ (mg/kg)			Ulcer rate in rat gastric injury model @200 mg/kg(%)
	Rat adjuvant-induced arthritis model	Rat carrageenan-induced paw edema model	Rat carrageenan-induced hyperalgesia model	
7	0.29	50%@30		0
26	0.07	5.4	6.6	0
34	0.37	7.1	34.5	0
27	0.63	13.0	7.7	0
35	0.35	2.4	37.3	0
32	0.01	13.7	6.0	100

(Continued)

TABLE 29.8 (Continued)

Compounds	ED$_{50}$ (mg/kg)			Ulcer rate in rat gastric injury model @200 mg/kg(%)
	Rat adjuvant-induced arthritis model	Rat carrageenan-induced paw edema model	Rat carrageenan-induced hyperalgesia model	
Compound 36	0.05	18.6	33.0	0
Compound 17	0.51	7.5	67.1	0
Indomethacin	0.11	1.15	4.1	UC$_{50}$ = 7 mg/kg
Piroxicam	0.15	2.4	52%@10	UC$_{50}$ = 2.9 mg/kg
Naproxen	0.94	1.6	66%@10	UC$_{50}$ = 255 mg/kg

comparable to traditional NSAIDs, but no acute gastrointestinal toxicity was observed in rats at a dose of up to 200 mg/kg. Furthermore, even with daily administration at a dose of 600 mg/kg for 10 days, Celecoxib showed no chronic gastrointestinal toxicity in rats, in contrast to traditional NSAIDs, which demonstrated severe toxicity at similar doses.

29.2.2.4 Metabolism of celecoxib

Celecoxib is well absorbed when administered on an empty stomach, reaching peak plasma concentration (C_{max}) within 2−3 hours. It is primarily eliminated as inactive metabolites through urine and feces, with only 3% of the drug directly excreted without metabolism. Metabolism primarily occurs in the liver, with the cytochrome CYP2C9 responsible for its oxidative metabolism. As depicted in Fig. 29.9, the in vivo metabolism of celecoxib involves the oxidation of the 4-methyl group to a hydroxymethyl intermediate. This intermediate is further oxidized to the carboxylic acid form and then excreted after esterification with glucuronic acid. None of the metabolites exhibit significant inhibitory activity against COX-1 or COX-2. Celecoxib can also inhibit CYP2D6, potentially affecting the pharmacokinetics of other drugs metabolized by this enzyme and leading to drug-drug interactions.

In summary, due to its excellent in vitro and in vivo antiinflammatory activity, good safety, and high bioavailability, celecoxib was ultimately selected as a candidate drug for further clinical trial research.

29.2.2.5 Clinical application and monitoring of celecoxib

In Phase I clinical trials, the average half-life of celecoxib in the human body was about 12 hours, and the blood concentration reached the C_{max} value at around 2 hours after administration. In an antiinflammatory analgesic experiment following tooth extraction, celecoxib demonstrated similar therapeutic effects to aspirin (at a dose of 100 mg), with an onset time of approximately 45 minutes [28,29].

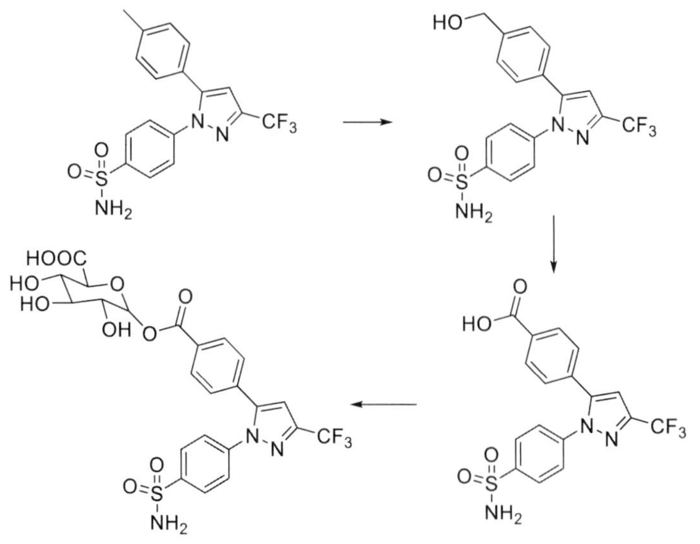

FIGURE 29.9 Metabolic pathways of celecoxib in vivo.

In multiple experiments treating osteoarthritis of the hip and knee over 2–12 weeks, standard oral doses of celecoxib (200 or 400 mg/day) were as effective as treatment regimens involving three daily doses of 50 mg of diclofenac sodium or daily doses of ibuprofen/naproxen. In dynamic verification experiments lasting 6–13 weeks, placebo-controlled daily doses of 200 or 400 mg of celecoxib demonstrated significant efficacy in treating symptoms of osteoarthritis in the hip and knee joints. In prolonged treatment for 13 or 26 weeks, daily intake of 200 mg of celecoxib demonstrated similar efficacy to other coxibs, such as 30 mg of etoricoxib and 100 mg of rofecoxib [27].

Concerned about the gastrointestinal adverse effects of COX-2 selective inhibitors, researchers conducted two clinical efficacy tracking and evaluation projects: the celecoxib long-term arthritis safety study (CLASS) for celecoxib and the Vioxx gastrointestinal outcomes research (VIGOR) for rofecoxib [30,31]. The CLASS study found that the incidence of gastrointestinal damage caused by celecoxib was lower than that of traditional NSAIDs such as ibuprofen, and the long-term use of celecoxib did not show a significant difference in the incidence of cardiovascular events compared to traditional NSAIDs. The VIGOR study revealed that rofecoxib resulted in fewer gastrointestinal adverse reactions than naproxen but increased the risk of cardiovascular disease with long-term, high-dose use, leading to the withdrawal of rofecoxib from the market (the infamous "Vioxx event"). Celecoxib, due to its good efficacy and high safety, continued to be used in humans.

29.2.2.6 Chemical synthesis of celecoxib

Numerous studies have been reported on the chemical synthesis of celecoxib, which involves condensation reactions, 1,3-dipolar cycloaddition reactions, coupling reactions, and C-H arylation reactions (Fig. 29.10).

29.2.2.6.1 Condensation reaction

The initial synthesis of celecoxib involved the condensation of a diketone intermediate (M2) with 4-methylsulfonylaminobenzene hydrazine hydrochloride salt (M3). As shown in Fig. 29.11, the process begins by dissolving 4-methylacetophenone (M1) in methanol, followed by the addition of a 25% sodium methoxide solution as a condensing agent, and then ethyl trifluoroacetate. Through the Claisen condensation reaction, the diketone intermediate (M2) is obtained. The dehydration cyclization of the 4-methylsulfonylaminobenzene hydrazine hydrochloride salt (M3) with the diketone intermediate (M2) ultimately yields celecoxib. The reaction produces celecoxib with a ratio of 99.5:0.05 compared to regioisomer 53, with yields ranging from 46% to 56%. However, this method suffers from poor regioselectivity, extended reaction times (20 hours), and a tendency to produce two isomers, which makes purification challenging in large-scale industrial synthesis [27,32].

Reddy et al. [33] optimized the synthetic route by employing ethyl acetate: water (1:1) as the reaction solvent to achieve the high-selectivity synthesis of the target compound (Fig. 29.12). The mixture of diketone intermediate (M3), 4-methylsulfonylaminobenzene hydrazine hydrochloride salt (M4), water, and ethyl acetate was heated under reflux for 2 hours. The reaction mixture was then cooled to 0°C–5°C and stirred for 1–1.5 hours. After filtration and washing with water, the filtrate was added to toluene and heated to 80°C–85°C. After the water layer was separated, the organic layer was cooled to 10°C–15°C, stirred for 1–1.5 hours, and then filtered to obtain celecoxib as a separated solid. The yield

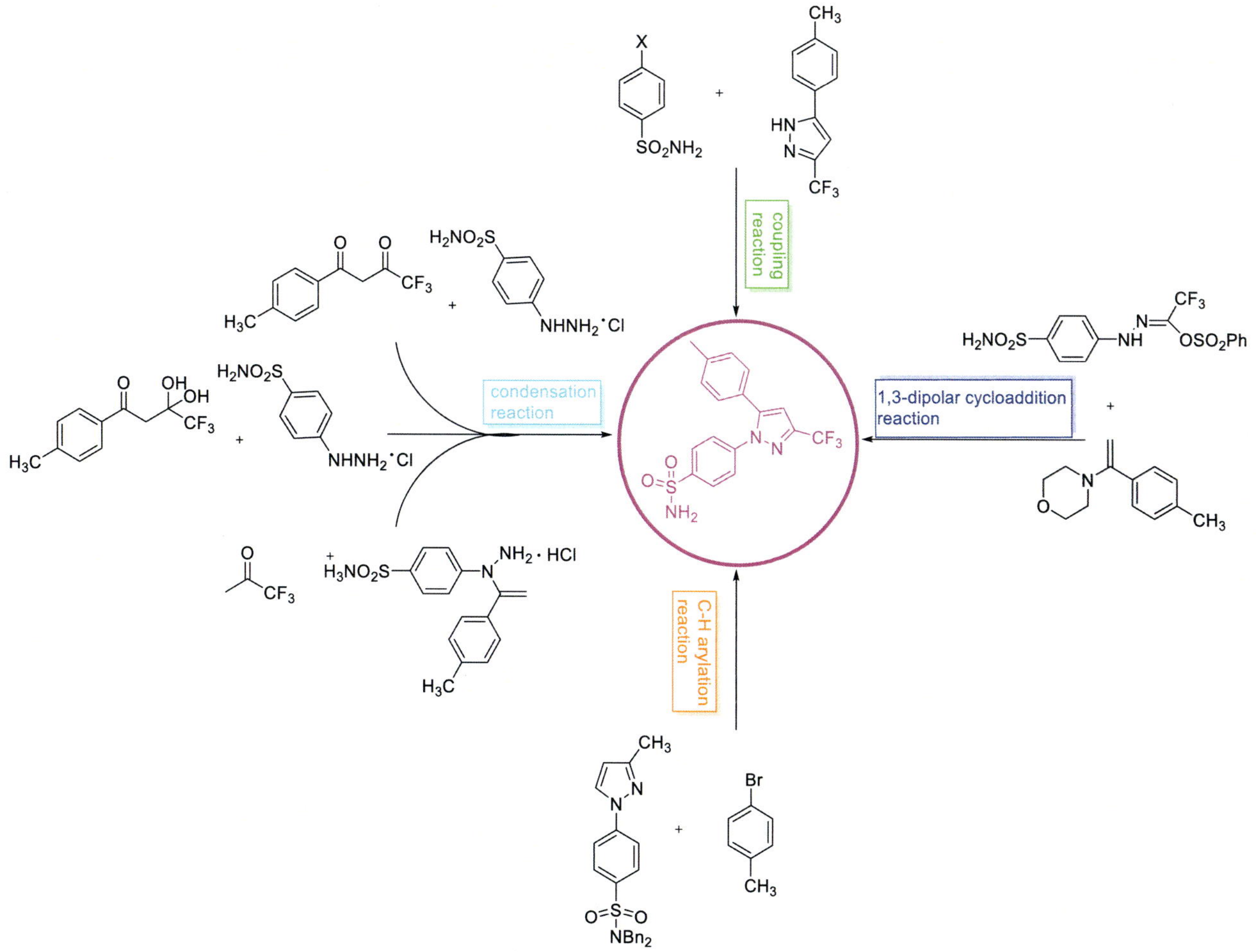

FIGURE 29.10 Synthesis study of celecoxib (□).

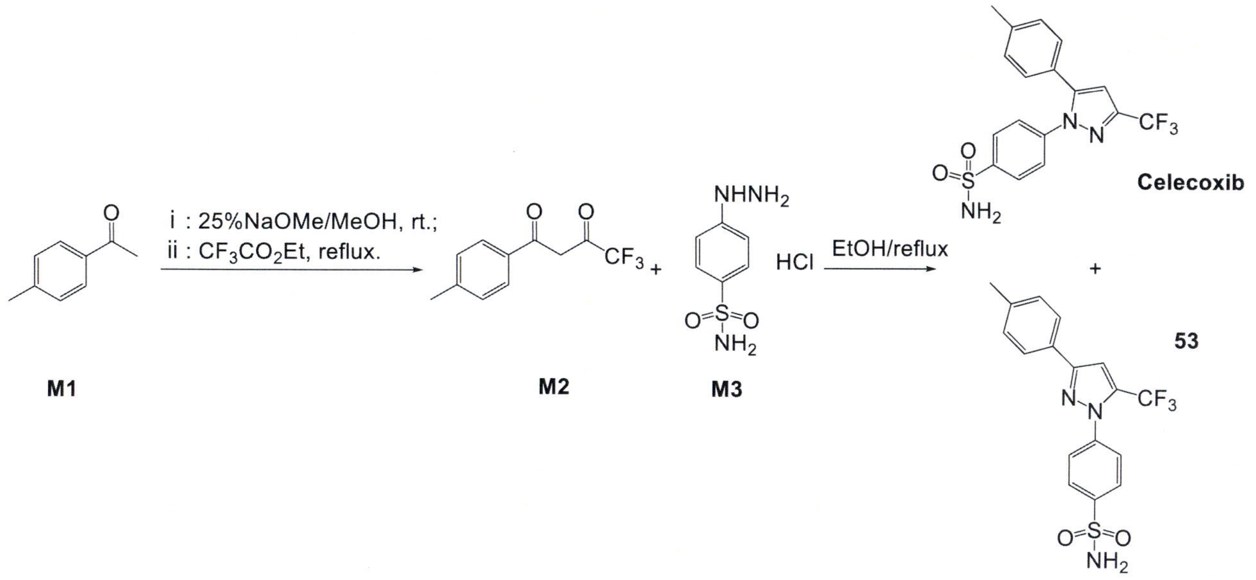

FIGURE 29.11 Chemical synthesis study of celecoxib (II).

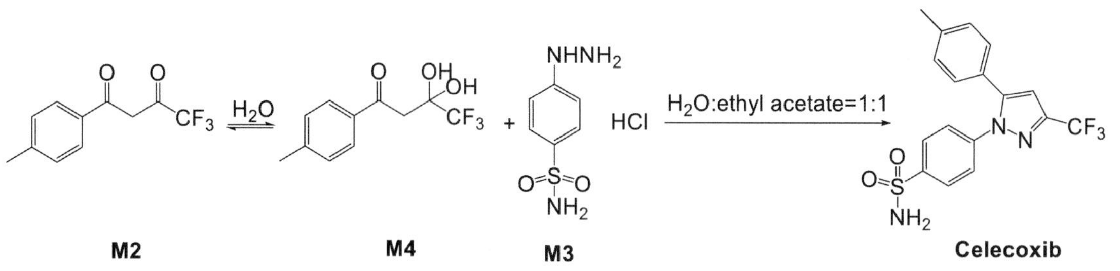

728 Medicinal Chemistry and Drug Development

FIGURE 29.12 Chemical synthesis study of celecoxib (III).

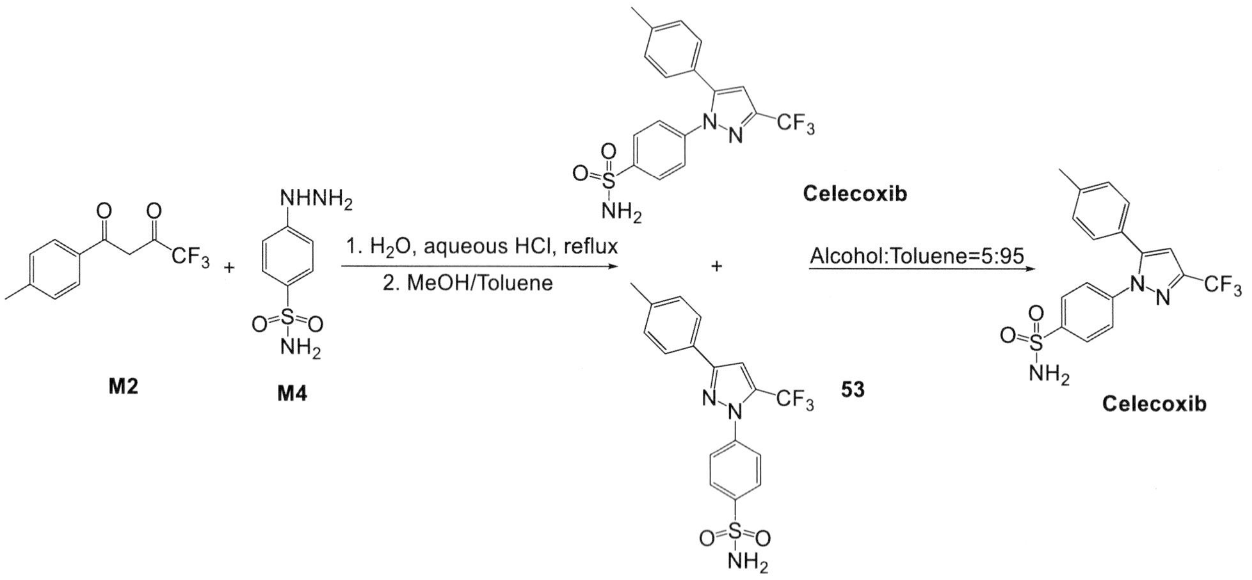

FIGURE 29.13 Chemical synthesis study of celecoxib (IV).

was approximately 84%, and the ratio of celecoxib to the isomer 53 was 99.97:0.03. While this method improves the yield and regioselectivity of celecoxib, it involves complex procedures and remains unsuitable for large-scale production.

Ambati et al. [34] reported a simpler, high-yielding, and environmentally friendly method for the large-scale synthesis of celecoxib (Fig. 29.13). In this method, the diketone intermediate (M2) reacted with 4-methylsulfonylaminobenzene hydrazine (M4) in the presence of hydrochloric acid and water under reflux conditions. The reaction mixture was then cooled and treated with a mixture of methanol and toluene, resulting in a crude product containing 2.5% isomer 53. Finally, recrystallization using a mixture of ethanol and toluene produced celecoxib with a purity of 99.8%.

In 2019, Liang et al. [35] reported a method for preparing celecoxib. As shown in Fig. 29.14, the reaction of 4-methylsulfonylaminobenzene hydrazine (M4) with acetaldehyde produced a reaction mixture containing an imine (M5). Subsequently, *p*-toluenesulfonyl chloride was added to the reaction mixture from the first step, yielding a reaction mixture that contained compound M6 through acylation. Then, hydrochloric acid in ethanol was added to the reaction mixture from the second step to produce the hydrochloride salt compound M7. Celecoxib was finally obtained through dehydration cyclization with 1,1,1-trifluoroacetone. This change in the cyclization method effectively avoided the generation of regioisomeric impurities. This preparation method integrates the steps of protection, condensation, and deprotection into a one-pot reaction, featuring mild conditions and convenient posttreatment operations, achieving a total yield of 95.8%. This method is better suited for large-scale industrial production.

29.2.2.6.2 1,3-Dipolar cycloaddition reaction

In addition, researchers discovered that the compound 1,1-disubstituted enamine amphiphilic dipole (M10) could be synthesized with high yield and 100% regioselectivity through a 1,3-dipolar cycloaddition reaction with a nitrile imine dipole to form celecoxib. As depicted in Fig. 29.15, acylation of 4-methylsulfonylaminobenzene hydrazine hydrochloride salt (M4) with trifluoroacetic anhydride produced the intermediate M8. Then, M8 was converted to its enol form

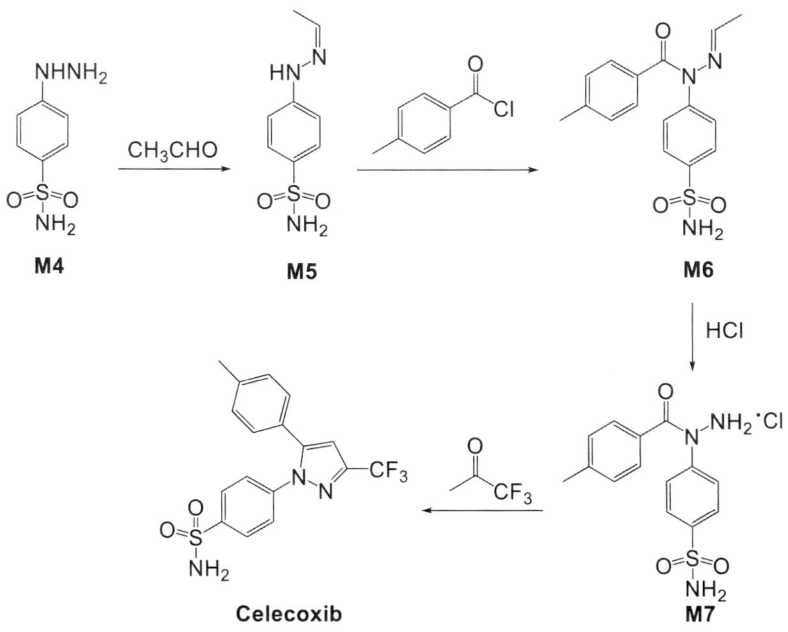

FIGURE 29.14 Chemical synthesis study of celecoxib (V).

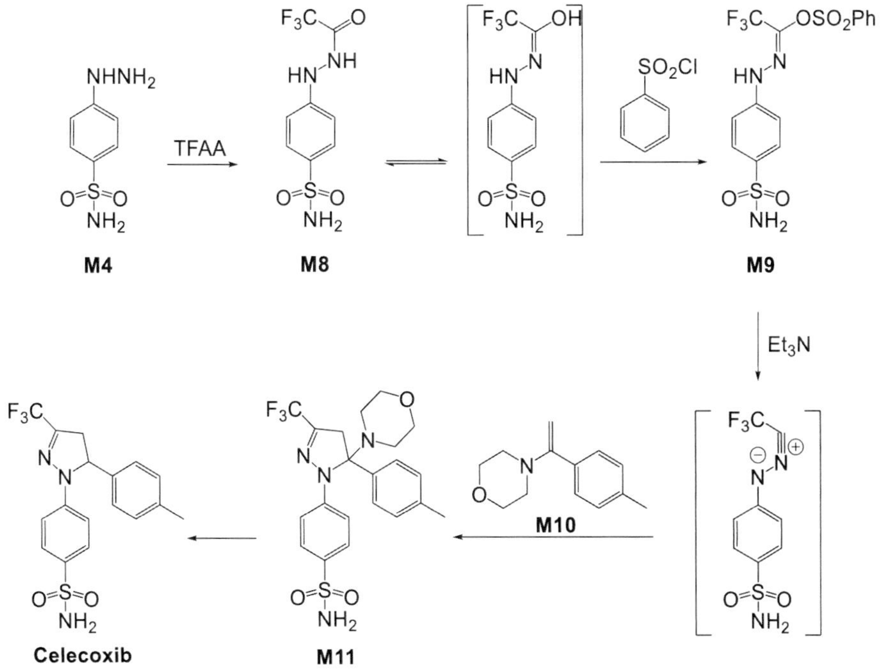

FIGURE 29.15 Chemical synthesis study of celecoxib (VI).

and reacted with benzenesulfonyl chloride to produce compound M9. Subsequently, the 1,3-dipolar cycloaddition between the nitrilimine dipole generated in situ by triethylamine and the 1,1-disubstituted alkene azomethine dipole (M10) yielded compound M11. Finally, the elimination of the morpholine group and β-H resulted in celecoxib, with a total yield of 52%. This method offers complete regioselectivity without generating isomers; however, the instability of intermediates during the reaction complicates control and renders it unsuitable for industrial production [36].

29.2.2.6.3 Coupling reaction

Another reported synthesis method for celecoxib involved a coupling reaction, as shown in Fig. 29.16. Upon heating, the diketone intermediate (M2) underwent dehydration cyclization with hydrazine hydrate to form compound M14.

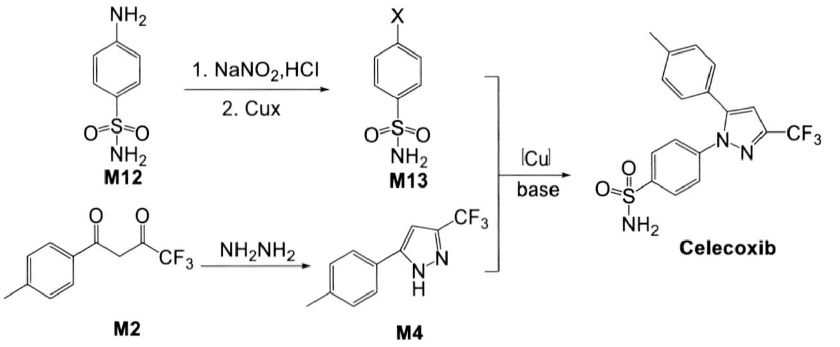

FIGURE 29.16 Chemical synthesis study of celecoxib (VII).

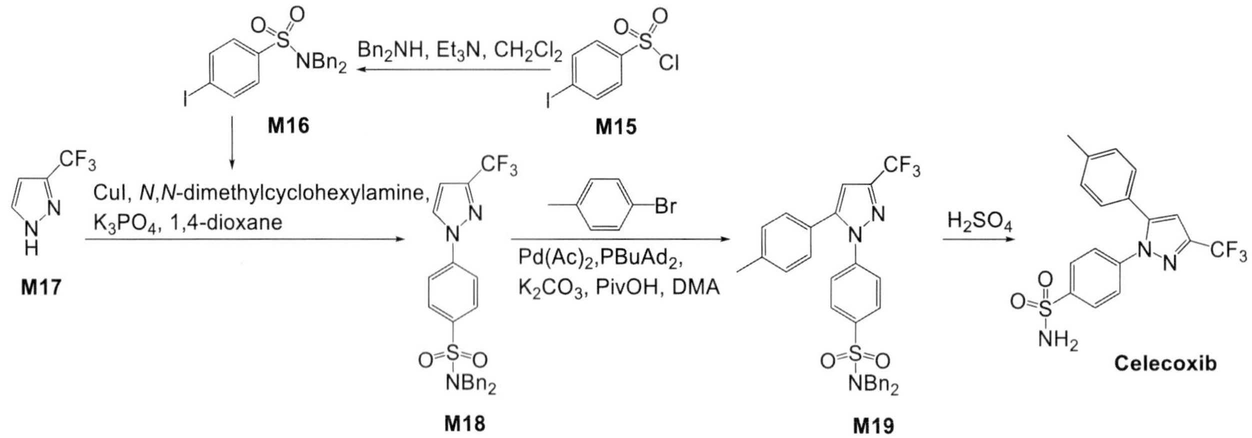

FIGURE 29.17 Chemical synthesis study of celecoxib (VIII).

Subsequently, p-aminobenzene sulfonamide (M12) was subjected to a Sandmeyer reaction by adding CuX in the presence of diazonium salt hydrochloride, where the diazo group was replaced by a halogen to generate p-halobenzene sulfonyl azide (M13). Finally, compounds M13 and M14 underwent a coupling reaction under alkaline conditions with CuI as a catalyst to yield celecoxib, with a final step yield of 72.6%. This method directly cyclizes the diketone intermediate with hydrazine to form a disubstituted pyrazole ring, effectively reducing regioisomer content, improving product quality, and achieving a high yield of 81.3% with only 0.01% regioisomer content [37].

29.2.2.6.4 C-H arylation reaction

Gaulier et al. introduced a new method for synthesizing celecoxib *via* a palladium-catalyzed C-H arylation reaction (Fig. 29.17) [38]. In this approach, 4-iodobenzenesulfonyl chloride (M15) and Bn$_2$NH react to form the intermediate *N,N*-dibenzyl-4-iodobenzenesulfonamide (M16). M16 then undergoes a Ullmann reaction with trifluoromethylpyrazole (M17) to produce the intermediate M18. Under palladium catalysis, M18 is subjected to a C-H arylation with 1-bromomethylbenzene, resulting in M19. Finally, deprotection using concentrated sulfuric acid produces celecoxib, achieving a total yield of 33% and a purity of over 95%. While innovative, the high cost of palladium acetate and the relatively low yield render this method unsuitable for large-scale production.

Given the widespread use and high demand for celecoxib, various synthetic methods have been developed. However, drawbacks including low yields, high impurity content, and inefficiencies necessitate further exploration of greener, more economical, and more efficient synthesis methods. Currently, the most commonly used method is the condensation of the diketone intermediate (M2) with 4-methylsulfonylaminophenylhydrazine hydrochloride (M3), which is the primary method for industrial synthesis. Research on novel strategies, such as 1,3-dipolar cycloaddition reactions, coupling reactions, and C-H arylation reactions, for the synthesis of celecoxib needs further exploration.

29.3 Other representative coxib drugs

Celecoxib, first approved in the United States in 1998 and in China in 2000 under the trade name "Xilebao," has played a pivotal role in ushering in a new era of antiinflammatory and pain-relieving drugs. By 2004, global sales of celecoxib had reached 3.3 billion dollars. Pharmaceutical companies and research institutes worldwide have invested significant resources in the NSAIDs field, leading to the development of several coxib drugs. New drugs from this class come onto the market almost every year (see Fig. 29.18).

Rofecoxib and celecoxib are both specific COX-2 inhibitors capable of blocking the synthesis and inflammatory effects of PGs in inflammatory tissues. In May 1999, rofecoxib, marketed as "Vioxx" by Merck Pharmaceuticals, was approved for sale by the US Food and Drug Administration (FDA). It was indicated for the treatment of osteoarthritis, rheumatoid arthritis, acute pain relief, and primary dysmenorrhea. After its launch, rofecoxib quickly achieved tremendous success, generating $2.5 billion in sales in 2003. However, due to the significantly higher COX-1/COX-2 selectivity inhibition index (38) of rofecoxib, compared to celecoxib (6.3), it decreased the production of prostacyclin PGI2 and led to platelet aggregation inhibition and vasodilation. Additionally, low COX-1 inhibition increased the risk of heart attack and stroke, according to VIGOR clinical tracking data. The use of high-dose Vioxx was associated with a significant increase in the risk of heart attacks and sudden cardiac deaths, obliging Merck to voluntarily withdraw rofecoxib from the market in September 2004. The announcement of the withdrawal resulted in a significant decline in Merck's stock price, which plummeted by over 25% and had a profound impact on the future development and clinical application prospects of COX-2 inhibitors. Following the disclosure of data from the VIGOR project, controversy arose over whether Merck-funded researchers had failed to disclose unfavorable data in articles published in *The New England Journal of Medicine*. There were concerns that the FDA, upon receiving associated information, did not immediately stop the clinical use of the drug but merely added black box warnings, sparking significant debate over drug regulation. In 2007, Merck agreed to pay $4.85 billion to settle thousands of drug liability lawsuits related to Vioxx causing heart attacks and other illnesses. This infamous "Vioxx" incident set extremely high standards for future drug development and regulatory practices.

Pfizer's valdecoxib, approved by the FDA in 2001 for treating pain caused by osteoarthritis and rheumatoid arthritis, faced a potential cardiovascular risk and stopped sale in the US market in April 2005. Pfizer researchers then performed the derivation of valdecoxib and acylated it with aminopropionyl; that work led to the creation of parecoxib as a sodium salt with better solubility. It received FDA approval in 2002 and became the only injectable selective COX-2 inhibitor. Although Pfizer's parecoxib entered the Chinese market later than celecoxib, recent sales data suggests that parecoxib has consistently been the top-selling drug among COX-2 inhibitors, with significant sales growth, particularly from 2018 to 2019 [39,40].

Etoricoxib, another highly selective COX-2 inhibitor, has shown time- and dose-dependent effects on COX-2 activity in clinical studies involving healthy individuals while having no significant impact on COX-1 activity. This characteristic significantly reduces the incidence of gastrointestinal side effects. Moreover, etoricoxib provides rapid analgesic relief, taking effect within 24 minutes and lasting for 24 hours.

Imrecoxib, developed by the Chinese Academy of Medical Sciences Institute of Medicinal Biotechnology and Jiangsu Hengrui Medicine Co., Ltd., was independently researched and received approval from the Chinese Food and Drug Administration in May 2011. Its development was guided by Professor Guo Zongru's strategy of "moderate inhibition" of COX-1/COX-2. Pharmacological studies have demonstrated that Imrecoxib's selectivity index, in terms of IC_{50} COX-1/IC_{50} COX-2, is 6.39, which correlates with a lower incidence of adverse reactions. The antiinflammatory activity and selectivity of its metabolites closely mirror those of Imrecoxib, making it an

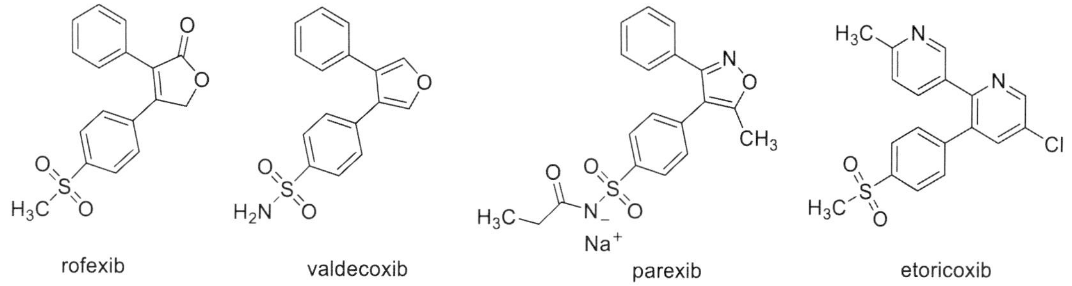

FIGURE 29.18 Molecular structures of representative coxibs.

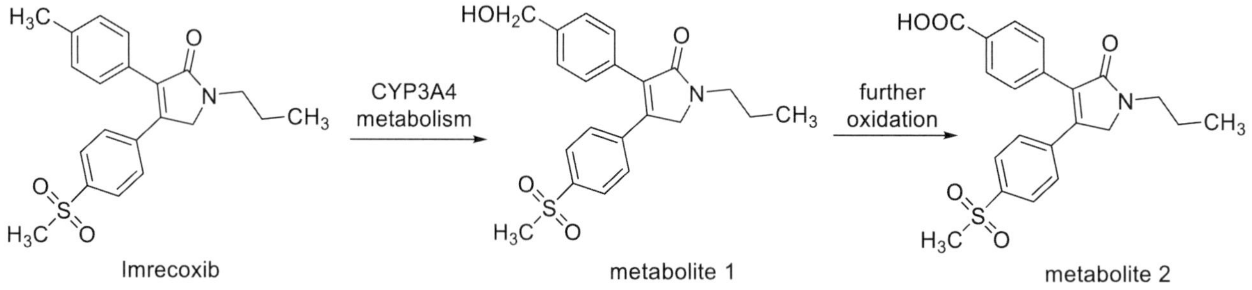

FIGURE 29.19 Chemical structures of Imrecoxib and its metabolites.

effective and safe treatment for osteoarthritis. In 2017, the innovative drug Imrecoxib was included in the new version of the health insurance catalog and recorded rapid growth and an increasing market share every year [41] (Fig. 29.19).

29.4 Summary and perspective

Early NSAIDs were discovered through animal phenotype/function experiments. From the discovery of COX enzymes in the 1970s to the successful commercialization of various selective COX-2 inhibitors like celecoxib around 2000, nearly 30 years of research and development have yielded several safe, effective, and controllable antiinflammatory and pain-relieving medications. Fundamental biological research breakthroughs related to inflammation have significantly propelled NSAID development. Vane's discovery in 1971 that COX is the therapeutic target of NSAIDs marked a milestone in studying the molecular biology mechanisms of these drugs. In the early 1990s, the identification of two COX isoenzymes laid the molecular groundwork for understanding the pharmacological effects and side effects of NSAIDs. Furthermore, high-throughput screening models for antiinflammatory compounds have been promoted through large-scale, rapid in vitro enzyme assays. In the mid-1990s, the protein crystal structures of COX-1 and COX-2 were used to elucidate the different modes of action between drugs and the two enzymes, allowing pharmacologists to accurately design and optimize COX-2 selective inhibitors.

The successful development of coxib-class NSAIDs also relies on the sophisticated chemical design of medicinal chemists, who discover drug candidates that are safe, effective, and controllable. Based on the differences in the amino acid sequences and structures of the catalytic sites of COX-1 and COX-2, as well as the different distribution of the two enzymes in various organs and tissues, researchers synthesized and screened tens of thousands of compounds to investigate the relationships between their structures and antiinflammatory activity, gastrointestinal toxicity, and metabolic distribution. Appropriate clinical candidate drugs were selected through a comprehensive analysis of the activity and drug-like properties of compounds. The development history of COX-2 selective inhibitors also suggests that sometimes excessive emphasis on high activity and high selectivity for a single target (particularly homologous proteins) may not always be ideal for medicinal chemists in designing and optimizing molecules. In the modern biotechnological context, the complexity and uniformity of the human body mean that most diseases are not caused by a single gene or target. In the drug development process, the impacts and effects of drugs on the entire disease process and multiple related functional pathways cannot be ignored. This is particularly important for defining molecular targets when the relevant physiological and pathological mechanisms are not completely clear.

After drugs are launched and widely applied in clinics, continuous monitoring and evaluation of clinical efficacy and safety are essential. The withdrawal of rofecoxib and valdecoxib mentioned in this chapter sounded an alarm for the global pharmaceutical community. Strengthening postmarketing adverse reaction monitoring is essential to ensure drug safety and minimize harm to patients.

References

[1] Winckler T, Schubert-Zsilavecz M, et al. Pharmazie Unserer Zeit 2010;38(1):3–3.
[2] Vane JR. Inhibition of prostaglandin synthesis as a mechanism of action for aspirin-like drugs. Nature 1971;231:232–5.
[3] Bakhle YS, Vane JR, Botting RM. Cyclooxygenases 1 and 2. Annu Rev Pharmacol Toxicol 2003;38(1):97–120.

[4] Charlier C, Michau C. Dual inhibition of cyclooxygenase-2 (cox-2) and 5-lipoxygenase (5-lox) as a new strategy to provide safer non-steroidal antiinflammatory drugs. Eur J Med Chem 2003;38(7-8):645—59.

[5] Fu JY, Masferrer JL, Seibert K, et al. The induction and suppression of prostaglandin H2 synthase (cyclooxygenase) in human monocytes. J Biol Chem 1990;265(28):16737—40.

[6] Warner TD, Giuliano F, Voinovic I, et al. Nonsteroid drug selectivities for cyclo-oxygenase-1 rather than cyclo-oxygenase-2 are associated with human gastrointestinal toxicity: a full in vitro analysis. Proc Natl Acad Sci USA 1999;96(13):7563—7563.

[7] Smith WL, Song I. The enzymology of prostaglandin endoperoxide H synthases-1 and 2. Prostagland Other Lipid Med 2002;68-69:115—28.

[8] Fukudome K, Esmon CT. Cloning and regulation of an endothelial cell protein C/activated protein C receptor. US, US6399064 1997;B1.

[9] Samad TA, Sapirstein A, Woolf CJ. Prostanoids and pain: unraveling mechanisms and revealing therapeutic targets. Trends Mol Med 2002;8(8):390—6.

[10] Kujubu DA. Tis10, a phorbol ester tumor promoter-inducible mrna from swiss 3t3 cells, encodes a novel prostaglandin synthase/cyclooxygenase homologue. J Biol Chem 1991;266(20):12866.

[11] Tazawa R, Xu XM, Wu KK, et al. Characterization of the genomic structure, chromosomal location and promoter of human prostaglandin H synthase-2 gene. Biochem Biophys Res Commun 1994;203(1):190—9.

[12] Williams CS, Dubois RN, Williams CS, Dubois RN. Prostaglandin endoperoxide synthase: why two isoforms? Am J Physiol 1996;270(3 Pt 1):G393—400.

[13] Konturek PC, Kania J, Burnat G, et al. Prostaglandins as mediators of COX-2 derived carcinogenesis in gastrointestinal tract. J Physiol Pharmacol 2005;56(Suppl 5):57—73.

[14] Thuresson E.D., Malkowski M.G., Lakkides K.M., et al. Substrate interactions in the cyclooxygenase-1 active site, 2001.

[15] Dannhardt G, Kiefer W. Cyclooxygenase inhibitors-current status and future prospects. Eur J Med Chem 2001;32(2):109—26.

[16] Kurumbail RG, Stevens AM, Glerse JK, et al. Structural basis for selective inhibition of cyclooxygenase-2 by anti-inflammatory agents. Nature 1996;384(6616):644—8.

[17] Chandrasekharan NV, Dai H, Roos K, et al. Cox-3, a cyclooxygenase-1 variant inhibited by acetaminophen and other analgesic/antipyretic drugs: cloning, structure, and expression. PNAS 2002;99(21):13926—31.

[18] Shaftel SS, Olschowka JA, Hurley SD, et al. Cox-3: a splice variant of cyclooxygenase-1 in mouse neural tissue and cells. Mol Brain Res 2003;119(2):213—15.

[19] Rial NS, Zell JA, Cohen AM, et al. Clinical end points for developing pharmaceuticals to manage patients with a sporadic or genetic risk of colorectal cancer. Expert Rev Gastroenterol Hepatol 2014;6(4):507—17.

[20] Picot, Daniel, Loll, et al. The x-ray crystal structure of the membrane protein prostaglandin H(2) synthase-1. Nature 1994;367:243—9.

[21] Gierse JK, Koboldt CM, Walker MC, et al. Kinetic basis for selective inhibition of cyclo-oxygenases. Biochem J 1999;339(3):607.

[22] Futaki N, Takahashi S, Yokoyama M, et al. NS-398, a new anti-inflammatory agent, selectively inhibits prostaglandin G/H synthase/cyclooxygenase (COX-2) activity in vitro. Prostaglandins 1994;47(1):55.

[23] Black WC, Li CS, Chan CC, et al. Cyclooxygenase-2 inhibitors. Synthesis and pharmacological activities of 5-methanesulfonamido-1-indanone derivatives. J Med Chem 1995;38(25):4897—905.

[24] Gans KR, Galbraith W, Roman RJ, et al. Anti-inflammatory and safety profile of DuP 697, a novel orally effective prostaglandin synthesis inhibitor. J Pharmacol Exp Thcrap 1990;254:180—7.

[25] Reitz DB, Li JJ, Norton MB, et al. Selective cyclooxygenase inhibitors: novel 1,2-diarylcyclopentenes are potent and orally active COX-2 inhibitors. J Med Chem 1994;37(23):3878.

[26] Seibert K, Yan Z, Leahy K, et al. Pharmacological and biochemical demonstration of the role of cyclooxygenase 2 in inflammation and pain. PNAS 1995,;91(25):12013—17.

[27] Penning TD, Talley JJ, Bertenshaw SR. Synthesis and biological evaluation of the 1,5-diarylpyrazole class of cyclooxygenase-2 inhibitors: identification of 4-[5-(4-methylphenyl)-3-(trifluoromethyl)-1H-pyrazol-1-yl]benzenesulfonamide (SC-58635, Celecoxib). J Med Chem 1997;40(9):1347—65.

[28] Magolda RL, Batt D, Covongton MB, et al. Structure-activity-relationships with a novel series of selective cyclooxygenase-2 inhibitors. Inflamm Res 1995;44(suppl. 3):A274.

[29] Hubbard RC, Mehlisch DR, Jasper DR, et al. Sc-58635, a highly selective inhibitor of cox-2, is an effective analgesic in an acute post-surgical pain model. J Investig Med 1996;44(3):293a.

[30] Silverstein FE, Faich G, Goldstin JL, et al. Gastrointestinal toxicity with celecoxib vs nonsteroidal anti-inflammatory drugs for osteoarthritis and rheumatoid arthritis: the CLASS study: a randomized controlled trial. JAMA 2000;284:1247—55.

[31] Bombardier C, Laine L, Reicin A, et al. Comparison of upper gastrointestinal toxicity of rofecoxib and naproxen in patients with rheumatoid arthritis. N Engl J Med 2000;343:1520—8.

[32] Abdellatif KR, Chowdhury MA, Dong Y, et al. Diazen-1-ium-1,2-diolated nitric oxide donor ester prodrugs of 5-(4-hydroxymethylphenyl)-1-(4-aminosulfonylphenyl)-3-trifluoromethyl-1H-pyrazole and its methanesulfonyl analog: synthesis, biological evaluation and nitric oxide release studies. Bioorg Med Chem 2009;17(14):5182—8.

[33] Reddy AR, Sampath A, Goverdhan G, et al. An improved and scalable process for celecoxib: a selective cyclooxygenase-2 inhibitor. Org Process Res Dev 2008;13(1):203—4.

[34] Ambati V., Garaga S., Mallela S., et al. An improved process for the prepartion of Celecoxib. 2010, WO, WO2010/095024A3.

[35] Liang SJ, Miao HM, Liang XY, et al. A method for the preparation of Celecoxib. 2022, CN, CN110526868B.
[36] Oh LM. Synthesis of celecoxib via 1,3-dipolar cycloaddition. Tetrahedron Lett 2006;47(45):7943–6.
[37] Zhang QH, Xu GY. Celecoxib and its preparation. 2014, CN, CN102558056B.
[38] Gaulier SM, Mckay R, Swain NA. A novel three-step synthesis of Celecoxib via palladium-catalyzed direct arylation. Tetrahedron Lett 2011;52(45):6000–2.
[39] Talley JJ, Brown DL, Carter JS, et al. 4-[5-methyl-3-phenylisoxazol-4-yl]-benzenesulfonamide, valdecoxib: a potent and selective inhibitor of COX-2. J Med Chem 2000;43(5):775–7.
[40] Talley JJ, Malecha JW, Bertenshaw S, et al. N-[[(5-Methyl- 3-phenylisoxazol-4-yl)-phenyl]sulfonyl]propanamide, sodium salt, parecoxib sodium: a potent and selective inhibitor of COX-2 for parenteral administration. J Med Chem 2000;43(9):1661–3.
[41] Guo ZR. Discovery of imrecoxib. Chin J New Drugs 2012;21(03):223–30.

Chapter 30

Case study of antisense oligonucleotides for duchenne muscular dystrophy

Xinyang Zhou, Yufei Pan and Zhenjun Yang

School of Pharmaceutical Sciences, Peking University, Beijing, P.R. China

Chapter outline

30.1 Introduction	735
30.2 Duchenne muscular dystrophy	737
30.2.1 Introduction to duchenne muscular dystrophy	737
30.2.2 Treatment and exon skipping in duchenne muscular dystrophy	737
30.3 Mechanism of action of antisense oligonucleotide drugs	739
30.3.1 RNase H	739
30.3.2 Alternative mechanisms	740
30.3.3 Exon skipping	740
30.4 The developmental trajectory of antisense oligonucleotide therapeutics targeting the DMD gene	741
30.4.1 Chemical modifications of antisense oligonucleotides	742
30.4.2 Oligonucleotide delivery techniques	745
30.4.3 Exon skipping therapy for DMD by ASO	749
30.5 Summary and outlook	752
References	752

30.1 Introduction

Nucleic acids are vital biomolecules capable of storing genetic information and participating in various biological processes, both intrinsically and through encoding functional proteins. Various functional oligonucleotides are currently a focal point of research for the regulation of genetic-level physiological processes and disease treatment, including antisense oligonucleotides (ASOs), small interfering ribonucleic acids (siRNAs), microRNAs, ribozymes, aptamers, messenger ribonucleic acids (mRNAs), plasmids, and cyclic dinucleotides (cDNs), among others. Due to their inherent negative charge under physiological conditions, overcoming the barriers presented by the intracellular environment and effectively delivering them to their targets is an urgent issue that needs to be addressed.

ASOs refer to a class of 15−20 nucleotide single-stranded deoxyribonucleic acids that are artificially synthesized or expressed by constructed carriers. They specifically bind to target mRNA and impede translation through steric hindrance effects or activate ribonuclease (RNase) H for degradation. ASOs can also reduce precursor mRNA stability and interfere with its splicing, leading to exon and intron skipping, among other effects. The first approved ASO, fomivirsen, a phosphorothioate (PS), was granted approval in 1998 for the treatment of cytomegalovirus retinitis in AIDS patients. Since 2016, several ASOs, including mipomersen for familial hypercholesterolemia; inotersen for hereditary transthyretin amyloidosis; volanesorsen for familial chylomicronemia syndrome; and eteplirsen, golodirsen, viltolarsen, and casimersen for Duchenne muscular dystrophy (DMD), have been approved. Numerous other ASOs are currently undergoing clinical trials.

The development of siRNA therapeutics has also garnered widespread international attention, with several companies actively involved. In 2018, an important milestone was reached with the Food and Drug Administration (FDA) approval of patisiran, the first siRNA therapeutic used to treat hereditary transthyretin amyloidosis (hATTR). Patisiran demonstrated superior safety compared to the related ASO inotersen. It utilized 2′-O-Me modifications and was delivered using DLin-MC3-DMA/Distearoylphosphatidylcholine (DSPC)/PEG-DMG (1,2-dimyristoyl-rac-glycero-3-methoxypolyethylene glycol-2000)/cholesterol lipid nanoparticles (LNP) with specific proportions (50/10/1.5/38.5; siRNA, 8%, w/w). Subsequent siRNA therapeutics, such as givosiran (GIVLAARI), inclisiran, and fitusiran, which have either obtained recent approvals or entered Phase III clinical trials, utilize a GalNAc (*N*-acetylgalactosamine) conjugate on the sense strand 3′-end and are administered subcutaneously to target the liver for the treatment of various metabolic and viral infectious diseases. These compounds feature 2′-F/2′-*O*-Me modifications, with some incorporating PS linkages. Notably, four GalNAc conjugates for hepatitis B treatment are currently in Phase II clinical trials, namely ALN-HBV02, JNJ3989, DCR-HBVS(siRNA therapeutics), and GSK3389404(ASO therapeutics).

Nucleic acid aptamers, typically composed of single-stranded deoxyribonucleic acid (DNA) or RNA with lengths ranging from 15 to 80 nucleotides, possess stable three-dimensional structures through self-folding. This structural stability allows them to engage in specific and induced fit interactions with target molecules. While only one aptamer, pegaptanib sodium (Macugen), has received approval for the treatment of wet age-related macular degeneration, there have been challenges in the clinical trials of other aptamers such as Fovista (anti-platelet derived growth factor (PDGF)) and Reg1 (anti-coagulation factor IXa (FIXa)) due to concerns regarding efficacy and safety. As a result, several nucleic acid aptamer candidates in Phase I–II trials have been discontinued.

By amplifying the mRNA of the antigen through in vitro methods, the formulation, upon administration, enters the bloodstream via capillaries within the muscle tissue. It subsequently reaches antigen-presenting cells and undergoes translation to obtain the antigen. The antigen is then presented by the MHC to activate T cells and initiate an immune response. The sequence design and production cycle of this process are relatively short. Two mRNA vaccines for prevention against Coronavirus 2019 (COVID-19) infection, namely Comirnaty (BNT162b2) from Pfizer-BioNTech and mRNA-1273 from Moderna, have received emergency use authorization from the FDA. Both vaccines carry mRNA encoding the COVID-19 S protein, incorporating pseudo-uridine (Ψ) nucleotides to enhance stability and intracellular translation efficiency while minimizing potential immunogenicity risks. Additionally, they incorporate the S-2P mutation to stabilize the conformation of the S protein before binding to receptors, thereby improving antibody neutralization effectiveness. The former utilizes LNP delivery with ALC-0325/DSPC/cholesterol/ALC-0159 (47.5/10/40.8/1.7; mRNA, 3%–4%, w/w), while the latter employs SM-102/DSPC/cholesterol/PEG2000-DMG (50/10/38.5/1.5; mRNA, 5%, w/w). Both vaccines exhibit high efficacy rates of 95% and 94.1%, respectively, ensuring complete prevention of severe infections. However, there have been reports of various adverse reactions associated with their administration.

Clustered regularly interspaced short palindromic repeats (CRISPR)/CRISPR-associated protein 9 (Cas9) has emerged as one of the most prominent gene editing tools in current research. It involves the introduction of sgRNA and the Cas9 nuclease into cells with the purpose of deleting or modifying specific gene loci, thereby correcting disease-causing genes. Cas9 is often delivered in conjunction with mRNA or plasmids through rational design, with viral vectors commonly employed for delivery. This technique is currently in Phase I/II clinical trials and actively recruiting participants. The gene editing process primarily focuses on T cells extracted from human blood, which are subjected to genetic modifications to express chimeric antigen receptors (CARs) that target specific antigens. These edited T cells are then reinfused into patients, allowing them to recognize tumor antigens and induce targeted cell death. Six CAR T-cell therapies have been approved overseas, including the first domestically approved axicabtagene ciloleucel by Fosun Kite Biotechnology for the treatment of various lymphomas.

Cyclic dinucleotides (CDNs) and their analogs (cDNs) belong to a class of pattern recognition receptor agonists that target the STING protein. They activate the cGAS-STING signaling pathway, resulting in the release of type I interferons and related cytokines, thus triggering immune responses. Several analogs of CDNs are currently undergoing Phase I/II clinical trials. Among them, one promising candidate is a biodegradable cationic polymer called poly(beta-amino ester). When loaded with cDNs (2 μg) and PD-1(20 μg) administration, this combination exhibits comparable therapeutic efficacy to naked cDNs. Remarkably, this treatment completely eliminates melanoma in mice models, showcasing its significant potential as an immunotherapeutic candidate for cancer treatment.

DMD is an X-linked recessive hereditary neuromuscular disease caused by a deficiency of the dystrophin protein. Affected children typically have short lifespans and poor quality of life, with no effective treatment currently available. However, the development of gene therapy has ignited hope for the treatment and potential cure of this disease. ASO drugs, which operate on the principle of exon skipping, can bypass one or two mutated exons to restore the disrupted reading frame. This promising approach provides treatment for 80% of patients. As of August 2021, the FDA has approved four ASO drugs for the treatment of DMD.

This chapter provides a brief overview of the characteristics of DMD and focuses on the research and development process of FDA-approved ASO drugs over the past five years. It delves into the principles, design strategies, and modification methods of these therapeutic agents. Furthermore, it provides an analysis of the technical principles, development process, and related advancements in nucleic acid therapeutics.

30.2 Duchenne muscular dystrophy

30.2.1 Introduction to duchenne muscular dystrophy

DMD, a rare condition, was first described by the French physician Duchenne in 1861. The genetic basis of the condition was identified in 1987. The global annual incidence of DMD is typically less than 100,000 cases, although the numbers vary across countries. This condition is caused by mutations in the DMD gene located on the X chromosome, making it an X-linked genetic disorder. The mutations predominantly manifest in boys, with an estimated incidence of approximately 1 in every 5000 births. In girls, it usually remains asymptomatic, with carriership of the gene being the only indication [1]. In China, around 400 cases of DMD are reported annually, and the total number of affected individuals has reached 70,000, making it the country with the highest incidence rate. Affected children typically exhibit noticeable developmental delays, including delayed motor skills, which become apparent around the ages of 3–5 years. As they grow older, the progressive deterioration of motor function becomes increasingly evident, often accompanied by respiratory impairments that frequently require mechanical support. Additionally, the disease progression can negatively impact brain development, leading to complications such as attention deficit, autism, and epilepsy. Due to the progressive and irreversible muscle degeneration and atrophy, patients lose their ability to walk independently after the age of 10 and become reliant on a wheelchair for mobility. Ultimately, they succumb to cardiorespiratory failure between the ages of 20 and 30. Currently, there are no available curative treatments for DMD, and clinical intervention primarily focuses on medication and physical measures to manage complications and control disease progression. The existing treatment options include the use of glucocorticoids and mechanical ventilators, which significantly extend patients' lifespans [2]. For instance, the administration of high-dose glucocorticoids (prednisone at 0.75 mg/kg/day) effectively slows down disease progression [3]. In addition, a nonaminoglycoside drug called ataluren (Translarna) and four ASO drugs, including EXONDYS 51, VYONDYS 53, AMONDYS 45, and VILTPSO, have been approved for the treatment of DMD. For diagnostic purposes, blood tests to detect muscle damage markers and genetic testing to identify specific mutations in the gene are performed on affected children in hospitals. Additionally, it is recommended that relatives of affected individuals undergo testing to determine their carrier status for the disease-causing gene (Fig. 30.1).

30.2.2 Treatment and exon skipping in duchenne muscular dystrophy

The structural integrity of muscle fibers is maintained by a complex system composed of cytoskeletal proteins and membrane proteins, which can withstand the physical forces exerted on the muscle membrane. These proteins are arranged in a specific manner to anchor the protein structures within the muscle cells to the basement membrane and extracellular matrix.

Dystrophin, an essential cytoskeletal protein (Fig. 30.2), is a highly organized contractile protein (427 kDa) that is primarily expressed in skeletal, cardiac, and smooth muscle cells. It is minimally expressed in the brain and retina, accounting for only 0.01% of the total muscle protein expression and 5% of the cytoskeletal proteins in muscle matrix cells. Dystrophin is located internally within the muscle membrane and is abundant at the tendon attachments and neuromuscular junctions, serving as a crucial component of the muscle cell's cytoskeleton. It bridges the contractile proteins within the muscle cell to the membrane, exhibiting a flexible rod-like structure and playing a pivotal role in stabilizing the muscle cell membrane during muscle contraction.

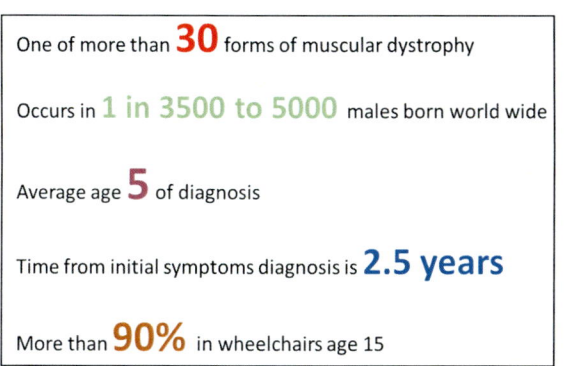

FIGURE 30.1 Numbers about DMD [4].

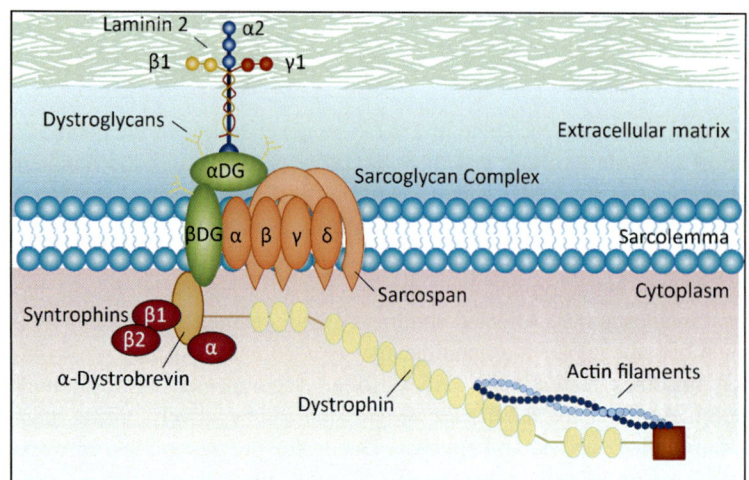

FIGURE 30.2 Dystrophin is an important link between intracellular actin (Actin filaments) and the extracellular matrix (Extracellular matrix) [5].

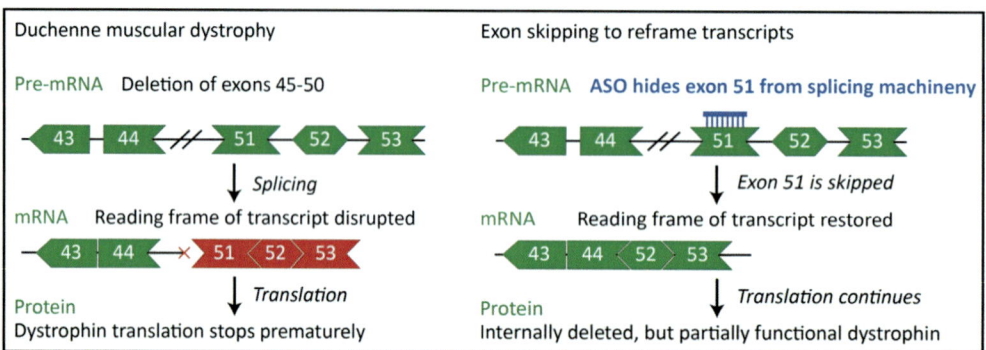

FIGURE 30.3 The restoration of dystrophin protein expression in patients with Duchenne muscular dystrophy through exon skipping [7].

The DMD gene, which encodes dystrophin protein, is the largest gene in the human genome (2.2 Mb) and consists of 79 exons. Approximately 65% of patients with DMD exhibit deletions and duplications of DNA fragments within the Xp21.22–Xp21.3 region of the X chromosome, which encompasses the dystrophin gene. Among these genetic alterations, exons 43–53 are particularly prone to mutations, causing disruptions in the open reading frame (ORF) and premature termination of normal protein translation. Various methods such as DNA probes targeting different regions of the Xp21 region, restriction enzyme analysis, and multiplex PCR can diagnose abnormalities in the dystrophin gene. In the absence of dystrophin, the contraction process of muscle fibers is susceptible to damage, leading to pathological changes characterized by fibrosis and replacement of fatty tissue, ultimately resulting in DMD. The deficiency of dystrophin in the brain is associated with a decline in cognitive function in patients [6].

The spliceosome is a ribonucleoprotein complex that plays a crucial role in excising introns from pre-mRNA molecules to generate mature mRNA. During this process, known as splicing, certain exons may be skipped, resulting in the production of truncated mRNA. The splicing process is tightly regulated to ensure the production of error-free mRNA. However, 90% of human genes are still prone to alternative splicing, which enriches gene and protein diversity. The most common form of alternative splicing is exon skipping, which is currently being applied in the development of antisense oligonucleotide drugs for DMD.

As depicted in Fig. 30.3, more than half of DMD patients experience exon deletions caused by genetic mutations. These mutations disrupt normal mRNA splicing and prevent the proper expression of dystrophin protein. The loss of protein function due to abnormal expression contributes to the development of DMD. Exon skipping therapy utilizes specific ASOs to exclude certain exons during the pre-mRNA splicing process of the DMD gene, thereby restoring the reading frame and enabling the theoretical production of truncated dystrophin protein with partial functionality in most patients. Approximately 80% of DMD gene mutations can be corrected by skipping 1–2 specific exons, with exon 51 skipping being able to treat approximately 13% of patients.

30.3 Mechanism of action of antisense oligonucleotide drugs

As pre-mRNA and mRNA are messenger molecules that carry all the information of the genome, they can undergo genetic information modification, splicing, and translation through base-pairing with themselves or other complementary molecules. They represent a distinct class of drug targets compared to proteins. ASO drugs are short nucleotide sequences typically consisting of 13–30 nucleotides that can complementarily bind to specific nucleic acid sequences (pre-mRNA or mRNA). Their unique feature is the sequence-specific binding, which allows them to regulate gene expression.

ASOs can exert their biological activity through various mechanisms, primarily by activating RNase H to degrade the intracellular hybrid molecules of ASO/mRNA. Additionally, through a steric hindrance effect, the complex formed by the binding of ASOs to the target mRNA can block the binding and translation of relevant enzymes (Fig. 30.4).

30.3.1 RNase H

RNase H is an endonuclease enzyme that cleaves RNA within DNA/RNA hybrid double-stranded molecules. It is primarily divided into two subtypes: RNase H1 and RNase H2 [9]. Eukaryotic RNase H1 possesses a high-affinity binding domain for its substrate, while RNase H2 consists of three distinct proteins, including a catalytic subunit (2A) and two additional subunits (2B and 2C) with unknown functions but necessary for catalysis. Despite having similar hydrolysis mechanisms, there are subtle differences between these two subtypes (Fig. 30.5). RNase H2 is more abundant in mammals compared to RNase H1, but only RNase H1 is involved in the cleavage of ASO/target RNA duplexes [10,11].

When the ASO reaches an effective concentration near the target mRNA, ASO enters the cell and forms a hybrid double-stranded structure. This hybrid structure then activates RNase H1. Subsequently, the target mRNA is cleaved and degraded. Experimental evidence has demonstrated that the molecular dynamics process of ASO activating RNase H1 is relatively sluggish [12]. Following transfection, it takes approximately 1 hour for the ASO to distribute within the cytoplasm or nucleus of the cell. Subsequently, it undergoes a search for and binding to homologous mRNA sites, recruiting proteins such as RNase H1 over a period of 20–40 minutes. Once the recruitment of the RNase H1 protein

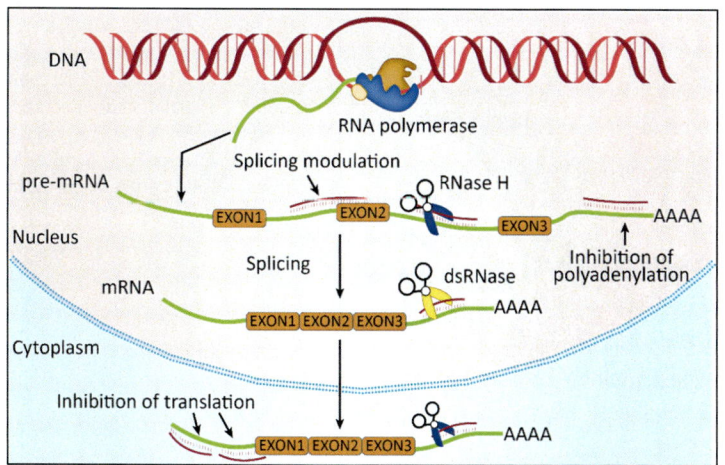

FIGURE 30.4 The mechanism of action of antisense oligonucleotides [8].

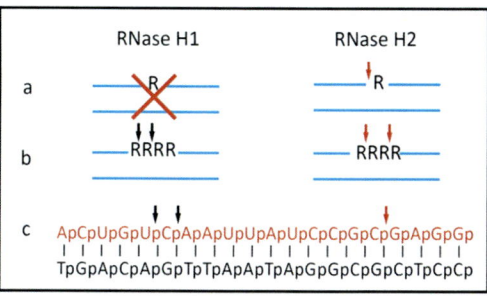

FIGURE 30.5 RNase H1 and RNase H2 exhibit different cleavage patterns at distinct substrate sites: a. RNase H2 can cleave single ribonucleotides within double-stranded DNA, whereas RNase H1 cannot; b/c. Cleavage sites for consecutive four ribonucleotides and RNA/DNA hybrid double-strands. Black arrows represent cleavage sites for RNase H1, while red arrows represent cleavage sites for RNase H2 [9].

complex is complete, efficient cleavage and degradation of the target gene take place. Importantly, the degradation rate of the target mRNA induced by RNase H1 is faster than the decay rate of normal mRNA [13].

30.3.2 Alternative mechanisms

In addition to activating RNase H for mRNA cleavage (Fig. 30.6A), ASOs can employ other strategies (Fig. 30.6B and C) to target the initiation sites or noncoding regions of mRNA. By forming complementary double-stranded structures, they can disrupt the binding of RNA-binding proteins, including ribosomal subunits, thereby interrupting the protein translation process. Furthermore, they can decrease the stability of pre-mRNA and interfere with pre-mRNA splicing, leading to exon skipping and intron retention (Fig. 30.6D). Moreover, they can also modulate the expression of upstream ORFs, thereby increasing the levels of protein translation from the main ORF (Fig. 30.6E).

30.3.3 Exon skipping

Genes are composed of fragments known as exons and introns. Exons are DNA segments that encode protein information and are interspersed with introns, which are often referred to as "DNA junk" as they are spliced out and discarded during protein production. During this process, if the gene encoding the protein in the target cell or tissue undergoes mutations, insertions and/or deletions, or splicing errors, it can lead to the generation of abnormal mature mRNA. Instead, the gene is transcribed into a nonsense mRNA, which is detected by stringent intracellular surveillance mechanisms and degraded. This process is also known as nonsense-mediated mRNA decay and can result in defects in the expression of normal proteins.

The principle of ASO-mediated exon skipping involves the specific binding of ASOs to aberrant exons during mRNA splicing, thereby regulating the maturation process of mRNA and correcting splicing abnormalities. ASO-induced exon skipping can be achieved through two main mechanisms [15]:

1. In the case illustrated in Fig. 30.7A, where rectangles represent exons and triangular edges represent exons carrying partial codons at the boundaries, a nonsense or frameshift mutation in the second exon can cause a shift in the

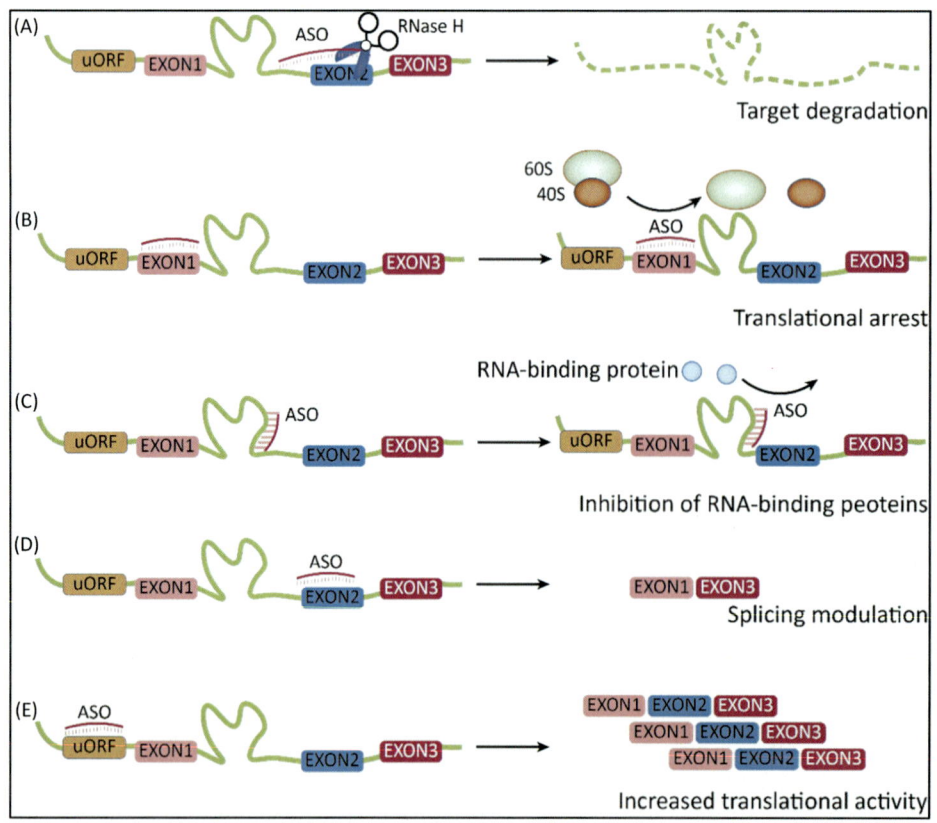

FIGURE 30.6 Mechanisms of ASO function: (A) mRNA degradation pathway; (B) Translation inhibition; (C) Spatial steric hindrance to prevent RNA-binding protein binding; (D) Splicing regulation; (E) Enhancement of protein translation capacity [14].

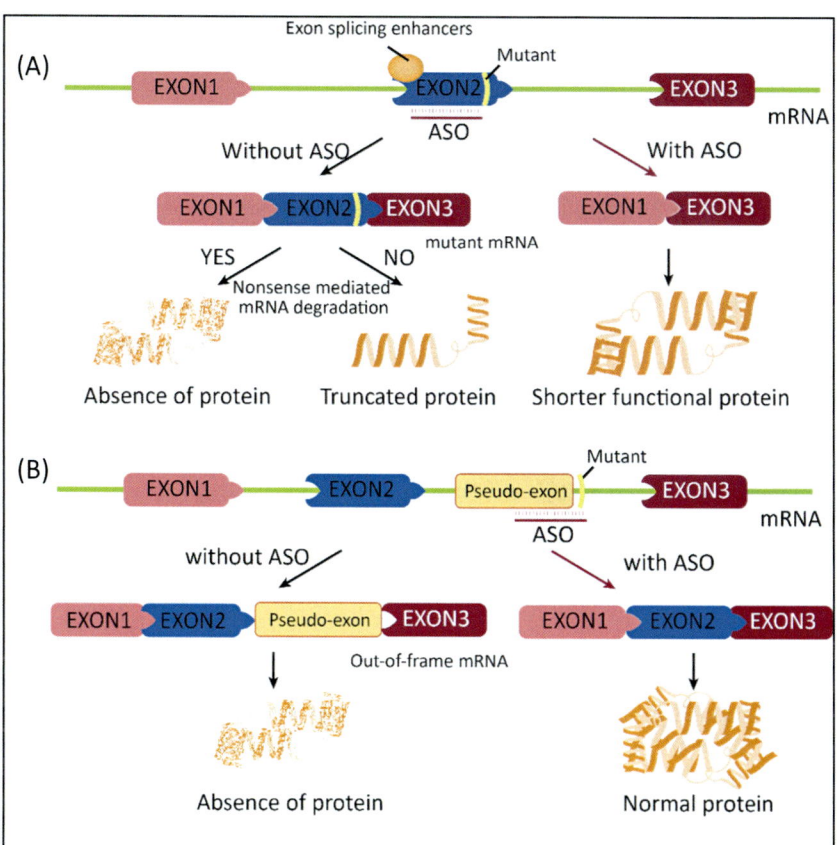

FIGURE 30.7 The schematic diagram of the principle of exon skipping rearrangement [15].

normal reading frame, resulting in premature transcription termination and no protein production. In this situation, ASOs can be designed to bind to the second exon, masking the mutation site and inducing exon skipping at the critical splice site. As a result, the mutated exon is hidden, and a shorter functional protein can be synthesized.

2. When a mutation in an intron creates a false reading frame, disrupting mRNA maturation by interfering with the normal reading frame at the exon boundary, ASOs can be applied to mask the mutation site and induce exon skipping. This process allows the skipping of the pseudoexon, resulting in the production of a normal protein (Fig. 30.7B).

Exon skipping is currently widely used in the treatment of DMD. The presence of milder allelic forms of the disease, such as Becker muscular dystrophy, has demonstrated that the restoration of partially truncated dystrophin protein can improve muscle function in DMD patients. This therapeutic approach has shown efficacy in over 80% of different mutation subtypes of DMD.

30.4 The developmental trajectory of antisense oligonucleotide therapeutics targeting the DMD gene

The current treatment for DMD primarily involves the use of corticosteroids, which can ameliorate symptoms and extend survival. However, it is merely symptomatic treatment that not only fails to cure the disease but also faces frequent questioning regarding its safety, as long-term use presents significant adverse reactions. Therefore, the development of specific drugs that restore the expression of antimuscle atrophy proteins is of paramount importance.

Despite significant advancements in studying the genetic aspects of the pathogenesis of DMD, the clinical management of this rare disease continues to present substantial challenges. Firstly, this disease is closely intertwined with the nervous system and possesses a high degree of concealment, as irreversible damage may occur before symptoms are reported to physicians. Secondly, traditional small-molecule drugs primarily target proteins, but DMD lacks specific protein targets, making it difficult to discover suitable drugs through traditional screening methods. Thirdly, neurodegenerative changes caused by neurological disorders in DMD lead to a cascade of downstream reactions, including protein misfolding, mitochondrial dysfunction, excitotoxicity, and oxidative stress. Consequently, single-target drugs have minimal potential for delaying disease progression.

The delivery of artificially synthesized mRNA to achieve the expression of specific proteins has been successful in the development of COVID-19 vaccines. However, due to the large size of the DMD gene, it is highly challenging to effectively deliver its mRNA in vivo.

Therefore, one of the most promising therapeutic approaches for DMD is exon skipping mediated by ASOs. Exon skipping therapy targets the pre-mRNA of the antimuscle atrophy protein using synthetic ASOs, thereby skipping at least one exon and restoring the reading frame, resulting in the production of truncated but partially functional antimuscle atrophy proteins.

In 1978, Zamecnik and Stephenson successfully inhibited the replication and cellular infection of Rous sarcoma virus by using a 13 nucleotide-long oligodeoxynucleotide that could complementarily pair with Rous sarcoma virus 35S RNA [16]. This novel oligonucleotide drug, known as the ASO, has entered the researchers' field of view. With the subsequent decoding of the human genome sequence, research on ASO drugs experienced a surge of interest. In 1998, the first ASO drug, fomivirsen, was approved by the FDA and launched for the treatment of cytomegalovirus retinitis in AIDS patients via intravitreal injection. The successful launch of fomivirsen provided a significant boost to the clinical development of ASO drugs.

However, over the next decade, a series of unsuccessful clinical studies dealt a heavy blow to both public and investor confidence in this drug class. The introduction of combination therapy for HIV infection led to effective treatment options, gradually reducing the market demand for fomivirsen. Consequently, it was withdrawn from the European and American markets in 2002 and 2006, respectively. Additionally, the limited effectiveness and notable side effects of the anticancer ASO drug G3239 led to the FDA rejecting its marketing application. Affinitak, a treatment for advanced nonsmall cell lung cancer developed by pharmaceutical giants Gilead and IONIS, failed to demonstrate a significant extension in patient survival during Phase III clinical trials. A series of inconclusive and controversial clinical results have cast a long shadow over the development process of ASO drugs.

The limited applicability of ASO drugs is closely associated with their inherent characteristics. Firstly, ASOs are prone to degradation by nucleases in both the bloodstream and cytoplasm, resulting in a short half-life and poor stability. Secondly, their negative charge and instability restrict the administration of these drugs, making it difficult to utilize conventional oral routes that generally exhibit better patient compliance. When administered intravenously, accumulation in target sites is relatively challenging, and the amount of drug detected in target cells often falls below 1% of the administered dose. Furthermore, during the process of circulation and cellular transportation in vivo, nucleic acid drugs are easily identified as exogenous RNA by the organism, leading to the activation of the immune system and nonspecific adverse reactions. Additionally, the large-scale synthesis of ASOs typically involves chemical methods, resulting in higher production costs.

However, with the continuous advancement of ASO drug development technologies, various challenges associated with in vivo applications have been effectively addressed through rational chemical modification, conjugation, and carrier delivery. The substantial increase in approved ASO drugs since 2016 further validates the effectiveness of these strategies.

30.4.1 Chemical modifications of antisense oligonucleotides

The limitations of nucleic acid drugs are primarily attributed to their inherent characteristics. One significant drawback is their strong negative charge and hydrophilicity, which hinders their ideal pharmacokinetic properties within the body. For instance, they face difficulties in crossing biological membrane barriers, resulting in very low cellular uptake efficiency and low drug delivery rates [17]. Additionally, nucleic acid drugs are susceptible to nucleases, leading to poor stability in serum and a short half-life, as unmodified ASOs are rapidly eliminated from human serum within 30 minutes [18]. Moreover, they are prone to uptake and accumulation by the reticuloendothelial system in the liver and spleen, causing potential hepatotoxicity and splenic toxicity [19].

Chemical modifications have provided effective means to enhance the pharmaceutical properties of nucleic acid drugs. Various modification strategies have been employed, such as phosphate backbone modifications, sugar ring 2'-O-methyl (2'-O-Me), 2'-O-methoxyethyl (2'-O-MOE), 2'-fluoro (2'-F), and locked nucleic acid (LNA) modifications, as well as base modifications [8]. The objective of these modifications is to enhance the resistance of oligonucleotides to nucleases, improve their binding affinity to the target, and reduce the immunogenicity of nucleic acid drug molecules (Fig. 30.8).

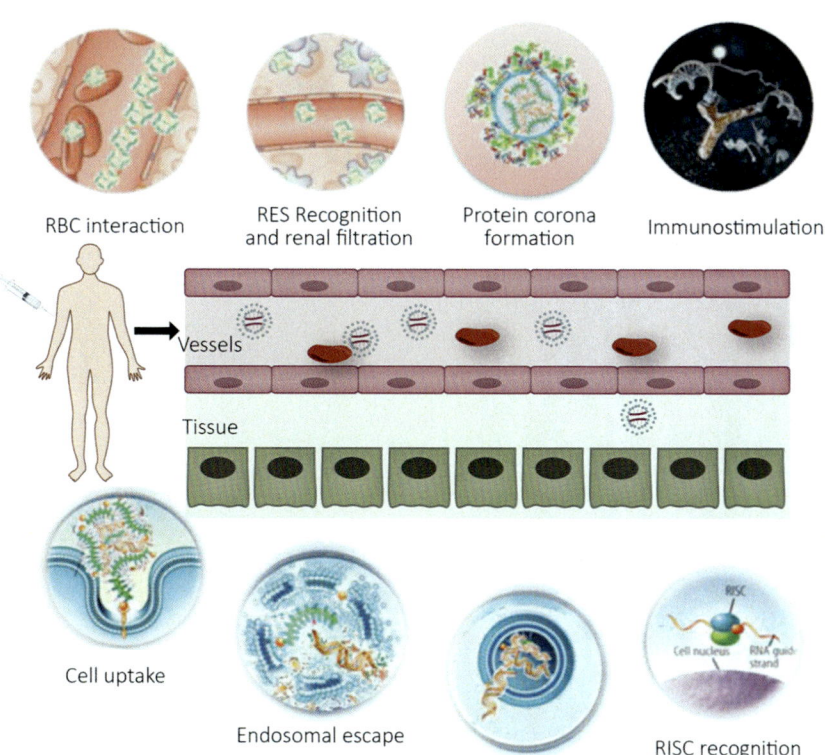

FIGURE 30.8 Schematic diagram of obstacles to systematic delivery of nucleic acid drugs [18].

30.4.1.1 Phosphorothioate modification

PS (Fig. 30.9) modification, also known as the "first-generation" method for chemical modification, is the earliest and most commonly used approach to modify ASOs. By replacing one of the nonbridging oxygen atoms with a sulfur atom in the phosphodiester bond, the ASO's resistance to nucleases is significantly enhanced, along with an increased binding capacity to serum proteins such as albumin. The introduction of PS modification extends the half-life of antisense nucleotides in serum to approximately 9 hours. This increased stability enables effective targeting of mRNA in human plasma, tissues, and cells. Consequently, it leads to improved tissue accumulation, cellular uptake efficiency, and overall bioavailability [20,21]. However, PS modification also has drawbacks, including increased toxicity and immunogenicity of the ASOs, interference with normal protein function, complement activation leading to immune reactions, and reduced affinity to target mRNA [22]. Additionally, the modified PS bonds have chiral centers, resulting in multiple stereoisomers of the fully phosphorothioated oligonucleotide. Each stereoisomer may have different pharmacological effects.

PS-modified ASOs, even when bound to mRNA, can still activate RNase H1 and facilitate target degradation. Furthermore, a modification strategy involving the replacement of the oxygen atom at the 3′-position of the sugar ring with a nitrogen atom in the PS backbone (thiophosphoramidate) can enhance the affinity to the target and increase resistance to enzymatic degradation [23]. However, this modified ASO cannot activate RNase H and can only regulate gene expression through other mechanisms [24].

30.4.1.2 Sugar ring modification strategies

Sugar ring modifications play a crucial role in altering the conformation of modified ASOs, affecting their affinity for complementary mRNA and their interaction with enzymatic tools. Chemical modifications at the 2′-position of the sugar ring are also known as second-generation modifications for ASOs. Among these, 2′-*O*-Me modification is widely utilized, as it improves the affinity for target mRNA to a certain extent and enhances enzymatic stability [25]. siRNAs with 2′-*O*-Me modifications have shown reduced immunogenicity. [26] Another common sugar ring modification is 2′-F(2′-fluoro) modification, which similarly enhances the affinity for target mRNA [27]. 2′-*O*-MOE modification also

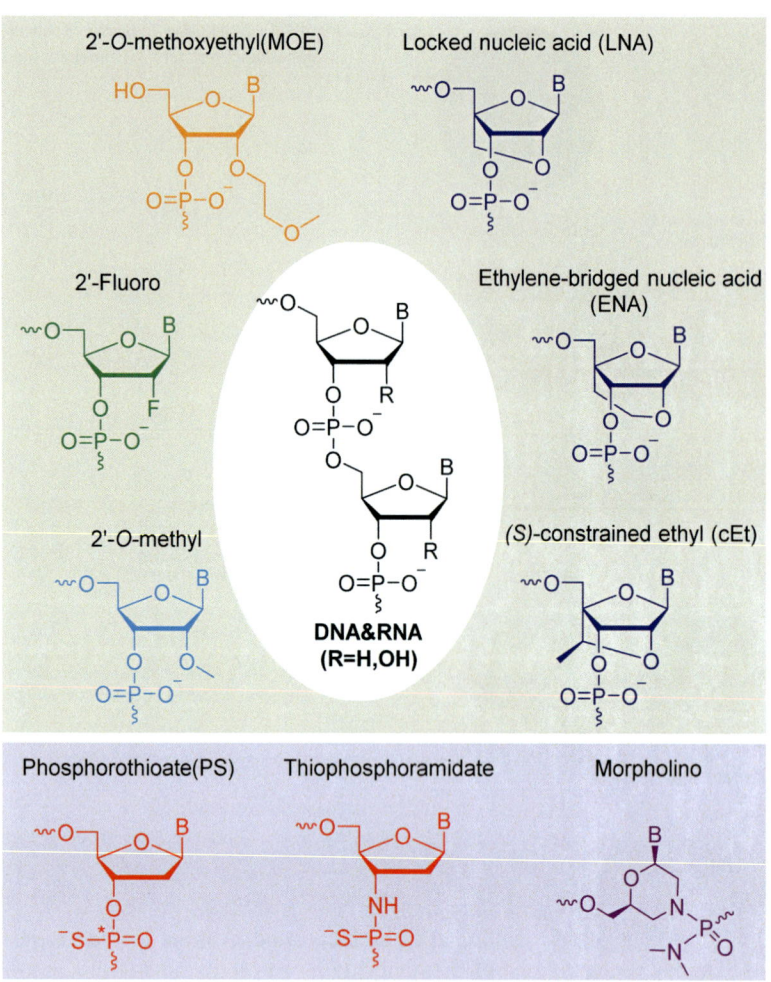

FIGURE 30.9 The nucleotide units used for the chemical modification of antisense oligonucleotides [8].

enhances target affinity and resistance to nucleases. Mipomersen, an approved ASO drug, utilizes both a combination of PS and 2'-O-MOE modification strategies.

Bridged nucleic acids connect the 2nd and 4th carbon atoms of nucleotides, forming a bicyclic nucleotide structure that restricts the nucleotide within a fixed conformation. Common bridging strategies include LNA, ethylene-bridged nucleic acid, and constrained ethyl (cEt). These modifications enhance resistance to nucleases and the affinity for the target. LNA modification, which connects the 2'-OH of the sugar ring to the C4' position with a methylene bridge, rigidifies the nucleotide into a bicyclic structure, resulting in increased stability and improved biological activity for ASOs [28]. cEt, an important monomer for 2.5th generation ASOs, significantly enhances the efficacy compared to 2'-O-MOE-modified ASOs, with approximately a tenfold increase. cEt was developed by Ionis, and the company has strict patent protection for its structure, preparation methods, and various forms of oligonucleotide molecules containing cEt.

Furthermore, applying sugar modifications to both flanks of PS ASOs (gapmers) has also demonstrated promising biological activity [29].

30.4.1.3 Nucleotide modifications

Morpholinos (PMOs) are nucleotide analogs that employ a modification method where a morpholine ring replaces the ribose sugar and is incorporated into the phosphorodiamidate backbone, converting the nucleic acid from negatively charged to electrically neutral. This modification strategy enhances the affinity for the target and resistance to nucleases [29]. Morpholino-modified ASOs lack the ability to activate RNase H and are thus used as translation inhibitors [27,30]. Peptide nucleic acids (PNAs) are another type of modification that utilizes a neutral charge backbone composed of N-(2-aminoethyl)glycine. Modified nucleotides with PNA show significant resistance to nucleases and proteases, as well as improved target affinity [31,32]. Similar to morpholino modifications, PNA-modified ASOs also do not activate RNase H for gene silencing activity. These two modifications significantly enhance the drug-like properties of ASOs and are referred to as third-generation modifications.

30.4.2 Oligonucleotide delivery techniques

30.4.2.1 Conjugation strategies for targeted delivery

Although chemical modifications improve the in vivo stability, membrane permeability, and affinity for targets and reduce immunogenicity of oligonucleotide therapeutics to some extent, challenges remain regarding poor targeting distribution (especially in nonhepatic tissues) and short half-life [33]. To overcome these therapeutic barriers, covalent conjugation and vector delivery strategies have emerged as new approaches to enhance gene delivery efficiency. Conjugation molecules, such as carbohydrate derivatives, peptides, antibodies, polymers, and lipids, have been utilized to achieve effective delivery of oligonucleotides to varying degrees (Fig. 30.10) [34—36].

Carbohydrate conjugation: The involvement of carbohydrate derivatives in various biological processes is well-documented, particularly in signaling transduction and cell surface recognition through lectins and carbohydrate-binding proteins [37,38]. One widely used carbohydrate derivative is N-Acetylgalactosamine (GalNAc), which exhibits a high affinity for asialoglycoprotein receptors present in liver cells [39]. This specificity makes GalNAc an effective targeting moiety for liver-directed delivery of nucleic acid therapeutics [40—42], including siRNA drugs such as givosiran, lumasiran, and inclisiran, which are commercially available. GalNAc-conjugated ASOs have demonstrated excellent safety and tolerability profiles when administered subcutaneously, with no significant local adverse reactions reported. Moreover, GalNAc conjugation allows for lower dosing frequencies due to improved liver uptake and sustained therapeutic effect. In clinical practice, a trivalent GalNAc cluster is commonly employed [43], although its applicability is limited to nonhepatic diseases. The general structure is depicted in Fig. 30.11.

GalNAc$_3$-conjugated ASOs have been well characterized for their pharmacokinetic properties in animals and humans. They exhibit stability in the bloodstream and specifically deliver the ASOs to parenchymal cells in the liver. Following internalization by liver cells, the GalNAc$_3$-conjugated ASOs undergo slow metabolism and release, resulting in an extended elimination half-life of 3—5 weeks. This allows for monthly administration and significantly improves safety. GalNAc$_3$ is rapidly metabolized in liver cells and subsequently excreted via the bile ducts and kidneys. Data suggests that the uptake of ASOs mediated by sialic acid glycoprotein receptors is nonlinear and can saturate at very high doses. However, the clinical doses of GalNAc$_3$-conjugated ASOs are typically lower, mostly below the level of 120 mg per month. After saturation of liver cell uptake, more drugs may be eliminated through the kidneys [44].

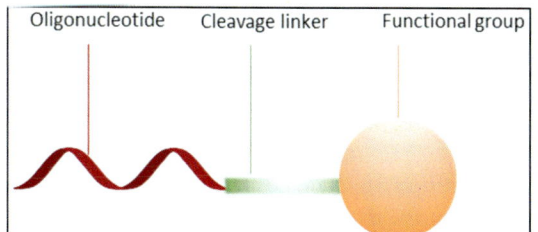

FIGURE 30.10 Typical modification strategies for oligonucleotide therapeutics.

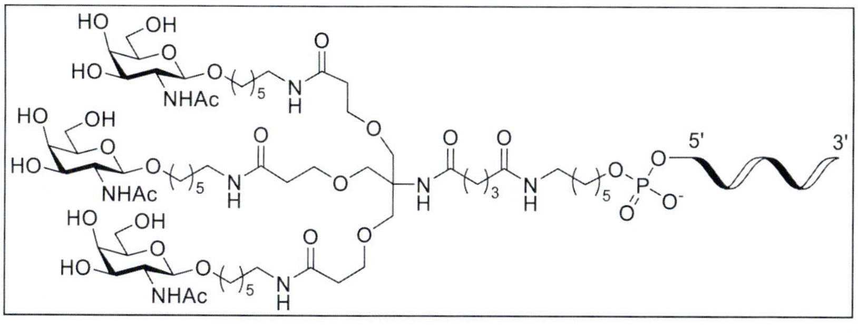

FIGURE 30.11 The structural composition of GalNAc$_3$-conjugated nucleic acid therapeutics.

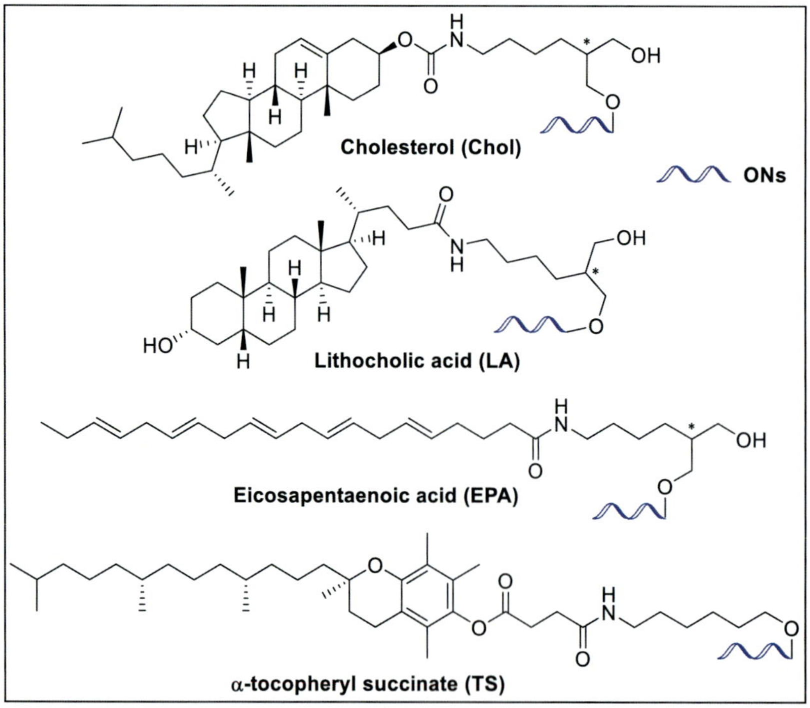

FIGURE 30.12 Lipid molecules used for nucleic acid conjugation.

Peptide conjugation: The attachment of specific peptide sequences covalently to the ends of ASOs can enhance their tissue targeting and transmembrane capabilities. Cell-penetrating peptides (CPPs) are a class of short-cationic peptides used for the transport of various small molecules and macromolecules (such as antibodies, proteins, or nucleic acids) [45]. Naturally or synthetically designed CPPs can traverse cellular membranes and blood-brain barriers. CPP-ASO conjugates administered intravenously can effectively spread to various locations in the brain without apparent toxicity. Most CPPs have positively charged guanidine salt groups on their side chains, which can interact electrostatically with various negatively charged groups (such as sulfate, phosphate, or carboxylate groups) on the cell membrane. This interaction creates a "channel" for the ASOs to enter cells, allowing them to be internalized through membrane diffusion without the need for transfection reagents. Preclinical studies in DMD have demonstrated improved tissue distribution characteristics of peptide-conjugated ASOs [46]. In this chapter, the authors coupled the peptide KALLAL to the 3'-ends of both the sense and antisense strands of mutant vraf murine sarcoma viral oncogene homolog B (BRAF) mRNA (siMB3). The resulting conjugates exhibited prolonged gene silencing in vitro and displayed improved serum stability with a 21-fold increase in half-life in vivo [47].

Lipid conjugation: Oligonucleotides are highly hydrophilic, large, and negatively charged molecules with poor pharmacological properties. Unmodified oligonucleotides typically do not bind to any serum proteins and are rapidly eliminated from the bloodstream through renal filtration. To increase their lipophilicity and impart "drug-like" properties, fatty acids, cholesterol, or other hydrophobic groups have been utilized as important lipid-soluble moieties to improve the properties of nucleic acids, such as cellular uptake, silencing activity, serum stability, and other pharmacokinetic characteristics (Fig. 30.12). Cholesterol was the first hydrophobic group used for oligonucleotide conjugation and can be attached to the 5', 3', or middle positions of ASOs. Smidt et al. synthesized a 16-mer oligonucleotide with cholesterol modification at the 5'-end (chol-oligodeoxynucleotide (ODN)) [48]. Compared to ODN, chol-ODN exhibited an increase in half-life from less than 1 minute to approximately 10 minutes. The resulting chol-ODN could further form chol-ODN-low-density lipoprotein (LDL) complexes by binding to LDL, enhancing stability against serum nucleases in rats. Additionally, docosahexaenoic acid, docosanoic acid, eicosapentaenoic acid, linoleic acid, retinoic acid, and α-tocopheryl succinate have also been used in the construction of ASO conjugates [49].

30.4.2.2 Vehicle delivery

Nucleic acid delivery systems can be broadly classified into viral and nonviral vectors. Viral vectors exploit the molecular mechanisms of viruses to deliver their genetic material into target cells and initiate infection. Common viral vectors include retroviral vectors, adenoviral vectors, adeno-associated viral vectors, herpes simplex viral vectors, and lentiviral vectors. Due to their high transfection efficiency, viral vectors have found wide application in gene therapy research [50]. However, viral vectors may also trigger host immune responses, thereby reducing the delivery efficiency upon subsequent administrations. Nonviral vectors encompass nanomaterials based on proteins and peptides, organic polymers, inorganic nanomaterials, and lipids. Among these, liposomes have been extensively studied and applied in gene delivery due to their excellent biocompatibility and ease of modification [51].

30.4.2.2.1 Cationic liposomes

Liposomes hold a crucial position in the field of drug delivery and have been widely explored for the transfection of oligonucleotide drugs. Despite the numerous challenges in achieving successful transfection, the pursuit of utilizing liposomes for nucleic acid delivery has never ceased [52]. Among the various types of liposomes, cationic lipids are currently the most commonly employed [53]. Cationic lipids refer to lipids with hydrophilic headgroups containing cationic moieties. They can electrostatically interact with negatively charged nucleic acids, facilitating their adsorption onto the surface or encapsulation into the interior of liposomes, thereby enhancing the transfection efficiency of nucleic acid drugs and reducing the required dosage (Fig. 30.13) [54,55]. The resulting complexes formed between cationic lipids and nucleic acids typically possess an excess of positive charges on their surface. This positive charge allows them to adsorb onto the negatively charged cell membrane and enter cells via endocytosis, followed by fusion with lysosomes [51]. Subsequently, the proton sponge effect leads to lysosomal swelling and the release of the complexes into the cytoplasm [56].

The siRNA drug patisiran, which was launched in 2018, employs a liposomal delivery strategy (Fig. 30.14). The delivery system utilizes cationic liposomes with DLin-MC3-DMA as the core and incorporates zwitterionic liposomes (DSPC) to enhance endosomal escape capability. The addition of cholesterol improves membrane fluidity and reduces cationic toxicity, while PEG-lipids are used to prolong the circulation time of the nanoparticles in vivo [57]. Despite the efficient cellular uptake of nucleic acid drugs by cationic liposomes, their toxicity issues cannot be overlooked. Specifically, the excessive positive charges of the complexes may nonspecifically bind to negatively charged proteins and other substances in the plasma, triggering immune responses and leading to self-deactivation [58]. Therefore, most ASO drugs currently under clinical investigation do not utilize liposomes for delivery.

30.4.2.2.2 Nucleotidyl lipids

In addition to the use of cationic lipids relying on electrostatic action, nucleotidyl lipids containing nucleotide heads have also gained widespread attention. These nucleotidyl lipids typically consist of a base, nucleoside, or nucleotide head and two lipid chains as hydrophobic tails. The base heads can interact with the bases of oligonucleotides through hydrogen bonding and π–π stacking interactions and then self-assemble to form nanoparticles or micelles for the

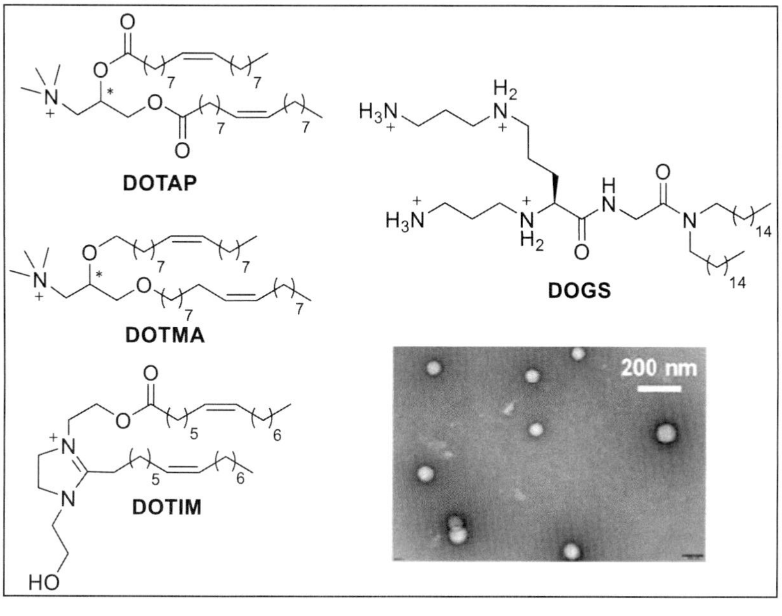

FIGURE 30.13 Common cationic lipid structures and typical electron microscopy microstructures of liposomes.

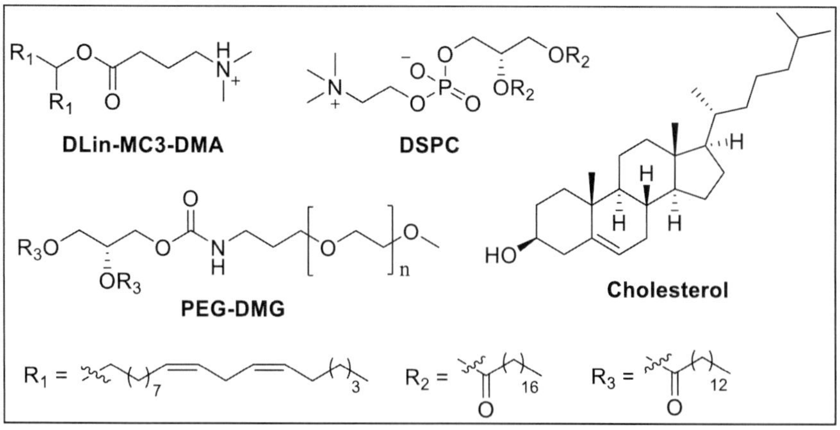

FIGURE 30.14 Nucleic acid delivery system: SNALP technology.

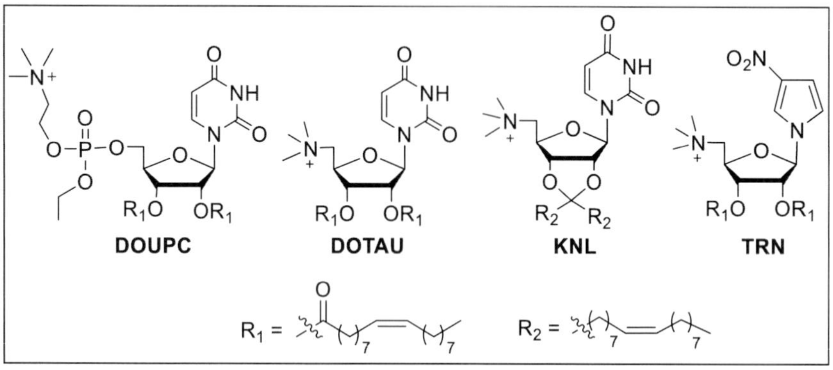

FIGURE 30.15 Structure of nucleotidyl lipids.

delivery of nucleic acid drugs. Because the nucleotidyl lipids are mainly composed of biodegradable nucleotides and lipid chains, they are safer in vivo and have lower toxicity. According to whether they have an electric charge or not, they can be divided into ionic and neutral nucleotidyl lipids. Ionic nucleotidyl lipids can further be divided into cationic, anionic, and zwitterionic nucleotidyl lipids.

Cationic nucleotidyl lipids enhance the binding affinity through the combination of their nucleotide heads and cationic groups, resulting in a dual interaction of hydrogen bonding and electrostatic forces. Barthélémy et al. designed a cationic nucleotidyl lipid called DOUPC (Fig. 30.15) [59], which can form nanoparticles ranging from 50 to 150 nm in size. Upon DNA incorporation, the structure of the lipid complex transitions from a monolayer to a multilayer. When the molar ratio of DOUPC/plasmid is 18/1, plasmid enhanced green fluorescent protein (pEGFP) can be transfected into cells. An improved version of DOUPC, called DOTAU, can form 60 nm nanoparticles and encapsulate DNA between the layers of the multilayered nanoparticles [60]. Subsequently, researchers designed and synthesized a novel cationic nucleotidyl lipid with ketones as hydrophobic tail-linking groups, referred as KNL (Fig. 30.15) [61]. KNL forms spherical complexes of 100 nm in size at $N/P = 10$ and efficiently delivers siRNA. In addition to using uracil as hydrophilic head, a cationic nucleotidyl lipid TRN with a nitro-pyrrole as the head can efficiently transfect siRNA. The lipid complexes have a wide particle size distribution ranging from 108 to 360 nm, and the particles carry a positive charge with a zeta potential of 37 mV [62]. Further studies have shown that the stereochemical structure of the base head influences the formation of siRNA-lipid complexes, with the β-isomer exhibiting the strongest affinity for siRNA [63]. In addition, anionic nucleotidyl lipids can also be used as delivery systems for oligonucleotides.

However, the precise role of the nucleotide base component in transfection remains unclear due to the presence of amino groups in the structure of cationic nucleotidyl lipids. In this chapter, the laboratory of the authors has successfully developed a series of neutral nucleotidyl lipids (DXBAs: DNCA, DNTA, DOCA, and DOTA, Fig. 30.16) that can encapsulate and deliver oligonucleotides, including ASOs, siRNAs, aptamers, and plasmids, through the utilization of hydrogen bonding and $\pi-\pi$ stacking interactions. This is achieved by coannealing the nucleotidyl lipid DXBAs and oligonucleotides to facilitate the self-assembly of nanoparticles [64]. Furthermore, the authors of this chapter designed and

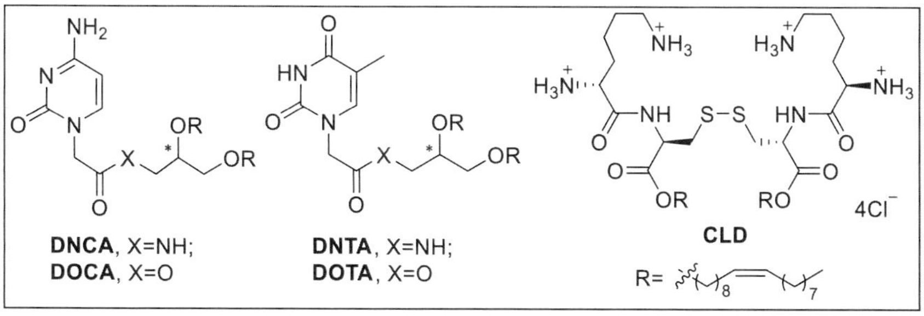

FIGURE 30.16 Nucleotidyl lipids DOTA/DOCA/DNTA/DNCA and cationic lipid CLD.

synthesized a cationic lipid CLD, which can effectively deliver siRNA at relatively low N/P ratios. The disulfide bonds in CLD can be cleaved intracellularly, enhancing endosomal escape capability and accelerating the release of oligonucleotides. CLD is a classical cationic lipid that possesses advantages such as high encapsulation efficiency and delivery efficacy. However, its toxicity at high concentrations remains a challenge for further applications (Fig. 30.16) [65–67]. Mixing DNCA with CLD in a specific ratio has been shown to efficiently and safely encapsulate and deliver chemically modified ASOs, aptamers, and siRNAs, demonstrating promising biological activities at the cellular and animal levels. This suggests the potential of the DNCA/CLD delivery platform in advancing the further development of oligonucleotides [68–72].

30.4.3 Exon skipping therapy for DMD by ASO

The DMD gene exhibits a significant number of exons susceptible to deletions. Approximately 20%, 13%, 12%, and 11% of patients can undergo correction through exon skipping of exons 51, 53, 45, and 44, respectively [73]. Currently, four ASOs have been approved for the treatment of the most common three types of exon deletions (Table 30.1). Despite the loss of several exons, the newly generated antidystrophin protein still retains the majority of the amino acid sequence, thereby preserving its essential biological functions. As a result, patients experience significant improvement in their symptoms.

The aforementioned medications belong to the category of orphan drugs, which have experienced a relatively sluggish development process. However, due to the advancements and maturation of modification strategies, four novel therapeutic varieties for the treatment of DMD have been approved in the past five years, thereby offering a greater array of clinical pharmacological options for patients' treatment.

30.4.3.1 Eteplirsen (EXONDYS 51, 2016)

Eteplirsen (EXONDYS 51, Sarepta Therapeutics Inc.) received accelerated approval from the US FDA in 2016, making it the first ASO drug for patients with DMD, suitable for approximately 13% of patients. Eteplirsen is indicated for the treatment of DMD patients with mutations amenable to exon 51 skipping and utilizes the PMO modification strategy.

However, the approval process for eteplirsen faced significant challenges. Due to the low prevalence of DMD and the relatively small patient population, only 12 children participated in the Phase II clinical study. The limited amount of data led the FDA to reject the drug's early approval and request additional Phase III clinical trials to gather more comprehensive evidence. However, the mothers of children who participated in the clinical study and benefited from the treatment publicly urged the FDA to grant early approval of eteplirsen. Such appeals from family members of patients with severe and life-threatening diseases often exert significant pressure on the FDA, leading to some relaxation of the approval standards for the drug.

In April 2016, an FDA expert panel voted (7:6) against the clinical efficacy of eteplirsen. Against the backdrop of BioMarin's similar drug, drisapersen, being denied approval due to failed Phase III clinical trials, the approval of eteplirsen represented the last hope for many children and their families. However, the Phase III clinical study demonstrated that there was no significant difference in antiatrophy protein levels between the treatment group and the placebo. Among the evaluable 12 patients, the pretreatment antiatrophy protein level was only 0.16% ± 0.12% of the levels observed in healthy subjects. After 48 weeks of treatment, this proportion increased to 0.44% ± 0.43%. In other words, even after almost a year of treatment, the increase in antiatrophy protein levels in patients was only 0.28% of the normal levels. Each FDA reviewer agreed that "there were significant flaws in the design and conduct of the Eteplirsen clinical trials." However, patients believed that the observed improvements in the treatment group should be attributed to eteplirsen and argued that

TABLE 30.1 Four antisense oligonucleotides have been approved for the treatment of Duchenne muscular dystrophy.

Name	Chemistry	Length	Administration	Targets (Exon)	Approved time
Eteplirsen	PMO	25	IV	51	2016
Golodirsen	PMO	25	IV	53	2019
Viltolarsen	PMO	21	IV	53	2020
Casimersen	PMO	25	IV	45	2021

"if it cannot be proven 100% ineffective, it should be approved." This viewpoint clearly contradicted the authority and scientific rigor of the FDA, and ultimately, the expert panel voted against its market approval.

However, Janet Woodcock, the director of the FDA's Center for Drug Evaluation and Research, insisted on using the agency's accelerated review pathway to approve the drug. The approval of eteplirsen seemed to employ a "rescue rule," with two perplexing reasons put forth. First, the rarity of the disease and the difficulty in recruiting patients made it impractical to follow the standard drug approval process. The second reason was that if not approved, Sarepta might go bankrupt, and the prospect of a new drug would be even more uncertain. This approval set a concerning precedent for future drugs targeting severe diseases, as scientific decision-making could face more emotional interference and potentially lead to the wasting of limited healthcare resources on ineffective therapies. Consequently, multiple insurance companies issued statements refusing to cover the cost of this drug, despite eteplirsen requiring at least $300,000 per year.

30.4.3.2 Golodirsen (VYONDYS 53®, 2019)

Golodirsen, developed by Sarepta Therapeutics, utilizes the PMO modification strategy (Fig. 30.17) and targets the antiatrophy protein pre-mRNA. Clinical trial results have demonstrated that golodirsen achieves biological endpoints in terms of safety, tolerability, pharmacokinetic properties, and expression of antiatrophy protein in a cohort of 25 confirmed eligible boys with DMD undergoing exon 53 skipping therapy. These endpoints include the correct transcription of RNA with exon skipping, increased expression of antiatrophy protein, and improved muscle strength. Following treatment for over 48 weeks, the average level of antiatrophy protein in patients increased from 0.1% of normal levels to 1.02%. Golodirsen received FDA approval in December 2019 for the treatment of DMD.

The approval process for golodirsen has been quite tumultuous. After submitting a new drug application and undergoing review by the FDA's Division of Neurology Products, the division recommended approval. However, the FDA's Office of Drug Evaluation issued a complete response letter (CRL) in August 2019, which essentially amounted to a rejection letter. The CRL raised concerns about golodirsen's renal toxicity and infection risks and also brought up the controversy surrounding eteplirsen, which was approved in 2016. Despite 469 patients using eteplirsen three years after its market release, Sarepta Therapeutics had yet to provide valid results from controlled clinical trials.

Following FDA guidelines, Sarepta Therapeutics subsequently filed a formal dispute resolution request. With support from the Division of Neurology Products, Dr. Peter Stein, Director of the FDA's Office of New Drugs, promptly assessed and addressed the issues raised in the response letter. Subsequently, Sarepta's appeal was approved, and the company resubmitted the new drug application to the Division of Neurology Products, which promptly reviewed and approved golodirsen. However, as part of the accelerated approval, the FDA has mandated that Sarepta Therapeutics conduct clinical trials to validate the clinical benefits of this therapy. If the results are insufficient to confirm clinical efficacy, the FDA may rescind its approval.

30.4.3.3 Viltolarsen (Viltepso, 2020)

Viltolarsen, developed by Japan New Drug Corporation, is a PMO-modified (Fig. 30.18) therapeutic agent that targets antiatrophy protein pre-mRNA. It has demonstrated effectiveness in patients with DMD who have deletions in exons 43–52, 45–52, 47–52, 48–52, 50–52, or 52. The recommended dosage for viltolarsen is 80 mg/kg, administered intravenously once weekly [74]. It is noteworthy that viltolarsen is the first and only exon 53 skipping therapy that has been confirmed to increase levels of dystrophin in children as young as 4 years old.

The FDA's conclusion states that the applicant's data indicate an increase in dystrophin production in patients with DMD, which may reasonably predict the clinical benefits of Viltepso. However, the clinical efficacy of this medication

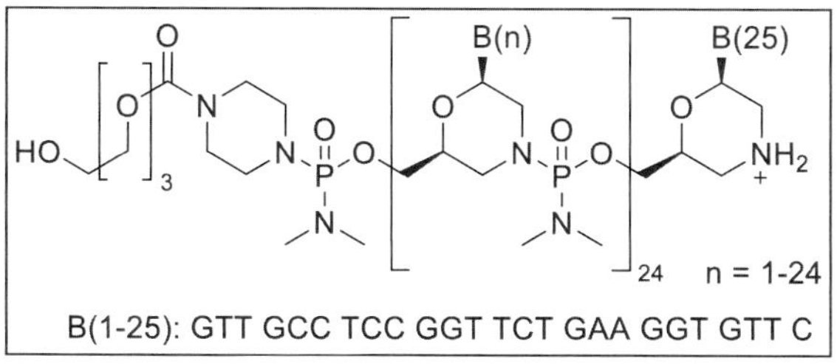

FIGURE 30.17 Structure of golodirsen.

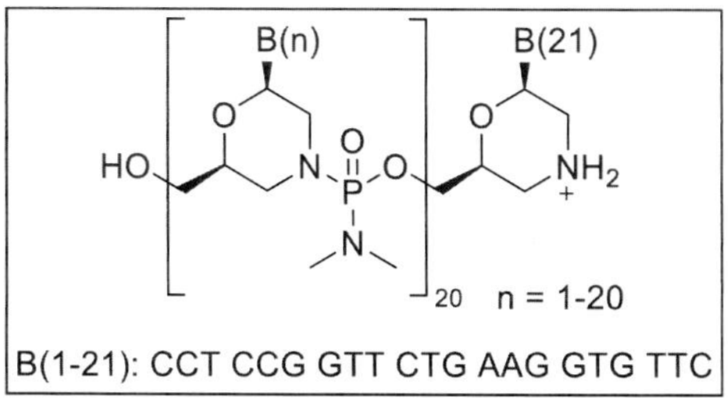

B(1-25): GTT GCC TCC GGT TCT GAA GGT GTT C

FIGURE 30.18 Structure of viltolarsen.

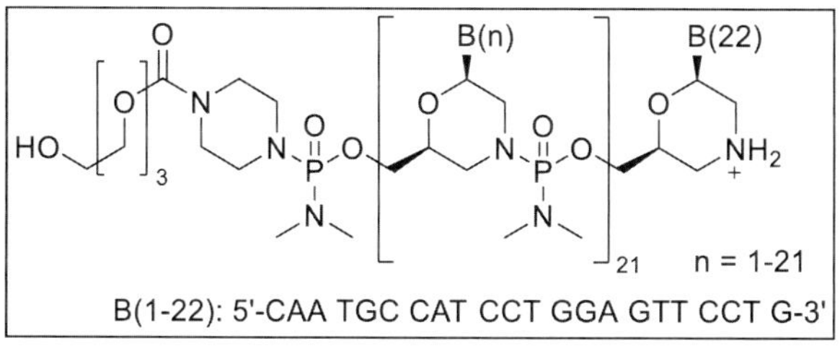

B(1-21): CCT CCG GTT CTG AAG GTG TTC

FIGURE 30.19 Structure of casimersen.

B(1-22): 5'-CAA TGC CAT CCT GGA GTT CCT G-3'

has not yet been confirmed. In making this determination, the FDA considered the potential risks associated with the drug, the life-threatening and debilitating nature of the disease, and the lack of available treatment options.

An increase in dystrophin, an antiatrophy protein, has been observed in the skeletal muscles of patients receiving viltolarsen treatment. Clinical trial data demonstrates a significant correlation between viltolarsen therapy, lasting for 20–24 weeks, and the average expression of dystrophin in 16 patients aged 4–10 years who are amenable to exon 53 skipping therapy. The 40 mg/kg/week and 80 mg/kg/week groups showed average baseline levels of dystrophin at 0.3% and 0.6%, respectively, which increased to 5.7% and 5.9% on average after the trial. Viltolarsen received approval from the PMDA in March 2020 and FDA approval in August 2020 for the treatment of DMD.

30.4.3.4 Casimersen (AMONDYS 45, 2021)

The FDA conditionally approved Sarepta Therapeutics' Casimersen in March 2021 as the first treatment option for confirmed DMD gene mutations suitable for exon 45 skipping in DMD patients. It is also the company's third approved ASO drug for DMD. However, full approval still requires more comprehensive data from the ongoing global Phase III ESSENCE study (NCT02500381), expected to conclude in 2024. Regarding this progress, Doug Ingram, President and CEO of Sarepta Therapeutics, stated that casimersen, together with other approved therapies, has the potential to treat nearly 30% of DMD patients in the United States.

Casimersen, modified with phosphorodiamidate morpholino oligomer (PMO) (Fig. 30.19), is recommended to be administered intravenously at a dose of 30 mg/kg once weekly. Although no renal toxicity has been observed in clinical studies, it is necessary to monitor patients' renal function during administration, including serum cystatin C, urine dipstick, and urine protein-to-creatinine ratio [75].

Within the dosage range of 4–30 mg/kg, the exposure to casimersen is roughly proportional to the dose. After a single intravenous infusion, peak plasma concentrations can be achieved at the end of the infusion. Casimersen exhibits a low binding affinity to human plasma proteins (8%–32%) and is independent of concentration. Following intravenous administration of casimersen at a dose of 30 mg/kg, the steady-state apparent volume of distribution is 367 mL/kg on average. The plasma clearance rate of casimersen is 180 mL/h/kg, with an elimination half-life of 3.5 hours. The majority (>90%) is excreted unchanged in the urine. Because casimersen does not undergo hepatic metabolism, its systemic clearance is not affected by impaired liver function, and the likelihood of clinical drug interactions is also low [76].

It is important to note that due to the variability of DMD gene mutations, the treatment methods approved by the FDA may not be applicable to every patient. Currently, there are still limited treatment options available that are universally applicable to all DMD patients. The FDA also strictly requires pharmaceutical companies not to overstate the indications in the labeling of marketed drugs.

30.5 Summary and outlook

One of the challenges in the field of orphan drugs is market share, which is also a pain point in orphan drug development. The diverse mutation types and unique characteristics of rare diseases make precise "one drug, one patient" treatment possible through the templated development of ASO drugs. However, this approach also leads to significantly increased costs in drug development. The cost of ASO therapy for rare diseases remains high. For example, Spinraza, used to treat spinal muscular atrophy, costs $750,000 in the first year and $375,000 per year thereafter for maintenance. Similarly, eteplirsen, used to treat Duchenne muscular dystrophy, can cost up to $1 million per year based on patient weight. Therefore, healthcare insurance companies, policymakers, and pharmaceutical companies urgently need to find ways to reduce the pricing of ASO drugs, allowing more drugs to enter the market and be affordable for patients.

Furthermore, the effectiveness of approved ASO drugs for treating DMD is still being questioned, and more clinical data is needed to scientifically validate the market approval of these drugs. At the same time, leveraging the latest chemical modifications and delivery strategies to further enhance drug efficacy is a reliable path out of the current predicament.

From the perspective of pharmaceutical companies involved in drug development, DMD falls under the category of rare diseases. Compared to common metabolic disorders or tumors, the number of patients is small and the market share is limited. Consequently, it becomes challenging to generate high profits and attract more new drug development companies. However, for diseases with a larger patient population, such as hypercholesterolemia, infectious hepatitis, and cancer, the market prospects are vast and can attract more drug developers. Compared with small molecule drug technology, antisense, RNA interference, and gene editing technologies are still in a new era, and it is firmly believed that there is great potential for extensive participation in research and development in these fields.

References

[1] Mendell JR, Shilling C, Leslie ND, et al. Evidence-based path to newborn screening for Duchenne muscular dystrophy. Ann Neurol 2012;71(3):304−23.

[2] Wein N, Alfano L, Flanigan KM. Genetics and emerging treatments for Duchenne and Becker muscular dystrophy. Pediatr Clin N Am 2015;62(3):723−42.

[3] Escolar DM, Hache LP, Clemens PR, et al. Randomized, blinded trial of weekend vs daily prednisone in Duchenne muscular dystrophy. Neurology 2011;77(5):444−52.

[4] Duchenne muscular dystrophy: the basics. https://www.duchenne.com/about-duchenne.

[5] Fairclough RJ, Wood MJ, Davies KE. Therapy for Duchenne muscular dystrophy: renewed optimism from genetic approaches. Nat Rev Genet 2013;14(6):373−8.

[6] Deisch JK. 135-Muscle and nerve development in health and disease. In: Swaiman KF;, Ashwal S;, Ferriero DM;, Schor NF;, Finkel RS;, Gropman AL, et al., editors. Swaiman's *Pediatric Neurology. 6th ed*. Elsevier; 2017. p. 1029−37.

[7] Aartsma-Rus A, Van Ommen G-JB. Less is more: therapeutic exon skipping for Duchenne muscular dystrophy. Lancet Neurol 2009;8(10):873−5.

[8] Bennett CF, Baker BF, Pham N, et al. Pharmacology of antisense drugs. Annu Rev Pharmacol Toxicol 2017;57(1):81−105.

[9] Cerritelli SM, Crouch RJ. Ribonuclease H: the enzymes in eukaryotes. FEBS J 2009;276(6):1494−505.

[10] Wu H, Lima WF, Zhang H, et al. Determination of the role of the human RNase H1 in the pharmacology of DNA-like antisense drugs. J Biol Chem 2004;279(17):17181−9.

[11] Lima WF, Murray HM, Damle SS, et al. ViableRNaseH1knockout mice show RNase H1 is essential for R loop processing, mitochondrial and liver function. Nucl Acids Res 2016;44(11):5299−322.

[12] Vickers TA, Crooke ST. The rates of the major steps in the molecular mechanism of RNase H1-dependent antisense oligonucleotide induced degradation of RNA. Nucl Acids Res 2015;43(18):8955−63.

[13] Liang XH, Sun H, Nichols JG, et al. RNase H1-dependent antisense oligonucleotides are robustly active in directing RNA cleavage in both the cytoplasm and the nucleus. Mol Ther 2017;25(9):2075−92.

[14] Rinaldi C, Wood MJA. Antisense oligonucleotides: the next frontier for treatment of neurological disorders. Nat Rev Neurol 2018; 14(1):9−21.
[15] Titeux M, Turczynski S, Pironon N, et al. Antisense-mediated splice modulation to reframe transcripts. Methods Mol Biol 2018;1828:532−52.
[16] Zamecnik PC, Stephenson ML. Inhibition of Rous sarcoma virus replication and cell transformation by a specific oligodeoxynucleotide. Proc Natl Acad Sci USA 1978;75(1):280−4.
[17] Reischl D, Zimmer A. Drug delivery of siRNA therapeutics: potentials and limits of nanosystems. Nanomedicine 2009;5(1):8−20.
[18] Cavallaro G, Sardo C, Craparo EF, et al. Polymeric nanoparticles for siRNA delivery: production and applications. Int J Pharm 2017;525(2):323−33.
[19] Blanco E, Shen H, Ferrari M. Principles of nanoparticle design for overcoming biological barriers to drug delivery. Nat Biotechnol 2015;33(9):941−51.
[20] Stein CA, Subasinghe C, Shinozuka K, et al. Physicochemical properties of phosphorothioate oligodeoxynucleotides. Nucl Acids Res 1988;16(8):3209−21.
[21] Campbell JM, Bacon TA, Wickstrom E. Oligodeoxynucleoside phosphorothioate stability in subcellular extracts, culture media, sera and cerebrospinal-fluid. J Biochem Bioph Meth 1990;20(3):259−67.
[22] Agrawal S, Kandimalla ER. Antisense therapeutics: is it as simple as complementary base recognition? Mol Med Today 2000;6(2):72−81.
[23] Chen JK, Schultz RG, Lloyd DH, et al. Synthesis of oligodeoxyribonucleotide N3'−>P5' phosphoramidates. Nucl Acids Res 1995;23(14):2661−8.
[24] Heidenreich O, Gryaznov S, Nerenberg M. RNase H-independent antisense activity of oligonucleotide N3'−> P5' phosphoramidates. Nucl Acids Res 1997;25(4):776−80.
[25] Rettig GR, Behlke MA. Progress toward in vivo use of siRNAs-II. Mol Ther 2012;20(3):483−512.
[26] Whitehead KA, Dahlman JE, Langer RS, et al. Silencing or stimulation? siRNA delivery and the immune system. Annu Rev Chem Biomol Eng 2011;2:77−96.
[27] Bennett CF, Swayze EE. RNA targeting therapeutics: molecular mechanisms of antisense oligonucleotides as a therapeutic platform. Annu Rev Pharmacol Toxicol 2010;50:259−93.
[28] Braasch DA, Corey DR. Locked nucleic acid (LNA): fine-tuning the recognition of DNA and RNA. Chem Biol 2001;8(1):1−7.
[29] Du L, Gatti RA. Potential therapeutic applications of antisense morpholino oligonucleotides in modulation of splicing in primary immunodeficiency diseases. J Immunol Methods 2011;365(1-2):1−7.
[30] Summerton J, Weller D. Morpholino antisense oligomers: design, preparation, and properties. Antisense Oligonucleotide Drug Dev 1997;7(3):187−95.
[31] Demidov VV, Potaman VN, Frank-Kamenetskii MD, et al. Stability of peptide nucleic acids in human serum and cellular extracts. Biochem Pharmacol 1994;48(6):1320−3.
[32] Montazersaheb S, Hejazi MS, Nozad Charoudeh H. Potential of peptide nucleic acids in future therapeutic applications. Adv Pharm Bull 2018;8(4):551−63.
[33] Khvorova A, Watts JK. The chemical evolution of oligonucleotide therapies of clinical utility. Nat Biotechnol 2017;35(3):238−48.
[34] Deleavey GF, Damha MJ. Designing chemically modified oligonucleotides for targeted gene silencing. Chem Biol 2012;19(8):937−54.
[35] Zhang S, Zhao Y, Zhi D, et al. Non-viral vectors for the mediation of RNAi. Bioorg Chem 2012;40(1):10−18.
[36] Ku SH, Jo SD, Lee YK, et al. Chemical and structural modifications of RNAi therapeutics. Adv Drug Deliv Rev 2016;104:16−28.
[37] Varki A. Biological roles of oligosaccharides - all of the theories are correct. Glycobiology 1993;3(2):97−130.
[38] Gabius HJ, Siebert HC, André S, et al. Chemical biology of the sugar code. ChemBioChem 2004;5(6):740−64.
[39] Shemesh CS, Yu RZ, Warren MS, et al. Assessment of the drug interaction potential of cnconjugated and GalNAc3-conjugated 2'-MOE-ASOs. Mol Ther Nucl Acids 2017;9:34−47.
[40] Ostergaard ME, Yu J, Kinberger GA, et al. Efficient synthesis and biological evaluation of 5'-GalNAc conjugated antisense oligonucleotides. Bioconjugate Chem 2015;26(8):1451−5.
[41] Cedillo I, Chreng D, Engle E, et al. Synthesis of 5'-GalNAc-conjugated oligonucleotides: a comparison of solid and solution-phase conjugation strategies. Molecules 2017;22(8):1356−67.
[42] Kinberger GA, Prakash TP, Yu J, et al. Conjugation of mono and di-GalNAc sugars enhances the potency of antisense oligonucleotides via ASGR mediated delivery to hepatocytes. Bioorg Med Chem Lett 2016;26(15):3690−3.
[43] Prakash TP, Yu J, Migawa MT, et al. Comprehensive structure-activity relationship of triantennary N-Acetylgalactosamine conjugated antisense oligonucleotides for targeted delivery to hepatocytes. J Med Chem 2016;59(6):2718−33.
[44] Wang Y, Yu RZ, Henry S, et al. Pharmacokinetics and clinical pharmacology considerations of GalNAc3-conjugated antisense oligonucleotides. Expert Opin Drug Metab Toxicol 2019;15(6):475−85.
[45] Fonseca SB, Pereira MP, Kelley SO. Recent advances in the use of cell-penetrating peptides for medical and biological applications. Adv Drug Deliv Rev 2009;61(11):953−64.
[46] Jirka SMG, T Hoen PAC, Parillas VD, et al. Cyclic peptides to improve delivery and exon skipping of antisense oligonucleotides in a mouse model for Duchenne muscular dystrophy. Mol Ther 2018;26(1):132−47.
[47] Fan XM, Zhang YF, Liu XJ, et al. Biological properties of a 3',3"-bis-peptide-siRNA conjugate in vitro and in vivo. Bioconjugate Chem 2016;27(4):1132−42.

[48] Lee CH, Lee SH, Kim JH, et al. Pharmacokinetics of a cholesterol-conjugated aptamer against the Hepatitis C Virus (HCV) NS5B protein. Mol Ther Nucleic Acids 2015;4(10):e254.
[49] Osborn MF, Coles AH, Biscans A, et al. Hydrophobicity drives the systemic distribution of lipid-conjugated siRNAs via lipid transport pathways. Nucl Acids Res 2019;47(3):1070–81.
[50] Ibraheem D, Elaissari A, Fessi H. Gene therapy and DNA delivery systems. Int J Pharm 2014;459(1-2):70–83.
[51] Zhou J, Shum KT, Burnett JC, et al. Nanoparticle-based delivery of RNAi therapeutics: progress and challenges. Pharmaceuticals(Basel) 2013;6(1):85–107.
[52] Alexander MY, Akhurst RJ. Liposome-medicated gene transfer and expression via the skin. Hum Mol Genet 1995;4(12):2279–85.
[53] Lee TW, Matthews DA, Blair GE. Novel molecular approaches to cystic fibrosis gene therapy. Biochem J 2005;387(Pt 1):1–15.
[54] Remy JS, Sirlin C, Vierling P, et al. Gene transfer with a series of lipophilic DNA-binding molecules. Bioconjugate Chem 1994;5(6):647–54.
[55] Morille M, Passirani C, Vonarbourg A, et al. Progress in developing cationic vectors for non-viral systemic gene therapy against cancer. Biomaterials 2008;29(24-25):3477–96.
[56] Creusat G, Rinaldi AS, Weiss E, et al. Proton sponge trick for pH-sensitive disassembly of polyethylenimine-based siRNA delivery systems. Bioconjugate Chem 2010;21(5):994–1002.
[57] Titze-De-Almeida R, David C, Titze-De-Almeida SS. The race of 10 synthetic RNAi-based drugs to the pharmaceutical market. Pharm Res 2017;34(7):1339–63.
[58] Yang JP, Huang L. Overcoming the inhibitory effect of serum on lipofection by increasing the charge ratio of cationic liposome to DNA. Gene Ther 1997;4(9):950–60.
[59] Moreau L, Barthelemy P, Li Y, et al. Nucleoside phosphocholine amphiphile for in vitro DNA transfection. Mol Biosyst 2005;1(3):260–4.
[60] Chabaud P, Camplo M, Payet D, et al. Cationic nucleoside lipids for gene delivery. Bioconjugate Chem 2006;17(2):466–72.
[61] Luvino D, Khiati S, Oumzil K, et al. Efficient delivery of therapeutic small nucleic acids to prostate cancer cells using ketal nucleoside lipid nanoparticles. J Control Rel 2013;172(3):954–61.
[62] Ceballos C, Prata CA, Giorgio S, et al. Cationic nucleoside lipids based on a 3-nitropyrrole universal base for siRNA delivery. Bioconjugate Chem 2009;20(2):193–6.
[63] Ceballos C, Khiati S, Prata CA, et al. Cationic nucleoside lipids derived from universal bases: a rational approach for siRNA transfection. Bioconjugate Chem 2010;21(6):1062–9.
[64] Ma Y, Zhu YJ, Wang C, et al. Annealing novel nucleobase-lipids with oligonucleotides or plasmid DNA based on H-bonding or pi-pi interaction: assemblies and transfections. Biomaterials 2018;178:147–57.
[65] Zheng Y, Guo YJ, Li YT, et al. A novel gemini-like cationic lipid for the efficient delivery of siRNA. N J Chem 2014;38(10):4952–62.
[66] Ma XF, Sun J, Qiu C, et al. The role of disulfide-bridge on the activities of H-shape gemini-like cationic lipid based siRNA delivery. J Control Rel 2016;235:99–111.
[67] Sun J, Qiu C, Diao YP, et al. Delivery pathway regulation of 3',3"-bis-peptide-siRNA conjugate via nanocarrier architecture engineering. Mol Ther Nucl Acids 2018;10:75–90.
[68] Ma Y, Zhao WT, Li YD, et al. Structural optimization and additional targets identification of antisense oligonucleotide G3239 encapsulated in a neutral cytidinyl-lipid combined with a cationic lipid in vitro and in vivo. Biomaterials 2019;197:182–93.
[69] Yang MY, Sun J, Wang C, et al. Transfection of 3',3"-bis-peptide-siRNA conjugate by cationic lipoplexes mixed with a neutral cytosin1yl lipid. J Chin Pharm Sci 2017;26(10):719–26.
[70] Zhang YF, Li SX, Zhou XY, et al. Construction of a targeting nanoparticle of 3',3"-bis-peptide-siRNA conjugate/mixed lipid with postinserted DSPE-PEG2000-cRGD. Mol Pharm 2019;16:4920–8.
[71] Zhou XY, Pan YF, Li Z, et al. siRNA packaged with neutral cytidinyl/cationic/PEG lipids for enhanced antitumor efficiency and safety in vitro and in vivo. ACS Appl Bio Mater 2020;3(9):6297–309.
[72] Zhou ZX, Liu S, Zhang YF, et al. Reductive nanocomplex encapsulation of cRGD-siRNA conjugates for enhanced targeting to cancer cells. Int J Nanomed 2017;12:7255–72.
[73] Flotats-Bastardas M, Hahn A. New therapeutics options for pediatric neuromuscular disorders. Front Pediatr 2020;8:583877.
[74] Dhillon S. Viltolarsen: first approval. Drugs 2020;80(10):1027–32.
[75] Casimersen. Am J Health Syst Pharm 2021;78(13):1149–50.
[76] Shirley M. Casimersen: first approval. Drugs 2021;81(7):875–9.

Index

Note: Page numbers followed by "*f*" and "*t*" refer to figures and tables, respectively.

A

Abacavir (ABC), 214
A-ring, 304, 480
 optimization of 4-sulfonylamino group in, 717, 718*t*
 substitution, 429
  derivatives of tamoxifen with, 429, 429*f*
AA. *See* Arachidonic acid (AA)
ABC. *See* ATP binding cassette (ABC)
Abelson (Abl), 362
Abnormal gastric acid secretion, 534
Abraxane, 291–292
Absorption, distribution, metabolism, and excretion studies (ADME), 369–370, 705, 721–722
Absorption, distribution, metabolism, excretion, and toxicity (ADME/T), 3
ABSSSI. *See* Acute bacterial skin and skin structure infections (ABSSSI)
ACE inhibitors. *See* Angiotensin-converting enzyme inhibitors (ACE inhibitors)
Acetyl coenzyme A (acetyl-CoA), 73
Acetylcholine (Ach), 532, 558
Acetylsalicylic acid. *See* Aspirin
Acid secretion by proton pumps, mechanism of, 539
Acidic proton, 119–120
Acinetobacter, 503–504
Acquired immunodeficiency syndrome (AIDS), 211–213, 247–249, 658
 discovery, transmission, and current status of, 211–212
 epidemic, 212
Acquired immunodeficiency syndrome-related virus (ARV), 247
Acrylamides, 394–396
 design of irreversible inhibitor PD with acrylamide-based electrophilic warhead, 395*f*
 fragments, 392
 structure-activity relationship of acylamide electrophilic warhead, 395*f*
Actinomycetes, 675
Activated coagulation, 142–143
Activation function 1 (AF-1), 421
Activation segment, 352–354
 active and inactive conformational transition of protein kinase, 353*f*
 hydrophobic residues in Abl catalytic domain, 353*t*

shell and regulatory spine of Abl, 354*f*
 structure of catalytic loop and, 353*f*
Active diastereomer
 characterization of, 201
 comparison of PSI-7851 diastereoisomers, 202*t*
 synthetic route towards fragment A, 202*f*
Active pharmaceutical ingredients (API), 12–13, 611
Activity-guided components, 287–288
Acute arterial embolism, 162
Acute bacterial skin and skin structure infections (ABSSSI), 471–472
Acute gastrointestinal bleeding, 7
Acute infections, 246
Acute lymphoblastic leukemia (ALL), 362
Acute myocardial infarction, 162
Acylation reactions, 491
Acyloxy group, 308–309
Adenosine binding pocket (AP), 376
Adenosine pocket (AP), 377–378
Adenosine triphosphate (ATP), 388
 ATP-citrate lyase inhibitors, 107
 ATP-competitive inhibitors, 356–360
  type I inhibitors, 357
  type I1/2 inhibitors, 358–359
  type II inhibitors, 359–360
  typical heterocyclic scaffolds of known PKIs, 357*f*
 ATP-competitive kinase inhibitors, 351
 binding pocket, 374
Adhesins, 533
Adjuvants, 707
ADME. *See* Absorption, distribution, metabolism, and excretion studies (ADME)
Adverse effects (AEs), 92–95, 144, 289
 of eribulin, 344–345
 of risperidone, 629
Adverse reactions, 67, 166, 284, 404, 407, 460, 629
AEs. *See* Adverse effects (AEs)
AF-1. *See* Activation function 1 (AF-1)
Afatinib, 387–388, 402–403, 408
 adverse reactions of, 406–407
 application of covalent strategy in development of small molecule EGFR inhibitors, 393–402
  3-aminopropanamides, 398–399
  α-substituted acetamides, 398

acrylamides, 394–396
 alkynyl thiophene rings, 398
 boric acids, 400–401
 butynamides, 396
 thiols and disulfides, 399–400
 vinylsulfonamides, 396–397, 397*f*
development of, 393–408
discovery of covalent irreversible EGFR inhibitor 2 afatinib, 402–406, 402*f*
pharmacokinetics, pharmacodynamics, and adverse reactions of afatinib, 406–407
structure-activity relationship of covalent EGFR inhibitor, 407–408, 408*f*
synthesis of, 408–411
 commercial synthetic route-sequential synthesis approach, 411
 Dimroth rearrangement, 409, 410*f*
 Horner-Wadsworth-Emmons reaction, 409, 410*f*
 laboratorial medicinal chemical synthetic route-modular synthesis approach, 409–410
 Mitsunobu reaction, 408
 retro-synthetic analysis, 409*f*
AIDS. *See* Acquired immunodeficiency syndrome (AIDS)
AIs. *See* Aromatase inhibitors (AIs)
Alanine (Ala), 45
Albiglutide, 49
Albumin-bound paclitaxel, 291–292
Alcohol, 593
Aldol condensation reaction, 96
Alectinib, 359
Alendronate, 699–701
Alfentanil, 616
Alkaline ammonia, 534
Alkaline phosphatase, 689–690
Alkyl chains, 171–173
Alkyl substitution, 396
Alkylamine, 229
Alkynes, 398–399
Alkynyl thiophene rings, 398
ALL. *See* Acute lymphoblastic leukemia (ALL)
Allergic reactions, 50
Allisartan isoproxil, 136
Allosteric inhibitors, 360
Allylamine antifungal drug, 454
 chemical structures of allylamine antifungal drugs, 454*f*
Almonertinib, 413–414

755

α,α-dichloropiperidone intermediate
    compound, 155–157
α-amino acids, 197
    α-amino acid-derived dipeptidyl peptidase
        inhibitors, 8–9
    early α-amino acid-derived dipeptidyl
        peptidase-4 inhibitors, 9f
    optimization of, 9f
α-aminoisobutyric acid (Aib), 47
α-glucosidase inhibitors, 57
    structures of representative drugs of, 58f
α-linolenic acid (LNA), 312–313
2'-α-methoxy substitution, 190–192
α-substituted acetamides, 398
α-subunit, 594
αC-helix$_{in}$ conformation, 352
AmB. See Amphotericin B (AmB)
Amelanchier alnifolia, 104
Amides, 119–120, 152
    bond, 117
    compound, 119–120
    derivative, 307
    group, 308–309
Amidinoisoxazole, 146–147
Amine, 524–525
Amino acids, 29, 391, 634
    molecular structure of
        insulin aspart, 30f
        insulin glargine, 31f
        insulin glulisine, 30f
        lispro insulin, 30f
        Novosol Basal, 31f
    mutations, 48
        comparison of sequence similarity
            between exendin-4 and GLP-1, 44f
        of peptide backbone, 44–45
    side chains, 206
    substitution, 29–31
Amino group, 500
6-amino-penicillanic acid (6-APA), 500–502
Aminobenzisoxazole, 149–150
Aminoethoxy side chain, alteration of, 429
Aminoglycoside antibiotics, 492, 494
Aminolysis, 157–158
3-aminopropanamides, 398–399
Aminothiazole moiety, 376
Ammonia, 533
Amphotericin B (AmB), 451
Amprenavir, 258
    to darunavir, 258–259
Anemia, 636–637, 639
    first-in-class antirenal anemia drug
        roxadustat
            development process of roxadustat,
                639–648
            medications for treatment of renal anemia,
                636–639
            renal anemia and pathogenesis, 633–635
Anesthesia, 585–586, 588–590
Anesthetic drugs, 585–586
Ang-I. See Angiotensin I (Ang-I)
Ang-III. See Angiotensin III (Ang-III)
Ang-IV. See Angiotensin IV (Ang-IV)
Angiotensin I (Ang-I), 111

Angiotensin II receptor antagonists, 113
    discovery of losartan, 114–131
    discovery of losartan analogs, 131–136
    hypertension and commonly used
        medications for treatment of
        hypertension, 109–110
    renin-angiotensin system, 110–113, 110f
    structures of saralasin and sarile, 113f
Angiotensin II receptor blockers (ARBs), 110,
    131
Angiotensin III (Ang-III), 111–112
Angiotensin IV (Ang-IV), 111–112
Angiotensin type 1 receptor (AT1), 111–112,
    127
Angiotensin type 2 receptor (AT2), 111–112
Angiotensin type 3 receptor (AT3), 111–112
Angiotensin type 4 receptor (AT4), 111–112
Angiotensin-converting enzyme inhibitors
    (ACE inhibitors), 110
Angiotensinogen, 111
1,6-anhydro cellobiose, 179
Anhydrous ethanol, 291
4-anilino-3-quinolinecarbonitrile derivative,
    377
4-anilinoquinazolines, 407
Animal toxicity experiments, 7
Anthropophilic fungi, 449–450
Anti-diabetic agents, 65
Anti-HIV drugs, 213–215
    classification of, 213–214
    drug resistance to, 214–215
Anti-HIV therapy, 212
Anti-HIV-1 activity
    of calanolides, 654–656
        cell culture assay, 654–655
        novel tetracyclic dipyranocoumarins in
            mouse hollow fiber model, 654–655
    of cordatolides, 657
    enantioselective total synthesis of optical 1,
        659
    of improved calanolides, 658–665
    of inophyllums, 656–657
    representative calanolide analogs, 659–665
        chemical resolution of racemic
            calanolides, 662f
        evolution of active calanolide analogs and
            identification of drug candidate, 664f
        modified analogs reported by Galinis, 661f
        optically active calanolide analogs
            produced through chemical resolution,
            663f
        representative calanolide analogs
            displaying, 661f
        synthetic route of 77 reported by Sharma,
            662f
        synthetic strategy used to construct
            chemical library based on scaffold, 663f
    total synthesis of (±)-1, 658–659, 658f
    synthetic route of racemic 1 reported by
        Kucherenko, 659f
Anti-HIV/AIDS drugs and novel treatment
    strategies, 260–263
    classification of anti-HIV/AIDS drugs, 260,
        261t

first-and second-line antiretroviral regimens,
    261t
new strategies for HIV/AIDS prevention and
    treatment, 261–263
Anti-*Mycobacterium tuberculosis* compound
    activities, 670–671
    natural product 1 as, 666–667, 667f
Antibacterial activity
    of linezolid
        in vitro, 472–473
        in vivo, 474–475
    molecule structures of compounds with
        fluorescence activity, 672f
    and stability, 505–506, 505f
    of tetrahydrobenzopyran nitrofuran
        derivatives, 670–671, 671f
Antibacterial agents, 475, 495
Antibacterial assays, 472
Antibacterial drugs, 475, 492
    antibacterial mechanisms of linezolid,
        477–479, 478f
    bioactivity and pharmacokinetics of
        antibacterial drug linezolid, 472–476
    development of antibacterial agents,
        465–467
    chemical structure of linezolid and
        oxazolidinone scaffold, 466f
    development of antibacterial agents, 466f
    discovery of antibacterial drug linezolid,
        467–472, 467f
    construction of S-configured
        oxazolidinone derivatives by Manninen
        reaction, 469f
    discovery of antibacterial drug linezolid,
        470f
    drug discovery flowchart for linezolid, 471f
    preliminary SAR summary of
        oxazolidinone derivatives, 468f
    representative oxazolidinone derivatives,
        469f
    structural modifications of dup 721 by
        Upjohn company, 468f
    research on synthesis process of linezolid,
        484–485
    study on structure-activity relationship of
        oxazolidinone antibiotics, 479–484
Antibacterial medications, 491
    chemical structures of vancomycin and
        polymyxin B1, 494f
    chemical structures
        penicillin and prontosil, 491f
        selected quinolone antibiotics, 493f
        telithromycin and tigecycline, 492f
    commonly used, 491–493
Antibacterial study, 474–475
Antibiotics, 493, 588–589
Antibody Fc segments fusion, 48–49
    dulaglutide, 49f
    structure of IgG antibody, 48f
Anticancer therapy
    bisphosphonate drugs and inhibitors in,
        706–707
    commercially available taxanes for,
        292–293

cabazitaxel, 293
docetaxel, 292–293
Anticoagulants, 163–165
drugs, 143
substances, 141–142
therapy, 182–183
Antidepressant medications, 629
Antidiabetic drugs, 3
based on sodium-glucose cotransporter 2 inhibitors
diabetes mellitus and antidiabetic drugs, 55–59
sodium-glucose cotransporter 2 inhibitors as anti-diabetic drugs, 59–67
successful experience in development of dapagliflozin, 67–69
Antifungal drug development, 454–455
Antifungal drugs, 452–455, 452f
allylamine, 454
antifungal antibiotics, 452–453, 452f
azole, 453
echinocandin, 454–455
Antigen, 736
Antiinfluenza drugs, 268–270
broad-spectrum antiviral drugs, 268–269
influenza virus inhibitors targeting polymerase complex, 269–270, 270f
M2 ion channel blockers, 268, 268f
neuraminidase inhibitors, 268, 269t
Antileukemic activity, 371
Antimicrobials, 477
resistance surveillance system, 495
Antineoplastic agents
classifications and design of PKIs, 354–362
composition and catalytic mechanism of protein kinase, 350–354, 351f
protein kinases, 350, 350f
and protein kinase inhibitors as, 349–362
Antiparasitic drugs, 510, 514
chemical structure, 511f
WHO-recommended antiparasitic medicines for use in preventive chemotherapy, 512t
Antiplatelet agents, 163
Antiplatelet aggregation drugs, 144
Antipsychotic drugs, 619–623
atypical, 620–621
classical, 619–620, 620f
and representative examples, 621t
multiple target drug design, 621–622, 622f
Antiretroviral drugs, 259
Antisense oligonucleotides (ASOs), 735, 742
ASO-mediated exon skipping, 740–741
chemical modifications of, 742–745
nucleotide modifications, 744–745
phosphorothioate modification, 743
sugar ring modification strategies, 743–744
developmental trajectory of antisense oligonucleotide therapeutics, 741–752
drugs, 736, 739, 742
Duchenne muscular dystrophy, 737–738
exon skipping therapy for DMD by, 749–752

mechanism of action of antisense oligonucleotide drugs, 739–741
alternative mechanisms, 740
exon skipping, 740–741
RNase H, 739–740, 739f
Antithrombin III (AT-III), 162, 168
Antithrombotic drugs, 143–146, 143f
Antitumor
action of mechanism, 288
activity, 293
drugs, 327
metastasis, 318
Antiulcer medications
classification and clinical applications of, 535–537
proton pump inhibitors on market, 536t
Antiviral drugs, 189, 214
Antiviral nucleoside drugs, 196
AP. See Adenosine binding pocket (AP); Adenosine pocket (AP)
API. See Active pharmaceutical ingredients (API)
Apidra. See Insulin glulisine
Apixaban, 143–144
clinical indications of, 158
medicinal chemistry of, 146–158
binding model of apixaban and FXa, 153–154
compounds during development, 146f
discovery of hit compound, 146–147
optimization of lead compound, 147–153
synthetic routes, 154–158, 156f, 157f, 158f
Apolipoproteins, 71
antisense oligonucleotides, 107
Arachidonic acid (AA), 712
Arbidol hydrochloride, 269
ARBs. See Angiotensin II receptor blockers (ARBs)
Area under concentration-time curve (AUC), 64, 232–233, 259–260, 573–575
Arginine (Arg), 29–31, 46–47, 634
Arixtra, 179
ARNT. See Aryl hydrocarbon receptor nuclear translocator (ARNT)
Aromatase, 443–444
Aromatase inhibitors (AIs), 422
Aromatic group, 121
Aromatic heterocycle, 218
Aromatic nucleophilic substitution, 224–225
Aromatic rings, 4
Artemisinin, 510
Arterial diseases, 141
Artificially synthesized mRNA, 742
ARV. See Acquired immunodeficiency syndrome-related virus (ARV)
Aryl hydrocarbon receptor nuclear translocator (ARNT), 634–635
Aryl iodide compound, 157
Aryl substituent, 719
4-arylamine group, 406
4-arylamine quinazoline, 410
Asciminib, 379
ASOs. See Antisense oligonucleotides (ASOs)

Asparagine (Asn), 30–31
Aspartate, 81–82
Aspartic acid, 352
Aspartyl amide residue, 253
Aspergillus, 449–450, 460
Aspirin, 711
Asthma, 106
AstraZeneca, 554
Asymmetric catalytic hydrogenation, 14
application of, 14–18
first generation process chemistry of sitagliptin, 15, 15f
green chemistry, 17–18
second-generation sitagliptin process chemistry, 15–16
third-generation sitagliptin process, 16–17
Asymmetric dihydroxylation reaction, 339–340
Asymmetric side chain synthesis methods, 99–102
(2 + 2) carbon unit introduction strategy in, 101f
(5 + 1) carbon unit introduction strategy in, 102f
retro-synthesis analysis of, 100f
Asymmetric synthesis of *trans*-tamoxifen, 437–438, 438f
AT-III. See Antithrombin III (AT-III)
AT1. See Angiotensin type 1 receptor (AT1)
AT2. See Angiotensin type 2 receptor (AT2)
AT3. See Angiotensin type 3 receptor (AT3)
AT4. See Angiotensin type 4 receptor (AT4)
Ataluren, 737
Atazanavir (ATV), 214
Atherosclerotic plaques, 75–76
Atorvastatin, 76–81
clinical indications, 80–81
discovery of, 76–79, 79f
blockbuster drug, 79
cerivastatin, rosuvastatin, and pitavastatin, 79
fluvastatin, 79
lovastatin, 79
mevastatin, 76–78
simvastatin and pravastatin, 79
drug–drug interactions of, 95
mechanism of action, 80–81
medicinal chemistry of, 81–102
HMG-CoA reductase, 81–82
interaction of statins with HMG-CoA reductase, 89–92
structure-activity relationship of statin drugs inhibiting HMG-CoA reductase, 82–89
total synthesis, 95–102
in vivo structure-activity, structure-metabolism, and structure-toxicity relationships of statin drugs, 92–95
optimization of structures with pyrrole as central ring, 83–89
2-position and 5-position substituents and compound activity, 87t
compounds with fixed 2-(4-fluorophenyl) and varied 5-position substituents, 86t

Atorvastatin (*Continued*)
    compounds with fixed 5-isopropyl and varied 2-position substituents, 86*t*
    compounds with fixed 5-methyl group and varied 2-position substituents, 85*t*
    compounds with varied 3-position and 4-position substituents, 88*t*
    safety of, 80–81
ATP. *See* Adenosine triphosphate (ATP)
ATP binding cassette (ABC), 460–461
Atypical antipsychotic drugs, 620–621
AUC. *See* Area under concentration-time curve (AUC)
Autoimmune diseases, 105
2-azido-substituted glucose, 179
Azido-substituted nucleoside analogs, 192
Azidothymidine (AZT), 206
Azilsartan medoxomil, 133
Azole antifungal agents, mechanism of action of, 457–458
Azole antifungal drugs, 453
    chemical structures of imidazole antifungal drugs, 453*f*
    chemical structures of triazole antifungal drugs, 454*f*
Azole drugs, 457–458
AZT. *See* Azidothymidine (AZT)

B

B-ring substituents
    optimization of, 719–721
    in vitro COX-1 and COX-2 inhibitory activity of 1,5-diarylpyrazole, 720*t*, 721*t*
Bacatin III, structure-activity relationship of C_1-and C_2-positions in, 303–304
Baccatin III as starting material, semisynthetic strategy involving, 301–302
    semisynthetic route proposed by Commercon, 301–302, 302*f*
Bacillus anthracis, 489–490
Bacillus calmette-Guérin (BCG), 670–671
Back pocket (BP), 355
Baclofen, 593–594
Bacteria, 489
Bacterial infections, 489–491, 490*f*
Bacterial resistance and special use level antibacterial drugs, 493–495
    bacterial resistance, 493–495
    special use level antibacterial drugs, 495
Baloxavir, 280
    antiinfluenza drugs, 268–270
    clinical study of, 283–284
        adverse reactions, 284
        drug administration, 283
        pharmacokinetics study, 283
        pharmacological action of, 283
        phase III clinical trial, 283–284
    development of, 270–285
        structure and function of endonuclease, 270–271
    discovery of, 271–279
        early structure-activity relationships of, 273*t*
        inverse synthesis analysis of, 279*f*
        structure-activity relationship analysis of, 275*t*
        influenza virus, 265–268
        inspiration from study of, 284–285
        synthesis of, 279–282, 281*f*
            fragment A, 280*f*, 281*f*
            preparation of chiral fragment, 282*f*
            preparation of fragment A' and, 282*f*
Baloxavir marboxil, 270–272
Barbiturate compounds, 587
Bark of Taxus tree, 296
Basal insulin, 26
Basic-helix-loop helix (bHLH), 635
BBB. *See* Blood–brain barrier (BBB)
BCG. *See* Bacillus calmette-Guérin (BCG)
Bcr gene. *See* Breakpoint cluster region gene (Bcr gene)
Bcr-Abl
    and CML, 362–363
    signaling pathway of, 363*f*
    structure, 363*f*
    fusion protein, 363
    kinase inhibitors, 381
BCRP. *See* Breast cancer resistance protein (BCRP)
Bempedoic acid, 107
Benzamide, 153–154, 620
Benzamidine
    analog, 149
    replacements, 149
Benzene ring modification, tamoxifen derivatives with, 429–430
Benzimidazole compounds, 544
    antihypertensive drug, 134
Benzodiazepines, 590–592
    drugs, 587, 595
    receptors, 594
Phenyltetrazole, 129
Benzoylation, 201–203, 301–302
Benzyl *para*-amide compounds, 116–117
Benzyl phenyl ring, 115–116
Benzyl-substituted phenyl group, 220–221
Best-in-class drug (BIC drug), 8
Betamipron, 498–499
β-amino acid series lead compounds
    discovery and optimization of hit compounds, 10*f*
    identification of, 9–10
    lead compounds, 11*f*
    optimization of, 10
    optimizing compound metabolism, permeability, and bioavailability, 11*f*
    preclinical candidate compounds 24 and JANUVIA™, 11*f*
β-amino acid-based DPP-4 inhibitors, 11
β-aminoethyl ketones, 398–399
β-blockers, 630
β-hairpin, 249
β-lactam antibiotics, 301, 494
β-lactamases, stability against, 505
β-tubulin isoforms, 290
β-α subunit interface, 602

β7
    second residue on, 352
Betrixaban, 144
bHLH. *See* Basic-helix-loop helix (bHLH)
Biapenem, 503–504
BIC drug. *See* Best-in-class drug (BIC drug)
Bicyclic piperazine derivatives, 10
Biguanides, 56, 58*f*
Bile acid sequestrants, 107
Binding free energy (ΔG), 91
Binding model of apixaban and FXa, 153–154, 156*f*
Bioactivity screening model, 241
Bioavailability, 253
Biologic therapeutic agents, 47
Biosteric approach, 336
Biphenyl compounds, 116–117, 128–129
1-(Biphenylmethyl)benzimidazole, 133
Bis-isopropylidene glucose, 179
Bisphosphonates, 691, 705–706
    drugs, 691–692, 706
    elucidating mechanisms of action of bisphosphonate drugs, 692–696
        isoprenoid biosynthesis pathway and farnesyl pyrophosphate synthase, 693–694
        molecular mechanisms of action of bisphosphonates on osteoclasts, 694–696
        osteoporosis and bisphosphonates, 692
    medicinal chemistry of nitrogen-containing bisphosphonates, 696–706
    novel applications of bisphosphonate inhibitors, 706–707
        bisphosphonate drugs and inhibitors in anticancer therapy, 706–707
        development of lipophilic bisphosphonate inhibitors as vaccine adjuvants, 707
    unveiling saga, 689–692
        discovery of bisphosphonate compounds and biological functions, 691, 700*t*
        historical progression of bisphosphonate drug development, 691–692
        pyrophosphate and hypophosphatasia, 689–691
    in vivo distribution and metabolism of, 705–706
    metabolic data of representative third-generation bisphosphonate drugs in human body, 706*t*
Blood clots, 162
Blood concentration-time curve, 95
Blood drug concentration, 225
Blood glucose control, 21
Blood pressure
    measurement, 109–110
    reduction, 67
Blood vessels, 141
Bloodborne transmission, 211
Blood–brain barrier (BBB), 5, 593–594
Bloodstream, 35
Boc-protected serine, 282
Boekelheide rearrangement reaction, 548
Bone marrow stem cells, 633

Bone marrow transplant, 262
Bone regeneration, 106
Bone resorption, 692
Boric acids, 393, 400–401
Boron atom, 393, 400–401
Boronic acid molecules, 34
Boronic glucose sensor, 33–34
　glucose-sensitive deglutinin hexamer, 34f
　glucose-sensitive insulin based on dual mechanisms of fatty acids and albumin, 35f
Bosutinib, 377
Bovine viral diarrhea virus model (BVDV model), 191–192
BP. See Back pocket (BP); British Pharmacopoeia (BP)
Bradykinin, 113
Breakpoint cluster region gene (Bcr gene), 362
Breast cancer resistance protein (BCRP), 5
Breast cancer, 419–422
　cells, 294, 434
　drugs targeting estrogen receptor pathway for, 443–444, 443f
　estrogen receptor-positive breast cancer and drug targets, 422
　estrogens and estrogen receptors, 420–421, 420f
　selective estrogen receptor modulators, 422, 423f
Bridged nucleic acids, 744
Bristol-Myers Squibb's class (BMS), 288, 295, 480
　taxane drugs, 295
British Pharmacopoeia (BP), 166–167
Broad-spectrum antiviral drugs, 268–269, 270f
5-bromo-2-chlorobenzoic acid, 65
BTN3A1 receptor. See Butyrophilin subfamily 3 member A1 receptor (BTN3A1 receptor)
Butenafine, 454
Butynamides, 396
　covalent irreversible EGFR inhibitors containing butynamide electrophilic warheads, 396f
　structure of covalent irreversible binding mechanism of EGFR inhibitors, 397f
Butyrophilin subfamily 3 member A1 receptor (BTN3A1 receptor), 693
BVDV model. See Bovine viral diarrhea virus model (BVDV model)

C

C protein. See Core protein (C protein)
C-H arylation reaction, 730, 730f
C-lobe, 352–354. See also N-lobe
　activation segment, 352–354
　catalytic loop, 352
　second residue on β7, 352
2-C-methyl-D-erythritol 4-phosphate (MEP), 693
C_1-and C_2-positions in bacatin III, structure-activity relationship of, 303–304
C_{13}-side chain, relationship between structure and effectiveness of, 305–306

C_4 position, relationship between structure and activity at, 304, 304f
C_7-to C_{10}-positions, relationship between structural modifications at, 304–305, 305f
Cabazitaxel, 293
Caco-2 cell model, 125
CADD. See Computer-aided drug design (CADD)
CagA. See Cytotoxin-associated protein A (CagA)
CagA pathogenicity island (CagPAI), 533
CagPAI. See CagA pathogenicity island (CagPAI)
(+)−Calanolide A
　and derivatives inhibit replicating and non-replicating Mycobacterium tuberculosis, 666–671
　mechanism of antibacterial activity of tetrahydrobenzopyran nitrofuran derivatives, 670–671
　natural product 1 as anti-Mycobacterium tuberculosis compound, 666–667, 667f
　preliminary structural modifications, 667, 667f
　evaluated compounds for preliminary SAR studies, 668f
　tetrahydropyranocoumarins derived from nitrofuran moiety potent activity, 668–670
(+)-calanolide, 651–654
Calanolides, anti-HIV-1 activity of, 654–656
Calcium salt, 97–98
Calophyllum, 651–654
　C. cordato-oblongum, 657
　C. inophyllum, 651–654
　C. lanigerum, 651–654
cAMP. See Cyclic adenosine monophosphate (cAMP)
cAMP response elements (CRE), 81
Camptothecin, 290
Canarypox virus-gp120 protein, 262
Cancer, 105, 287, 327, 349
　cells, 312
　　targeting cancer cells overexpressing receptors, 312, 313f
　　targeting hypoxic microenvironment of, 312
　drug resistance, 373
Candesartan cilexetil, 133
Candesartan's benzimidazole ring, 133–134
Candida, 449–450, 454–455, 460
　C. albicans, 451, 670
Candidate drugs
　full of twists and turns, 541–543
　selection of celecoxib as, 721–725
CAP. See Community-acquired pneumonia (CAP)
Cap-dependent endonuclease (CEN), 278
CAP-snatching, 270
Captopril, 114
Carbapenem antibiotics, 499, 502, 504–505, 507
　discovery of, 497

meropenem
　antibacterial activity and stability, 505–506, 505f
　bacterial infections, 489–491, 490f
　bacterial resistance and special use level antibacterial drugs, 493–495
　biapenem, 503–504
　case of meropenem, 495–502
　chemical structure features and structure-activity relationship, 505–506
　commonly used antibacterial medications, 491–493
　development of novel β-lactamase inhibitors for combinational use, 507
　development of oral drugs, 507
　doripenem, 504
　enhancement of activity against MRSA, 507
　ertapenem, 503
　mechanisms of carbapenem antibiotic resistance, 506
　progress on carbapenem antibiotics, 502–507
　prolonging half-life of drugs and reducing frequency of administration, 507
　recently marketed carbapenem antibiotics, 502–505, 503f
　relationship between structure and toxicity, 506
　research features of carbapenem antibiotics, 506–507
　stability against DHP-I, 506
　stability against β-lactamases, 505
　tebipenem pivoxil, 504–505
　structural optimization of, 497–499
Carbapenems, 496–497, 506
Carbohydrate conjugation, 745
Carbohydrate drugs, 183
Carbohydrate-based chemical monomers, 183
14-carbon monocarboxylic acid, 46–47
[2 + 2]carbon unit introduction method, 100–101
Carbons, 98–99
Carbonyl groups, 173, 436, 643–644
Carboxyl side chain, 614
Carboxylesterase, 278–279
Carboxylic acid, 115–119
4-carboxylic acid derivative, 114–115
Carcinoid tumors, 545
Cardiac repolarization process, 126
Cardiovascular diseases, 71–76, 141
　cholesterol metabolic regulation and hypercholesterolemia, 72–76
　lipid metabolism, 71–72
Cardiovascular safety, 126
Cardiovascular system, 109–110
Cardiovascular toxicity, 289
CARs. See Chimeric antigen receptors (CARs)
Cas9, 736
Casimersen, 751–752
Catalytic core domain (CCD), 215
Catalytic dehydrogenation, 524
Catalytic domain (CD), 351, 374, 558–559
Catalytic hydrogenation, 178, 368

Catalytic hydrophobic pocket, 374–375
Catalytic loop, 352
　catalytic mechanism of protein kinase, 352f
Catalytic mechanism of protein kinase
　C-lobe, 352–354
　composition and, 350–354
　hinge, 351
　N-lobe, 351–352
Cationic lipids, 747–748
Cationic liposomes, 747, 747f
Cationic nucleotidyl lipids, 748
CBR. See Clinical benefit rate (CBR)
CbzCl. See Condensation reaction with benzyl chloroformate (CbzCl)
CCD. See Catalytic core domain (CCD)
CD. See Catalytic domain (CD)
CD4 T-lymphocytes, 211–212
cDNA. See Complementary DNA (cDNA)
cDNs. See Cyclic dinucleotides (cDNs)
Celecoxib, 725–726, 731
　chemical synthesis of, 726–730
　clinical application and monitoring of, 725–726
　metabolism of, 725, 726f
　selection of celecoxib as candidate drug, 721–725
　　pharmacokinetic data of selected pyrazole compounds in rats, 723t
　　in vivo pharmacodynamic evaluation of selected pyrazole compounds, 724t
Celecoxib long-term arthritis safety study (CLASS), 726
Cell culture assay
　activities of calanolides against viral resistant to HIV-1-specific inhibitors, 656t
　anti-HIV-1 activity in, 654–655, 655t
　CEM-SS cells infected with viruses, 656t
Cell division, 328, 349
Cell membrane, 6, 703
Cell mitosis, 288
Cell rRNA synthesis, 197
Cell surface serine protease, 2
Cell wall, 492
Cell-based screening model, 223
Cell-penetrating peptides (CPPs), 746
Cellular antiviral screening models, 223
Cellular enzyme polymerization, 189–190
Cellular oxygen-sensing pathway, 634–635
Cellular toxins, 533
CEN. See Cap-dependent endonuclease (CEN)
Centers for Disease Control and Prevention, 247
Central nervous system, 42–43
Central ring
　structure and activity data of representative statin drugs, 83f
　substitutions of, 83
Cephalosporins, 495–496
Cephalosporium acremonium, 465–466
Cerebrospinal fluid (CSF), 369
Cerebrovascular diseases, 141
Ceritinib, 359
Cerivastatin, 79

C–Glycosides, 63
cGMP. See Cyclic guanosine monophosphate (cGMP)
Chemical drug development, 3
Chemical modifications, 742
Chemical reactions, efficiency of, 13
Chemical science, 526
Chemical synthesis
　of celecoxib, 726–730
　　1,3-dipolar cycloaddition reaction, 728–729
　　C-H arylation reaction, 730, 730f
　　condensation reaction, 726–728
　　coupling reaction, 729–730
　　synthesis study of celecoxib, 727f
　of fondaparinux sodium, 179
　　retrosynthetic analysis route for fondaparinux sodium, 180f
　method, 168–169
Chemo-enzymatic synthesis, 179
　of fondaparinux sodium, 179–181
　mimics, 183
Chemotherapy, 288, 317–318
Chemotherapy resistance induced by tumor microenvironment, 290
Chimeric antigen receptors (CARs), 736
Chinese Food and Drug Administration, 136
Chiral compound, 515
Chiral drugs, 515–516
　brief description of, 515–516
Chiral hydrogenation
　catalysts, 14
　process synthesis, 15–16
Chiral introduction method, 98–99
Chiral isomers, 431
Chiral separation method, 98
CHL. See Cholesterol (CHL)
Chlamydia, 492
Chlamydophila pneumoniae, 493
Chlorine atom, 132–133, 716
3-chloro-4-fluoroaniline group, 404–405
4-chloroacetoacetic acid ethyl ester, 102–103
2-chloromethyl-4-methoxy-3,5-dimethylpyridine hydrochloride (II), 547
5-chlorovaleryl chloride, 157–158
Cholesterol (CHL), 71, 692, 746
　atorvastatin
　　additional effects of statins, 105–106
　　apolipoprotein antisense oligonucleotides, 107
　　atorvastatin, cholesterol-lowering drug, 76–81
　　ATP-citrate lyase inhibitors, 107
　　bile acid sequestrants, 107
　　cholesterol-lowering drugs and targets, 106–107
　　HMG-CoA reductase inhibitors, 106
　　hypercholesterolemia and cardiovascular diseases, 71–76
　　intestinal cholesterol absorption inhibitors, 106
　　medicinal chemistry of atorvastatin, 81–102

　　microsomal triglyceride transfer protein inhibitors, 107
　　novel molecules targeting HMG-CoA reductase, 103–104
　　PCSK9 monoclonal antibodies, 107
　CHL-lowering drug, 76
　metabolic regulation, 72–76
　　biosynthesis of cholesterol, 73f
　　cholesterol biosynthesis and regulation, 73–74, 74f
　　cholesterol transport and regulation, 74, 75f
　　pathogenesis of hypercholesterolemia, 75–76
Cholesterol synthesis inhibition screening (CSI screening), 82
Chromene compound, 658
Chronic disease, 8, 55, 109
Chronic hepatitis C, 205
Chronic kidney disease (CKD), 633
Chronic myeloid leukemia (CML), 349–350
　clinical efficacy of imatinib in treatment of, 371–372, 372t
Chronic schizophrenia, 627
CIAT. See Crystallization-induced asymmetric transformation (CIAT)
Cilastatin, 498, 506
Ciprofol, 609–610
Ciprofol disodium, emergence of, 603–610
1,2-cis glycosidic bond, 176
Cis isomers, 423, 499–500
CKD. See Chronic kidney disease (CKD)
Claisen condensation reaction, 96, 726
Clarithromycin, 95
CLASS. See Celecoxib long-term arthritis safety study (CLASS)
Clinical benefit rate (CBR), 344
Clinical proof of concept (cPOC), 6
Clonorchiasis, 510
CMB. See Complete mitotic block (CMB)
CML. See Chronic myeloid leukemia (CML)
CMN131, 540
CoA reductase inhibition screening (COR inhibition screening), 82
Coagulant substances, 141–142
Coagulation cascade, 142–143
Coagulation System Abnormalities, 162
Coca leaves, 587
Cocaine, 587
Cocktail therapy, 214–215
Cocrystallization analysis, 579–580
Column chromatography, 128
Combination principles, 625
Combination therapy, 233, 261, 292, 296, 664
　of statins with agents, 104
Community-acquired pneumonia (CAP), 466–467
Complementary DNA (cDNA), 41
Complete mitotic block (CMB), 333–335
Complete response letter (CRL), 750
Computer-aided drug design (CADD), 114
Condensation reaction with benzyl chloroformate (CbzCl), 484

Condensation reactions, 96, 155–157, 726–728
  chemical synthesis study of
    celecoxib, 727f
    celecoxib (III), 728f
    celecoxib (IV), 728f
    celecoxib (V), 729f
Conjugated long-chain fatty acids, 31–33
  molecular structure of
    insulin degludec, 32f
    insulin detemir, 32f
    structural modification strategies for insulin analogs, 33f
  variations in absorption and onset rates, 33t
Conmutaxel, 316
Constrained ethyl (cEt), 744
Contezolid, 472
Conventional dosage form, 291
Conventional prodrug technologies
  application of, 194–195
    comparative data for PSI-6130 and Prodrug RG7128, 195t
Coordination bonds, 400–401
Copper catalyst, 157
COR inhibition screening. See CoA reductase inhibition screening (COR inhibition screening)
Cordatolides, anti-HIV-1 activity of, 657
Core pocket (Q pocket), 579
Core protein (C protein), 187
Corynebacterium diphtheria, 489–490
Coumarins, 651–654
Coupling reaction, 729–730
Covalent binding mechanisms, 392, 400
Covalent inhibition strategies, 390–392
  chemical structure of electrophilic warhead used in covalent inhibitor design, 391f
  drug design based on, 390–393
  mechanism of covalent inhibitors, 391f
Covalent inhibitors, 361–362, 390–391, 406
  representatives of, 361f
  warheads targeting specific residues in kinases and reaction mechanisms, 362t
Covalent irreversible drugs, 361
Covalent kinase inhibitors, 362
Covalent small molecule kinase inhibitors, 373
Covalent strategies
  based on addition-elimination, 392
  based on mechanism of Michael reaction, 392
  based on reversible covalent mechanisms, 392–393
COX. See Cyclooxygenase (COX)
Coxib drugs, 716–717
  discovery of, 716–717, 716f, 718f
  representative, 731–732
    chemical structures of Imrecoxib and metabolites, 732f
  structural optimization of, 717–721
    optimization of 3-and 4-position substituents of pyrazole ring, 718, 719t
    optimization of 4-sulfonylamino group in A-ring, 717, 718t
    optimization of B-ring substituents, 719–721

CP5609, 505–506
cPOC. See Clinical proof of concept (cPOC)
CPPs. See Cell-penetrating peptides (CPPs)
Crizotinib, 359
CRL. See Complete response letter (CRL)
Cryptococcus neoformans, 451
Crystalline bovine insulin, 22
Crystallization-induced asymmetric transformation (CIAT), 577
CSF. See Cerebrospinal fluid (CSF)
CSI screening. See Cholesterol synthesis inhibition screening (CSI screening)
Cyan model, 696
Cyano derivatives, 152
Cyclic adenosine monophosphate (cAMP), 42–43, 544, 558
Cyclic dinucleotides (cDNs), 735–736
Cyclic guanosine monophosphate (cGMP), 558
Cyclic sulfite compound, 201–203
[3 + 2]cycloaddition pyrrole synthesis, 98–99
  chiral introduction strategy in, 100f
  chiral separation strategy in, 99f
  retro-synthesis analysis of, 99f
[3 + 2]cycloaddition reaction, 96
Cyclohexyl-substituted carboxylic ester, 200
Cyclohexylcarbonyloxy group, 133–134
Cyclooxygenase (COX), 712–714, 714f, 715f
  activity, 715–716
  COX-1, 711–712
  COX-2, 712, 715–716
  cyclooxygenase-2 selective inhibitor celecoxib, 716–730
    chemical synthesis of celecoxib, 726–730
    clinical application and monitoring of celecoxib, 725–726
    discovery of coxib lead compounds, 716–717, 716f
    metabolism of celecoxib, 725, 726f
    selection of celecoxib as candidate drug, 721–725
    structural optimization of coxib drugs, 717–721
  inhibiting synthesis of prostaglandins by, 534–535
  inhibitors, 715–716, 716f
  nonsteroidal antiinflammatory drugs, 711–714
  mechanism of action, 712–714
  pharmacology, 714
  selective cyclooxygenase-2 inhibitor celecoxib, 715–730
Cyclopropyl substitution, 197, 278
Cyclopropylmethyl group, 294
Cyclotriene derivatives, 469–470
CYP2D6, 435
CYP450 enzymes. See Cytochrome P450 enzymes (CYP450 enzymes)
Cytidine monophosphate, 192
Cytochrome enzymes, 406
Cytochrome P450 enzymes (CYP450 enzymes), 3, 5–6, 8, 93, 125, 203, 232, 616
Cytochrome P450 monooxygenase, 443–444
Cytokines, 534

Cytoplasm, 215, 450
Cytosine, 192
Cytoskeletal proteins, 737
Cytotoxic drugs, 293
Cytotoxicity, 304–305
Cytotoxin-associated protein A (CagA), 533

D

D-glucuronic acid-δ-lactone, 65
D-glucuronolactone, 337
D-glyceraldehyde, 201–203
D-tryptophan methyl ester, 577
DA. See Dopamine (DA)
DAAs. See Direct-acting antivirals (DAAs)
Dalteparin sodium, 167
Damage-associated molecular patterns (DAMPs), 317–318
DAMPs. See Damage-associated molecular patterns (DAMPs)
Danishefsky total synthesis route, 299–300
Dapagliflozin, 64
  efficacy and action of, 67
  SGLT2 inhibitors and successful development of, 60–65
    C-glucosides exhibiting SGLT2 inhibitory activity, 63f
    discovery of compound 17, 64f
    phlorizin and structural modifications, 61f
    SGLT2 inhibitors of O-glucosides, 62f
    structural features of O-glycosides and C-glycosides, 63f
  successful experience in development of, 67–69
    development process of dapagliflozin, 69f
  synthetic process of, 65–67
    initial synthetic route, 66f
    optimized synthetic route, 66f
Darbepoetin alfa, 637
Darunavir, 259
  amprenavir to darunavir, 258–259, 258f
  binding mode of amprenavir with HIV-1 protease, 256f
  discovery of, 256–260
  pharmacokinetic properties of darunavir, 259–260
  side-chain targeting to backbone targeting, 257–258
Dasatinib, 375, 379–380
DBD. Deoxyribonucleic acid binding domain (DBD)
dCK. See Deoxycytidine kinase (dCK)
DCR. See Disease control rate (DCR)
DD model. See Drug discrimination model (DD model)
ddC. See Dideoxycytidine (ddC)
ddI. See Dideoxyinosine (ddI)
DDIs. See Drug–drug interactions (DDIs)
10-deacetylated analog, 292
10-deacetylbaccatin III (10-DAB), 296–297
  Holton semisynthesis route, 301, 302f
  Potier semisynthesis route, 301, 301f
  semisynthetic strategy starting from, 301
DEAD. See Diethyl azodicarboxylate (DEAD)

Decahydroisoquinoline, 252−253, 255−256
Deep vein thrombosis, 167
Deep-seated mycoses, 450
Defense cells, 490−491
Dehydrogenation reaction endpoint, 525
Dehydropeptidase-I (DHP-I), 498
　stability against, 506
Dementia, 106
Deoxycytidine kinase (dCK), 192
Deoxyribonucleic acid (DNA), 421
　polymerases, 203
　synthesis, 349
Deoxyribonucleic acid binding domain (DBD), 421
Depolymerization process, 329−330
Deprotection, 97−98
DES. See Trans-diethylstilbestrol (DES)
Dess−Martin oxidation reaction, 333
Desulfation, 170−171
Deuterated drugs, 517
Deuterated praziquantel, pharmacokinetics of, 517−518
Deuterium (D), 517
Development Therapeutics Program (DTP), 651−654
Dexlansoprazole, 537−538
DHP-I. See Dehydropeptidase-I (DHP-I)
Diabetes mellitus, 8, 21−26, 55−59, 105
　biological basis of SGLT2 as therapeutic target for, 59−60
　　molecular mechanisms underlying glucose absorption by SGLT1 and SGLT2, 61f
　　vital organs and tissues of regulating blood glucose balance, drugs and targets, 60f
　classification, and current status of, 55
　clinical anti-diabetic medications, and targets and mechanisms, 56−59
　　α-glucosidase inhibitors, 57
　　biguanides, 56
　　dipeptidyl peptidase-4 inhibitors, 58−59
　　GLP-1 receptor agonists, 58
　　insulin and insulin analogs, 56
　　insulin secretagogues, 56
　　insulin sensitizers, 58
　factors related to onset of diabetes, 55−56
Diamidine compound, 146−147
Diastereoisomers, 280−282
Diastereomers, 305−306
Diazepam, 595
Dibenzyl ketone derivative, 117
2,3-dicyano-5,6-dichlorobenzoquinone (DDQ), 524
Dideoxycytidine (ddC), 654
Dideoxyinosine (ddI), 654
Diels−Alder reaction, 13, 298
Diethyl azodicarboxylate (DEAD), 408
3,4-difluorobenzoic acid, 279−280
Digoxin, 95
Dihydrodibenzocycloheptenene, 274−278
Dihydroxy pyrimidine lead compound, 221, 241
　optimization of, 226−232
　　pharmacokinetic parameters of compound, 232t

　　SAR and SPR of 2-position of
　　　dihydroxy pyrimidine compounds, 228t
　　　N-methyl pyrimidone compounds, 229t, 230t
　　SAR of 2-position of
　　　dihydroxy pyrimidine compounds, 227t
　　　N-methyl pyrimidone compounds, 231t
7,10-dihydroxymethyl derivative, 293
3′,5′-dihydroxypentanoic acid segment, 90
Dihydroxypentanoic acid side chain, 82−83, 89−90
2,6-diisubstituted phenolic compound, 607
Diketo acid
　compounds, 241
　structure, 218
Dimethyl 2-butynedioate, 234
Dimethyl oxalylglycine (DMOG), 643
Dimethylallyl carbocation, 696−698
Dimethylallyl pyrophosphate (DMAPP), 73, 693
Dimethylamino, 152
Dimethylformamide (DMF), 221−223
Dimroth rearrangement reaction, 409, 410f
Dipeptide Phe-Pro to lead compound 3, 251−252, 251f
Dipeptidyl peptidase-7 (DPP-7), 7−8
Dipeptidyl peptidase−4 inhibitors (DPP−4 inhibitors), 1−3, 43, 58−59
　chemical structures of, 59f
　early pharmacological effects of, 6−8
　　early dipeptidyl peptidase-4 inhibitors, 6f
　early toxicity studies of, 6−8
　　selectivity of early dipeptidyl peptidase-4 inhibitors, 7f
　optimization strategies for, 8
　secretion, function, and degradation of intestinal proinsulin, 3f
Diphenyl tert-butyldimethylsilyl group, 337
1,3-dipolar cycloaddition reaction, 728−729, 729f
Direct-acting antivirals (DAAs), 186−187
Discovery process, 467
Disease control rate (DCR), 413−414
Disulfides, 399−400
Disulfur heterocycles, 400
DMAPP. See Dimethylallyl pyrophosphate (DMAPP)
DMD. See Duchenne muscular dystrophy (DMD)
DMOG. See Dimethyl oxalylglycine (DMOG)
DNA. See Deoxyribonucleic acid (DNA)
Docetaxel, 292−293
　commercially available taxane-based antineoplastic drugs, 292−293
Docosahexaenoic acid (DHA), 312−313
Dolutegravir (DTG), 214, 271−272
Dopamine (DA), 619
Doripenem, 504
Dosage form
　albumin-bound paclitaxel, 291−292
　alternative formulations, 292
　issues about, 291−292
　paclitaxel injection, 291
　paclitaxel liposomes, 291

Dose tolerance issues, 289
　hypersensitivity reactions, 289
　myelosuppression, 289
　neurotoxicity, 289
Dose-limiting toxicities, 292
Double bond-reduced tamoxifen derivatives, 431
　structure-activity relationship of tamoxifen, 432f
　tamoxifen derivatives with reduced double bond, 432f
Double tetrahydrofuran (Bis-THF), 258
Double-bonded immobilized tamoxifen derivatives, 430−431
DOUPC, 748
DPP-7. See Dipeptidyl peptidase-7 (DPP-7)
DPP−4 inhibitors. See Dipeptidyl peptidase−4 inhibitors (DPP−4 inhibitors)
Drug discrimination model (DD model), 624
Drug−drug interactions (DDIs), 5, 125, 177−178, 233, 371
　of atorvastatin, 95
Drugs target, 1, 57, 104, 163, 268, 435, 467, 553, 589, 629
　administration, 283
　　baloxavir for adults and adolescents, 283t
　based on SGLT2 inhibitors, 67, 68t
　in clinical anesthesia, 586−588
　　inhalation anesthetics, 586−587, 586f
　　intravenous anesthetics, 587, 588f
　　local anesthetics, 587−588
　common factors influencing ADME/T properties of, 4−6
　design, 250−251, 625
　　addition-elimination or oxidation mechanisms, 392
　　based on covalent inhibition strategies, 390−393
　　covalent inhibition strategies, 390−392
　　mechanism of Michael reaction, 392
　　reversible covalent mechanisms, 392−393
　strategy, 284
　development, 194
　discovery process, 114, 218−219
　drug-resistant TB, 668
　estrogen receptor-positive breast cancer and, 422
　identification of, 544
　molecules, 4−5, 92
　permeability, 5
　plasma exposure, 232
　production, 484−485
　for renal anemia treatment, 636−637, 637t
　resistance, 256, 442, 514
　　of fluconazole, 460−461
　　to HIV, 214−215
　safety
　　assessment, 370
　　and drug-drug interaction, 370−371
　sensitivity
　　experiments, 259
　　utilization of compound 125 as innovative fluorescent diagnostic reagent, 677−678

targeting estrogen receptor pathway for breast cancer treatment, 443−444
toxicities, 5
DTP. See Development Therapeutics Program (DTP)
DU. See Duodenal ulcer (DU)
Duchenne muscular dystrophy (DMD), 735−738
  developmental trajectory of antisense oligonucleotide therapeutics targeting, 741−752
    chemical modifications of antisense oligonucleotides, 742−745
    exon skipping therapy for DMD by ASO, 749−752
    oligonucleotide delivery techniques, 745−749
  gene, 738, 749
  numbers, 737f
  treatment and exon skipping in, 737−738, 738f
Duodenal ulcer (DU), 531
DuPont Pharmaceuticals, 114, 471
Dystrophin, 737

E

Ebola hemorrhagic fever, 247
Echinocandin antifungal drugs, 454−455, 455f
ECL cells. See Enterochromaffin-like cells (ECL cells)
ED. See Erectile dysfunction (ED)
EDF. See Endoxifen (EDF)
Edoxaban, 144
EDTA. See Ethylenediaminetetraacetic acid (EDTA)
Efavirenz (EFV), 214, 234
EGFR. See Epidermal growth factor receptor (EGFR)
Electron cloud density, 88
Electron-withdrawing groups, 719
Electronegativity, 195−196
Electrophilic warheads, 392
1,8-elimination electron cascade reaction, 312
Elvitegravir (EVG), 214
EM. See Extensive metabolizer (EM)
EMB. See Ethambutol (EMB)
EMEA. See European Agency for Evaluation of Medicines (EMEA)
Emtricitabine (FTC), 214
Enantiomers, 515
Enantioselective total synthesis of optical 1, 659
  chiral synthesis of 1 and 2, 660f
  chiral synthesis of 15 and 1, 660f
Endocrine metabolic disorder, 55
Endocrine substance, 22
Endocrine therapy, 420, 439−440
Endocytic vesicles, 266−268
Endogenous estrogens, 420
Endogenous peptide, 114−115
Endogenous substrates, 360
Endonuclease
  PA inhibitor, 284

structure and function of, 270−271
  crystal structure of PA and structure, 271f
  graphic illustration of CAP-snatching process, 271f
Endothelial cells, 166
Endothelial Injury, 162
Endoxifen (EDF), 432
4-enepyranosuronic acid, 167
Energy homeostasis, 2
ENF. See Enfuvirtide (ENF)
Enfuvirtide (ENF), 214
Enterobacteriaceae, 506
Enterochromaffin-like cells (ECL cells), 532
Enterococcus, 489−490
  E. faecalis, 471−472
Enteroendocrine L cells, 41
Enthalpy, 91
Environmental fungi. See Geophilic fungi
Enzymatic catalysis, 22
Enzymes, 272−274, 371, 634
  catalysis, 16−17
  enzyme-based ST inhibition assay, 223
  enzyme-mediated conversion methods, 22
  kinetics studies, 81−82
  proteins in tumor tissue as target, 311
EoE. See Eosinophilic esophagitis (EoE)
Eosinophilic esophagitis (EoE), 550
Epidemiology and virus genotyping, 186
Epidermal growth factor receptor (EGFR), 350, 387−388
  cellular signaling mediated by EGFR, 389f
  development of covalent irreversible EGFR inhibitor 2 afatinib, 393−408
  drug design based on covalent inhibition strategies, 390−393
  knowledge expansion, 411−414
    emergence of EGFR$^{T790M/C797S}$ double mutations and design strategies for allosteric inhibitors, 414
    research progress on selective small molecule inhibitors for EGFR^{T790M} mutation, 412−414
  and quinazoline-based small molecule inhibitors, 388−390
  resistance mutations for, 390
  schematic diagram of structure of epidermal growth factor receptor, 389f
  synthesis of afatinib, 408−411
Epidermophyton, 449−450
Epithelial cells, weakening defensive capabilities of, 535
EPO. See Erythropoietin (EPO)
Epogen, 637
Epoxides, 393
Eprosartan, 131−132
ER. See Estrogen receptor (ER)
Eradication treatment, 550
  therapy, 531−532
Erectile dysfunction (ED), 557
  approval of second and third-generation highly selective phosphodiesterase type 5A inhibitors, 565−576
  improvement in, 565

molecular mechanisms of phosphodiesterase type 5A inhibitors, 578−580
  interaction between sildenafil or vardenafil and phosphodiesterase type 5A proteins, 579−580
  protein structure of phosphodiesterase type 5A, 578−579, 579f
nitric oxide-cyclic guanosine monophosphate signaling pathway, 557−559
sildenafil for management of male erectile dysfunction, 559−565
synthesis of selective phosphodiesterase type 5A inhibitors, 576−577
Ergosterol, 453
Eribulin
  antitumor mechanism of, 328−330
    mechanism of action, 329−330
    structure and function of microtubules, 328−329, 329f
    tubulin inhibitors, 329, 330f
  clinical research, 343−344
    adverse effects of eribulin, 344−345
    phase I clinical study, 343
    phase II clinical study, 344
    pivotal phase III clinical study, 344
    and safety evaluation, 343−345
  development process of, 330−342
    discovery and chemical synthesis of antitumor natural product halichondrin B, 330−333
    late-stage synthesis of eribulin, 340−342, 342f
    process chemistry, 336−342
    structure-activity relationship of halichondrin B-discovery process of eribulin, 333−336
    synthesis of fragment 22, 336−337, 337f, 338f
    synthesis of fragment 23, 337−340, 339f
    synthesis of fragment 24, 340, 341f
  pharmacological characteristics of, 342−343
    pharmacodynamics of eribulin, 342−343
    pharmacokinetics and toxicology of eribulin, 343
  structure and fundamental information, 328f
Eribulin, 327
Eribulin methylate, 336
Erosive esophagitis, 550
Ertapenem, 503
Erythro-1,3-diol intermediate, 97
Erythropoiesis-stimulating agents (ESAs), 637
Erythropoietin (EPO), 633
  gene expression, 634−635, 638
  production, 633, 645
ESAs. See Erythropoiesis-stimulating agents (ESAs)
ESBL. See Extended-spectrum β-lactamase (ESBL)
Escherichia coli, 22, 489, 670
Esomeprazole, 536−537, 551−552, 554
ESR1 genome and structural mutations in estrogen receptor, alterations in, 440−441
Ester pro-drugs, 123
Ester type local anesthetics, 587−588

Estradiol, 420
Estrogen receptor (ER), 419–422
  alterations in ESR1 genome and structural mutations in, 440–441
  conversion of tamoxifen metabolites to, 439
  ERα, 421, 441
  ERα36, 441–442
  estrogen receptor-positive breast cancer and drug targets, 422
  estrogens and estrogen receptors, 420–421, 420f
  loss of, 439–440
  mechanism of tamoxifen binding to, 425–427, 426f
  selective estrogen receptor modulators, 422, 423f
Estrogens, 420–421
  antagonists, 424
  resistance due to activation of estrogen membrane receptor pathway, 441–442
  signaling pathway, 422
Estrone, 420
Eteplirsen, 749–750, 751f
Ethambutol (EMB), 666–667
Ethoxy diphenylmethane, 65
Ethyl group, 430
Ethyl-modified tamoxifen derivatives, 430
Ethylenediaminetetraacetic acid (EDTA), 503–504
Etoricoxib, 731
Etravirine (ETR), 214
Eukaryotic RNase H1, 739
European Agency for Evaluation of Medicines (EMEA), 565
Evaluation process, 196–197
Excretion, 94
Exenatide-4, 43
Exogenous insulin, 27–28
Exon skipping, 740–741
  therapy for DMD by ASO, 738, 749–752
    casimersen, 751–752
    eteplirsen, 749–750, 751f
    golodirsen, 750
    viltolarsen, 750–751
  treatment and exon skipping in Duchenne muscular dystrophy, 737–738, 738f
  restoration of dystrophin protein expression in patients, 738f
Exons, 740
Extended-spectrum β-lactamase (ESBL), 494–495
Extensive metabolizer (EM), 552
Extrapyramidal system, 619
Extrinsic coagulation, 162
Ezetimibe, 106

F

Factor Xa (FXa), 142–143
  active structure, 164f
  binding model of, 153–154
  functions of, 163
  mechanism of action of fondaparinux sodium, 164f

Farnesyl pyrophosphate (FPP), 692
Farnesyl pyrophosphate synthase (FPPS), 692–694
  crystallographic depiction, 697f
  cylindrical model depiction, 697f
  as molecular target of nitrogen-containing bisphosphonates, 696–698
Fatty acid, 31–32
  acylation, 46
  conjugation, 45–48
    antibody Fc segments fusion, 48–49
    human serum albumin fusion, 49
    liraglutide, 45–47
    semaglutide, 47–48
FBS. See Fetal bovine serum (FBS)
Fc-fusion technology, 48
FDA. See US Food and Drug Administration (FDA)
Feasible model cell assays, 363
Fetal bovine serum (FBS), 217
FFC. See Fluorescent fold change (FFC)
FG-2216, 644–645
Fibrinolytic enzymes, 141–142
FibroGen, 639, 643, 646
Fimasartan, 135
First generation process chemistry of sitagliptin, 15, 15f
First-generation nitrogen-free bisphosphonates, 694–695
First-generation PPIs, 535
First-generation reversible EGFR inhibitors, 390
First-generation synthetic process, 236–238
  coordination of magnesium salt with intermediate, 237f
  optimization of, 234–236
  selectivity in methylation reaction, 237f
FIs. See Fusion inhibitors (FIs)
Flagella, 533
Fluconazole, 453, 460
  antifungal drugs, 452–455, 452f
  developmental history, 455–461
    clinical application, 460
    discovery of lead compounds, 455–457
    drug resistance, 460–461
    mechanism of action of azole antifungal agents, 457–458
    optimizing lead compounds, 457
    protein binding mode and structure-activity relationships, 458–459
    research on synthesis process, 459–460, 459f
  fungal infections, 449–451
  molecule resides, 458–459
  structure optimization, 461–463
    development of isavuconazole, 462, 462f
    development of voriconazole, 461–462
    future development of triazole drugs, 463
Fluorescent activity of nitrofuran derivatives, 672–682
  action of mycothiol, 675–676
  implementing single-cell diagnostic technology for nitrofuran compounds, 678–682, 678f

nitrofuran compounds interact with Rv2466c and mycothiol, 673f, 674–675
  relationship between structure and molecular fluorescence activity, 672–674
  utilization of compound 125 as innovative fluorescent diagnostic reagent, 677–678
Fluorescent fold change (FFC), 672–674
Fluoride compounds, 427
Fluorine atom, 396
2′-fluoro (2′-F), 742
4-fluorobenzylamine, 223, 226–227
4-fluorophenyl group, 8–9
Fluorophore, 680
Fluvastatin, 79
fMet degron pathway. See Formylmethionine degron pathway (fMet degron pathway)
Fondaparinux sodium, 168–178
  chemical process of, 168–169
    chemical synthesis of fondaparinux sodium, 179
    chemo-enzymatic synthesis of fondaparinux sodium, 179–181, 182f
    synthesis challenges of fondaparinux sodium, 178
  development strategy for, 161–163
    chemical process of fondaparinux sodium, 168–169
    development of small-molecule carbohydrate drugs, 162
    development strategy for fondaparinux sodium, 161–163
    development trends in heparin-like anticoagulants, 161–162
    discovery and history of anticoagulant drug, 168–178
    functions of factor Xa, 163
    thrombotic disorders, 161–163
    treatment of thrombotic disorders, 163–168
  genesis of, 170–176
  lead compound, 168–169
  mechanism of action of, 176
  pharmacokinetics and safety of, 176–178, 178t
Foodborne parasitic diseases, 509
Foodborne pathogenic bacteria, 489
Formaldehyde, 610
Formylmethionine degron pathway (fMet degron pathway), 634
Fortovase, 254
Fosamprenavir, 256
Fospropofol disodium, emergence of, 603–610
Fospropofol sodium, 610
FP. See Front pocket (FP)
FPP. See Farnesyl pyrophosphate (FPP)
FPPS. See Farnesyl pyrophosphate synthase (FPPS)
Fragment 22
  synthesis of, 336–337
Fragment 23
  synthesis of, 337–340
Fragment 24
  synthesis of, 340

Fragment crystallizable (Fc), 48
Fragment-based screening, 380–381
Free amino group, 505–506
Friedel-Crafts acylation reaction, 65
Friedel-Crafts alkylation, 612
Front pocket (FP), 355
Fungal cells, 450
Fungal CYP51 protein, 458
Fungal infections, 449–451
   current status and challenges of fungal infections, 451
   fungal cell structure and pathogenic mechanisms, 450–451
   human pathogenic fungi, 449–450, 450f
Fungi, 449, 451
   fundamental structure of, 450, 451f
   pathogenic mechanisms of, 451
Furan aminobenzenesulfonamide, 256
Furapromide, 510–511
Fusion inhibitors (FIs), 214, 260
Fusion process, 262

G
G protein-coupled receptor family, 42–43
G proteins, 706–707
GABA. See Gamma-aminobutyric acid (GABA)
Gag gene, 248
Gamma-aminobutyric acid (GABA), 498, 593–594
   $GABA_A$ receptor agonists, 589–595, 590f, 593f
     anesthesia, 585–586
     common drugs in clinical anesthesia, 586–588
     discovery of barbiturates, 594f
     discovery of benzodiazepines, 595f
     medicinal chemistry of general intravenous anesthetic propofol and analogs, 588–616
   GABAergic system, 589–593, 590f, 592f
     crystal structure of endogenous GABA bound to $GABA_A$ receptor, 591f
     general anesthetics bind to different sites on $GABA_A$ receptor, 591f
     receptors, 590
γ-hydroxybutyric acid (GHB), 593–594
Gas anesthetics, 586–587
Gastric acid, 532–534, 532f
Gastric cancer, 535
Gastric hormone secretion, 21
Gastric parietal cells, 539
Gastric pepsinogen, 533
Gastric proteases, 532–533
Gastric ulcer (GU), 531
Gastrin, 532
Gastroesophageal reflux disease (GERD), 550
Gastrointestinal hormone, 41–42
Gastrointestinal stromal tumor (GIST), 369
Gastrointestinal system, 194–195
Gatekeeper residue, 352
GC. See Guanylate cyclase (GC)
General anesthesia, 586, 592–593

Genes, 740
   editing process, 262, 736
   expression, 712–714
   recombinant technology, 28
Genesis of fondaparinux sodium, 170–176, 171f
Genetic bone disease, 689–690
Genetic engineering, 296–297
Genotype, 195, 204–205
Genotype 1 hepatitis C, 195
Genotyping of hepatitis C, 186
Geophilic fungi, 449–450
Geranyl pyrophosphate (GPP), 693
Geranylgeranyl pyrophosphate (GGPP), 693
Geranylgeranyl pyrophosphate synthase (GGPPS), 693
GERD. See Gastroesophageal reflux disease (GERD)
Gestational diabetes, 55
GFR. See Glomerular filtration rate (GFR)
GGPP. See Geranylgeranyl pyrophosphate (GGPP)
GGPPS. See Geranylgeranyl pyrophosphate synthase (GGPPS)
GIP. See Glucose-dependent insulinotropic polypeptide (GIP)
GIST. See Gastrointestinal stromal tumor (GIST)
GlaxoSmithKline (GSK), 131–132, 567–568, 639
Gleevec, 362
Glivec, 362
Glomerular filtration rate (GFR), 67
GLP-1. See Glucagon—like peptide-1 (GLP-1)
Glucagon—like peptide-1 (GLP-1), 1, 41–43
   analogs, 50
   development of GLP-1 therapeutics, 43–49
     limitations of native GLP-1 as therapeutic agent, 43
   developmental history of GLP-1 medications, 41–42
   milestones in historical progression of GLP-1 drug therapy, 42f
   receptor agonists, 58
   strategies for extending GLP-1 analogs time action, 44–49
     amino acid mutation of peptide backbone, 44–45
     fatty acid conjugation, 45–48
   structure and physiology, 42–43
     GLP-1 related peptide amino acid sequence, 42–43
     physiological and pharmacological effects of GLP-1 in organs, 43t
   unsuccessful case in GLP-1 drug R&D and implications and lessons, 49–50
   taspoglutide, 50f
Glucocorticoid antiinflammatory drugs, 711
Glucosamine, 164, 170–171
Glucosamine monophosphate, 206
Glucose, 60
   homeostasis, 59–60
   metabolism, 21

Glucose transporters (GLUTs), 60, 311
Glucose-dependent insulin biosynthesis and secretion, 2
Glucose-dependent insulinotropic polypeptide (GIP), 2, 41
Glucose-dependent insulin secretion, 1
Glucose-sensitive insulin, 33
Glucose-stimulated insulin secretion. See Glucose-dependent insulin secretion
Glucuronidation reaction, 123, 134
Glucuronosyltransferase (UGT), 616
Glutamate, 81–82
Glutamic acid, 352
GLUTs. See Glucose transporters (GLUTs)
Gly. See Glycine (Gly)
Glycan-modifying enzymes, 179–181
Glycated hemoglobin (HbA1c), 12, 47
Glycine (Gly), 45
Glycoprotein (GP), 25, 144, 212, 248
Glycosaminoglycans, 143, 166
Glycosidic indirect FXa inhibitor, 163
Glycosylation reactions, 179
Glycosyltransferases, 179–181
GMP. See Good manufacturing practice (GMP)
Golgi apparatus, 74
Golodirsen, 750
Good manufacturing practice (GMP), 611
GP. See Glycoprotein (GP)
GPP. See Geranyl pyrophosphate (GPP)
Gram-negative bacilli, 492
Gram-negative bacteria, 493, 495, 506–507
Gram-positive bacteria (G+), 466–467, 499
Green chemistry, 526
   characteristics of today's and tomorrow's chemical sectors, 527f
   promising pathway toward sustainability, 17–18
Green process for praziquantel and levoisomer, 518–526
   green chemistry, 518–519
   levorotatory praziquantel synthesis, 522–526
   praziquantel synthesis, 519–522, 520f
Grignard reagent, 128–129
GSK. See GlaxoSmithKline (GSK)
GTP. See Guanosine triphosphate (GTP)
GU. See Gastric ulcer (GU)
Guanosine triphosphate (GTP), 558
Guanylate cyclase (GC), 558

H
1H-1,3-benzimidazole, 549–550
H^+, K^+-ATPase o0095, 535, 538
H12. See Helix12 (H12)
HA. See Hemagglutinin (HA)
Haemophilus influenzae, 472, 481
Halaven. See Eribulin 1
Halichondria okadai, 330–331
Halichondrin B, 330–331
   discovery and chemical synthesis of, 330–333
   Kishi's synthetic strategy for halichondrin B and key reactions, 332f

Halichondrin B (*Continued*)
  structure and activity of halichondrin B and homologs, 332*f*
  structure-activity relationship of halichondrin B-discovery process of eribulin, 333–336
    SAR study of halichondrin B, 335*f*
    total synthesis of halichondrin B, 334*f*
Halogen atoms, 197, 224–225
5-halomethyl-3-phenyl-2-oxazolidinone derivatives, 467
Haloperidol, 623
HAP. *See* Hospital-acquired pneumonia (HAP)
Harvoni, 205
HCV. *See* Hepatitis C virus (HCV)
HDL. *See* High-density lipoproteins (HDL)
Heart diseases, 103
Helicobacter pylori (Hp), 531–534
  abnormal gastric acid secretion, 534
  colonization and toxin-mediated damage, 533, 533*f*
  immune response, 534
  infection, 550
Helix12 (H12), 427
Hemagglutinin (HA), 266
Hematological stem cell disorder, 362
Hemiacetal form, 170
Hemolytic streptococcus, 489
Hemostatic system, 162
Heparin, 143, 164–165
  development trends in heparin-like anticoagulants, 161–162
  discovery of heparin pentasaccharide sequence, 168–169
    binding mode of pentasaccharide fragment in heparin sequence with AT-III, 170*f*
    minimal effective structural unit of heparin, 169*f*
  fragment, 168–169
  heptasaccharide analogs, 179–181
  representative structure, 166*f*
  structure-activity relationship studies based on, 170–176
Heparin-Induced Thrombocytopenia (HIT), 166
Hepatic fluoriasis, 510
Hepatitis C virus (HCV), 185–187
  biology, 187–188
  discovery and development of therapeutic drugs, 186–187
  epidemiology and genotyping of, 186
  polymerase inhibitors, 220
  RNA domains, 188*f*
  structure, 187, 188*f*
  structure of hepatitis C virus NS5B protein, 187–188
    X-ray structures of NS5B polymerase, 189*f*
  symptoms, causes, and transmission, 185–186
  stages of HCV infection, 185*f*
Hepatocytes, 198–200
HER2. *See* Human epidermal growth factor receptor-2 (HER2)
Heteroaromatic rings, 230–231

Heterocyclic core, 357
Heterocyclic oxygen-containing tetrahydropyran, 297
Heterocyclic scaffold compounds, 388–389
Heterocyclic tetrahydrofuran ring, 287–288
Heterogeneous metabolic disorder, 21
Hexahydronaphthalene ring, replacement of, 79
Hexamer, 23–25
HIF. *See* Hypoxia-inducible factor (HIF)
High-boiling solvents, 524
High-density lipoproteins (HDL), 71
High-performance liquid chromatography (HPLC), 664
Highest occupied molecular orbital (HOMO), 672–674
Highly active antiretroviral therapy, 261–262
  national free AIDS antiviral drug treatment guidelines, 262*t*
Hinge, 351
HINT1. *See* Histidine triad nucleotide-binding protein 1 (HINT1)
Histamine, 532
Histidine triad nucleotide-binding protein 1 (HINT1), 200–201
HIT. *See* Heparin-Induced Thrombocytopenia (HIT)
Hit compounds, 146–147
  design and optimization of diaryl diketone derivatives, 219*f*
  diaryl diketone compounds to 1,6-naphthyridine compounds, 220*f*
  diketo acid derivatives with HIV-1 integrase, 219*f*
  discovery and optimization of, 216–221
  hit compounds of HCV polymerase inhibitor, 220*f*
  HIV-1 integrase inhibitors with diverse scaffolds, 221*f*
  identification and optimization of, 643, 643*f*
  molecular structure of 5-CITEP and its crystal structure in complex, 219*f*
  SAR of diketo acid derivatives, 218*f*
  screening model and Merck screening model for HIV-1 integrase inhibitors, 217*f*
HIV. *See* Human immunodeficiency virus (HIV)
HMG-CoA reductase, 81–82
  affinity and thermodynamic characteristics, 91–92
  catalytic mechanism of HMG-CoA reductase, 82*f*
  catalytic steps of HMG-CoA reductase, 82*f*
  degradants, 104
  inhibitors, 106
  interaction modes, 89–90
    four statin drugs with HMG-CoA reductase, 91*t*
  interaction of statins with, 89–92
  novel molecules targeting, 103–104
    combination therapy of statins with agents, 104
    HMG-CoA reductase degradants, 104
    novel HMG-CoA reductase inhibitors, 103–104, 103*f*, 104*f*

  structural representation of, 82*f*
  structure-activity relationship of statin drugs inhibiting, 82–89
    optimization of structures with pyrrole as central ring, 83–89
    substitutions of central ring, 83
Hodgkin's lymphoma, 262–263
Holton semisynthesis route, 301
Holton total synthesis route, 299
HOMO. *See* Highest occupied molecular orbital (HOMO)
Hormone receptors (HR), 419–420
Hormone therapy. *See* Endocrine therapy
Hormone-based antibreast cancer drugs, 424–425
Horner-Wadsworth-Emmons reaction (HWE reaction), 339–340, 409, 410*f*
Hospital-acquired pneumonia (HAP), 466–467
Host cells, 245, 248–249
HPLC. *See* High-performance liquid chromatography (HPLC)
HR. *See* Hormone receptors (HR)
HREs. *See* Hypoxia response elements (HREs)
HSA. *See* Human serum albumin (HSA)
HT-29 cells, 430
5-HT2 receptor, 620
HTLV-III. *See* Human T-cell lymphotropic virus type III (HTLV-III)
Huisgen reaction, 96
Human antiviral warfare, 247
Human blood vessels, 142
Human DNA polymerases, 221
Human epidermal growth factor receptor-2 (HER2), 349–350, 419–420
Human Ether-a-go-go-Related Gene (*h*ERG), 3, 126
Human immunodeficiency syndrome, 211
Human immunodeficiency virus (HIV), 185–186, 211–213, 247–249. *See also* Influenza virus
  drug resistance to, 214–215
  integrase inhibitors, 216–217, 224
  mechanisms of HIV infection and HIV life cycle, 248–249
  new strategies for HIV/AIDS prevention and treatment, 261–263
    dawn of humanity's conquest of AIDS, 262–263
    developments in HIV prevention and treatment strategies, 262
    highly active antiretroviral therapy, 261–262
  protease and inhibitor saquinavir, 249–254
    design and discovery of saquinavir, 251–253
    design of HIV protease inhibitors, 250–251
    pharmacokinetic properties and deficiencies of saquinavir, 253–254
    structural characteristics of HIV proteases, 249
    structure and mechanism of action of, 215–216

protein sequence diagram of HIV-1
  integrase and tertiary structure, 215f
viral DNA and host DNA catalyzed by
  HIV-1 integrase, 216f
structure and replication of, 212–213, 212f,
  213f, 248, 248f
Human melanoma, 336
Human pathogenic fungi, 449–450, 450f
Human serum albumin (HSA), 31
  albiglutide, 49f
  fusion, 49
Human T-cell lymphotropic virus type III
  (HTLV-III), 247
Human-sequence insulin drugs, 28
Humanity's conquest of AIDS, dawn of,
  262–263
HWE reaction. See Horner-Wadsworth-
  Emmons reaction (HWE reaction)
Hybrid chemoenzymatic synthesis, 179
Hydrochloric acid (HCl), 532, 728
Hydrogen (H), 517
  bonds, 253, 257–258, 609–610
Hydrolysis, 15, 250
Hydrophilic peptide, 43
Hydrophilic small molecule moieties as
  carriers, prodrug utilizing, 310–320
Hydrophilicity, 92–95
Hydrophobic group, 569–570
Hydrophobic interactions, 23–25
Hydrophobic pocket (H pocket), 120, 579
Hydrophobic segments, 92
Hydrophobic skeletons, 353
Hydrophobic structural segment, 82–83
Hydrophobic tert-butyl group, 252
Hydrophobicity, 87–88
Hydroxy group, 426–427
2-hydroxy-3-benzamido-phenylpropionic acid,
  301
3-hydroxy-3-methylglutaryl coenzyme A
  (HMG-CoA), 73
Hydroxyapatite, 689–690
Hydroxyethylamine, 251
Hydroxyisopropyl group, 135
Hydroxyl apixaban, 158
Hydroxyl groups, 171–173, 190–192, 659
4-hydroxytamoxifen (4-OHT), 422, 432–434
Hypercalcemic rat model, 691
Hypercholesterolemia, 71–76
  cholesterol metabolic regulation and, 72–76
  lipid metabolism, 71–72
  pathogenesis of, 75–76
    formation and progression of
      atherosclerosis, 75f
Hyperlipidemia treatment, 81
Hypersensitivity reactions, 289
Hypertension, 109
  and commonly used medications for
    treatment, 109–110
Hypoglycemia, 27–28
Hypoglycemic adverse reactions, 27
Hypophosphatasia, 689–691
  schematic representation of structure, 690f
  zoledronate structural formula and 3D ball-
    and-stick model, 690f

Hypoxia response elements (HREs), 635
Hypoxia-inducible factor (HIF), 634–635, 636f
  HIF-1α protein, 635
  HIF-2α, 635
  HIF-α, 638, 641–642
  HIF-β subunit, 634–635
Hypoxic microenvironment of cancer cells
  prodrug targeting hypoxic cancer cells, 313f
  targeting, 312

I

ICAAC. See Interscience Conference on
  Antimicrobial Agents and
  Chemotherapy (ICAAC)
ICI. See Imperial Chemical Industries (ICI)
ICTV. See International Committee on
  Taxonomy of Viruses (ICTV)
IDE. See Insulin-degrading enzymes (IDE)
Idiopathic peptic ulcer, 535
IDL. See Intermediate-density lipoproteins
  (IDL)
Idraparinux, 171–173
IDV. See Indinavir (IDV)
IFNα. See Interferon alpha (IFNα)
IGF-I. See Insulin-like growth factor-I (IGF-I)
IgG. See Immunoglobulin G (IgG)
Ilaprazole, 537
Imatinib
  Bcr-Abl and CML, 362–363
  clinical efficacy and expansion of
    indications, 371–373
    clinical efficacy of imatinib in treatment
      of CML, 371–372, 372t
    expansion of clinical indications,
      372–373
  clinical mechanisms of imatinib resistance,
    373–374
    activation loop, 374
    ATP binding pocket, 374
    catalytic domain, 374
    phosphate binding loop, 374
  drug safety and drug-drug interaction,
    370–371
  medicinal chemistry of, 362–373
  molecular design and structure optimization,
    363–366
    conformation of H-bonding part of PAPs,
      365f
    optimization process for imatinib, 364f
    selectivity and analysis of conformation,
      365f
  next-generation drugs to overcome imatinib
    resistance, 374–381
  pharmacokinetics and pharmacodynamics,
    369–370
  resistance and solutions, 373–381
  structure-activity relationship, 366–367
  synthesis, 367–368, 368f
Imidazole antifungal drugs, 453
Imidazole-5-acetic acids, 113
Imidazoles to triazoles, 455–457
Imipenem, 506
Immune response, 534

Immunoglobulin G (IgG), 48
Immunotherapeutic agents, 290
Imperial Chemical Industries (ICI), 595–596
Imrecoxib, 731–732
In situ-generated vinylstannane reagent, 337
In vitro antimicrobial susceptibility testing, 678
In vitro antiviral activity, 195
In vitro binding, 176
In vitro compound evaluation processes,
  196–197
In vitro experiments, 200, 329–330
In vitro proliferation inhibition toxicity, 253
In vitro receptor, 625
In vivo antiviral activity experiments, 223–224
In vivo compound evaluation processes,
  196–197
In vivo distribution of bisphosphonates,
  705–706
In vivo efficacy, 92–95
In vivo metabolic characteristics of tamoxifen,
  432–435
  4-hydroxytamoxifen, 434
  metabolites of tamoxifen in body, 433t
  N,N-didesmethyl tamoxifen and metabolite
    Y, 435, 435f
  N-desmethyl-4-hydroxytamoxifen, 434
  N-desmethyltamoxifen, 434
  in vivo pharmacokinetics of tamoxifen with
    two SERMs drugs, 433t
In vivo metabolic stability, 151
In vivo pharmacological studies, 722
In vivo structure-activity, structure-metabolism,
  and structure-toxicity relationships of
  statin drugs, 92–95
Incretins, 2–3, 58–59
IND. See Investigational new drug (IND)
Indinavir (IDV), 654
Industrial synthesis, 614
Infectious nucleic acid, 245
Inflammation diseases, 105
Influenza A virus (H1N1 virus), 265–266
Influenza vaccination, 268
Influenza virus, 265–268, 270. See also
  Human immunodeficiency virus (HIV)
  endonuclease inhibitor molecules, 239–240
  inhibitors targeting polymerase complex,
    269–270
  life cycle of, 266–268, 267f
  structure, function, and classification of,
    265–266, 266f
    genome-encoded proteins of influenza A
      virus and functions, 267t
  transmission and status quo of, 265
  typical influenza pandemic events, 266t
Inhalation anesthetics, 586–587, 586f
  chemical structure of partial, 587f
Inhibitors in anticancer therapy,
  bisphosphonate drugs and, 706–707
Injectable paclitaxel, 289
  application limitations of, 289–292
  dose tolerance issues, 289
  issues about dosage form, 291–292
  resistance issue, 289–290
    β-tubulin isoforms, 290

Injectable paclitaxel (*Continued*)
   chemotherapy resistance induced by tumor microenvironment, 290
   multiple drug resistance, 290
   response rate to monotherapy is limited combination therapy, 290
Injection site
   discomfort reactions, 50
   reactions, 50
Innate immune cells, 313−314
Inophyllums, anti-HIV-1 activity of, 656−657
Inorganic phosphate (Pi), 539
Inorganic pyrophosphate (PPi), 689−690
INSTIs. *See* Integrase strand transfer inhibitors (INSTIs)
Insulin, 21−26
   analogs, 21
   clearance mechanism, 26
   degludec, 32
   detemir, 31−32
   glulisine, 29−30
   injections, 56
   and insulin analogs, 56
   mechanism of action of, 25
      SAR of insulin obtained through alanine scanning, 25f
   monomers, 22
   peptide chain, 30
   receptors, 26
   secretagogues, 56
      nonsulfonylurea secretagogues, 58f
      sulfonylurea secretagogues, 57t
   secretion, 42−43
   sensitizers, 58
      medications, 58
      representative structures of thiazolidinedione medications, 59f
   structure, 22−25, 23f
      monomeric insulin exists in distinct conformations, 24f
      three-dimensional structure of insulin molecule, 24f
   therapy, 26
Insulin pharmaceuticals, 46
   development of, 26−37
   development process of insulin medications, 27−28
      1921 to late 1970s, 27−28
      early 1980s to pre-approval of insulin lisprо in 1996, 28
      FDA approval of insulin lispro in 1996, 28
      panel illustrates physiological range of blood glucose concentration, 31f
   structural modification strategies for insulin analogs, 28−37
      amino acid substitution, 29−31
      boronic glucose sensor, 33−34
      competitive interference with mannose receptor and lectin degradation strategy, 34−37
      conjugated long-chain fatty acids, 31−33
      pharmacokinetic and pharmacodynamic characteristics of, 29t
Insulin-degrading enzymes (IDE), 26

Insulin-like growth factor-I (IGF-I), 25
Integrase inhibitors, 214−215
Integrase strand transfer inhibitors (INSTIs), 260
Interferon, 204−205
Interferon alpha (IFNα), 186
Interferon regulatory factor 3 (IRF3), 313−314
Interferon regulatory factor 7 (IRF7), 313−314
Intermediate-density lipoproteins (IDL), 71
International Committee on Taxonomy of Viruses (ICTV), 246
Interscience Conference on Antimicrobial Agents and Chemotherapy (ICAAC), 497
Intestinal cholesterol absorption inhibitors, 106
   chemical structures of cholesterol-lowering drugs, 106f
Intestinal hormone, 41−42
Intravenous anesthetics, 586−587, 588f
Intravenous heparin product, 164−165
Intravenous injection, 295
Introns, 740
Invasive fungal diseases. *See* Deep-seated mycoses
Investigational new drug (IND), 13, 127
Ion exchange process, 539
IPP. *See* Isopentenyl pyrophosphate (IPP)
Irbesartan, 132−133
Iridium (Ir), 14
Irreversible covalent bonds, 361
Isavuconazole, 462
   development of, 462, 462f
Isavuconazonium sulfate, 462
Islets of Langerhans, 22
Isobutyrylacetic acid methyl ester, 97
Isoleucine 5 (Ile5), 131−132
Isomerization to obtain trans-tamoxifen, 437
Isoniazid (INH), 666−667
Isopentenyl pyrophosphate (IPP), 73, 693
Isoprenoid biomolecules, 94−95
Isoprenoid biosynthesis pathway, 693−694, 693f
Isoprenyl groups, 105
Isotopes, 517
Isoxazolidine ring derivatives, 480

J

JANUVIATM, preclinical candidate compounds 24 and, 11f
Japp-Klingemann reaction, 154
JGA. *See* Juxtaglomerular apparatus (JGA)
Juxtaglomerular apparatus (JGA), 67

K

K^+−ATPas, 535, 538
Ketoconazole, 453
Kidneys, 59−60, 498, 633
Kinases, 350
   catalytic domain, 356
   domain, 405
   inhibitor, 372−373
   mutations, 373

Klebsiella pneumoniae, 472
Klebsiella pneumoniae carbapenemase (KPC), 507
KPC. *See Klebsiella pneumoniae* carbapenemase (KPC)
KRAS mutation, 707

L

L-arabinose, 336−337
L-arginine (L-Arg), 558
L-citrulline (L-Cit), 558
Laboratorial medicinal chemical synthetic route-modular synthesis approach, 409−410
   synthesis of
      4-arylamine quinazoline core 52, 410f
      afatinib according to original research, 411f
      afatinib based on Horner-Wadsworth-Emmons, 411f
Lactam, 279
Lamivudine (3TC), 214
Lansoprazole, 535
Larotaxel, 293, 294f
LAV. *See* Lymphadenopathy associated virus (LAV)
LBD. *See* Ligand-binding domain (LBD)
LDL. *See* Low-density lipoproteins (LDL)
LDL-C. *See* Low-density lipoproteincholesterol (LDL-C)
LDLR. *See* Low-density lipoprotein receptor (LDLR)
Lead compounds, 10, 168−169
   confirmation of, 8−10
      α-amino acid-derived dipeptidyl peptidase inhibitors, 8−9
      ideal lead compound, 8
      identification of β-amino acid series of lead compounds, 9−10
   discovery of, 455−457
   evolution of lead compounds in early stage, 114−116
      N-benzyl para-amide analogs, 116f
      para-carboxylated *N*-benzyl derivatives, 115f
   optimization of, 147−153
   optimization of lead compound 3, 252−253
      derivative structures and activity characteristics based on, 252f
   optimizing, 457
      developmental history of fluconazole, 457f
Lead discovery and optimization of prolyl hydroxylase domain inhibitors, 643−645
Lead optimization, 3, 116−117
   representative sulfonamides as carboxylic acid bioisosteres, 117f
   SAR of different connecting groups between phenyl rings, 118f
Lectin degradation strategy
   competitive interference with, 34−37
   TPEs with distinct chemical structures, 36f
Legionella, 492−493
   L. pneumophila, 472
Lentivirus, 212

Levoisomer, green process for, 518–526
Levopantoprazole, 537
Levopraziquantel, 515–517
  brief description of chiral drugs, 515–516
Levorotatory praziquantel
  acemization of 7 in presenceof styrene, 525f
  dehydrogenation of 7, 524f, 524t
  possible mechanism for palladium-catalyzed dehydrogenation, 525f
  racemization of 6 by dehydrogenation, 523f
  resolution of praziquanamine, 523f
  synthesis of, 522–526
  two-stage dehydrogenation of 7, 525f
Lewis acid (AlCl$_3$), 279–280
Life cycle of influenza virus, 266–268
Ligand-binding domain (LBD), 427
Linezolid, 466–467, 470–472, 475, 485
  antibacterial mechanisms of, 477–479, 478f
  antimicrobial mechanisms of common antibiotics, 477f
  bioactivity of antibacterial drug, 472–476
    antibacterial activity of Linezolid in vitro, 472–473
    antibacterial activity of linezolid in vivo, 474–475, 474t
    clinical efficacy of linezolid, 476
    pharmacokinetic properties of linezolid, 475–476
  clinical efficacy of, 476
  pharmacokinetic properties of, 475–476
  research on synthesis process of, 484–485
    optimization of synthesis process of linezolid, 485f
    original synthetic route of linezolid, 484f
  in vitro, antibacterial activity of, 472–473
  in vivo, antibacterial activity of, 474–475, 474t
Lipid nanoparticles (LNP), 735–736
Lipidation, 45–48
Lipids, 71
  conjugation, 746
  emulsions, 610
  lipid-insoluble gas molecule, 558
  metabolism, 71–72
    LDL and HDL in cholesterol metabolism, 72f
    physicochemical parameters of plasma lipoproteins, 72t
Lipinski's rule, 596–597
Lipophilic anticoagulant, 164
Lipophilic biphenyl system, 117–119
Lipophilic bisphosphonate inhibitors as vaccine adjuvants, development of, 707
Lipophilic compounds, 596
Lipophilic statins, 95
Lipophilic sulfonamide bioisosteres, 116
Lipophilic thioamide group, 135
Lipophilicity, 92–95
Lipopolysaccharide (LPS), 313–314
Liposomes, 291, 747
Liraglutide, 45–47
  interaction between secondary structure of GLP-1 and ECD, 46f
  structure, 46f

Lispro insulin, 29
Listeria, 489
Liver, 195–196
  cells, 196
  design of liver-targeted nucleoside prodrugs, 195–197
    design and screening cascade of liver-targeted nucleoside prodrugs, 196f
  disease, 185–186
  extraction rates, 92
  microsomes, 259
  structure-activity relationship of liver-targeting prodrug molecule pharmasset small-molecule inhibitor-7851, 197–201
    biological activity, stability, and PK properties of phosphoramidate prodrugs, 199t
    metabolic pathway of phosphoramidate prodrug PSI-7851, 201f
    pharmacokinetic data of phosphoramidate prodrugs in dog and monkey, 200t
    effect of R1 and R2 on inhibitory activity and cytotoxicity, 198t
    effect of R1 and R3 on inhibitory activity and cytotoxicity, 198t
    structure of phosphoramidate prodrug, 197f
LMWHs. See Low-molecular-weight heparins (LMWHs)
LNA. See Locked nucleic acid (LNA)
LNP. See Lipid nanoparticles (LNP)
Local anesthetics, 587–588
  chemical structures of partial local anesthetics, 588f
  investigation of local anesthetic agents, 539–540
Local irritation symptoms, 615
Locked nucleic acid (LNA), 742
Lomitapide, 107
Long-chain fatty acids, 31
Longest linear steps (LLS), 333
LORR model. See Loss of righting reflex model (LORR model)
Losartan
  discovery of, 114–131
    carboxylic acid group on terminal phenyl ring on activity, 118f
    evolution of lead compounds in early stage, 114–116
    lead optimization, 116–117
    metabolites of losartan and corresponding pro-drugs, 123–125
    properties and actions of losartan, 127
    safety profile of losartan, 125–127
    SAR of representative bioisosteric analogs of carboxylic acid, 119f
    impact of substituents at 2-position of imidazole ring on activity, 121f
    impact of substituents at 4-position of imidazole ring on activity, 122f
    impact of substituents at 5-position of imidazole ring on activity, 122f
    synthesis of losartan, 128–130

    terminal phenyl ring on activity, 120f
  discovery of losartan analogs, 131–136
    allisartan isoproxil, 136f
    candesartan cilexetil and azilsartan medoxomil, 133f
    irbesartan and design rationale, 133f
    olmesartan and olmesartan medoxomil, 135f
    structure of fimasartan, 135f
    structures of losartan and valsartan, 131f
    telmisartan and compound, 134f
  metabolites of losartan and corresponding pro-drugs, 123–125
    properties of losartan and compound, 125t
    impact of substituent at 4-position of imidazole ring on activity, 124f
  potassium, 127
  properties and actions of, 127
  safety profile of, 125–127
    inhibitory activity of losartan on certain CYP450 enzymes, 126t
  synthesis of, 128–130
    medicinal chemistry synthesis route of losartan, 128f
    process route for production of losartan, 129f
Loss of righting reflex model (LORR model), 603
Lovastatin, 79
Low-density lipoprotein receptor (LDLR), 71–72
Low-density lipoproteincholesterol (LDL-C), 71–72
Low-density lipoproteins (LDL), 71, 746
Low-molecular-weight heparins (LMWHs), 166–167
  classification of, 167t
Lower clearance rate (CL), 607–608
Lowest unoccupied molecular orbital (LUMO), 672–674
LPS. See Lipopolysaccharide (LPS)
LSD model. See Lysergic acid diethylamide model (LSD model)
LUMO. See Lowest unoccupied molecular orbital (LUMO)
Lung adenocarcinoma, 707
Lung cancer, 112–113, 388
Lymphadenopathy associated virus (LAV), 247
Lysergic acid diethylamide model (LSD model), 624
Lysine (K), 81–82, 352

M
M2 ion channel blockers, 268
Macrocyclic domain, 333–335
Macrolide antibiotics, 492
Macromolecules, 194
Magnesium salt, 235–236
Major facilitator superfamily (MFS), 460–461
Malassezia, 449–450
Male erectile dysfunction, sildenafil for management of, 559–565
Mammalian aspartic proteases, 250

Mannich bases, 398–399
Manninen reaction, 469
Mannose receptors, 34–35
    competitive interference with, 34–37
MAPKs. *See* Mitogen-activated protein kinases (MAPKs)
Maraviroc (MVC), 214
Mass spectrometry, 147
Maturation, 213, 249
Maximum tolerated dose (MTD), 343
MBC. *See* Minimum bactericidal concentration (MBC)
MBD. *See* Membrane-binding domain (MBD)
MBG. *See* Metal-binding group (MBG)
McMurry coupling reaction, 436
    synthesis of tamoxifen by, 436
MDP. *See* Muramyl dipeptide (MDP)
MDR. *See* Median duration of response (MDR); Multiple drug resistance (MDR)
MDR-TB. *See* Multidrug-resistant tuberculosis (MDR-TB)
MDRSP. *See* Multidrug-resistant *Streptococcus pneumoniae* (MDRSP)
Mechanism of action (MOA), 144
    of eribulin, 329–330
        antitumor mechanism of action, 331*f*
    of fondaparinux sodium, 176
        binding mode of fondaparinux sodium with AT-III, 177*f*
        in vivo activity, 176*t*
    of insulin, 25
    of nonsteroidal antiinflammatory drugs, 712–714
        biological functions of prostaglandins, 712
        cyclooxygenase, 712–714, 714*f*
        thrombosis, 143–144
Median duration of response (MDR), 344
Median overall survival (mOS), 344
Median progression-free survival (mPFS), 344, 413–414
Medication regimen, 262
Medicinal chemistry, 3, 221–223, 596–597, 639
    of apixaban, 146–158
    of atorvastatin, 81–102
    of general intravenous anesthetic propofol and analogs, 588–616
        clinical application and metabolism of propofol in vivo, 615–616
        GABA$_A$ receptor agonists, 593–595, 593*f*
        GABA$_A$ receptor and GABAergic system, 589–593, 590*f*
        optimization of candidate, 600–602, 601*t*
        pharmaceutical manufacturing technology, 611–615
        phenolic compounds, 596–599
        propofol analogs, 603–610
        story of propofol, 595–596
    of imatinib, 362–373
    of nitrogen-containing bisphosphonates, 696–706
        chemical structure and structure-activity relationships of lipophilic bisphosphonates, 704*t*
        comparison of cellular activity between zoledronic acid and lipophilic bisphosphonates, 705*t*
        design and development of next-generation lipophilic bisphosphonate inhibitors, 703–705
        farnesyl pyrophosphate synthase as molecular target of nitrogen-containing bisphosphonates, 696–698
        structure-activity relationships of nitrogen-containing bisphosphonates, 698–703
        in vivo distribution and metabolism of bisphosphonates, 705–706
    of omeprazole, 546–550
        structural characteristics of omeprazole, 546
        structure-activity relationship of proton pump inhibitors, 549–550
        synthesis process of omeprazole, 546–549
    of praziquantel, 514–518
        levopraziquantel, 515–517
        pharmacokinetics of praziquantel and deuterated praziquantel, 517–518
        structure-activity relationship of praziquantel, 514–515
    research, 219–220
    of risperidone, 623–627
        chemical structure of risperidone, 623*f*
        discovery of risperidone, 624–625, 624*f*
        pharmacological basis of risperidone, 623–624
        synthesis of risperidone, 626–627
    of selective estrogen receptor modulator tamoxifen, 423–438
        discovery of tamoxifen—serendipity and opportunity, 423–425, 424*f*
        mechanism of action and structure-activity relationship of tamoxifen, 425–427
        structure-activity relationship of tamoxifen, 427–431
        synthesis and process of tamoxifen, 435–438
        tamoxifen drug interactions, 435
        in vivo metabolic characteristics of tamoxifen, 432–435
    synthesis of sitagliptin, 14
        α-amino acid to β-amino acid in drug synthesis pathway of sitagliptin, 15*f*
    synthetic route in, 234
Membrane depolarization, 42–43
Membrane proteins, 441–442, 737
Membrane-binding domain (MBD), 714
Membrane-bound homodimer, 2
Mental illnesses, 619
Merck's acquisition, 34–35
Merck's process, 15
Meropenem, 495–502
    chemical structures of penicillin and carbapenem antibiotics, 496*f*
    discovery and structural features, 499–500, 499*f*
    discovery of carbapenem antibiotics, 497
    mechanism of action, 500
    pharmacodynamics and pharmacokinetics, 500
    process synthesis, 500–502, 501*f*
    structural optimization of carbapenem antibiotics, 497–499
Messenger RNA (mRNA), 213
Metabolic disorders, 105
Metabolic processes, 26
Metabolism, 94, 123, 253
    of bisphosphonates, 705–706
    of celecoxib, 725
    clinical application and metabolism of propofol in vivo, 615–616
    process, 200–201
Metabolites of losartan and corresponding pro-drugs, 123–125
Metadiazonium derivatives, 304
Metal-binding group (MBG), 271–272, 463
Metal-binding site (M site), 579
Metal-catalyzed coupling reactions, 224–225
Metamethoxy derivatives, 304
Metformin, 56
Methanol, 282
Methicillin-resistant *Staphylococcus aureus* (MRSA), 466, 492–493, 507
    enhancement of activity against, 507
Methicillin-resistant *Staphylococcus epidermidis* (MRSE), 466
Methoxy alkene ether, 340
Methoxy compound, 115–116
5-methoxy-2-((4-methoxy-3,5-dimethyl-2-pyridinyl)methyl)-sulfinyl-1*H*-benzimidazole, 546
4-methoxyaniline, 154
Methoxymethyl, 121
Methyl amino formate ester, 121
Methyl ethyl ether substituent, 278–279
Methyl group, 366–367
Methyl sulfonyl linker, 550
Methylation reaction, 238–239
2-(1-methylbutyl) phenol 3, 597–598
Methyloxadiazole-substituted compound, 230–231
2-methylpropenyl, 305–306
Methylsulfonyl, 152
Mevalonate (MVA), 692
Mevastatin, 76–78
MFS. *See* Major facilitator superfamily (MFS)
MGIT 960 method, 678
MIC. *See* Minimum inhibitory concentration (MIC)
Michael addition reaction, 235
Michael reaction, covalent strategies based on mechanism of, 392
Michael–Stetter reaction, 96
Microenvironments, 290, 349
Microscopic heterogeneity, 164
Microsomal triglyceride transfer protein (MTTP), 74, 107
Microtubules, 288, 328
    assembly, 303
    polymerization, 303
    structure and function of, 328–329
    system, 290
Microvilli, 539
Midazolam, 616

Milataxel, 293, 294f
Minimum bactericidal concentration (MBC), 496
Minimum inhibitory concentration (MIC), 496
 range, 666
 values, 461, 468–469
Minodronic acid, 696
Mipomersen, 107, 743–744
Mitochondrial respiratory chain, 105
Mitogen-activated protein kinases (MAPKs), 25
Mitosis, 328
Mitsunobu reaction, 15, 408
MOA. See Mechanism of action (MOA)
Moffat oxidation reaction, 339–340
Molecular binding, 114–115
Molecular biology technologies, 262
Molecular docking studies, 399–400
Molecular fluorescence activity, relationship between structure and, 672–674
Molecular target of nitrogen-containing bisphosphonates, farnesyl pyrophosphate synthase as, 696–698
Molecular weight (MW), 10
Molecule inhibitors, 388–389
Monooxygenases, 5–6, 125
Monotherapy, 12, 290
Morpholinos, 744–745
mOS. See Median overall survival (mOS)
Mouse hollow fiber model, anti-HIV-1 activity of novel tetracyclic dipyranocoumarins in, 654–655
Mouse lymphoma mutation assay, 343
mPFS. See Median progression-free survival (mPFS)
MRL41, 424
mRNA, 736, 739
mRNA. See Messenger RNA (mRNA)
MRSA. See Methicillin-resistant *Staphylococcus aureus* (MRSA)
MRSE. See Methicillin-resistant *Staphylococcus epidermidis* (MRSE)
MSH. See Mycothiol (MSH)
MTD. See Maximum tolerated dose (MTD)
Mucous-bicarbonate barrier, 533
Multidrug-resistant *Streptococcus pneumoniae* (MDRSP), 475
Multidrug-resistant tuberculosis (MDR-TB), 466, 678
Multiple drug resistance (MDR), 290
Multiple drugs, 595–596
Multiple target drug design, 621–622, 622f
Multiplex PCR, 738
Muramyl dipeptide (MDP), 313–314
Muscle fibers, 737
Mutations, 25, 256–257, 374, 737
MVA. See Mevalonate (MVA)
MVC. See Maraviroc (MVC)
MW. See Molecular weight (MW)
Mycobacteriaceae, 680
Mycobacterium tuberculosis (*Mtb*), 481, 492–493, 666
Mycoplasma, 492
 M. pneumoniae, 493

Mycothiol (MSH), 674–675
 action of, 675–676
 nitrofuran compounds interact with, 674–675
 structure activity relationships of compound 160 and derivatives, 675–676, 677f
 mechanism of reduction of NFC 125 by Rv2466c, 677f
 synthesis of 160 and derivatives, 674f, 675
Myelosuppression, 289

N

N,N-desdimethyl tamoxifen and metabolite Y, 435, 435f
N,N-dimethylamino modification, 403
N,N-dimethylformamide-diethylacetal, 368
N-acetyl substituent, 152–153
N-acetylgalactosamine (GalNAc), 745
N-acetylglucosamine (NAG), 316, 477
N-acetylmuramic acid, 477
N-desmethyl tamoxifen, 434
N-desmethyl-4-hydroxytamoxifen, 434
N-desmethyltamoxifen (*N*-DES-TAM), 432–434
N-lobe, 351–352. See also C-lobe
 gatekeeper residue, 352
 glutamic acid, 352
 lysine, 352
 phosphate-binding loop, 352
N-methyl-D-aspartate receptors (NMDA receptors), 590
N-methylacetamide-substituted compound, 152–153
N-methylformamide group, 226
N-methylmorpholine, 236
N-methylpiperazine group, 367, 377–378
N-oxalylglycine (NOG), 643
N-terminal regulatory domain, 558–559
N-terminus hydrophobicity enhancement, 252
NA. See Neuraminidase (NA)
Nadroparin calcium, 167
NAG. See *N*-acetylglucosamine (NAG)
NAIs. See Neuraminidase inhibitors (NAIs)
NANC nerves. See Noncholinergic nerves (NANC nerves)
Nanoscale microorganisms, 246
Nanosized colloidal suspension composed of paclitaxel, 291–292
Naphthalene ring, 197
1,6–naphthyridine compounds, 221, 226–227
 optimization of, 221–226
 SAR and SPR of 5-position, 224t, 225t
 SAR of 5-position, 222t
 SAR of amine fragments in amide group, 222t
National Cancer Institute (NCI), 287, 330–331, 651–654
National Institutes of Health (NIH), 218–219
National Medical Products Administration (NMPA), 647
Natural heparin, 164
Natural nonnucleoside reverse transcriptase inhibitor (NNRTI), 651–654

Natural paclitaxel
 extracting directly from bark of Taxus tree, 296
 method of obtaining, 296–297
 milestones in development of paclitaxel, 297
 semisynthesis and total synthesis, 296–297
Natural pentasaccharide, 170
Natural product, simple modification of, 79
Natural sterols, 104
Natural tetracyclic dipyranocoumarin
 (+)-calanolide A and derivatives inhibit replicating and non-replicating *Mycobacterium tuberculosis*, 666–671
 anti-HIV-1 activity of improved calanolides, 658–665
 discovery and structural diversity of, 651–654, 652t
 fluorescent activity of nitrofuran derivatives, 672–682
 natural nonnucleoside reverse transcriptase inhibitors, 654–658
 anti-HIV-1 activity of calanolides, 654–656
 anti-HIV-1 activity of cordatolides, 657
 anti-HIV-1 activity of inophyllums, 656–657
 investigation of 1 in clinical trial, 657–658
NCI. See National Cancer Institute (NCI)
Nelfinavir (NFV), 654
Neonatal Fc receptor (FcRn), 48
NEP. See Nuclear export protein (NEP)
Nephrotoxicity, 506
NERD. See Nonerosive reflux disease (NERD)
Neuraminidase (NA), 266
Neuraminidase inhibitors (NAIs), 268
Neurodegenerative diseases, 106
Neuronal cell membranes, 589–590
Neurons, 43
Neurotoxicity, 289, 506
Neutral protamine Hagedorn (NPH), 27–28
Neutral protamine lispro, 29
Neutrophil count, 289
Nevirapine (NVP), 214, 654
New Delhi metallo-beta-lactamase-1 (NDM-1), 493
New drug sitagliptin, clinical studies of, 11–12
Next-generation drugs to overcome imatinib resistance, 374–381
 chemical structure of GNF-2 and GNF-5, 380f
 chemical structure of olverembatinib, 379f
 cocrystal structure and binding mode of Abl with
  asciminib and nilotinib, 379f
  dasatinib, 376f
  ponatinib, 378f
 optimization process for
  bosutinib, 377f
  dasatinib, 376f
  nilotinib, 375f
  ponatinib, 378f
NFV. See Nelfinavir (NFV)

NHK reaction. *See* Nozaki−Hiyama−Kishi reaction (NHK reaction)
NHS. *See* Normal human serum (NHS)
Niacinamide, 29
Nicolaou total synthesis route, 298, 299f
NIH. *See* National Institutes of Health (NIH)
Nilotinib, 374−375
Nitrates, 562
Nitric oxide (NO), 535, 558
   nitric oxide-cyclic guanosine monophosphate signaling pathway, 557−559
      molecular biological mechanisms of priapism, 558, 559f
      phosphodiesterase protein structure and mechanism of action, 558−559, 560f
      physiological mechanisms of penile erection, 557−558
Nitro-containing compounds, 677−678
Nitrofuran compounds
   implementing single-cell diagnostic technology for, 678−682, 678f
   conjugates of novel tuberculosis fluorescence probe molecule NFC with trehalose, 679f
   correlation of integrated fluorescence, 681f
   diagnosing *Mtb* in patients with TB using 175, 682f
   fluorescent-specific labeling of bacteria by compound 173, 679f
   imaging phagocytosed *Mtb*, 682f
   imaging with 175, 681f
   structure and fluorescence activity of Compound 174, 680f
   structure-fluorescence activity relationship of NFC compounds, 680f
   structures of probes 175, 681f
   interact with Rv2466c and mycothiol, 673f, 674−675
Nitrofuran derivatives, fluorescent activity of, 672−682
Nitrofuran moiety exhibit potent activity, 668−670
   antimicrobial activity of compound 123, 669f
   antimicrobial activity of nitrofuran-based tetracyclic coumarin derivatives, 670f
   structural optimization of compound 123 and corresponding SARs, 669f
2-nitrofuran-based structures, 392
Nitrogen (N), 470
   atom, 153−154, 366−367, 407, 643, 698
   modifications on nitrogen atom, 427−431, 428f
      alteration of aminoethoxy side chain, 429
      derivatives of tamoxifen with A-ring substitution, 429, 429f
      double bond-reduced tamoxifen derivatives, 431
      double-bonded immobilized tamoxifen derivatives, 430−431
      ethyl-modified tamoxifen derivatives, 430
      modification of *N*, *N*-dimethyl moiety in tamoxifen, 428t
      tamoxifen derivatives with benzene ring modification, 429−430

nitrogen-containing bisphosphonates, 699
   binding mode of zoledronic acid with FPPS, 698f
   compounds, 707
   drugs, 698
   farnesyl pyrophosphate synthase as molecular target of, 696−698
   general formula for structure of nitrogen-containing bisphosphonates, 699f
   medicinal chemistry of, 696−706
   structure-activity relationships of, 698−703, 702t
nitrogen-methylated product, 238−239
2-nitroimidazole derivatives, 401−402
NMDA receptors. *See* N-methyl-D-aspartate receptors (NMDA receptors)
N−methyl pyrimidone, 229, 240−241
NMPA. *See* National Medical Products Administration (NMPA)
NNRTI. *See* Natural nonnucleoside reverse transcriptase inhibitor (NNRTI)
NNRTIs. *See* Nonnucleoside reverse transcriptase inhibitors (NNRTIs)
No effect level (NOEL), 12
Nocturnal hypoglycaemia, 31
NOD1/2. *See* Nucleotide-binding oligomerization domain 1/2 (NOD1/2)
NOEL. *See* No effect level (NOEL)
NOG. *See* *N*-oxalylglycine (NOG)
Non-replicating *Mycobacterium tuberculosis* (NR-Mtb), 666, 668
   (+)-calanolide A and derivatives inhibit replicating and, 666−671
   discovered and optimized tetrahydropyranocoumarins derived from nitrofuran moiety, 668−670
Non-sulfonylurea drugs, 56
Noncholinergic nerves (NANC nerves), 557
Nonerosive reflux disease (NERD), 550
Nonnucleoside compounds, 189
Nonnucleoside reverse transcriptase inhibitors (NNRTIs), 214, 260
Nonreceptor tyrosine kinases (NRTKs), 350
Nonsense-mediated mRNA, 740
Nonsmall cell lung cancer (NSCLC), 387−388
Nonsteroidal antiinflammatory drugs (NSAIDs), 534−535, 711−712, 713f
   inhibit mitochondrial oxidative phosphorylation process, 535
   inhibit synthesis of prostaglandins by cyclooxygenase enzymes, 534−535
   mechanism of action of, 712−714
   mode of action of aspirin, 712f
   nonsteroidal antiinflammatory drug-related gastrointestinal injury, 550
   and cyclooxygenase, 711−714
   representative coxib drugs, 731−732
   selective cyclooxygenase-2 inhibitor celecoxib, 715−730
   weakening defensive capabilities of epithelial cells, 535
Nonsterol isoprenoid compounds, 105
Nonstructural protein 1 (NS1), 266
Nonvalvular atrial fibrillation (NVAF), 144

Normal human serum (NHS), 223
Novel drug discovery, 544
Novel fungal CYP51 inhibitor, 463
Novel lipophilic bisphosphonates, 698
Novel oligonucleotide drug, 742
Novel tetracyclic dipyranocoumarins in mouse hollow fiber model, anti-HIV-1 activity of, 654−655
Novel β-lactamase inhibitors for combinational use with carbapenem drugs, development of, 507
NovoLog, 29
NovoRapid, 29
Nozaki−Hiyama−Kishi reaction (NHK reaction), 333
NP. *See* Nucleoprotein (NP)
NPH. *See* Neutral protamine Hagedorn (NPH)
NRTIs. *See* Nucleoside Reverse Transcriptase Inhibitors (NRTIs)
NRTKs. *See* Nonreceptor tyrosine kinases (NRTKs)
NS1. *See* Nonstructural protein 1 (NS1)
NSAIDs. *See* Nonsteroidal antiinflammatory drugs (NSAIDs)
NSCLC. *See* Nonsmall cell lung cancer (NSCLC)
Nuclear export protein (NEP), 266
Nucleic acids, 245−246, 735, 746
   delivery systems, 746−747
   drugs, 742
   endonuclease, 271−272
Nucleophile, 216
Nucleophilic addition, synthesis of tamoxifen by, 436
Nucleophilic groups, 392, 394−396
Nucleophilic substitution, 398
   synthesis of tamoxifen by, 436
Nucleoprotein (NP), 265−266
Nucleoside
   analogs, 189, 451
   compound favipiravir, 268
   drugs, 253
   mechanism of nucleoside antiviral drugs, 189−190
      nucleotide molecules inhibit viral replication, 190f
      Pharmasett anti-HCV hit compounds, 190f
      structure-activity relationship of nucleoside antiviral drugs, 191t
   molecules, 198−200
   nucleoside-based drugs, 206
   structure-activity relationship of nucleoside scaffold, 190−194
      metabolic pathways and metabolites of PSI-6130, 193f
      reported nucleoside inhibitors targeting HCV, 191f
   triphosphate metabolite of compound, 189−190
Nucleoside Reverse Transcriptase Inhibitors (NRTIs), 214, 260
Nucleotide-binding oligomerization domain 1/2 (NOD1/2), 313−314

Nucleotides polymorphism, 216, 694–695
    modifications, 744–745
    polymorphism, 552
Nucleotidyl lipids, 747–749, 748f
NVAF. *See* Nonvalvular atrial fibrillation (NVAF)
Nystatin, 452–453

O

O-demethyl apixaban, 158
O-glycosidic bond, 62
2′-O-methoxyethyl (2′-O-MOE), 742
2′-O-methyl (2′-O-Me), 742
OAT1. *See* Organic anion transporter 1 (OAT1)
OAT3. *See* Organic anion transporter 3 (OAT3)
Objective response rate (ORR), 344, 407
OCT2. *See* Organic cation transporter 2 (OCT2)
Ojima coupling reaction, 297
Oligonucleotides, 746
    conjugation strategies for targeted delivery, 745–746, 745f
    delivery techniques, 745–749
    vehicle delivery, 746–749
Oligosaccharide, 183
Olmesartan, 135
Olmutinib, 412–413
Omega-3 fatty acids, 104
Omeprazole, 535, 538–547
    clinical applications of, 550–552
    clinical indications, 550–551
        eosinophilic esophagitis, 550
        functional dyspepsia, 551
        gastroesophageal reflux disease, 550
        Helicobacter pylori infection, 550
        nonsteroidal antiinflammatory drug-related gastrointestinal injury, 550
        peptic ulcer, 550
        prevention of stress ulcers, 551
        safety of omeprazole, 551
        Zollinger-Ellison syndrome, 551
    clinical indications and safety, 550–551
    development process, 539–545
        full of twists and turns, 541–543
        initiation, 539–540
        new starting point, 540, 541f
        novel drug discovery, 544
        patent controversy, 541
        rescued from desperation, 544–545, 544t
        subsequent development, 545
    launch of, 544–545, 544t
    mechanism of action, 545–546, 545f
    medicinal chemistry of, 546–550
    omeprazole and esomeprazole, 551–552
    patent portfolio, 553–554
        patent network strategy, 553–554
        product line extension strategy, 554
    physiological functions and structural characteristics of proton pumps, 538–539
    structural characteristics of, 546

synthesis process of, 546–549
    oxidation of thioether, 549
    synthesis of thioether, 547–548
treatment, 550
OMPs. *See* Outer membrane proteins (OMPs)
Once-daily dosing (QD dosing), 12
Open reading frame (ORF), 187, 738
Optimization
    of 1,6-naphthyridine lead compound, 221–226
    of dihydroxy pyrimidine lead compound, 226–232
    of first-generation synthetic process, 234–236
    of lead compound, 147–153
        3-position substituent of pyrazole, 154f
        bicyclic pyrazoles to reduce probability of amide hydrolysis, 151f
        compounds optimization of bicyclic series, 153f
        exploration of bicyclic scaffold, 152f
        insert methyl substitution to positions of pyrazole, 148f
        optimization from HTS to diamidine compound, 146f
        optimization of aminobenzisoxazole series, 150f
        optimization of substitutions on isooxazoline, 147f
        P4 substituent connected with nitrogen atom, 155f
        pharmacokinetic properties of compound, 150t
        pharmacokinetic properties of compounds, 151t
        scaffold hopping of core structure, 148f
        in vitro and in vivo profiles of compounds, 155t
    of lead compound 3, 252–253
    of second-generation synthetic process, 236–239
Oral absorption, 629
Oral antihypertensive compound, 123
Oral bioavailability, 5, 259–260
Oral drugs, development of, 507
Oral peptide, 35–36
Oral sustained-release formulation, 631
ORF. *See* Open reading frame (ORF)
Organic anion transporter 1 (OAT1), 64–65
Organic anion transporter 3 (OAT3), 64–65
Organic cation transporter 2 (OCT2), 64–65
Organic reactions, 470
Organic solvents, 369
Organic synthesis, 13
Organon Pharmaceuticals, 170
Orphan drugs, 749
ORR. *See* Objective response rate (ORR)
Ortataxel, 295, 296f
Ortho-substituted arylmethyl aglycone, 63
Ortho-substituted compounds, 599
Orthomyxoviridae, 265–266
OS. *See* Overall survival (OS)
Oseltamivir group, 284
Oseltamivir phosphate, 278–279

Osimertinib, 412
Osteoclasts, molecular mechanisms of action of bisphosphonates on, 694–696
    binding mode of minodronic acid to FPPS, 696f
    cytotoxicity of first-generation nitrogen-free bisphosphonates, 695f
    general structural formulae and representative molecular structures, 694f
    schematic representation of catalytic mechanism, 695f
Osteoporosis, 166, 692
Outer membrane proteins (OMPs), 506
Ovarian cancer, 439
Overall survival (OS), 412
Overt infection, 246
Oxadiazole fragment, 234
Oxazolidinones, 467–468
    derivatives, 467–468, 479, 484
    study on structure-activity relationship of, 479–484, 483f
Oxazolinone compound, 128–129
Oxidation
    mechanisms, 392
    reactions, 299
    of thioether, 549
Oxidative cleavage, 337
Oxime, 121
2-oxoglutarate (2OG), 635
Oxygen (O), 400–401
    anion, 200–201
    atoms, 307–308, 691
    heterocycle, 308–309
    oxygen-containing D-ring, 298
    single bond, 641–642

P

P-glycoprotein gene (P-gp gene), 3, 64–65, 125, 289
P-gp gene. *See* P-glycoprotein gene (P-gp gene)
p-RIP2. *See* Phosphorylation of RIP2 (p-RIP2)
P450 enzymes, 587–588
PA. *See* Polymerase acidic protein (PA)
Paal–Knorr pyrrole synthesis, 97–98
    method, 101–102
    reaction, 95–96
    retro-synthesis analysis of, 97f
PABA. *See* Para-aminobenzoic acid (PABA)
Paclitaxel, 287
    conjugates, 310
    design strategy for, 310–320
        prodrug utilizing hydrophilic small molecule moieties as carriers, 310–320, 310f
    injection, 291
    liposomes, 291
    milestones in development of, 297
    paclitaxel–unsaturated fatty acid conjugates, 312–313, 314f
    pharmaceutical chemistry of, 297–309
    prodrug targeting inflammatory microenvironment of tumors, 313–320, 314f

Paclitaxel (*Continued*)
   chemical library constructed with paclitaxel and MDP\covalent compounds, 316*f*
   first-generation conjugate of paclitaxel with MDP, 315*f*
   mechanism of action of Conmutaxel as prodrug molecule, 317*f*
   molecular structure of docetaxel, 317*f*
   synthesis of nonhydrolyzable paclitaxel and MDP conjugate, 318*f*
   prodrugs of paclitaxel utilizing water-soluble polymers as carriers, 310
   resistance, 290
   semisynthesis of paclitaxel, 300–302
     semisynthetic strategy involving Baccatin III as starting material, 301–302
     semisynthetic strategy starting from 10-deacetylbaccatin III, 301
   study on structure-activity relationship of paclitaxel, 302–309, 303*f*
   total synthesis of paclitaxel, 297–300, 298*f*
     analysis of structure and synthetic strategies of paclitaxel, 297, 298*t*
     Danishefsky total synthesis route, 299–300, 300*f*
     Holton total synthesis route, 299, 300*f*
     Nicolaou total synthesis route, 298, 299*f*
PAE. *See* Post-antibiotic effect (PAE)
Palladium (Pd), 14
Pamidronate, 699–701
Pancreatic duct, 22
Pancreatic hyperplasia, 50
Pancreatic protease, 149–150
Pancreatic β-cells, 56
Pancreatitis, 50
Pantoprazole, 536
PAP compounds. *See* Phenylaminopyrimidine compounds (PAP compounds)
Para-aminobenzenesulfonamide, 256
Para-aminobenzoic acid (PABA), 491
para-hydroxyphenyl group, 62
para-methoxybenzyl (PMB), 333
Para-substituted removal reactions, 612
Parasitic diseases, 509–510
   antiparasitic drugs, 510
Parasympathetic system, 557
Partial response (PR), 344
Patent term extension system (PTE system), 554
Pathogen vectors, 510
Pathogenic bacteria, 493
Pathogenic mechanisms, 451
   fundamental structure of fungi, 450, 451*f*
   fungal cell structure and, 450–451
   pathogenic mechanisms of fungi, 451
Pathogens, 465, 494–495
Pattern recognition receptors (PRRs), 313–314
PB1. *See* Polymerase basic protein 1 (PB1)
PB2. *See* Polymerase basic protein 2 (PB2)
PBPs. *See* Penicillin-binding proteins (PBPs)
PCOS. *See* Polycystic ovary syndrome (PCOS)
PCSK9 monoclonal antibodies, 107

PCSK9. *See* Proprotein convertase subtilisin/kexin 9 (PCSK9)
PD. *See* Progressive disease (PD)
PDC. *See* Peptide-drug conjugate (PDC)
PDE. *See* Phosphodiesterase (PDE)
PDGFR. *See* Platelet-derived growth factor receptor (PDGFR)
Pegylated interferon alpha (PEG-IFNα), 186–187
PEGylation. *See* Polyethylene glycosylation (PEGylation)
Penicillin, 465–466, 491, 495–496
Penicillin-binding proteins (PBPs), 492, 494, 496
Penicillin-resistant *Streptococcus pneumoniae* (PRSP), 466
Penicillium, 449–450
   P. citrium, 76
   P. terreus, 79
Penile erectile function
   nitric oxide-cyclic guanosine monophosphate signaling pathway associated with, 557–559
   physiological mechanisms of, 557–558
Pentacyclic triterpenes, 104
Pentanoic acid methyl ester, 129–130
Pentasaccharide, 170–171, 176
Peptic ulcer (PU), 531–537, 550
   classification and clinical applications of antiulcer medications, 535–537
   pathogenesis of, 531–535
     gastric acid and gastric proteases, 532–533, 532*f*
     Helicobacter pylori, 533–534
     idiopathic peptic ulcer, 535
     nonsteroidal antiinflammatory drugs, 534–535
Peptide backbone, amino acid mutation of, 44–45
Peptide conjugation, 746
Peptide nucleic acids (PNAs), 744–745
Peptide-drug conjugate (PDC), 311
Peptide-paclitaxel conjugate, 311
Peptides-based molecules stems, 35
Per/ARNT/Sim (PAS), 635
Peripheral arterial thrombotic diseases, 161
PET effect. *See* Photo-induced electron transfer effect (PET effect)
PF4. *See* Platelet Factor 4 (PF4)
Pfizer's valdecoxib, 731
PFS. *See* Progression-free survival (PFS)
PGG2. *See* Prostaglandin G2 (PGG2)
PGH2. *See* Prostaglandin H2 (PGH2)
PGs. *See* Prostaglandins (PGs)
Pharmaceutical manufacturing technology, 611–615
   chemical synthesis method 1 of ciprofol, 612*f*
   chemical synthesis method 2 of ciprofol, 613*f*
   industrial synthesis method 1 of ciprofol, 613*f*
   industrial synthesis method 1 of propofol, 611*f*

   industrial synthesis method 2 of ciprofol, 614*f*
   industrial synthesis method 2 of propofol, 612*f*
   industrial synthesis method 3 of ciprofol, 614*f*
Pharmacodynamics (PD), 1–2, 406–407, 645
   evaluation, 1–2
   of imatinib, 369–370
     ADME, 369–370
   of meropenem, 500
   of roxadustat, 645–646
Pharmacokinetics (PK), 92–95, 406–407
   of antibacterial drug linezolid, 472–476
     antibacterial activity of Linezolid in vitro, 472–473
     antibacterial activity of linezolid in vivo, 474–475, 474*t*
     clinical efficacy of linezolid, 476
     pharmacokinetic properties of linezolid, 475–476
   data, 201
   drug-drug Interaction of risperidone, 629–630
   evaluation, 1–2
   of imatinib, 369–370, 369*t*
     ADME, 369–370
     pharmacokinetics in special groups, 370
   of meropenem, 500
   of praziquantel and deuterated praziquantel, 517–518
     deuterated praziquantels, 518*f*
     main metabolites of praziquantel, 518*f*
   of risperidone, 629
     metabolism of risperidone, 630*f*
   of roxadustat, 645–646
   and safety of fondaparinux sodium, 176–178, 178*t*
   studies, 475, 573–575
Pharmacological basis of risperidone, 623–624
   chemical structure of haloperidol, 623*f*
   classification of classical antipsychotic drugs and representative examples, 621*t*
Pharmacological characteristics of risperidone, 627–629
   adverse effects of risperidone, 629
   indications of risperidone, 627–629
   pharmacological mechanism of risperidone, 627
Pharmacologists, 590, 716
Pharmacophore, 220–221, 239–240, 514
Pharmasett, 194
   small-molecule inhibitor, 190
   small-molecule inhibitor-6130, 190–194
     application of conventional prodrug technologies, 194–195
     characterization of active diastereomer, 201
     design of liver-targeted nucleoside prodrugs, 195–197
     pharmacokinetic study of, 194–201
     structure-activity relationship of liver-targeting prodrug molecule pharmasset small-molecule inhibitor-7851, 197–201
   small-molecule inhibitor-7977, 201

PHD. See Prolyl hydroxylase domain (PHD)
Phenformin, 56
Phenol, 436
Phenolic compounds, 596–599
  structure-activity relationship of
    2,6-dialkyl phenol derivatives, 600t
    multisubstituted para-alkylated phenol
      derivatives, 598t
    phenol, 597t
Phenolic hydroxyl group, 220, 609
Phenotypic drug discovery, 716–717
Phenyl group, 308–309
Phenyl rings, 88, 116–117, 227, 305–306
Phenylalanine 8 (Phe8), 131–132, 356
Phenylaminopyrimidine compounds (PAP
  compounds), 364
Phenylsulfonyl group, 255–256
Philadelphia chromosome (Ph-chromosome),
  362
Phlorizin, 60–61
Phosphate binding loop, 374
Phosphate ester, 197, 558–559
Phosphate-binding loop (P-loop), 352
Phosphatidylinositide-3-kinase (PI3K), 25
Phosphatidylinositol-3,4,5-triphosphate, 25
3'-phosphoadenosine-5'-phosphosulfate,
  179–181
Phosphodiesterase (PDE), 558
  approval of second and third-generation
    highly selective phosphodiesterase type
    5A inhibitors, 565–576
    phosphodiesterase type 5A inhibitor
      activity, PK properties, and efficacy,
      572–576, 574t
    second-generation selective
      phosphodiesterase type 5A inhibitor,
      565–568
    tadalafil, third-generation selective
      phosphodiesterase type 5A inhibitor,
      568–572
  molecular mechanisms of interaction
    between sildenafil or vardenafil and
    phosphodiesterase type 5A proteins,
    579–580
    crystal structure of PDE5A-GMP
      complex, 580f
    molecular binding pattern of PDE5A-
      sildenafil complex, 580f
    molecular binding pattern of PDE5A-
      vardenafil complex, 581f
  molecular mechanisms of phosphodiesterase
    type 5A inhibitors, 578–580
  protein structure and mechanism of action,
    558–559, 560f
    representative four marketed
      phosphodiesterase type 5A inhibitors,
      561t
    schematic diagram of distribution of
      PDE5A, 560f
  protein structure of, 578–579
  synthesis of selective phosphodiesterase type
    5A inhibitors, 576–577
    sildenafil citrate synthesis, 576
    tadalafil synthesis, 577

vardenafil hydrochloride synthesis,
  576–577
Phosphoramidate prodrug, 201–203
Phosphorodiamidate morpholino oligomer
  (PMO), 751
Phosphorothioate (PS), 735
  modification, 743
Phosphorus atom, 201, 691
Phosphorylation, 352–353
Phosphorylation of RIP2 (p-RIP2), 318
Photo-induced electron transfer effect (PET
  effect), 672–674
Phylogenetic analysis, 81
Phytohormones, 693
PI3K. See Phosphatidylinositide-3-kinase
  (PI3K)
PIC. See Preintegration complex (PIC)
Picoprazole, 543
Pictet-Spengler reaction, 577
Pinworm disease, 510
Pioglitazone, 58
Piperazine ring, 481
2-piperidone, 157
Pirenperone, 625
PIs. See Protease inhibitors (PIs)
Pitavastatin, 79
PKA. See Protein kinase A (PKA)
PKB. See Protein kinase B (PKB)
PKC. See Protein kinase C (PKC)
PKIs. See Protein kinase inhibitors (PKIs)
Planar isoxazole series, 146
Planar pyrazole ring, 153
Plasma, 198–200
Plasma protein binding (PPB), 5, 150–151,
  223, 310, 343
Plasma proteins, 93–94, 166, 226, 500
Plasmalemmasome, 450
Plasmin, 311
Platelet aggregation, 176
Platelet Factor 4 (PF4), 166
Platelet-derived growth factor receptor
  (PDGFR), 366
Platinum–based chemotherapy, 412
PM. See Poor metabolizer (PM)
PMF. See Potential of mean force (PMF)
PMO. See Phosphorodiamidate morpholino
  oligomer (PMO)
PNAs. See Peptide nucleic acids (PNAs)
POC. See Proof-of-concept (POC)
Polar aprotic solvents, 235
Polar surface area (PSA), 4
Pollution, 518
Poly L-glutamic acid–paclitaxel conjugate, 311
Poly(beta-amino ester), 736
Polycystic ovary syndrome (PCOS), 439
Polyethylene glycol (PEG), 44, 50, 310
Polyethylene glycol-loxenatide (PEG-
  loxenatide), 50
Polyethylene glycosylation (PEGylation),
  636–637
Polygenic process, 55–56
Polymerase acidic protein (PA), 266
Polymerase basic protein 1 (PB1), 266
Polymerase basic protein 2 (PB2), 266

Polymerase-targeted pimodivir, 269–270
Polymerized microtubules, 304–305
Polyoxyethylene castor oil, 291
Polypeptide, 23
Polyphosphate salts, 690
Polyproline, 44
Ponatinib, 377–378
Poor metabolizer (PM), 552
7-position methylthiomethyl ether, 295
Post-antibiotic effect (PAE), 498
Potassium-competitive acid blockers, 537
Potential of mean force (PMF), 602
Potier semisynthesis route, 301
PPB. See Plasma protein binding (PPB)
PPIs. See Proton pump inhibitors (PPIs)
PR. See Partial response (PR)
Pradaxa, 143–144
Pravastatin, 79, 94
Praziquanamine 7, 523
Praziquantel, 510–514, 516–517, 519–520
  brief history of antischistosomal drugs,
    510–513
  dosage and treatment duration of, 513–514
  dosage and treatment duration of
    praziquantel, 513–514
  green process for, 518–526
  insecticidal mechanism of action of, 513, 514f
  insecticidal mechanism of action of
    praziquantel, 513, 514f
  medicinal chemistry of, 514–518
  pharmacokinetics of, 517–518
  resistance to, 514
  structure-activity relationship of, 514–515
  synthesis of, 519–522, 520f, 521f, 522f
  tablets, 513
Pre-mRNA, 739
Precision-driven process, 249
Preclinical pharmacokinetic studies, 406
Prednisone, 630
Preintegration complex (PIC), 213
Priapism, molecular biological mechanisms of,
  558, 559f
Pro degron pathway. See Proline degron
  pathway (Pro degron pathway)
Procaine, 587–588
Prodrugs, 194
  design and application of, 194–201
  utilizing hydrophilic small molecule moieties
    as carriers, 310–320
    paclitaxel prodrug targeting inflammatory
      microenvironment of tumors, 313–320
    paclitaxel–unsaturated fatty acid
      conjugates, 312–313
    peptide-paclitaxel conjugate, 311
    poly L-glutamic acid–paclitaxel
      conjugate, 311, 311f
    polyethylene glycol–paclitaxel
      conjugates, 310, 310f, 311f
    prodrugs designed for targeted tissue
      delivery, 311
    prodrugs of paclitaxel utilizing water-
      soluble polymers as carriers, 310
    targeting cancer cells overexpressing
      receptors, 312

Prodrugs (Continued)
  targeting hypoxic microenvironment of cancer cells, 312
Proglucagon, 41–42
Progression-free survival (PFS), 407
Progressive disease (PD), 344
Proline degron pathway (Pro degron pathway), 634
Prolonged hyperglycemia, 55
Prolyl hydroxylase, 634–635, 636f
  inhibitors, 638–639, 638f
  structure and mechanism of, 639–642, 641f
    crystal structure of PHD2 in complex with endogenous, 641f
Prolyl hydroxylase domain (PHD), 635
  lead discovery and optimization of, 643–645
Prontosil, 465
Proof-of-concept (POC), 6
Propofol ($C_{12}H_{18}O$), 600–602, 611–612, 615–616
  analogs, 603–610
  candidates from 2,6-diisubstituted phenolic compound series, 609f
  clinical application and metabolism of propofol in vivo, 615–616
    intravenous use and dosage of propofol, 615t
  2,6-diisubstituted phenolic compounds, 606t
  impact of compound 71, 608f
  compounds of benzocyclobutene series, 604t
  fat emulsion, 596
  hydrogen bond between phenol hydroxyl group and $GABA_A$ receptor, 609f
  MM/GBSA calculations of propofol, 610t
  optimization of benzocyclobutene series compounds, 605t
  prodrug design of fospropofol sodium, 611f
  propofol and compound 65 with 2,6-diisobutyl substitution, 606f
  separation of 2,6-diisubstituted phenolic compounds, 608t
  story of, 595–596
Proprotein convertase subtilisin/kexin 9 (PCSK9), 74
Prostacyclin, 141–142
Prostaglandin G2 (PGG2), 712
Prostaglandin H2 (PGH2), 712
Prostaglandins (PGs), 534–535, 711
  biological functions of, 712
  inhibition of synthesis of prostaglandins by cyclooxygenase enzymes, 534–535
PROTACs. See Protein hydrolysis targeting chimeras (PROTACs); Proteolysis targeting chimeras (PROTACs)
Protease inhibitors (PIs), 95, 186–187, 214
Protein, 374, 674–675
  binding mode and structure-activity relationships of fluconazole, 458–459
  coat, 245
  crystallography, 388–389
  degradation, 444
  drugs, 35–36
  mass spectrometry, 394–395
  structure of phosphodiesterase type 5A, 578–579, 579f

Protein hydrolysis targeting chimeras (PROTACs), 444
Protein kinase A (PKA), 350
Protein kinase B (PKB), 25
Protein kinase C (PKC), 126, 364
Protein kinase inhibitors (PKIs), 349–350
  as antineoplastic agents, 349–362
  classifications and design of, 354–362
    allosteric inhibitors, 360
    ATP-competitive inhibitors, 356–360
    covalent inhibitors, 361–362
    drug-binding pocket of PKA, 355f
    ligand-binding pockets within PK catalytic domain, 355t, 356f
Protein kinases, 350
  as antineoplastic agents, 349–362
  composition and catalytic mechanism of, 350–354, 351f
Proteolysis targeting chimeras (PROTACs), 382
Proteusbacillus vulgaris, 489
ProTide technology, 206–207
  application, 207f
  development, 207t
Proton pump inhibitors (PPIs), 531
  methyl sulfonyl linker, 550
  structure-activity relationship of, 549–550
  substituted benzimidazole ring, 549–550
  substituted pyridine ring, 549
Proton pumps, 535, 538
  mechanism of acid secretion by proton pumps, 539
  molecular structure of proton pumps, 538, 538f
  physiological functions and structural characteristics of, 538–539
Proximal tubular reabsorption, 26
PRRs. See Pattern recognition receptors (PRRs)
PRSP. See Penicillin-resistant Streptococcus pneumoniae (PRSP)
PS. See Phosphorothioate (PS)
PSA. See Polar surface area (PSA)
Pseudomonas aeruginosa, 489, 670
Psychogenic ED, 558
PTE system. See Patent term extension system (PTE system)
PU. See Peptic ulcer (PU)
Pulmonary arterial hypertension, 575–576
Pulmonary embolism (PE), 141
Purification process, 22, 65, 178
Pyrazino[2,1-a]isoquinoline ring, 515
5-pyrazole amide linker, 151
Pyrazole ring, 148, 718
  optimization of 3-and 4-position substituents of, 718, 719t
Pyridine ring, 380–381, 549
2-(2-pyridyl) thioacetamide, 540, 541f
Pyrimidine ring, 364
Pyrophosphate, 689–691
  schematic representation of structure, 690f
  zoledronate structural formula and 3D ball-and-stick model, 690f
Pyrrole as central ring, 83–89

Q

QPP. See Quiescent cell proline peptidase (QPP)
QT interval prolongation syndrome, 126
Quiescent cell proline peptidase (QPP), 7–8
Quinazoline, 410
  epidermal growth factor receptor, 388
  epidermal growth factor receptor and quinazoline-based small molecule inhibitors, 388–390
  quinazoline-based small molecule epidermal growth factor receptor inhibitors, 388–390, 390t
  resistance mutations for epidermal growth factor receptor, 390
  structure, 405
Quinolones, 477, 493

R

R&D process. See Research and development process (R&D process)
(R)-tetrahydrofuran-2-carboxylic acid, 279
Rabeprazole, 536
Racemization methods, 524
Radioactive marker detection, 283
Raloxifene, 426–427
Raltegravir (RAL), 214
  discovery journey of, 215–234, 239–241, 240f
  clinical investigation of raltegravir, 232–234
  crystal structure of prototype, 242f
  discovery and optimization of hit compounds, 216–221
  optimization of 1,6-naphthyridine lead compound, 221–226
  optimization of dihydroxy pyrimidine lead compound, 226–232
  structure and mechanism of action of HIV-1 integrase, 215–216
  RAL-based combination therapy, 234
  research on synthetic process of, 234–239
    optimization of first-generation synthetic process, 234–236, 236f
    optimization of second-generation synthetic process, 236–239, 239f
    synthetic route in medicinal chemistry, 234, 235f
Raney nickel-catalyzed hydrogenation, 97
Rapid-acting insulin analogs, 30
Rat aortic smooth muscle cells (RSMCS), 569
Ravuconazole, 462
Razaxaban, 151
RBV. See Ribavirin (RBV)
Recognition motifs, 634
Recombinant DNA technology, 22, 28
Recombinant human erythropoietin (rhEPO), 636–637
Red blood cells, 126–127, 162
Remogliflozin, 62–63
Renal anemia, 633, 636–637
  medications for treatment of, 636–639
    commonly used drugs for renal anemia treatment, 636–637, 637t

prolyl hydroxylase inhibitors, 638–639, 638f
and pathogenesis, 633–635
  hypoxia-inducible factor and prolyl hydroxylase, 634–635, 636f
  proteolytic degradation and degron, 633–634
  renal anemia, 633, 634f
Renal cell injury, 634–635
Renal glucose threshold elevation, 60
Renal hypertensive rats (RHR), 116
Renal protection, 67
Renal-controlling blood glucose, 60
Renin-angiotensin system, 110–113
  conversion of bradykinin by ACE, 113f
  and launched time of list of ACE inhibitors, 112t
  relationship between RAS and elevation of blood pressure, 111f
  structure of aliskiren, 112f
Replication process, 214, 266–268
Representative drugs, 56, 453
Research and development process (R&D process), 154
Residual drugs, 677–678
Resistance antibodies, 28
Resolution to obtain *trans*-tamoxifen, 437, 437f
Respiratory disorders, 106
Restriction enzyme analysis, 738
Reverse transcriptase (RT), 212
Reverse transcription process, 214
Reversible covalent bonds, 361
Reversible covalent mechanisms, covalent strategies based on, 392–393
Reversible covalent reactions, 392
Reversible EGFR inhibitors, 393–394
Reversible PPIs, 537
Rhabdomyolysis, 79, 94–95
rhEPO. *See* Recombinant human erythropoietin (rhEPO)
Rhodium (Rh), 14
RHR. *See* Renal hypertensive rats (RHR)
Ribavirin (RBV), 186–187
Ribonuclease (RNase), 213
Ribonucleic acid (RNA), 186, 265–266
Ribosomal cycling, 478
Rickettsia, 492
RIF. *See* Rifampicin (RIF)
Rifampicin (RIF), 630, 677–678
Rifampin, 95
Risedronate, 699–701
Risperidone, 625, 627, 629–630
  adverse effects of, 629
  antipsychotic drugs, 619–622
  characteristics of risperidone's effects, 627–631
    drug-drug Interaction of, 629–630
    pharmacokinetics of risperidone, 629
    pharmacological characteristics of risperidone, 627–629
    progress of risperidone, 630–631
  discovery of, 624–625, 624f
    affinity of risperidone, 626t
    benorilate, 626f

combination methods of combination principle, 626f
  design concept of risperidone, 625f
  indications of, 627–629
  medicinal chemistry of risperidone, 623–627
  pharmacological basis of, 623–624
  pharmacological mechanism of, 627
  synthesis of, 626–627
    industrial synthesis routes of risperidone, 628f
    structure of risperidone, 627f
  tablets, 631
Ritonavir (RTV), 254–255, 654
Rivaroxaban, 143–144
RNA. *See* Ribonucleic acid (RNA)
RNA interference, 262
RNA polymerase, 189, 203, 265–266
RNA-related viruses, 192
RNase. *See* Ribonuclease (RNase)
RNase H, 739–740, 739f
RNase H2, 739
Rociletinib, 412
Rosiglitazone, 58
Rosuvastatin, 79, 95
Roxadustat, 646–647
  clinical research on, 645–647
    pharmacodynamics and pharmacokinetics, 645–646
    phase II and phase III clinical trials, 646–647
  development process of, 639–648
  identification and optimization of hit compounds, 643, 643f
  lead discovery and optimization of prolyl hydroxylase domain inhibitors, 643–645
  structure and mechanism of prolyl hydroxylase, 639–642, 641f
  synthetic process of, 647–648
RSMCS. *See* Rat aortic smooth muscle cells (RSMCS)
RT. *See* Reverse transcriptase (RT)
RTV. *See* Ritonavir (RTV)
Ruthenium (Ru), 14
Rv2466c, nitrofuran compounds interact with, 674–675
Rv2466c-MSH-NFC (RvMN), 674–675
RvMN. *See* Rv2466c-MSH-NFC (RvMN)

S

16S ribosomal RNA (rRNA), 492
Salmonella, 489
Salt bridge, 696
Salutaxel prototype, 319
Sanfetrinem cilexetil, 507
Sanofi Pharmaceuticals, 170
Sanofi's mature process, 179
Saquinavir (SQV), 253, 654
  design and discovery of, 251–253
  development of, 254–260
  dipeptide Phe-Pro to lead compound 3, 251–252

discovery of darunavir, 256–260
discovery of saquinavir, 253
enhancement of pharmacokinetic properties, 254–256
  first-generation HIV protease inhibitors after saquinavir, 255f
  molecular structures of compounds, 255f
  optimization of lead compound 3, 252–253
  pharmacokinetic properties and deficiencies of, 253–254
  interaction between saquinavir and HIV-1 protease, 254f
SARs. *See* Structure-activity relationships (SARs)
SC-57666, 717
SC-58125, 717
SCAP. *See* SREBP cleavage-activating protein (SCAP)
Schistosoma mansoni, 514
Schistosomiasis, 510
Schizophrenia, 627
SD. *See* Stable disease (SD)
Seasonal influenza, 265
Second-generation sitagliptin process chemistry, 15–16
  second-generation sitagliptin process synthesis route, 16f, 17f
Second-generation synthetic process optimization of, 236–239
  research on nitrogen methylation reaction of intermediate, 238f
  synthetic process of intermediate, 238f
Secondary alcohol, 121
Secreted protein acidic and rich in cysteine (SPARC), 291
Secretory canaliculus, 539
Selective ER downregulators (SERDs), 422
Selective estrogen receptor modulators (SERMs), 420, 422, 423f
  medicinal chemistry of, 423–438
Selective FXa inhibitor, specificity and advantages of, 144–146
Self-aggregation process, 29
Semaglutide, 47–48
  structure, 47f
Sensory stimuli, 532
Separation process, 178
Sequence analysis, 696–698
SERDs. *See* Selective ER downregulators (SERDs)
Serine proteases, 145–146
Serine proteinase, 2
SERMs. *See* Selective estrogen receptor modulators (SERMs)
Serotonin, 620
Severe acute respiratory syndrome, 247
Severe adverse reactions, 127
Sexual stimulation, 558
Sexual transmission, 211
SGLT1/2. *See* Sodium-glucose co transporter (SGLT1/2)
SGLTs. *See* Sodium-dependent glucose transporters (SGLTs)
Shigella, 489

778 Index

Side-chain targeting to backbone targeting
   backbone targeting, 257–258
   inhibitory activity of Saquinavir against mutant HIV protease, 257–258
Sildenafil, 565, 575–576
   for management of male erectile dysfunction, 559–565
     discovery of sildenafil and structure-activity relationship study, 562–564, 563f
     structural-activity relationships of 3-propylpyrazolo, 564t
     unexpected findings of sildenafil in clinical trials, 565
     molecular mechanisms of interaction between sildenafil and phosphodiesterase type 5A proteins, 579–580
   synthesis of sildenafil citrate, 576, 576f
Simian immunodeficiency virus (SIV), 654
Simvastatin, 79
Single *trans* isomer, 436
Single *trans* tamoxifen
   asymmetric synthesis of *trans*-tamoxifen, 437–438, 438f
   isomerization to obtain trans-tamoxifen, 437
   separation to obtain *trans*-tamoxifen, 437, 437f
   synthesis of, 436–438
Single-crystal X-ray diffraction, 201
Single-stranded RNA viruses, 187, 246
Single-target drugs, 621–622
siRNAs. *See* Small interfering RNAs (siRNAs)
Sitagliptin, 12–18
   application of asymmetric catalytic hydrogenation, 14–18
   clinical studies of new drug sitagliptin, 11–12
   common factors influencing ADME/T properties of drugs, 4–6, 4t
   confirmation of lead compounds, 8–10
   early pharmacological effects of dipeptidyl peptidase IV inhibitors, 6–8
   early toxicity studies of dipeptidyl peptidase IV inhibitors, 6–8
   efficiency of chemical reactions, 13
   enterostatin and degrading enzyme dipeptidyl peptidase-4, 2–3
   first generation process chemistry of, 15, 15f
   medicinal chemistry synthesis of, 14, 14f
   optimization of β-amino acid series lead compounds, 10
   optimization strategies for DPP-4 inhibitors, 8
   process chemistry, 12–18
   property-based drug design, 3–4
   type 2 diabetes drug sitagliptin, 1–2
SIV. *See* Simian immunodeficiency virus (SIV)
Skin and skin structure infections (SSSI), 476
Skin or soft tissue infections (SSTI), 466–467
Small interfering RNAs (siRNAs), 735
   patisiran, 747
   therapeutics, 735–736
Small molecule inhibitors, 216–217

Small molecule prodrug, 283
Small-molecule carbohydrate drugs, development of, 162
Small-molecule drugs, 26
Sodium cyanide, 520
Sodium N-[8-(2-hydroxybenzoyl)amino] caprylate (SNAC), 47–48
Sodium-dependent glucose transporters (SGLTs), 60–61
Sodium-glucose co transporter (SGLT1/2), 68
   as anti-diabetic drugs, 59–67
   biological basis of SGLT2 as therapeutic target for diabetes, 59–60
   drugs based on SGLT2 inhibitors, 67, 68t
   efficacy and action of dapagliflozin, 67
   SGLT2 inhibitors and successful development of dapagliflozin, 60–65
   synthetic process of dapagliflozin, 65–67
Sofosbuvir
   clinical studies of, 203–205
   clinical trial results of sofosbuvir, 203–204, 204f
   discovery of, 189–203
   mechanism of nucleoside antiviral drugs, 189–190
   pharmacokinetic study of pharmasset small-molecule inhibitor-6130, 194–201
   preclinical studies of sofosbuvir, 203
   ProTide technology, 206–207
   structure-activity relationship of nucleoside scaffold, 190–194, 192f
   synthesis of, 201–203, 203f
   synthesis of fragment B, 203f
   treatment regimens with sofosbuvir, 204–205
     EMA suggested treatment regimens containing sofosbuvir for different genotypes, 205t
Solid-phase peptide synthesis (SPPS), 42
Solid-phase synthesis methods, 314–316
Somatostatin, 532
Sorafenib, 360
SPARC. *See* Secreted protein acidic and rich in cysteine (SPARC)
Spike proteins, 246
Spirochetes, 492
Spliceosome, 738
Splicing process, 738
SPPS. *See* Solid-phase peptide synthesis (SPPS)
SQV. *See* Saquinavir (SQV)
SREBP. *See* Sterol regulatory element binding protein (SREBP)
SREBP cleavage-activating protein (SCAP), 73–74
SSSI. *See* Skin and skin structure infections (SSSI)
SSTI. *See* Skin or soft tissue infections (SSTI)
ST. *See* Strand transfer (ST)
Stable disease (SD), 319–320, 344
Staphylococcus, 491
   S. aureus, 489, 670
   S. epidermidis, 489–490
   strains, 472

Statins, 105
   additional effects of, 105–106
     bone regeneration, 106
     cancer, 105
     diabetes and metabolic disorders, 105
     inflammation and autoimmune diseases, 105
     neurodegenerative diseases, 106
     respiratory disorders, 106
   beginning of, 76–78
   development of statin drugs, 77t
   combination therapy of statins with agents, 104
   drugs, 103
     drug–drug interactions of atorvastatin, 95
     hydrophilicity/lipophilicity and in vivo efficacy, pharmacokinetics, and adverse effects, 92–95, 93t
     inhibiting HMG-CoA reductase, structure-activity relationship of, 82–89
     target of, 81–82
     vivo structure-activity, structure-metabolism, and structure-toxicity relationships o in f, 92–95
   interaction of statins with HMG-CoA reductase, 89–92
Stereoisomers, 654
Sterol regulatory element binding protein (SREBP), 73–74
Sterols, 457
Stetter reaction, 96
Strand transfer (ST), 215–216
Strecker reaction, 234
Streptococcus
   S. agalactiae, 471–472
   S. anginosus, 471–472
   S. pyogenes, 471–472
Streptomyces
   S. cattleya, 497
   S. noursei, 452–453
Stress ulcers, prevention of, 551
Structural-functional relationship based on ring D, 307–308
Structure-activity relationships (SARs), 25, 68–69, 79, 84, 115–116, 147–148, 218, 251, 297, 331, 363, 366–367, 468
   active conformation and inactive conformation of Abl, 366f
   based on ring A, 307
   based on ring A, 307, 307f
   based on ring C, 307
   based on ring C, 307, 308f
   based on ring D, 307–308, 308f
   of C_1- and C_2-positions in bacatin III, 303–304, 303f
   cocrystal structure and binding mode of Abl, 367f
   conversion of heparin pentasaccharide binding fragment, 171f
   of covalent EGFR inhibitor, 407–408, 408f
   of halichondrin B-discovery process of eribulin, 333–336
   of liver-targeting prodrug molecule pharmasset small-molecule inhibitor-7851, 197–201

of methyl glycoside derivatives at O-sulfate
  positions, 172t, 174t
  and O-alkyl positions, 175t
of nucleoside scaffold, 190–194
of paclitaxel, 302–309, 303f, 309f
relationship between structural
  modifications at C_7-to C_{10}-positions,
  304–305
relationship between structure and activity at
  C_4 position, 304
relationship between structure and
  effectiveness of C_{13}-side chain,
  305–306, 306f
of statin drugs inhibiting HMG-CoA
  reductase, 82–89
structure-activity relationship of open-ring
  methyl glycoside derivatives of sugars
  E and G, 173t
studies based on Heparin pentasaccharide
  sequence, 170–176
of tamoxifen, 427–431
  mechanism of action and, 425–427
Sugar ring modification strategies, 743–744
Sulfonamides, 119–120
  drugs, 493
  moieties, 258
Sulfonyl oxime, 121
4-sulfonylamino group in A-ring, optimization
  of, 717
Sulfotransferase (SULT), 616
Sulfur (S), 400–401
SULT. See Sulfotransferase (SULT)
Sunitinib, 360
Sustainable chemistry, 17–18
Sustained virological response rate (SVR),
  186–187
Suzuki coupling reaction, 129–130
SVR. See Sustained virological response rate
  (SVR)
Synthetic bovine insulin, 22
Synthetic fragment A, 280
Synthetic routes, 155–158, 459
  of apixaban, 154–158, 156f
Systematic screening process, 16

T

t-butyl ester, 239
T4SS. See Type IV secretion system (T4SS)
T790M mutation, 390
TAD. See Transcription activation domains
  (TAD)
Tadalafil, 568–569, 575
  modification of hydantoin ring, 572f
  PDE5A inhibitory potency of C-5 Aromatic
    or heterocyclic derivatives, 569t
  phosphodiesterase type 5A inhibition and
    cellular activity of N-substituted
    hydantoins, 571t
  synthesis of, 577, 578f
  synthesis of PDE5A inhibitors, 568f
  third-generation selective
    phosphodiesterase type 5A inhibitor,
    568–572

Tamoxifen, 422, 428–434, 438–439, 442
  adverse reactions of tamoxifen, 442
  clinical indications of tamoxifen, 438–439
  clinical investigations of, 438–442
  derivatives of tamoxifen with A-ring
    substitution, 429
  derivatives with benzene ring modification,
    429–430
  drug interactions, 435
  estrogen receptors and breast cancers,
    419–422
  historical significance of, 442–443
  knowledge expansion, and references,
    442–444
    drugs targeting estrogen receptor pathway
      for breast cancer treatment, 443–444,
      443f
    historical significance of tamoxifen,
      442–443
  mechanism of action and structure-activity
    relationship of, 425–427
  mechanism of tamoxifen binding to estrogen
    receptors, 425–427, 426f
  medicinal chemistry of selective estrogen
    receptor modulator tamoxifen, 423–438
  serendipity and opportunity, discovery of,
    423–425, 424f
    development history of tamoxifen, 425t
    early nonsteroidal antiestrogen drugs, 424f
  structure-activity relationship of, 427–431
    modifications on nitrogen atom, 427–431,
    428f
  studies on tamoxifen resistance, 439–442
    alterations in ESR1 genome and structural
      mutations in estrogen receptor,
      440–441
    conversion of tamoxifen metabolites to
      estrogen receptor agonists, 439
    loss of estrogen receptors, 439–440
    resistance due to activation of estrogen
      membrane receptor pathway, 441–442
    resistance due to activation of pathways
      estrogen receptors, 442
  synthesis of mixture of two isomers of
    tamoxifen, 435–436
    synthesis of tamoxifen by McMurry
      coupling reaction, 436
    synthesis of tamoxifen by nucleophilic
      addition, 436
    synthesis of tamoxifen by nucleophilic
      substitution, 436
  synthesis of single trans tamoxifen, 436–438
  in vivo metabolic characteristics of,
    432–435
Target protein, 391, 444
Targeted delivery, conjugation strategies for,
  745–746, 745f
Targeted drugs, 290
Targeted therapies, 349
Targeted tissue delivery
  enzymes or transport proteins overexpressed
    in tumor tissue as target, 311, 312f
  prodrugs designed for, 311
Taspoglutide, 49–50

Tau protein, 290
Taxane-based drug candidates studied in
  clinical trials, 293–296
  BMS series taxane drugs, 295
  larotaxel, 293, 294f
  milataxel, 293, 294f
  ortataxel, 295, 296f
  tesetaxel, 296, 296f
  TL-310, 294, 295f
  TPI-287, 294, 294f
Taxanes for anticancer therapy, commercially
  available, 292–293
Taxol, discovery and development of, 287–297
  antitumor action of mechanism, 288
  application limitations of
    injectable paclitaxel, 289–292
  clinical research on paclitaxel, 288, 288f
  commercially available taxanes for
    anticancer therapy, 292–293
  discovery of paclitaxel, 287–288
  method of obtaining natural paclitaxel,
    296–297
  taxane-based drug candidates studied in
    clinical trials, 293–296
Taxus tree
  bark of, 296
  resources, 296
TBS. See Tert-butyldimethylsilyl (TBS)
Tebipenem pivoxil, 504–505, 507
Telmisartan, 134
Tenofovir (TDF), 214
Terpenes, 693
3′-tert-butoxycarbonyl amide derivative, 292
Tert-butyl-substituted phenyl group, 295
Tert-butyldimethylsilyl (TBS), 333
TES. See Triethylchlorosilane (TES)
Tesetaxel, 296, 296f, 297t
2,3,4,6-tetra-O-trimethylsilyl-D-glucuronic acid-
  δ-lactone, 65
Tetracyclines, 492–493
Tetrahydro-β-carboline hydantoin, 569
Tetrahydrobenzopyran nitrofuran derivatives,
  mechanism of antibacterial activity of,
  670–671
3-tetrahydrofuran (THF), 255
Tetrahydropyran ring, 335
Tetrasaccharides, 168–169
Tetrazoles, 119–120, 134, 463
TG. See Triglycerides (TG)
Therapeutic drugs
  discovery of hepatitis C and development of,
    186–187
  structures of anti-HCV drugs, 188f
Therapeutic methods, 449
Thiazole compound nitazoxanide, 269
Thienamycin, 497
Thioether
  oxidation of, 549
  synthesis of, 547–548
    compound I, 547
    compound II, 547–548
    compound III, 548
Thiols, 399–400
Thiopental sodium, 587

Thiourea-based antithyroid drugs, 541
Third-generation irreversible EGFR inhibitors, 414
Third-generation sitagliptin process, 16–17, 18f
Threonine (Thr), 45
Thrombin generation, 176
Thromboembolic diseases, 165
Thromboembolism, 161, 163
Thrombolytic drugs, 144
Thrombolytics, 163
Thrombosis, 141, 161
　dangers of, 141
　pathogenesis of, 141–143
　　coagulation cascade, 142f
　　coagulation factors, 142t
　　specificity and advantages of selective FXa inhibitor, 144–146, 145f
　treatment of, 143–146
　　antithrombotic drugs and mechanisms of action, 143–144
Thrombotic diseases, 163
Thrombotic disorders, 161–163
　factors and mechanisms of thrombosis formation, 162
　　coagulation cascade and involved coagulation factors, 163f
　and hazards, 161–162
　treatment of, 163–168
　　anticoagulants, 164–165
　　antiplatelet agents, anticoagulants, and thrombolytics, 163
　　low-molecular-weight heparin, 166–167
　　marketed drugs for thrombotic disorders, 165t
　　ultra-low-molecular-weight heparins, 168
　　unfractionated heparin, 165–166
Thromboxanes (TXs), 711–712
Thrombus, 141
Timoprazole, 535, 541
　birth of, 541
TK. *See* Tyrosine kinase (TK)
TL-310, 294, 295f
TLR4. *See* Toll-like receptor 4 (TLR4)
TLRs. *See* Toll-like receptors (TLRs)
Toll-like receptor 4 (TLR4), 313–314
Toll-like receptors (TLRs), 533–534
Total synthesis of atorvastatin, 95–102
　[3 + 2] cycloaddition pyrrole synthesis, 98–99
　asymmetric side chain synthesis methods, 99–102
　Paal–Knorr pyrrole synthesis, 97–98
Toxic reagents, 522
Toxic solvent chloroform, 235
TPC. *See* Treatment of physician's choice (TPC)
TPI-287, 294, 294f
Traditional chemical industry, 526
Traditional chiral resolution, 523
Traditional NSAIDs, 722–725
Traditional prodrug molecule, 198–200
Traditional small-molecule drugs, 741–742
Trans isomers, 423

Trans-acrylic acid, 131–132
Trans-diethylstilbestrol (DES), 426–427
Transaminase-catalyzed new process, 17
Transcription activation domains (TAD), 635
Transfer RNA (tRNA), 694–695
Transmembrane glycoprotein tissue factor, 162
Transport proteins overexpressed in tumor tissue as target, 311
Trapping theory, 535
Trastuzumab, 349–350
Treatment of physician's choice (TPC), 344
Triazoles, 119–120
　antifungal drugs, 453
　　development of new generation, 461–463
　compound 14, 8–9
　drugs, 462–463
　　future development of, 463
　elucidating pharmacophore of triazole-difluorophenyltertiary alcohol, 457
　imidazoles to, 455–457
　to tetrazoles, 463
Tricyclic carbon ring, 307–308
Triethylchlorosilane (TES), 301
Trifluoromethyl, 152
Trifluoromethyl group, 718–719
Trifluoromethyl isopropyl group, 278–279
Triglycerides (TG), 71
Trimethyl acetic acid, 97–98
3-trimethylsilyl-4-pentenoate, 340
Triphenylethylene, 423–424
Triphenylmethyl phenyltetrazole, 129
Triphenylphosphine (PPh$_3$), 408
Triphosphate nucleotides, 187
Triple-negative breast cancer, 420
Tritium (T), 517
tRNA. *See* Transfer RNA (tRNA)
Tuberculosis diagnosis, utilization of compound 125 as innovative fluorescent diagnostic reagent for drug sensitivity testing in, 677–678
Tuberoinfundibular pathway, 619
Tubulin, 329
　inhibitors, 329
　tubulin-binding site, 305
Tumor cells, 312, 329
Tumor microenvironment, chemotherapy resistance induced by, 290
Tumor necrosis factor-α (TNF-α), 313–314
Tumor tissues, 310
　enzymes or transport proteins overexpressed in, 311
Tumors, paclitaxel prodrug targeting inflammatory microenvironment of, 313–320
Two polyethylene glycol molecules and γ-glutamic acid (2OEG-γGlu), 47
TXs. *See* Thromboxanes (TXs)
Type 1 diabetes, 55
Type 2 diabetes, 49–50, 55–56, 105
　drug sitagliptin, 1–2, 2f
　treatment, 43
Type I inhibitors, 357
　binding mode of, 357f
　representatives of, 358f

Type I1/2 inhibitors, 358–359
　binding mode of, 358f
　representatives of, 359f
Type II inhibitors, 359–360
　binding mode of, 360f
　representatives of, 360f
Type IV secretion system (T4SS), 533
Tyr4. *See* Tyrosine 4 (Tyr4)
Tyrosine 4 (Tyr4), 131–132
Tyrosine kinase (TK), 350, 387–388

U

Ubiquitin-proteasome system, 634
Ubiquitinated protein, 634
UFH. *See* Unfractionated heparin (UFH)
UGT1A9. *See* Uridine diphosphate-glucuronosyltransferase 1A9 (UGT1A9)
Ullmann reaction, 157
ULMWH. *See* Ultralow molecular weight heparin (ULMWH)
Ultralow molecular weight heparin (ULMWH), 168
Unfractionated heparin (UFH), 165–166
Unsaturated olefins, 398–399
Urease, 533
Uric acid reduction, 67
Uridine diphosphate-glucuronosyltransferase 1A9 (UGT1A9), 65
Uridine molecule, 195–196
US Food and Drug Administration (FDA), 1, 126, 186–187, 268, 288, 349, 516, 647, 731, 735–736

V

Vabomere, 507
VacA. *See* Vacuolating cytotoxin A (VacA)
Vaccines, 262
　development of lipophilic bisphosphonate inhibitors as, 707
Vaccinia virus, 246
Vacuolating cytotoxin A (VacA), 533
Valine (Val), 45
Valopicitabine, 191–192
Valsartan, 131
Van der Waals interactions, 377–378
Vancomycin-resistant *Enterococcus* (VRE), 466
Vardenafil, 565–568, 575–577
　discovery of vardenafil with imidazo, 567f
　in vitro enzyme inhibition activity of phosphodiesterase type 5A inhibitors, 567t
Vardenafil and phosphodiesterase type 5A proteins, molecular mechanisms of interaction between, 579–580
Vardenafil hydrochloride
　synthesis of, 576–577
　synthetic process route of vardenafil, 577f
Vehicle delivery, 746–749
　cationic liposomes, 747, 747f
　nucleotidyl lipids, 747–749, 748f
Veins, 162

Venous thromboembolism (VTE), 141
Very-low-density lipoproteins (VLDLs), 71
VHL. *See* Von Hippel-Lindau (VHL)
Viagra, 559–562
Vibrio parahaemolyticus, 489
VIGOR. *See* Vioxx gastrointestinal outcomes research (VIGOR)
Viltolarsen, 750–751
Vinylsulfonamides, 396–397, 397*f*
Vioxx gastrointestinal outcomes research (VIGOR), 726
Viral DNA, 215, 241
Viral infection, 55–56
Viral membrane protein, 212, 248
Viral RNA (vRNA), 270
Viral RNA ribonucleoprotein (vRNP), 266–268
Viridans streptococci, 489–490
Virus, 194, 212, 245–247
   classification and nomenclature of, 246
   human antiviral warfare, 247
   infection and pathogenic properties, 246
   nomenclature, 246
   nucleocapsid, 246
   particles, 245
   structure and biological functions, 245–246
   virus-resistant strains, 664
Vitamin K antagonists, 143

VLDLs. *See* Very-low-density lipoproteins (VLDLs)
Volatile anesthetics, 586–587
Von Hippel-Lindau (VHL), 635
Voriconazole, 461
   development of, 461–462
VRE. *See* Vancomycin-resistant Enterococcus (VRE)
vRNA. *See* Viral RNA (vRNA)
vRNP. *See* Viral RNA ribonucleoprotein (vRNP)
VT-1161, 463
VTE. *See* Venous thromboembolism (VTE)

W

Warheads, 390–391
Water molecules, 253, 639–641
Water solubility, 5
Water-soluble conjugate carrier, 311
Water-soluble groups, 396
Water-soluble paclitaxel prodrug, 311
Water-soluble phosphate ester prodrug, 610
Water-soluble polymers as carriers, prodrugs of paclitaxel utilizing, 310
Waterborne parasitic diseases, 509
WBC. *See* White blood cells (WBC)
Weight reduction, 67

White blood cells (WBC), 162, 371
WHO. *See* World Health Organization (WHO)
Wieland–Miescher ketone, 299
World Health Organization (WHO), 162, 205, 247, 265, 494–495
Worrisome, 285
Wyeth Pharmaceuticals, 403–404

X

X chromosome, 738
X-ray crystallographic study, 153–154, 380
X-ray diffraction crystal, 163

Y

Y181C mutation, 654

Z

ZDV. *See* Zidovudine (ZDV)
ZES. *See* Zollinger-Ellison syndrome (ZES)
Zidovudine (ZDV), 213–214, 260, 654
ZOL. *See* Zoledronic acid (ZOL)
Zoledronate, 689
Zoledronic acid (ZOL), 698, 706–707
Zollinger-Ellison syndrome (ZES), 535, 551

Printed in the United States
by Baker & Taylor Publisher Services